INGENIX®
*e*solutions

S0-BAB-338

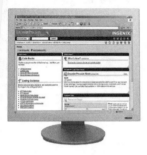

Electronic coding, billing and reimbursement products.

Ingenix provides a robust suite of eSolutions to solve a wide variety of coding, billing and reimbursement issues. As the industry moves to electronic products, you can rely on Ingenix to help support you through the transition.

← Web-based applications for all markets

← Dedicated support

← Environmentally responsible

Key Features and Benefits

Using eSolutions is a step in the right direction when it comes to streamlining your coding, billing and reimbursement practices. Ingenix eSolutions can help you save time and increase your efficiency with accurate and on-time content.

SAVE UP TO 20%
with source code FB11B

 Visit **www.shopingenix.com** and enter the source code to save 20%.

 Call toll-free **1.800.INGENIX** (464.3649), option 1 and save 15%.

- **Simplify ICD-10 transition.** ICD-10 mapping tools provide crosswalks between ICD-9-CM and ICD-10 codes quickly and easily

- **Save time and money.** Ingenix eSolutions combine the content of over 37 code books and data files

- **Increase accuracy.** Electronic solutions are updated regularly so you know you're always working with the most current content available

- **Get the training and support you need.** Convenient, monthly webinars and customized training programs are available to meet your specific needs

- **Rely on a leader in health care.** Ingenix has been producing quality coding products for over 26 years. All of the expert content that goes into our books goes into our electronic resources

- **Get Started.** Visit **shopingenix.com/ eSolutions** for product listing

---

Ingenix | Information is the Lifeblood of Health Care | Call toll-free 1.800.INGENIX (464.3649), option 1.

100% Money Back Guarantee If our merchandise ever fails to meet your expectations, please contact our Customer Service Department toll-free at 1.800.INGENIX (464.3649), option 1, for an immediate response. Software: Credit will be granted for unopened packages only.

Also available from your medical bookstore or distributor.   FB11B

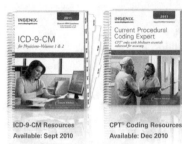
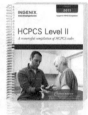
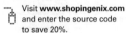

INGENIX®

2011 Specialty References

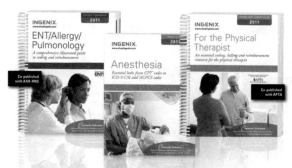

Simplify a coder's job with quick-find reference guides.

Increase cash flow in your specialty practice with the all-in-one solutions equipped with specialty-specific information your practice needs for accurate and efficient coding and billing.

← Essential CPT® code information, customized to specialty

← Links from CPT® codes to appropriate ICD-9-CM and HCPCS codes

← Industry-leading content available in over 20 specialties

To view our full line of specialty resources, please visit www.shopingenix.com/specialty.

SAVE UP TO 20%

with source code FB11C

 Visit www.shopingenix.com and enter the source code to save 20%.

 Call toll-free **1.800.INGENIX** (464.3649), option 1 and save 15%.

Key Features and Benefits

Boost your coders' efficiency with these specialty-specific books that offer the most up-to-date coding information in a quick-search format.

2011 Coding Companion® and Coding and Payment Guides
- *New for 2011!* Medicare Modifiers, MUEs, and status indicators
- Specialty-specific CPT® code sets with clear, concise definitions, coding tips, terminology, crosswalks, and more, all in a quick-find, single page format
- Receive quarterly CCI edits, RVUs and MUEs, via email

2011 Billing Companion for OB/GYN
- Practical guidance for billing OB/GYN services
- Boost accuracy before claim submission
- CMS-1500 claim form alerts

2011 Cross Coders
- Essential links between CPT®, ICD-9-CM, and HCPCS code sets
- Appendix offers a complete listing of add-on and unlisted codes, as well as CPT® and HCPCS modifiers

2011 Coders' Desk References for Specialty Diagnoses
- Easy to understand clinical information provides the foundation for correct diagnosis coding
- Essential for ICD-10 preparation

Ingenix | Information is the Lifeblood of Health Care | Call toll-free 1.800.INGENIX (464.3649), option 1.

INGENIX®
Coder Education

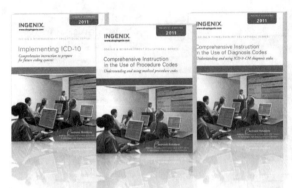

Information is what keeps an expert an expert.

Ingenix Coder Education Series provides comprehensive education and training programs that provide opportunities for health care professionals to increase their knowledge, enhance their skills and keep pace with industry trends. The result is a more capable workforce that enables health care organizations to continually improve their services.

← Convenient and self-paced

← Deep and diverse industry expertise

← Comprehensive coding curriculum

SAVE UP TO 20%
with source code FB11A

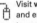 Visit **www.shopingenix.com** and enter the source code to save 20%.

 Call toll-free **1.800.INGENIX** (464.3649), option 1 and save 15%.

Key Features and Benefits

Ingenix Coder Education Series provides a robust curriculum with a variety of courses that focus on urgent coding and claims review training needs.

- **Satisfy your coding needs by creating your own coder.** Customized curriculum to meet your individual practice needs

- **Keep up-to-date with coding and regulatory changes.** Ingenix experts develop new content based on current guidelines and rules so you and your staff are always up-to-date and prepared in case of an audit

- **Streamline your revenue cycle with knowledgeable coding professionals.** Quickly reap the benefits of knowledgeable coding professionals: fewer denied claims, faster reimbursements and increased revenue

- **Save time and money.** Reduce overall training costs by eliminating travel expenses and reducing costs associated with instructor time and salary

For our full curriculum, visit Training and Education on www.shopingenix.com.

Ingenix | Information is the Lifeblood of Health Care | Call toll-free 1.800.INGENIX (464.3649), option 1.

100% Money Back Guarantee If our merchandise ever fails to meet your expectations, please contact our Customer Service Department toll-free at 1.800.INGENIX (464.3649), option 1, for an immediate response. Software: Credit will be granted for unopened packages only.

Also available from your medical bookstore or distributor.

Are You Ready to Make a Successful Transition to ICD-10?

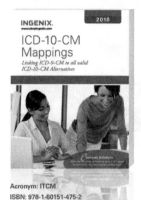

INGENIX. 2010

ICD-10-CM Mappings

Linking ICD-9-CM to all valid ICD-10-CM Alternatives

Acronym: ITCM
ISBN: 978-1-60151-475-2
Item Number: ITCM10
Available: Sep 2010
Price: $129.95

SAVE UP TO 20%

with source code FB11L

Visit **www.shopingenix.com** and enter the source code to save 20%.

Call toll-free **1.800.INGENIX** (464.3649), option 1 and save 15%.

2010 ICD-10-CM Mappings

It's not too early to start improving documentation habits now in preparation for increased documentation requirements under ICD-10. This new tool will help you focus your ICD-10 training without learning the entire code set. By mapping the most frequently used ICD-9-CM codes for your practice or facility to their corresponding ICD-10-CM codes, you can identify areas needing increased documentation and evaluate how additional specificity may impact your revenue.

← Simplify your transition

← Get ready for future documentation and coding needs

← Verify code choices in the new code system

Key Features and Benefits

Jump-start your implementation plan. Start improving documentation habits now in preparation for increased documentation requirements under ICD-10.

- Perform impact analysis to identify and focus on high priority coding issues. Using the ICD-9-CM codes you already know as your guide, you'll be able to quickly identify the ICD-10-CM codes that are pertinent to your office or facility and zero-in on codes to focus on for training and system transition

- Easily identify documentation issues

- Update super bills, forms, reports, and EHRs/PHRs that meet your specific clinical and coding criteria

- Verify software accuracy, evaluate new software, and assist in conversion planning

- Easy-to-use table format lists ICD-9-CM codes with titles and the corresponding ICD-10-CM codes with titles

Also available....

New ICD-10 Draft Code Set Resources

Ease into the new classification system with the most current and complete drafts of the official ICD-10 code sets. Redesigned with the familiar look and feel of an Ingenix ICD-9-CM code book with hallmark color and additional character required symbols.

ICD-10-CM & ICD-10-PCS versions available as printed code books or CD eBooks.

NEW Hallmark color coding and symbols

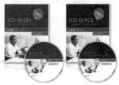

ICD-10-CM	ICD-10-PCS
Book	*Book*
Item# ITEN10	Item# ITPC10
Price: $99.95	Price: $99.95
eBook	*eBook*
Item# 1780	Item# 1781
Price: $119.95	Price: $119.95

Used by the AAPC for ICD-10 training

INGENIX.

Create Your Own Package

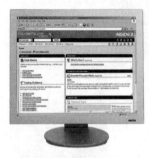

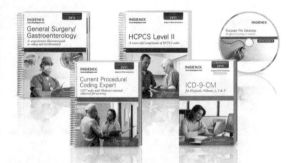

SAVE UP TO 30%

with source code FB11E

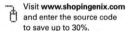

Visit **www.shopingenix.com** and enter the source code to save up to 30%.

Call toll-free **1.800.INGENIX** (464.3649), option 1.

Build your own coding library with the resources you need.

Ingenix resources are tailored to meet your specific needs. Now, you can combine the resources you want—nothing more, nothing less.

← Buy 2–3 items – save 20%

← Buy 4–5 items – save 25%

← Buy 6 or more – save 30%

Key Features and Benefits

Imagine how much time you could save if you could get to the code information you needed, faster. Our resources are designed to shave time off the coding process so you can work smarter, not harder. In addition, we have a dedicated team of experts who research changes in codes and regulations so our resources are updated with the most current information to help you stay compliant.

Buy more and save on the following product categories:

- 2011 Essential Code Books
- 2011 Specialty Reference
- 2011 Desk References
- Coding, Billing and Payment
- Training
- Electronic Resources

Visit www.shopingenix.com/packages2 to determine what products apply.

INGENIX®

2010 Evaluation and Management Coding Advisor

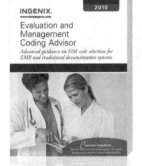

Acronym: EMCA
ISBN: 978-1-60151-473-8
Item Number: EMCA10
Available: Now
Price: $129.95

SAVE UP TO 20%

with source code FB11I

 Visit **www.shopingenix.com** and enter the source code to save 20%.

 Call toll-free **1-800-INGENIX** (464.3649), option 1 and save 15%.

Advanced guidance for E/M code selection

Evaluation and Management (E/M) coding is notoriously difficult, mainly because coders have trouble accurately selecting a code from among a range of seemingly appropriate choices. Consequently, providers make more mistakes with E/M coding than coding for any other item or service. This new resource offers detailed and advanced guidance on selecting the appropriate EM codes, with helpful resources designed for difficult E/M coding situations.

← Review of the E/M rules and protocols

← E/M template examples for EMRs

← Review codes targeted by auditors

Key Features and Benefits

- Helpful advice designed for difficult E/M coding situations such as well-patient exams, H1N1 flu, and other common, but problematic coding scenarios

- E/M template examples for EMRs promote accurate code selection with guidelines for using templates to avoid over-coding

- Review what auditors are targeting, such as critical care

- Compiles payer and specialty association guidance on E/M coding issues

- Documentation guidance and key factors for proper E/M code selection, plus advice to help clinicians make an objective review of subjective information

- E/M code selection benchmarking tool with "Bell Curve" data that shows the range of code selection by specialty

---

Ingenix | Information is the Lifeblood of Health Care | Call toll-free 1.800.INGENIX (464.3649), option 1.

INGENIX.

Ingenix CareTracker EHR

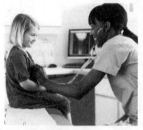

Ready to make the move to EHR? We can help.

Ingenix CareTracker is a web-based CCHIT®-certified EHR that is fully integrated with all the operational functions of a practice. Our unique solution requires **no IT hardware, no license fees,** and **no maintenance costs**. And with our affordable monthly subscription, you only pay for the components you use – to help ensure you enjoy a positive ROI sooner.

With CareTracker you can depend on:

● **Time:** Quick and easy implementation and online training

● **Simplicity:** A web-based solution that does not require hardware

● **Value:** Predictable subscription pricing with no minimum commitment and always current

FOR PRICING DETAILS

 Visit **www.ingenix.com/ehr**

 Call toll-free **1.800.EHR.0845** and mention source code **FB11G**

Meaningful Use Guarantee

■ **Ingenix CareTracker is guaranteed to meet federal meaningful use requirements and qualify for ARRA reimbursements**

Interest-free financing, no out-of-pocket costs

We believe so strongly in Ingenix CareTracker's value to physicians that we're offering them a quick-start financing program to help cover its cost until stimulus incentive payments arrive. Physicians can apply for a no-interest loan to cover:

■ **Implementation**

■ **Monthly license fees**

■ **Training**

■ **Conversion fees**

■ **Setup**

The AMA selects Ingenix CareTracker

The American Medical Association (AMA) has selected Ingenix CareTracker as the first electronic health records (EHR) system offered through the AMA's new online health information solutions platform for physicians. The AMA platform will enable physicians to assess and meet their clinical and practice needs. It will provide physicians access to information, products and services with a single, secure sign-on.

Ingenix | Information is the Lifeblood of Health Care | Call toll-free 1.800.EHR.0845.

Ingenix CareTracker Version 6.2 from Ingenix is a CCHIT Certified® product for CCHIT Ambulatory EHR 2007

INGENIX®

Coders' Dictionary

2011

Notice

Coders' Dictionary is designed to be an authoritative source of information about coding and reimbursement terminology. Every effort has been made to verify accuracy and all information is believed reliable at the time of publication. Absolute accuracy cannot be guaranteed, however. This publication is made available with the understanding that the publisher is not engaged in rendering legal or other services that require a professional license. If you identify a correction or wish to share information, please email the Ingenix customer service department at customerservice@ingenix.com or fax us at 801.982.4033.

American Medical Association Notice

CPT only © 2010 American Medical Association. All rights reserved.

Fee schedules, relative value units, conversion factors and/or related components are not assigned by the AMA, are not part of CPT, and the AMA is not recommending their use. The AMA does not directly or indirectly practice medicine or dispense medical services. The AMA assumes no liability for data contained or not contained herein.

CPT is a registered trademark of the American Medical Association.

Our Commitment to Accuracy

Ingenix is committed to producing accurate and reliable materials. To report corrections, please visit www.ingenixonline.com/accuracy or email accuracy@ingenix.com. You can also reach customer service by calling 1.800.INGENIX (464.3649), option 1.

Copyright

ISBN 978-1-60151-370-0

Acknowledgments

The following staff contributed to the development and/or production of this book:

Mike Grambo, *Product Manager*
Karen Schmidt, BSN, *Technical Director*
Stacy Perry, *Manager, Desktop Publishing*
Lisa Singley, *Project Manager*
LaJuana Green, RHIA, CCS, *Clinical/Technical Editor*
Nannette Orme, CCS-P, CPC, CPMA, CEMC
   Clinical/Technical Editor
Karen Prescott, CMM, CPC, CPC-I, CCS-P, *Clinical Technical Editor*
Tracy Betzler, *Desktop Publishing Specialist*
Hope M. Dunn, *Desktop Publishing Specialist*
Kimberli Turner, *Editor*

Clinical/Technical Editor

Nannette Orme, CCS-P, CPC, CPMA, CEMC

Ms. Orme has more than 15 years of experience in the health care profession. She has extensive background in CPT/HCPCS and ICD-9-CM coding. Her prior experience includes physician clinics and healthcare consulting. Her areas of expertise include physician audits and education, compliance and HIPAA legislation, litigation support for Medicare self-disclosure cases, hospital chargemaster maintenance, workers' compensation and emergency department coding. Ms. Orme has presented at national professional conferences and contributed articles for several professional publications. She is a member of the American Academy of Professional Coders.

Karen M. Prescott, CMM, CPC, CPC-I CCS-P

Ms. Prescott has more than 16 years of experience in the health care profession. She has an extensive background in professional component coding and billing. Her prior experience includes establishing and maintaining a coding and billing service, directing physician practice start ups, functioning as director of physician credentialing, negotiating insurance contracts, and functioning as a health care consultant. Her areas of expertise include coding and reimbursement, documentation education, compliance, practice management, and revenue cycle management. Ms. Prescott is a member of the American Academy of Professional Coders, the American Health Information Management Association (AHIMA), and the Professional Association of Health Care Office Management (PAHCOM).

Introduction

Congratulations on your decision to purchase the *Coders' Dictionary*, the only medical dictionary designed exclusively for medical coders, billers, and reimbursement professionals. It was created when our own clinical editors discovered traditional medical dictionaries often did not provide answers to their coding questions. Unlike more traditional medical dictionaries, *Coders' Dictionary* lays the groundwork for understanding medical terminology from a coding perspective, enhancing the ability to interpret a medical record and more accurately code a claim.

The intention of *Coders' Dictionary* is not to provide definitions for all conceivable medical terms, but to provide definitions for those terms in the medical record that may confound a coder or biller. Readers should not expect to find a definition for "femur" in this book, as a certain basic level of medical terminology knowledge is presumed of a coder. A reader will, however, find in *Coders' Dictionary* a definition for "WIT," an acronym for water-induced thermotherapy, a minimally invasive treatment for benign prostatic hyperplasia. WIT is not defined in most medical dictionaries.

To create *Coders' Dictionary*, Ingenix coding experts generated a list of ambiguous or vexing words found in the medical record or in billing and reimbursement communications. The words may be acronyms, eponyms, or abbreviations, or they may represent generic or brand name medical devices or pharmaceuticals. Unusual procedural, anatomical, or epidemiological terminology from the medical record is also included. The goal of *Coders' Dictionary* is to provide specific definitions and sometimes instructions that accommodate the narrow focus of the medical coder or biller. In some cases, the definition may direct the reader to a single, specific code. In other cases, only a general clinical definition is necessary to provide a road map to appropriate code selection.

Contents

Coders' Dictionary is comprised of different segments, including anatomical illustrations, the main body of alphabetically ordered terms with coding information for ICD-9-CM, CPT, and HCPCS Level II coding, and Appendixes of tables for metric conversions.

Organization

Terms and Definitions

The entries in the main body of the book are organized in numeric and alphabetic order, with numeric entries preceding the alphabetic entries. The term being defined will appear in bold, at the beginning of the entry.

Compound nouns will appear in their natural language order:

radiotherapy afterloading

rather than:

afterloading, radiotherapy

Following the bolded term will be a definition appropriate to coding and reimbursement and sometimes coding instructions. If the term being defined is an acronym, the first words of the definition will provide the acronym's actual meaning:

TCD Transcranial Doppler. Noninvasive ultrasound technology used to evaluate blood flow in the major intracranial arteries. TCD done with contrast is performed by intravenous microbubble injection, in which the bubbles serve to enhance ultrasound signals, thereby producing better visualization. TCD procedures are reported with a CPT code from range 93886–93893.

Prefixes and Suffixes

Prefixes and suffixes used in medical terminology are incorporated alphabetically into the main body of the book. These are not complete words; only the beginning (prefix) or end (suffix) of a word appears with its meaning. Each partial word has a meaning:

cyst- Relating to the urinary bladder or a cyst. (prefix)

-ectomy Excision, removal. (suffix)

These partial words can be put together to define a complete word:

cystectomy *1)* Excision or removal of the urinary bladder. *2)* Excision or removal of a cyst on any anatomical site.

Prefixes and suffixes are typically not seen in medical documentation as stand-alone words.

Multiple Definitions

Some definitions in the main body of the book have multiple meanings. These are presented in two ways in the *Coders' Dictionary*. The first way in which terms with multiple meanings are listed is as one term followed by different numbered definitions:

trephine *1)* Specialized round saw for cutting circular holes in bone, especially the skull. *2)* Instrument that removes small disc-shaped buttons of corneal tissue for transplanting.

The second way in which terms with multiple meanings are presented is with the main term followed by additional concepts containing the main term. The main term is not listed again; instead, only the first letter of the main term appears in its place within the sequence of words for the additional terms:

ganglion Fluid-filled, benign cyst appearing on a tendon sheath or aponeurosis, frequently found in the hand, wrist, or foot and connecting to an underlying joint. *gasserian g.* Large group of nerve cells at the root of the trigeminal nerve (cranial nerve V). *geniculate g.* Group of nerve cell bodies of the facial nerve where the fibers turn sharply at the lateral end of the internal acoustic meatus.

Cross References

Cross references are indicated with a "See." It will refer the user to the term where they can find the definition:

conjugated estrogen See estrogen.

estrogen Group of estrus-stimulating hormones produced by the ovaries, possibly the adrenal cortex and testes, that have different functions in both sexes. They are the main female sex hormones (estradiol, estrone, and estriol) responsible for the maturation and development of female secondary characteristics and act on the reproductive organs to prepare for fertilization, implantation, and nourishment of the embryo. Estrogens also have nonreproductive actions such as minimizing calcium loss from bones by antagonizing the effects of parathyroid hormone and promoting blood clotting.

Coding Information

Many definitions include the ICD-9-CM diagnosis and/or procedural, CPT procedural, and/or HCPCS Level II supply and service codes associated with the term being defined. These codes guide the user to the appropriate code set and sometimes the code for claim reporting purposes. These codes are not to be used directly out of the *Coders' Dictionary*. Always refer to the appropriate code book to identify the best choice of code to be reported. Do not code directly from this book. Some codes listed will not be complete codes; this book is only a map to help the user identify the definitions of

medical terms found in medical documentation, and possibly, the coding usage for those terms.

Illustrations

The anatomical illustrations located among the main terms consist of anatomical areas or body parts and procedures commonly found in medical documentation and operative reports. Not all of the illustrations are listed in the main body of the book; some will be located in the Anatomical Illustrations chapter at the front of the book.

Anatomical Illustrations

The front of the book contains detailed anatomical illustrations to help the user in identifying anatomical sites seen in medical documentation.

Appendixes

Metric Conversion Tables

These tables convert metric measurements into the standard measuring system used in the United States. Metric system measurements are used in many of the code descriptions, such as:

In ICD-9-CM:

Other Conditions Originating in the Perinatal Period (764–779)

The following fifth-digit subclassification is for use with category 764 and codes 765.0 and 765.1 to denote birthweight:

0 unspecified [weight]
1 less than 500 grams
2 500-749 grams
3 750-999 grams
4 1,000-1,249 grams
5 1,250-1,499 grams
6 1,500-1,749 grams
7 1,750-1,999 grams
8 2,000-2,499 grams
9 2,500 grams and over

In CPT:

58260 Vaginal hysterectomy, for uterus 250 grams or less

The notes in the medical documentation may indicate the weight in ounces and/or pounds. These charts assist the user in converting the weight to match the documentation.

How to Use Coders' Dictionary

In the main body of the *Coders' Dictionary*, terms are listed alphabetically and numerically. They include a term and definition and may have coding information for ICD-9-CM, CPT, and/or HCPCS Level II. Not all terms include coding, billing, and reimbursement information, especially the anatomical sites. Coding, billing, and/or reimbursement information, if listed, helps direct the user to the most appropriate code or have billing or reimbursement information that may be useful when submitting claims.

This book is not to be used as a coding book but as a resource to help direct the user to the appropriate code set. From there, the user should reference the CPT, ICD-9-CM, and/or HCPCS Level II book or electronic product for further direction on the use of the code(s). The *Coders' Dictionary* provides definitions to diseases, conditions, procedures, medical or surgical devices, eponyms, anatomical sites, acronyms, modifiers, reimbursement terms, medical terminology, prefixes, suffixes, and drug names (both brand names and generic names). These terms are defined in the *Coders'*

Dictionary mainly because they can be found in medical documentation and operative reports.

Unable to Locate a Term

Coders' Dictionary is an ambitious project and already represents thousands of hours of clinical coding research and documentation. In subsequent editions, users will find an expansion of terms as our database of difficult terms and concepts from the medical record continues to grow. If you seek information on a term not found in *Coders' Dictionary*, forward that information to Ingenix for inclusion in the next edition. Please email your term to customerservice@ingenix.com or mail to Customer Service, *Coders' Dictionary*, Ingenix; 2525 Lake Park Boulevard; Salt Lake City, Utah, 84120.

Anatomical Illustrations

Body Planes and Movements

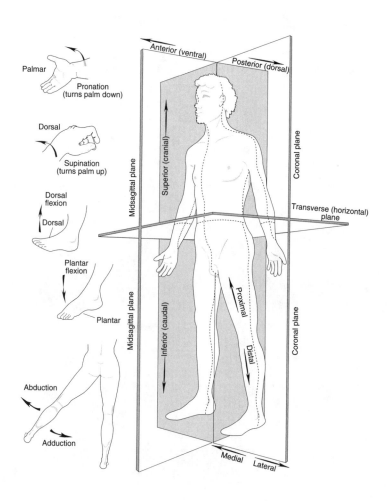

Anatomy

Musculoskeletal System

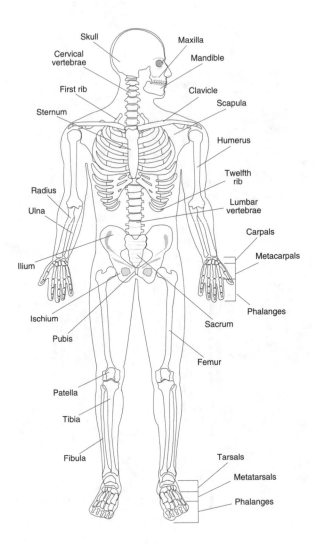

Skull
Cervical vertebrae
First rib
Sternum
Radius
Ulna
Ilium
Ischium
Pubis
Patella
Tibia
Fibula

Maxilla
Mandible
Clavicle
Scapula
Humerus
Twelfth rib
Lumbar vertebrae
Carpals
Metacarpals
Phalanges
Sacrum
Femur
Tarsals
Metatarsals
Phalanges

Musculoskeletal System

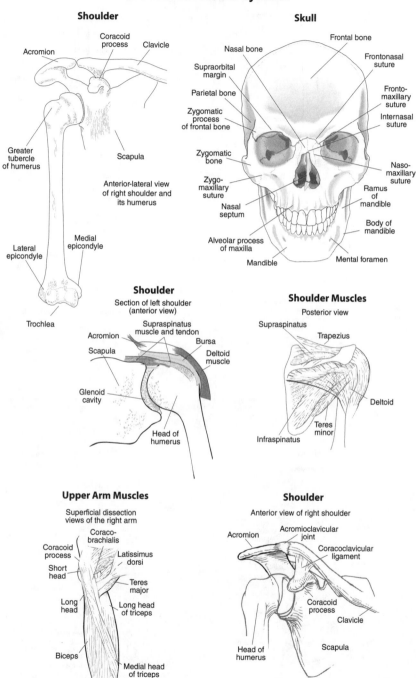

Shoulder

Coracoid process
Clavicle
Acromion
Greater tubercle of humerus
Scapula

Anterior-lateral view of right shoulder and its humerus

Lateral epicondyle
Medial epicondyle
Trochlea

Skull

Frontal bone
Nasal bone
Frontonasal suture
Supraorbital margin
Fronto-maxillary suture
Parietal bone
Internasal suture
Zygomatic process of frontal bone
Zygomatic bone
Naso-maxillary suture
Zygo-maxillary suture
Ramus of mandible
Nasal septum
Body of mandible
Alveolar process of maxilla
Mental foramen
Mandible

Shoulder

Section of left shoulder (anterior view)

Supraspinatus muscle and tendon
Acromion
Bursa
Scapula
Deltoid muscle
Glenoid cavity
Head of humerus

Shoulder Muscles

Posterior view

Supraspinatus
Trapezius
Supraspinatus
Deltoid
Teres minor
Infraspinatus

Upper Arm Muscles

Superficial dissection views of the right arm

Coraco-brachialis
Coracoid process
Latissimus dorsi
Short head
Teres major
Long head
Long head of triceps
Biceps
Medial head of triceps

Shoulder

Anterior view of right shoulder

Acromioclavicular joint
Acromion
Coracoclavicular ligament
Coracoid process
Clavicle
Head of humerus
Scapula

Musculoskeletal System

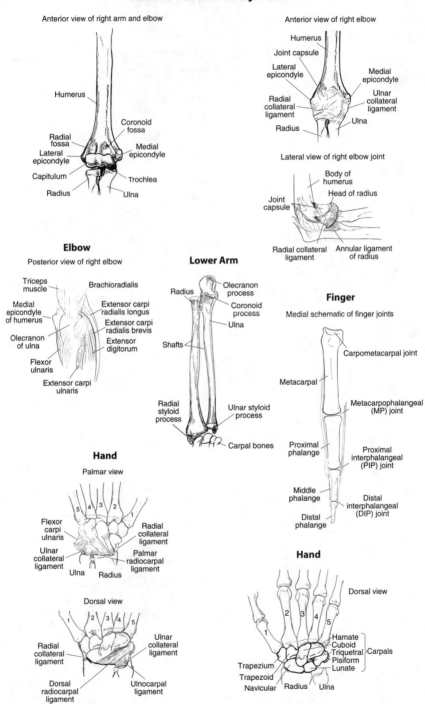

Anterior view of right arm and elbow

Humerus

Coronoid fossa

Radial fossa

Lateral epicondyle

Capitulum

Radius

Medial epicondyle

Trochlea

Ulna

Anterior view of right elbow

Humerus

Joint capsule

Lateral epicondyle

Radial collateral ligament

Radius

Medial epicondyle

Ulnar collateral ligament

Ulna

Lateral view of right elbow joint

Body of humerus

Head of radius

Joint capsule

Radial collateral ligament

Annular ligament of radius

Elbow

Posterior view of right elbow

Triceps muscle

Medial epicondyle of humerus

Olecranon of ulna

Flexor ulnaris

Extensor carpi ulnaris

Brachioradialis

Extensor carpi radialis longus

Extensor carpi radialis brevis

Extensor digitorum

Lower Arm

Radius

Shafts

Radial styloid process

Olecranon process

Coronoid process

Ulna

Ulnar styloid process

Carpal bones

Finger

Medial schematic of finger joints

Carpometacarpal joint

Metacarpal

Metacarpophalangeal (MP) joint

Proximal phalange

Middle phalange

Distal phalange

Proximal interphalangeal (PIP) joint

Distal interphalangeal (DIP) joint

Hand

Palmar view

Flexor carpi ulnaris

Ulnar collateral ligament

Ulna

Radius

Radial collateral ligament

Palmar radiocarpal ligament

Dorsal view

Radial collateral ligament

Dorsal radiocarpal ligament

Ulnar collateral ligament

Ulnocarpal ligament

Hand

Dorsal view

Hamate
Cuboid
Triquetral } Carpals
Pisiform
Lunate

Trapezium
Trapezoid
Navicular

Radius

Ulna

Musculoskeletal System

Ankle

Lateral and posterior views of right ankle

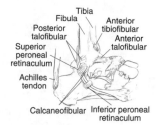

Achilles tendon not shown

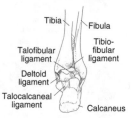

Foot

Select extensors of the foot

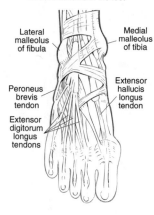

Foot

Tarsals, excluding talus and
calcaneus (dark), superior view

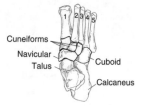

Foot

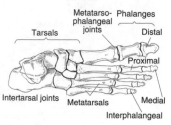

Anatomy

Musculoskeletal System

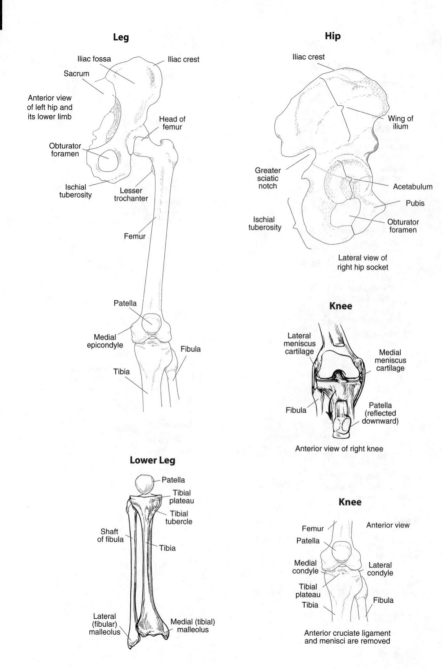

Leg

Iliac fossa
Iliac crest
Sacrum
Anterior view
of left hip and
its lower limb
Head of
femur
Obturator
foramen
Ischial
tuberosity
Lesser
trochanter
Femur
Patella
Medial
epicondyle
Fibula
Tibia

Hip

Iliac crest
Wing of
ilium
Greater
sciatic
notch
Acetabulum
Pubis
Ischial
tuberosity
Obturator
foramen

Lateral view of
right hip socket

Knee

Lateral
meniscus
cartilage
Medial
meniscus
cartilage
Fibula
Patella
(reflected
downward)

Anterior view of right knee

Lower Leg

Patella
Tibial
plateau
Tibial
tubercle
Shaft
of fibula
Tibia
Lateral
(fibular)
malleolus
Medial (tibial)
malleolus

Knee

Femur
Anterior view
Patella
Medial
condyle
Lateral
condyle
Tibial
plateau
Tibia
Fibula

Anterior cruciate ligament
and menisci are removed

Rule of Nines for Burns (Adults)

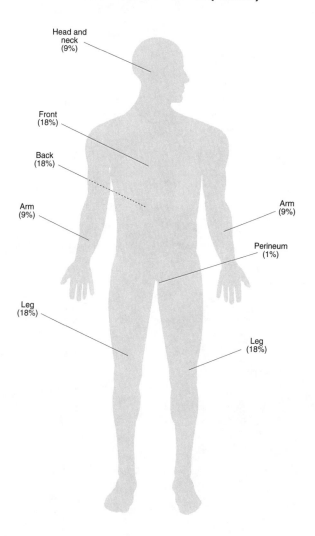

Head and
neck
(9%)

Front
(18%)

Back
(18%)

Arm
(9%)

Arm
(9%)

Perineum
(1%)

Leg
(18%)

Leg
(18%)

First-degree burns involve surface layers only and
tissue destruction is minimal.

Second-degree burns damage deeper epidermal layers
and upper layers of the dermis; damage to sweat glands, hair
follicles, and sebaceous glands may occur.

Third-degree burns include destruction of both epidermis
and dermis and tissue death extends below the hair
follicles and sweat glands.

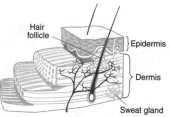

Hair
follicle

} Epidermis

Dermis

Sweat gland

Anatomy

Digestive System

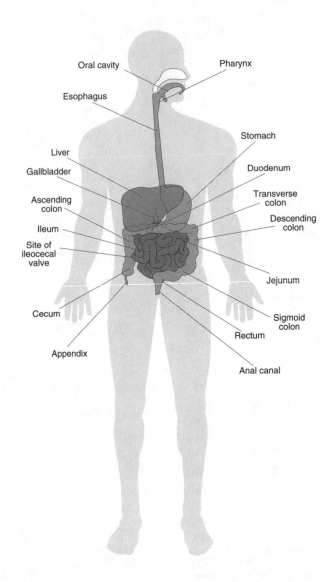

Oral cavity

Pharynx

Esophagus

Stomach

Liver

Duodenum

Gallbladder

Transverse colon

Ascending colon

Descending colon

Ileum

Site of ileocecal valve

Jejunum

Cecum

Sigmoid colon

Rectum

Appendix

Anal canal

Digestive System

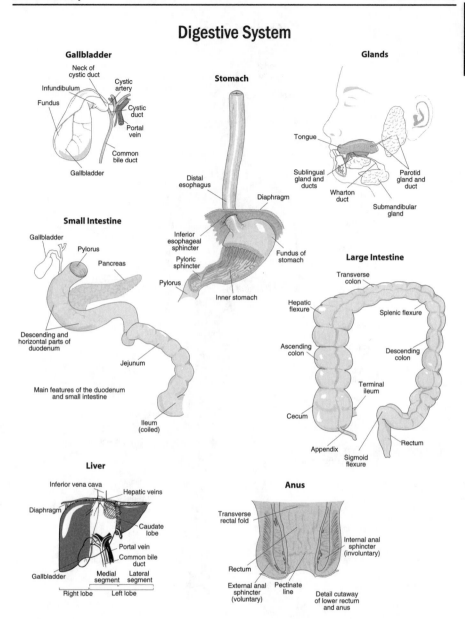

Gallbladder

Neck of cystic duct
Infundibulum
Fundus
Cystic artery
Cystic duct
Portal vein
Common bile duct
Gallbladder

Stomach

Distal esophagus
Diaphragm
Inferior esophageal sphincter
Pyloric sphincter
Pylorus
Inner stomach
Fundus of stomach

Glands

Tongue
Sublingual gland and ducts
Wharton duct
Parotid gland and duct
Submandibular gland

Small Intestine

Gallbladder
Pylorus
Pancreas
Pylorus
Descending and horizontal parts of duodenum
Jejunum
Main features of the duodenum and small intestine
Ileum (coiled)

Large Intestine

Transverse colon
Hepatic flexure
Splenic flexure
Ascending colon
Descending colon
Terminal ileum
Cecum
Appendix
Sigmoid flexure
Rectum

Liver

Inferior vena cava
Hepatic veins
Diaphragm
Caudate lobe
Portal vein
Common bile duct
Gallbladder
Medial segment
Lateral segment
Right lobe
Left lobe

Anus

Transverse rectal fold
Internal anal sphincter (involuntary)
Rectum
External anal sphincter (voluntary)
Pectinate line
Detail cutaway of lower rectum and anus

Anatomy

Arterial System

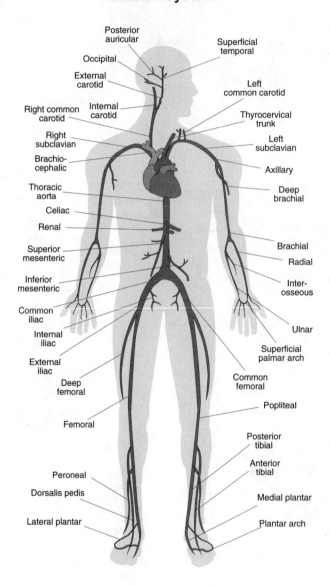

Anatomy

Arterial System

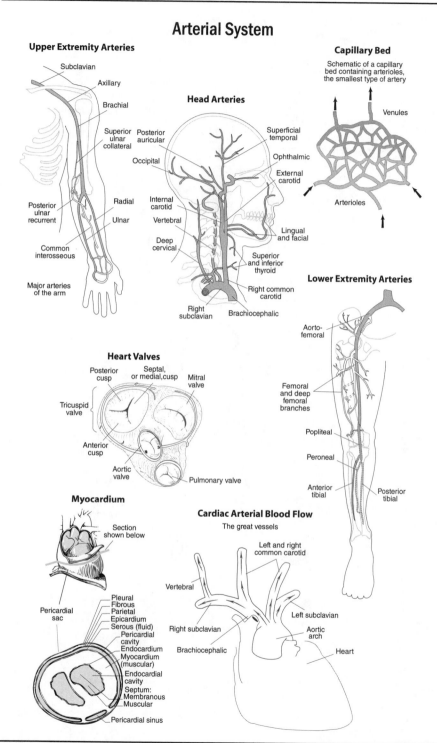

Upper Extremity Arteries

Subclavian
Axillary
Brachial
Superior ulnar collateral
Posterior auricular
Occipital
Internal carotid
Radial
Ulnar
Vertebral
Deep cervical
Posterior ulnar recurrent
Common interosseous
Major arteries of the arm

Head Arteries

Superficial temporal
Ophthalmic
External carotid
Lingual and facial
Superior and inferior thyroid
Right common carotid
Right subclavian
Brachiocephalic

Capillary Bed

Schematic of a capillary bed containing arterioles, the smallest type of artery

Venules
Arterioles

Lower Extremity Arteries

Aorto-femoral
Femoral and deep femoral branches
Popliteal
Peroneal
Anterior tibial
Posterior tibial

Heart Valves

Posterior cusp
Septal, or medial, cusp
Mitral valve
Tricuspid valve
Anterior cusp
Aortic valve
Pulmonary valve

Myocardium

Section shown below
Pericardial sac
Pleural
Fibrous
Parietal
Epicardium
Serous (fluid)
Pericardial cavity
Endocardium
Myocardium (muscular)
Endocardial cavity
Septum:
Membranous
Muscular
Pericardial sinus

Cardiac Arterial Blood Flow

The great vessels

Left and right common carotid
Vertebral
Right subclavian
Brachiocephalic
Left subclavian
Aortic arch
Heart

Venous System

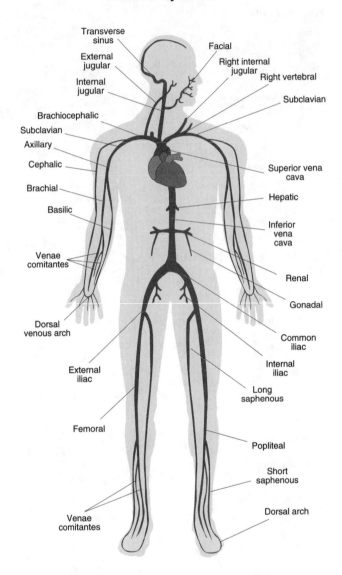

Transverse sinus

External jugular

Internal jugular

Brachiocephalic

Subclavian

Axillary

Cephalic

Brachial

Basilic

Venae comitantes

Dorsal venous arch

External iliac

Femoral

Venae comitantes

Facial

Right internal jugular

Right vertebral

Subclavian

Superior vena cava

Hepatic

Inferior vena cava

Renal

Gonadal

Common iliac

Internal iliac

Long saphenous

Popliteal

Short saphenous

Dorsal arch

Venous System

Upper Extremity Veins

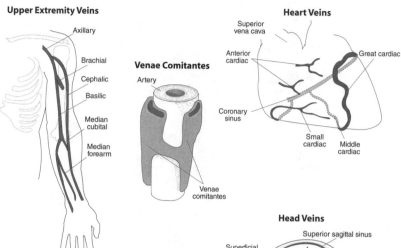

- Axillary
- Brachial
- Cephalic
- Basilic
- Median cubital
- Median forearm

Venae Comitantes

- Artery
- Venae comitantes

Heart Veins

- Superior vena cava
- Anterior cardiac
- Great cardiac
- Coronary sinus
- Small cardiac
- Middle cardiac

Head Veins

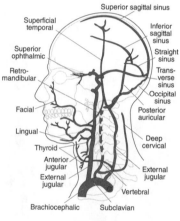

- Superior sagittal sinus
- Superficial temporal
- Inferior sagittal sinus
- Superior ophthalmic
- Straight sinus
- Retro-mandibular
- Transverse sinus
- Occipital sinus
- Facial
- Posterior auricular
- Lingual
- Deep cervical
- Thyroid
- Anterior jugular
- External jugular
- External jugular
- Vertebral
- Brachiocephalic
- Subclavian

Venous Blood Flow

Venous blood flow is assisted by valves in the lumen of the vessels

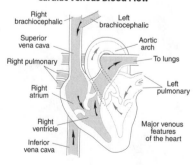

- Valve cusps in closed position
- Valve cusps in open position

Cardiac Venous Blood Flow

- Right brachiocephalic
- Left brachiocephalic
- Superior vena cava
- Aortic arch
- Right pulmonary
- To lungs
- Right atrium
- Left pulmonary
- Right ventricle
- Major venous features of the heart
- Inferior vena cava

Abdominal Veins

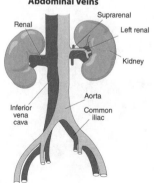

- Renal
- Suprarenal
- Left renal
- Kidney
- Inferior vena cava
- Aorta
- Common iliac

Nervous System

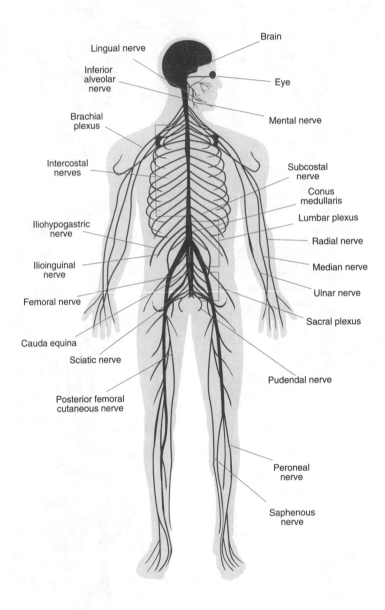

Lingual nerve

Inferior alveolar nerve

Brachial plexus

Intercostal nerves

Iliohypogastric nerve

Ilioinguinal nerve

Femoral nerve

Cauda equina

Sciatic nerve

Posterior femoral cutaneous nerve

Brain

Eye

Mental nerve

Subcostal nerve

Conus medullaris

Lumbar plexus

Radial nerve

Median nerve

Ulnar nerve

Sacral plexus

Pudendal nerve

Peroneal nerve

Saphenous nerve

Anatomy

Nervous System

Brain

Corpus callosum
Cerebrum
Hypothalamus
Interventricular foramen
Fornix
Third ventricle
Pineal body
Optic chiasm
Hypophysis
Pons
Mamillary body
Peduncle
Medulla oblongata
Spinal cord
Corpora quadrigemina
Cerebral aqueduct
Vermis
Fourth ventricle
Median aperture

Cranial Nerves

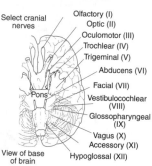

Select cranial nerves
Olfactory (I)
Optic (II)
Oculomotor (III)
Trochlear (IV)
Trigeminal (V)
Abducens (VI)
Facial (VII)
Pons
Vestibulocochlear (VIII)
Glossopharyngeal (IX)
Vagus (X)
Accessory (XI)
Hypoglossal (XII)
View of base of brain

Spinal Cord

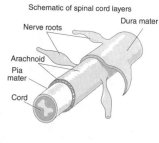

Schematic of spinal cord layers

Nerve roots
Dura mater
Arachnoid
Pia mater
Cord

Spinal Column

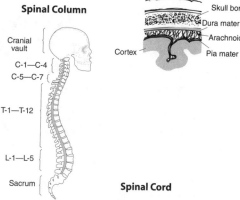

Cranial vault
C-1—C-4
C-5—C-7
T-1—T-12
L-1—L-5
Sacrum

Cranial Layers

Skin
Skull bone
Dura mater
Arachnoid
Cortex
Pia mater

Spinal Cord

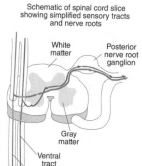

Schematic of spinal cord slice showing simplified sensory tracts and nerve roots

White matter
Posterior nerve root ganglion
Gray matter
Ventral tract
Lateral tract

Spinal Cord

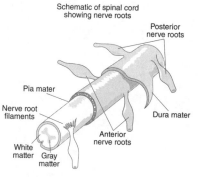

Schematic of spinal cord showing nerve roots

Posterior nerve roots
Pia mater
Nerve root filaments
Dura mater
White matter
Gray matter
Anterior nerve roots

Lymphatic System

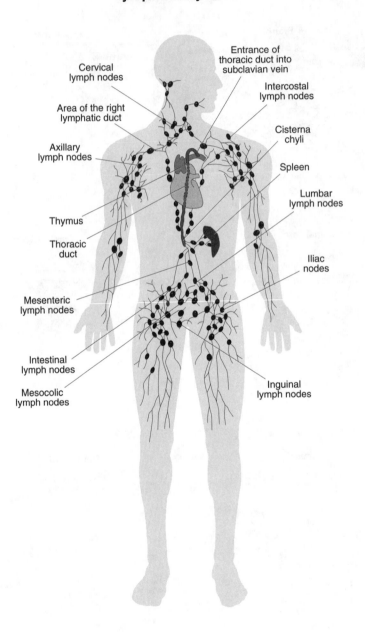

Cervical
lymph nodes

Entrance of
thoracic duct into
subclavian vein

Intercostal
lymph nodes

Area of the right
lymphatic duct

Cisterna
chyli

Axillary
lymph nodes

Spleen

Lumbar
lymph nodes

Thymus

Thoracic
duct

Iliac
nodes

Mesenteric
lymph nodes

Intestinal
lymph nodes

Inguinal
lymph nodes

Mesocolic
lymph nodes

Anatomy

Lymphatic System

Axillary Lymph Nodes

Parasternal nodes
Sternum
Clavicle
Deltoid
Brachialis
Lateral nodes
Subscapular nodes
Pectoral nodes
Axillary lymph nodes
Central lymph nodes
Latissimus dorsi muscle
Rectus abdominis

Lymphatic Capillaries

Schematic of lymphatic capillaries

Tissue cells
Valves
Endothelial cells

Fluids and particles can enter the capillary through overlapping valves

Lymphatic Drainage

Lymphatic drainage of the colon follows blood supply

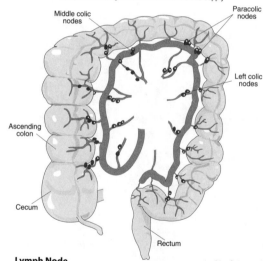

Middle colic nodes
Paracolic nodes
Left colic nodes
Ascending colon
Cecum
Rectum

Lymph Node

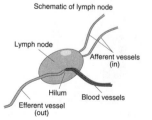

Schematic of lymph node

Lymph node
Afferent vessels (in)
Hilum
Blood vessels
Efferent vessel (out)

Neck Lymph Nodes

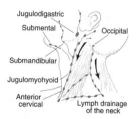

Jugulodigastric
Submental
Occipital
Submandibular
Jugulomyohyoid
Anterior cervical
Lymph drainage of the neck

Endocrine System

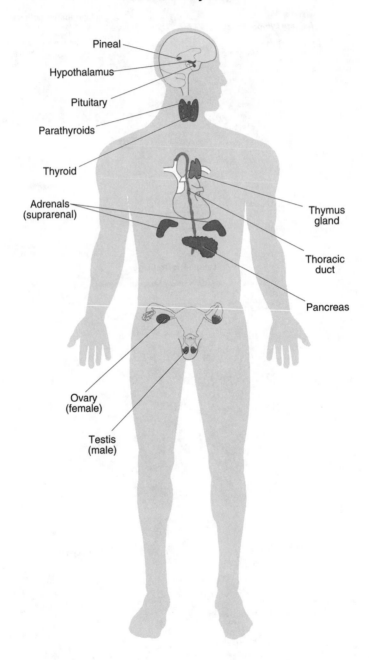

Pineal

Hypothalamus

Pituitary

Parathyroids

Thyroid

Adrenals
(suprarenal)

Thymus
gland

Thoracic
duct

Pancreas

Ovary
(female)

Testis
(male)

Endocrine System

Thyroid Glands

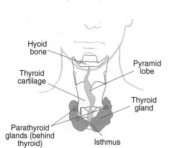

Pituitary Glands

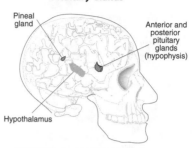

The pituitary gland and its controller, the hypothalamus, control body growth and stimulate and regulate other glands

Thyroid

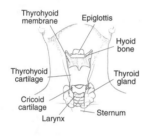

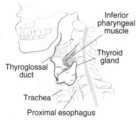

Thyroid

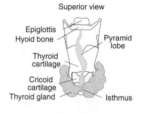

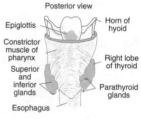

Placenta

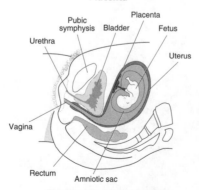

The placenta is considered part of the endocrine system, secreting chorionic gonadotropin, estrogen, progesterone, and somatomammotropin

Anatomy

Genitourinary System

Kidney

Cutaway detail of right kidney

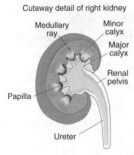

Medullary ray
Minor calyx
Major calyx
Renal pelvis
Papilla
Ureter

Nephron

Schematic of nephron, the tiny filtering mechanism of the kidney

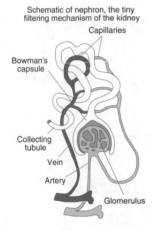

Capillaries
Bowman's capsule
Collecting tubule
Vein
Artery
Glomerulus

Urinary

Posterior view showing location of kidneys and ureters

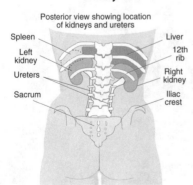

Spleen
Left kidney
Ureters
Sacrum
Liver
12th rib
Right kidney
Iliac crest

Male Urinary

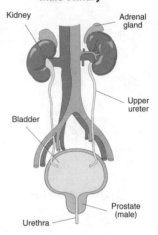

Kidney
Adrenal gland
Upper ureter
Bladder
Prostate (male)
Urethra

Male Genitourinary

Posterior view of male bladder and prostate

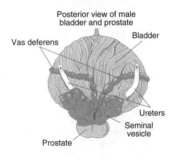

Vas deferens
Bladder
Ureters
Seminal vesicle
Prostate

Male Reproductive

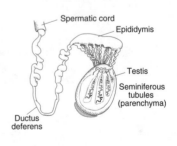

Spermatic cord
Epididymis
Testis
Seminiferous tubules (parenchyma)
Ductus deferens

Genitourinary System

Female Genitourinary

Sideview schematic of
female urogenital system

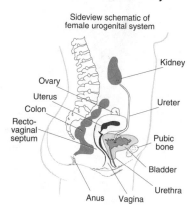

Kidney
Ovary
Uterus
Ureter
Colon
Recto-
vaginal
septum
Pubic
bone
Bladder
Anus   Vagina   Urethra

Female Rectoperineal

Lateral schematic showing
the female rectoperineal area

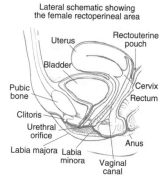

Uterus
Rectouterine
pouch
Bladder
Pubic
bone
Cervix
Rectum
Clitoris
Urethral
orifice
Anus
Labia majora Labia
minora   Vaginal
canal

Female Bladder

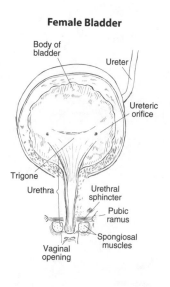

Body of
bladder
Ureter
Ureteric
orifice
Trigone
Urethra
Urethral
sphincter
Pubic
ramus
Spongiosal
muscles
Vaginal
opening

Female Reproductive

Uterine
tube
Uterine cavity
Ovary
Fimbriae
of tube
Ovarian
ligament
Broad
ligament
Vaginal canal
Cervix

Female Reproductive

Sideview schematic
of female breast

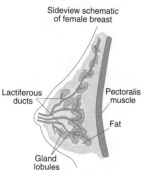

Lactiferous
ducts
Pectoralis
muscle
Fat
Gland
lobules

Anatomy

Respiratory System

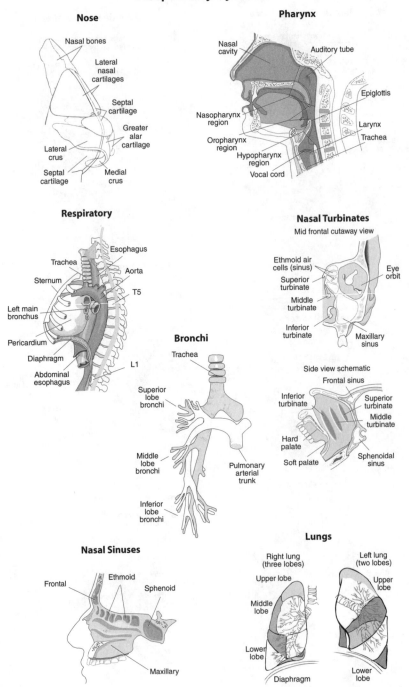

Eye

Eye

Muscles of the right eye

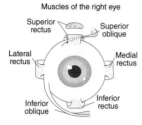

Superior rectus
Superior oblique
Lateral rectus
Medial rectus
Inferior oblique
Inferior rectus

Lacrimal System

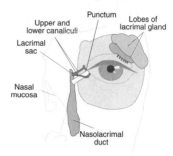

Upper and lower canaliculi
Punctum
Lobes of lacrimal gland
Lacrimal sac
Nasal mucosa
Nasolacrimal duct

Eye

Anterior and posterior chambers of the eye

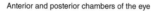

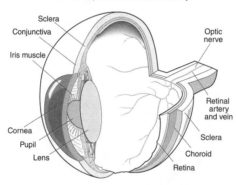

Sclera
Conjunctiva
Iris muscle
Optic nerve
Retinal artery and vein
Cornea
Sclera
Pupil
Lens
Choroid
Retina

Ear

Ear

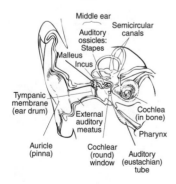

Middle ear
Semicircular canals
Auditory ossicles: Stapes
Malleus
Incus
Tympanic membrane (ear drum)
External auditory meatus
Cochlea (in bone)
Pharynx
Auricle (pinna)
Cochlear (round) window
Auditory (eustachian) tube

Middle Ear

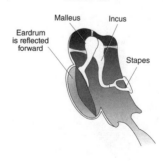

Malleus
Incus
Eardrum is reflected forward
Stapes

/ Or.

< Less than.

<= Less than or equal to.

> Greater than.

>= Greater than or equal to.

@ At.

13 syndrome Variable symptoms in newborns with an extra chromosome in group D. Condition is usually fatal within two years and includes mental retardation and malformed ears, cardiac defects, convulsions, and others. Report this disorder with ICD-9-CM code 758.1. *Synonym(s): D1, Patau's, trisomy D.*

16-18 syndrome Congenital malformations in which extra chromosome is group E. Includes mental retardation, abnormal skull shape, malformed ears, small mandible, cardiac defects, short sternum, and other symptoms. Report this disorder with ICD-9-CM code 758.2. *Synonym(s): E3, Edward's, trisomy E.*

2-D Two-dimensional or cross-sectional view produced by reconstructed B-mode ultrasound scanning or multiple angled x-ray images, such as from computed tomography, for diagnostic purposes.

2-LINT Second lumbrical interosseous technique. Nerve conduction test comparing conduction speed of segments of the median and ulnar nerves. The tests are conducted for various diagnoses but indicate the presence of lesions on either nerve.

2nd Skin Brand name hydrogel dressing to promote healing and protect against infection.

21 CPT modifier deleted in 2009. Prolonged services codes 99354-99357 may be used to report a face-to-face or hospital floor service that is prolonged or otherwise greater than that required for the level of E/M service documented. A report should be submitted when appropriate.

21 syndrome Retardation with numerous markers varying from one person to another. Symptoms include retarded growth, flat face with short nose, epicanthic skin folds, protruding lower lip, rounded ears, thickened tongue, pelvic dysplasia, broad hands and feet, stubby fingers, and absence of Moro reflex. Report this disorder with ICD-9-CM code 758.0.

22 CPT modifier, for use with CPT or HCPCS Level II codes, that identifies when a service provided is greater than that usually required for the listed procedure. Surgical procedures that require additional physician work due to complications or medical emergencies may warrant the use of this modifier. Claims that are submitted with this modifier should have attached supporting documentation that demonstrates the unusual distinction of the service(s).

22 syndrome Retardation with numerous markers varying from one person to another. Symptoms include retarded growth, flat face with short nose, epicanthic skin folds, protruding lower lip, rounded ears, thickened tongue, pelvic dysplasia, broad hands and feet, stubby fingers, and absence of Moro reflex. Report this disorder with ICD-9-CM code 758.0.

23 CPT modifier, for use with CPT anesthesia codes, that identifies when a procedure must be done under general anesthesia when it would otherwise require no anesthesia or local anesthesia.

24 CPT modifier, for use with CPT evaluation and management (E/M) codes, that identifies when an E/M service was performed by the same physician during a postoperative period for a reason(s) unrelated to the original procedure. For Medicare, this modifier can be used for CPT codes 92012-92014 and 99201-99499.

25 CPT modifier, for use with CPT evaluation and management (E/M) codes, that identifies when the patient's condition requires a significant, separately identifiable E/M service above and beyond the other service provided or above and beyond the usual preoperative and postoperative care associated with the procedure that was performed. Medicare will allow separate payment for two office visits provided on the same day by the same physician when each visit is rendered for an unrelated problem. Both visits must be at different times of the day and must be medically necessary.

26 CPT modifier, for use with CPT and HCPCS Level II codes, that identifies when a procedure is reported for the professional component only. This is assigned for the physician portion of a procedure that is a combination of a physician component and a technical component. It is used when the physician is providing the interpretation of the diagnostic study or laboratory test.

27 CPT modifier, for use with CPT and HCPCS codes, that identifies when a provider has performed multiple separate E/M services in an outpatient facility on the same patient during the same day.

3DCRT Three-dimensional conformal radiation therapy.

3DXRT Three-dimensional external radiation therapy.

32 CPT modifier, for use with CPT evaluation and management (E/M) codes, that identifies when the services performed are related to mandated consultation and/or related services (e.g., third-party payer, governmental, legislative, or regulatory requirement).

33 CPT modifier to identify mandated preventive services performed in order to comply with the Patient Protection and Affordable Care Act.

47 CPT modifier, for use with CPT and HCPCS Level II codes, that identifies when regional or general anesthesia

1-99
66

is provided by the physician. This modifier does not include local anesthesia.

5-alpha reductase Prostate enzyme that converts testosterone into dihydrotestosterone (DHT). Blockage of the action of 5-alpha reductase results in a slowing of DHT production, which in turn slows or stops the growth of benign prostate tumors.

50 CPT modifier, for use with CPT and HCPCS Level II codes, that identifies when a procedure is performed bilaterally. The modifier is used only when the exact same service/code is reported for each bilateral anatomical site. For Medicare claims, this modifier is reported as a single line item; only one code is reported with 50 appended to the end of the code. Other payers may require reporting the CPT code twice, with 50 appended to the second procedure.

51 CPT modifier, for use with CPT and HCPCS Level II codes, that identifies when multiple procedures (other than evaluation and management services) are performed at the same session by the same provider. The first code is reported without a modifier, any subsequent procedures are reported with modifier 51 appended to the end of the code.

52 CPT modifier, for use with CPT and HCPCS Level II codes, that identifies when a procedure or service is reduced or eliminated at the physician's discretion. Documentation should be present in the medical record indicating the reason(s) for the reduction in the procedure or service. This modifier may affect payment.

53 CPT modifier, for use with CPT and HCPCS Level II codes for physician claims, that identifies when a procedure was started but terminated due to extenuating circumstances or circumstances that threaten the well-being of the patient. If the procedure was discontinued after anesthesia was induced, report the aborted procedure using the appropriate CPT code, appending modifier 53 to the end of the code.

54 CPT modifier, for use with CPT and HCPCS Level II codes, that identifies when the physician performs only the surgical portion of a procedure. Another physician(s) has provided or will provide the preoperative and postoperative care of the patient. There must be a transfer of care between patients. Transfer of care is determined by the date of the transfer order.

55 CPT modifier, for use with CPT and HCPCS Level II codes, that identifies when a physician performs only postoperative care of the patient. Another physician has performed the surgical procedure and has transferred postoperative care to the physician reporting this modifier.

56 CPT modifier, for use with CPT and HCPCS Level II codes, that identifies when the physician performs only the preoperative care of a patient. This modifier is not typically used on Medicare claims; it is usually included in the payment for the surgical/diagnostic procedure.

57 CPT modifier, for use with CPT evaluation and management (E/M) codes that identifies an E/M service that resulted in the initial decision to perform surgery. This modifier should be used only on procedure codes with a 90-day postoperative period (major surgery).

58 CPT modifier, for use with CPT and HCPCS Level II codes, that identifies when a procedure or service was planned prospectively at the time of the original procedure (staged procedure), more extensive than the original procedure, or is reported for therapy following a diagnostic surgical procedure.

59 CPT modifier, for use with CPT codes, that indicates that a procedure or service was distinct or independent from other services performed on the same day. This modifier is used to report procedures/services that are not normally reported together but that are appropriate under the circumstances. This may represent a different session or patient encounter, different procedure or surgery, different site or organ system, separate incision/excision, separate lesion or separate injury not ordinarily encountered or performed on the same day by the same physician.

62 CPT modifier, for use with CPT codes, that identifies a procedure performed by two surgeons who work together as primary surgeons performing distinct part(s) of the procedure. Each surgeon should report his/her distinct operative work by adding this modifier to the procedure code and any associated add-on code(s) for that procedure as long as both surgeons continue to work together. Each surgeon should report the cosurgery once using the same procedure code.

63 CPT modifier, for use with CPT codes, that identifies procedures performed on neonates and infants up to a present body weight of 4 kilograms, which may involve significantly increased complexity and physician work commonly associated with these patients. In the CPT book, this modifier should not be used if the parenthetical statement notes exclude its use.

66 CPT modifier, for use with CPT codes, that identifies highly complex procedures that require the skills of several physicians, often of different specialties, under the surgical team concept. Each participating physician will report the basic procedure, with this modifier appended.

72-hour rule CMS and private payer standard stating that procedures for outpatient diagnostic services or other services related to the admission that occur within the three calendar days immediately preceding a patient's admission to a hospital for a related condition are included in the charges for the admission.

73 CPT modifier, for use with CPT codes on ambulatory surgery center and outpatient hospital claims, that identifies a discontinued procedure prior to the administration of anesthesia (local, regional block(s) or general). This procedure may be discontinued due to extenuating circumstances or those that threaten the well-being of the patient. Discontinuation may be subsequent to the patient's surgical preparation, including sedation (when provided).

74 CPT modifier, for use with CPT codes on ambulatory surgery center and outpatient hospital claims, that identifies a discontinued procedure after the administration of anesthesia (local, regional block(s) or general). The procedure may have been started by intubation, incision, and/or scope insertion. This procedure may be discontinued due to extenuating circumstances or those that threaten the well-being of the patient.

76 CPT modifier, for use with CPT or HCPCS Level II codes, that identifies that a procedure or service was repeated subsequent to the original procedure or service by the same physician or other qualified health care professional with the same CPT or HCPCS Level II code. If the procedure is performed in the same day, the procedure code is reported twice with this modifier appended to the second code(s).

77 CPT modifier, for use with CPT or HCPCS Level II codes, that indicates that a basic procedure or service performed by a different physician or other qualified health care professional was a repeated procedure.

78 CPT modifier, for use with CPT codes, that identifies a patient return to the operating room (OR) for a related procedure by the same physician or other qualified health care professional during the postoperative period of the initial procedure. This modifier is reported when a procedure requires a return to the OR due to complications that arise from the original surgery and/or when any related surgical procedures are performed in the OR.

79 CPT modifier, for use with CPT or HCPCS Level II codes, that indicates that the performance of a procedure or service by the same physician during the postoperative period was unrelated to the original procedure. With this modifier, a different diagnosis should be reported.

80 CPT modifier, for use with CPT codes, that indicates that the physician assisted with the surgery. For Medicare Part B, this modifier may be used with only certain CPT codes. Check with the Medicare physician fee schedule for a list of those procedures.

81 CPT modifier, for use with CPT codes, that identifies minimal surgical assistant services. Medicare rarely recognizes this modifier (except in extreme cases).

82 CPT modifier, for use with CPT codes, that identifies an assistant surgeon when a qualified resident surgeon is unavailable. Medicare Part B allows payment for this

modifier only when the services are performed by a physician not in a residency or fellowship program.

837i Approved HIPAA transaction set for institutional electronic claims submission. Also known as the X096 or ASC X12N 837.

837p HIPAA compliant standardized electronic transaction format for the transmission of professional claims.

90 CPT modifier, for use with CPT codes, that identifies when laboratory procedures are performed by a party other than the treating or reporting physician. When appending this modifier, the physician office is indicating that the laboratory procedures were performed by an outside laboratory. Medicare does not allow the physician office to bill for tests unless it actually performs them.

91 CPT modifier, for use with CPT codes, that identifies a repeated diagnostic laboratory test on the same day to obtain subsequent (multiple) test results.

92 CPT modifier, for use with CPT codes, that identifies laboratory tests that are specific to HIV tests performed using a kit or portable instrumentation. This modifier is used with CPT codes 86701-86703.

99 CPT modifier, for use with CPT and HCPCS Level II codes, that indicates when two or more modifiers are used to completely describe the procedures performed. This modifier should be added to the basic procedure, and the other applicable modifiers may be listed as part of the description of the service.

A *1)* Assessment. *2)* Blood type.

a- Without, away from, not.

a (ante) Before.

a fib Atrial fibrillation.

a flutter Atrial flutter.

A&Ox3 Alert and oriented to person, place, and time. Description of the patient's mental status at the time of the encounter. Documentation of x1 or x2 indicates disorientation. In some cases, the documentation will state x4, which indicates the patient is also oriented to the cause of the immediate medical emergency.

A&P Auscultation and percussion.

a.a. Of each.

a.c. Before eating.

a.d. *1)* Right ear. *2)* To, up to.

a.m. Morning.

a.s. Left ear.

a.u. Each ear, both ears.

A/G Albumin-globulin ratio.

A/S, A.S., or AS Administrative simplification.

A2 Aortic second sound.

AA *1)* Anaplastic astrocytoma. High-grade brain tumor. AAs are usually aggressive and require intensive therapy. *2)* HCPCS Level II modifier for use with CPT or HCPCS Level II codes, identifying anesthesia services performed personally by an anesthesiologist. This modifier affects Medicare payment. *3)* Anesthesiology assistant. Individual with specialized training to assist anesthesiologists with anesthesia administration. *4)* Alcoholics Anonymous. *5)* Arytenoid adduction. Placement of a suture to reposition the vocal cord and its cartilage. AA is reported with CPT code 31400 if an external approach is used, and 31560 if performed endoscopically. *Synonym(s): arytenoidopexy vocal cord paralysis.*

AAA: Abdominal Aortic Aneurysm

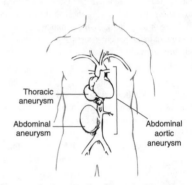

AAA Abdominal aortic aneurysm. Dilation or sac-like outpouching of the abdominal aorta, usually associated with severe atherosclerosis. This is a dangerous and life-threatening condition because of the risk of aortic rupture. Repair of an abdominal aneurysm may be endovascular or direct, open repair through incision. AAA without rupture is reported with ICD-9-CM code 441.4; with rupture, 441.3. *NCD Reference: 20.23.*

AAASF American Association for the Accreditation of Ambulatory Surgery Facilities. Regulatory organization that sets the standards for ambulatory surgery centers.

AABB American Association of Blood Banks.

AAC American Academy of Cardiology. Professional organization for cardiology medical specialty.

AACD Aging-associated cognitive decline, reported with ICD-9-CM code 797.

AACG Acute angle-closure glaucoma, reported with ICD-9-CM code 365.22.

AACR American Association for Cancer Research. Organization that provides information about causes and diagnosis of cancer, as well as prevention and treatment.

AAFP American Academy of Family Physicians. Professional organization for family practice medical specialty.

AAHomecare American Association for Homecare. Association for the home care industry, including home IV therapy, home medical services and manufacturers, and home health providers. AAHomecare was created through the merger of the Health Industry Distributors Association's Home Care Division (HIDA Home Care), the Home Health Services and Staffing Association (HHSSA), and the National Association for Medical Equipment Services (NAMES).

AAHP American Association of Health Plans. National association of health plans created by the merger of the

Group Health Association of America (GHAA) and the American Managed Care and Review Association (AMCRA).

AAI Acute alcohol intoxication. ICD-9-CM code selection is determined by whether the patient is dependent upon alcohol or simply abusing alcohol, and also whether the AAI is continuous or episodic.

AAL Anterior axillary line.

AAMT American Association for Medical Transcription.

AAN American Academy of Neurology. Professional organization for neurology medical specialty.

AAOS American Academy of Orthopaedic Surgeons. Nonprofit organization for orthopaedic surgeons and allied health professionals

AAPA American Academy of Physician Assistants.

AAPC American Academy of Professional Coders. National organization for coders and billers offering certification (CPC, CPC-H, and CPC-P) based upon physician-, outpatient facility-, or payer-specific guidelines.

AAPCC Adjusted average per capita cost. Estimated average cost of Medicare benefits for an individual, based upon criteria including age, sex, institutional status, Medicaid, disability, and end-stage renal failure.

AAPPO American Association of Preferred Provider Organizations.

AAROM Active assistive range of motion. AAROM is used in physical therapy. The physical therapist moves the patient's limbs in range of motion exercises.

AAT Alpha-1 antitrypsin. Plasma protein inhibitor of elastase activity and other enzymes, such as trypsin and cathepsin G, that digests various proteins. AAT is produced primarily in the liver and a deficiency of this protein has been connected with emphysema.

AAV AIDS-associated virus. Report AAV with the appropriate ICD-9-CM code for HIV: asymptomatic infection, V08; exposure, V01.79; nonspecific serologic evidence, 795.71; or symptomatic infection, 042.

AAW Anterior aortic wall.

ab Abortion.

AB Blood type.

ab- From, away from, absent.

ABA Allergic bronchopulmonary aspergillosis. Noninvasive hypersensitivity reaction caused by an allergy to aspergillus fumigatus (mold), a fungus normally found growing in stored grain, decaying vegetation, bird feces, or dead leaves. Symptoms include exacerbation of asthma symptoms, wheezing, and hemoptysis. Report ABA with ICD-9-CM code 518.6.

abarelix Injectable gonadotropin-releasing hormone (GnRH) antagonist approved for the treatment of advanced symptomatic prostate cancer under certain conditions. Abarelix may be sold under the brand name Plenaxis. *NCD Reference: 110.19.*

abarognosis Loss of the ability to sense or consciously perceive weight, such as the weight of hand-held objects, reported with ICD-9-CM code 781.99. *Synonym(s): baragnosis.*

abasia Inability to walk due to impaired muscular coordination. Code assignment is dependent upon underlying cause. If muscular incoordination is the underlying cause, report ICD-9-CM code 781.3; if it is a psychogenic cause, report 300.11 or 307.9.

abatacept Chemotherapeutic agent used in the treatment of rheumatoid arthritis. Infusion of abatacept is reported with CPT code 96413, 96415, or 96417 or for inpatient facilities, ICD-9-CM procedure code 99.29. May be sold under the brand name Orencia. Report supply with HCPCS Level II code J0129.

abattoir fever Disease caused by infection with Coxiella burnetii, a rickettsial bacteria spread by inhaling contaminated dust or aerosols, contact with infected livestock, or articles such as wool, hair, and hides. It most often affects workers in stockyards, textile plants, or meat packing plants. Symptoms are usually mild and flu-like, but may manifest with high fever, muscle pain, and severe headache and may require antibiotic treatment. Report this condition with ICD-9-CM code 083.0. *Synonym(s): Balkan grippe, Q fever, query fever.*

Abbe-Estlander Procedure

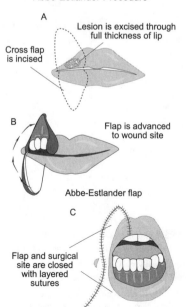

A

Lesion is excised through full thickness of lip

Cross flap is incised

B

Flap is advanced to wound site

Abbe-Estlander flap

C

Flap and surgical site are closed with layered sutures

Abbe-Estlander procedure Reconstructive lip procedure in which a full-thickness portion of the lip is removed. A skin flap from the opposing lip is incised, cross-advanced to the surgical site, and sutured with a layered closure. This procedure is utilized to fill defects of the lip due to cleft deformities, cancer, or trauma. Report this procedure with CPT code 40527.

ABBI Advanced breast biopsy instrumentation. Method of percutaneous needle biopsy that employs a motorized oscillating blade, developed to increase the volume of tissue harvested in a breast biopsy. It is used with stereotactic visualization of a nonpalpable lesion localized with injected dye. An ABBI biopsy is reported with CPT code 19103.

Abbokinase Brand name of urokinase, a thrombolytic enzyme that dissolves large pulmonary emboli, especially indicated in conditions of unstable vascular dynamics. This drug is also used for coronary artery thrombosis and venous catheter occlusion. Supply is reported with HCPCS Level II code J3364 or J3365.

abd Abdomen.

abdominal lymphadenectomy Surgical removal of the abdominal lymph nodes grouping, with or without para-aortic and vena cava nodes.

abdominoplasty Excision of excess skin, fat, and subcutaneous tissue in the abdominal area, with repair. Report abdominoplasty with CPT code 15830 or 15847.

Abduction

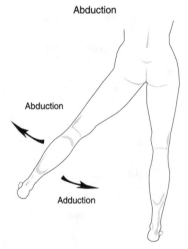

Abduction

Adduction

abduction Pulling away from a central reference line, such as moving away from the midline of the body.

abduction pillow Device that immobilizes the hips and legs of hip surgery patients postoperatively.

abductor hallucis Muscle that pulls the great toe away from the second digit or from the midline of the foot.

ABE Acute bacterial endocarditis. Reported with ICD-9-CM code 421.0.

Abercrombie's syndrome One of a group of syndromes characterized by accumulation of insoluble fibrillar proteins in various organs and tissues of the body. Report this disorder with ICD-9-CM code 277.39.

aberrant Deviation or departure from the normal or usual course, condition, or pattern.

abetalipoproteinemia Genetic disorder of lipoprotein metabolism in which the body fails to produce low density and very low density lipoproteins, affecting the way in which fats are utilized in the body. This deficiency is associated with hypocholesterolemia, progressive ataxic neuropathy, lack of fat-soluble vitamins, pigmentary retinal degeneration, and faulty intestinal absorption. Report this disorder with ICD-9-CM code 272.5. **Synonym(s):** *Bassen-Kornzweig syndrome.*

ABG Arterial blood gas. Diagnostic service used to evaluate the gas exchange in the lungs. Measurements include partial pressure of oxygen (PaO2), partial pressure of carbon dioxide (PaCO2), pH to measure the acid-base level of the blood or the hydrogen ion (H+) concentration, oxygen content (O2CT), oxygen saturation (O2Sat), and bicarbonate (HCO3-). Correct code assignment is dependent upon the number and type of analytes; reported with CPT codes 82803-82810.

ABI Auditory brainstem implant. Aid to restore some hearing in people who become deaf after surgery to remove auditory nerve tumors that have damaged the nerves. The system includes both surgically implanted and externally worn components. The system consists of a receiver/stimulator, a pocket sized speech processor worn on the body, and the microphone/headset. The device is implanted in teenagers and adults who have neurofibromatosis type 2, in which tumors growing on cranial nerves need to be surgically removed.

Abilify Brand name of aripiprazole, an antipsychotic medication indicated for the treatment of schizophrenia and bipolar disorder. Report supply of the intramuscular injection with HCPCS Level II code J0400.

AbioCor Brand name total replacement heart system, reported with ICD-9-CM procedure code 37.52.

abiotrophy Strength deficit with deterioration of tissues and cells without any apparent injury, reported with ICD-9-CM code 799.89.

ablation Removal or destruction of a body part or tissue or its function. Ablation may be performed by surgical means, hormones, drugs, radiofrequency, heat, chemical application, or other methods.

ABLB test Alternate binaural loudness balance test, reported with CPT code 92562.

ablepharia Congenital anomaly in which there is partial or complete absence of the eyelid, reported with ICD-9-CM code 743.62.

ablepharon Congenital absence of an eyelid, reported with ICD-9-CM code 743.62.

ablutomania Fixated preoccupation with cleanliness and bathing, often seen in obsessive-compulsive disorders and often accompanied by rituals of a compulsive nature. Report ablutomania with ICD-9-CM code 300.3.

ABN Advance beneficiary notice.

abn. Abnormal.

ABO ABO incompatibility, an immune system reaction that occurs if two different and incompatible blood types are combined. Blood is typed as A, AB, B, and O groups. This is determined by certain molecules on the surface of blood cells, which function as antigens, or immune system triggers. Type O lacks any molecule. Each person has a combination of two surface molecules, resulting in blood type A (AA or AO), type B (BB or BO), type AB, or type O. In order to avoid an ABO incompatibility reaction, blood types must be matched when patients receive blood transfusions or organ transplants. Since type O lacks surface molecules, it can be given to patients with any blood type. However, patients with type O blood can receive only type O.

abocclusion Condition in which the upper and lower teeth do not make contact when biting, reported with ICD-9-CM code 524.20.

abortion Premature expulsion or extraction of the products of conception. *NCD Reference: 140.1.*

aboulomania Condition of being pathologically indecisive, reported with ICD-9-CM code 301.6. *Synonym(s): abulomania.*

ABPM Ambulatory blood pressure monitoring.

ABR Auditory brainstem response, reported with CPT codes 92585 and 92586.

abrachia Congenital abnormality in which the arms are absent, reported with ICD-9-CM code 755.20.

abrachiocephalus Congenital abnormality in which the head and arms are absent in a developing fetus, reported with ICD-9-CM code 759.89. *Synonym(s): abrachiocephalia, acephalobrachia.*

abrasion Removal of layers of the skin. This term can be a diagnosis occurring as a superficial injury, or a procedure for removal of problematic skin or skin lesions. *Synonym(s): friction burn, rug burn, scrape.*

ABS Agitated Behavior Scale. Measurement for assessing agitated behaviors during the acute recovery period in acquired brain injury.

abs. fev. Without fever.

abscess Circumscribed collection of pus resulting from bacteria, frequently associated with swelling and other signs of inflammation. Abscesses may be either punctured or aspirated or the physician may perform an incision and drainage. Diagnosis codes for abscesses are based upon anatomical location and type of tissue.

absorbable sutures Strands prepared from collagen or a synthetic polymer and capable of being absorbed by tissue over time. Examples include surgical gut and collagen sutures; or synthetics like polydioxanone (PDS), polyglactin 910 (Vicryl), poliglecaprone 25 (Monocryl), polyglyconate (Maxon), and polyglycolic acid (Dexon). For wound repair, see CPT codes 12001-13160. Correct code assignment is dependent upon the type of closure performed (i.e., simple, intermediate, or complex), the anatomical site, and the wound size.

abstractor Person who selects and extracts specific data from the medical record and enters the information into computer files.

abulia Lack of will or impairment in the ability to make decisions, sometimes as a result of damage to the frontal lobes of the brain, reported with ICD-9-CM code 799.89.

abuse In medical reimbursement, an incident that is inconsistent with accepted medical, business, or fiscal practices and directly or indirectly results in unnecessary costs to the Medicare program, improper reimbursement, or reimbursement for services that do not meet professionally recognized standards of care or which are medically unnecessary. Examples of abuse include excessive charges, improper billing practices, billing Medicare as primary instead of other third-party payers that are primary, and increasing charges for Medicare beneficiaries but not to other patients.

abutment Tooth or implant fixture supporting a prosthesis.

abutment crown Artificial tooth cap for the retention and/or support of a dental prosthesis.

AC *1)* Anterior cephalic. *2)* Antecubital. *3)* Acromioclavicular. *4)* Anticoagulant. *5)* Autologous cell. *6)* Alternating current.

ac Before meals. *Synonym(s): preprandial.*

academic underachievement disorder Failure to achieve in most school tasks despite adequate intellectual capacity, supportive environment, and apparent effort.

acanthoma Tumor of the outer skin layer composed of epidermal or squamous cells. The tumor can be benign or malignant and can affect any body site. *Synonym(s): basal cell carcinoma, squamous cell carcinoma.*

acanthosis nigricans Skin disease where gray, wart-like patches are apparent.

A-C

acapnia Condition in which blood carbon dioxide levels are abnormally low, often as a result of hyperventilation. Report this condition with ICD-9-CM code 276.3. *Synonym(s): hypocapnia.*

acarbia Condition in which there is decreased blood plasma bicarbonate concentration and an increase in acid, reported with ICD-9-CM code 276.2.

acarbose Oral medication exclusive to lowering blood glucose in Type II diabetics. May be sold under the brand name Precose.

Acat 1 Brand name intraaortic balloon pump used during cardiac procedures.

acatalasemia Hereditary condition in which there is a deficiency of catalase in the blood. Recurrent infections and ulcerations of the gums and other oral structures are often the manifestations. Report this condition with ICD-9-CM code 277.89. *Synonym(s): acatalasia, Takahara's disease.*

acathisia State of motor restlessness manifested by an inability to sit or lie still, fidgeting, pacing, and feelings of muscular quivering and agitation. When specified as a side effect of medication, often from neuroleptic drugs, report this condition with ICD-9-CM code 333.99, otherwise report 781.0. *Synonym(s): akathisia.*

ACB Albumin cobalt binding. Test to determine cardiac ischemia, designed to rule out myocardial infarction (MI) in patients with chest pain. ACB is reported with CPT code 82045.

ACBE Air contrast barium enema. Diagnostic procedure to detect abnormalities of the large intestine in which the patient receives a barium enema followed by the infusion of air. The air allows the intestinal walls to be better visualized in x-ray, which is part of the air contrast barium enema, CPT code 74280. This code also includes the optional injection of glucagon to facilitate reflux of the air through the ileocecal valve. *Synonym(s): double contrast barium enema.*

ACBG Aortocoronary bypass graft.

ACC Adenoid cystic carcinoma. Uncommon and slow-growing malignancy forming from secretory glands, most commonly salivary glands. Diagnostic code selection would depend on the site.

access control Method of restricting access to resources, allowing access only to privileged entities.

accessory bone Anomalous extra bone or ossicle that develops in the carpal or tarsal bones. Removal of one carpal bone is reported with CPT code 25210. CPT code 28116 reports removal of tarsal coalition, an anomaly of the foot in which an extra bar or bridge of fused bone has grown between normally separated bones. Report ICD-9-CM code 755.56 for accessory bone of the carpus and 755.67 for tarsal coalition.

accommodation Adjustment the lens of the eye makes for focusing at different distances.

accommodation revenue code Three-digit code that identifies a specific accommodation or ancillary charge on the bill. This revenue code identifies routine hospital or skilled nursing facility (SNF) beds, room accommodations (e.g., private, ward) and/or board charges (including charges for nursing services) for general care, coronary care, and intensive care. It is used by facilities when billed to a third-party payer.

ACCORD Action to Control Cardiovascular Risk in Diabetes. Clinical study sponsored by the National Heart, Lung and Blood Institute.

accreditation Evaluative process in which a health care organization undergoes an examination of its policies, procedures, and performance by an external organization to ensure it is meeting predetermined criteria. It usually involves both on- and off-site surveys.

accredited record technician Former AHIMA certification describing medical records practitioners; now known as a registered health information technician (RHIT). *Synonym(s): ART.*

Accredited Standards Committee Organization accredited by the American National Standards Institute (ANSI) for the development of American national standards. *Synonym(s): ASC.*

accrual Amount of money set aside to cover a health care benefit plan's expenses based upon estimates using a combination of data, including the claims system and the plan's prior history.

AccuDEXA Brand name diagnostic tool used to measure bone density for monitoring and diagnosing osteoporosis.

AccuLase Brand name laser used in transmyocardial revascularization (TMR), reported with CPT codes 33140 and 33141. Laser energy is directed into the heart muscle through an incision in the chest, creating small channels in the heart muscle that restore the flow of blood and oxygen. TMR relieves severe angina in patients who are not candidates for bypass surgery.

Acculink Brand name carotid stent.

ACD Absolute cardiac dullness.

ACE *1)* Angiotensin converting enzyme. *2)* Adrenal cortical extract.

Ace bandage Brand name for a nonadhesive elastic wrap used to support an injured limb or hold other dressings or splints in place. Supply is reported with HCPCS Level II codes A6448-A6452.

ACEP American College of Emergency Physicians. Professional organization for emergency medicine medical specialty.

acetabular Relating to the acetabulum, the cup-shaped socket of the hip bone. *a. line* Anatomical reference point

A-C

drawn from the superolateral tips of both acetabuli, used in radiographic diagnostics. An interrupted line is an indicator of femoral disease. This reference line is also used as a means for measuring a prosthetic femoral head and estimating the size of the acetabular implant for preventing prosthetic migration. Seen in operative notes and radiograph readings, it may lend support for the diagnosis but has no coding implications. *a. notch* Defect found just above the acetabulum in the lateral iliac wall, shaped like a cup and most often seen in infants with hip dysplasia. There is no specific diagnosis code for acetabular notch. Acetabular notch is reported with ICD-9-CM code 755.63 Other congenital deformity of hip (joint). *a. rim syndrome* Condition occurring in developmental dysplasia of the hip marked by pain and impaired function, such as subluxation and locking of the hip, and unequal leg length. Degeneration of the acetabular labrum and roof also occur. Often seen in young adults and sometimes with tears of the labrum, it is reported as juvenile osteochondrosis of hip and pelvis, ICD-9-CM code 732.1. Pelvic or femoral osteotomy and hip debridement is often attempted first before total hip arthroplasty is ultimately needed.

acetabuloplasty Surgical repair or reconstruction of the large cup-shaped socket in the hipbone (acetabulum) with which the head of the femur articulates. Report this procedure with CPT code 27120 or 27122.

acetabulum Cup-shaped socket in the hipbone into which the head of the femur fits, forming a ball-and-socket joint. *Synonym(s): acetabular bone, cotyloid cavity, os acetabuli.*

acetaldehyde blood test Converted form of ethanol (alcohol) metabolized by alcohol dehydrogenase in the liver and tested for in blood serum by gas-liquid chromatography. Once alcohol is metabolized, its blood level decreases to zero. Measuring acetaldehyde as the by-product of alcohol metabolism helps in determining what caused symptoms of intoxication. The serum chemistry test for blood acetaldehyde is reported with CPT code 82000.

acetaminophen Pain and fever relieving drug that can cause acute liver failure when given in high levels. Report CPT code 82003 for serum chemistry, and E935.4 for adverse affect of therapeutic acetaminophen. May be sold under the brand name Tylenol.

acetazolamide sodium Multifunctional drug used to lower intraocular pressure, as an adjunctive therapy for patients suffering from open angle glaucoma, and as a perioperative treatment for acute closed angle glaucoma. It is also effective in treating seizures and controlling intracranial pressure, reducing edema in heart failure or drug-induced edema, preventing altitude sickness, and correcting periodic paralysis. Supply is reported with HCPCS Level II code J1120. May be sold under the

brand names Acetazolam, Apo-Acetazolamide, Diamox, Diamox Sequels.

acetohexamide Oral medication exclusive to lowering blood glucose in Type II diabetics. May be sold under the brand name Dymelor.

acetone Derivative of fatty acid metabolism that is elevated in starvation/carbohydrate depletion. When the body has insufficient food to metabolize, it uses fatty acids for fuel but the ketone bodies are not taken up at the cellular level and remain in circulation until excreted in the urine, causing metabolic acidosis. Serum positive for acetone without severe acidosis, while the anion gap, bicarbonate, and glucose are in normal range may indicate rubbing alcohol (isopropanol) intoxication. Report CPT codes 82009-82010 for serum chemistry. *Synonym(s): ketone bodies.*

acetonuria Presence of ketone bodies in the urine seen with diabetes mellitus or starvation. Report acetonuria with ICD-9-CM code 791.6. *Synonym(s): ketonuria.*

acetylcholinesterase Enzyme found in red blood cells specific for hydrolyzing acetylcholine, used primarily to look for toxicity caused by systemic insecticides. It is collected in a heparinized tube and processed by calorimetry, spectrometry, or fluorometry. Amniotic fluid that tests positive test for acetylcholinesterase along with elevated alpha-fetoprotein is indicative of a neural tube defect. Report CPT code 82013 for a chemistry test on blood. *Synonym(s): true cholinesterase.*

acetylcysteine Amino acid derivative used to treat pulmonary congestion as an inhaled mucolytic. It is also given by mouth or intravenously to patients with Tylenol overdose as an antidote to prevent liver failure. Be certain to assign an E code to report circumstances of an overdose. Acetylcysteine is also used as a prophylaxis against kidney failure related to radiographic contrast. Supply is reported with HCPCS Level II code J0132, J7604, or J7608. Note: This drug may be given via nasogastric tube (B4081or B4082) if the patient is unconscious. May be sold under the brand names Mucomyst, Mucomyst-10, Mucosil-10, Mucosil-20, and Parvolex.

ACG 1) Ambulatory care group. 2) American College of Gastroenterologists. Professional organization for gastroenterology medical specialty.

ACH Automated clearinghouse. Entity that processes or facilitates the processing of information received from another entity in a nonstandard format or containing nonstandard data content into standard data elements or a standard transaction, or that receives a standard transaction from another entity and processes or facilitates the processing of that information into nonstandard format or nonstandard data content for a receiving entity. *Synonym(s): health care clearinghouse.*

achalasia Failure of the smooth muscles within the gastrointestinal tract to relax at points of junction; most commonly referring to the esophagogastric sphincter's failure to relax when swallowing. This condition is reported with ICD-9-CM code 530.0.

Achard-Thiers syndrome Aranodactyly with small, receding mandible, broad skull, and laxity of joints in hands and feet. Report this disorder with ICD-9-CM code 255.2.

acheilia Condition present at birth in which one or both lips are absent, reported with ICD-9-CM code 750.26.

acheiria Congenital absence of one or both hands, reported with ICD-9-CM code 755.21.

Achilles Of or relating to the ankle. *A. bulge sign* Diagnostic sign that helps determine joint stability of the ankle. A special maneuver is done by pulling the foot forward and pushing the leg backwards with the knee flexed. The ankle is considered unstable when the Achilles tendon bulges during the maneuver. Testing for this sign may be part of a musculoskeletal system review performed in an E/M exam. *A. squeeze test* Diagnostic maneuver performed during an orthopedic exam to determine Achilles tendon rupture. The calf muscle is squeezed to see if the ankle fails to flex in the plantar or downward direction, which is positive for a rupture. This test may be part of a musculoskeletal system review performed in an E/M exam. *A. tendon* Tendon attached to the back of the heel bone (calcaneus) that flexes the foot downward.

achillodynia Pain in Achilles tendon caused by bursal inflammation, reported with ICD-9-CM code 726.71. *Synonym(s): achillobursitis.*

achlorhydria Absence of free hydrochloric acid in the stomach, reported with ICD-9-CM code 536.0, unless the condition is secondary to a vagotomy in which case it is reported with 564.2.

acholia Condition in which there is obstructed bile flow into the digestive tract or abnormally low bile secretion. Report this condition with ICD-9-CM code 575.8.

achondroplasia Congenital anomaly of bone growth and cartilage development in which the arms and legs are abnormally short while the trunk is near normal size. The head is generally large, with a prominent forehead and flat nose. Achondroplasia is reported with ICD-9-CM code 756.4.

achromatopsia Complete color blindness or total inability to distinguish colors with all hues appearing as lighter or darker shades of grey. Achromatopsia is reported with ICD-9-CM code 368.54. *Synonym(s): achromatism, monochromatism.*

Achromycin Brand name for tetracycline, a broad-spectrum antibiotic used to treat various bacterial

infections including respiratory tract infections, urethritis, gastrointestinal infections, acne, and biliary tract infections. Supply is reported with HCPCS Level II code J0120.

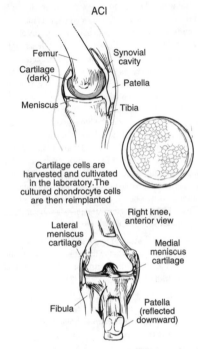

ACI

Cartilage cells are harvested and cultivated in the laboratory. The cultured chondrocyte cells are then reimplanted

Right knee, anterior view

ACI Autologous chondrocyte implantation. Staged surgical procedure for treatment of knee defects caused by damage to the hyaline cartilage in which some of the patient's own cartilage is obtained arthroscopically. Chondrocytes are separated and cultured for several weeks until 5 to 10 million healthy chondrocytes have grown. At the time of implantation, a small portion of periosteum is removed from the patient's tibia and inserted over the defect. The cultured chondrocytes are then injected under the periosteum, where they will expand and mature, eliminating the defect. Report the arthroscopic removal of the chondrocyte cells with CPT code 29870 and the implantation with CPT code 27412.

acid etching Process of using an acidic chemical substance to prepare a tooth surface for bonding.

acid pulmonary aspiration syndrome Pulmonary disorder resulting from aspirating the contents of stomach following vomiting or regurgitation. Report this disorder with ICD-9-CM code 997.39. *Synonym(s): Mendelson's syndrome.*

acid reflux test Monitoring of esophageal pH to detect esophageal reflux. A tube inserted into the patient's esophagus measures the acidity level by a sensor on the tip of a probe. Report this test with a code from CPT range 91034-91038.

ACL Anterior cruciate ligament. Strong band of connective tissue located in the middle of the knee that connects the lateral condyle of the femur to the tibia, controls rotation, and provides stability.

ACLE Acute cutaneous lupus erythematosus.

ACLF Adult congregate living facility.

ACLS Advanced cardiac life support. Certification for health care professionals who have achieved proficiency in providing emergent care of cardiac and respiratory systems and medication management.

aclusion Condition in which there is no contact between the biting surfaces of the upper and lower teeth; absence of occlusion, reported with ICD-9-CM code 524.4.

ACMCS American College of Medical Coding Specialists.

ACMI Age-consistent memory impairment.

acne Inflammatory skin disease affecting the sebaceous glands and hair follicles resulting in comedones, papular, and pustular skin eruptions.

ACOG American College of Obstetrics and Gynecology. Professional organization for obstetrical and gynecologic or women's health medical specialty.

acoustic reflex decay test Middle ear measurement of the acoustic reflex. In a normal ear, the acoustic reflex persists for 10 seconds. In an abnormal ear, it diminishes at least 50 percent in the first five seconds. When performed in conjunction with tympanometry, report this test with CPT code 92570.

acoustic reflex testing Middle ear measurement of stapedius muscle response to a loud sound. This test is reported with CPT code 92568.

acoustic rhinometry Technique using sound wave analysis as the waves are reflected from the nasal cavities in order to evaluate nasal obstruction and assess the geometry of the nasal cavity. Acoustic rhinometry is used prior to nasal surgery and to compare the decongestive action of corticosteroids and antihistamines. Report acoustic rhinometry with ICD-9-CM procedure code 89.12 and CPT code 92512. *Synonym(s): rhinomanometry.*

ACP Acid phosphatase.

acq. Acquired.

acquired Produced by outside influences and not by genetics or birth defect.

acquired immune deficiency syndrome Contagious retroviral disease resulting from infection with human immunodeficiency virus (HIV) that can, in severe cases, suppress vital immunity. Several opportunistic infections, such as Kaposi's sarcoma and pneumocystitis pneumonia, are associated with this syndrome. Report this disorder with ICD-9-CM code 042. *Synonym(s): AIDS, ARC, symptomatic HIV.*

ACR *1)* American College of Radiology. *2)* Adjusted community rate, calculation of what premium the plan charges to provide Medicare-covered benefits for greater frequency of use by participants.

ACRF Acute-on-chronic respiratory failure.

acro- Extremity, top, highest point.

acrocephalosyndactylism syndrome Chromosomal condition with webbing of digits and a pointed head and variety of defects. Often associated with other chromosomal abnormalities. Report this disorder with ICD-9-CM code 755.55. *Synonym(s): Apert's syndrome.*

acrocephaly Congenital condition in which the top of the skull is pointed or conical, reported with ICD-9-CM code 756.0.

acromegaly Chronic condition caused by overproduction of the pituitary growth hormone that results in enlarged skeletal parts and facial features. Acromegaly is reported with ICD-9-CM code 253.0.

Acromioclavicular Joint

Acromioclavicular joint
Clavicle
Sternoclavicular joint
Coracoid process
Glenohumeral joint
Scapula

acromioclavicular joint Junction between the clavicle and the scapula. The acromion is the projection from the back of the scapula that forms the highest point of the shoulder and connects with the clavicle. Trauma or injury to the acromioclavicular joint is often referred to as a dislocation of the shoulder. This is not correct, however, as a dislocation of the shoulder is a disruption of the glenohumeral joint. *Synonym(s): AC joint.*

acromioclavicular separation Disruption in the acromioclavicular (AC) joint secondary to tears in the acromioclavicular and coracoclavicular ligaments, resulting in the upper limb falling or separating from the clavicle. Traumatic impact on the tip of the shoulder is often the cause. Acromioclavicular separation is often classified by the Rockwood system, which classifies the degree of the separation and the associated need for surgery. Separations are described as Type I through VI. ICD-9-CM directs the coder to see dislocation for separation, acromioclavicular. Pathological fractures of the AC joint are coded to 718.21.

acromion process Highest point and outer most projection of the shoulder joint, formed from a lateral projection of the spine of the scapula. Fracture of the acromion process is reported with ICD-9-CM code 811.01, closed and 811.11, open.

acromionectomy Surgical treatment for acromioclavicular arthritis in which the distal portion of the acromion process is removed. Acromioplasty or acromionectomy is reported with CPT code 23130. Check the mutually exclusive rules in the Correct Coding Initiative before assigning this code with another procedure, as it is often unbundled. CPT codes 23415, 23420, and 29826 include acromionectomy by definition.

acromioplasty Repair of the part of the shoulder blade that connects to the deltoid muscles and clavicle.

acronym Word formed from the initial letters of a name or by combining initial letters or parts of a series of words.

acronyx Ingrowing fingernail or toenail, for which surgical treatment may be required. Report this condition with ICD-9-CM code 703.0.

acrophobia Abnormal fear of heights often successfully treated with behavioral therapy. Report acrophobia with ICD-9-CM code 300.29.

AcrySof ReSTOR Brand name posterior chamber intraocular lens.

ACSV Aortocoronary saphenous vein.

ACSW Academy of Certified Social Workers.

ACTH Adrenocorticotropic hormone. Hormone secreted by the anterior pituitary that acts on the adrenal cortex and its secretion of corticosteroids. ACTH is used in hormone replacement therapy and as a diagnostic aid. Supply is reported with HCPCS Level II code J0800. May be sold under the brand name Acthar.

Acthar Adrenocorticotropic hormone.

ACTHIB Brand name haemophilus influenzae type B vaccine provided in a single-dose vial. Code selection for ACTHIB is dependent upon the patient's immunization schedule. The number of doses specified does not necessarily have to be given; for children who start the Hib series late, fewer doses may be required. For children who start the schedule on time, CPT code 90648 would be reported. Administration is reported separately. Need for vaccination is reported with ICD-9-CM code V03.81.

ACTHREL See corticorelin ovine triflutate.

Acticon Brand name artificial anal sphincter consisting of a cuff placed around the anal canal, a pressure regulating balloon placed in the abdomen, and a control pump secured in the labium or scrotum. The procedure to implant this system is reported with CPT code 46762. It is performed to treat severe fecal incontinence, reported with ICD-9-CM code 787.60.

actigraphy Science of monitoring activity levels, particularly during sleep. In most cases, the patient wears a wristband that records motion while sleeping. The data are recorded, analyzed, and interpreted to study sleep/wake patterns and circadian rhythms. A minimum of three days worth of recording, with analysis and interpretation, is reported with CPT code 95803.

ACTIMMUNE Brand name drug used to modify or delay disease progression in patients with chronic granulomatous diseases or malignant osteoporosis. ACTIMMUNE contains interferon gamma-1b. Supply is reported with HCPCS Level II code J9216.

actinic keratosis Flat, scaly precancerous lesions appearing on dry, sun-aged, and overexposed skin, including the eyelids. Actinic keratosis is identified by ICD-9-CM code 702.0. Treatment often includes photodynamic therapy, cryotherapy, dermabrasion, or chemical peel. *Synonym(s): solar keratosis.* **NCD Reference:** *250.4.*

actinic porokeratosis Autosomal skin disease appearing on sun-exposed skin with discolored lesions with depressed centers surrounded by a keratotic rim.

actinotherapy Use of ultraviolet light to treat various skin ailments, reported with CPT code 96900. *Synonym(s): phototherapy.*

Activa Brand name implanted brain stimulator to suppress symptoms of Parkinson's disease. A pulse generator implanted under the skin of the abdomen or collarbone sends a steady electrical impulse through a series of wires to electrodes in selected areas of the brain. The electrical impulses block Parkinson's tremors unilaterally. Two separate systems are necessary to relieve symptoms bilaterally. Implants are reported with CPT codes 61850-61888; programming is reported with 95970-95975.

Activase See alteplase recombinant.

activities of daily living Self-care activities often used to determine a patient's level of function such as bathing, dressing, using a toilet, transferring in and out of bed or a chair, continence, eating, and walking.

Actiwatch Brand name device for monitoring activity levels, particularly during sleep.

ACTSEB Anterior chamber tube shunt to encircling band. An implant for the treatment of glaucoma. Insertion of the shunt is reported with CPT code 66180; revision with 66185; removal with 67120.

actual charge Charge a physician or supplier bills for a service rendered or a supply item.

actuarial assumptions Characteristics used in calculating the risks and costs of a plan, including age, sex, and occupation of enrollees; location; utilization rates; and service costs.

Acu-Form Brand name penile prosthesis, implanted as a treatment for erectile dysfunction. The Acu-Form is not inflatable. Its placement is reported with CPT code 54400 or ICD-9-CM procedural code 64.95.

acupressure Chinese massage providing deep pressure over key meridian points to relieve pain. Acupressure is often administered in the course of other therapeutic modalities in physical therapy, such as massage or manual therapy (CPT codes 97124 and 97140), or osteopathic or chiropractic manipulative treatment (CPT codes 98925-98943). Acupressure cannot be coded separately.

acupuncture Method of producing analgesia by inserting tiny needles into specific sites on the body along channels, called meridians, and twirling, energizing, or warming the needles. Acupuncture is reported with CPT codes 97810-97814. *NCD References: 30.3, 30.3.1, 30.3.2.*

acute Sudden, severe. Documentation and reporting of an acute condition is important to establishing medical necessity.

acute alcohol intoxication Psychic and physical state resulting from alcohol ingestion characterized by slurred speech, unsteady gait, poor coordination, flushed face, nystagmus, sluggish reflexes, strong smell of alcohol, loud speech, emotional instability (e.g., jollity followed by gloominess), excessive socializing, talkativeness, and poorly inhibited sexual and aggressive behavior.

acute alcoholism Psychic and physical state resulting from alcohol ingestion characterized by slurred speech, unsteady gait, poor coordination, flushed face, nystagmus, sluggish reflexes, strong smell of alcohol, loud speech, emotional instability (e.g., jollity followed by gloominess), excessive socializing, talkativeness, and poorly inhibited sexual and aggressive behavior. *NCD References: 130.1, 130.2, 130.4, 130.5.*

acute apical periodontitis Severe inflammation of the oral tissue surrounding the root of a tooth, caused by infection or necrosis of the dental pulp and periapical abscesses. This condition is reported with ICD-9-CM code 522.4.

acute care facility Health care institution primarily engaged in providing treatment to inpatients and diagnostic and therapeutic services for medical diagnosis, treatment, and care of injured, disabled, or sick persons who are in an acute phase of illness.

acute coronary syndrome Any group of clinical symptoms compatible with acute myocardial ischemia.

acute fractures Complicated limb fracture with severe bony comminution, extensive soft tissue damage, or multiple trauma. External fixation may be required.

acute lymphadenitis Sudden, severe inflammation, infection, and swelling in lymphatic tissue.

acute lymphoblastic leukemia Malignant disease of blood-forming organs, that is progressive, with symptoms of thrombocytopenia, hepatosplenomegaly, anemia, fatigue, and bruising easily. May spread to the central nervous system or other organs. *Synonym(s): ALL.*

acute megakaryocytic leukemia Malignant disease of the blood and blood-forming organs characterized by predominating numbers of megakaryocytes and platelets in the blood. A type of acute myelogenous leukemia that can occur at any age and is often seen with fibrosis, acute megakaryocytic leukemia is reported with ICD-9-CM codes 207.20-207.22. *Synonym(s): acute megakaryoblastic leukemia.*

acute monocytic leukemia Malignant disease of the blood and blood-forming organs characterized by predominating numbers of monocytes and monoblasts in the blood, sometimes with a few myelocytes. An uncommon type of acute myelogenous leukemia affecting any age group, acute monocytic leukemia is reported with ICD-9-CM codes 206.00-206.02. *Synonym(s): acute Schilling's leukemia.*

acute myeloblastic leukemia Malignant disease of the blood and blood-forming organs characterized by predominating numbers of myeloblasts in the blood. A common type of acute myelogenous leukemia affecting infants and middle-aged or older adults, acute myeloblastic leukemia is reported with a code from ICD-9-CM range 205.00-205.02. *Synonym(s): acute myeloid leukemia.*

acute myelocytic leukemia One of two major categories of acute leukemia (myelogenous/myelocytic and lymphocytic) that includes several types identified by the stage in which abnormal proliferation begins: acute myeloblastic, acute myelomonocytic, acute monocytic, acute erythroleukemia, and acute megakaryocytic leukemia. Symptoms include anemia, bruising, fatigue, weight loss, thrombocytopenia, and prolonged bacterial infections. *Synonym(s): acute myelogenous leukemia, AML.*

acute myocardial infarction Sudden, severe death of heart muscle due to decreased coronary blood flow. Classification is based on the location of the affected tissue, when known.

acute myocardial ischemia Chest pain due to insufficient blood supply to the heart muscle as a result of coronary artery or heart disease.

acute psycho-organic syndrome Describes a mental health patient who chooses not to participate in day-to-day activities or therapy as a result of emotional, organic or chemical causes. Report this disorder with ICD-9-CM code 293.0.

acute Schilling's leukemia Malignant disease of the blood and blood-forming organs characterized by predominating numbers of monocytes and monoblasts

A-C

in the blood, sometimes with a few myelocytes. An uncommon type of acute myelogenous leukemia affecting any age group, acute Schilling's leukemia is reported with ICD-9-CM codes 206.00-206.02. **Synonym(s):** *acute monocytic leukemia.*

acute swimmer's ear Inflammation of the external auditory canal as a result of irritation caused by ocean water or other seaside environmental factors. Report this condition with ICD-9-CM code 380.12. **Synonym(s):** *beach ear, otitis externa, tank ear.*

ACVB Aortocoronary venous bypass.

ACVD Acute cardiovascular disease.

acyclovir Na Antiviral used to treat mucocutaneous Herpes Simplex Virus-1 (HSV-1) and Herpes Simplex Virus 2 (HSV-2) infections. It is also used to treat any episode of HSV-1 and HSV-2 in immunosuppressed patients and to treat severe initial episodes of HSV-2 (genitalis) in patients with healthy immune systems, as well as long-term therapy for genital herpes. Supply is reported with HCPCS Level II code J0133. May be sold under the brand name Acihexal, Avirax, Zovirax.

ad- Toward, adherence to, or increase.

AD HCPCS Level II modifier, for use with CPT or HCPCS Level II codes, that indicates medical supervision by a physician for more than four concurrent anesthesia procedures. This modifier affects Medicare payment.

ad lib As desired, at pleasure.

ad part. dolent. To the aching parts.

ad. hib. To be administered.

ad. lib. As desired.

ad. us. ext. For external use.

ADA *1)* American Diabetes Association. *2)* Americans with Disabilities Act. *3)* American Dental Association.

Adacel Brand name tetanus, diphtheria, acellular pertussis vaccine, for patients ages 11 to 64, provided in a single-dose vial. Supply of Adacel is reported with CPT code 90715; administration is reported separately. The need for vaccination is reported with ICD-9-CM code V06.1.

Adair-Dighton syndrome Hereditary condition with symptoms including blue sclera, little growth, brittle bones, and deafness. Report this disorder with ICD-9-CM code 756.51. **Synonym(s):** *van der Hoeve's syndrome.*

ADAM Androgen deficiency/decline in aging male. Symptomatic ADAM is reported with ICD-9-CM code 608.89. **Synonym(s):** *andropause, male climacteric, viropause.*

Adams-Stokes (-Morgagni) syndrome Heart block often causing slow or absent pulse, vertigo, syncope, convulsions, and sometimes Cheyne-Stokes respiration. Report this disorder with ICD-9-CM code 426.9.

Synonym(s): *Morgagni's disease, Spens syndrome, Stokes-Adams syndrome.*

Adaptation reaction Abnormal or maladaptive reaction with emotional or behavioral characteristics as a result of a life event or stressor that is usually temporary.

ADAS-L Alzheimer's Disease Assessment Scale - Late. Survey reviewing patient's memory, word knowledge, and activities of daily living to assess Alzheimer's status. Alzheimer's is reported with ICD-9-CM code 331.0 and a code for the dementia: 294.10 without behavioral disturbance or 294.11 with behavioral disturbance.

Addis test Test to determine the specific gravity of the urine after administering a dry diet for 24 hours.

Addison's disease Adrenocortical insufficiency caused by destruction of the adrenal cortex from an autoimmune response or tuberculosis, resulting in failure of the adrenal glands to produce aldosterone and cortisol. Addison's disease is fatal without hormone replacement and presents with hypotension, anorexia, weakness, and discoloration of the skin. This disease is reported with ICD-9-CM code 255.41.

Addisonian syndrome Acute adrenal insufficiency caused by illness, trauma, or large amounts of hormones used as therapy. Symptoms include hypotension, hyperthermia, hyponatremia, hyperkalemia, hypoglycemia, nausea, and vomiting. Report this disorder with ICD-9-CM code 255.41. **Synonym(s):** *Bernard-Sergent syndrome.*

additional development request Formal request from a Medicare contractor for additional information needed to determine if a claim is covered and/or payable.

additional documentation request When contractors cannot make a coverage or coding determination based upon the information on the claim and its attachments, the contractors may solicit additional documentation from the provider by issuing an ADR. Contractors must ensure that all records requested are from the period under review. Contractors must specify in the ADR the specific pieces of documentation needed (and ONLY those pieces needed) to make a coverage or coding determination. **Synonym(s):** *ADR.*

add-on code CPT code representing a procedure performed in addition to the primary procedure and designated with a + in the CPT book. Add-on codes are never reported for stand-alone services but are reported secondarily in addition to the primary procedure.

Adduction

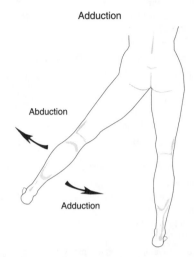

adduction Pulling toward a central reference line, such as toward the midline of the body.

Adductor Longus and Adductor Brevis

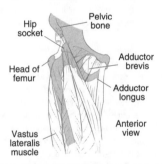

adductor Muscle with a pulling function. a. brevis Short muscle connected to the outer, lower surface of the pubic bone and the femur that acts to pull the thigh inwards toward the midline of the body, to rotate, and flex the thigh. a. gracilis Adductor muscle of the thigh connected to the inferior ramus of the pubic bone and medial shaft of the tibia that flexes the knee joint and pulls the thigh inwards toward the midline of the body.

ADE Acute disseminated encephalomyelitis. Neurological disorder with brain and spinal cord inflammation. It typically occurs two to three weeks following an infection or immunization. ADE is reported with the ICD-9-CM code for the initial infection, and 323.6 secondarily. *Synonym(s): ADEM.*

ADEM Acute disseminated encephalomyelitis. Inflammation of the brain and spinal cord caused by

damage to the myelin sheath, reported with ICD-9-CM code 323.61.

Aden fever Acute, self-limiting disease lasting up to a week, spread by the Aedes mosquito infected with one of four dengue virus serotypes of the Flavivirus genus. The disease is found in the tropics and subtropics and causes fever, headache, muscle and joint pain, generalized aches, prostration, rash, enlarged lymph nodes, and leukopenia. The muscle and joint pain experienced can be so severe the bones feel as if they are breaking. Report Aden fever with ICD-9-CM code 061. *Synonym(s): breakbone fever, dandy fever, dengue fever.*

adenitis Inflammation of one or several lymph nodes, related lymphoid tissues, or specific gland. Report according to site, type, and/or infectious agent involved. Unspecified adenitis is reported with ICD-9-CM code 289.3.

adeno- Relating to a gland.

adenocarcinoma Malignant tumor of a gland.

Adenocard Brand name for adenosine, an injectable drug used as an antiarrhythmic in patients with paroxysmal supraventricular tachycardia, Wolfe-Parkinson-White syndrome, and wide-complex tachycardia. Supply is reported with HCPCS Level II code J0150.

Adenoidectomy

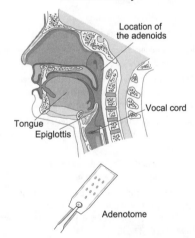

The adenoids are removed in an oral surgical procedure

adenoidectomy Surgical procedure in which the adenoids (the lymphoid tissue in the back wall and roof of the nasopharynx) are removed, often in conjunction with other procedures such as tonsillectomy or placement of tympanostomy tubes, most often in pediatric patients. When performed alone, report primary removal with ICD-9-CM procedure code 28.6 and CPT code 42830 or 42831. Report removal of recurrent adenoids with CPT code 42835 or 42836.

adenoma Epithelial tumor, often benign, in which the cells are derived from glandular tissue or have a glandular structure

adenomyosis Abnormal presence of endometrial glands and tissue within the myometrium, the smooth muscle walls of the uterus, causing hypertrophy of the myometrium. At menses, blood is trapped within the muscle of the uterus, causing pain and cramping. Report adenomyosis with ICD-9-CM code 617.0. *Synonym(s): endometriosis interna.*

adenopathy Disease process resulting in enlargement of the lymph glands. Generalized adenopathy is a symptom and not a primary diagnosis, reported with ICD-9-CM code 785.6. Procedures on lymph glands are found in CPT code range 38300-38999 and also referenced in physical examination in the course of an E/M service under a review of the lymphatic system. *Synonym(s): adenomegaly, lymphadenopathy.*

adenosine 5-mono-phosphate Cyclic nucleotide that carries messages from the cell surface to proteins in the cell such as the parathyroid hormone (PTH). The serum test is used to identify pseudohypoparathyroidism and to target organ resistance to PTH. Report CPT code 82030 for serum chemistry test. May be sold under the brand name cAMP, Cyclic AMP.

ADG Ambulatory diagnostic group.

ADH Antidiuretic hormone.

adherent leucoma Dense corneal opacity or scarring attached to the iris.

adhesion Abnormal fibrous connection between two structures, soft tissue or bony structures, that may occur as the result of surgery, infection, or trauma.

adhesion of pupillary membranes Retention of the fetal membrane that traverses the pupil, resulting in vision loss.

adhesive capsulitis Excessive scar tissue in the shoulder, causing stiffness and pain.

Adie (-Holmes) syndrome Paralysis of conjugate movement of eyes without paralysis of convergence. Caused by lesions of midbrain. Report this disorder with ICD-9-CM code 379.46.

adip(o)- Relating to fat.

adipectomy Surgical excision of fatty tissue. Adipectomy can be performed with or without suction-assistance. Correct code selection is dependent upon the anatomical site. *Synonym(s): lipectomy.*

adiposalgia Painful areas of subcutaneous fat, reported with ICD-9-CM code 272.8.

adipose tumor Benign tumor consisting of fat cells that can occur subcutaneously or in any organ system. *Synonym(s): angiolipoma, fibrolipoma, hibernoma, lipoma, myelolipoma, myxolipoma.*

adiposity Site or organ that is fatty in nature.

adiposogenital syndrome Obesity and hypogonadism in adolescent boys. Rare accompanying dwarfism is thought to indicate hypothyroidism. Report this disorder with ICD-9-CM code 253.8. *Synonym(s): Babinski-Fröhlich syndrome, Fröhlich syndrome.*

adjacent tissue transfer Rotation or advancement of skin from an adjacent area to repair or fill in a defect while maintaining attachment to original blood supply.

adjudication Processing and review of a submitted claim resulting in payment, partial payment, or denial. In relationship to judicial hearings, it is the process of hearing and settling a case through an objective, judicial procedure.

adjusted average per capita cost Estimated average cost of Medicare benefits for an individual, based upon criteria including age, sex, institutional status, Medicaid, disability, and end-stage renal failure. *Synonym(s): AAPCC.*

adjusted community rate Calculation of what premium the plan charges to provide Medicare-covered benefits for greater frequency of use by participants. *Synonym(s): ACR.*

adjustment reaction or disorder Abnormal or maladaptive reaction with emotional or behavioral characteristics as a result of a life event or stressor that is usually temporary. *a. with brief depression* Short-term depressive symptoms following a life event or stressor. *a. with depression* State of depression associated with an abnormal or maladaptive reaction with emotional or behavioral characteristics as a result of a life event or stressor that is usually temporary. *a. with emotional disturbance* Abnormal or maladaptive reaction with emotional disturbance as a result of a life event or stressor that is usually temporary. *a. with mixed conduct and emotional disturbance* Abnormal or maladaptive reaction with emotional and behavioral (conduct) characteristics as a result of a life event or stressor that is usually temporary. *a. with prolonged depression* Depressive symptoms following a life event or stressor that continue over an extended period of time.

adjuvant technique Additional procedure, such as placing a vein patch graft or creating an arteriovenous fistula during surgery, that may be necessary for a newly created lower extremity bypass graft to ensure its patency. CPT codes 35685-35686 for adjuvant techniques are add-on codes only and should be reported with the primary procedure.

A-C

adjuvant therapy Therapy intended to enhance the primary therapy.

ADKC Atopic dermatitis with keratoconjunctivitis.

ADL Activities of daily living.

adm Admission, admit.

ADM Alcohol, drug, or mental disorder.

administrative code sets Code sets that characterize a general business situation, rather than a medical condition or service. Under HIPAA, these are sometimes referred to as nonclinical or nonmedical code sets.

administrative law judge Hearing officer who presides over appeal conflicts between Medicare contractors and providers, physicians, suppliers, or beneficiaries.

administrative services only Contractual agreement between a self-funded plan and an insurance company in which the insurance company assumes no risk and provides administrative services only. *Synonym(s): ASO.*

administrative simplification Title II, subtitle of HIPAA, that gives HHS the authority to mandate the use of standards for the electronic exchange of health care data; to specify what medical and administrative code sets should be used within those standards; to require the use of national identification systems for health care patients, providers, payers (or plans), and employers (or sponsors); and to specify the types of measures required to protect the security and privacy of personally identifiable health care information. This is also the name of Title II, subtitle F, part C of HIPAA. *Synonym(s): A.S., A/S, AS.*

admission Formal acceptance of a patient by a health care facility. *A. date* Date the patient was admitted to the health care facility for inpatient care, outpatient service, or for the start of care.

ADMX Adrenal medullectomy.

adnexa Appendages, adjunct parts, or connecting structures, related by functionality.

ADP *1)* Adenosine diphosphate. *2)* ALAD porphyria. Inherited hepatic porphyria with symptoms of nausea and fatigue due to a deficiency in delta-aminolevulinic acid dehydratase (ALAD) and increased secretion of delta-aminolevulinic acid in the urine. ADP is reported with ICD-9-CM code 277.1.

ADPKD Autosomal dominant polycystic kidney disease. Congenital condition in which multiple cysts form on the kidneys found in both children and adults, often not becoming symptomatic until middle age. This condition is reported with ICD-9-CM code 753.13.

ADR Additional development request.

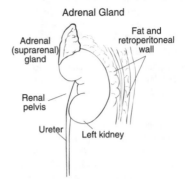

Adrenal Gland

The adrenal glands rest atop each kidney and are imbedded in fat along the retroperitoneal wall

adrenal gland Specialized group of secretory cells located above the kidneys that produce hormones that regulate the metabolism, maintain fluid balance, and control blood pressure. The adrenal glands also produce slight amounts of androgens, estrogens, and progesterone.

adrenalin chloride Bronchodilator and vasopressor used to treat hypersensitivity reactions, acute asthma, and bronchospasm. Adrenaline chloride is also used for its cardiac stimulant properties in cases of cardiac arrest to restore heart rhythm. It extends the effect of local anesthesia when mixed with the anesthetic agent and acts as an antihemorrhagic when applied topically. Supply is reported with HCPCS Level II code J0171. May be sold under the brand names Adrenalin, Ana-guard, AsthmaHaler Mist, Bronitin Mist, Bronkaid Mist, Bronkaid Mist Suspension, Bronkaid Mistometer, Epi Pen Auto-Injector, Epi Pen Jr Auto-Injector, Epinephrine, Medihaler-Epi, Primatene Mist, Primatene Mist Suspension, Sus-Phrine.

adrenocorticotropic hormone Hormone secreted by the anterior pituitary that acts on the adrenal cortex and its secretion of corticosteroids. ACTH is used in hormone replacement therapy and as a diagnostic aid. Supply is reported with HCPCS Level II code J0800. *Synonym(s): ACTH.*

adrenogenital disorders Congenital or acquired disorders of the genitals due to adrenal dysfunction.

adriamycin PFS/RDF See doxorubicin HCl.

Adrucil See fluorouracil.

ADS Alternative delivery system. Any health care delivery system other than traditional fee-for-service.

Adson test Physiological assessment for thoracic outlet syndrome.

adst. feb. Fever is present.

adult maltreatment syndrome Maltreatment (abuse) of an adult with emotional or physical violence. Most often committed against spouses and elders. Report this disorder with a code from ICD-9-CM range 995.80-995.85.

adult respiratory distress syndrome Respiratory distress following surgery, shock or trauma. Report this disorder with ICD-9-CM code 518.5.

advance Move away from the starting point.

advance beneficiary notice Written communication with a Medicare beneficiary given before Part B services are rendered, informing the patient that the provider (including independent laboratories, physicians, practitioners, and suppliers) believes Medicare will not pay for some or all of the services to be rendered. Form CMS-R-131 form may be used for all situations where Medicare payment is expected to be denied. This revised form has been effective since March 1, 2009 and replaces the ABN-G (Form CMS-R-131G), ABN-L (Form CMS-R-131L), and NEMB (Form CMS-20007). (Note: Skilled nursing facilities (SNF) must use the revised ABN for items/services expected to be denied under Medicare Part B only.)

advance directive Legal documents, such as living wills and durable powers of attorney for health care decisions, stating medical preferences in the event the patient should become incapable of voicing his or her opinion.

advanced cardiac life support Certification for health care professionals who have achieved proficiency in providing emergent care of cardiac and respiratory systems and medication management. *Synonym(s): ACLS.*

advanced determination of Medicare coverage Request by a supplier or beneficiary that a determination be made in advance of delivery of an item as to whether or not it is a covered item. ADMC requests are limited to items that are customized or items that have been specified as "not inexpensive" by the secretary. This is a voluntary program. Suppliers and beneficiaries are not required to obtain an ADMC prior to delivery of supplies, but may wish to request an ADMC when the item is customized or when the item is on the "not inexpensive" list. *Synonym(s): ADMC.*

adventitia Outermost layer of connective tissue covering an organ or other tissue. *Synonym(s): tunica adventitia.*

adverse effect or reaction Correct administration of a drug, therapeutically or prophylactically, that causes an adverse response in a patient.

adverse selection In health care contracting, the risk of enrolling members who are sicker than assumed and who will utilize expensive services more frequently.

Advicor Brand name combination of niacin and lovastatin used for lowering cholesterol levels.

adynamia Loss or lack of strength, vitality, or energy, that may occur sporadically, result from disease, or occur as a hereditary condition. Report adynamia with ICD-9-CM code 359.3.

adynamic ileus Intestinal obstruction due to loss of bowel motility or paralysis, usually as a result of localized or generalized peritonitis or shock. Report adynamic ileus with ICD-9-CM code 560.1. *Synonym(s): paralytic ileus.*

AE *1)* Above the elbow. *2)* HCPCS Level II modifier used to denote a service provided by a registered dietician.

AED Antiepilepsy drug.

aero- Relating to gas or air.

Aerobacter aerogenes Part of a former classification system of organisms. Currently, it refers to a genus of bacteria now under the family Enterobacteriaceae. Aerogenes has been assigned to the genus Enterobacter. Infection is reported with ICD-9-CM code 008.2. *Synonym(s): enterobacter aerogenes.*

aerobe Bacteria that can grow in the presence of oxygen. Aerobe is frequently seen on laboratory reports but does not directly drive code selection. It does, however, dictate treatment decisions.

AeroBid See flunisolide.

aerodontalgia Tooth pain resulting from changes in atmospheric pressure, such as occurs in mountain climbing, decompression chambers, or flying, that causes expansion of the air in the maxillary cavities. Report aerodontalgia with ICD-9-CM code 993.2. Assign an additional E code to describe the causative environmental factor.

aerophagia Excessive swallowing of air, usually unconsciously done in relation to anxiety, causing excess gas, abdominal bloating, and belching. Report aerophagia with ICD-9-CM code 306.4.

AERS Adverse event reporting system.

AESOP Automated Endoscopic System for Optimal Positioning.

AF *1)* Atrial fibrillation. *2)* HCPCS Level II modifier used to denote a service provided by a specialty physician.

AFB Acid fast bacilli. Bacteria, such as Mycobacterium tuberculosis, that have long chains of mucolytic acids in their cell walls, making them high in lipids and impermeable to most basic dyes unless those dyes are combined with Phenol. Once a dye is applied, acid fast bacilli resist decolorization when treated with acidified organic solvents and retain the dye coloring.

AFDC Aid to families with dependent children.

AFEHCT Association for Electronic Health Care Transactions. Organization that promotes the use of electronic data interchange (EDI) in the health care industry.

affective NEC syndrome Organic disorder in which the patient exhibits a number of changes in personality such as amotivation, depression, outbursts, and poor social judgment. Report this disorder with ICD-9-CM code 293.83.

affective psychosis Severe disturbance of mood or emotion that adversely affects the thinking process and may be accompanied by delusions or hallucinations. *a. bipolar* Manic-depressive psychosis that has appeared in both the depressive and manic form, alternating or separated by an interval of normality. *a. bipolar atypical* Episode of affective psychosis with some, but not all, of the features of the one form of the disorder in individuals who have had a previous episode of the other form of the disorder. *a. bipolar depressed* Manic-depressive psychosis, circular type, in which the depressive form is currently present. *a. bipolar manic* Manic-depressive psychosis, circular type, in which the manic form is currently present. *a. bipolar mixed* Manic-depressive psychosis, circular type, in which both manic and depressive symptoms are present at the same time. *a. depressed type* Manic-depressive psychosis in which there is a widespread depressed mood of gloom and wretchedness with some degree of anxiety, reduced activity, or restlessness and agitation. There is a marked tendency to recurrence; in a few cases this may be at regular intervals. *a. depressed type, atypical* Affective depressive disorder that cannot be classified as a manic-depressive psychosis, depressed type or chronic depressive personality disorder, or as an adjustment disorder. *a. manic type* State of elation or excitement out of keeping with the individual's circumstances and varying from enhanced liveliness (hypomania) to violent, almost uncontrollable, excitement. Aggression and anger, flight of ideas, distractibility, impaired judgment, and grandiose ideas are common. *a. mixed type* Manic-depressive psychosis syndrome corresponding to both the manic and depressed types that cannot be classified more specifically.

afferent Moving or carrying toward. *a. loop syndrome* Distended afferent loop with illness and pain caused by acute or chronic obstruction of the duodenum and jejunum proximal to a gastrojejunostomy. Report this disorder with ICD-9-CM code 537.89. *Synonym(s): gastrojejunal loop obstruction. a. nerve* Nerve that transports impulses toward the central nervous system (i.e., from the tissues to the spinal cord and brain).

AFI Amniotic fluid index. Scale for measuring the volume of amniotic fluid. The maternal abdomen is divided into four quadrants. Using an ultrasound transducer, a pocket of amniotic fluid in each quadrant is identified and measured. The numbers from each quadrant are then added, with the sum being the AFI. An AFI of less than or equal to 5 cm is considered decreased amniotic fluid, while an AFI of greater than or equal to 24 cm is considered increased amniotic fluid. Measurement testing is reported with ICD-9-CM procedure code 88.78 and CPT code 76815.

AFO

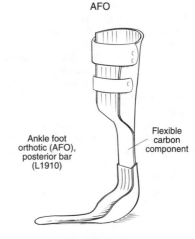

Ankle foot orthotic (AFO), posterior bar (L1910)

Flexible carbon component

Foot component may fit inside shoe

AFO Ankle foot orthosis. Orthotic device functioning like a type of brace, applied externally to the foot and ankle. It is designed to support, control, and correct a limb in order to avoid deformity. Commercially available braces can assist or resist motion, provide corrective measures, and/or reduce the weight load to a specific area of the body. Some common AFOs include Charcot restraint orthotic walker (CROW), floor reaction orthosis, patellar tendon bearing (PTB) orthosis, spring wire orthosis, and thermoplastic orthosis. These are considered supplies and are coded with HCPCS Level II codes L1900-L1990.

AFP Alpha-fetoprotein. Plasma protein produced by the fetus that crosses the placenta and appears in the mother's blood. AFP is useful in screening for fetal disorders such as spina bifida, anencephaly, and Down syndrome. While AFP testing is most often associated with antenatal testing for defects and the serum protein levels decline by age 1, it may also be used to detect other disorders such as viral hepatitis, cirrhosis, or primary liver tumors, in which case the serum levels may elevate again. Serum AFP is reported with CPT code 82105. Amniotic AFP is reported with 82106. *Synonym(s): fetal alpha globulin. NCD Reference: 190.25.*

African macroglobulinemia syndrome Earmarked by an increase in macroglobulins in the blood with symptoms of hyperviscosity such as weakness, fatigue, bleeding disorders, and visual disturbances. Report this disorder with ICD-9-CM code 273.3. **Synonym(s):** *Waldenström's syndrome.*

African tickbite fever Acute, febrile, rickettsial disease transmitted by tick bites and causing a primary lesion at the site of the bite, with rash, muscle and joint pain, headache, chills, fever, and sensitivity to light. It is commonly found in the Mediterranean and around the Black and Caspian Seas, having many names depending on the geographical region. This condition is reported with ICD-9-CM code 082.1. **Synonym(s):** *Boutonneuse fever, Indian tick typhus, Kenya tick typhus, Marseilles fever, Mediterranean tick fever.*

after-cataract Cataract that can occur in the posterior capsule following extracapsular cataract extraction (ECCE). In ECCE, the posterior shell of the lens remains in the eye. If this becomes clouded, the condition is called an after-cataract. An after-cataract is reported with ICD-9-CM codes 366.50-366.53.

AG HCPCS Level II modifier used to denote a service performed by a primary physician.

ag. feb. Increase in fever.

AGA Appropriate (average) for gestational age.

against medical advice Discharge status of patients who leave the hospital before completion of medical treatment and release by a physician who may or may not have signed a release document. **Synonym(s):** *AMA.*

agalactia Failure or cessation of milk secretion from the maternal breasts following childbirth, reported with a code from ICD-9-CM subcategory 676.4.

agalsidase beta Recombinant form of the defective enzyme found in Fabry syndrome. Fabry syndrome patients do not process lipids in the body due to a lack of this enzyme. Research suggests that the vascular damage resulting from improper storage of lipids in a variety of cell types ultimately manifests in multi-system damage. The FDA has recently approved Agalsidase beta for use in patients with Fabry disease to reduce globotriaosylceramide (GL-3) deposits in renal capillaries and certain other cell types.

AGB Adjustable gastric banding. **NCD Reference:** *100.1.*

age restriction In health care contracting, limitation of benefits when a patient reaches a certain age.

age/sex rating In health care contracting, structuring capitation payments based on members' ages and genders.

agenesis Absence of an organ due to developmental failure in the prenatal period.

Aggrastat Brand name drug prevalently used in the medical management of acute coronary syndrome and to treat patients who have had percutaneous transluminal coronary angioplasty (PTCA) and/or atherectomy. Report supply with HCPCS Level II code J3246.

aggregate amount Contracted maximum for which a member is insured for any single event in a health plan.

aggressive personality Personality disorder characterized by instability of mood with uncontrollable outbursts of anger, hate, violence, or affection demonstrated by words or actions.

AgNO3 Silver nitrate.

agoraphobia Profound anxiety or fear of leaving familiar settings like home, or being in unfamiliar locations or with strangers or crowds; almost always preceded by a phase during which there are recurrent panic attacks.

-agra Severe pain.

agraphia Loss or impairment in the ability to write. Agraphia may occur with alexia or alone, and may be the result of a developmental or neurological disorder or trauma. Code assignment depends upon the underlying condition.

AGV Ahmed glaucoma valve. Eponymous implant to mitigate glaucoma. Insertion of the valve is reported with CPT code 66180; revision with 66185; removal with 67120.

AH HCPCS Level II modifier, for use with CPT or HCPCS Level II codes, that indicates a service that is performed by a clinical psychologist. This modifier is required on claims when services are performed by a clinical psychologist.

AHA American Hospital Association. Health care industry association that represents the concerns of institutional providers. The AHA hosts the National Uniform Billing Committee (NUBC), which has a formal consultative role under HIPAA. The AHA also publishes *Coding Clinic for ICD-9-CM.*

AHC Alternative health care.

AHIMA American Health Information Management Association. Association of health information management professionals that offers professional and educational services, providing these certifications: RHIA, RHIT, CCS, CCS-P, CCA, CHDA, and CHPS.

Ahmed glaucoma valve Aqueous drainage device implanted to reduce intraocular pressure in a patient with glaucoma. It is implanted in the anterior segment of the eye to facilitate drainage of aqueous. Insertion of the valve is reported with CPT code 66180; revision with 66185; and removal with 67120. **Synonym(s):** *AGV.*

AHRQ Agency for Healthcare Research and Quality. Federal agency providing evidence-based information on outcomes, costs, and utilization in health care.

Ahumada-Del Castillo syndrome Lactation and amenorrhea not following pregnancy characterized by hyperprolactinemia and pituitary adenoma. Report this disorder with ICD-9-CM code 253.1. *Synonym(s): Argonz-Del Castillo syndrome.*

A-Hydrocort Brand name glucocorticoid used to treat severe inflammation and adrenal insufficiency (adrenocorticoid replacement). It is also used as an adjunctive treatment for ulcerative colitis and proctitis. Supply is reported with HCPCS Level II code J1710.

AI *1)* Aortic insufficiency. *2)* HCPCS Level II modifier denoting the principal physician of record.

AICC Anti-inhibitor coagulant complex. Drug utilized in the treatment of hemophilia in patients with factor VIII inhibitor antibodies. *NCD Reference: 110.3.*

Automatic Implantable Cardioverter-defibrillator (AICD)

Schematic showing epicardial ICD leads and electrodes

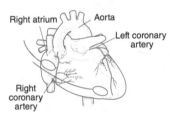

Right atrium
Aorta
Left coronary artery
Right coronary artery

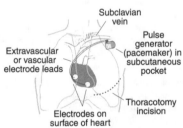

Subclavian vein
Pulse generator (pacemaker) in subcutaneous pocket
Extravascular or vascular electrode leads
Thoracotomy incision
Electrodes on surface of heart

AICD Automatic implantable cardioverter-defibrillator. Device much like a pacemaker, but used to administer defibrillating, low-energy electric shocks with a combination of antitachycardia pacing to treat ventricular arrhythmias. This device consists of the pulse generator with a battery and the electrodes, or leads, which are placed in single or dual chambers of the heart, usually transvenously. Leads that are placed epicardially require a thoracotomy. An extra lead may be used for biventricular pacing of the left ventricle. The generator

is placed in a subcutaneous pocket below the clavicle or in an abdominal location. Biventricular pacing is one key to differentiating between code choices, in addition to leads placed transvenously or epicardially. Some procedures may also be done on the leads alone or the generator alone. CPT provides codes for reporting implantation or replacement, removal, repair, and repositioning. *NCD Reference: 20.4.*

AID *1)* Acute infectious disease. *2)* Artificial insemination donor.

AIDS Acquired immunodeficiency syndrome. *NCD Reference: 190.9.*

AIED Autoimmune inner ear disease. Progressive hearing loss and dizziness caused by the immune system attacking the auditory nerve. Report AIED with ICD-9-CM code 279.49 and the appropriate codes for manifestations.

AIH Artificial insemination by husband.

AIN Anal intraepithelial neoplasia. AIN is usually the result of a sexually-transmitted infection of human papilloma virus. AIN I: low-grade abnormality; mild dysplasia. AIN II: high-grade abnormality; moderate dysplasia. AIN III: carcinoma in situ; severe dysplasia. Report AIN I and AIN II with ICD-9-CM code 569.44. Report AIN III with 230.5 or 230.6.

AION Anterior ischemic optic neuropathy. Common cause of vision loss in older people as a shortage of blood supply to the optic nerve head damages the nerve and creates a loss in vision. AION is reported with ICD-9-CM code 377.41.

AIP Acute intermittent porphyria. Rare genetic disease caused by a deficiency in porphobilinogen deaminase. AIP is a hereditary hepatic porphyria and is one of the porphyrias that does not have dermal symptoms. Symptoms include nausea, vomiting, constipation, pain in back/arms/legs, muscle weakness, urinary retention, heart palpitations, elevated blood pressure, confusion, hallucination, and seizures. AIP is reported with ICD-9-CM code 277.1. *Synonym(s): hydroxymethylbilane synthase.*

air ambulance service One-way conventional air services reported with HCPCS Level II code A0430 for fixed wing and A0431 for rotary wing.

air conditioner lung Allergic alveolitis caused by inhalation of a variety of agents passed through contaminated ventilating equipment and humidifiers, causing an acute febrile illness with muscle aches and pains and mild shortness of breath. This does not include infection caused by the Legionella pneumophila organism (482.84). Report with ICD-9-CM code 495.7. *Synonym(s): humidifier fever, ventilation pneumonitis.*

air conduction Transportation of sound from the air, through the external auditory canal, to the tympanic membrane and ossicular chain. Air conduction hearing is tested by presenting an acoustic stimulus through earphones or a loudspeaker to the ear.

air contrast barium enema Diagnostic procedure to detect abnormalities of the large intestine in which the patient receives a barium enema followed by the infusion of air. The air allows the intestinal walls to be better visualized in x-ray, which is part of the air contrast barium enema, CPT code 74280. This code also includes the optional injection of glucagon to facilitate reflux of the air through the ileocecal valve. *Synonym(s): ACBE, double contrast barium enema.*

air embolism Blockage of an artery by air bubbles that have entered the bloodstream during surgery, after an injury, or through an IV line. Report an air embolism with ICD-9-CM code 958.0.

air puff device Instrument that measures intraocular pressure by evaluating the force of a reflected amount of air blown against the cornea.

Airet See albuterol.

air-fluidized bed Durable medical equipment used for patients with pressure sores in which small ceramic beads are circulated by pressurized warm air, simulating fluid movement and producing a floating sensation in the patient, whose weight is evenly distributed. Supply is reported with HCPCS Level II code E0194. *NCD Reference: 280.8.*

AIS Androgen insensitivity syndrome. X-linked recessive condition in which individuals who are chromosomally male fail to develop normal male external genitalia due to an abnormality on the X chromosome that prohibits the body, completely or in part, from recognizing the androgens produced. This failure may be complete (CAIS) or partial (PAIS). Female external genitalia are found in individuals with CAIS, while internally the patient may have a short vagina, but absence of internal female organs, and testicles that may require surgical removal due to possible cancer risk. Those with PAIS may exhibit decreased penis size, female external genitalia, or both to some degree. In either case, there may be testes and normal testosterone production. Report androgen insensitivity syndromes with a code from ICD-9-CM subcategory 259.5.

AJ HCPCS Level II modifier for use with CPT or HCPCS Level II codes, that indicates a service performed by a clinical social worker. This modifier is required on claims when services are performed by a clinical social worker. These services are limited to CPT codes 90801-90899 or as limited by the state practice set. Medicare reimbursement is 75 percent of the physician fee schedule allowable.

AK Above the knee.

AKA 1) Also known as. 2) Antikeratin antibodies. Seen in roughly half of rheumatoid arthritis patients, AKA is considered a marker for the disease.

akamushi disease Acute infectious disease resembling typhus, caused by rickettsia bacteria and transmitted by the bite of infected larval mites, called chiggers. This disease occurs chiefly in Asia and the Pacific and is manifested by a specific telltale lesion or eschar at the site of the bite, fever, regional lymphadenopathy, and skin lesions and rashes. Report this disease with ICD-9-CM code 081.2. *Synonym(s): inundation fever, island fever, Japanese flood fever, Japanese river fever, kedani fever, mite-borne typhus, Mossman fever, scrub typhus, shimamushi disease, tropical typhus, tsutsugamushi disease.*

Akineton Anticholinergic drug that acts as an antagonist to acetylcholine, used to treat Parkinson's disease. Supply is reported with HCPCS Level II code J0190.

ALA Aminolevulinic acid.

Alagille syndrome Inherited liver disease with noted renal, cardiovascular, and ocular abnormalities. Report this syndrome with ICD-9-CM code 759.89.

Al-Anon, Alateen Alcoholic support groups.

ALARA As low as reasonably achievable.

alb. (albus) White.

Albarran test Test that screens for colibacilluria, a bacteria found in the intestine.

Albers-Schönberg disease Rare congenital condition in which the bones are excessively dense, resulting from a discrepancy in the formation and breakdown of bone. This disease manifests in various types and severity and can cause optic atrophy and deafness, hepatosplenomegaly, fractures, and depleted bone marrow and nerve foramina in the skull. This condition is reported with ICD-9-CM code 756.52. *Synonym(s): marble bones, osteopetrosis.*

albinism Absence of pigment in skin, hair, and eyes. This genetic condition is often accompanied by astigmatism, photophobia, and nystagmus. Albinism is reported with ICD-9-CM code 270.2.

Albright's hereditary osteodystrophy Rare genetic disease in which there is sufficient amount of parathyroid hormone produced, but the body is unable to respond to it, due to a defective type of protein required for the hormone's signal transduction. This results in low blood calcium levels and high phosphate levels. Physical characteristics include a short physique, round face, obesity, and short hand bones. Report this disorder with ICD-9-CM code 275.49. *Synonym(s): Bantam-Albright-Martin disease, Martin-Albright-Bantam disease, pseudohypoparathyroidism.*

Albright-McCune-Sternberg syndrome Patchy skin pigmentation, endocrine dysfunctions and polyostotic fibrous dysplasia. Report this disorder with ICD-9-CM code 756.59. **Synonym(s):** *Albright's hereditary osteodystrophy syndrome, McCune-Albright syndrome.*

albumin Most prevalent protein in blood plasma, synthesized in the liver, serving as a transport protein for larger anions, like bilirubin and fatty acids, and also for some hormones. Decreased levels in serum samples can indicate malnutrition, acute inflammation, and serious liver and kidney disease. Microalbumin is used to detect early signs of proteinuria in diabetes and suspected preeclampsia. Report CPT codes 82040-82045 for albumin chemistry tests.

albuterol Bronchodilator taken by inhalation when airways are restricted and breathing becomes difficult. A nebulizer or handheld inhaler may be used. Albuterol acts to relax the smooth muscle and open up the constricted airways in the lungs. Albuterol may also be mixed with ipratropium bromide, a medication used to treat bronchospasm. This mixed compound is used to treat chronic obstructive pulmonary disease (COPD) and other obstructive airway diseases. May be sold under the brand names Adrenergic Accuneb, Airomir, Combivent, Duoneb, Proventil, Proventil HFA, Proventil Repetabs, Ventolin, Ventolin HFA, Volmax.

alcohol dependence syndrome Chronic, progressive state of dependence upon alcohol that is both psychological and physical with periodic or continuous episodes impairing health and the ability to function emotionally, socially, and occupationally.

alcohol septal ablation Alcohol injected into a targeted artery of the heart during endoscopic surgery to induce a small myocardial infarction (MI) that will cause tissue shrinkage over time as a treatment for hypertrophic obstructive cardiomyopathy, reported with ICD-9-CM code 425.1. This procedure is reported with CPT code 93799.

alcohol withdrawal syndrome Absence of alcohol in an alcohol-dependent individual with physiological and psychological symptoms. Severity may result in death. Report this disorder with ICD-9-CM code 291.81.

alcoholic amnestic syndrome Prominent and lasting reduction of memory span, including striking loss of recent memory, disordered time appreciation, and confabulation, occurring in alcoholics as the sequel to an acute alcoholic psychosis or, more rarely, in the course of chronic alcoholism. It is usually accompanied by peripheral neuritis and may be associated with Wernicke's encephalopathy. Report this disorder with ICD-9-CM code 291.1.

alcoholic cardiomyopathy Heart disease, damage, or failure caused by excessive intake of alcohol, reported with ICD-9-CM code 425.5.

alcoholic psychoses Organic psychotic states due mainly to excessive consumption of alcohol that may be exacerbated by nutritional defects. ***a. abstinence syndrome*** Cessation of prolonged heavy drinking of alcohol that results in tremor of hands, tongue, and eyelids that can also include nausea and vomiting, dry mouth, headache, heavy perspiration, fitful sleep, acute anxiety attacks, mood depression, feelings of guilt and remorse, and irritability. ***a. amnestic syndrome*** Prominent and lasting reduction of memory span, including striking loss of recent memory, disordered time appreciation, and confabulation, occurring in alcoholics as the sequel to an acute alcoholic psychosis or, more rarely, in the course of chronic alcoholism. It is usually accompanied by peripheral neuritis and may be associated with Wernicke's encephalopathy. ***a. dementia*** Nonhallucinatory dementias occurring in association with alcoholism, but not characterized by the features of alcohol withdrawal delirium (delirium tremens) or alcohol amnestic syndrome (Korsakoff's alcoholic psychosis). ***a. hallucinosis*** Psychosis usually of less than six months' duration, with slight or no clouding of consciousness and much anxious restlessness in which auditory hallucinations, mostly of voices uttering insults and threats, predominate. ***a. jealousy*** Chronic paranoid psychosis characterized by delusional jealousy and associated with alcoholism. ***a. paranoia*** Chronic paranoid psychosis associated with alcoholism. ***a. polyneuritic psychosis*** Disturbance of long- and short-term memory that is attributed to alcohol use or dependence and affects emotional, social, and occupational function. ***a. withdrawal delirium (delirium tremens)*** Acute or subacute organic psychotic states in alcoholics, characterized by clouded consciousness, disorientation, fear, illusions, delusions, hallucinations of any kind, notably visual and tactile, restlessness, tremor, and sometimes fever. ***a. withdrawal hallucinosis*** Psychosis usually of less than six months' duration, with slight or no clouding of consciousness and much anxious restlessness in which auditory hallucinations, mostly of voices uttering insults and threats, predominate. ***a. withdrawal syndrome*** Cessation of prolonged heavy drinking of alcohol that results in tremor of hands, tongue, and eyelids that can also include nausea and vomiting, dry mouth, headache, heavy perspiration, fitful sleep, acute anxiety attacks, mood depression, feelings of guilt and remorse, and irritability.

Aldesleukin Genetically engineered chemotherapy drug created using recombinant DNA technology to produce a pure protein analog of human Interleukin 2, also referred to as a lymphokine. It stimulates the body's natural defenses at the cellular level to attack and destroy cancer cells and is used to treat metastatic renal cell carcinoma and melanoma. Supply is reported with HCPCS Level II code J9015. This drug is usually

A-C

administered only in a hospital setting due to harsh side effects. May be sold under the brand name Proleukin.

aldolase Enzyme that breaks down larger aldehyde compounds into smaller ketone or aldehyde molecules, tested for to differentiate between progressive muscle dystrophies and diseases affecting the muscles of neurogenic origin. Aldolase is 10 to 15 times higher than normal in the early stages of diseases such as muscular dystrophy and dermatomyositis, while muscle mass is still largely intact. Levels of this enzyme to not change in muscle diseases of neurogenic origin. Report CPT code 82085 for serum chemistry test. *Synonym(s): ALD.*

Aldomet Brand name drug given as antihypertensive therapy or in response to a hypertensive crisis. This drug may be given initially intravenously to gain control of blood pressure and then given orally. Supply is reported with HCPCS Level II code J0210. Aldomet contains methyldopate HCl.

aldosterone Major mineralocorticoid hormone secreted from the adrenal cortex that promotes the retention of sodium, excretion of potassium, and retention of water. It is used to diagnose primary hyperaldosteronism in patients who present with hypertension when high levels of aldosterone are present in blood and/or urine with low levels of plasma renin. Report CPT code 80408 for aldosterone suppression evaluation and 82088 for serum chemistry levels.

Aldrich (-Wiskott) syndrome Inherited immunodeficiency with eczema, thrombocytopenia, recurrent pyogenic infection, and increased susceptibility to infection with encapsulated bacteria. Report this disorder with ICD-9-CM code 279.12. *Synonym(s): Wiskott-Aldrich syndrome.*

ALDs Assistive listening device. Directed hearing aid. ALDs include microphones placed near a teacher, transmitting the sound to a receiver with the patient, or amplifiers attached to a phone, television set, or radio. The advantage of ALDs is that unlike traditional hearing aids, only one source of sound is amplified, without amplification of background noise. Supply of ALDs is reported with HCPCS Level II codes V5268-V5274.

Ale-Calo syndrome Congenital defect characterized by a combination of mental retardation and deformities including peculiar faces with bulb-like nose, small head, little hair, redundant skin, multiple exostoses, and joint laxity. Report this syndrome with ICD-9-CM code 759.89. *Synonym(s): Langer-Giedion syndrome.*

alefacept Immunosuppressive drug given to adult patients with moderate to severe plaque psoriasis, who are candidates for systemic or phototherapy. It inhibits lymphocyte activation at the cellular level. Supply is reported with HCPCS Level II code J0215. May be sold under the brand name Amevive.

alemtuzumab Antineoplastic drug given for chemotherapy to treat B-cell chronic lymphocytic leukemia (B-CLL). Alemtuzumab is reserved for patients treated with alkylating drugs and for whom fludarabine therapy has failed. Supply is reported with HCPCS Level II code J9010. May be sold under the brand name Campath.

Aleppo boil Dry or urban cutaneous leishmaniasis, one form of Old World cutaneous leishmaniasis. This parasitic skin disease is caused by the protozoa Leishmania tropica, spread by the bite of sand flies, and occurring in large urban areas in the Middle East, especially Iran and Iraq, the Mediterranean, and India. Manifestation is mainly a single, large developing boil or furuncle type lesion that persists over a year. Lymphadenopathy may be present. Report this condition with ICD-9-CM code 085.1. *Synonym(s): Baghdad boil, Biskra boil, Delhi boil, Gafsa boil, Jericho boil.*

Alexander's operation Uteral displacement repaired by shortening round ligaments.

alexia Impairment of the ability to comprehend written words that may be acquired as a result of a cerebral lesion, reported with ICD-9-CM code 315.01, or a developmental disorder, reported with 784.61.

Alferon-N. See interferon.

Alfi's syndrome Rare congenital defect with a complex of disorders including mental retardation and muscle weakness, caused by a defect on the ninth chromosome. Report this syndrome with ICD-9-CM code 759.89. *Synonym(s): monosomy 9P-minus syndrome.*

-algia Pain.

alglucerase Enzyme used in the treatment of Type I Gaucher disease with severe symptoms. Gaucher disease is the most common lipid-storage disorder, due to lack of the enzyme glucocerebrosidase. Alglucerase is a modified form of the enzyme beta-glucocerebrosidase and catalyzes the hydrolysis of the glycolipid, glucocerebroside, into glucose and ceramide as it would normally degrade. Supply is reported with HCPCS Level II code J0205. May be sold under the brand name Ceredase.

alglucosidase alfa Injectable pharmaceutical indicated for the treatment of Pompe disease (GAA deficiency). May be sold under the brand name Myozyme. Report supply with HCPCS Level II code J0220.

algology *1)* Medicinal study of pain and pain management. *2)* Botanical study of algae.

algoneurodystrophy Neuropathy of the peripheral nervous system.

Alibert-Bazin syndrome Malignant neoplasm resembling a fungus and growing outside of the body. Report this disorder with a code from ICD-9-CM code range 202.10-202.18.

Alice in Wonderland syndrome Organic disorder with patient presenting an illusion of dreams, feelings of levitation, and alteration of passage of time. Associated with epilepsy, migraines, and other problems of the parietal part of brain. Report this disorder with ICD-9-CM code 293.89.

ALIF Anterior lumbar interbody fusion. Surgical procedure done on the spine to fuse two or more lumbar vertebrae. Lumbar fusion is often done for cases of degenerative disease affecting the intervertebral discs. The intervertebral discs are removed at the same time for decompression. Anterior fusion is accomplished by approaching the lower spine though the abdomen, or front of the body, and not directly from the back. CPT codes 22558-22585 include a small clearing of the intervertebral disc to make room for the bone graft material. If a concomitant discectomy for decompressing nerve roots or spinal cord is documented, code also the appropriate procedure done for nerve root decompression as described in the nervous system section of CPT, as well as any appropriate grafting codes. Modifier 51 is applied to each separately identifiable procedure (except add-on codes) in addition to the primary procedure. The primary procedure is the one with the highest dollar value, or relative value units.

alignment Establishment of a straight line or harmonious relationship between structures.

Alimta Brand name for pemetrexed, an injectable chemotherapeutic drug approved for treatment of malignant pleural mesothelioma. Supply is reported with HCPCS Level II code J9305.

ALJ Administrative law judge.

ALK Automated lamellar keratoplasty. Surgical procedure for vision correction utilizing a device called a microkeratome to excise a narrow sliver of the cornea from the eye in order to reshape it. An incomplete flap is first cut across the outer layer of the cornea, but left attached, exposing the sublayers of cornea. The exact depth of the corrective cut from sublayers is calculated and made with the microkeratome. The outer flap is re-laid into position and as healing occurs, myopia is corrected. Report ALK with ICD-9-CM procedure code 11.62 and CPT code 65710.

alk. phos. Alkaline phosphatase.

Alkaban-AQ See vinblastine.

Alkeran IV or PO See melphalan HCl.

ALL Acute lymphocytic leukemia. **Synonym(s):** *acute lymphoblastic leukemia.*

all- Another, other, or different.

All patient diagnosis-related group 3M HIS made revisions and adjustments to the DRG system, now referred to as the All Patient DRGs (AP-DRGs). Early features of AP-DRGs included MDC 24, specifically

devoted to HIV, and restructuring of the MDC governing newborns.

Allen test Test often done as part of a patient examination prior to invasive surgery on arteries of the wrist. The patient closes the hand into a tight fist to force blood out from the skin of the fingers and palm. The examiner then occludes both the radial and ulnar arteries by applying pressure over each. The arteries are released one at a time and the hand is opened. Capillary refill or Doppler pulse to the fingers is observed to determine if blood is returning to the hand and fingers. Failure indicates an obstruction in the artery currently released from digital pressure. Refer to CPT codes 99201-99350 and their guidelines for determining the level of exam completed and key components met, as this is a part of an E/M service.

Allen-Masters syndrome Pelvic pain resulting from old laceration of broad ligament received during delivery. Report this disorder with ICD-9-CM code 620.6.

allergen Substance that produces an immediate hypersensitivity (allergic) reaction upon contact, such as pollen or animal dander. For allergen bronchial provocation tests, report CPT codes 95070-95071. a. immunotherapy Introduction of an antigen into the body to induce sensitivity and trigger an immune response with the production of antibodies. Report CPT codes 95115-95199.

allergic rhinitis Inflammation of the mucous membranes of the nose due to allergy.

allergy Immune system mediated hypersensitivity reaction to an allergen. An allergen can be almost anything, including food, drug, plant, animal, or environmental agent. Allergies are treated with immunotherapy. Report CPT codes 95004-95075 for testing and 95115-95199 for immunotherapy. Allergy skin tests with bacterial, viral, or fungal extracts are reported with codes from CPT range 86485-86580 and 95028.

all-inclusive rate In health care contracting, a flat fee charged by a facility on a daily basis (per diem) or for a total stay. The all-inclusive reimbursement rate usually pertains to state psychiatric hospitals. The UB-04 is used for billing all-inclusive rate accommodations and/or ancillary services. The only billable revenue codes under this rate are 0100 (all-inclusive room and board plus ancillary) and 0101 (all-inclusive room and board).

Allis sign Diagnostic sign that helps determine if a femoral neck fracture is present. The patient lies supine with the hips and knees flexed. When an unequal upper leg length is noted and the knees are not at the same level, it indicates relaxation of the fascia between the iliac crest and the greater trochanter in a femoral neck fracture. This test may be part of a musculoskeletal system review during an E/M exam. Refer to CPT codes

A-C

99201-99350 and their guidelines for determining the level of exam completed and key components met.

allo- Difference or divergence from the norm.

Alloderm Brand name cultured epidermal allograft that is a permanent replacement for skin or other tissue, created from a culture of donor skin cells and used in skin grafting and plastic reconstruction. Skin graft procedures associated with Alloderm can be reported with CPT codes 15340-15341. Report supply with HCPCS Level II code Q4116.

allodynia Condition in which ordinary, non-painful stimuli evoke a pain response.

allograft Graft from one individual to another of the same species. *Synonym(s): allogeneic graft, homograft.*

allograft, morselized Small pieces of bone from a donor other than the patient.

allograft, structural Segment of bone from other than the patient that is machined into the space.

allopathy Traditional medical approach to illness in which a disease is treated through the application of agents or treatments that are incompatible with a particular antagonist. Doctors of Medicine (MD) are allopaths and graduates of programs accredited by the American Association of Medical Colleges (AAMC) or equivalent overseas schools.

alloplastic Inert, nonbiological material, such as plastic or metal, implanted into tissues to construct, augment, or reconstruct a body part. A. dressing: Synthetic materials applied immediately following an excisional procedure to enable the wound to generate new skin without the physician having to perform additional autografting procedures. Alloplastic dressings are reported with CPT codes 15002-15005.

alloplastic dressing Synthetic materials applied immediately following an excisional procedure to enable the wound to generate new skin without the physician having to perform additional autografting procedures. Alloplastic dressings are reported with CPT codes 15002-15005.

allowable charge Fee schedule amount for a medical service as determined by the physician fee schedule methodology as published annually by CMS. *Synonym(s): approved charge.*

alopecia Congenital abnormality in which the scalp hair fails to grow or develop, and affected children are bald. Alopecia is reported with ICD-9-CM code 757.4. a. areata Patchy hair loss of the beard or scalp that is usually reversible from inflammatory causes, reported with ICD-9-CM code 704.01. a. totalis Lack of hair, especially on the scalp. Hair loss may be partial or total and can occur at any age, reported with ICD-9-CM code 704.00. *Synonym(s): baldness, ophiasis.*

ALOS Average length of stay. Utilization benchmark average compiled from the actual number of inpatient days calculated using factors such as geographical location and diagnosis.

Aloxi Brand name for palonosetron, an injectable drug for treatment of chemotherapy-induced nausea and vomiting. Supply is reported with HCPCS Level II code J2469.

ALP Alkaline phosphatase.

alpha-1-antitrypsin deficiency Insufficient production of the antibody glycoprotein alpha-1 antitrypsin, or AAT. This reactive protein protects tissue from the destructive proteolytic action of enzymes, particularly limiting the effects of neutrophil elastase, a natural enzyme that helps clean up dead tissue in the lungs. AAT is produced in the liver and secreted into the bloodstream in response to infection or injury. This enzyme deficiency is a genetic defect that causes an abnormal form of the protein to be produced, which cannot be secreted by the liver. This genetic metabolic disorder is linked to both lung and liver disease and is a major genetic cause of transplantation. Report with ICD-9-CM code 273.4.

AlphaNine SD See factor IX complex.

Alport's syndrome Inherited, progressive sensorineural hearing loss, ocular defects, and glomerulonephritis, or pyelonephritis. Report this disorder with ICD-9-CM code 759.89.

alprostadil Potent vasodilator given by IV infusion to children with patent ductus arteriosus to improve cardiac circulation until surgery can be performed. It is also injected directly into the penis to correct erectile dysfunction via vasodilation. Supply is reported with HCPCS Level II code J0270. May be sold under the brand names Caverject, Edex, Prostin PR Pediatric.

alprostadil urethral suppository Potent vasodilator inserted into the urethra of the penis to correct erectile dysfunction via vasodilation. Supply is reported with HCPCS Level II code J0275. May be sold under the brand name Muse.

ALS Advanced life support.

ALT Alanine aminotransferase.

alt. dieb. Every other day.

alt. hor. Every other hour.

alt. noc. Every other night.

Altemeier procedure Removal of a rectal prolapse through a perineal approach (CPT code 45130) or through a combined abdominal and perineal approach (45135).

alteplase recombinant Thrombolytic agent used to dissolve clots in coronary arteries, peripheral bypass grafts, central venous access devices, and the lungs through its action of initiating local fibrinolysis. It is also

A-C

used to manage acute ischemic cerebrovascular accidents. Supply is reported with HCPCS Level II code J2997. May be sold under the brand names Actilyse, Activase.

altering patient records   Inappropriately changing or amending patient records, usually to obtain reimbursement or because of pending audits and legal review of records.

alternative delivery system   Any health care delivery system other than traditional fee-for-service. **Synonym(s):** *ADS.*

aluminum   Lightweight silvery metal element often presenting as aluminum silicate, causing toxicity in high concentrations that result in microcytic hypochromic anemia, progressive dementia, and osteodystrophy. Patients at higher risk for toxicity include those on parenteral nutrition, patients with chronic renal failure who collect aluminum through dialysate, and those with industrial exposure. Report serum chemistry level with CPT code 82108. **Synonym(s):** *Al.*

Alupent   Bronchodilator administered by oral inhalation, used to treat asthma, bronchitis, or emphysema by relaxing the airway muscles in order to improve breathing. Supply is reported with HCPCS Level II code J7668 or J7669. Alupent contains metaproterenol sulfate.

alveolar capillary block syndrome   Chronic inflammation and progressive fibrosis of pulmonary alveolar walls, with progressive dyspnea leading to death by oxygen deprivation or right heart failure. Report this disorder with ICD-9-CM code 516.3. **Synonym(s):** *Hamman-Rich syndrome.*

alveolar process   Bony part of the maxilla or mandible that supports the tooth roots and into which the teeth are implanted.

alveolectomy   Partial or total excision of the maxillary or mandibular alveolar process.

alveoloplasty   Surgical recontouring of the bone to which a tooth is attached, usually performed prior to the fitting of prosthesis.

alveoplasty   Procedure in which the physician alters the contours of the alveolus by removing sharp areas or undercuts of alveolar bone.

Alzheimer's disease   Diffuse atrophy of the cerebral cortex, causing a progressive decline in intellectual and physical functions, including memory loss, personality changes, and profound dementia. Alzheimer's disease is reported with ICD-9-CM code 331.0, with an additional code from subcategory 294.1 to identify associated dementia when applicable.

AM   HCPCS Level II modifier, for use with CPT or HCPCS Level II codes, that identifies a physician who provides a service as part of a team.

AMA   *1)* Against medical advice. Discharge status of patients who leave the hospital before completion of medical treatment and release by a physician who may or may not have signed a release document. *2)* American Medical Association. Professional organization for physicians. The AMA is the secretariat of the National Uniform Claim Committee (NUCC), which has a formal consultative role under HIPAA. The AMA also maintains the Current Procedural Terminology (CPT) coding system.

amalgam   Alloy that is used for dental restorations including fillings.

Amaryl   Brand name oral medication exclusive to lowering blood glucose in Type II diabetics. Amaryl contains glimepiride.

amaurotic familial idiocy   Inherited disorder in which the body stores excessive amounts of lipofuscin, the pigment that remains after damaged cells are broken down and digested, resulting in progressive nervous tissue damage. This term actually denotes a group of genetic lipidoses, named for the type by age, all characterized by continual neurodegeneration manifesting in muscle incoordination, vision loss, retardation, seizures, and fatality. Report this disorder with ICD-9-CM code 330.1. **Synonym(s):** *ceroid lipofuscinosis, neuronal ceroid lipofuscinosis.*

amb   Ambulate.

ambi-   *1)* Both sides. *2)* About or around. **Synonym(s):** *amphi-.*

AmbioDry   Brand name amniotic membrane allograft for use in ophthalmic surgery. Supply of AmbioDry is reported with HCPCS Level II code V2790. Transplant of AMT to the ocular surface is reported with CPT code 65780.

Ambisome   Brand name for amphotericin B liposome, Ambisome is used to treat systemic fungal infections in patients who are refractory or intolerant to Amphotericin B. Ambisome is also used to treat visceral Leishmaniasis in immunocompromised patients as well as cryptococcal meningitis in HIV infected patients. Supply is reported with HCPCS Level II code J0289.

amblyopia ex anopsia   Decreased or impaired vision in one or both eyes without detectable anatomic damage to the retina or visual pathways, brought on by disuse, often as a result of esotropia. Usually not correctable by eyeglasses or contact lenses. Report amblyopia ex anopsia with a code from ICD-9-CM subcategory 368.0. **Synonym(s):** *lazy eye.*

ambulance fee schedule   Final rule published on February 27, 2002, established a fee schedule for the payment of ambulance services under the Medicare program effective on or after April 1, 2002. The rule established a five-year transition during which payment is based on a blended amount - part fee schedule and

A-C

part provider reasonable cost or suppliers' reasonable charge.

ambulatory patient group Reimbursement methodology developed for the Centers for Medicare and Medicaid Services.

ambulatory payment classification Cost-containment tool developed by CMS and the basis for the outpatient prospective payment system (OPPS). Outpatient services are grouped into multiple payment classifications based on resource utilization. Facilities are paid a fixed rate dependent on the service classification. *Synonym(s): APC.*

ambulatory surgery Surgical procedure in which the patient is admitted, treated, and released on the same day.

ambulatory surgery center Any distinct entity that operates exclusively for the purpose of providing surgical services to patients not requiring hospitalization. To receive reimbursement for treatment of Medicare patients, an ASC must have an agreement with the Centers for Medicare and Medicaid Services (CMS) and meet certain required conditions. *Synonym(s): ASC.*

Amcort Brand name injectable corticosteroid used to treat asthma, Addison's disease, allergic reactions, and various skin conditions. It is also used to reduce swelling in cases of arthritis, bursitis, or tendonitis. Supply is reported with HCPCS Level II code J3302. Amcort contains triamcinolone diacetate.

AMCRA American Managed Care Review Association.

AMD Age-related macular degeneration. Deterioration of the central portion of the retina (macula), causing blurring of central vision. There are two forms. The more advanced, wet AMD, results from the formation of abnormal blood vessels behind the retina that grow under the macula. These fragile vessels leak blood and fluid and displace the macula from its normal position at the back of the eye. Central vision loss occurs quickly. Dry AMD results from deterioration of the light-sensitive cells in the macula causing gradually blurring central vision. As AMD progresses, central vision can be lost. Report wet AMD with ICD-9-CM code 362.52; dry with 362.51. *Synonym(s): ARMD, macular degeneration.*

amebiasis Infection with a single cell protozoan known as the amoeba. Transmission occurs through ingestion of feces, contaminated food or water, use of human feces as fertilizer, or person-to-person contact. Entamoeba is a genus of naked ameboid protozoan organisms that are parasitic in vertebrates including humans. Entamoeba histolytica is the only species with the potential to produce human amebiasis, classified to ICD-9-CM category 006. Amoebae in the active feeding stage of their life cycle feed on the lining of the intestine, causing ulcers and destroying it. They may invade the blood vessels of the large intestines and subsequently spread to the liver (006.3), brain (006.5), lung (006.4), and skin (006.6). If the protozoal intestinal disease is caused by amebiasis other than E. histolytica, report 007.8. Diagnosis is made by demonstrating the presence of cysts or trophozoites in stool, see CPT code 87177.

amelia Congenital absence of one or more limbs.

amendments and corrections Amendment to a record indicates that the data are in dispute while the original information is retained; correction to a record alters or replaces the original record.

amenorrhea Absence of menstruation. Primary amenorrhea is the failure of menstruation to begin by age 16. Secondary amenorrhea is menstruation that ceases once it has begun. Primary or secondary amenorrhea is reported with ICD-9-CM code 626.0.

American Academy of Orthopaedic Surgeons Nonprofit organization for orthopaedic surgeons and allied health professionals. *Synonym(s): AAOS.*

American Academy of Professional Coders National organization for coders and billers offering certification based upon physician-, facility- or payer-specific guidelines, providing CPC, CPC-H, CPC-P and CIRCC, as well as a variety of specialty credentials.

American Association for Homecare Association for the home care industry, including home IV therapy, home medical services and manufacturers, and home health providers. AAHomecare was created through the merger of the Health Industry Distributors Association's Home Care Division (HIDA Home Care), the Home Health Services and Staffing Association (HHSSA), and the National Association for Medical Equipment Services (NAMES). *Synonym(s): AAHomecare.*

American Association of Health Plans National association of health plans created by the merger of the Group Health Association of America (GHAA) and the American Managed Care and Review Association (AMCRA). *Synonym(s): AAHP.*

American College of Medical Coding Specialists National organization for coders, billers, and payers offering certification based upon physician-, facility-, or payer-specific guidelines, providing PCS, FCS, and CSP credentials and education.

American Dental Association Professional organization for dentists. The ADA maintains a hardcopy dental claim form and the associated claim submission specifications, and also maintains the Current Dental Terminology (CDT-2005) medical code set. The ADA and the Dental Content Committee (DeCC), which it hosts, have formal consultative roles under HIPAA. *Synonym(s): ADA.*

American Health Information Management Association Association of health information management professionals that offers professional and educational services. *Synonym(s): AHIMA.*

American Hospital Association Health care industry association that represents the concerns of institutional providers. The AHA hosts the National Uniform Billing Committee (NUBC), which has a formal consultative role under HIPAA. It also publishes ICD-9-CM Coding Clinic. *Synonym(s): AHA.*

American Hospital Association Central Office Central office of the AHA works in partnership with the National Center for Health Statistics (NCHS), American Health Information Management Association (AHIMA), and Centers for Medicare and Medicaid Services (CMS) to maintain the integrity of and develop education regarding the ICD-9-CM coding system.

American Medical Association Professional organization for physicians. The AMA is the secretariat of the National Uniform Claim Committee (NUCC), which has a formal consultative role under HIPAA. The AMA also maintains the Physician's Current Procedural Terminology (CPT) coding system. *Synonym(s): AMA.*

American Medical Informatics

Association Professional organization that promotes the development and use of medical informatics for patient care, teaching, research, and health care administration. *Synonym(s): AMIA.*

American mucocutaneous leishmaniasis Form of leishmaniasis endemic in Mexico, Central America, and South America in which lesions from cutaneous leishmaniasis spread chronically and progressively months to years after the initial lesion, causing destructive, ulcerative sores associated with mutilation of the nasal septum, palate, pharynx, larynx, and buccal mucosa. Report American mucocutaneous leishmaniasis with ICD-9-CM code 085.5.

American National Standards Standards developed and approved by organizations accredited by the American National Standards Institute (ANSI). *Synonym(s): ANS.*

American National Standards Institute Organization that accredits various standards-setting committees and monitors their compliance with the open rule-making process that they must follow to qualify for ANSI accreditation. HIPAA prescribes that the standards mandated under it be developed by ANSI-accredited bodies whenever practical. *Synonym(s): ANSI.*

American Society for Testing and Materials Standards group that has published general guidelines for developing standards, including those for health care identifiers. ASTM Committee E31 on Health Care Informatics develops standards on information used within health care. *Synonym(s): ASTM.*

American Society of Anesthesiologists National organization for anesthesiology that maintains and publishes the guidelines and relative values for anesthesia coding. *Synonym(s): ASA.*

A-methaPred Brand name glucocorticoid used primarily to treat severe inflammation and for immunosuppression purposes. A-methaPred is frequently used to treat shock, acute exacerbation of multiple sclerosis, severe cases of lupus nephritis, and spinal cord injury in an effort to decrease motor and sensory deficits. This glucocorticoid is also used as an adjunct therapy in the treatment of moderate to severe Pneumocystis carinii pneumonia. Supply is reported with HCPCS Level II code J2930. A-MethaPred contains methylprednisone acetate.

Amevive See alefacept.

AMI Acute myocardial infarction. Interruption of blood flow to heart muscle caused by an arterial blockage. AMI is reported with an ICD-9-CM code from category 410. Code selection is based on the site of the infarct and the episode of care.

AMIA American Medical Informatics Association. Professional organization that promotes the development and use of medical informatics for patient care, teaching, research, and health care administration.

amifostine Drug used to decrease the cumulative toxic affects of repeated Cisplatin doses. Amifostine is administered to patients receiving Cisplatin for non-small-cell lung cancer and advanced ovarian cancer who exhibit renal toxicity. It has also been shown to reduce moderate to severe xerostomia in patients undergoing postoperative treatment with radiation for head and neck cancer. Supply is reported with HCPCS Level II code J0207. May be sold under the brand name Ethyol.

amikacin sulfate Drug that kills susceptible gram negative aerobic bacteria, especially specific for *Pseudomonas aeruginosa, E. Coli, Proteus, Klebsiella, Serratia, Enterobacter, Acinetobacter, Providencia, Citrobacter,* and *Staphylococcus* (meningitis). Supply is reported with HCPCS Level II code J0278.

Amikin See amikacin sulfate.

aminocaproic acid Antithrombolytic used as a prophylaxis against hemorrhage for dental procedures or surgery in patients who have hemophilia or other platelet disorders. Supply is reported with HCPCS Level II code S0017. May be sold under the brand names Amikar, Cyklokapron.

aminolevulinic acid HCl Chemical used in conjunction with photodynamic therapy for treatment of actinic keratoses (precancerous skin lesions) of the face or scalp. Supply is reported with HCPCS Level II code J7308. May be sold under the brand names Levulan Kerastick.

aminolevulinic acid test Test for abnormal urine concentrations of ALA that can accumulate in the acute neurologic forms of the porphyrias, as well as increased levels in blood and urine from lead poisoning. This test

A-C

is reported with CPT code 82135. *Synonym(s): ALA, Delta (5) aminolevulinic acid.*

aminophyllin Bronchodilator used to provide relief of symptoms and reverse airflow obstruction associated with chronic lung disorders. Supply is reported with HCPCS Level II code J0280. May be sold under the brand names Ethylenediamine, Phyllocontin, Somophyllin, Somophyllin-DF, Theophylline, Truphylline.

amiodarone HCl Drug used to treat ventricular and supraventricular arrhythmias. Supply is reported with HCPCS Level II code J0282. May be sold under the brand names Cordarone, Cordarone X, Pacerone.

amitriptyline Antidepressant used not only to treat depression, but also to treat eating disorders, and as an adjunct therapy for neurogenic pain. Amitriptyline is used for elderly and adolescent patients in addition to the adult population. Supply is reported with HCPCS Level II code J1320. Route can be IM or PO. Amitriptyline comes in a syrup as well as a pill form, however the J code is for injection only. May be sold under the brand names Apo-Amitriptyline, Elavil, Endep, Tryptanol.

AML Acute myelogenous or myelocytic leukemia. One of the two major categories of acute leukemia (myelogenous/myelocytic and lymphocytic) that includes several types identified by the stage in which abnormal proliferation begins: acute myeloblastic, acute myelomonocytic, acute monocytic, acute erythroleukemia, and acute megakaryocytic leukemia. Symptoms include anemia, bruising, fatigue, weight loss, thrombocytopenia, and prolonged bacterial infections. *Synonym(s): acute myeloid leukemia.*

AMLOS Arithmetic mean length of stay. Average number of days patients within a given DRG stay in the hospital. The AMLOS is used to determine payment for outlier cases and to predict occupancy rates. *Synonym(s): average length of stay.*

AMML Acute myelomonocytic leukemia.

ammonia dermatitis Nonallergic skin irritation in infants in the area that has contact with the diaper. It can be caused by extended contact with feces, urine, soaps, and ointments, and by friction and the irritating effects of ammonia by-products in urine. The rash is often accompanied by secondary yeast or bacterial infection. Report this condition with ICD-9-CM code 691.0. *Synonym(s): diaper dermatitis, diaper rash, Jacquet's dermatitis, Jacquet's erythema, napkin rash.*

ammonia rash Contact dermatitis affecting the thighs and buttocks as a result of exposure to urine and feces, usually affecting young children. Report this condition with ICD-9-CM code 691.0. *Synonym(s): diaper rash, napkin rash.*

amnestic syndrome Amnestic dementia in which the patient has no short-term or long-term memories but is not delirious. Report this disorder with ICD-9-CM code 294.0.

amniocentesis Surgical puncture through the abdominal wall, with a specialized needle and under ultrasonic guidance, into the interior of the pregnant uterus and directly into the amniotic sac to collect fluid for diagnostic analysis or therapeutic reduction of fluid levels. Report cases of newborns affected by amniocentesis with ICD-9-CM code 760.61. Amniocentesis is reported with CPT codes 59000 and 59001. These procedures are excluded from the maternity care global package. *Synonym(s): diagnostic amniocentesis, therapeutic amniotic fluid reduction.*

amniotic band syndrome In-utero entanglement of body parts of the fetus by fibrous bands caused by a rupture of the amnion. The resulting intrauterine constrictions cause a range of symptoms ranging from soft tissue depressions on the extremities, limbs, neck, or chest to intrauterine amputation of the affected extremity. *Synonym(s): ABS, constriction band syndrome.*

amniotomy Artificial rupture of the amniotic sac in order to induce or enhance labor, to check for fetal stool, or to place a fetal monitor. If performed for induction of labor, amniotomy is reported with ICD-9-CM procedure code 73.01; if amniotomy is performed after labor has begun, it is reported with 73.09. In CPT, it is included in the code for maternity care and should not be reported separately. *Synonym(s): AROM, breaking of waters, surgical induction of labor.*

amobarbital Barbiturate causing central nervous system depression with sedative hypnotic and anticonvulsant properties as well. Amytal is the trade name. Injectable amobarbital described by HCPCS Level II code J0300 is for the parenteral drug administered by IV and is frequently used as an IV sedative preoperatively or in abreaction psychotherapy. May be sold under the brand name Amytal.

A-mode Implies one-dimensional procedure.

amoral personality Personality disorder characterized by disregard for social obligations, lack of feeling for others, and impetuous violence or callous unconcern and self-rationalization of behavior.

amotivational syndrome Nonparticipation in day-to-day activities or therapy as a result of emotional, organic, or chemical causes. Report this disorder with ICD-9-CM code 292.89.

AMP *1)* Adenosine monophosphate. *2)* Ampule.

amphetamine Schedule II controlled substance that acts as a stimulant on both the central nervous and peripheral nervous systems. It relaxes bronchial muscle and suppresses appetite and is used to treat narcolepsy, obesity, and hyperkinetic syndromes. Amphetamines are often abused as a street drug and can cause dependence. Most often tested for in urine. Report CPT code 82145 for quantitative analysis and 80100-80103 for drug screening. **Synonym(s):** *methamphetamine.*

Amphocin   See amphotericin B.

Amphotec   Brand name for amphotericin B cholesteryl sulfate complex, Amphotec is a lipid form of amphotericin B used primarily for the treatment of invasive aspergillosis in patients where renal impairment or toxicity precludes the use of amphotericin B deoxycholate in effective doses or where prior amphotericin B deoxycholate has failed. Supply is reported with HCPCS Level II code J0285.

amphotericin B   Antifungal used to fight systemic infections of histoplasmosis, coccidioidomycosis, blastomycosis, cryptococcosis, disseminated candidiasis, aspergillosis, and mucormycosis. The drug is also used for fungal infections of the endocardium and as a prophylaxis against fungal infections in bone marrow transplant patients. Candidal infections of the GI tract, mouth, and bladder are also treated with Amphotericin B. Supply is reported with HCPCS Level II code J0285. May be sold under the brand names Fungalin, Fungizone.

amphotericin B lipid complex   Drug used to treat the systemic fungal infections in patients who are refractory or intolerant to Amphotericin B. The lipid complex form is also used to treat visceral Leishmaniasis in immunocompromised patients as well as cryptococcal meningitis in HIV infected patients. Supply is reported with HCPCS Level II code J0287. May be sold under the brand name Abelcet.

ampicillin sodium   Antibiotic that prohibits cell wall synthesis in microbes as they reproduce, often given to patients in labor prior to delivery to prevent neonatal group B streptococcal infection. This antibiotic is also used to treat meningitis, gonorrhea, and enterococcal endocarditis and can be used as a prophylaxis against endocarditis resulting from dental procedures. Supply is reported with HCPCS Level II code J0290. May be sold under the brand names Ampicin, Ampicyn, Omnipen-N, Penbritin, Polycillin-N, Totacillin-N.

ampicillin sodium/sulbactam sodium   Antibiotic ampicillin with the added properties of sulbactam, which inactivates the enzyme that bacteria produce to render them ampicillin resistant. Used primarily to treat intra-abdominal, skin, and skin structure infections, and pelvic inflammatory disease. Supply is reported with HCPCS Level II code J0295. May be sold under the brand name Unasyn.

AmpliChip   Brand name technology used in pharmacogenetic assay for cytochrome P450 genotype. It is used to evaluate a patient's genetics as they relate to metabolization of medication, so that the correct treatment can be determined.

amplitude   Size, extent, abundance, fullness, or amount of movement.

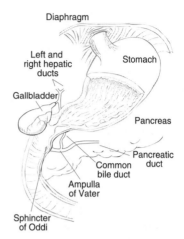

Ampulla of Vater

Diaphragm

Left and right hepatic ducts

Stomach

Gallbladder

Pancreas

Pancreatic duct

Common bile duct

Ampulla of Vater

Sphincter of Oddi

Location of the gallbladder in relation to select surrounding structures

ampulla of Vater   Tubular structure with flask-like dilation where the common bile and pancreatic ducts join before emptying into the duodenum. **Synonym(s):** *hepatopancreatic ampulla.*

amputation   Removal of all or part of a limb or digit through the shaft or body of a bone. Amputation can be the diagnosis in cases of accidental injury or the procedure in cases of surgery.

AMS Sphincter 800   Brand name implanted prosthesis that mimics the function of the urinary sphincter, providing incontinent patients with control of urination following prostate surgery. The device consists of a fluid-filled cuff that surrounds the urethra, a pump implanted near the testicles, a balloon implanted in the abdomen, and tubing to connect these parts. To urinate, the patient squeezes the pump in the scrotum. This causes fluid to drain from the cuff, which opens the urethra. The cuff automatically refills several minutes later, closing the urethra. CPT codes that report implant or removal of this system include 53444-53449.

Amsler grid   Chart used to diagnose or follow macular disease or macular degeneration.

Amsler's sign   Hemorrhage in a patient with Fuchs' heterochromic iridocyclitis, following cataract surgery or applanation tonometry.

AMT   Amniotic membrane transplant. AMT is used as graft material in eye surgery. Supply of AMT is reported with HCPCS Level II code V2790. Transplant of AMT to the ocular surface is reported with CPT code 65780.

Amussat's operation Long transverse incision made to expose the colon.

amyelia Congenital condition in which the spinal cord is absent, reported with ICD-9-CM code 742.59.

amyelotrophy Atrophy of the spinal cord.

amygdalohippocampectomy Surgical removal of all or part of the amygdala, hippocampus, and parahippocampal gyrus of the brain to treat medically refractive temporal lobe epilepsy with sparing of unaffected brain tissue and reduced effects of the more conventional anterior temporal lobectomy. Amygdalohippocampectomy is reported with CPT code 61566. **Synonym(s): mesial temporal lobectomy, SAH.**

amyloidosis Condition in which insoluble, fibril-like proteins (amyloid) build up in one or more organs and tissues within the body. The material cannot be broken down and interferes with the normal function of the organ. The disease may be inflammatory, hereditary, or neoplastic in nature. Report this condition with ICD-9-CM codes 277.30-277.39.

amyostatic syndrome Accumulation of copper in the brain, cornea, kidney, liver, and other tissues causing cirrhosis of the liver and deterioration in the basal ganglia of the brain. Report this disorder with ICD-9-CM code 275.1.

Amytal See amobarbital.

an- Without, away from, not.

ANA 1) American Nursing Association. 2) Antinuclear antibodies. Immunoglobulins produced against the body's own cellular nuclei as the antigen. ANA is found in diseases such as rheumatoid arthritis and systemic lupus erythematosus.

anaerobe Bacteria growing in the total or partial absence of oxygen, frequently seen on laboratory report. Although it does not directly drive code selection, it does drive treatment decisions.

anal fissure Slit, crack, or tear of the anal mucosa that can cause pain, bleeding, and infection. This condition may also occur with hemorrhoids and is reported with ICD-9-CM code 565.0.

anal fistula Abnormal opening on the skin surface near the anus, which may connect with the rectum. This condition is reported with ICD-9-CM code 565.1.

anal papilla Skin tag protruding up from the area between the skin and the inside lining of the anus. Anal papillae frequently occur with anal fissures and are often detected during a digital examination of the anus or with a scope.

analgesia Absence of a normal sense of pain without loss of consciousness.

analgesic Agent that relieves pain without causing loss of consciousness.

analysis Study of body fluid, tissue, section, or parts.

analyte Any material or chemical substance subjected to analysis.

anancastic (anankastic) neurosis Feeling of subjective compulsion to carry out an action, dwell on an idea, recall an experience, or ruminate on an abstract topic or to perform a quasiritual that may result in anxiety or inner struggle as the individual tries to cope with the behavior.

anancastic (anankastic) personality Feeling of subjective compulsion to perform an action or a thought process that causes anxiety if there is interruption or discontinuance of the action or thought by the self or others.

Anastomosis

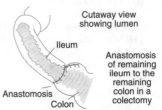

Cutaway view showing lumen

Ileum

Anastomosis of remaining ileum to the remaining colon in a colectomy

Anastomosis

Colon

anastomosis Surgically created connection between ducts, blood vessels, or bowel segments to allow flow from one to the other.

anatomic narrow angle Defect restricting aqueous drainage.

anatomic snuff box Landmark used as a diagnostic indicator to identify scaphoid fractures. When the thumb is abducted and extended, the area on the radial border of the dorsum of the wrist creates a triangular depression defined by the extensor and abductor tendons of the thumb. Tenderness or effusion within the snuff box is often indicative of a fracture. This test may be part of a musculoskeletal system review performed in an E/M exam. See the E/M section of CPT to determine the level of examination and key component criteria met when selecting the appropriate code.

anatomical crown Portion of a tooth covered by enamel.

anatomy Science of body structures and relationships among structures.

ANC Absolute neutrophil count. Automated cell count blood test with cell differential for evaluation of immunity. Neutrophils are a type of white blood cell, and ANC may be indicated for a patient prior to chemotherapy, following transplant, in the otherwise immunosuppressed, or in other specific illnesses. ANC is reported with CPT code 85048.

Ancef See cefazolin sodium.

ancillary services Services, other than routine room and board charges, that are incidental to the hospital stay. These services include operating room; anesthesia; blood administration; pharmacy; radiology; laboratory; medical, surgical, and central supplies; physical, occupational, speech pathology, and inhalation therapies; and other diagnostic services.

Anderson tibial lengthening Tibia is severed and screws are affixed to plates supporting the bone across the gap in this technique to lengthen the patient's leg.

ANDI Aberrations of normal development and involution. Diagnostic term used to describe benign conditions of the breast, including fibrocystic changes, duct ectasia, or fibroadenoma.

Andro-Estro 90-4 Brand name hormone combination drug of estrogen and testosterone used to prevent breast fullness after childbirth and for relief of menopausal symptoms such as sweating, hot flashes, chills, faintness, and dizziness. It restores estrogen balance in tissues and stimulates cells that produce male sex characteristics, to replace normal levels of androgens lost in menopausal women. This class of drug is exempt from consideration as an anabolic steroid in most states and may not be considered medically necessary by CMS for hormone replacement unless used as an adjunct to chemotherapy. Supply code reported with HCPCS Level II code J0900.

androgen Male sex hormone. Testosterone is the primary androgen. In the fetus, androgens cause the formation of external male genitalia.

androgen insensitivity syndrome X-linked recessive condition in which individuals who are chromosomally male fail to develop normal male external genitalia due to an abnormality on the X chromosome that prohibits the body, completely or in part, from recognizing the androgens produced. This failure may be complete (CAIS) or partial (PAIS). Female external genitalia are found in individuals with CAIS, while internally the patient may have a short vagina, but absence of internal female organs, and testicles that may require surgical removal due to possible cancer risk. Those with PAIS may exhibit decreased penis size, female external genitalia, or both to some degree. In either case, there may be testes and normal testosterone production. Report androgen insensitivity syndromes with a code from ICD-9-CM subcategory 259.5. *Synonym(s): AIS.*

anecortave acetate Injectable drug to treat subfoveal neovascularization due to macular degeneration. The injection of anecortave acetate is reported with CPT code 0124T, with modifier RT or LT. Supply of anecortave acetate is reported with HCPCS Level II code J3490. May be sold under the brand name Retaane.

anemia Deficiency in the blood whether in red blood cells, hemoglobin, or total blood count.

anemia of chronic disease Anemia occurring as a result of chronic illnesses, such as end stage renal disease, chronic infections, inflammatory disorders, malignancies, or other chronic diseases. Report this disease with a code from ICD-9-CM subcategory 285.2.

anencephalus Fatal brain defect of a newborn caused by closure of the neural groove early in the first trimester of pregnancy. It may present as absence of the cranial vault, abnormally shaped brain, or missing or malformed cerebral hemispheres. Anencephalus is reported with ICD-9-CM code 740.0. *Synonym(s): acrania, amyelencephalus, hemianencephaly, hemicephaly.*

anesthesia Loss of feeling or sensation, usually induced to permit the performance of surgery or other painful procedures.

anesthesia dolorosa Spontaneous pain perceived in an anesthetized area.

anesthesia formula Reimbursement formula consisting of base units plus time units plus modifying units (e.g., physical status and qualifying circumstances) plus other allowed unit/charges that is multiplied by a conversion factor.

anesthesia time Time period factored into anesthesia procedures beginning with the anesthesiologist preparing the patient for surgery and ending when the patient is turned over to the recovery department.

AneuRx AAAdvantage Brand name abdominal aortic aneurysm stent grafting system.

Aneurysm

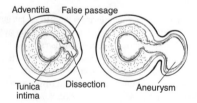

An aneurysm is a weakening and swelling of the arterial wall

aneurysm Circumscribed dilation or outpouching of an artery wall, often containing blood clots connecting directly with the lumen of the artery. *NCD Reference: 20.23.*

aneurysmal bone cyst Solitary bone lesion that bulges into the periosteum, marked by a calcified rim.

Angelchik Brand name large silastic "C" shaped ring placed around the esophagus near the sphincter as an antireflux device in the treatment of GERD, an alternative to fundal plication, or to reduce a sliding hiatal hernia. It is considered a new technology.

Angelman syndrome Emergence in early childhood of a pattern of interrupted development, stiff, jerky gait, absence or impairment of speech, excessive laughter, and seizures. Report this disorder with ICD-9-CM code 759.89.

Anghelescu sign Diagnostic sign that helps determine the presence of vertebral tuberculosis or other spinal destructive processes. While lying supine, the patient attempts to lift his or her body upward with weight on his head and heels, to bend the spine and rest on the head and heels alone. An ongoing disease process is indicated by an inability to bend the spine.

angi- Relating to a vessel.

angiectasis Abnormal expansion and lengthening of a blood or lymphatic vessel, reported with ICD-9-CM code 459.89.

angina Chest pain that occurs secondary to the inadequate delivery of oxygen to the heart muscle and may be described as a heavy or squeezing pain in the midsternal area of the chest.

angina cruris syndrome Number of symptoms in a moving limb including pain, tension, and weakness but absent at rest. Caused by occlusive arterial diseases of the limbs. Report this disorder with ICD-9-CM code 443.9. *Synonym(s): Charcot's syndrome.*

angina syndrome Acute, choking pain most notable in the pectoral region of the chest and implying the onset of a heart attack. Report this disorder with ICD-9-CM code 413.9.

angiodysplasia Vascular abnormalities, with or without bleeding.

angiogram Radiographic image of the arteries. Imaging may be performed to study the vasculature of any given organ, body system, or area of circulation such as the brain, heart, chest, kidneys, limbs, gastrointestinal tract, aorta, and pulmonary circulation to visualize the formation and the function of the blood vessels to detect problems such as a blockage or stricture. A catheter is inserted through an accessible blood vessel and the artery is injected with a radiopaque contrast material after which x-rays are taken. Code selection is determined by the specific anatomical site. *NCD Reference: 220.9.*

angiography Radiographic imaging of the arteries. Imaging may be performed to study the vasculature of any given organ, body system, or area of circulation such as the brain, heart, chest, kidneys, limbs, gastrointestinal tract, aorta, and pulmonary circulation to visualize the formation and the function of the blood vessels to detect problems such as a blockage or stricture. A catheter is inserted through an accessible blood vessel and the artery is injected with a radiopaque contrast material after which x-rays are taken. Code

selection is determined by the specific anatomical site. *Synonym(s): angiogram. NCD Reference: 220.9.*

angioma Benign tumor made up of blood or lymph vessels. *Synonym(s): hemangioma, lymphangioma.*

Angiomax See bivalirudin.

angion Segment of lymphatic vessel between two lymphatic valves, acting to push the lymphatic fluid in one direction. *Synonym(s): lymphangion.*

angioplasty Reconstruction or repair of a diseased or damaged blood vessel. *A. balloon:* Balloon-tipped medical device used to clear the blockage of an artery. After insertion into the clogged artery, the balloon is inflated to expand a narrowing arterial section.

angioplasty balloon Balloon-tipped medical device used to clear the blockage of an artery. After insertion into the clogged artery, the balloon is inflated to expand a narrowing arterial section.

angioscopy Visualization of capillary blood vessels with a microscope, or the inside of a blood vessel with a fiberoptic-equipped catheter. *Synonym(s): cardiac "scope."*

Angio-Seal Brand name for a mechanical and biochemical closure device used to seal arterial puncture wounds from diagnostic and therapeutic catheterization procedures such as PTCA, angiography, and stent placement. Supply is reported with HCPCS Level II code G0269.

angiotensin II Hormone that acts as a powerful vasopressor to raise blood pressure and reduce fluid loss, and also stimulates the release of aldosterone; used to assess hyper aldosteronism. Report CPT code 82163 for chemistry test.

angle closure Blockage in aqueous drainage.

angle closure glaucoma Progressive optic disease associated with high intraocular pressure that can lead to irreversible vision loss. The aqueous humor is the clear fluid filling the chambers of the eye that is continually drained and renewed, produced by the ciliary body and passing out through the pupil and trabecular meshwork. Angle closure glaucoma causes an increase in intraocular pressure due to an impairment of aqueous outflow caused by a narrowing or closing of the anterior chamber angle as the iris comes into contact with the trabecular meshwork. This type of glaucoma is identified in four stages: latent, intermittent, acute, and chronic. In the latent and intermittent phases, minor or transient attacks of varying severity, duration, and frequency occur in which intraocular pressure (IOP) rises with accompanying pain and edema. Acute angle closure glaucoma is a grave medical emergency as IOP rises, the cornea swells, and excruciating pain radiates through the eye. Visual acuity falls rapidly as the eye swells and blindness may result if the IOP is not lowered. The chronic stage manifests as irreversible IOP increases from progressive damage and scar tissue closing the anterior angle. Angle-closure glaucoma is reported with ICD-9-CM codes 365.20-365.24. **Synonym(s):** *closed angle glaucoma, narrow angle glaucoma, pupillary block glaucoma.*

angle's classification System of classifying malocclusion of the teeth based on the relationship of the first molars. Class I malocclusion is manifested by a faulty line of occlusion but a normal molar relationship. In Class II malocclusion there is an overbite, or the upper molar is placed over the lower molar. In Class III malocclusion, or underbite, the lower molar is positioned forward to the upper molar. Report these conditions with a code from ICD-9-CM range 524.21-524.23.

anhedonia Inability to experience pleasure from experiences that are normally pleasurable. Anhedonia is a clinical feature of various mental illnesses, including depression and schizophrenia, and is reported with ICD-9-CM code 780.99.

aniridia Congenital anomaly in which there is incomplete formation or absence of the iris, resulting in loss of vision. Aniridia is typically bilateral and other health or developmental problems may be present. Aniridia is reported with ICD-9-CM code 743.45.

aniseikonia Visual defect in which the size and shape of an image as seen by one eye differs from that seen by the other. This condition is reported with ICD-9-CM code 367.32.

aniso- Dissimilar, unequal, or asymmetrical.

anisocoria Congenital anomaly in which the pupils are unequal in diameter, reported with ICD-9-CM code 743.46.

anisometropia Visual defect in which there are different focal lengths in the lenses of the two eyes, causing the refractive power to differ. Different corrective prescriptions for each eye are necessary for good vision. Report this condition with ICD-9-CM code 367.31.

anisospondyly Vertebral bodies of varying abnormal shapes found in several inherited or genetic diseases, such as spondyloepimetaphyseal dysplasia. There is no specific diagnostic code supplied for this condition, which is reported with ICD-9-CM code 756.19. Treatment could include any spinal procedure related to the specific problem requiring correction.

anistreplase Drug used to dissolve clots in blood vessels and in central venous catheters that is given intravenously under direct physician supervision. Supply is reported with HCPCS Level II code J0350. May be sold under the brand name Eminase.

ankle brachial index Common test to evaluate lower extremity arterial blood flow in which the systolic blood pressure of the upper extremity is compared to the systolic pressure at the ankle. The index is found by dividing the lower extremity pressure by the upper extremity pressure. An index of 0.9 or less indicates arterial insufficiency of the lower extremities. This test is part of the review of systems or physical exam in an office visit and is not reported separately. **Synonym(s):** *ABI.*

ankylo- Bent, crooked, or two parts growing together.

ankylodactylia Condition defined by fingers or toes adhering or fusing to one another, resulting in restricted motion. The index in ICD-9-CM directs the coder to see syndactylism 755.10 when looking up ankylodactylism. CPT codes relating to surgical correction of syndactyly include 26560-26562.

ankylosing spinal hyperostosis Arthritic disorder manifested by osteophytes on opposite sides of the spine fusing two or more vertebral bodies together.

ankylosing spondylitis Rheumatic inflammation of the joints of the hips, spine, and pelvis most commonly affecting young men. This arthritic disease of the joints can lead to fusion and deformity of the spine. The cause is unknown. Report this condition with ICD-9-CM code 720.0. **Synonym(s):** *Marie Strumpell disease, rheumatoid spondylitis.*

ankylosis Abnormal union or fusion of bones in a joint, which is normally moveable. Choose the code based on the joint affected, see ICD-9-CM subcategory 718.5 or for teeth, 521.6.

annuloplasty Surgical plicaton of weakened tissue of the heart, to improve its muscular function. Annuli are thick, fibrous rings and one is found surrounding each of the cardiac chambers. The atrial and ventricular muscle fibers attach to the annuli. In annuloplasty, weakened annuli may be surgically plicated, or tucked, to improve muscular functions.

anodontia Partial or complete absence of teeth due to a congenital defect involving the tooth bud, reported with ICD-9-CM code 520.0, or acquired as a result of caries, trauma, extraction, or periodontal disease, coded to causality within ICD-9-CM subcategory 525.1. The causal code is used in addition to a code for the class of edentulism: 525.40-525.44 (complete edentulism) or 525.50-525.54 (partial edentulism). **Synonym(s):** *adontia, anodontism, edentia, edentulism.*

anomalous atrioventricular excitation Pre-excitation associated with paroxysmal tachycardia or atrial fibrillation with a short P-R interval on EKG and an early delta wave. The normal conduction pathway is bypassed. This syndrome is reported with ICD-9-CM code 426.7. **Synonym(s):** *pre-excitation syndrome, Wolff-Parkinson-White syndrome, WPW syndrome.*

anomaly Irregularity in the structure or position of an organ or tissue.

anomia Inability to remember words or names of common objects, without loss of comprehensive or repetitive faculties, reported with ICD-9-CM code 784.69. *Synonym(s): anomic aphasia.*

anonychia Absence of toenails. Nails arise from the same embryogenic layer as hair, skin, and teeth-the ectoderm. There is no specific diagnosis code assigned for anonychia and it is subsequently reported with ICD-9-CM code 782.9. When the loss of nails is due to a disease process, assign 703.8.

anophthalmia Absence of eyes due to a congenital anomaly.

anophthalmos Congenital absence of an eye, reported with ICD-9-CM code 743.00.

anopia Absence or loss of vision.

anorchism Congenital condition in which one or both testes are absent. This condition is reported with ICD-9-CM code 752.89.

anorectal anometry Measurement of pressure generated by anal sphincter to diagnose incontinence.

anorexia nervosa Psychological eating disorder characterized by an intense fear of gaining weight, an unrealistic perception of body image that perpetuates the feeling of being fat or having too much fat, even though the body is emaciated, and an accompanying refusal to maintain normal body weight. This condition typically affects young women in adolescent years and also manifests with amenorrhea, depression, denial, and peculiar behaviors or obsessions over food. Report anorexia nervosa with ICD-9-CM code 307.1.

anoscope Short speculum for examining the anal canal and lower rectum.

anoscopy Endoscopic diagnostic procedure in which an anoscope is inserted through the anus and advanced. The anal canal and distal rectal mucosa are visualized and brushings or washings may be obtained.

anosognosia Inability or refusal of an individual to recognize his or her own disability, illness, functional defect, or handicap. Anosognosia is reported with ICD-9-CM code 780.99.

anotia Congenital absence of the auricle of the ear. Anotia is reported with ICD-9-CM code 744.09.

anovular menstruation Menstruation that occurs without ovulation. The egg remains within the ovary and deteriorates normally, associated with infertility. On rare occasions the egg may be fertilized, resulting in an ectopic ovarian pregnancy.

anovulation Abnormal condition in which an ovum is not released each month. Anovulation is a prime factor in female infertility and is reported with ICD-9-CM code 628.0. Polycystic ovaries are a common cause of anovulation.

anoxic brain damage Injury sustained to the brain due to lack of oxygen.

ANP Atrial natriuretic peptide. Hormone involved in maintaining homeostasis of renal and cardiovascular functions. Muscle cells of the atrium manufacture the prohormone and release it into circulation as the atrial wall responds to dilation or increased fluid volume. ANP regulates blood pressure and volume by causing diuresis and the excretion of salt, and reducing concentrations of antidiuretic hormone and aldosterone. Elevated blood levels of ANP are indicative of heart failure. *Synonym(s): atriopeptin.*

ANS *1)* Autonomic nervous system. *2)* American National Standards. Standards developed and approved by organizations accredited by the American National Standards Institute (ANSI).

ANSI American National Standards Institute. Organization that accredits various standards-setting committees and monitors their compliance with the open rule-making process that they must follow to qualify for ANSI accreditation. HIPAA prescribes that the standards mandated under it be developed by ANSI-accredited bodies whenever practical.

ANSI/HISB ANSI Health Information Standards Board.

ant Anterior.

Antagon See ganirelix acetate.

antalgic gait Abnormal walk due to pain upon placing weight on the affected foot, resulting in less time spent bearing weight on the affected side. Such a finding during the course of an E/M service exam would be part of a musculoskeletal system review.

ante- In front of, before.

antebrachium Part of the upper limb between the wrist and elbow. *Synonym(s): forearm.*

antepartum Period of pregnancy between conception and the onset of labor.

anterior Situated in the front area or toward the belly surface of the body; an anatomical reference point used to show the position and relationship of one body structure to another.

Anterior Chamber

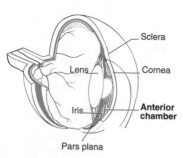

Sclera

Lens

Cornea

Iris

Anterior chamber

Pars plana

anterior chamber Space in the eye located between the cornea and the lens that contains aqueous humor. The anterior chamber is bounded by the sclera and cornea in front and the ciliary body, iris, and pupillary portion of the lens in the back. *Synonym(s): camera anterior bulbi, camera oculi anterior.*

anterior chamber lenses Lenses inserted into the anterior chamber following intracapsular cataract extraction.

anterior compartment One of four muscle compartments found in the leg. The anterior compartment houses a group of muscles that includes the tibialis anterior, extensor hallucis longus, extensor digitorum longus, and the peroneus tertius. Together these muscles help provide dorsiflexion of the ankle and all five toes.

anterior cranial fossa Supports the frontal lobes of the brain and is composed of the frontal bone (anteriorly), the ethmoid bone (in the middle), and the body and lesser wings of the sphenoid bone (posteriorly).

anterior cruciate instability test Specific maneuver to test instability of the anterior cruciate ligament in the knee. The patient lies down with the knee flexed and as the knee is extended slowly with the foot on the table, a sudden anterior shift of the tibia may occur. This test may be part of a musculoskeletal system review performed in an E/M exam.

anterior cruciate ligament Ligament composed of two parts: anteromedial and posterolateral bundle. It helps hold the tibia and femur together deep within the knee joint. When this tears or ruptures, it creates instability of the knee. Repair can be done either open or arthroscopically.

anterior symblepharon Adhesions between the eyelid and the eyeball.

anterior synechiae Adhesion binding the iris to the cornea.

anterior teeth Six upper and six lower front teeth; the upper and lower incisors and cuspids.

antero- Before, front, anterior.

anterolateral Situated in the front and off to one side.

anteromedial Situated in the front and to the side of the central point or midline.

anteroposterior Front to back. *a. x-ray* Radiography taken from the front of the body to the back. *Synonym(s): AP.*

anteroposterior and lateral Two projections, front to back and side, are included in this examination.

anthrax Infection caused by bacillus anthracis, a gram positive, rod-shaped, motile bacterium that forms spores. Most cases are cutaneous (ICD-9-CM code 022.0), occurring by direct contact with the bacterium. Inhaled spores can cause pulmonary anthrax (022.1) in which the spores get into the lungs and multiply, entering into the lymph system and producing a strong and lethal toxin. The bacteria cause gastrointestinal problems when ingested in poorly cooked meat contaminated with B. anthracis (022.2). Use 795.31 to report nonspecific positive findings for anthrax (e.g., positive findings per nasal swab).

anti- In opposition to, against.

antiandrogens Drugs that inhibit the ability of the body to utilize androgens. Antiandrogens are frequently used with orchiectomy and LHRH analogs (manmade hormone that impedes the production of testosterone) in the treatment of prostate cancer. Antiandrogens include bicalutamide, Casodex, Eulexin, flutamide, Nilandron, nilutamide.

antibody Immunoglobulin or protective protein encoded within its building block sequence to interact only with its specific antigen.

anticoagulant Substance that reduces or eradicates the blood's ability to clot. *NCD Reference: 190.11.*

antigen Substance inducing sensitivity or triggering an immune response and the production of antibodies.

antiinhibitor coagulant complex Medication used to prevent and control hemorrhage in Hemophilia A patients who have developed antibodies to antihemophilic factor and in patients with acquired hemophilia who have developed inhibitors to factor VIII. Supply is reported with HCPCS Level II code J7198. May be sold under the brand names Autoplex T, Feiba VH Immune.

Antikickback Act National legislation which prohibits knowing or willful solicitation or receipt of remuneration in return for referring, recommending, or arranging for the purchase, lease, or ordering of items or services for which payment will be made from any federal or state health care program. *Synonym(s): Stark.*

antimongolism syndrome Mental and growth retardation, hypertonia, high-arched palate, micrognathia, microcephaly and an antimongoloid obliquity of the palpebral fissures. Report this disorder with ICD-9-CM code 758.39.

antineoplastic Any agent with the ability to inhibit the growth of new tumors by keeping the proliferation of malignant cells in check.

antinuclear antibodies Immunoglobulins produced against the body's own cellular nuclei as the antigen. ANA is found in diseases such as rheumatoid arthritis and systemic lupus erythematosus. *Synonym(s): ANA.*

antiphospholipid antibody syndrome Immune disorder distinguished by the presence of abnormal antibodies in the blood that are directed against phosphorous-containing fats (phospholipids). This disorder is associated with abnormality in blood clotting, thrombocytopenia (low blood platelet counts), migraine headaches, and repeated spontaneous abortions. It can be a primary disorder (occurring alone) or secondary to another underlying condition. Approximately a third of patients with the primary form have abnormal heart valves. Report this disorder with ICD-9-CM code 289.81. *Synonym(s): APLS.*

Antispas See dicyclomine HCl.

antithrombin III Glycoprotein used as a replacement in patients with antithrombin III deficiency. It acts as an anticoagulant or antithrombolytic by inhibiting reactions in the coagulation cascade. Supply is reported with HCPCS Level II code J7197.May be sold under the brand names Atnativ, Thrombate III.

Antizol See fomepizole.

Antley-Bixler syndrome Rare congenital disorder primarily manifested by craniofacial and other skeletal abnormalities. Craniosynostosis is typically present, as well as a prominent forehead, underdeveloped midface, protruding eyes, and radiohumeral and/or radioulnar fusion. The thighbones may be bowed and there may be joint contractures. This syndrome is reported with ICD-9-CM code 759.89. *Synonym(s): Trapezoidocephaly-synostosis syndrome.*

Anton (-Babinski) syndrome Form of cortical blindness caused by damage to the occipital lobe in which the patient denies the visual impairment. Report this disorder with ICD-9-CM code 307.9.

antro- Relating to a chamber or cavity.

antrum Chamber or cavity, typically with a small opening.

ANUG Acute necrotizing ulcerative gingivitis. *Synonym(s): fusospirochetosis, trench mouth, Vincent's angina.*

anuria Suppression, cessation, or failure of the kidneys to secrete urine.

anvil test Test to indicate diseased vertebrae or early disease of the hip joints in which the leg is extended and

the sole of the foot is struck with a closed fist. Disease is indicated if pain is produced in the vertebrae or hip.

anxiety hysteria Neurotic state with abnormally intense dread of certain objects or specific situations that would not normally affect the individual.

anxiety state Apprehension, tension, or uneasiness that stems from the anticipation of danger, the source of which is largely unknown or unrecognized. *atypical a.* Anxiety disorder that does not fulfill the criteria of generalized or panic attack anxiety. *generalized a.* Disorder of at least six months' duration manifested by diffuse and persistent anxiety without the specific symptoms that characterize phobic disorders, panic disorder, or obsessive-compulsive disorder. *panic attack a.* Episodic and often chronic, recurrent disorder manifested by discrete periods of sudden onset, intense apprehension, fearfulness, or terror often associated with feelings of impending doom.

any willing provider Provider who meets the network's usual selection criteria as defined in statues requiring a provider network. *Synonym(s): AWP.*

AOA American Osteopathic Association.

AOD Arterial occlusive disease.

AODM Adult onset diabetes mellitus.

aortic dissection Pathologic process characterized by splitting of the wall of the aorta, caused by blood entering a tear in the vessel intima or an interstitial hemorrhage, leading to formation of a dissecting aneurysm. Report aortic dissection with ICD-9-CM codes 441.00-441.03.

aortic insufficiency Malfunction of the aortic valve resulting in backflow of blood into the ventricle.

aortic stenosis Narrowing of the aortic valve resulting in backflow of blood into the ventricle.

aortic valve Heart valve, comprising three cusps, that divides the left ventricle and the aorta.

aortic valve disorders Various types of aortic valve dysfunction, two main types being stenosis and insufficiency.

aortofemoral bypass Surgically created conduit from the aorta to the femoral artery to bypass occlusion and/or disease in the lower aorta or iliac artery.

aortography Radiographic visualization of the aorta and its branches by injecting contrast medium through percutaneous puncture or catheterization technique. *Synonym(s): angiogram, aortogram.*

aortopexy Surgical suturing of the aorta and right subclavian artery to the sternum. This suspension is done to open a compressed trachea and restore airflow in cases of tracheomalacia, either congenital or acquired.

aortopulmonary transposition Transposition of the great vessels. A life-threatening congenital malformation of the two main vessels of the cardiovascular system in which the pulmonary artery branches from the left ventricle and the aorta branches from the right ventricle. This condition causes the blood being returned from the extremities to be shunted back into the systemic circulation without being oxygenated. This condition may appear in differing forms: complete or classical transposition; double outlet right ventricle in which there is incomplete transposition of the vessels, or both vessels arise from the right ventricle; and corrected transposition of the great vessels in which a developmental cardiac anomaly inverts the ventricles and valves to compensate for the transposed vessels by producing mirror-image blood flow through the heart. Study the documentation to select the code that accurately reflects which form of transposition is present. Aortopulmonary transposition should be reported with a code from ICD-9-CM category 745. **Synonym(s):** *TGV.*

AOSD Adult onset Still's disease. Type of systemic arthritis characterized by a transient rash and spiking fevers. AOSD may resolve or develop into a chronic condition and may affect internal organs, as well as joints. There is no ICD-9-CM code specific to AOSD but may be reported with 714.2.

AP *1)* Anteroposterior. Front to back. *2)* Antepartum. *3)* Apical. *4)* HCPCS Level II modifier, for use with CPT or HCPCS Level II codes, indicating that refraction was not performed in the course of diagnostic ophthalmological examination. This modifier has no effect on reimbursement.

A-P Anterior posterior.

APA *1)* American Psychiatric Association. *2)* Antiphospholipid syndrome. Autoimmune disorder associated with the development of arterial and venous thromboses. APA can be seen secondary to another disease, prominently lupus. It can also occur without an underlying disorder. It is reported with ICD-9-CM code 795.79.

APACHE II Acute physiology and chronic health evaluation score. System to measure the severity of illness in intensive care patients, based on age, previous health status, lab values, and physiologic measurements.

APAP Auto-titrating continuous positive airway pressure. Sleep apnea system used in some patients with obstructive airway sleep apnea. APAP contains sensors that trigger automatic decreases or increases in air pressure.

APB Abductor pollicis brevis. Short abductor muscle of the thumb.

APBI Accelerated partial breast irradiation. Radiation therapy that targets a portion of the breast surrounding the tumor rather than the whole breast. Treatment typically lasts four to five days, with the radiation being delivered in fewer fractions at larger doses than whole-breast external beam radiation therapy. Placement of the single or multichannel radiotherapy afterloading expandable catheter in the breast is reported with a code from CPT range 19296-19298.

APC Ambulatory payment classification. Cost-containment tool developed by CMS and the basis for the outpatient prospective payment system (OPPS). Outpatient services are grouped by CPT code into multiple payment classifications based on resource utilization. Facilities are paid a fixed rate dependent on the service classification.

AP-DRG All patient diagnosis-related group. 3M HIS made revisions and adjustments to the DRG system, now referred to as the All Patient DRGs. Early features of AP-DRGs included MDC 24, specifically devoted to HIV, and restructuring of the major diagnostic categories governing newborns.

APEC Asymmetrical periflexural exanthem of childhood. Nonspecific, benign, and self-limiting disorder including viral rash, mild fever, diarrhea, and lymphadenopathy seen in childhood.

Apert's syndrome Congenital condition that involves premature fusion of the cranial sutures, asymmetrical facies, webbed hands and feet, and progressive calcification and fusion of the bones of the hands and feet. Other features common to this condition are visual disturbances, hearing loss, acne, and cardiac and gastrointestinal malformations. This syndrome is reported with ICD-9-CM code 755.55.

Apert-Gallais syndrome Type I acrocephalosyndactyly with a peaked head, fusion of digits (specifically the second through fifth digits), and severe acne vulgaris of forearms. Report this disorder with ICD-9-CM code 255.2.

apertognathia Abnormal condition in which some of the teeth do not touch when the jaws are biting or closing. This abnormality most often occurs in the front teeth and is generally the result of an overgrowth of the back part of the upper jaw or improper growth of the lower jaw. Apertognathia is reported with ICD-9-CM code 524.20. **Synonym(s):** *open-bite deformity.*

apex Highest point of a root end of a tooth, or the end of any organ.

apexification In dentistry, a method of bringing about root development.

apexogenesis Procedure performed to remove a portion of the pulp of a tooth; medication is then applied to encourage root growth and vitality.

APG Ambulatory patient group. Reimbursement methodology developed for the Centers for Medicare and Medicaid Services.

aphakia Condition in which the crystalline lens of the eye is absent, usually as a result of cataract surgery or trauma, resulting in the inability of the eye to adjust its

A-C

focus for viewing at different distances. Report acquired aphakia with ICD-9-CM code 379.31. If specified as congenital, report with 743.35.

aphalangia Absence of a fully developed finger or toe or a phalange or phalanges of a finger or toe. This anomaly is categorized as a congenital reduction deformity. The diagnosis codes for these conditions are based on the limb involved (upper vs. lower) and the direction of the deficiency (longitudinal vs. transverse). Aphalangia is a longitudinal deficiency reported with ICD-9-CM code 755.29 for the congenital absence of a finger and 755.39 for a toe. Transverse deficiencies, or complete absence of all five digits, are coded with 755.21 for the fingers and 755.31 for the toes.

aphasia Partial or total loss of the ability to comprehend language or communicate through speaking, the written word, or sign language. Aphasia may result from stroke, injury, Alzheimer's disease, or other disorder. Common types of aphasia include expressive, receptive, anomic, global, and conduction. Aphasia is reported with ICD-9-CM code 784.3. Other codes apply when specified as developmental, late effect, or from tertiary syphilis. **Synonym(s):** *logagnosia, logamnesia, logasthenia.*

aphasia-apraxia-alexia syndrome Sensory aphasic condition with alexia and apraxia associated with lesions in the left parietal lobe. Report this disorder with ICD-9-CM code 784.69. **Synonym(s):** *Bianchi's syndrome.*

Apheresis

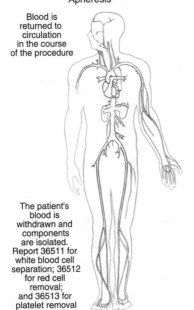

Blood is returned to circulation in the course of the procedure

The patient's blood is withdrawn and components are isolated. Report 36511 for white blood cell separation; 36512 for red cell removal; and 36513 for platelet removal

apheresis Process of extracting blood from a donor, centrifuging or separating the desired part of the blood, and transfusing the remainder back into the donor. **NCD Reference:** *110.14.*

aphthae Small ulcers of the oral mucosa that resemble a grayish canker-type lesion within a red ring, commonly seen in patients on chemotherapy. Aphthae is reported with ICD-9-CM code 528.2. **Synonym(s):** *recurrent aphthous stomatitis.*

apical ballooning syndrome Acute but reversible cardiomyopathy mimicking myocardial infarct or coronary syndrome. Described as "stunned myocardium," it occurs in women who have recently suffered a traumatic event. The syndrome is reported with ICD-9-CM code 429.89.

apical-aortic conduit Channel created between the tip of the left ventricle and the aorta, above the coronary arteries, with a valve allowing blood to flow out of the heart only. Creation of this conduit is done to correct transposition of the great vessels (TGV) and allow oxygenated blood to be circulated through the body. **Synonym(s):** *TGV correction.*

apicoectomy Removal of the root tip of an abscessed tooth along with the diseased tissue that surrounds it. It may be performed in conjunction with root canal therapy and is reported with ICD-9-CM procedure code 23.72 or 23.73 or HCPCS Level II codes D3410-D3426. **Synonym(s):** *root end resection.*

APL Abductor pollicis longus. Long abductor muscle of the thumb.

aplasia Incomplete development of an organ or tissue. Aplasia may be congenital (present at birth) or acquired. ICD-9-CM provides multiple codes to report this condition depending on site and underlying etiology.

aplasia axialis extracorticalis Inherited degenerative brain disease manifested by gradually advancing white matter sclerosis of the frontal lobes, mental deficits, and vasomotor disorders. Report this disease with ICD-9-CM code 330.0. **Synonym(s):** *hereditary cerebral leukodystrophy, Merzbacher-Pelizaeus disease, Pelizaeus-Merzbacher disease.*

aplastic anemia Failure of the bone marrow to produce sufficient red blood cells. Underlying causes can include neoplasm, toxic exposure, infections, certain drugs, or radiation. Report aplastic anemia with a code from ICD-9-CM category 284.

apleuria Congenital absence of one or more ribs, reported with ICD-9-CM code 756.3.

Apley test Diagnostic maneuver used to help differentiate injury to ligaments from injury of the meniscus. The patient lies prone with the knee flexed and the tibia is compressed into the femur, pulled from the femur (distracted), and rotated internally and externally. Pain with compression suggests meniscal injury, while pain with distraction and compression suggests ligament injury.

Apligraf Brand name bioengineered skin for treatment of skin ulcers. Its application is reported with CPT codes 15340 and 15341. Supply is reported with HCPCS Level II code Q4101.

APLS Antiphospholipid antibody syndrome.

APM Arterial pressure monitoring.

apnea Absence of breathing or breath.

apnea monitor Device used to monitor breathing during sleep that sounds an alarm if breathing stops for more than the specified amount of time.

apodia Congenital absence of one or both feet, reported with ICD-9-CM code 755.31.

apolipoprotein Constituent of lipoproteins (e.g., LDL, VLDL) synthesized in the liver and released as part of the low-density lipoprotein particle. It participates in delivery of cholesterol to the cells and is measured in relation to coronary risk factors. *Synonym(s): Apo B, Apolipoprotein B.*

aponeurectomy Excision of an aponeurosis, the flat, white, stringy tissue that extends from a tendon to connect a muscle to its moving part. CPT does not address this directly, as this is usually performed in the course of other tendon and muscle work.

aponeurorrhaphy Surgical repair of an aponeurosis, the flat, white, stringy tissue that extends from a tendon to connect a muscle to its moving part. CPT does not address this directly, as this is usually performed in the course of other tendon and muscle work.

aponeurosis Flat expansion of white, ribbon-like tendinous tissue that functions as the connection of a muscle to its moving part.

apophyseal fracture Avulsion fracture in which a bony prominence, such as a process or tuberosity, is removed from its bone. Code this type of fracture for the bone or location on the bone involved.

appeal Specific request made to a payer for reconsideration of a denial or adverse coverage or payment decision and potential restriction of benefit reimbursement.

appeal process Steps required for appealing negative decisions related to payer denials such as denied authorization for requested services or denied charges.

appendectomy Surgical removal of the appendix by either an incision into the right lower abdominal quadrant (CPT code 44950) or by laparoscopy (CPT code 44970). If an appendectomy is performed for suspected appendicitis and none is found, code the symptom(s), such as abdominal pain. If an appendectomy is

performed at the same time as another intraabdominal surgery, it should not be reported separately.

appendicitis Inflammation and infection of the appendix. In the acute stage of the disease, common symptoms include severe pain in the right lower quadrant of the abdomen, nausea, and vomiting. The acute form of the condition is reported with ICD-9-CM code 540.9.

appendiclausis Withering or blockage of the appendix.

appendico-vesicostomy Surgical procedure in which a stoma is created from the vermiform appendix in order to directly divert the flow of urine. The vermiform appendix is dissected and then connected to the bladder. The distal end is brought through an incision in the skin to form the stoma for direct emptying of urine. Report this procedure with ICD-9-CM procedure code 57.21 and CPT code 50845.

applanation tonometer Instrument that measures intraocular pressure by recording the force required to flatten an area of the cornea.

appliance Device providing function to a body part.

applicant In health care, an individual or group that is applying for a health insurance policy.

applicator Device for placing a substance into or onto the body, such as radioactive materials for cancer treatment.

approach Method or anatomical location used to gain access to a body organ or specific area for procedures. The approach is not coded separately although it may be a specified component of the procedure, such as laparoscopic vs. incisional, or spinal procedures in which the amount of dissection required to expose the spine significantly alters with the site of approach.

appropriateness of care Proper setting of medical care that best meets the patient's care or diagnosis, as defined by a health care plan or other legal entity.

approx Approximately.

appy. Appendectomy.

APR Average payment rate. Amount of money CMS could pay an HMO for services provided to Medicare recipients under a risk contract.

Apraxia Impaired sequencing of motor skills. Apraxia can be used to describe a variety of symptoms, from an awkward gait to anomalous speech.

APR-DRG All Patient Refined Diagnosis Related Group. Grouping system developed by 3M HIS that takes into account the severity of inpatient illness and the risk of mortality.

Apresoline See hydralazine HCl.

aprotinin Drug used to inhibit fibrinolysis during cardiopulmonary bypass. This decreases bleeding and

A-C

the need for transfusion. Supply is reported with HCPCS Level II code J0365. May be sold under the brand name Trasylol.

APT Admissions per thousand.

AQ HCPCS Level II modifier used to denote services provided by a physician in an unlisted health professional shortage area.

aq. Water (aqua).

aquatic therapy Therapeutic exercises performed in an aquatic environment, such as a swimming pool or whirlpool, requiring skilled intervention by a clinician. This therapy is reported with CPT code 97113.

aqueous humor Fluid within the anterior and posterior chambers of the eye that is continually replenished as it diffuses out into the blood. When the flow of aqueous is blocked, a build-up of fluid in the eye causes increased intraocular pressure and leads to glaucoma and blindness.

Aqueous Misdirection

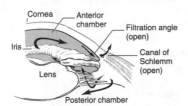

aqueous misdirection Form of glaucoma that occurs when aqueous humor flows into the posterior chamber of the eye (vitreous) rather than through the normal recycling channels into the anterior chamber. This condition is reported with ICD-9-CM code 365.83.

aqueous misdirection syndrome Increase in intraocular pressure that is accompanied by a shallow anterior chamber and forward displacement of the iris and lens.

aqueous shunt Silicone tube inserted into the anterior chamber of the eye and connected to a reservoir plate behind the pars plana to enhance drainage in the eye's anterior chamber and improve aqueous flow. This procedure is reported with CPT code 66180 or 66185 for a revision.

AR Acoustic reflex. Measure of contraction of the stapedius muscle that occurs with loud sound.

arachidic Related to or caused by peanuts or another member of the genus Arachis.

arachnidism Condition resulting from a venomous spider bite, often characterized by necrosis and ulcerating lesions at the bite site. Report this condition with ICD-9-CM code 989.5, with an additional E code to identify the venomous spider. **Synonym(s):** *arachnoidism, araneism.*

arachnodactyly Abnormally long, thin fingers and toes that have a spider-like appearance. Arachnodactyly is a former synonym for Marfan's syndrome.

Aralen See chloroquine HCl.

Aramine Brand name vasopressor that constricts peripheral blood vessels and has a positive inotropic effect on the heart, increasing the strength of contractions. Aramine is indicated for prevention and reversal of acute hypotension associated with spinal anesthesia and is also used as an adjunctive treatment for hypotension secondary to hemorrhage, reactions to medications, surgical complications, and shock from brain trauma or tumor. Supply is reported with HCPCS Level II code J0380. Aramine contains metaraminol bitartrate.

Aran's cancer Disorder manifested by numerous malignant tumors produced by bony infiltrates in myelogenous leukemia. The masses are most often found in the skull, but may occur in any part of the skeleton. The tumors appear green colored, due to pigment effects of myeloperoxidase. Report with a code from ICD-9-CM category 205.3. **Synonym(s):** *Balfour's disease, chloroleukemia, chloroma, chloromyeloma, chlorosarcoma, granulocytic sarcoma, green cancer, Naegeli's disease.*

Aranesp See darbepoetin alfa.

ARB Angiotensin receptor blocker. Oral medication that lowers blood pressure, often used in the treatment of hypertension and heart failure, and to prevent kidney failure in diabetic patients.

arbitration Settling of a dispute through a designated individual, group, or committee that is assigned to hear both sides of the story and has the authority to make a binding decision.

arc *1)* AIDS-related complex. *2)* Radiation beam that is not stationary but moves around an axis in a curved path. **Synonym(s):** *rotation, segment.*

Arcalyst See rilonacept.

arch- Beginning, first, principal. **Synonym(s):** *arche-, archi-.*

arch syndrome Progressive obliteration of brachiocephalic trunk and left subclavian and left common carotid arteries above their source in the aortic arch. Symptoms include ischemia, transient blindness, facial atrophy, and many others. Report this disorder with ICD-9-CM code 446.7. **Synonym(s):** *Martorell-Fabre syndrome, Raed-Harbitz syndrome, Takayasu-Onishi syndrome.*

archo- Relating to the rectum or anus.

arcuate ligament syndrome Compression of the celiac artery by the median arcuate ligament in the diaphragm. Report this disorder with ICD-9-CM code 447.4.

arcus cornealis Opaque, grayish ring at the periphery of the cornea just within the sclerocorneal junction, frequently seen in patients older than 50 but sometimes present at birth. Arcus cornealis results from cholesterol deposits associated with ocular defects or inherited hyperlipidemia, reported with ICD-9-CM code 371.41 (senilis) or 743.43 (juvenilis). *Synonym(s): arcus adiposus.*

arc-welders' syndrome Temporary or permanent spot blindness resulting from observing bright light with unprotected eyes. Report this disorder with ICD-9-CM code 370.24.

ARD Acute respiratory disease.

ARDS Adult respiratory distress syndrome. Lung inflammation or injury resulting in a build-up of fluid in the air sacs, preventing the passage of oxygen from the air into the bloodstream. There is no specific code for ARDS in ICD-9-CM. ARDS is reported as other pulmonary insufficiency (ICD-9-CM code 518.82) or pulmonary insufficiency following trauma or surgery (518.5).

Aredia Brand name for injectable pamidronate disodium, which is used to treat moderate to severe hypercalcemia. Supply is reported with HCPCS Level II code J2430.

ARF *1)* Acute respiratory failure. *2)* Acute renal failure. Abrupt failure of the kidneys' abilities to rid the blood of wastes and concentrate urine. Potential causes are numerous and can include dehydration, injury, hypotension, septic shock, and autoimmune disorders. Common laboratory indications include abnormal urinalysis, increased serum creatinine, BUN, serum potassium, and decreased creatinine clearance. Generalized swelling is common. ARF is reported with a code from ICD-9-CM category 584, with additional codes to indicate causative conditions.

argatroban Drug that prevents the formation of blood clots, given to patients on heparin therapy and patients suffering from heparin-induced thrombocytopenia. Argatroban is also used as an anticoagulant during percutaneous cardiac interventions in patients at risk for heparin-induced thrombocytopenia. Supply is reported with HCPCS Level II code C9121.

argentaffin, argentaffinoma syndrome Carcinoid tumors causing severe attacks of cyanotic flushing of the skin, diarrhea watery stools, bronchoconstrictive attacks, hypotension, edema, and ascites. Report this disorder with ICD-9-CM code 259.2.

argentous Containing silver. Argentous deposits within the cornea are reported with ICD-9-CM code 371.16.

argon laser Laser light energy that uses ionized argon as the active source, has a radiation beam between the visible green-blue spectrum, and is effective in coagulating blood-rich tissue with heat (photocoagulation).

Argonz-Del Castillo syndrome Lactation and amenorrhea not following pregnancy and characterized by hyperprolactinemia and pituitary adenoma. Report this disorder with ICD-9-CM code 253.1. *Synonym(s): Ahumada-Del Castillo syndrome.*

ARGUS User-friendly personal computer software package developed by the Office of Inspector General (OIG) both to access provider claims data and to limit the need for the OIG to submit multiple requests to carriers for claims data. ARGUS is a useful tool for reviewing relationships of data that carriers have available. The billing practices of physicians, for example, can be compared to that of their peers as a means of detecting aberrant behavior.

Argyll Robertson pupil Absence of light reflex in the pupil, with no change in the pupil's focus functions.

Argyll Robertson syndrome Condition where the pupil of the eye is small and unresponsive to changes in light intensity. Report this disorder with ICD-9-CM code 094.89 when this condition is syphilitic, report 379.49 for non-syphilitic.

Aries-Pitanguy mammaplasty Procedure to reduce breast size.

aripiprazole Antipsychotic medication indicated for the treatment of schizophrenia and bipolar disorder. Report supply of the intramuscular injection with HCPCS Level II code J0400. *Synonym(s): Abilify.*

arithmetic mean length of stay Medicare calculation of the average number of days patients within a given DRG stay in the hospital. The AMLOS is used to determine payment for outlier cases. *Synonym(s): AMLOS, average length of stay.*

Arlt procedure Ciliary transplant as a treatment for distichiasis.

Arlt's line Conjunctival scarring that occurs as a late effect of trachoma, reported with ICD-9-CM code 139.1. Arlt's line can lead to ocular complications including entropion, trichiasis, or dry eye, which would be reported in addition to the late effect code.

ARMD Age-related macular degeneration. Deterioration of the central portion of the retina (macula), causing blurring of central vision. There are two forms. The more advanced, wet ARMD, results from the formation of abnormal blood vessels behind the retina that grow under the macula. These fragile vessels leak blood and fluid and displace the macula from its normal position at the back of the eye. Central vision loss occurs quickly. Dry ARMD results from deterioration of the light-sensitive cells in the macula causing gradually blurring central vision. As ARMD progresses, central vision can be lost. Report wet ARMD with ICD-9-CM code 362.52; dry with 362.51. **Synonym(s):** *AMD, macular degeneration.*

arm-shoulder syndrome Disorder following a heart attack with pain and stiffness in the shoulder and swelling and pain in the hand. Report this disorder with ICD-9-CM code 337.9. **Synonym(s):** *Claude Bernard-Homer syndrome, Reilly's syndrome, Steinbrocker's syndrome.*

Arnold-Chiari syndrome Congenital malformation of the brain in which the cerebellum protrudes through the foramen magnum into the spinal canal. There are three types of official Chiari malformation, classified by the severity of herniation. Type II is referred to as the syndrome. This malformation is seen with hydrocephalus, mental defects, and always with a lumbosacral myelomeningocele. For ICD-9-CM classification purposes, type I is not coded as a congenital anomaly, but as a nervous system disorder of compression or herniation of the brain stem, 348.4. Type II is coded to 741.0 Spina bifida with hydrocephalus and requires a fifth digit to specify the region. Type III, which is a complete herniation of the cerebellum forming an encephalocele, is coded to encephalocele, 742.0. In ICD-9-CM, there is also a Type IV classified as a reduction deformity of the brain, 742.2.

Arnozan's syndrome Miliary abscesses in the scalp's hair follicles, resulting in scars and bald patches. Arnozan's syndrome is reported with ICD-9-CM code 704.09. **Synonym(s):** *acne decalvans, Brocq's lupoid sycosis, Quinquaud's syndrome.*

AROM *1)* Active range of motion. *2)* Artificial rupture of membranes.

Aromasin See exemestane.

ARPKD Autosomal recessive polycystic kidney disease. Congenital condition in which the kidneys develop many fluid-filled cysts and the liver becomes fibrotic, leading to renal and hepatic failure in childhood and adolescence. Lungs are also often underdeveloped with a high rate of infant death. ARPKD is reported with ICD-9-CM code 753.14. **Synonym(s):** *Infantile PKD.*

ARRA American recovery and reinvestment act of 2009.

arrhythmia induction Heart disorder of rhythm or rate, due to an electrical conduction system malfunction. A. induction: Intentional performance of cardiac pacing into arrhythmic states at different rates by the introduction of critically timed electrical impulses. This is usually included as part of an intracardiac electrophysiological study to determine where the disruption of the heart's normal pattern of conduction occurs, and help identify the proper treatment or its effectiveness for the patient's rhythm abnormalities.

arrhythmogenic focus Point of origin causing a rhythm disturbance in the heart. Known as the root of an arrhythmia, this electrical impulse causes the heart to beat in irregular patterns. Some codes describe the identification and mapping of the focal aberration, such as add-on code 93609. Other codes describe the ablation of the arrhythmogenic focus (93651).

Arrillaga-Ayerza syndrome Cyanosis and hypertension resulting from sclerosis of the pulmonary arteries. Report this disorder with ICD-9-CM code 416.0. **Synonym(s):** *arteriosclerosis.*

arsenic Heavy metal toxic by inhalation and ingestion that can be found in a patient's serum, plasma, or hair and nails. Acute poisoning may cause skin eruptions, vomiting, abdominal pain, cramping, and swelling of the hands and feet, and may result in shock and death. Chronic poisoning from long periods of ingestion causes scaling and pigmented skin, hyperkeratosis on the palms and soles, peripheral neuropathy, confusion, and transverse white lines on the fingernails. Report chemistry test with CPT code 82180 and heavy metal screening with 83015.

arsenic trioxide Chemotherapy drug that kills promyelocytic leukemic cells by causing breaks in their DNA. It is used to treat relapsed patients with acute promyelocytic leukemia or those who are refractory to other accepted chemotherapy treatments. Supply is reported with HCPCS Level II code J9017. May be sold under the brand name Trisenox.

ART *1)* Arterial. *2)* Accredited record technician. Former AHIMA certification describing medical records practitioners; now known as a registered health information technician (RHIT).

art. Artery, arterial.

arterio- Relating to an artery.

arteriogram Radiograph of arteries.

arteriomesenteric duodenum occlusion syndrome Distended afferent loop with illness and pain caused by acute or chronic obstruction of the duodenum and jejunum proximal to a gastrojejunostomy. Report this disorder with ICD-9-CM code 537.89. **Synonym(s):** *gastrojejunal loop obstruction.*

arteriosclerosis depressive syndrome Organic disorder in which the patient exhibits changes in personality such as amotivation, depression, outbursts, poor social judgment, etc. Caused by constriction of the arteries to the brain. Report this disorder with ICD-9-CM code 293.83.

arteriosclerotic dementia Dementia attributable, because of physical signs (confirmed by examination of the central nervous system), to degenerative arterial disease of the brain.

arteriotomy Incision into an artery.

arteriovenous fistula Connecting passage between an artery and a vein.

arteriovenous malformation Connecting passage between an artery and a vein.

artery Vessel through which oxygenated blood passes away from the heart to any part of the body.

artery compression syndrome Compression of the celiac artery by the median arcuate ligament in the diaphragm. Report this disorder with ICD-9-CM code 447.4.

arthrectomy Surgical excision or resection of a joint. Multiple codes exist in ICD-9-CM and CPT to report arthrectomy, depending upon site.

arthritis Inflammation of the joints often accompanied by swelling, stiffness, pain, and deformity.

arthro- Relating to a joint.

arthrocentesis Puncture and aspiration of fluid from a joint for diagnostic or therapeutic purposes. Anesthetics or corticosteroids may also be injected into the joint during this procedure. Report arthrocentesis with ICD-9-CM procedure code 81.91 and CPT codes 20600-20610.

arthrodesis Surgical fixation or fusion of a joint to reduce pain and improve stability, performed openly or arthroscopically. Multiple codes exist in ICD-9-CM and CPT to report arthrodesis, depending upon site.

arthrodiastasis Controlled joint separation (distraction) using external fixators, applied following injury or infection as an alternative to joint fusion or replacement.

arthrodysplasia Congenital condition of joint deformity from abnormal development, reported with ICD-9-CM code 755.9.

arthrogram X-ray of a joint after the injection of contrast material.

arthrography Radiographic study of a joint and its internal structures. Air or contrast medium is injected into the joint just before the images are taken. Report arthrography with ICD-9-CM procedure code 88.32. In CPT, the injection procedure is reportedly separately from the radiological supervision and interpretation by site.

arthropathy Disease of the joints.

arthroplasty Surgical reconstruction of a joint to improve function and reduce pain. Arthroplasty may involve partial or total joint replacement. Coding depends upon site and method.

arthroscopy Use of an endoscope to examine the interior of a joint (diagnostic) or to perform surgery on joint structures (therapeutic).

arthrotomy Surgical incision into a joint that may include exploration, drainage, or removal of a foreign body. Coding depends upon site and intent.

articular Relating to a joint or the involvement of joints.

articular cartilage Smooth living tissue that covers and protects moving surfaces resulting in the reduction of friction.

articulate Comprised of separate segments joined together, allowing for movement of each part on the other.

articulation disorder Developmental disorder of the inability to correctly produce speech sounds (phonemes) because of imprecise placement, timing, pressure, speed, or flow of movement of the lips, tongue, or throat. Report this disorder with ICD-9-CM code 315.39.

articulator Functional or anatomical device on which dental study models or casts are mounted that mimic the hinge movements of the temporomandibular joint. Dental articulators are used to aid in diagnosis and procedure planning for assuring proper occlusion with restorations or complete or partial dentures.

artificial crown In dentistry, a ceramic or metal restoration made to cover or replace a major part of the top of a tooth.

ARTISS Fibrin sealant made from pooled human plasma. Used in adult and pediatric burn patients to adhere autologous skin grafts to surgically prepared wound beds. ARTISS is reported with HCPCS Level II code C9250.

arytenoid Cartilage located at the back of the larynx attached to the vocal cords.

A-C

Arytenoidpexy

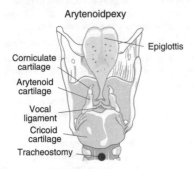

Corniculate cartilage
Epiglottis
Arytenoid cartilage
Vocal ligament
Cricoid cartilage
Tracheostomy

(Posterior cutaway view)

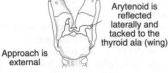

Arytenoid is reflected laterally and tacked to the thyroid ala (wing)

Approach is external

arytenoidopexy Fixation of the arytenoid cartilage tacked against the thyroid to open the glottis and improve the airway. Arytenoidopexy may alter voice quality. This procedure is reported with CPT code 31400.

AS *1)* Administrative simplification. Title II, subtitle of HIPAA, which gives HHS the authority to mandate the use of standards for the electronic exchange of health care data; to specify what medical and administrative code sets should be used within those standards; to require the use of national identification systems for health care patients, providers, payers (or plans), and employers (or sponsors); and to specify the types of measures required to protect the security and privacy of personally identifiable health care information. This is also the name of Title II, subtitle F, part C of HIPAA. *2)* HCPCS Level II modifier, for use with CPT or HCPCS Level II codes, when a physician assistant, nurse practitioner, or clinical nurse specialist acts as an assistant at surgery. The provider should report the procedure(s) using his/her own provider identification number. *3)* Aortic stenosis. *4)* Associate of Science.

ASA American Society of Anesthesiologists. National organization for anesthesiology that maintains and publishes the guidelines and relative values for anesthesia coding.

ASAP As soon as possible.

asbestosis Lung disease caused by long-term inhalation of asbestos particles. Asbestos exposure has been linked to lung cancer, most commonly mesothelioma and is reported with ICD-9-CM code 501.

ASC *1)* Accredited Standards Committee. Organization accredited by the American National Standards Institute (ANSI) for the development of American national standards. *2)* Ambulatory surgery center. Any distinct entity that operates exclusively for the purpose of providing surgical services to patients not requiring hospitalization. To receive reimbursement for treatment of Medicare patients, an ASC must have an agreement with the Centers for Medicare and Medicaid Services (CMS) and meet certain required conditions.

ASC anesthesia standards Standards set up by the American Association for Accreditation of Ambulatory Surgery Facilities for classifying facilities based on the type of anesthesia performed. *Class A:* All surgical procedures are performed under local or topical anesthesia. *Class B:* Surgical procedures are performed under local, topical, or regional anesthesia, parenteral sedation, or dissociative drugs (excluding propofol). The use of endotracheal intubation or laryngeal mask airway anesthesia, inhalation general anesthesia (including nitrous oxide), spinal or epidural anesthesia, and propofol are prohibited in a Class B facility. *Class C-M:* Surgical procedures are performed under local, topical, or regional anesthesia, parenteral sedation, or dissociative drugs (including propofol). The use of endotracheal intubation or laryngeal mask airway anesthesia, inhalation general anesthesia (including nitrous oxide), and spinal or epidural anesthesia are prohibited in a Class C-M facility. *Class C:* Surgical procedures may be performed using local, topical, or regional anesthesia, parenteral sedation, dissociative drugs (including propofol), epidural or spinal anesthesia, and general anesthesia with or without endotracheal intubation or laryngeal mask airway anesthesia. The standards also specify the level of personnel required to administer these agents.

ASC payment group rate Facility payment received by an ASC when a covered surgical procedure is performed on a Medicare beneficiary. This rate is adjusted for geo-economic variation. ASCs are currently in a four-year transition period to phase in APC reimbursement.

ASC surgical procedure One of the designated surgical procedures performed on an outpatient basis in an ambulatory surgical center.

A-scan Method of diagnostic ophthalmic ultrasound that produces one-dimensional measurements using straight-line, high frequency sound waves from a transducer placed on the eye. The images are seen as vertical spikes that vary according to tissue density. A-scans are used to image intraocular anatomy to define a lesion's structure and identify its borders and also to measure the axial length of the eye or calculate the power required for an intraocular lens. A-scans are reported with CPT codes 76510-76511 and 76516-76519.

Ascension MCP Brand name two-piece artificial finger metacarpophalangeal joint. One piece has a ball-shaped end and a stem, and the other piece has a cup-shaped receptacle and stem. The implant is a treatment for severe osteo- or rheumatoid arthritis or posttraumatic repair.

ascites Abnormal accumulation of free fluid in the abdominal cavity, causing distention and tightness, in addition to shortness of breath, as the fluid accumulates. Ascites is usually an underlying disorder. Ascites is indexed to several ICD-9-CM codes, but the most common is an accumulation of clear, serous fluid, reported with 789.59. If ascites is specified as malignant, report 789.51 in addition to a code for the malignancy. Ascites can be a manifestation of any number of diseases, including lymphoma, liver disease, heart failure, nephritic syndrome, or hypoalbuminemia. **Synonym(s):** *hydroperitoneum, hydrops abdominis.*

ascorbic acid Essential micronutrient used in collagen synthesis, carnitine biosynthesis, and stimulation of neutrophil chemotaxis, lipid and protein metabolism, and wound healing. Serum chemistry test is reported with CPT code 82180. **Synonym(s):** *ascorbate, vitamin C.*

ASCVD Arteriosclerotic cardiovascular disease.

ASCX12N American Standard Committee standard for claims and reimbursement.

ASD Atrial septal defect.

-ase Denoting an enzyme.

aseptic necrosis Death of bone tissue resulting from a disruption in the vascular supply, caused by a noninfectious disease process, such as a fracture or the administration of immunosuppressive drugs. Aseptic necrosis is often found in adults at the femoral head following trauma. In children, this is often referred to as epiphyseal ischemic necrosis or epiphyseal avascular necrosis. Osteonecrosis is reported with an ICD-9-CM code from subcategory 733.4. Code selection is based on the bone involved, not the age of the patient. **Synonym(s):** *osteonecrosis.*

ASH Asymmetric septal hypertrophy. Genetic disorder causing myocardial hypertrophy carrying a risk of sudden death due to arrhythmia in children and adolescents. ASH is reported with ICD-9-CM code 746.84. **Synonym(s):** *HCM.*

ASHD Arteriosclerotic heart disease.

Asherman's syndrome Irritation of the uterine lining and formation of scar tissue that causes abnormal adherence in parts of the uterus. Females who are affected with Asherman's syndrome undergo a gradual decline in menstrual flow, an increase in abdominal cramps and pain, ultimate cessation of menstruation, and infertility. Asherman's syndrome is reported with ICD-9-CM code 621.5. **Synonym(s):** *intrauterine synechiae syndrome.*

ASIS Anterosuperior iliac spine. Anatomical landmark on the iliac crest, often noted in hip surgery. ASIS was previously used as a landmark for femoral resection during total knee arthroplasty, until studies proved this to be unreliable. ASIS is often seen in an operative report with no direct bearing on code selection.

ASN Associate of Science, Nursing.

ASO Administrative services only. Contractual agreement between a self-funded plan and an insurance company in which the insurance company assumes no risk and provides administrative services only.

asocial personality Personality disorder characterized by disregard for social obligations, lack of feeling for others, and impetuous violence or callous unconcern and self-rationalization of behavior.

asparaginase Antineoplastic used to treat acute lymphocytic leukemia. It kills leukemia cells by destroying the amino acid asparagine, which is needed for protein synthesis in the cell. Supply is reported with HCPCS Level II code J9020. May be sold under the brand name Elspar, Kidrolase.

aspergillosis Infection by *Aspergillus* species, mainly *A. Fumigatus, A. flavus* group, or *A. terreus* group. This condition is classifiable to ICD-9-CM subcategory 117.3.

aspermia Rare condition in which seminal fluid is not produced or ejaculated, reported with ICD-9-CM code 606.0.

asphyxia Insufficient intake of oxygen, resulting in pathological changes brought on by a lack of oxygen perfusion to the tissues or excessive carbon dioxide in the blood. Correct code assignment is dependent upon a number of factors including age and cause.

aspirate To withdraw fluid or air from a body cavity by suction.

aspiration Drawing fluid out by suction.

aspiration syndrome Intrauterine fetal aspiration of amniotic fluid contaminated by meconium. Report this disorder with ICD-9-CM code 770.18.

ASPIRE AFEHCT's Administrative Simplification Print Image Research Effort work group.

asplenia Congenital absence of the spleen. A serious condition associated with congenital heart anomalies. Asplenia is reported with ICD-9-CM code 759.0.

ASR Age/sex rate.

assay Test of purity.

assessment Process of collecting and studying information and data, such as test values, signs, and symptoms.

A-C

assigned claim Claim from a physician or supplier who has agreed to accept the Medicare allowable amount as payment in full for the services rendered. Reimbursement is made directly to the provider of the service.

assignment In medical reimbursement, the arrangement in which the provider submits the claim on behalf of the patient and is reimbursed directly by the patient's plan. By doing so, the provider agrees to accept what the plan pays.

assignment of benefits Authorization from the patient allowing the third-party payer to pay the provider directly for medical services. Under Medicare, an assignment is an agreement by the hospital or physician to accept Medicare's payment as the full payment and not to bill the patient for any amounts over the allowance amount, except for deductible and/or coinsurance amounts or noncovered services.

assistant-at-surgery Physician or other appropriate health care provider who assists another provider during performance of a surgery.

assistive devices Variety of implements or equipment used to aid patients in performing actions, activities, movements, or tasks.

Association for Electronic Health Care Transactions Organization that promotes the use of electronic data interchange (EDI) in the health care industry. *Synonym(s): AFEHCT.*

ASST *1)* Autologous serum skin test. Injection of the patient's own blood serum as a test for autoimmune disorder, usually performed in cases of chronic idiopathic urticaria. There is no CPT code specific to ASST, but CPT unlisted antigen skin test code 86486 may be used. *2)* Assistance (min = minimal; mod = moderate).

AST Aspartate aminotransferase.

astasia-abasia, hysterical Form of conversion hysteria in which the individual is unable to stand or walk although the legs are otherwise under control.

astereognosis Type of tactile agnosia in which the ability to understand or distinguish the shape, form, or nature of objects being touched is lost or diminished. This condition is reported with ICD-9-CM code 780.99. *Synonym(s): astereocognosy, stereoagnosis, tactile amnesia.*

asthenic personality Personality disorder characterized by passive compliance with the wishes of elders and others and a weak, inadequate response to the demands of daily life. Those with the disorder may be intellectual or emotional with little capacity for enjoyment.

asthma Narrowing or inflammation of the airway causing obstructed, labored breathing. Asthma is reported with ICD-9-CM category 493 and is classified as different types: Extrinsic or allergic asthma is a transient stricture of bronchial diameters due to environmental factors. Intrinsic asthma is due to pathophysiological disturbances within the body.

astigmatism Bending or diffusing of light rays in the eye that cannot be brought to a point of focus on the retina, due to unequal curvature on the refractive surface of the eye. Astigmatism produces visual irregularities and blurring.

ASTM American Society for Testing and Materials. Standards group that has published general guidelines for developing standards, including those for health care identifiers. ASTM Committee E31 on Health Care Informatics develops standards on information used within health care.

astragalectomy Surgical removal of the astragalus (talus), the bone that forms the ankle joint by articulating with the tibia and fibula, reported with ICD-9-CM procedure code 77.98 and CPT code 28130. Indications include trauma, congenital abnormalities, severe fractures, chronic infection, or tumors. *Synonym(s): talectomy.*

astragalus Highest tarsal bone that forms the ankle joint by articulating with the fibula and tibia.

astro- Star-like or shaped.

astrovirus Only genus in the family Astroviridae. Ribonucleic acid (RNA) virus that causes gastroenteritis in humans and a number of other animals, named for the star shape in the middle of the virus. Report with ICD-9-CM code 008.66.

asymmetry Lack of symmetry over unevenness in corresponding parts.

AT HCPCS Level II modifier that should be used when reporting acute treatment services, CPT codes 98940, 98941, 98942. This modifier has no effect on Medicare reimbursement.

at risk In medical reimbursement, a type of contract between Medicare and a payer or a payer and a provider in which the payer (in the case of Medicare) and the provider (in the case of the payer contracts) gets paid a set amount for care of a patient base. If costs exceed the amount the payer or provider were paid, the patients still receive care during the term of the contract.

ataxia Defect in muscular coordination, seen especially when voluntary muscular movements are attempted.

ataxiaphasia Speech deficit in which some necessary grammatical elements for coherent sentences are lacking. *Synonym(s): syntactical aphasia.*

ataxia-telangiectasia syndrome Gonadal hypoplasia, insulin resistance and hyperglycemia, liver function problems, increased sensitivity to ionizing radiation, ataxia, and nystagmus. Report this disorder with ICD-9-CM code 334.8. *Synonym(s): Boder-Sedgwick syndrome, Louis-Bar syndrome.*

atelectasis Collapse of lung tissue affecting part or all of one lung, preventing normal oxygen absorption to healthy tissues. Report atelectasis with ICD-9-CM code 518.0 or 770.4-770.5 for newborns.

atelo- Incomplete or imperfect.

atelomyelia Congenital condition in which there is incomplete development of the spinal cord, reported with ICD-9-CM code 742.59.

atherectomy Surgical removal of arterial plaque from inside an artery. The procedure may be performed percutaneously, using a special catheter with a high-speed burr at the tip to bore through the sclerotic deposits, or transluminally by open incision. The procedure is coded not only by the method employed, but also specifically to the vessel or branches on which it is performed.

atherosclerosis Buildup of yellowish plaques composed of cholesterol and lipoid material within the arteries.

athetosis Nervous disorder visible by monotonous slow movement.

athlete's foot Dermatophytic fungal infection on the plantar (bottom) surface of the feet, extending to the nails and between the toes. The condition manifests itself with intense itching, scaling, and cracking of the foot with areas of erosion between the toes. Athlete's foot is reported with ICD-9-CM code 110.4. *Synonym(s): dermatophytosis of foot, tinea pedis.*

Ativan See lorazepam.

ATLL Adult T-cell leukemia/lymphoma. Aggressive non-Hodgkin's lymphoma caused by HTLV-1. ATLL presents with bone and skin lesions, enlarged lymph nodes, high calcium levels, and enlarged liver and spleen.

atony Absence of normal muscle tone and strength.

atopic dermatitis Inflammation of the skin caused by a hypersensitivity reaction to environmental allergens. This includes such conditions as diaper rash (ICD-9-CM code 691.0) and acute eczema (692.9). *Synonym(s): eczema.*

ATP Adenosine triphosphate.

atresia Congenital closure or absence of a tubular organ or an opening to the body surface.

atria Two upper chambers of the heart. The left and right atria are divided by the septum, a muscular wall.

atrial ectopic beat Interruption in normal heart rhythm due to a premature electrical impulse to the atrial muscle, causing a premature atrial contraction, reported with ICD-9-CM code 427.61. *Synonym(s): PAC.*

atrial fibrillation Cardiac arrhythmia caused by small areas of muscle fibers becoming erratically and spontaneously activated through multiple circuits in uncoordinated phases of depolarization and repolarization. This causes the atria to quiver in a continuously erratic pattern instead of contracting in the regular rhythm. Report atrial fibrillation with ICD-9-CM code 427.31.

atrial flutter Form of cardiac arrhythmia in which the upper chambers (atria) of the heart experience well-organized but exceedingly rapid contractions. Many impulses begin and spread through the atria, but occur so rapidly that the atria cannot fully empty their contents into the ventricles of the heart. Report atrial flutter with ICD-9-CM code 427.32.

atrial myxoma Primary, benign cardiac neoplasm arising most commonly in the left atrium attached by a stalk to the septum. Symptoms may include cardiac murmurs, which change with alteration of body position. Signs of mitral stenosis or insufficiency may also be noted. Atrial myxoma is reported with ICD-9-CM code 212.7.

atrial septal defect Cardiac anomaly consisting of a patent opening in the atrial septum due to a fusion failure, classified as ostium secundum type, ostium primum defect, or endocardial cushion defect. An atrial septal defect may also include the complete absence of the atrial septum. This type of defect allows oxygenated blood to return to the lungs instead of circulating throughout the rest of the body and can increase pulmonary blood flow, causing pulmonary hypertension if the defect is not closed. Not all septal defects are congenital. The patient may present with an acquired cardiac septal defect that was not present at birth, in which case the correct ICD-9-CM code is found in the circulatory system chapter, 429.71. *Synonym(s): ASD.*

atrioventricular block Condition in which there is a disturbance of electrical conduction, such as a delay, intermittence, or absence in the transmission of an impulse from the atria to the ventricles and categorized according to degree of severity.

Atrixtra See fondaparinux sodium.

atrophy Reduction in size or activity in an anatomic structure, due to wasting away from disease or other factors.

atropic macular degeneration Age-related pigmentary disturbance in the macula with no scarring or hemorrhaging.

atropine Drug used in inhalation therapy as a bronchodilator. Supply is reported with HCPCS Level II codes J7635-J7636.

atropine sulfate Anticholinergic used to treat bradycardia and to block cardiac vagal reflexes preoperatively. By inhibiting the acetylcholine at the neurofunction, it enhances conduction through the atrioventricular node and increases the heart rate. It is also used as an antidote for anticholinesterase insecticide poisoning and as treatment for peptic ulcers and gastrointestinal function disorders. Supply is reported with HCPCS Level II code J0461. May be sold under the brand names Atropen and Sal-Tropine.

Atrovent See ipratropium bromide.

ATT Attached.

attained age In medical reimbursement, the age of the member as of the last birthday.

attended surveillance Ability of a technician at a remote surveillance center or location to respond immediately to patient transmissions regarding rhythm or device alerts as they are produced and received at the remote location. These transmissions may originate from wearable or implanted therapy or monitoring devices.

attention deficit disorder Syndrome characterized by short attention span, distractibility, and overactivity without significant disturbance of conduct or delay in specific skills.

attenuation correction Application of a mathematical equation required to correct the scatter and absorption of photons that are emitted from a radioactive tracer introduced into the body. The calculation tries to account for distortion that renders the results unreliable. For example, when performing myocardial perfusion imaging, attenuation correction calculations provide a more accurate diagnostic image by raising the importance of radioactivity distribution counts arising from certain areas like the anterior wall, which may reduce or impede photon emission detection because of the presence of the breast. This factor varies depending on the test being performed (e.g., PET, SPECT, CT).

Attenuvax Brand name measles vaccine provided in a single-dose vial. Supply of Attenuvax is reported with CPT code 90705; administration is reported separately. The need for vaccination is reported with ICD-9-CM code V04.2.

atticotomy Surgical opening of the tympanic attic of the ear. This procedure is performed at the time of other services such as a tympanoplasty.

attrition In dentistry, wearing away or erosion of tooth surface from abrasive food or grinding teeth.

AU HCPCS Level II modifier, for use with HCPCS Level II codes for an item(s) furnished in conjunction with a urological, ostomy, or tracheostomy supply. Used with HCPCS Level II codes A4450, A4452, and A4217.

audiology services Services provided for evaluation and treatment of congenital or acquired speech, language, and hearing deficits by a qualified speech-language pathologist or audiologist.

audiometry Measurement of hearing that can employ a number of methods to help diagnose the cause and type of hearing loss.

audit Examination or review that establishes the extent to which performance or a process conforms to predetermined standards or criteria. An audit may target utilization, quality of care, coding, or reimbursement.

AUDIT Alcohol use disorder identification test. Report this assessment with intervention using HCPCS Level II codes G0396 and G0397.

auditing and monitoring Regular review of an organization's claim development and submission process from the point where service for a patient is initiated to the submission of a claim for payment. Monitoring involves a system of checks of and controls over, as well as a method of reporting, all areas of compliance, including regulations and audits.

auditor Professional who evaluates a provider's utilization, quality of care, or level of reimbursement.

Audry's syndrome Increased thickening of the skin on extremities and face with clubbing of fingers and deformities in bone of the limb. Report this disorder with ICD-9-CM code 757.39.

Aufrecht's sign Decrease in breathing sounds above the jugular fossa seen in tracheal stenosis.

augment Add to or increase.

augmentation Add to or increase the substance of a body site, usually performed as plastic reconstructive measures. Augmentation may involve the use of an implant or prosthesis, especially within soft tissue or grafting procedures, such as bone tissue. Correct code assignment is dependent upon the anatomical location, such as the chin, breast, cheek, or jawbones.

AUR Ambulatory utilization review.

aura Warning symptoms, usually visual, that may sometimes occur shortly before a migraine headache or seizure begins. Aura comes from the Greek word for wind. An aura may precede a migraine or seizure as a strong wind may precede a storm.

auricle External ear, which is a single elastic cartilage covered in skin and normal adnexal features (hair follicles, sweat glands, and sebaceous glands), shaped to channel sound waves into the acoustic meatus.

auricular prosthesis Ear prosthesis that artificially restores the appearance of an outer ear lost to radical surgery, amputation, burns, and/or congenital defects. The surgeon inserts the prosthesis and covers it with highly sensitive skin. The prosthetic ear helps to direct sound waves into the auditory canal and maintain a proper environment for the inner ear, improving hearing up to 20 percent.

auriculotemporal syndrome Localized sweating and flushing of the cheek and ear in response to chewing. Report this disorder with ICD-9-CM code 350.8. *Synonym(s): Frey's syndrome.*

aurothioglucose Gold salt with antiinflammatory effects used to treat the signs and symptoms of rheumatoid arthritis and pemphigus. Supply is reported with HCPCS Level II code J2910. May be sold under the brand names Gold-50, Solganal.

AuSCT Autologous stem cell transplantation. *NCD Reference: 110.8.1.*

Austin procedure Surgical treatment generally used for a large bunion deformity in which there is minimal angulation of the great toe, and involves a resection of the medial eminence of the first metatarsal. A "V," or chevron shaped cut, is made near the end of the bone, which allows the surgeon to slide the head of the bone laterally, or toward the little toe. Report this procedure with CPT code 28296. *Synonym(s): chevron procedure, Mitchell procedure.*

authentication Characteristic of electronic signature. Under HIPAA, authentication is the product of a technology that, when it affixes a signature to a document, also includes a means of establishing that the person or entity signing the document is who he or she claims to be.

authorization Verbal or written agreement indicating that a third-party payer will pay for services rendered by the provider as set forth in the authorization.

authorized official Appointed official to whom the provider or supplier has granted the legal authority to enroll it in the Medicare program, to make changes and/or updates to its status in the Medicare program (e.g., new practice locations, change of address, etc.) and to commit the provider/supplier to fully abide by the laws, regulations, and program instructions of Medicare. The authorized official must be the providerⓈs or supplierⓈs general partner, chairman of the board, president, chief financial officer, or chief executive officer, or must hold a position of similar status and authority within the provider or supplier. An authorized official can also be anyone who is a direct owner of 5 percent or more of the provider or supplier. An entity can have only one designated authorized official at one time.

auto- Relating to the self.

autofluorescence Special light source that allows physicians to distinguish between normal and abnormal tissue, such as finding abnormal bronchial tissue in patients with known or suspected lung cancer. Tissue that looks suspicious under the light is biopsied to confirm findings.

autogenous transplant Tissue, such as bone, that is harvested from the patient and used for transplantation back into the same patient. Unlike other transplants, post-autograft status is not clinically significant and its status is not classified in ICD-9-CM.

Autograft

Example of structural autograft with plate

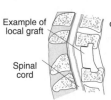

Example of local graft

Lateral cutaway views

Spinal cord

Local autograft is harvested, processed, and placed

autograft Any tissue harvested from one anatomical site of a person and grafted to another anatomical site of the same person. Most commonly, blood vessels, skin, tendons, fascia, and bone are used as autografts and codes specific to harvest and graft are found in many sections of the CPT code book and Volume 3 of ICD-9-CM. In some cases, harvest is reported separately; in others, it is bundled into the main graft code. The description of the code will usually identify if that is the case. For post surgical skin transplant status, report ICD-9-CM code V42.3. *Synonym(s): autochthonous graft, autogenic graft; autologous graft, autotransplant.*

autologous Tissue or structure derived from the same individual. A. cultured chondrocytes: Mature cartilage cells derived first from the patient's own normal, articular cartilage and then cultured in a laboratory setting to grow a higher volume of cells needed for transplant. Cells are taken from the lesser-weight bearing area of the knee and used to repair knee defects from damage to the hyaline cartilage. Supply is reported with HCPCS Level II code J7330. Implantation is reported with CPT code 27412 and harvesting with 29870. May be sold under the brand name Carticel.

autologous cultured chondrocytes Mature cartilage cells derived first from the patient's own normal, articular cartilage and then cultured in a laboratory setting to grow a higher volume of cells needed for transplant. Cells are taken from the lesser-weight bearing area of the knee and used to repair knee defects from damage to the hyaline cartilage. Supply is reported with HCPCS Level II code J7330. Implantation is reported with CPT code 27412 and harvesting with 29870. May be sold under the brand name Carticel.

automated clearinghouse Entity that processes or facilitates the processing of information received from another entity in a nonstandard format or containing

A-C

nonstandard data content into standard data elements or a standard transaction, or that receives a standard transaction from another entity and processes or facilitates the processing of that information into nonstandard format or nonstandard data content for a receiving entity. *Synonym(s): ACH, health care clearinghouse.*

automatic renewal clause Clause in a contract that allows the contract to automatically renew with the same terms for another stated period of time.

automatism syndrome Infarction of the postero-inferior thalamus causing transient hemiparesis, severe loss of sensation with crude pain in the limbs, or vasomotor or trophic disturbances. Report this disorder with ICD-9-CM code 348.89.

autonomic nervous system Portion of the nervous system that controls involuntary body functions. The fibers of the autonomic nervous system regulate the iris of the eye and the smooth-muscle action of the heart, blood vessels, lungs, glands, stomach, colon, bladder, and other visceral organs that are not under conscious control by the individual. The autonomic nerve fibers exit from the central nervous system and branch out into the sympathetic and parasympathetic nervous systems.

AutoPap Brand name advanced computerized review technique to evaluate Pap or vaginal smears that were interpreted as normal in the initial screening. Abnormal samples will be manually rescreened. AutoPap is performed on the original specimen and does not require additional tissue sampling. It is reported with CPT code 88152.

autophony Condition in which one is abnormally aware of one's own voice, often seen in patients with diseases of the middle ear. Autophony is reported with ICD-9-CM code 388.40.

Autoplex T See anti-inhibitor coagulant complex.

autotopagnosia Inability to locate or orient the various parts of one's own body, usually due to a thalamic lesion. Report this condition with ICD-9-CM code 780.99. *Synonym(s): body image, posture agnosia.*

autotransplantation Excising tissue from the patient and transplanting it into another location in the same patient.

auxiliary personnel Individual acting under a physician's supervision. It may be an employee, leased employee, or independent contractor of the physician (or other practitioner) or of the same entity that employs or contracts with the physician (or other practitioner).

AV HCPCS Level II modifier, for use with HCPCS Level II codes for an item or items furnished in conjunction with a prosthetic or orthotic device. Used with HCPCS Level II codes A4450, A4452, and A4217.

A-V Arteriovenous.

Avandia Brand name oral medication exclusive to lowering blood glucose in Type II diabetics. Avandia contains rosiglitazone maleate.

Avastin Brand name of bevacizumab, an injectable antiangiogenic agent used to treat neovascular (wet) age-related macular degeneration. Avastin may also be used in combination with chemotherapeutic drugs in the treatment of patients with certain cancers, such as colon, rectum, and lung. Report supply with HCPCS Level II code J9035.

Avaulta Brand name biosynthetic mesh for treatment in pelvic organ prolapse. Insertion of mesh during pelvic floor repair is reported with CPT add-on code 57267 or ICD-9-CM procedure code 59.72.

Avellis' syndrome Paraplegia and anesthesia over part of the body caused by lesions in the brain or spinal cord. Report this disorder with ICD-9-CM code 344.89.

average length of stay Average number of inpatient days within a given diagnostic-related group (DRG, the inpatient prospective payment system for Medicare patients). The average length of stay is based on factors such as geographical location and diagnosis and is also used to determine payment for outlier cases.

average payment rate Amount of money CMS could pay an HMO for services provided to Medicare recipients under a risk contract. *Synonym(s): APR.*

average resources Relative volume and types of diagnostic, therapeutic, and bed services used in managing a particular illness.

average wholesale price Pharmaceutical price based on common data that is included in a pharmacy provider contract. *Synonym(s): AWP.*

AVF Arteriovenous fistula.

AVM Arteriovenous malformation. Clusters of abnormal blood vessels that grow in the brain comprised of a blood vessel "nidus" or nest through which arteries and veins connect directly without going through the capillaries. As time passes, the nidus may enlarge resulting in the formation of a mass that may bleed. AVMs are more prone to bleeding in patients ages 10 to 55. Once older than age 55, the possibility of bleeding is reduced dramatically.

avoidant personality Excessive social inhibitions and shyness, a tendency to withdraw from opportunities for developing close relationships, and a fearful expectation of being belittled and humiliated.

Avonex See interferon.

avulse Tear away from, whether in an accidental injury or as a surgical procedure.

avulsion Forcible tearing away of a part, by surgical means or traumatic injury.

AW HCPCS Level II modifier, for use with HCPCS Level II codes for an item or items furnished in conjunction with a surgical dressing. Used with HCPCS Level II codes A4450, A4452, and A4217.

awl Pointed instrument for piercing small holes.

AWP *1)* Average wholesale price. Pharmaceutical price based on common data that is included in a pharmacy provider contract. *2)* Any willing provider. Describing statutes requiring a provider network to accept any provider who meets the network's usual selection criteria.

AX *1)* HCPCS Level II modifier, for use with HCPCS Level II codes for an item or items furnished in conjunction with dialysis services. Used with HCPCS Level II codes A4651, A4652, A4657, A4660, A4663, A4670, A4927, A4928, A4930, A4931, E1632, E1637, and E1639. *2)* Auxiliary.

Axenfeld's syndrome Dysgenesis of the eye marked through widened trabecular meshwork, large iridial bands, and glaucoma. Report this disorder with ICD-9-CM code 743.44.

axillary Area under the arm. *a. block* Regional anesthesia that is administered to create a loss of sensation in the distal two-thirds of an upper extremity by injecting an anesthetic into the axillary nerve trunk. *a. region* Area immediately surrounding the armpit.

axio- Relating to an axis. *Synonym(s): axo-.*

axon Extension from a neuron that carries impulses to receiving terminal branches.

AY HCPCS Level II modifier denoting an item or service furnished to an ESRD patient that is not for the treatment of ESRD.

Ayerza (-Arrillaga) syndrome Cyanosis and hypertension, resulting from sclerosis of the pulmonary arteries. Report this disorder with ICD-9-CM code 416.0.

AZ HCPCS Level II modifier denoting a physician who is providing a service in a dental health professional shortage area for the purpose of an electronic health record incentive payment.

azathioprine Immunosuppressant given to kidney transplant patients beginning on the day of surgery. It is also used for refractory or severe rheumatoid arthritis. Supply is reported with HCPCS Level II code J7500 for the oral form and J7501 for the parenteral form. May be sold under the brand names Azasan, Imuran, Thioprine.

AZH Assisted zonal hatching. Small opening created in the zona pellucida (the outer layer of an embryo) using mechanical or chemical means. This technique is used in cases of in vitro fertilization in which the patient has produced an embryo with a thickened zona, which may prevent the embryo from implanting in the uterus. This procedure is performed just prior to embryo replacement in order to allow the embryo to hatch more easily and improve the chances for implantation. AZH is reported with CPT code 89253.

azidothymine Oral or intravenous antiviral for the treatment of human immunodeficiency virus (HIV) that causes AIDS. Azidothymine is used with other antiretrovirals to prevent HIV transmission by pregnant women to the baby, for health care workers with needle stick exposure, and in some rape cases. Its supply is reported with HCPCS Level II code J3485 or S0104. May be sold under the brand name Retrovir.

azithromycin Antibiotic that acts against both gram negative and gram positive anaerobic and aerobic bacteria. When it is supplied in oral powder or capsule form, it is reported with HCPCS Level II code Q0144. When it is supplied as an injectable, report J0456. May be sold under the brand name: Zithromax.

azoospermia Failure of the development of sperm or the absence of sperm in semen. Azoospermia is one of the most common factors in male infertility and is reported with ICD-9-CM code 606.0. *Synonym(s): Del Castillo's syndrome, Sertoli cell syndrome.*

AZT Asidothymidine. Oral or intravenous antiviral for the treatment of human immunodeficiency virus (HIV) that causes AIDS. AZT is used with other antiretrovirals to prevent HIV transmission by pregnant women to the baby, for health care workers with needle stick exposure, and in some rape cases. Its supply is reported with HCPCS Level II code J3485 or S0104.

aztreonam Bacteriocidal agent to kill susceptible bacteria systemically, such as in cases of septicemia and skin infections. It is also used against bacteria commonly infecting the urinary tract and lower respiratory tract and for gynecological and post-surgical infections. Supply is reported with HCPCS Level II code S0073. May be sold under the brand name Azactam.

b Small balloon catheter placed in the Bartholin's gland cavity during treatment of a Bartholin's cyst or abscess, as an alternative to marsupialization, to promote healing. The placement of a Word catheter follows incision and drainage of the abscess or excision of the cyst, and would be bundled into CPT code 56420 (abscess) or 56740 (cyst).

B&B Bowel and bladder.

b.i.d. Two times a day.

b.i.n. Twice a night.

b.i.s. Twice.

BA *1)* Business associate. Person or organization that performs a function or activity on behalf of a covered entity but that is not part of the covered entity's workforce. A business associate can also be a covered entity in its own right. *Synonym(s): BP, business partner.* *2)* HCPCS Level II modifier, for use with HCPCS Level II codes for an item or items furnished in conjunction with parenteral enteral nutrition (PEN) services. This modifier is appended to HCPCS Level II code E0776, for an IV pole. *3)* Barium.

Baader's syndrome   Necrolysis of the skin caused by toxins. Report this disorder with ICD-9-CM code 695.19. *Synonym(s): erythema multiforme exudativum.*

Baastrup's syndrome   Malformation of the spine in which kyphosis becomes so great nonadjacent vertebrae touch. Report this disorder with ICD-9-CM code 721.5. *Synonym(s): kissing spine.*

Babcock operation   Varicose veins are eliminated using a long probe and tying the end of the vein to it to draw out the vein by invagination.

babesiosis   Tick-borne illness similar to malaria and characterized by fever, fatigue, severe hemolytic anemia, and hemoglobinuria. Babesiosis is reported with ICD-9-CM code 088.82.

Babington's disease   Post-pubescent appearing genetic disorder with small telangiectasia and dilated venules developing slowly on the skin and mucus membranes of the lips, nasopharynx, and tongue with recurrent bleeding occurring. Report this disorder with ICD-9-CM code 448.0. *Synonym(s): hereditary hemorrhagic telangiectasia, Rendu-Osler-Weber disease.*

Babinski sign   Deep tendon reflex elicited by taking the handle of the reflex hammer and running it up the bottom of the foot. The big toe will dorsiflex or extend up as a normal reaction in infants. This is considered an abnormal finding in older patients, indicating a lesion in the central nervous system, usually in the pyramidal tract. Babinski testing is included in an office visit physical exam. *Synonym(s): Babinski's phenomenon, toe phenomenon, toe sign.*

Babinski's syndrome   Late manifestations of syphilis with associated disorders of the heart and arteries. Manifestations may include tabes dorsalis, paralytic dementia, and syphilitic meningitis. Babinski's syndrome is reported with ICD-9-CM code 093.89. *Synonym(s): Babinski-Vaquez syndrome.*

Babinski-Fröhlich syndrome   Obesity and hypogonadism in adolescent boys with rare accompanying dwarfism, thought to indicate hypothyroidism. Report this disorder with ICD-9-CM code 253.8.

Babinski-Nageotte syndrome   Paraplegia and anesthesia over part of the body caused by lesions in the brain or spinal cord. Report this disorder with ICD-9-CM code 344.89.

BAC   Blood alcohol content or concentration. Measurement of alcohol in the blood, used in law enforcement to diagnose intoxication and to provide a measure for impairment. Elevated BAC is reported with

ICD-9-CM code 790.3. Codes in ICD-10-CM report specific ranges of elevated BAC.

backbench preparation   Procedures performed on a donor organ following procurement to prepare the organ for transplant into the recipient. Excess fat and other tissue may be removed, the organ may be perfused, and vital arteries may be sized, repaired, or modified to fit the patient. These procedures are done on a back table in the operating room before transplantation can begin. *Synonym(s): backtable prep.*

backlog   In medical reimbursement, the queue of claims that have not been adjudicated.

baclofen   Muscle relaxant to reduce painful muscle spasms from multiple sclerosis or injury. Intrathecal injection is given for patients who can't tolerate oral dosing. This medication is also frequently delivered through an implantable pump. May be sold under the brand names Clofen, Kemstro, Lioresal.

bacteremia   Nonspecific laboratory finding of bacteria in the blood in the absence of signs of illness; not to be confused with septicemia, the more acute infectious illness progressing from bacteremia, or with urosepsis, the presence of pus or bacteria found in the urine. Bacteremia is reported with ICD-9-CM code 790.7.

bacteriuria   Bacteria in the urine. The presence of large amounts may be a sign of infection in the urinary tract. Bacteriuria alone is reported with ICD-9-CM code 791.9. *Synonym(s): bacturia.*

bacteroides fragilis   Most common bacteria found in the human intestinal tract, also found in the mouth, throat, and vaginal tract, and the most commonly encountered species in clinical specimens. These are gram-negative, antibiotic resistant species of anaerobes. A subspecies of this group is most often responsible for abdominal infections, bacteremia, and abscesses. Report intestinal infection with ICD-9-CM code 008.46 under other anaerobes and infections of other sites with ICD-9-CM code 041.82. Report CPT codes 87075 and 87076 for anaerobic stool cultures.

Bactocill   See oxacillin sodium.

Bactrim IV   Injectable combination antibacterial drug used in the treatment and prevention of Pneumocystis carinii. It is also used to treat certain other bacterial infections including UTI, bronchitis, gastrointestinal infection, and otitis media infections. Supply is reported with HCPCS Level II code S0039.

bad trip   Acute intoxication from hallucinogen abuse, manifested by hallucinatory states, typically lasting only a few days or less.

BAE   Bi-atrial enlargement.

Baehr-Schiffrin disease   Thrombocytopenia with thrombi formation in the small arterioles and capillaries causing hemolytic anemia, purpura, azotemia, fever, and central nervous system disorders manifested by bizarre neurological effects. Report this disease with ICD-9-CM code 446.6. **Synonym(s):** *microangiopathic hemolytic anemia, Moschcowitz disease, thrombotic microangiopathy, thrombotic thrombocytopenic purpura.*

Baelz's disease One of the three types of cheilitis glandularis, an uncommon disease of the lower lip in which it becomes larger and then turns inside out. Characteristics of Baelz's include painless swelling, hardening, crusting, and lip ulcers. Report this condition with ICD-9-CM code 528.5. **Synonym(s):** *superficial suppurative cheilitis glandularis.*

BAEP Brainstem auditory evoked potential, reported with CPT codes 92585 and 92586.

BAER Brainstem auditory evoked response. Measurement of response to auditory stimulus measured using electrodes attached to the scalp, especially useful in testing hearing in infants and children, or as a diagnostic tool in cases of neoplasms or multiple sclerosis. BAER is reported with CPT code 92585 or 92586. **Synonym(s):** *BAEP, brainstem auditory evoked potential.*

Baerveldt Eponym for an eye implant used to mitigate glaucoma. Insertion is reported with CPT code 66180; revision with 66185; and removal with 67120.

bagassosis Pulmonary disease caused by breathing bagasse dust, the residue from sugar cane after extraction of the sugar. This condition is reported with ICD-9-CM code 495.1.

Baghdad boil Dry or urban cutaneous leishmaniasis, one form of Old World cutaneous leishmaniasis. This parasitic skin disease is caused by the protozoa Leishmania tropica, spread by the bite of sand flies, and occurring in large urban areas in the Middle East, especially Iran and Iraq, the Mediterranean, and India. Manifestation is mainly a single, large developing boil or furuncle type lesion that persists over a year. Lymphadenopathy may be present. Report this condition with ICD-9-CM code 085.1.

Bagratuni's syndrome Temporal arteritis. Giant cells and inflammation in large arteries, usually the temporal artery. May lead to occlusion of the artery. Report this disorder with ICD-9-CM code 446.5. **Synonym(s):** *giant cell arteritis, Horton's syndrome.*

BAHA

BAHA is the acronym for bone-anchored hearing aid

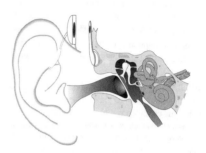

The electromagnetic bone conduction hearing device is placed or replaced

BAHA Bone anchored hearing aid. Implanted bone conduction hearing aid for patients with conductive and mixed hearing loss. Surgical placement of BAHA is reported with CPT code 69710.

Baker tube Tube placed into the small bowel for decompression. Enterotomy with placement of Baker tube for decompression is reported with CPT code 44021.

Baker's cannula Flexible cannula used on the trachea.

Baker's Cyst

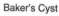

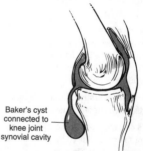

Baker's cyst connected to knee joint synovial cavity

Baker's cyst Sac filled with clear synovial fluid in adults, usually secondary to disease inside the joint, located on the back of the knee in the popliteal fossa area. In children, the cyst usually represents a ganglion of one of the tendons in the knee. Diagnosis of Baker's cyst is reported with ICD-9-CM code 727.51. Removal of a Baker's cyst is reported with CPT code 27345.

BAL Bronchoalveolar lavage. Procedure performed by a bronchoscope with sterile saline solution pumped into the bronchus and removed to recover both fluid and cells from the epithelial surface of the bronchioles and alveoli for diagnostic analysis.

BAL in Oil See dimercaprol.

bal. Bath.

balan(o)- Relating to the glans penis or glans clitoridis.

balance billing Arrangement prohibited in Medicare regulations and some payer contracts whereby a provider bills the patient for charges not reimbursed by the payer.

Balanced Budget Act of 1997 Legislation to cut federal spending and balance the federal budget. *Synonym(s): BBA.*

balanitis Inflammation of the glans penis, most often affecting uncircumcised males. The most common underlying condition is diabetes, although balanitis is also associated with poor hygiene, chemical irritation, and allergies. This condition is reported with ICD-9-CM code 607.1

balano- Relating to the glans penis or glans clitoridis.

balanoposthitis Inflammation and/or infection of the glans penis and prepuce.

balanoposthomycosis Infection thought to be due to a spirochetal infection in which there is rapid erosion and destruction of the glans penis and sometimes the entire external genitalia. Balanoposthomycosis is reported with ICD-9-CM code 607.1. *Synonym(s): Corbus' disease, gangrenous balanitis.*

balantidiasis Infection with a ciliated protozoan of the genus balantidium coli, found in the intestines of vertebrates and causing diarrhea, dysentery, and ulcers in the intestinal mucosa. Report B. coli infection with ICD-9-CM code 007.0.

balbutio Speech impediment characterized by stuttering, stammering, or numerous repetitions of words or portions of words. This impairment is reported with ICD-9-CM code 315.35 if unspecified or childhood onset and with 307.0 if adult onset.

Baldy-Webster operation Ligaments may be used to correct displacement of the uterus.

Balfour's disease Disorder manifested by numerous malignant tumors produced by bony infiltrates in myelogenous leukemia. The masses are most often found in the skull, but may occur in any part of the skeleton. The tumors appear green colored, due to pigment effects of myeloperoxidase. Report this disease with a code from ICD-9-CM category 205.3. *Synonym(s): Aran's cancer, chloroleukemia, chloroma, chloromyeloma, chlorosarcoma, granulocytic sarcoma, green cancer, Naegeli's disease.*

Balint's syndrome Cortical paralysis of visual fixation, optic ataxia, and disturbance of visual attention with normal eye movements. Report this disorder with ICD-9-CM code 368.16. *Synonym(s): Holmes' syndrome, Riddoch's syndrome.*

Balkan grippe Disease caused by infection with Coxiella burnetii, a rickettsial bacteria spread by inhaling contaminated dust or aerosols or contact with infected livestock or articles such as wool, hair, and hides. It most often affects workers in stockyards, textile plants, or meat packing plants. Symptoms are usually mild and flu-like, but may manifest with high fever, muscle pain, and severe headache and may require antibiotic treatment. Report this condition with ICD-9-CM code 083.0. *Synonym(s): abattoir fever, Q fever, query fever.*

Ballantyne (-Runge) syndrome Placental dysfunction occurring in postmature fetuses. Report this disorder with ICD-9-CM code 766.22.

ballistocardiogram Graphic recording of the movements of the body caused by cardiac contractions and blood flow, used to evaluate cardiac function. Ballistocardiogram is reported with HCPCS Level II code S3902.

balloon angioplasty Procedure for treating blockages and plaque build-up within blood vessels. A small balloon-tip catheter is inflated inside an artery to open clogged or narrowed areas, stretching the intima and breaking up the plaque deposit.

balloon assist device Circulation assist device consisting of a balloon placed in the thoracic aorta that inflates and deflates in coordination with the beating of the heart.

balloon catheter Any catheter equipped with an inflatable balloon at the end to hold it in place in a body cavity or to be used for dilation of a vessel lumen.

ballooning posterior leaflet syndrome "Mid-late" systolic click of the heart due to massive protrusion of the mitral valvular leaflet in the left atrial cavity. Report this disorder with ICD-9-CM code 424.0. *Synonym(s): Barlow's syndrome.*

ballottement test Physical exam to evaluate joint stability between the lunate and triquetrum bones of the wrist. The lunate is stabilized with one hand and the triquetrum with the other, then one is pushed down while the other is lifted up. If there is pain and crepitus this test is positive for instability. *Synonym(s): shuck test.*

Baló's concentric sclerosis Rare disorder affecting the white matter of the brain, occurring in childhood in both sexes and manifested by increased mental deterioration, spastic paralysis, blindness, and deafness. The portion of the brain that is affected determines the signs and symptoms of the neurological disorder. This condition is reported with ICD-9-CM code 341.1. *Synonym(s): Baló's disease, Balo's concentric sclerosis, chronic leukoencephalopathy, Schilder's disease.*

bamboo hair Condition in which small, white nodules appear in the hair shafts where the hair shaft cortex has broken and split apart, causing the hair to break off, usually after growing only an inch or two. **Synonym(s):** *clastothrix, trichoclasia, trichorrhexis nodosa.*

bamboo spine Rigidity of the spine as a result of advanced ankylosing spondylitis, which produces a bamboo-like appearance on x-rays. Bamboo spine is reported with ICD-9-CM code 720.0.

bandemia CBC laboratory finding in which there is an increase in early neutrophil cells, or band cells. The nucleus is not segmented but forms a continuous band. In normal circumstances, less than 5 percent of neutrophils are bands. An increased number of band cells may be suggestive of a bacterial infection and indicate increased granulocytopoiesis. Further testing or workup, such as a culture to confirm infection, may be warranted. The code for bandemia (ICD-9-CM code 288.66) is assigned when bandemia is present, but a definitive diagnosis of infection has not yet been established.

Bandl's ring Complication of labor in which the ridge that normally forms between the upper and lower portions of the uterus due to contractions (retraction ring) becomes exaggerated and visible through the abdomen above the pubic joint. This may be indicative of cephalopelvic disproportion or unstable lie, and signals pending uterine rupture if left untreated. This condition is reported on the mother's chart with a code from ICD-9-CM category 661.4. If specified as affecting the fetus or newborn, report 763.7. **Synonym(s):** *pathologic retraction ring.*

band-shaped keratopathy Horizontal bands of superficial corneal calcium deposits.

Banflex Muscle relaxant used for stiff and sore muscles secondary to injury or trauma.

Bang's disease Infectious disease caused by a species of Brucella bacteria, a gram-negative, aerobic coccobacilli, transmitted from cattle to humans by direct or indirect contact. Seldom fatal, symptoms include fever, weakness, sweating, and aching. Treatment consists of antibiotics. Bang's disease is reported with ICD-9-CM code 023.1. **Synonym(s):** *Brucella abortus.*

Bankart *1)* Deformity osteochondral fracture or detachment of the inferior glenoid labrum, the ring of fibrocartilage attached to the rim of the glenoid cavity of the scapula, occurring with anterior shoulder dislocation. *2)* Procedure done to repair the labrum with capsulorrhaphy, reported with CPT code 23455. **Synonym(s):** *Bankart lesion.*

Bankart procedure Procedure used to treat recurrent dislocation of the shoulder requiring reconstruction of the avulsed capsule and labrum at the glenoid lip. **Synonym(s):** *capsulolabral reconstruction.*

bankruptcy When a provider or supplier files for protection in a federal bankruptcy court, it may choose, with the permission of the court, to cease operations (chapter 7) or reorganize (chapter 11). When a provider or supplier files under chapter 7, it liquidates its assets and ceases operations and must notify the contractor of this fact. When the assets are sold to a different entity, that entity must enroll with the contractor if it wishes to bill the Medicare program

Bantam-Albright-Martin disease Rare genetic disease in which there is sufficient amount of parathyroid hormone produced, but the body is unable to respond to it due to a defective type of protein required for the hormone's signal transduction. This results in low blood calcium levels and high phosphate levels. Physical characteristics include a short physique, round face, obesity, and short hand bones. Report this disorder with ICD-9-CM code 275.49. **Synonym(s):** *Albright's hereditary osteodystrophy, Martin-Albright-Bantam disease, pseudohypoparathyroidism.*

baragnosis Loss of the ability to sense or consciously perceive weight, such as the weight of hand-held objects, reported with ICD-9-CM code 781.99. **Synonym(s):** *abarognosis.*

Barany caloric test Extent of nystagmus is determined by irrigating the external auditory meatus with hot or cold water.

barbiturate abuse Cases in which an individual has taken barbiturates to the detriment of his/her health or social functioning in doses above or for periods beyond those normally regarded as therapeutic.

Bardenheurer operation Arterial fistula in the chest is repaired by ligation and sutures.

Bard-Pic syndrome Signs and symptoms associated with cancer of the head of the pancreas, including jaundice, a palpable gallbladder with common bile duct blockage, and cachexia. This syndrome is reported with ICD-9-CM code 157.0.

bariatric Describing supplies, services, or diagnoses assigned to the treatment of obesity. Bariatric surgery seeks to reduce the patient's weight by restricting the amount of food that can be held in the stomach and/or by reducing the body's ability to absorb nutrients. There are specific CPT and ICD-9-CM procedure codes to describe these surgeries, and also specific HCPCS Level II codes to describe supplies required to accommodate bariatric patients. The most common diagnosis associated with these supplies and procedures is morbid obesity, reported with ICD-9-CM code 278.01. Bariatric surgery may complicate the care of a patient and postsurgical status should be reported with ICD-9-CM code V45.86. **NCD Reference:** *100.1.*

baritosis Type of pneumoconiosis. Chronic nonmalignant respiratory disease caused by the

A-C

inhalation of barium dust. Report this condition with ICD-9-CM code 503.

barium enema   Radiology exam for viewing the intestine that utilizes a suspension of barium sulfate, a chalk-like substance that appears white on x-ray, to delineate the lining of the colon and rectum. The barium is administered via the rectum and held inside the colon while x-rays are taken. Barium enema may also be performed therapeutically in order to relieve intussusception or intestinal obstructions. Report barium enema with ICD-9-CM procedure codes 87.64, 96.29, and 96.38-96.39 and CPT codes 74270-74283 according to therapeutic or diagnostic purpose.

barium sulfate   Contrast agent used for enhancing x-rays of the digestive tract. It is ingested as a chalky liquid. *Synonym(s): blanc fixe, synthetic baryta.*

Barkan's operation   Technique corrects glaucoma by opening Schlemm's canal.

Barker operation   Incision of the dorsal area of the foot.

Barlow's syndrome   "Mid-late" systolic click of the heart due to massive protrusion of the mitral valvular leaflet in the left atrial cavity. Report this disorder with ICD-9-CM code 424.0.

baro-   Relating to weight or heaviness.

Baron Munchausen syndrome   Chronic, factitious illness with physical, but psychosomatic symptoms. Report this disorder with ICD-9-CM code 301.51.

barotrauma   Pain or damage caused to tissue by changes in pressure that constrict or expand the gas contained in various parts of the body such as lungs, sinuses, or middle ear. Report this condition with ICD-9-CM codes 993.0-993.2.

Barr procedure   Correction of talipes equinovarus that may result from polio, and includes the anterior transfer of the tibialis posterior tendon.

Barré-Guillain syndrome   Disorder of the immune system with paraplegia of limbs, flaccid paralysis, ophthalmoplegia, ataxia, and areflexia. Report this disorder with ICD-9-CM code 357.0. *Synonym(s): Fisher's syndrome, Guillain-Barre syndrome, Landry syndrome, Miller-Fisher's syndrome, Strohl syndrome.*

barrel chest   Acquired deformity of the chest in which it appears rounded or bulging, resembling a barrel shape with little movement noticed upon respiration. Underlying causative conditions may include asthma, COPD, emphysema, kyphosis, and osteoarthritis. Report this condition with ICD-9-CM code 738.3.

Barré-Liéou syndrome   Irritation of the nerve roots emanating from the posterior cervical spinal cord. Report this disorder with ICD-9-CM code 723.2.

Barrett's esophagus   Complication of gastroesophageal reflux disease causing peptic ulcer and stricture in the lower part of the esophagus due to columnar epithelial cells from the lining of the stomach and intestine replacing the natural esophageal lining made of normal squamous cell epithelium. Barrett's esophagus is linked to an elevated risk of esophageal cancer, and is sometimes followed by esophageal adenocarcinoma. Diagnosis is made by endoscopic biopsy. Treatment consists of acid suppressive drugs or proton pump inhibitors. Report Barrett's esophagus with ICD-9-CM code 530.85. *Synonym(s): Barrett's syndrome.*

Barsky's procedure   Cleft hand repaired by closing the cleft, bringing the ring and index fingers closer together, and correcting webbing between the fingers.

Bársony-Polgár syndrome   Strong, uncoordinated contraction of the esophagus evoked by deglutition in the elderly. Appears as a series of concentric spirals on an x-ray. Report this disorder with ICD-9-CM code 530.5. *Synonym(s): Barsony-Teschendorf syndrome, corkscrew esophagus.*

Barth syndrome   X-linked genetic disorder that includes a weakened immune system, heart and muscle weakness, extreme fatigue, and growth retardation. Early diagnosis is key to survival for patients with Barth. Mortalities are due to cardiomyopathy and systemic infection. Cardiac improvement is seen in the majority of treated cases of Barth syndrome, which is very rare in the United States. Report this syndrome with ICD-9-CM code 759.89.

Bartholin's gland   Mucous-producing gland found in the vestibular bulbs on either side of the vaginal orifice and connected to the mucosal membrane at the opening by a duct. *Synonym(s): greater vestibular gland.* **B. abscess** Pocket of pus and surrounding cellulitis caused by infection of the Bartholin's gland and causing localized swelling and pain in the posterior labia majora that may extend into the lower vagina. Report this abscess with ICD-9-CM code 616.3.

Bartter's syndrome   Cluster of symptoms caused by a defect in the ability of the kidney to reabsorb potassium. This is indicated by signs and symptoms such as alkalosis, increased aldosterone and plasma renin levels, normal blood pressure, muscle cramping, weakness, constipation, and frequent urination. This syndrome is reported with ICD-9-CM code 255.13. *Synonym(s): juxtaglomerular cell hyperplasia, urinary potassium wasting.*

base   In dentistry, material utilized beneath a filling to take the place of lost tooth structure.

base rate   Calculation assigned to a hospital used to calculate diagnosis-related group (DRG) reimbursement. Base rates vary from hospital to hospital. The base rate adjusts reimbursement to allow for such individual characteristics of the hospital as geographic location, status (urban/rural, teaching), and local labor costs.

base unit Relative weighted value based upon the usual anesthesia services and the relative work or cost of the specific anesthesia service assigned to each anesthesia-specific procedure code. *Synonym(s): basic value.*

baseball finger Injury to the distal portion of the finger, usually caused by a blow resulting in hyperextension. The majority of these injuries require conservative treatment, such as splinting. Report this injury with ICD-9-CM code 842.13.

Basedow syndrome Toxic diffuse goiter. Enlargement of the thyroid gland seen mostly in women, stemming from an autoimmune process, and causing excessive secretion of thyroid hormone, goiter, and bulging eyes. The syndrome seen with hyperplasia of the thyroid and excessive hormone production consists of fatigue, nervousness, emotional lability and irritability, heat intolerance and increased sweating, weight loss, palpitations, and tremor of the hands and tongue. If there is no documentation of a thyrotoxic crisis or storm, report ICD-9-CM code 242.00; with thyrotoxic crisis or storm, report 242.01. *Synonym(s): Begbie's disease, Flajani disease, Graves' disease, Marsh's disease, Parry's disease, toxic diffuse goiter.*

baseline Starting point or place of reference from which to base progression or treatment of a condition.

basi(o)- Relating to the base or foundation.

basic coverage Insurance providing coverage for hospital care.

basic health services Defined set of benefits all federally qualified HMOs must offer enrollees.

basic value Relative weighted value based upon the usual anesthesia services and the relative work or cost of the specific anesthesia service assigned to each anesthesia-specific procedure code. *Synonym(s): base unit.*

basilar artery syndrome Quadriplegia, anesthesia, and nystagmus due to obstruction of twigs of the basilar artery, and causing lesions in the pontine region. Report this disorder with ICD-9-CM code 435.0.

basiliximab Drug used as one part of an immunosuppressive medication regimen specifically to prevent organ rejection in kidney transplant patients. Supply is reported with HCPCS Level II code J0480. May be sold under the brand name Simulect.

basofrontal syndrome Meningioma of the optic nerve, marked by central scotoma and contralateral choked disk. Report this disorder with ICD-9-CM code 377.04. *Synonym(s): Foster-Kennedy syndrome, Gowers-Paton-Kennedy syndrome.*

Bassen-Kornzweig syndrome Genetic disorder of lipoprotein metabolism in which the body fails to produce low density and very low density lipoproteins, affecting the way in which fats are utilized in the body. This deficiency is associated with hypocholesterolemia, progressive ataxic neuropathy, lack of fat-soluble vitamins, pigmentary retinal degeneration, and faulty intestinal absorption. Report this syndrome with ICD-9-CM code 272.5. *Synonym(s): abetalipoproteinemia.*

Bassett's operation Dissection of the inguinal glands for a radical resection of the vulva.

BAT Brightness acuity test. Evaluation of glare caused by opacities in the eye. BAT is used in evaluating subjective halo disturbances in a patient's vision.

Batch-Spittler-McFaddin operation Leg is severed at the knee joint, which offers an alternative to severing a long bone.

bathophobia Aberrant fear of depths, reported with ICD-9-CM code 300.23. Symptoms may include exacerbation of feelings of fright and apprehension.

Batista procedure Partial left ventriculectomy performed to reduce an enlarged heart and to improve its function, named for Brazilian surgeon Randas Batista. This procedure is reported with unlisted CPT code 33999. The Batista procedure differs from left ventricular restoration (reported with 33548) in that the Batista reduces only the muscle mass of the heart, not the capacity of the chamber.

Batten-Mayou disease Juvenile type of neuronal ceroid lipofuscinosis or amaurotic familial idiocy. This disease is an inherited disorder in which the body stores excessive amounts of lipofuscin, the pigment that remains after damaged cells are broken down and digested, resulting in progressive nervous tissue damage, vision loss, and fatality. Batten disease or Batten-Mayou disease is used to mean Vogt Spielmeyer juvenile type as well as the genetically-induced retinal dystrophy that occurs in neuronal ceroid lipofuscinosis. This disease is reported with ICD-9-CM codes 330.1 and 362.71.

Batten-Steinert syndrome Condition in which the peritoneal cover of the liver converts to a white mass resembling cake icing. Report this disorder with ICD-9-CM code 359.21. *Synonym(s): Curschmann (-Batten) (-Steinert) syndrome.*

Battle's operation Appendectomy in which the rectus muscle is temporarily retracted.

battle's sign Sign appearing with fracture of the skull base consisting of bruising, ecchymosis, or discoloration immediately behind the ears.

Baumgarten-Cruveilhier syndrome Cirrhosis of the liver with patent paraumbilical, varicose periumbilical or umbilical veins. Report this disorder with ICD-9-CM code 571.5.

BayGam See gamma globulin.

Bayonet sign Test that looks at the extensor function and patellar stability of the knee. With the patient

A-C

supine, the knee is turned outward and a pattern produced by the patella, patellar tendon, and tibial tubercle is observed that resembles a bayonet found on the end of a rifle. This is caused by the tibial tubercle being in a lateral position and consequently pulling the patella sideways.

BB Blow bottles.

BBA Balanced Budget Act of 1997. Legislation to cut federal spending and balance the federal budget.

BBB *1)* Blood brain barrier. *NCD Reference: 110.20. 2)* Bundle branch block. Intraventricular conduction disorder due to interruption of electrical impulses in one of the two main branches of the His bundle and manifested in the EKG by markedly prolonged QRS complex.

BBRA Balanced Budget Refinement Act of 1999.

BCBS Blue Cross Blue Shield.

BCBSA Blue Cross and Blue Shield Association. Association that represents the common interests of Blue Cross and Blue Shield health plans. The BCBSA serves as the administrator for the Health Care Code Maintenance and also helps maintain the HCPCS Level II coding system.

BCC Basal cell carcinoma.

BCG live intravesical vaccine Bacillus Calmette-Guerin bladder vaccine. Chemotherapy agent, in a live vaccine form, instilled into the bladder to decrease the occurrence of superficial tumors. Supply is reported with HCPCS Level II code J9031. May be sold under the brand name: Immucyst, Pacis, Theracys, TICE BCG.

BCP Birth control pill.

BCT Breast-conservation therapy.

BDAE Boston Diagnostic Aphasia Examination. Standardized diagnostic test for aphasia.

BE *1)* Barium enema. *2)* Below the elbow.

beach ear Inflammation of the external auditory canal as a result of irritation caused by ocean water or other seaside environmental factors. Report this condition with ICD-9-CM code 380.12. *Synonym(s): acute swimmer's ear, otitis externa, tank ear.*

Beals syndrome Congenital contractural arachnodactyly. Rare congenital condition related to Marfan syndrome and characterized by abnormally long and slender digits, scoliosis, contractures of the joints, underdeveloped muscles, and abnormally shaped ears. Treatment normally consists of physical therapy or bracing. Report this disorder with ICD-9-CM code 759.82.

beam Usually referring to focused, unidirectional stream of electromagnetic radiation emissions, either photons or electrons.

beam offset Radiation beam not centered on the central ray, accomplished by using a physical block or asymmetric collimation.

beam splitter Microscope attachment that splits light.

Bearn-Kunkel (-Slater) syndrome Chronic hepatitis with autoimmune manifestations. Report this disorder with ICD-9-CM code 571.49.

Beau's syndrome Degeneration of the muscles of the heart. Report this disorder with ICD-9-CM code 429.1.

becaplermin gel Topical medication that aids in wound repair and helps to build granulation tissue, used to treat diabetic ulcers. Supply is reported with HCPCS Level II code S0157. May be sold under the brand name Regranex.

Bechterew-Strümpell-Marie syndrome Rheumatoid inflammation of the vertebrae. Report this disorder with ICD-9-CM code 720.0.

Beck's cannula Butterfly-shaped cannula used for blood transfusion.

Beck's clamp Vascular clamp for partial dilation of the aortic wall.

Beck's syndrome Occlusion of the spinal artery as a result of injury, disk damage, or cardiovascular disease. Report this disorder with ICD-9-CM code 433.80 or 433.81.

Beckwith (-Wiedemann) syndrome Congenital disorder with macroglossia, gigantism, dysplasia of the renal medulla, visceromegaly, adrenocortical cytomegaly, and exophthalmos. Report this disorder with ICD-9-CM code 759.89.

beer potomania Severe hyponatremia accompanied by mental status changes occurring as a rare syndrome associated with binge beer ingestion and inadequate dietary intake.

beer-drinker's heart Disorder caused by excessive alcohol use in which the heart muscle is weakened and fails to pump blood effectively, resulting in heart failure. Report this condition with ICD-9-CM code 425.5. *Synonym(s): alcoholic cardiomyopathy.*

Begbie's disease Enlargement of the thyroid gland seen mostly in women, stemming from an autoimmune process and causing excessive secretion of thyroid hormone, goiter, and bulging eyes. The syndrome seen with hyperplasia of the thyroid and excessive hormone production consists of fatigue, nervousness, emotional lability and irritability, heat intolerance and increased sweating, weight loss, palpitations, and tremor of the hands and tongue. If there is no documentation of a thyrotoxic crisis or storm, report ICD-9-CM code 242.00; with thyrotoxic crisis or storm, report 242.01. *Synonym(s): Basedow syndrome, Flajani disease, Graves'* *disease, Marsh's disease, Parry's disease, toxic diffuse goiter.*

behavior management   Education and modification techniques or methodologies aimed at helping a patient change undesirable habits or behaviors.

Behçet's syndrome   Chronic condition linked to disturbances in the immune system where small blood vessels become locally inflamed, causing ulcerations of the oral and pharyngeal mucous membranes, skin lesions, and inflammation of joints Report this disorder with ICD-9-CM code 136.1.

bejel   Disease closely related to syphilis but transmitted by nonsexual skin contact. It normally begins as a latent infection followed by a more aggressive disease. Characteristics include oral lesions, blisters on the trunk and extremities, and infection of the leg bones at later stages. Bejel is reported with ICD-9-CM code 104.0. *Synonym(s): endemic syphilis.*

Bekesy audiometry   Automatic hearing-threshold measuring technique utilizing interrupted or continuous tones in which the patient presses a button to increase or decrease the intensity of the tone to trace monaural thresholds to detect hearing loss. Reported with CPT codes 92560-92561.

Bekhterev-Strümpell-Marie syndrome   Rheumatoid inflammation of the vertebrae. Report this disorder with ICD-9-CM code 720.0.

Bell's palsy   Facial paralysis or weakness resulting from facial nerve damage. The muscles on one side of the face are affected, causing the face to sag on the side involved. Bell's palsy usually occurs abruptly and often resolves spontaneously within a few weeks. It is usually idiopathic (without a known cause) and reported with ICD-9-CM code 351.0. If occurring in an infant due to birth trauma, report 767.5. If specified as syphilitic, report 094.89. *NCD Reference: 160.15.*

Bellise bra   Brand name, compressor comfort bra designed to treat breast and chest edema, usually a late effect of breast cancer treatment. Supply of the Bellise bra may be reported with HCPCS Level II code S8429; check with individual payers and provide documentation.

Benadryl   See diphenhydramine HCl.

Bender-Gestalt test   Psychological test gauges perceptual-motor coordination to assess personality dynamics, review organic brain impairment, and measure neurological maturity.

bends   Decompression sickness caused by rapid reduction in atmospheric pressure in deep-sea divers and caisson workers who return to normal air pressure environments too quickly or pilots flying at high altitudes. This disease causes joint pain, respiratory problems, neurologic symptoms, and skin lesions, and is reported with ICD-9-CM code 993.3. *Synonym(s):*

Caisson disease, compressed air disease, diver's palsy, dysbarism.

Benedict test for dextrose   Test using sodium or potassium citrate and sodium carbonate in a reagent to determine dextrose content of urine.

Benedikt's syndrome   Paraplegia and anesthesia over part of the body caused by lesions in the brain or spinal cord. Report this disorder with ICD-9-CM code 344.89. *Synonym(s): Avellis syndrome, Babinski-Nageotte syndrome, Benedikt's paralysis, Brown-Sequard syndrome, Cestan-Chenais syndrome, Cestan's syndrome, Foville's syndrome, Gubler-Millard syndrome, Jackson's syndrome, Weber-Leyden syndrome.*

beneficiary   Person entitled to receive Medicare or other payer benefits who maintains a health insurance policy claim number.

benefit   Services an insurance program agrees to cover under a contractual arrangement. *b. period* Period of time during which medical benefits are available to the patient. Under Medicare Part A, 60 full days of hospitalization plus 30 coinsurance days represent the benefit period. The period is renewed when the beneficiary has not been in the hospital or SNF for a period of 60 days.

benign   Mild or nonmalignant in nature.

benign lesion   Neoplasm or change in tissue that is not cancerous (nonmalignant).

benign mammary dysplasias   Noncancerous fibrous or cystic growths in the breast.

benign prostatic hyperplasia   Benign enlargement of the prostate caused by proliferation of fibrostromal elements of the gland and commonly affecting men older than age 50. BPH is often characterized by urination difficulties such as slow start, weak stream, dribbling, nocturia (night-time urination), and urinary obstruction as the urethra is compressed as the gland enlarges. Report benign prostatic hyperplasia with a code from ICD-9-CM category 600, depending upon the specified type of hyperplasia and whether or not urinary obstruction is present. *Synonym(s): BPH.*

Bennett fracture   Intra-articular fracture/dislocation at the base of the first metacarpal bone (thumb) on the ulnar side. A small fragment of metacarpal continues to articulate with the trapezium with lateral retraction of the metacarpal shaft by the abductor pollicis longus. Assign ICD-9-CM code 815.01 for a closed fracture and 815.11 for an open fracture. Fracture care is reported based on type with CPT codes 26645-26665.

Bentyl   See dicyclomine hydrochloride.

benztropine mesylate   Drug that acts on the central nervous system used to treat acute dystonic reactions and Parkinson's disease. Supply is reported with HCPCS

Level II code J0515. May be sold under the brand names Apo-Benztropine, Cogentin.

beriberi Disease caused by a lack of vitamin B1 (thiamine) causing cardiac damage, polyneuritis, and edema. The disease is found mostly in areas where white, polished rice is the main staple of the diet. Report this disorder with ICD-9-CM code 265.0. *Synonym(s): dietetic neuritis, endemic polyneuritis, rice disease.*

berloque dermatitis Form of phytophotodermatitis that appears as brown-pigmented patches occurring after application of perfumed products containing bergamot oil followed by exposure to sunlight. Report this condition with ICD-9-CM code 692.72.

Berman locator Small, sensitive tool used to detect the location of a metallic foreign body in the eye.

Bernard-Horner syndrome Disorder following a heart attack with pain and stiffness in the shoulder, and swelling and pain in the hand. Report this disorder with ICD-9-CM code 337.9. *Synonym(s): Claude Bernard-Horner syndrome, Reilly's syndrome, Steinbrocker's syndrome.*

Bernard-Sergent syndrome Acute adrenal insufficiency caused by illness or trauma or by large amounts of hormones used as therapy. Symptoms include hypotension, hyperthermia, hyponatremia, hyperkalemia, hypoglycemia, nausea, and vomiting. Report this disorder with ICD-9-CM code 255.41.

Bernhardt-Roth syndrome Tingling, paresthesia, itching, and other symptoms on the outer side of the lower part of the thigh caused by lateral femoral cutaneous nerve compression. Report this disorder with ICD-9-CM code 355.1. *Synonym(s): Bernhardt-Roth disease.*

Bernheim's syndrome Right heart failure accompanied by enlarged liver, distended neck veins, and edema without pulmonary congestion, caused by hypertrophied septum. Report this disorder with ICD-9-CM code 428.0.

Bernstein test Acid perfusion test used to differentiate substernal chest pain due to gastroesophageal reflux disease (GERD).

Bertolotti's syndrome Fusion of the bottom lumbar vertebra to the top sacral vertebra, making a sixth sacral vertebra accompanied by sciatica and scoliosis. Report this disorder with ICD-9-CM code 756.15.

Berubigen See cyanocobalamin.

berylliosis Hypersensitivity reaction to beryllium compounds affecting the skin and subcutaneous tissues, liver, lymph nodes, and lungs when imbedded in the skin or inhaled. Acute pulmonary disease is seen as toxic fulminating or allergic pneumonitis with rhinitis, pharyngitis, and tracheobronchitis. Chronic pulmonary disease is the common form of berylliosis, characterized by a progressive, immunologically mediated, diffuse inflammatory reaction to the formation of beryllium granulomas. Report berylliosis with ICD-9-CM code 503.

Best's disease Rare autosomal dominant form of macular degeneration, with symptoms occurring in early childhood, anywhere from ages 3 to 15. A mass of fatty material appears as a striking yellowish, orange yolk-like (vitelline) lesion under the retinal pigment epithelium in the macula, which then progresses through different stages over years. The break-up of this mass, which often ruptures, is referred to as the scrambled-egg stage and causes vision loss. Fluid and yellow deposits from the ruptured cyst spread throughout the macula. The macula and the underlying retinal pigment epithelium begin to atrophy, with possible development of a choroidal neovascular membrane, causing vision loss as central vision deteriorates to about 20/100 late in life. Best's disease does not always affect both eyes equally. This disease is reported with ICD-9-CM code 362.76. *Synonym(s): vitelliform dystrophy, vitelliform macular degeneration.*

bestiality Sexual relations between humans and animals.

beta blocker Drugs (such as propranolol) that combine with and block the activity of a beta-receptor to decrease the heart rate and force of contractions to lower high blood pressure, used especially to treat hypertension, angina pectoris, and ventricular and supraventricular arrhythmias.

betamethasone Corticosteroid available in different forms and combinations used to treat severe inflammation that requires immunosuppression. The topical form is used to treat inflammation and itching of dermatological conditions. The inhalant form helps control asthma. Supply is reported with HCPCS Level II code J0702.

Betaseron See interferon.

Bethesda system Standardized staging and nomenclature system for classifying cytopathological diseases from cervical and vaginal pap smear results, developed by the Centers for Disease Control and the National Institute for Health. This method utilizes three components: adequacy of specimen taken, general categorization, and descriptive diagnosis. Nomenclature used to report diagnostic results include atypical squamous cells cannot exclude high-grade squamous intraepithelial lesion (ASC-H); atypical squamous cells of undetermined significance (ASC-US); low-grade squamous intraepithelial lesion (LGSIL); and high-grade squamous intraepithelial lesion (HGSIL). Diagnostic results are reported with a code from ICD-9-CM subcategory 795.0.

Betke-Kleihauer test Venipuncture blood test taken to determine the amount of Rh immune globulin an Rh-negative woman should receive in order to prevent formation of antibodies against her fetus. *Synonym(s): fetal-maternal erythrocyte distribution, K-B stain, Kleihauer-Betke stain.*

bevacizumab Injectable antiangiogenic agent used to treat neovascular (wet) age-related macular degeneration. Bevacizumab may also be used in combination with chemotherapeutic drugs in the treatment of patients with certain cancers, such as colon, rectum, and lung. May be sold under the brand name Avastin. Report supply with HCPCS Level II code J9035 or C9257.

Bevan's operation Relocation of an undescended testicle down into the scrotum.

Bexxar Brand name radioimmunotherapeutic agent for treatment of non-Hodgkin's lymphoma. Supply of Bexxar is reported with HCPCS Level II code A9544 or A9545. Bexxar contains tositumomab with iodine 1-131 tositumomab.

bezoar Accumulation of foreign matter, such as hair or undigestible fibers, within the stomach or intestines that fails to pass through the intestines and may require surgical removal. Report a bezoar with ICD-9-CM codes 935.2, 936, and 938, dependent upon its location in the digestive tract.

Bezold's sign Swelling near the ear, seen in patients diagnosed with mastoiditis. Mastoiditis is reported with a code from ICD-9-CM category 383.

BFLS Borjeson-Forssman-Lehmann syndrome. Rare congenital complex of mental and physical disorders, reported with ICD-9-CM code 759.89.

BHR Birmingham Hip Resurfacing system. Metal-on-metal resurfacing artificial hip replacement system surgically implanted in the hip joint. It is called "resurfacing" because only the surface of the femoral head is removed to implant the new metal ball. The system contains a socket and a ball head. Patients receiving this hip replacement are generally younger and more active.

BI Biopsy.

bi- Double, twice, two.

Bianchi's syndrome Sensory aphasic condition with alexia, apraxia, and lesions in the left parietal lobe. Report this disorder with ICD-9-CM code 784.69.

bib. Drink.

biceps femoris One of three hamstring muscles found in the posterior thigh, this is the outer hamstring. The contraction of these muscles helps the knee to flex. CPT code 27097 is used to report a release of one of the hamstring muscles.

Bicillin C-R Antibiotic used to inhibit cell wall synthesis during multiplication. It is used to treat susceptible strains of gram-positive and gram-negative aerobic cocci,

spirochetes, and some strains of gram-positive and negative aerobic and anaerobic bacteria.

bicipital tendonitis Inflammatory condition affecting the biceps muscle where the tendon inserts into the shoulder. Report this condition with ICD-9-CM code 726.12.

bicipital tenosynovitis Inflammatory condition affecting the bicipital tendon.

BiCNU See carmustine.

bicompartmental knee replacement Repair of the femoral condyles and the tibial plateaus in both the medial and lateral compartments. When both compartments are done, with or without any patella resurfacing, it is considered a total knee arthroplasty and is reported with CPT code 27447.

bicornuate uterus Most common congenital anomaly of the uterus, in which it is heart shaped with two horns. This condition may affect the ability to reproduce, and is associated with a higher rate of cervical incompetence, spontaneous abortion, premature labor, breech presentation, and trapped or retained placenta. In pregnancy, it is reported with a code from ICD-9-CM category 654.0; in a nonpregnant female, report this condition with ICD-9-CM code 752.34. *Synonym(s): double uterus, uterus bicornis.*

BICROS Bilateral routing of signals.

bicuspid Tooth with two cusps or a premolar tooth.

bicuspid aortic valve Common congenital abnormality in which the aortic valve has only two cusps due to incomplete separation of two of the three. Bicuspid aortic valve is often asymptomatic in early years, but can cause calcification and stenosis in later years. Surgical intervention is often required. Bicuspid aortic valve is reported with ICD-9-CM code 746.4.

BID/b.i.d. Twice daily.

Biedl-Bardet syndrome Mental retardation, pigmentary retinopathy, obesity, polydactyly, and hypogonadism. Report this disorder with ICD-9-CM code 759.89. *Synonym(s): Biemond's syndrome.*

Bielschowsky's head tilt test Test for damage to the fourth cranial nerve, as evidenced by a palsy in the superior oblique muscle.

Biemond's syndrome Mental retardation, pigmentary retinopathy, obesity, polydactyly, and hypogonadism. Report this disorder with ICD-9-CM code 759.89. *Synonym(s): Biedl-Bardet syndrome.*

Bier block Form of regional anesthesia performed by injecting an anesthetic agent intravenously into a limb. A double tourniquet system is used, one above and one below the area to be worked on. Anesthesia is produced in the limb below the proximal tourniquet. The distal tourniquet keeps the anesthesia from circulating

A-C

systemically. Report with CPT code 64999 for procedures on the upper or lower extremity. A separate code for regional block anesthesia used in dental procedures is reported with HCPCS Level II code D9211.

Biesenberger mammaplasty Reduction procedure for transposition of the nipple with excision of the side of the mammary gland and rotation of the remaining glandular pedicle to form a skin brassiere.

bifurcated Having two branches or divisions, such as the left pulmonary veins that split off from the left atrium to carry oxygenated blood away from the heart.

bifurcation Point of division into two separate branches or structures, such as the site where the trachea divides into the right and left main bronchi or the common carotid artery becomes the external and internal carotid arteries. For diagnostic purposes, a bifurcation is a congenital anomaly that results in an imperfect closure of an organ or other anatomical structure, such as the ureter, renal pelvis, hard or soft palate, lip, etc.

bifurcation syndrome Obstruction of the terminal aorta causing fatigue in the hips, thighs, or calves and pallor of lower extremities and impotence in exercising males. Report this disorder with ICD-9-CM code 444.0. **Synonym(s):** *Leriche's syndrome.*

big spleen syndrome Enlarged spleen caused by cirrhosis of the liver or portal or splenic vein thrombosis causing anemia and hyperplasia of marrow precursors of deficient cell type. Report this disorder with ICD-9-CM code 289.4. **Synonym(s):** *hypersplenism.*

bigeminy Arrhythmia consisting of one premature beat followed by one normal sinus beat repeating in sequence on a regular basis. Bigeminy may be atrial or ventricular, and may be associated with acute myocardial infarction, drug overdose, ischemic heart disease, or lack of oxygen. Report this condition with ICD-9-CM code 427.89.

bilateral Consisting of or affecting two sides.

bilateral polycystic ovarian syndrome Acute adrenal insufficiency caused by illness, trauma, or by large amounts of hormones used as therapy with hypotension, hyperthermia, hyponatremia, hyperkalemia, hypoglycemia, nausea, and vomiting. Report this disorder with ICD-9-CM code 256.4.

bilharziasis Parasitic infection caused by blood flukes of the genus Schistosoma, a worm that is typically found in infested waters. The larva enters through the skin and eggs from the parasite lodge in various places such as portal venules, liver, mesenteric vein, intestines, and urinary tract, causing inflammatory response in the organ, fibrosis, abdominal pain, diarrhea, bloody stools, and hematuria. Report bilharziasis with a code from ICD-9-CM rubric 120. **Synonym(s):** *schistosomiasis.*

bilirubinuria Condition in which bilirubin is present in the urine, reported with ICD-9-CM code 791.4. **Synonym(s):** *biliuria.*

Bill's bar Bony crest or anatomic "beak" in the superior internal ear canal, separating the facial nerve canal anterior to Bill's bar, from the superior vestibular nerve posterior to it. Bill's bar is important in differentiating between the two nerves.

biller Person who submits claims for services provided by a health care provider or supplier to payers.

billing agency Company the applicant contracts with to prepare or edit the content of the claim.

Billroth operation Anastomosis of the stomach to the duodenum or jejunum.

bilocular Containing two cells, compartments, or chambers.

bimalleolar fracture Break of both sides of the ankle that includes the rounded projection of the lower tibia (medial malleolus) and of the fibula (lateral malleolus). This fracture is reported with ICD-9-CM code 824.4 if closed and 824.5 if open.

binder Broad bandage that supports a body part.

Binet test Psychological measurement of the ability to think and reason. The Binet test is a precursor to the development of today's IQ tests. The subject performs tasks such as following commands, copying patterns, naming things, and putting things in order.

Bing-Horton syndrome Idiopathic, unilateral headaches that recur in brief, sudden attacks that may disappear entirely over time. Report this disorder with ICD-9-CM code 339.00. **Synonym(s):** *histamine cephalgia.*

Binswanger's disease Rare type of dementia manifested by deep white-matter brain lesions, memory loss, loss of cognitive ability, and alteration in mood. This is a slowly progressive condition often manifested by strokes and partial recovery. Treatment is symptomatic and consists of medication to control hyper- and hypotension, depression, and arrhythmia. Report this condition with ICD-9-CM code 290.12. **Synonym(s):** *subcortical arteriosclerotic encephalopathy, subcortical dementia.*

BioArc Brand name urethral sling for treatment of female stress incontinence and cystocele. The sling may be inserted using a suprapubic or transobturator approach.

Biobrane Brand name biosynthetic wound dressing made of silicon and collagen. When the dressing is applied in the physician's office, supply of the wound dressing is reported separately with HCPCS Level II codes A6021-A6024.

BioDome Brand name processed human scleral shell for use as a wrapping of an orbital implant during enucleation surgery, reported with CPT code 67550.

BioElevation Brand name processed fascia lata slings, derived from human donors, for eyelid correction. BioElevation is used to correct ptosis, lower lid ectropion, and facial palsy. Surgery to correct eyelid ptosis using BioElevation is reported with CPT code 67901. Supply of fascia lata in outpatient facilities is reported with HCPCS Level II code C1762.

biofeedback Process by which a person learns to influence autonomic or involuntary nervous system responses and physiologic responses normally regulated voluntarily, but whose control has been affected by trauma or disease. The patient learns through monitoring to associate body responses with related stimuli and how to control those responses. Biofeedback helps regulate vital signs such as heart rate, blood pressure, temperature, and muscle tension and is considered to be effective in the treatment of migraine headaches, high blood pressure, incontinence, Raynaud's syndrome, and anticipatory nausea due to chemotherapy. Report biofeedback with CPT codes 90875, 90876, and 90911. *NCD References: 30.1, 30.1.1.*

bioimpedance Noninvasive, continuous measurement of blood flow, respiration, and other cardiopulmonary dynamics, using a patient's thorax as an impedance transducer. Bioimpedance is reported with CPT code 93701.

biometric identifier Identifier based on some physical characteristic, such as a fingerprint.

biometry Statistical analysis of biological data.

biopsy Tissue or fluid removed for diagnostic purposes through analysis of the cells in the biopsy material.

Biörck (-Thorson) syndrome Carcinoid tumors that cause cyanotic flushing of the skin, diarrhea, watery stools, bronchoconstrictive attacks, hypotension, edema, and ascites. Report this disorder with ICD-9-CM code 259.2. *Synonym(s): Cassidy-Scholte syndrome, Hedinger's syndrome.*

BIPA Benefits Improvement and Protection Act of 2000. BIPA affects Medicare, Medicaid, and State Children's Health Insurance Program.

BiPAP Noninvasive mechanical ventilation. BiPAP consists of both continuous positive airway pressure (CPAP) and pressure support ventilation. According to CPT guidelines, since a component of BiPAP includes CPAP, CPT code 94660 is appropriate for the initiation and follow-up management of the service.

biparietal diameter Ultrasound measurement of the fetus that measures the distance between the two parietal bones of the skull, which is correlated to the gestational age of the fetus. *Synonym(s): BPD.*

biperiden lactate Used to treat Parkinson's disease, this anticholinergic drug acts as an antagonist to acetylcholine. Supply is reported with HCPCS Level II code J0190. May be sold under the brand name Akineton.

bird breeders' lung Allergic inflammation of the lung caused by exposure to bird droppings. When exposure ceases, the symptoms, which may include chills, fever, cough, and shortness of breath, also subside. This condition is reported with ICD-9-CM code 495.2. *Synonym(s): bird-fanciers' lung, budgerigar-fancier's disease, pigeon-fancier's lung.*

bird face Congenital anomaly in which the lower jaw is abnormally short or recessed, reported with ICD-9-CM code 756.0. *Synonym(s): brachygnathia.*

Bird's Nest Filter

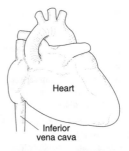

Heart

Inferior
vena cava

The inferior vena cava (or IVC) is the major return vessel of the lower body. It extends from the right atrium of the heart down to the bifurcation of the iliac veins

An intravascular "umbrella" device in the IVC. Such devices are intended to entrap clots and prevent clot passage into the pulmonary arteries

Bird's nest filter Permanent, umbrella-shaped filter implanted in the vena cava and designed to trap small clots of blood or plaque before they reach the lungs and cause pulmonary embolism. The filter is inserted intraluminally, usually through the femoral or jugular veins. Placement of a Bird's nest filter is reported with CPT code 37620. Radiological supervision and interpretation of filter placement is reported with CPT code 75940.

birthing room Comfortable home-like hospital room where both labor and delivery take place and in which the mother and baby usually remain during the hospital stay.

Bishop score Evaluation method to determine if induction of labor should be attempted based upon fetal position and cervical consistency, effacement, dilation, and position in relation to the vaginal axis.

Biskra boil Dry or urban cutaneous leishmaniasis, one form of Old World cutaneous leishmaniasis. This parasitic skin disease is caused by the protozoa Leishmania tropica, spread by the bite of sand flies, and occurring in large urban areas in the Middle East, especially Iran and Iraq, the Mediterranean, and India. Manifestation is mainly a single, large developing boil or furuncle type lesion that persists over a year. Lymphadenopathy may be present. Report this condition with ICD-9-CM code 085.1.

bite block Device placed in the patient's mouth to assist in the positioning of oral structures.

bitewing x-ray Radiograph of the coronal portion of the tooth.

bitolterol mesylate Generic name for Tornalate, a bronchodilator used to treat bronchospasms in asthma, emphysema, and chronic bronchitis. Supply is reported with HCPCS Level II code J7628 or J7629.

Bitot's spots Superficial, gray, triangular spots on the conjunctiva, consisting of keratinized epithelium. Bitot's spots are associated with vitamin A deficiency, reported with ICD-9-CM code 264.1.

bivalirudin Drug used to prevent blood clots in patients with unstable angina who are undergoing percutaneous transluminal coronary angioplasty (PTCA). Supply is reported with HCPCS Level II code J0583. May be sold under the brand name Angiomax.

bivalve cast Cast that is split into two halves by cutting on opposite sides either to relieve pressure or allow for removal and re-application in physical therapy.

biventricular pacing Placing of an additional electrode in the left ventricle when inserting a cardiac pacemaker or cardioverter-defibrillator system. In dual chamber systems, the right ventricle and atrium are fixed with electrodes. The placement of an additional electrode in the left ventricle is accomplished through the cardiac venous system and is reported separately using CPT code 33224 or 33225.

Bjerrum scotoma Visual field defect common in glaucoma and reported with ICD-9-CM code 368.43.

BK Below the knee.

BKA Below-the-knee amputation. Report BKA with ICD-9-CM procedure code 84.15 or CPT code 27598, 27880, 27881, or 27882.

BL HCPCS Level II modifier used to denote a special acquisition of blood and blood products.

black death Highly contagious, most common form of plague, caused by infection of Yersinia pestis. It is characterized by onset of fever, chills, headache, and swollen, tender, inflamed lymph glands called buboes, which develop intravascular coagulation, turning necrotic and gangrenous. Report this condition with ICD-9-CM code 020.0. *Synonym(s): bubonic plague, glandular plague, pestis bubonica.*

black hairy tongue Condition in which the papillae do not shed normally from the tongue, resulting in collections of debris, bacteria, and a dark fuzzy appearance. Report this condition with ICD-9-CM code 529.3. *Synonym(s): lingua nigra.*

Black Lung Program Federal workers compensation (WC) plan administered by the U.S. Department of Labor (DOL) that provides workers compensation coverage to federal civil service employees and certain other categories of employees not covered or not adequately covered under state WC programs; e.g., coal miners totally disabled due to pneumoconiosis.

black lung syndrome Blockage of bronchioles by "coal macules" brought about by aspiration of coal dust. Report this disorder with ICD-9-CM code 500. *Synonym(s): coal miners' pneumoconiosis.*

Blackfan-Diamond syndrome Congenital anemia that manifests during infancy and requires a number of blood transfusions to maintain life. Report this disorder with ICD-9-CM code 284.01.

blackwater fever One of the most dangerous complications of malaria, having a high mortality rate, and occurring almost exclusively with infection from the parasite Plasmodium falciparum. Symptoms include rapid pulse, high fever and chills, extreme prostration, rapidly developing anemia, and the passage of urine that is black or dark red in color. Report black water fever with ICD-9-CM code 084.8. *Synonym(s): malarial hemoglobinuria.*

bladder hypertonicity Abnormal tension in the muscular walls of the bladder, or prolonged muscle spasms, and hypersensitivity or hyperreflexia of the detrusor sphincter muscle. Bladder hypertonicity is reported with ICD-9-CM code 596.51.

bladder instillation Introduction by drops of an anticarcinogenic agent into the bladder to treat cancer. Bacillus Calmette Guerin is the agent used in treating bladder cancer, introduced through a catheter and held in the bladder for a certain period of time. Report this procedure with CPT code 51720.

blade plate General class of internal fixation devices that consist of a plate with a right angle or nearly right angle flange. This may be encountered in an operative note for open reduction internal fixation (ORIF) procedures.

Blair arthrodesis Procedure that treats avascular necrosis or other degeneration of the ankle joint where inadequate bone remains for proper functioning. Fusion of the tibia to the talus bone is performed using an anterior sliding tibial graft through an anterolateral approach. Separate bone harvest may be indicated. Report CPT code 27870 for an open approach or 29899 for an arthroscopic approach.

Blair fusion   Arthrodesis of the ankle following avascular collapse or talar neck fracture.

Blalock-Hanlon procedure   Excision of a segment of the right atrium, creating an atrial septal defect.

Blalock-Taussig procedure   Anastomosis of the left subclavian artery to the left pulmonary artery or the right subclavian artery to the right pulmonary artery in order to shunt some of the blood flow from the systemic to the pulmonary circulation. This is a palliative procedure done to treat Tetralogy of Fallot or insufficient pulmonary arterial flow from congenital anomalies. Report with CPT code 33750. *Synonym(s): TGV repair.*

Blasius Duct

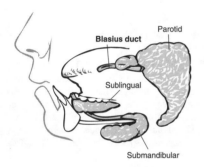

Synonym for parotid gland duct

Blasius duct   Duct extending from the parotid gland to an opening in the cheek, adjacent to the maxillary second molar. The Blasius duct drains saliva from the parotid gland into the oral cavity. *Synonym(s): parotid papilla, Steno's duct, Stensen's duct.*

-blast   Incomplete cellular development.

blast cell   Incomplete formed cell. A number of these cells in the blood can be evidence of a blood disorder.

blasto-   Relating to an early, formative, or primitive stage of a cell or embryonic element or layer.

Blatt capsulodesis   Procedure done for instability of the carpal bones in which a flap of the proximal wrist capsule is fixed to the distal part of the scaphoid bone in order to prevent downward movement of the scaphoid

during radial deviation of the wrist. Report with CPT code 25320. *Synonym(s): dorsal capsulodesis.*

BLDS   Brachmann-de Lange syndrome. Congenital disorder presenting with impaired prenatal and postnatal development, mental retardation, microcephaly, and palmar crease, reported with ICD-9-CM code 759.89. *Synonym(s): de Lange's syndrome.*

BLEED   Bleeding, low systolic blood pressure, elevated prothrombin time, erratic mental status, and disease as a comorbidity. BLEED is used to classify patients presenting to the emergency department with gastrointestinal (GI) hemorrhage. The acronym identifies variables that will affect outcomes. These data points can be used to determine whether patients should be admitted to an intermediate care or intensive care unit.

blended payment rate   Blend of federal and local area wage indexes used to phase in a prospective payment system or reimbursement methodology.

blenn-   Relating to mucus.

blenn(o)-   Relating to mucus.

Blenoxane   See bleomycin sulfate.

bleomycin sulfate   Antineoplastic used to treat lymphomas, HIV-related Kaposi sarcoma, and also to treat malignant pleural effusion in AIDS-related pneumothorax or Pneumocystis carinii. May be sold under the brand name Blenoxane.

blepharelosis   Inversion of the eyelid, turning the edge in toward the eyeball and causing irritation from contact of the lashes with the surface of the eye. Blepharelosis is classified to ICD-9-CM subcategory 374.0, unless specified as congenital (743.62). For repair of an entropion, see CPT codes 67921-67924. *Synonym(s): entropion.*

blepharo-   Relating to the eyelid.

blepharochalasis   Loss of elasticity and relaxation of skin of the eyelid, thickened or indurated skin on the eyelid associated with recurrent episodes of edema, and intracellular atrophy. Blepharochalasis is reported with ICD-9-CM code 374.34 if acquired and with ICD-9-CM code 743.62 if congenital. *Synonym(s): pseudoptosis.*

blepharoclonus   Rapid, uncontrolled contraction or spasm of the orbicularis oculi muscle (one of the muscles of the eyelid), resulting in a winking or blinking movement. This condition is reported with ICD-9-CM code 333.81.

blepharophimosis   Displacement of the inside of the canthi of the eye laterally, causing abnormal horizontal narrowing of the palpebral fissure. If the condition is acquired, report ICD-9-CM code 374.46; if congenital, report 743.62. *Synonym(s): ankyloblepharon.*

blepharoplasty   Plastic surgery of the eyelids to remove excess fat and redundant skin weighting down the lid.

The eyelid is pulled tight and sutured to support sagging muscles. Blepharoplasty is reported with CPT codes 15820-15823. **Synonym(s):** *canthoplasty, eyelid lift.*

blepharoplegia Condition in which the eyelid muscles are paralyzed, reported with ICD-9-CM code 374.89.

blepharoptosis Droop or displacement of the upper eyelid, caused by paralysis, muscle problems, or outside mechanical forces. For acquired blepharoptosis, see ICD-9-CM codes 374.30-374.33. For congenital blepharoptosis, see 743.61. **Synonym(s):** *ptosis.*

blepharopyorrhea Infection and inflammation of the eye manifested by a discharge of pus, normally as a result of a gonorrheal infection. Report this condition with ICD-9-CM code 098.49. **Synonym(s):** *purulent ophthalmia.*

blepharorrhaphy Suture of a portion or all of the opposing eyelids to shorten the palpebral fissure or close it entirely.

blepharospasm Continuous, tonic spasm of the orbicularis oculi muscle, resulting in the eyelids being completely closed. Blepharospasm can be classified as essential, in which there is no abnormality of the eye or of the trigeminal nerve, or symptomatic, in which there is an associated eye lesion or trigeminal nerve abnormality. Report either with ICD-9-CM code 333.81.

blighted ovum Fertilized egg that fails to develop into a full-term fetus due to abnormality or degeneration of the zygote. Positive diagnosis consists of a positive pregnancy test, as well as identification of a blighted ovum on ultrasound. Blighted ovum is reported with ICD-9-CM code 631 as an abnormal product of conception. The blighted tissue may pass normally or require surgical intervention. **Synonym(s):** *anembryonic pregnancy.*

blind hypertensive eye Vision loss due to painful, high intraocular pressure.

blind loop syndrome Stasis of the intestine from many different causes that results in an overgrowth of bacteria in the small intestine. This can result from strictures, fistulae, diverticula, surgery, motility and acid secretion disturbances, or a chronic blockage in the intestine. It causes diarrhea, steatorrhea, weight loss, multiple vitamin deficiencies, and anemia. This syndrome is reported with ICD-9-CM code 579.2. **Synonym(s):** *bacterial overgrowth syndrome, stagnant loop syndrome, stasis syndrome.*

Bloch-Siemens syndrome Pigmented lesions appearing in linear, zebra stripe, and other configurations, preceded by vesicles and bullae and followed by verrucal lesions. Report this disorder with ICD-9-CM code 757.33. **Synonym(s):** *Block-Sulzberger syndrome.*

Block Device made of some form of heavy metal, such as Cerrobend, that is placed between the radiation beam

and a part of the patient's body for protection from the radiation beam.

Blocq's disease Type of hysterical ataxia in which the patient is able to move the legs normally when sitting or lying but is unable to walk or stand, reported with ICD-9-CM code 307.9. **Synonym(s):** *abasia-astasia.*

blood clot Semisolidified, coagulated mass of mainly platelets and fibrin in the bloodstream.

blood deductible Number of unreplaced pints of whole blood or units of packed red blood cells furnished to the patient for which the patient is responsible. The beneficiary is responsible for paying for the first three pints of blood used each calendar year unless they are replaced. The three-pint deductible applies to both Part A and Part B benefits. The Part A blood deductible is reduced to the extent that the blood deductible under Part B is satisfied.

blood patch Injection of a person's blood to close a cerebrospinal fluid leak in the dura of the spine. Report CPT code 62273 for the procedure and 01991 for anesthesia. **Synonym(s):** *clot patch.* **NCD Reference:** *10.5.*

blood transfusion Introduction of blood or blood products from another source into a vein or artery. **NCD References:** *110.7, 110.8.*

blood type Classification of blood by group.

Bloodgood's disease Multiple, benign cysts of the breast, colored brown or blue, caused by hyperplasia of the ductal epithelium. Occurs in women, usually after the age of 30. Bloodgood's disease is reported with ICD-9-CM code 610.1. **Synonym(s):** *Phocas' disease, Reclus syndrome, Schimmelbusch disease, Tillaux-Phocas disease.*

Bloom (-Machacek) (-Torre) syndrome Butterfly-shaped lesions on the face and hands, dolichocephalic skull and narrow face, and dwarfism with normal body proportions. Report this disorder with ICD-9-CM code 757.39.

Blount osteotomy Surgery to arrest unequal growth in the lower limbs. Epiphyseal arrest is accomplished by stapling across the growth plate. There are several CPT codes used to report this procedure based on how epiphyseal arrest is accomplished. See CPT codes 27455 and 27475-27485.

Blount plate Blade plate used in fixation surgery of the hip. The plate is easily bendable to adjust to the needed shape and angle of the hip. This term may be encountered in an operative note for reconstructive procedures of the hip.

Blount's disease Disease in children causing a lesion of the medial proximal epiphysis of the tibia. A lateral bowing or varus deformity of the tibia results in a bowlegged appearance. Report this condition with

ICD-9-CM code 732.4. **Synonym(s):** *osteochondrosis deformans tibia, tibia vara.*

Blount-Barber syndrome Bow-legs in children. Report this disorder with ICD-9-CM code 732.4.

blowout fracture Fracture of the orbital floor caused by a blow to the globe leaving the rim intact.

BLS *1)* Basic life support. *2)* Bureau of Labor Statistics.

blue baby Infant born with bluish discoloration due to cyanosis.

Blue Cross and Blue Shield Association Association that represents the common interests of Blue Cross and Blue Shield health plans. The BCBSA serves as the administrator for the Health Care Code Maintenance and also helps maintain the HCPCS Level II coding system. **Synonym(s):** *BCBSA.*

blue diaper syndrome Rare hereditary disorder of metabolism in which the nutrient, tryptophan, is not broken down completely or absorbed in the digestive tract. Bacterial action on the tryptophan in the intestines causes a bluish discoloration to appear in the urine, accompanied by fever, gastrointestinal (GI) disturbances, and visual disorders. Report this condition with ICD-9-CM code 270.0. **Synonym(s):** *Drummond's syndrome, tryptophan malabsorption.*

blue nevus Benign, usually solitary, dark blue to black neoplasm made up of melanocytes that presents as a somewhat firm, well defined, and rounded nodule. **Synonym(s):** *dermal melanocytoma, Jadassohn-Tièche nevus.*

blue toe syndrome Complication of pancreatitis characterized by tissue ischemia secondary to cholesterol crystal or atherothrombotic embolization, which leads to occlusion of small vessels that may present as cyanosis of digits, such as the toes. Report this disorder with ICD-9-CM code 445.02.

Blumensaat's line Normal, linear shadow on lateral x-rays of the knee evaluated in relation to the relative position of the patella.

blunt dissection Surgical technique used to expose an underlying area by separating along natural cleavage lines of tissue, without cutting. A blunt instrument or fingers are used to do this. This term is found in most surgery notes with no bearing on code selection.

BM Bowel movement.

BMAC Breath methylated alkane contour. Chemical marker in the breath that may indicate rejection of a transplanted heart. Testing for BMAC is reported with CPT code 0085T.

BMI Body mass index. Tool for calculating weight appropriateness in adults. The Centers for Disease Control and Prevention places adult BMIs in the following categories: below 18.5, underweight; 18.5-24.9, normal;

25.0-29.9 overweight; 30.0 and above, obese. BMI may be a factor in determining medical necessity for bariatric procedures, and can be reported with ICD-9-CM codes from the V85 rubric.

B-mode Implies two-dimensional procedure with two-dimensional display.

BMP Bone morphogenetic protein. Allograft typically used in treatment of long bone nonunion, for acceleration of fresh fracture repair, and for promoting bone growth in spinal fusions.

BMR Basal metabolic rate.

BMT

BMT is the acronym for bilateral myringotomy and tubes

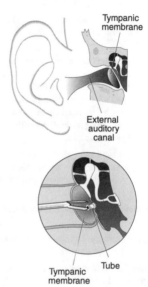

Tympanic membrane

External auditory canal

Tympanic membrane   Tube

BMT *1)* Bilateral myringotomy and tubes. Small tube placed through each eardrum to equalize pressure within the eustachian tube. BMT is reported with CPT code 69433 or 69436. These codes are considered bilateral, so no modifier should be appended. *2)* Bone marrow transplant.

BNO Bladder neck obstruction.

BO Body odor.

board certification Certification in a particular specialty based on the physician's demonstration of expertise and experience.

boarder Individual who receives lodging, such as a parent, caregiver, or other family member, who is not a patient but may wish or need to be near the patient.

boarder baby *1)* Newborn that remains in the nursery following discharge because the mother is still hospitalized. *2)* Premature infant who no longer needs intensive care but who remains for observation or to reach developmental milestones.

Bockhart's impetigo Superficial inflammation of the hair follicles most commonly caused by Staph aureus that manifests as rounded, sphere-shaped, pustular eruptions in the areas of the scalp, beard, underarms, extremities, and buttocks. This condition is reported with ICD-9-CM code 704.8. *Synonym(s): superficial folliculitis.*

Boder-Sedgwick syndrome Gonadal hypoplasia, insulin resistance and hyperglycemia, liver function problems, increased sensitivity to ionizing radiation, ataxia and nystagmus. Report this disorder with ICD-9-CM code 334.8. *Synonym(s): Louis-Bar syndrome.*

body casts Plaster mold that circumferentially encloses the trunk of the body. Report with CPT codes 29035-29046.

body mass index Tool for calculating weight appropriateness in adults. The Centers for Disease Control and Prevention places adult BMIs in the following categories: below 18.5, underweight; 18.5-24.9, normal; 25.0-29.9 overweight; 30.0 and above, obese. BMI may be a factor in determining medical necessity for bariatric procedures. *Synonym(s): BMI.*

body-rocking Disorders in which voluntary repetitive stereotyped movements, which are not due to any psychiatric or neurological condition, constitute the main feature.

Bohler reduction Traction method treats a closed fracture of the heel bone.

bonding In dentistry, two or more components connected by chemical adhesion or mechanical means.

bone conduction Transportation of sound through the bones of the skull to the inner ear. A bone conduction hearing aid consists of a typical hearing aid as well as an oscillator, which vibrates. The oscillator is placed against the mastoid bone and the sound vibration is then carried through the skull to both inner ears. For hearing aid examination and selection services, report CPT codes 92590-92595.

bone graft Bone that is removed from one part of the body and placed into another bone site without direct re-establishment of blood supply. Bone grafting is used in a variety of situations to help in healing and stabilizing surgical sites. Bone grafts are reported separately with CPT codes from 20900-20902 and 20930-20938 only when the grafting is not included as part of the primary procedure.

bone marrow Soft tissue found filling the cavities of bones, consisting of two types: yellow and red. Red bone marrow is a hematopoietic tissue that manufactures various cellular components of blood, such as platelets and red and white blood cells. Yellow marrow consists mostly of fat cells and is found in the medullary cavities of large bones. Bone marrow is a network of connective tissue of branching fibers forming a frame-like structure, filled with marrow cells. Bone marrow is harvested and transplanted for its progenitor or stem cells in cases of leukemia and other diseases. Marrow is used in spinal fusion to provide osteoprogenitor cells to mix with the allograft and form strong bone fusion. Bone marrow is biopsied to help diagnose many diseases of the blood, based on the distribution and formation of various blood cells. Bone marrow procedures are reported with CPT codes 38204-38242.

bone mass measurement Radiologic or radioisotopic procedure or other procedure approved by the FDA for identifying bone mass, detecting bone loss, or determining bone quality. The procedure includes a physician's interpretation of the results. Qualifying individuals must be an estrogen-deficient woman at clinical risk for osteoporosis with vertebral abnormalities. *NCD Reference: 150.3.*

bone spur Abnormal bony growth.

bones Hard, rigid tissue of the skeletal system made of both living organic cells and inorganic mineral components.

Bonnevie-Ullrich syndrome Short stature, webbed neck, congenital heart disease, and mental retardation. Report this disorder with ICD-9-CM code 758.6.

Bonnier's syndrome Ocular disturbances, deafness, nausea, thirst, anorexia, and symptoms resulting from a lesion of Deiters' nucleus and its connections. Report this disorder with ICD-9-CM code 386.19.

book of business Payer's list of clients and contracts.

BOOP Bronchiolitis obliterans with organizing pneumonia. Interstitial lung disease that often follows bronchiolitis obliterans. This condition is classified to ICD-9-CM code 516.8. An additional code for the organism may be identified if it is known.

Boostrix Brand name tetanus, diphtheria, acellular pertussis vaccine, for patients ages 10 to 18, provided in a single-dose vial or syringe. Supply of Boostrix is reported with CPT code 90715; administration is reported separately. The need for vaccination is reported with ICD-9-CM code V06.1.

boot top fracture Fracture involving the lower third of the tibia, occurring where the top of a ski boot would rest. Report ICD-9-CM code 823.20 for a closed fracture and 823.30 for an open fracture. *Synonym(s): skier's injury.*

borborygmus Abdominal gurgling sounds attributable to the passage of gas and fluids through the intestine.

Lactose intolerance, celiac disease, and irritable bowel syndrome are among the conditions that can cause excessive borborygmus.

borderline personality Disorder that is characterized by instability in behavior, mood, self-image, and interpersonal relationships that are intense, unstable, and may shift dramatically. The disorder is manifested by impulsive and unpredictable behavior or expressions of boredom, emptiness, or fear of being alone.

borderline psychosis of childhood Atypical infantile psychosis manifested by stereotyped repetitive movements, hyperkinesis, self-injury, retarded speech development, echolalia, or impaired social relationships, and is particularly common in those with mental retardation and is not as severe as infantile autism.

borderline schizophrenia Condition of eccentric or inconsequent behavior and anomalies of affect that give the impression of schizophrenia though no definite and characteristic schizophrenic anomalies, present or past, have been manifested.

Bornholm disease Illness caused by infection with the coxsackie virus, affecting children and young adults. Symptoms include fever, abdominal pain, headache, and paroxysmal chest pain typically worsened by breathing or coughing. Report this disease with ICD-9-CM code 074.1. *Synonym(s): epidemic pleurodynia.*

bortezomib Injectable chemotherapeutic drug used as a third-line treatment for multiple myeloma and in treatment of non-small cell lung cancer. Supply of bortezomib is reported with HCPCS Level II code J9041 and its administration is reported with CPT code 96409 or ICD-9-CM procedure code 99.25. Note that the volume of medication covered in the supply code is 0.1 mg. For a typical 3.5 mg single-dose vile of bortezomib, the total number of billing units would be 35. May be sold under the brand name VELCADE.

Boston exanthema Mild, febrile illness causing skin eruptions and rashes, caused by echovirus 16, named for an epidemic which occurred in Boston, Mass. Report this condition with ICD-9-CM code 048.

Bosworth fracture Fracture of the distal fibula and dislocation of the ankle due to external rotation of the supinated foot. Bosworth fracture is reported with the appropriate diagnostic code for the fibular fracture.

botryoid Shaped like a bunch of grapes, botryoid is a form of rhabdomyosarcoma that occurs in hollow organs, such as the bladder, vagina, and uterus, often seen in infants and toddlers. Report this disease with malignant neoplasm codes for connective tissue of the affected site. *Synonym(s): botryoid rhabdomyosarcoma.*

botulinum toxin Neurotoxin of the bacterium clostridium botulinum, used therapeutically in small doses to produce temporary paralysis of muscles to stop involuntary muscle contractions in conditions like blepharospasm, spasmatic torticollis, strabismus, and oromandibular and cervical dystonia. It works by inhibiting neurotransmission across nerve synapses. It is also used cosmetically to smooth wrinkles and off-label to treat hyperhidrosis. Because it is gradually broken down, injections need to be repeated every few months. Botox provides chemodenervation but is not a neurolytic. Supply is reported with HCPCS Level II code J0585. May be sold under the brand name Botox, Myobloc Botox.

botulism Uncommon but serious neuromuscular poisoning caused by the toxin *Clostridium botulinum.* Botulism occurs in three forms. Food-borne botulism is a result of ingesting foods containing the botulism toxin and is reported with ICD-9-CM code 005.1. Wound botulism, caused by a toxin produced from a wound infected with *Clostridium botulinum,* is frequently the result of a traumatic injury or a deep puncture wound. Often caused by abscess formation due to self-injected illegal drugs, its manifestations include neurologic symptoms with onset typically two weeks following the initial wound or trauma. Wound botulism is reported with ICD-9-CM code 040.42. Infant botulism is a result of consuming the spores of the botulinum bacteria, and occurs most often in infants less than six months of age. The spores colonize in the large intestine, frequently resulting in constipation and progressing to neuromuscular paralysis. Infant botulism is reported with ICD-9-CM code 040.41. All forms of botulism can be fatal, with life-threatening impairment of respiratory function one of the greatest complications.

botulism food poisoning Muscle-paralyzing neurotoxic disease caused by ingesting pre-formed toxin from the bacterium *Clostridium botulinum.* It causes vomiting and diarrhea, vision problems, slurred speech, difficulty swallowing, paralysis, and death. Report this disease with ICD-9-CM code 005.1.

Bouffée délirante Paranoid states apparently provoked by some emotional stress such as imprisonment, immigration, or strange and threatening environments; frequently manifested as an attack or threat.

bougie Probe used to dilate or calibrate a body part.

bounty system Situation in which individuals who report prohibited conduct on the part of a provider receive a percentage of any fines or penalties assessed against the provider.

Boutonneuse fever Acute, febrile, rickettsial disease transmitted by tick bites and causing a primary lesion at the site of the bite, with rash, muscle and joint pain, headache, chills, fever, and sensitivity to light. It is commonly found in the Mediterranean and around the Black and Caspian Seas, having many names depending on the geographical region. This condition is reported with ICD-9-CM code 082.1.

A-C

boutonniere defect Finger deformity that presents as flexion of the proximal interphalangeal joint and extension of the distal interphalangeal joint. Report with ICD-9-CM code 736.21.

boutonniere deformity Finger deformity with hyperextension of the distal joint and flexion of the interphalangeal joint.

boutonniere reconstruction Reconstruction of the central slip extensor tendon in the affected finger to allow extension of the proximal interphalangeal joint. Report with CPT codes 26426-26428. **Synonym(s):** *Fowler procedure, Littler procedure, Matav procedure.*

Bouveret (-Hoffmann) syndrome Rapid action of the heart with sudden onset and cessation. Report this disorder with ICD-9-CM code 427.2.

BOW Bag of waters.

bowel distress syndrome Abdominal pain, watery stools, and gas. Report this disorder with ICD-9-CM code 536.9.

bowel syndrome Hypoglycemia and malabsorption following surgery. Report this disorder with ICD-9-CM code 579.3.

Bower's arthroplasty Joint repair of the wrist done to treat rheumatoid arthritis or trauma of the distal radioulnar joint. The articular surface of the distal radius, as well as the ulna if it is severely involved, is removed, and a prosthetic piece is interposed. Report with CPT code 25332. **Synonym(s):** *hemi-resection interposition arthroplasty.*

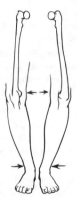

Bowleg

Genu vara (bowleg)

bowleg Condition in which the thighs and/or legs are bowed in an outward curve with an abnormally increased space between the knees. Report this condition with ICD-9-CM code 736.42 if acquired and 754.44 if congenital. **Synonym(s):** *genu varum, tibia vara.*

bowler's thumb Irritation of the lateral side of the thumb from holding the bowling ball. Results in flexor tendon irritation. Report the diagnosis with ICD-9-CM code 727.05.

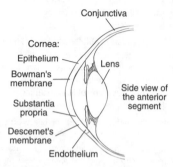

Bowman's Membrane

Conjunctiva

Cornea:
Epithelium
Bowman's membrane
Substantia propria
Descemet's membrane
Endothelium
Lens
Side view of the anterior segment

Bowman's membrane Corneal layer just under the epithelium and above the corneal stroma.

boxer's elbow Chip fracture (closed) on the tip of the olecranon process resulting from a fast extension of the elbow in a missed punch. Report the diagnosis with ICD-9-CM code 813.01.

boxer's fracture Fracture resulting from punching a hard surface, causing a break of the head of the fifth metacarpal with volar angulation. Report treatment as appropriate with CPT codes 26600-26615. Diagnosis is reported with ICD-9-CM code 815.04 for a closed fracture and 815.14 for an open fracture.

Boyd amputation Removal of the foot at the ankle level with fusion of the tibia and calcaneal bones. See CPT amputation codes 27880-27889 for appropriate selection.

Boyer cyst Cyst or enlargement within the subhyoid bursa, found in the tissue posterior to the hyoid bone in the throat. Boyer cyst is reported with ICD-9-CM code 478.79.

BP *1)* Blood pressure *2)* Business partner. Person or organization that performs a function or activity on behalf of a covered entity but that is not part of the covered entity's workforce. A business associate can also be a covered entity in its own right. **Synonym(s):** *BA, business associate.*

BPD *1)* Biliopancreatic diversion. Treatment for obesity in which three-quarters of the stomach is removed to restrict food intake and reduce acid output. The small intestine is divided, with one end attaching to the newly-reduced stomach. A biliopancreatic limb allows digestive juices to flow into the intestine for digestion. **Synonym(s):** *Scopinaro procedure.* **NCD Reference:** *100.1. 2)* Bronchopulmonary dysplasia. Complication seen in premature infants reported with ICD-9-CM code 770.7.

BPH Benign prostatic hyperplasia.

BPPV Benign positional paroxysmal vertigo. Common cause of dizziness that may be idiopathic or caused by neuritis, stroke, or trauma. BPPV is reported with ICD-9-CM code 386.11.

Br Breastfeeding.

brace Orthotic device that supports, in correct position, any moveable body part, and allows for limited movement. Medicare has a strict definition of a brace that includes only rigid or semirigid devices.

brachi(o)- Relating to the arm.

brachial plexus Large bundle of nerves originating in the C5 to T2 spinal segments, located in the neck, axilla, and subclavicular area, and an anatomic landmark and site of administration of medication for pain management. CPT codes 64415-64416, 64713, and 64861 pertain to services specific to the brachial plexus.

brachial plexus lesions Acquired defect in tissues along the network of nerves in the shoulder, causing corresponding motor and sensory dysfunction.

brachial plexus syndrome Anesthesias and vascular contraction in extremities caused by pressure of the brachial plexus and subclavian artery against the first thoracic rib. Report this disorder with ICD-9-CM code 353.0. *Synonym(s): Naffziger's syndrome.*

Brachmann-de Lange syndrome Congenital disorder presenting with impaired prenatal and postnatal development, mental retardation, microcephaly, and palmar crease, reported with ICD-9-CM code 759.89. *Synonym(s): de Lange's syndrome.*

brachy- Short.

brachycephaly Congenital deformity in which there is an abnormally broad head and a high forehead, associated with early closure of the coronal sutures. Brachycephaly is present in many syndromal abnormalities and is reported with ICD-9-CM code 756.0.

brachydactyly Congenital anomaly where digital underdevelopment results in short fingers. Brachydactyly can affect any component of a digit and can occur alone or with other anomalies. Report the diagnosis with ICD-9-CM code 755.29.

brachygnathia Congenital anomaly in which the lower jaw is abnormally short or recessed, reported with ICD-9-CM code 756.0. *Synonym(s): bird face.*

BrachySil Brand name liquid suspension injected into inoperable liver malignancy using a fine gauge needle. BrachySil is in clinical trials and has no specific codes assigned for supply or injection.

brachytherapy Form of radiation therapy in which radioactive pellets or seeds are implanted directly into the tissue being treated to deliver their dose of radiation in a more directed fashion and over a longer period of time. Brachytherapy provides radiation to the prescribed body area while minimizing exposure to normal tissue. The most common indications are for treatment of cancers of the prostate.

brady- Slow or prolonged.

bradycardia Slowed heartbeat, usually defined as a rate fewer than 60 beats per minute. Heart rhythm may be slow as a result of a congenital defect or an acquired problem.

bradycardia-tachycardia syndrome Rapid action of the heart followed by protracted or transient stopping of the heart. Report this disorder with ICD-9-CM code 427.81.

bradyphagia Abnormal slowness in eating.

bradypnea Abnormally slow respiratory rate, reported with ICD-9-CM code 786.09.

Braes PV10 Brand name device for delivering continuous positive airway pressure for treatment of obstructive sleep apnea. Supply is reported with HCPCS Level II code E0601.

Brailsford-Morquio syndrome Accumulation of mucopolysaccharide sulfates affecting the eye, ear, skin, teeth, skeleton, joints, liver, spleen, cardiovascular system, respiratory system, and central nervous system. Report this disorder with ICD-9-CM code 277.5.

brain ventricles Normally occurring communicating brain cavities: two lateral ventricles, third ventricle, and fourth ventricle.

Brandt's syndrome Zinc metabolism defect in young children with blisters, crusting, oozing eruptions, loss of hair, and diarrhea. Report this disorder with ICD-9-CM code 686.8. *Synonym(s): Danbolt syndrome.*

Brandt-Daroff exercise Self-therapy prescribed for benign positional paroxysmal vertigo. In Brandt-Daroff exercise, the patient systematically sits and lies on his side to displace canaliths in the inner ear. The canaliths may be the source of dizziness in the patient.

BRAO Branch retinal artery occlusion. Ocular stroke that presents with painless loss of vision in one eye, usually affecting only one segment of the visual field. A medical emergency, BRAO can lead to permanent vision loss. BRAO is reported with ICD-9-CM code 362.32. *Synonym(s): branch RAO.*

brass-founders' ague Fever caused by the vapors of certain metals, particularly zinc, copper, or magnesium. This condition is reported with ICD-9-CM code 985.8. *Synonym(s): braziers' chill, braziers' fever.*

brassy cough Respiratory illness in children that causes a hoarse voice and a brassy, barking cough. Doctors sometimes call it croup laryngotracheitis because it

A-C

usually involves inflammation of the larynx (voice box) and trachea (windpipe). Report this illness with ICD-9-CM code 464.20, 464.21, or 464.4. **Synonym(s):** *croup laryngotracheitis.*

BRAT diet Bananas, rice, applesauce, and toast. Diet commonly recommended for children suffering from diarrhea once solid foods can be tolerated.

Braun procedure Shoulder operation that consists of a tenotomy of the subscapularis tendon. Multiple tendons may be involved, in which the subscapularis and pectoralis major are released. Report CPT code 23405 for one tendon and 23406 for multiple tendons.

Bravelle Brand name fertility medication. Administered by injection, its active ingredient is urofollitropin. Supply of the drug is reported with HCPCS Level II code J3355.

Bravo pH-monitoring system used primarily for evaluating esophageal reflux, consisting of a capsule that is temporarily implanted into the esophageal mucosa using endoscopic or manometric guidance, which then records pH levels for up to 48 hours. Data are transmitted to a receiver worn by the patient and uploaded to a computer for professional analysis.

Braxton-Hicks contractions False form of labor, characterized by irregular, normally painless tightening of the uterine muscles that begin lightly and increase in frequency and intensity. The contractions are more regular and rhythmic during the late part of the last trimester and are sometimes mistaken for labor. **Synonym(s):** *false labor, Hicks sign, prelabor contractions.*

braziers' fever Fever caused by the vapors of certain metals, particularly zinc, copper, or magnesium. This condition is reported with ICD-9-CM code 985.8. **Synonym(s):** *brass-founders' ague, braziers' chill.*

BRBPR Bright red blood per rectum.

BrC Breast care.

BRCA 1 Gene that identifies the patient as at risk to develop breast cancer, ovarian cancer, or prostate cancer. A complete gene sequence analysis of BRCA 1 is reported with HCPCS Level II code S3818. Codes S3819-S3823 report other BRCA 1 and BRCA 2 analyses. CPT modifier 0A identifies genetic testing for BRCA 1.

BRCA 2 Gene that identifies the patient as at risk to develop breast cancer or ovarian cancer. A complete gene sequence analysis of BRCA 2 is reported with HCPCS Level II code S3819. Codes S3818 and S3820-S3823 report other BRCA 1 and BRCA 2 analyses. CPT modifier 0B identifies genetic testing for BRCA 2.

breakbone fever Acute, self-limiting disease lasting up to a week, spread by the Aedes mosquito infected with one of four dengue virus serotypes of the Flavivirus genus. The disease is found in the tropics and subtropics and causes fever, headache, muscle and joint pain, generalized aches, prostration, rash, enlarged lymph nodes, and leukopenia. The muscle and joint pain experienced can be so severe the bones feel as if they are breaking. Report breakbone fever with ICD-9-CM code 061. **Synonym(s):** *Aden fever, dandy fever, dengue fever.*

Breast Lift

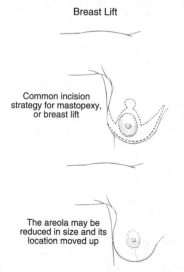

Common incision strategy for mastopexy, or breast lift

The areola may be reduced in size and its location moved up

breast lift Surgical procedure on the breast in which the nipple and areola are relocated to a higher position and the excess skin below the nipple and above the lower breast crease is excised. Report this procedure with ICD-9-CM procedure code 85.6 or CPT code 19316. **Synonym(s):** *mastopexy.*

breast microcalcification Tiny build-up of calcium in the breast. It cannot be felt but it can be seen on a mammogram. A cluster of these very small specks of calcium may mean that cancer is present. Report this condition with ICD-9-CM code 793.81.

breast moulage Configuration and molding of a breast model used to construct a custom breast implant.

Breech Presentation

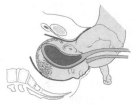

Obstetric forceps provide traction, rotation, or both to the birthing head and designs vary to accomplish specific tasks (e.g., Kielland forceps to rotate the head). Low forceps is application when the skull is at station plus 2 or lower; mid forceps is application above station plus 2; high forceps is application at point of engagement

breech presentation Abnormal condition in which the fetal buttocks present first. In frank breech, the legs of the fetus extend over the abdomen and thorax so that the feet lie beside the face. In complete breech, the legs are flexed and crossed, while incomplete breech presents with one or both lower legs and feet prolapsed into the vagina. If the fetus is not successfully converted to a cephalic (head-first) position before delivery, it is reported with an ICD-9-CM code from subcategory 652.2. When successful version occurs, it is reported with a code from subcategory 652.1. When occurring in multiple gestations, report with a code from subcategory 652.6. A breech extraction without mention of indication is reported with a code from subcategory 669.6. Breech pregnancies are often delivered by cesarean section. *Synonym(s): buttocks presentation, footling presentation.*

Brennemann's syndrome Lymphadenitis in the mesentery and retroperitoneal area as a sequela of throat infection. Report this disorder with ICD-9-CM code 289.2.

Brethine Brand name for terbutaline sulfate, a bronchodilator administered for treatment of bronchospasms associated with asthma, bronchitis, and emphysema. Supply of Brethine when injected subcutaneously is reported with HCPCS Level II code J3105.

brevicollis Congenital condition in which fusion of existing cervical vertebrae and the absence of at least one cervical vertebra result in a short, wide neck. Associated with a high rate of malformations or syndromes, brevicollis is reported with ICD-9-CM code 756.16.

brick dust urine Presence of precipitated urates in acidic urine.

bridge Connection between two parts of an organ or body part.

Brinkerhoff speculum Device inserted into the rectum for viewing its interior walls.

Briquet's (Brissaud-Marie) syndrome Personality disorder involving concurrent alcoholism and somatization whereby the patient reports physical complaints absent of medical indication, more prevalent among women Report this disorder with ICD-9-CM code 300.81.

Briquet's disorder Chronic, but fluctuating, neurotic disorder that begins early in life and is characterized by recurrent and multiple somatic complaints for which medical attention is sought but that are not due to any apparent physical illness.

brisement injection Dilute anesthetic infused into a tendon sheath to break up adhesions. It is performed under ultrasonic guidance. The injection is reported with CPT code 20550 or 20551; ultrasound guidance would be reported separately.

Brissaud-Meige syndrome Hypothyroidism resulting from acquired injury of thyroid gland or presence of cretinism. Report this disorder with ICD-9-CM code 244.9.

Bristow procedure Anterior capsulorrhaphy prevents chronic separation of the shoulder. In this procedure, the bone block is affixed to the anterior glenoid rim with a screw.

BRM Biological response modifier.

broad ligament Fold of peritoneum extending from the side of the uterus to the wall of the pelvis.

Broca's aphasia Telegraphic, slow, and labored speech due to an abnormality in the circle of Willis.

Brock's operation Surgical relief of pulmonary valvular stenosis by passing a valvulotome through the wall of the right ventricle into the pulmonary artery .

Brock's syndrome Incomplete expansion of the right middle lobe of a lung with chronic pneumonitis. Report this disorder with ICD-9-CM code 518.0.

Brocq's lupoid sycosis Miliary abscesses in the scalp's hair follicles, resulting in scars and bald patches. Brocq's lupoid sycosis is reported with ICD-9-CM code 704.09. *Synonym(s): acne decalvans, Arnozan's syndrome, Quinquaud's syndrome.*

bromhidrosis Chronic condition in which the skin emits an excessive odor that is typically unpleasant. Most commonly originating in the axillary region, bromhidrosis may also occur in the regions of the genitals or feet. Report bromhidrosis with ICD-9-CM code 705.89. *Synonym(s): body odor, bromidrosis.*

bromocriptine Drug that lowers the level of prolactin to increase fertility. Bromocriptine may also be used to treat Parkinson's disease and to reduce or prevent the production of breast milk. May be sold under the brand name Parlodel.

brompheniramine maleate Antihistamine used to treat hay fever, pruritic rashes, or allergic reactions to insect bites. Supply is reported with HCPCS Level II code J0945. May be sold under the brand name Nasahist B.

bronchial murmur Breath sounds with a high pitch like that of blowing through a tube. Bronchial murmur may indicate areas of consolidated or compressed lung.

bronchiectasis Dilation of the bronchi due to infection or chronic conditions. Bronchiectasis causes diminished lung capacity and frequent infections of the lung. Report this condition with ICD-9-CM category 494.

bronchiolitis Inflammation of the finer subbranches of the bronchial tree due to infectious agents or irritants. Most commonly a disease of children, symptoms include cough with differing productions of sputum, fever, and lung rales. Bronchiolitis is reported with a code from ICD-9-CM subcategory 466.1.

bronchiolitis obliterans Interstitial lung disease characterized by a chronic scarring process in which connective tissue from the wall of the terminal bronchioles encroaches out into the airspace, obstructing the lumen. The process is usually irreversible and may occur with heart-lung transplants, organizing pneumonia, or after an acute case of pneumonia in children. Report this condition with ICD-9-CM code 491.8, 516.8, or 996.84. *Synonym(s): bronchiolitis fibrosa obliterans.*

bronchitis Inflammation of the main branches of the bronchial tree. Symptoms include cough, production of sputum, fever, and lung rales, unspecified bronchitis is reported with ICD-9-CM code 490. Acute bronchitis is reported with ICD-9-CM code 466.0.

broncho- Relating to the trachea.

bronchogenic carcinoma Large group of carcinomas of the lung, originating from the epithelium of the bronchial tree, with four primary subtypes: adenocarcinoma of the lung, large cell carcinoma, small cell carcinoma, and squamous cell carcinoma. Report bronchogenic carcinoma with a code from ICD-9-CM category 162.

bronchography Radiography of the lung.

bronchoplasty Reconstruction or plastic repair of the bronchus.

bronchoscope Endoscopic instrument used for the diagnosis, inspection, and treatment of the tracheobronchial tree.

bronchoscopy Endoscopic procedure used for the diagnosis, inspection, and treatment of the tracheobronchial tree. The diagnostic procedure alone is reported with CPT code 31622 and includes the use of fluoroscopic guidance. Report other bronchoscopy services with CPT codes 31623-31656.

bronchospirochetosis Chronic bronchitis occurring with the coughing up of blood, caused by a spirochetal infection. Report this condition with ICD-9-CM code 104.8. *Synonym(s): bronchopulmonary spirochetosis, Castellani's bronchitis, hemorrhagic bronchitis.*

Brooke's disease Benign skin disease most commonly occurring on the face, around the eyelids, and on the scalp. The lesions form firm, flesh-colored, translucent papules with slight surface telangiectasia; small lesions may coalesce to form a solid sheet tumor. This is reported as a benign neoplasm of the skin.

broom-stick cast Special type of hip spica cast applied specifically for Legg-Perthes disease or osteochondrosis of the femoral epiphysis. It holds the leg in abduction to assist with ambulation. Application is reported with CPT code 29305 for one leg or 29325 for both legs or 1 12 hip spica. *Synonym(s): Petrie spica cast.*

Brostrom procedure Surgical repair of a sprained ankle.

brow presentation Extension of the neck with presentation of the brow or face of the fetus first during delivery, rather than the top of the head presenting with face down. This condition is reported with a code from ICD-9-CM subcategory 652.4. *Synonym(s): mentum presentation.*

Brown set Brand name trigeminal ganglion microcompression set using a balloon catheter for the treatment of trigeminal neuralgia.

brown spot syndrome Patchy skin pigmentation, endocrine dysfunctions and polyostotic fibrous dysplasia. Report this disorder with ICD-9-CM code 756.59. *Synonym(s): Albright syndrome, Albright's hereditary osteodystrophy.*

Brown's tendon sheath syndrome Limited elevation of eye, marked by paresis of inferior oblique muscle. Report this disorder with ICD-9-CM code 378.61.

Browne's operation Hypospadias is repaired with a strip of epithelium left on the top of the penis to form a top of the urethra. Margins of the incision are used to form the bottom.

Brown-Séquard syndrome Paraplegia and anesthesia over part of the body caused by lesions in the brain or spinal cord. Report this disorder with ICD-9-CM code 344.89. *Synonym(s): Avellis syndrome, Babinski-Nageotte syndrome, Benedikt's syndrome, Cestan-Chenais syndrome, Cestan's syndrome, Foville's syndrome, Gubler-Millard syndrome, Jackson's syndrome, Weber-Leyden syndrome.*

BRP *1)* Bathroom, private. *2)* Bathroom privileges.

brucellosis Infection in humans caused by the bacterium brucella, a gram-negative, aerobic, coccobacilli microorganism, conveyed by contact with infected animals via infected meat and unpasteurized milk or cheese. Symptoms include fever, chills, sweating, weakness, fatigue, weight loss, aches, and abdominal pain. The various species or sub-classes of brucellosis are based on the host animal: sheep, goat, cattle, pigs, or dogs. Brucellosis is reported with a code from ICD-9-CM category 023. *Synonym(s): cyprus fever, malta fever, Mediterranean fever, rock fever, undulant fever.*

Bruch's membrane Transparent inner layer of the choroid that comes in contact with the pigmented layer of the retina. *Synonym(s): basal lamina, complexus basalis choroideae, lamina basalis choroideae, vitreal lamina.*

Bruck-de Lange syndrome Congenital cerebral condition involving dwarfism, mental deficiency, and brachycephaly. Report this disorder with ICD-9-CM code 759.89.

Brudzinski's sign Indication of meningitis wherein neck flexion often results in flexion of the hip and knee.

Brugada syndrome Congenital heart anomaly in which the hypertrophy (enlargement) is localized to the left ventricle. Report this disorder with ICD-9-CM code 746.89.

Brugsch's syndrome Increased thickening of the skin on extremities and face with clubbing of fingers and deformities in bones of the limb. Report this disorder with ICD-9-CM code 757.39.

bruising syndrome Bruising occurring easily, involving surrounding tissues resulting in pain, frequently found in women. Report this disorder with ICD-9-CM code 287.2.

brush Tool used to gather cell samples or clean a body part.

Brushfield spots Small, elevated, white spots on the periphery of the iris arranged in a ring concentric with the pupil. These spots are sometimes present in children with Down syndrome. As an asymptomatic sign, Brushfield spots are not reported separately. Down syndrome is reported with ICD-9-CM code 758.0. *Synonym(s): speckled iris.*

bruxism Involuntary clenching or grinding of the teeth, usually while asleep, often stemming from repressed anger, tension, stress, fear, or frustration. Bruxism results in symptoms of temporomandibular joint disease such as jaw pain, headaches, earaches, and damaged teeth. Report bruxism with ICD-9-CM code 306.8.

Bryant traction Application of a pulling force along the main axis of a body structure. Bryant traction is overhead vertical traction applied for the treatment of femoral shaft fractures, especially in infants and young children at risk of limb ischemia from lack of perfusion.

BS *1)* Bachelor of surgery. *2)* Bowel sounds. *3)* Breath sounds.

BSA Body surface area.

BSC Bedside commode.

B-scan Method of diagnostic ultrasound using two-dimensional scanning to produce two-dimensional measurements and display of images. For instance, in ophthalmic ultrasound, high-frequency sound waves from a transducer placed directly on the eye are used. The two-dimensional images created of the internal eye help to locate structures that may be obscured by cataract, hemorrhages, or opacities, as well as provide information about a lesion's shape and relation to neighboring structures. B-scan may be used in diagnostic imaging on many different areas of the body and is coded accordingly.

BSD Bedside drainage.

BSE Bovine spongiform encephalopathy. *Synonym(s): mad cow disease.*

BSN Bachelor of Science, Nursing.

BSS Balanced salt solution. Solution used in ocular surgery. Its use is inherent in many anterior segment procedures and may also be used for irrigation in various ear, nose, or throat procedures.

BTE Behind the ear.

BTT Bridge to transplant. Transplant or assist device that represents an interim therapy until a permanent transplant can be made. For example, an artificial heart can be a BTT until a donor heart can be found for a patient. The FDA has separate rules for clinical trials for BTTs than for permanent devices. *NCD Reference: 20.9.*

bubbly lung syndrome Intrauterine fetal aspiration of amniotic fluid contaminated by meconium. Report this disorder with ICD-9-CM code 770.7.

bubonic plague Highly contagious, most common form of plague, caused by infection of Yersinia pestis. It is characterized by onset of fever, chills, headache, and swollen, tender, inflamed lymph glands called buboes, which develop intravascular coagulation, turning necrotic and gangrenous. Report this condition with ICD-9-CM code 020.0. *Synonym(s): black death, glandular plague, pestis bubonica.*

buccal Relating to or toward the cheek. *b. frenum* Band of mucosal membrane that connects the alveolar (dental) ridge to the cheek, separating the lip vestibule from the cheek vestibule. *b. mucosa* Tissue from the mucous membrane on the inside of the cheek. *b. vestibule* Space in the mouth between the cheek and the teeth and gums.

Buchem's syndrome Multiple fractures and bowing of all extremities, thickening of skull bones, and osteoporosis beginning in childhood. Report this disorder with ICD-9-CM code 733.3.

Buck traction Type of skin traction of the extremities maintained by using an apparatus such as a special splint, applied by dressings to the affected body part.

Buck traction may be used on burn patients to hold the arm in a suspended upward position to prevent swelling, reduce skin shrinkage, and allow for greater range of motion with healing.

bucket-handle fracture Break of the anterior pubis and the opposite ilium in a vertical shear. This type of fracture is coded to multiple fractures of the pelvis with disruption of the pelvic circle, reported with ICD-9-CM code 808.43 if closed or 808.53 if open or individual fractures of the pubis and ilium. See ICD-9-CM codes 808.2 and 808.3 for the pubis and 808.41 and 808.51 for the ilium.

Bucket-Handle Tear

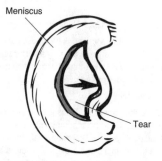

Meniscus

Tear

bucket-handle tear Disruption in the meniscus of the knee that resembles the half circle curvature of a bucket handle. Current tears on the lateral meniscus are reported with ICD-9-CM code 717.41 while old tears of this type in the medial meniscus or unspecified cartilage are reported with 717.0.

Budd-Chiari syndrome Thrombus or other obstruction of the hepatic vein, with an enlarged liver, intractable ascites, portal hypertension, and the growth of extensive collateral vessels. This syndrome is reported with ICD-9-CM code 453.0. *Synonym(s): hepatic vein thrombus.*

budesonide Respiratory and nasal antiinflammatory corticosteroid used to treat seasonal rhinitis and to prevent nasal polyp regrowth after surgery. It is also used as a prophylactic for asthma treatment. Supply is reported with HCPCS Level II codes J7626, J7627, and J7633. May be sold under the brand name Pulmicort Turbohaler, Rhinocort Aqua.

Büdinger-Ludloff-Läwen syndrome Old disruption of ligaments in the knee. Report this disorder with ICD-9-CM code 717.89.

bulbar syndrome Paralysis-based symptoms from defects in the medulla oblongata. Report this disorder with ICD-9-CM code 335.22. *Synonym(s): Duchenne's syndrome.*

bulbourethral glands Periurethral glands on each side of the prostate gland that secrete a component of the seminal fluid and are connected to the urethra by ducts. *Synonym(s): Cowper's glands.*

bulimia Episodic pattern of overeating (binge eating) followed by purging or extreme exercise accompanied by an awareness of the abnormal eating pattern with a fear of not being able to stop eating.

bulla Large, elevated, membranous sac or blister on the skin containing serous or seropurulent fluid. Assign ICD-9-CM code 709.8 for this condition. Bullae are usually treated by incision and drainage or puncture aspiration; report with CPT code 10160.

bullet Under the 1997 E/M guidelines, each physical examination element is commonly referred to as a bullet point or bullet.

Bullis fever Tick-borne, rickettsial disease transmitted by the tick Amblyomma americanum, observed in soldiers who had been at Camp Bullis, Texas. Marked by very low leukocyte count with neutropenia, headache, and constant lymphadenitis. Report Bullis fever with ICD-9-CM code 082.8. *Synonym(s): Lone Star fever.*

bullous keratopathy Corneal degeneration characterized by recurring epithelial blisters that rupture and expose corneal nerves, causing extreme pain. This can occur in conditions such as glaucoma, iridocyclitis, and Fuchs' epithelial dystrophy. Bullous keratopathy is reported with ICD-9-CM code 371.23.

Bumex Brand name for bumetanide, a diuretic indicated in the treatment of hypertension and heart and liver disease. Supply is reported with HCPCS Level II code S0171.

bumper fracture Break resulting from direct force to the tibial tuberosity such as that exerted by a car bumper hitting the leg. The force can result in a fracture of the tibia or femur. Code selection is based on the bone sustaining the fracture.

BUN Blood urea nitrogen. Blood test performed on a venipuncture sample to measure the amount of urea nitrogen in the blood. The primary indication for this test is to evaluate kidney function. An elevated BUN level can indicate kidney disease, although elevations may also be caused by dehydration, congestive heart failure, myocardial infarction, or intestinal bleeding.

bundle of His Bundle of modified cardiac fibers that begins at the atrioventricular node and passes through the right atrioventricular fibrous ring to the interventricular septum, where it divides into two branches. Bundle of His recordings are taken for intracardiac electrograms. *NCD Reference: 20.13.*

bundle of Kent syndrome Muscular bundle forming a direct connection between the ventricle and atrial walls. Report this disorder with ICD-9-CM code 426.7.

bundled *1)* Gathering of several types of health insurance policies under a single payer. *2)* Inclusive grouping of codes related to a procedure when submitting a claim.

bundling Including all services provided on the day of outpatient surgery on one bill. These services typically include nursing, technical personnel, facility use, drugs, biologicals, surgical dressings, supplies, splints, casts, appliances, equipment, diagnostic or therapeutic items and services, blood and blood plasma, platelets, and materials for anesthesia.

Bunion

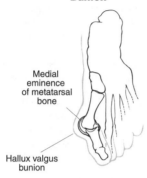

Medial eminence of metatarsal bone

Hallux valgus bunion

bunion Displacement of the first metatarsal bone outward with a simultaneous displacement of the great toe away from the mid-line toward the smaller toes. This causes a bony prominence of the joint of the great toe on the inside (medial) margin of the forefoot, termed a bunion. A large inflamed bursa is often noted and can be accompanied by osteophytes. Bunion is reported with ICD-9-CM code 727.1. A bunion is not synonymous with hallux valgus; there are separate diagnosis codes for hallux valgus, depending on whether it is acquired or congenital. CPT does not make this distinction for correctional procedures and classifies all bunion repairs as correction of hallux valgus; report with CPT codes 28290-28299 per technique.

bunionectomy Surgical removal of a bony prominence (exostosis) on the head of the first metatarsal. Simple bunionectomy or exostectomy is referred to as a Silver procedure and is reported as a correction of hallux valgus, CPT code 28290.

bunionette Deformity of the fifth metatarsal head resulting in lateral enlargement of the little toe or a dorsal malposition of the first metatarsal. This deformity is reported with ICD-9-CM code 727.1.

bunkbed fracture Intra-articular fracture that occurs in children at the base of the first metatarsal. Report the diagnosis with ICD-9-CM code 825.25 if the fracture is closed and 825.35 if open.

Bunnell procedure Surgical procedure that restores active flexion of the elbow by transferring the latissimus dorsi muscle to the arm and anchoring it to the radial head. Report with CPT code 24301.

Bunnell suture Common technique used for tendon repair that resembles a figure-eight zigzag.

buphthalmos Congenital glaucoma resulting in distended and enlarged fibrous coatings of the eye from the increased intraocular pressure. Buphthalmos is reported with a code from ICD-9-CM subcategory 743.2. *Synonym(s): hydrophthalmos, megophthalmos.*

bupivacaine HCl Anesthetic agent used to produce local or regional anesthesia for surgical and dental procedures. Supply is reported with HCPCS Level II code S0020. May be sold under the brand name Marcaine, Sensorcaine.

buprenorphine HCl Schedule V controlled narcotic used to relieve pain and as an adjunct to surgical anesthesia. Supply is reported with HCPCS Level II code J0592. May be sold under the brand name Buprenex, Subutex.

bupropion HCl Drug used to treat depression and as an aide to smoking cessation. Supply is reported with HCPCS Level II code S0106. May be sold under the brand name Wellbutrin, Wellbutrin SR, Wellbutrin XL, Zyban.

BUR Back-up rate (ventilator).

Burch Procedure

1. A common approach involves placing sutures from pubic bone to paraurethral tissues

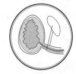

2. The urethrovesical angle is elevated and continence restored

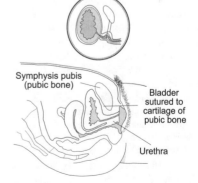

Symphysis pubis (pubic bone)

Bladder sutured to cartilage of pubic bone

Urethra

Burch procedure Surgical procedure to correct urinary stress incontinence in which the bladder is suspended

A-C

A-C

by placing several sutures through the tissue surrounding the urethra and into the vaginal wall. The sutures are pulled tight so that the tissues are tacked up to the symphysis pubis and the urethra is moved forward. This procedure is normally reported with CPT code 51840; if the procedure is performed for the second time or if some other factor increases the time or level of complexity, report with 51841.

Bürger-Grütz syndrome Abdominal pain, hepatosplenomegaly, pancreatitis, and eruptive xanthomas in a genetic condition. Report this disorder with ICD-9-CM code 272.3.

Burgess amputation Long posterior flap is preserved to cover the incision to amputate the leg below the knee.

buried bumper syndrome Peritubal leakage, infection, abdominal pain, or resistance to infusion related to a percutaneous gastrostomy tube. The symptoms are caused by partial or complete overgrowth of gastric mucosa over the internal flange, or bumper, of the feeding tube. Buried bumper syndrome is reported with ICD-9-CM code 536.49.

buried suture Continuous or interrupted suture placed under the skin for a layered closure.

Burke's syndrome Chronic neutropenia with pancreatic insufficiency resulting in obstruction of mucosal passageways, poor growth, chronic bronchitis, recurrent pneumonia, emphysema, clubbing of fingers, and salt depletion with abnormal secretions in exocrine glands. Report this disorder with ICD-9-CM code 577.8. *Synonym(s): Clarke-Hadfield syndrome.*

Burkitt's lymphoma Malignancy of the lymphatic system, most often seen as a large bone-deteriorating lesion within the jaw or as an abdominal mass. The Epstein-Barr herpes virus is known to be associated with this type of lymphoma. *Synonym(s): Burkitt's tumor, malignant lymphoma.*

Burnett's syndrome Disorder of the kidneys induced by ingestion of large amounts of alkali and calcium. Reversible in the early stages, but can lead to renal failure. Report this disorder with ICD-9-CM code 275.42.

Burnier's syndrome Dwarfism resulting from malfunction of the pituitary gland. Report this disorder with ICD-9-CM code 253.3. *Synonym(s): Levi syndrome, Lorain-Levi syndrome.*

burning feet syndrome Severe discomfort of the feet and other extremities with excessive sweating and elevated skin temperature, and believed to be caused by a riboflavin deficiency. Report this disorder with ICD-9-CM code 266.2. *Synonym(s): Gopalan's syndrome.*

burr Specialized surgical drill used to shape or make holes in bones or gain access into the cranium. Use of a burr has no bearing on coding, as this is a surgeon's instrument.

Burrow's operation In a skin flap procedure, triangles of skin at the base of the pedicle of the flap are excised to achieve advancement.

burrowing flea disease Disease spread by the parasitic flea, Tunga penetrans, the pregnant female of which burrows into the host's skin, often the lower limbs and under nails, causing inflammation, swelling, and cyst formation that turns ulcerative. Gas gangrene, bacteremia, or tetanus may occur in cases of severe infestation, as well as spontaneous loss of a digit. Report this condition with ICD-9-CM code 134.1. *Synonym(s): chigoe disease, jigger disease, sand flea disease.*

bursa Cavity or sac containing fluid that occurs between articulating surfaces and serves to reduce friction from moving parts. An anatomical structure frequently referenced in orthopedic notes as it may become diseased or need removal.

bursectomy Surgical excision of a bursa, a fluid-filled cavity or sac that reduces friction between neighboring, moving parts. A variety of bursectomies are listed in CPT by site (e.g., 24105 olecranon, 25115-25116 wrist, 27060-27062 hip, and 27340 knee).

bursitis Inflammation of the fluid-filled cavity or sac that reduces friction between neighboring, moving parts. Diagnosis codes for this are reported based on the involved area.

bursolith Concentration of minerals, such as calcium deposits, or a calculus within the bursa of a joint. Report the diagnosis with ICD-9-CM code 727.82.

bursotomy Incision into the bursa of a joint, the fluid-filled cavity or sac that reduces friction between neighboring, moving parts. A bursotomy is usually included in all intra-articular surgery and is not reported separately. When performed alone to drain an infected joint bursa, select the CPT code for incision and drainage of bursa by joint.

bursting fracture Fracture resulting in multiple bone fragments and most often seen in the first cervical vertebra.

Burton sign Blue streak seen along the gum line in patients with lead poisoning. If the sign is present, but there is no notation of poisoning, do not code lead toxicity based on a positive sign alone. Documentation of the diagnosis must be made. Lead toxicity is reported with the appropriate ICD-9-CM code from 984.0-984.9. *Synonym(s): lead line.*

BUS Bartholin urethra Skene's.

Buschke's disease Systemic disease characterized by excess fibrotic collagen build-up, turning the skin thickened and hard. Fibrotic changes also occur in various organs and cause vascular abnormalities and affect more women than men. Report this condition with ICD-9-CM code 710.1.

business associate Person or organization that performs a function or activity on behalf of a covered entity but that is not part of the covered entity's workforce. A business associate can also be a covered entity in its own right. *Synonym(s): BA, BP, business partner.*

business coalition Employers who form a cooperative to purchase health care less expensively.

business model Model of a business organization or process.

business partner Person or organization that performs a function or activity on behalf of a covered entity but that is not part of the covered entity's workforce. A business associate can also be a covered entity in its own right. *Synonym(s): BA, BP, business associate.*

business relationships "Agent" is often used to describe a person or organization that assumes some of the responsibilities of another one. This term has been avoided in the final rules so that a more HIPAA-specific meaning could be used for business associate. The term "business partner (BP)" was originally used for business associate. A third-party administrator (TPA) is a business associate that performs claims administration and related business functions for a self-insured entity. Under HIPAA, a health care clearinghouse is a business associate that translates data to or from a standard format on behalf of a covered entity. The HIPAA security NPRM used the term "chain-of-trust agreement" to describe the type of contract that would be needed to extend the responsibility to protect health care data across a series of subcontractual relationships. While a business associate is an entity that performs certain business functions, a trading partner is an external entity, such as a customer, with which one does business. This relationship can be formalized via a trading partner agreement. It is quite possible to be a trading partner of an entity for some purposes, and a business associate of that entity for other purposes.

busulfan Alkylating antineoplastic used to treat chronic myelocytic leukemia as part of a conditioning regime prior to hematopoietic progenitor cell transplantation in patients with chronic myelogenous leukemia. Oral supply is reported with HCPCS Level II code J8510. May be sold under the brand name Myleran.

butorphanol tartrate Schedule IV controlled substance used to relieve pain and to enhance anesthesia. It is also given to patients in labor. Supply is reported with HCPCS Level II codes J0595 and S0012. May be sold under the brand names Butorphanol Tartrate Nasal Spray, Stadol NS.

butterfly fracture Comminuted fracture in which a piece of bone breaks from either side of a main fragment, resembling a butterfly and coded to the specific fracture site based on radiographic evidence.

buttress Device used for stabilization or support that is built out from a structure.

bx Biopsy.

bypass Auxiliary or diverted route to maintain continuous flow. *b. graft:* Surgically created alternative blood vessel used to reroute blood flow around an area of obstruction or disease.

Bywaters' syndrome Traumatic anuria (lack of urinary secretion) following crushing injury, especially of kidneys. Report this disorder with ICD-9-CM code 958.5.

c With.

C *1)* Centigrade. *2)* Cervical vertebrae. *3)* Complements.

C&S Culture and sensitivity.

c.m. Tomorrow morning.

c.n. Tomorrow night.

C/A/Ox3 Conscious, alert, and oriented to person, place, and time. Description of the patient's mental status at the time of the encounter. Documentation of x1 or x2 indicates disorientation. In some cases, the documentation will state x4, which indicates the patient is also oriented to the cause of the immediate medical emergency.

c/m Counts per minute.

c/o Complaints of.

C/S Cesarean section.

CA *1)* Cancer. *2)* Calcium. *3)* HCPCS Level II modifier, for use with CPT codes, that indicates when a procedure payable only in the inpatient setting is performed emergently on an outpatient who expires before admission. The procedure reported must be considered an inpatient service, as identified with status indicator C in the outpatient prospective payment system. The patient must have died without being admitted as an inpatient.

ca in situ Malignant neoplasm arising from the vessels, glands, and organs that has not spread to neighboring tissues.

CA15-3 Tumor marker consisting of oncofetal antigen expressed by carcinomas, including breast cancer. It is a common focus of testing for recurrence of breast cancer and prognosis. Non-cancerous conditions associated with elevated CA15-3 include benign breast or ovarian disease, endometriosis, pelvic inflammatory disease, and hepatitis. *NCD Reference: 190.29.*

CA19-9 Tumor marker consisting of oncofetal antigen expressed most commonly by gastrointestinal tract cancers. It is a common focus of testing for recurrence of tumors and to determine prognosis. *NCD Reference: 190.30.*

A-C

CABG

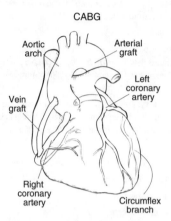

Labels on diagram: Aortic arch, Arterial graft, Left coronary artery, Vein graft, Right coronary artery, Circumflex branch

Schematic of a single vein graft bypass

Venous grafts typically are harvested from the saphenous vein, although other sites may also be used. Harvest and vein preparation is included in this series of codes

CABG Coronary artery bypass graft. Diversion of the blood supply to the heart around an occluded portion of a coronary artery by anastomosing a section of harvested vein, artery, combined arterial-venous graft, or prosthetic conduit. The graft is placed between the aorta and the blocked coronary artery, distal to the obstruction in the coronary artery to permit revascularization of the heart. Grafting codes for coronary artery bypass are reported under subcategory 36.1 in ICD-9-CM. ICD-9-CM procedure codes are selected based on the number of coronary arteries being bypassed and the type of graft used. These bypass codes are found in CPT range 33510-33536. CPT codes are selected by the type and number of grafts used. Combined arterial venous grafting requires that two codes be reported: one for the combined graft and one for the arterial graft. Harvesting of veins or arteries is included in the work description for the bypass procedure with a few exceptions: harvesting an upper extremity vein or artery, or a femoropopliteal vein segment are reported in addition to the bypass.

cabulance Taxicab that also functions as an ambulance.

CAC Certified alcoholism counselor.

cac(i)/(o)- Diseased or bad.

cachexia Severe state of wasting manifested by malnutrition, weakness, and loss of weight and muscle mass. Cachexia is often indicative of an underlying disease such as cancer, autoimmune disorder, or infectious disease. Cachexia alone is reported with ICD-9-CM code 799.4.

CACI Computer-assisted continuous infusion.

CAD *1)* Computer aided detection. Traditional radiology replaced with digitized images and software searches for abnormalities within the images. *2)* Coronary artery disease.

cadaver Dead body.

Cafcit See caffeine citrate.

café au lait spots Hyperpigmented skin lesions that are often the initial signs of neurofibromatosis. Lesions vary in size, number, and color, and may have even or asymmetrical borders. The spots typically develop in early infancy. Report this condition with ICD-9-CM code 709.09.

cafeteria plan Employer's offer of various services of many payers as separate elements in a health care plan.

caffeine citrate Drug used to treat apnea in premature infants 28-33 weeks gestation at birth. Caffeine is a bronchodilator, smooth muscle relaxant, central nervous system and cardiac stimulant, and diuretic. Supply is reported with HCPCS Level II code J0706. May be sold under the brand name Cafcit.

Caffey's syndrome Soft tissue swelling over the affected bones, irritability, and fever, and running periods of exacerbation and remission. Report this disorder with ICD-9-CM code 756.59.

CAH Critical Access Hospital, as designated by CMS.

caisson disease Decompression sickness caused by rapid reduction in atmospheric pressure in deep-sea divers and caisson workers who return to normal air pressure environments too quickly or pilots flying at high altitudes. This disease causes joint pain, respiratory problems, neurologic symptoms, and skin lesions, reported with ICD-9-CM code 993.3. *Synonym(s): bends, compressed air disease, diver's palsy, dysbarism.*

cake kidney Urogenital abnormality present at birth in which the two kidneys never separated, but fused into a single entity and drain through a single ureter. Report this abnormality with ICD-9-CM code 753.3. *Synonym(s): clump kidney.*

caked breast Engorgement problem occurring in early lactation causing a painful lump in the organ and may affect multiple lobes of the breast. Report this condition with a code from ICD-9-CM subcategory 676.2. *Synonym(s): stagnation mastitis.*

calcaneal apophysitis Inflammation of the calcaneus at the point of Achilles tendon insertion usually occurring in boys ages 8 to 14. Pain, tenderness, and localized swelling are present. Report this condition with ICD-9-CM code 732.5. *Synonym(s): epiphysitis of the calcaneus, Sever's disease.*

calcaneal spur Overgrowth of the calcaneus bone from calcium deposits and chronic avulsion of the plantar fascia from the heel bone. A bone spur forms at the attachment points of tendons in the mid and hind foot region on the lower surface of the calcaneus and causes pain and tenderness with walking. ICD-9-CM code 726.73 reports the calcaneal spur and CPT code 28119 reports the removal.

calcaneonavicular bar Congenital abnormality in which there is a bony, cartilaginous, or fibrous connection between the calcaneus and navicular tarsal bones, resulting in pain and limitation upon movement. If conservative treatment fails, surgical intervention may be required. Report this condition with ICD-9-CM code 755.67.

Calcaneus

Lateral view of right ankle

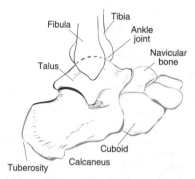

calcaneus Largest tarsal bone in the foot, also referred to as the heel bone.

calcicosis Lung disease caused by the inhalation of calcium-containing dust, often seen in those exposed to lime, limestone, or marble dust. This condition is reported with ICD-9-CM code 502.

calcification Normal process of calcium salts deposition in bone. Calcification can also occur abnormally in fibroconnective soft tissues. This has no direct bearing on CPT or ICD-9-CM coding.

calcifying tendinitis Inflammation and hardening of tissue due to calcium salt deposits, occurring in the tendons and areas of tendonomuscular attachment.

Calcijex See calcitriol.

Calcimar See calcitonin-salmon.

calcitonin-salmon Drug that decreases osteoclastic activity as well as the resorption of calcium in bone and renal tubules, used to treat menopausal osteoporosis, Paget's disease of the bone, and hypercalcemia. Supply is reported with HCPCS Level II code J0630. May be sold under the brand names Miacalcin, Salmonine.

calcitriol Drug that raises calcium levels by stimulating calcium absorption from the gastrointestinal tract and promoting calcium secretion from bone to the

bloodstream. Supply is reported with HCPCS Level II code J0636. May be sold under the brand names Calcijex, Rocaltrol.

calcium disodium versenate Chelating agent given to reduce the blood levels and stored amounts of lead in patients with lead poisoning and lead encephalopathy. Supply is reported with HCPCS Level II code J0600. May be sold under the name Calcium EDTA.

calcium gluconate Calcium replacement used to maintain normal calcium levels in the body, indicated in the treatment of hypocalcemic emergency with hypocalcemic tetany. Calcium gluconate is also used as an adjunct treatment in cardiac arrest. Supply is reported with HCPCS Level II code J0610.

calcium pyrophosphate deposition disease Deposition of calcium pyrophosphate dihydrate primarily in and around fibrocartilage and articular joints of the wrist, hips, and knees causing metabolic arthropathy and may lead to secondary metabolic osteoarthritis. Report this disease with ICD-9-CM codes in subcategory 712.2.

calculus Abnormal, stone-like concretion of calcium, cholesterol, mineral salts, or other substances that forms in any part of the body.

Caldwell view Posteroanterior projection for x-ray views of the head where the central beam enters the head from the back but at a superior angle. It is used to visualize the frontal and anterior ethmoid sinuses.

Caldwell-Luc operation Intraoral antrostomy approach into the maxillary sinus for the removal of tooth roots or tissue, or for packing the sinus to reduce zygomatic fractures by creating a window above the teeth in the canine fossa area.

calicivirus Enteritis from a subgroup of picornaviruses that causes vomiting in children and diarrhea in adults, generally not treated unless the patient becomes dehydrated and requires IV fluids. It is contracted by contaminated water and spread by the fecal-oral route and has also been known to come from raw oysters. Calicivirus is reported with ICD-9-CM code 008.65.

caliectasis Condition in which the calices of the kidney are dilated, often due to infection or obstruction. Caliectasis is reported with ICD-9-CM code 593.89.

caliper Gauge with a calibrated micrometer screw for the measurement of thin objects, such as microscope cover glasses and slides.

Callander knee disarticulation Patella is removed and the long anterior and posterior skin flaps of the tibia are retained to enhance healing.

callosities Localized, hardened patches of overgrowth on the epidermis caused by friction or pressure.

caloric vestibular test Test to induce nystagmus, uncontrolled rapid movement of the eyeball appearing in vestibular disturbances, in order to measure the difference between the patient's right and left vestibular function. Each ear is irrigated separately first with cool, then warm water. In some tests, the physician may observe without an electrical recording, or ENG/PENG recordings may be made. The test is useful in patients with dizziness, difficulty with balance, or sensorineural hearing loss of unknown cause. This test is reported with CPT codes 92533 and 92543.

calvaria Skullcap or rounded top portion of the cranium. The calvaria is made up of the frontal and parietal bones and the squamous portions of the occipital and temporal bones. *Synonym(s): cranial concha, skull cap.*

Calvé-Legg-Perthes syndrome Disease of the growth centers, especially the top of the femur, in which the epiphyses is replaced by new calcification. Report this disorder with ICD-9-CM code 732.1.

calycoplasty Surgery on the calyx, the cup-shaped recess of the renal pelvis, usually to increase its lumen at the infundibulum. Report this procedure with CPT code 50405.

CAM Continuous active motion. Manual therapy to improve range of motion in patients recovering from joint surgery, applied prior to the weight-bearing stage of recovery. The joint is conditioned and the patient's muscles are exercised in CAM.

camelback sign Unusually prominent infrapatellar fat pad of the knee with concomitant hypertrophy of the vastus lateralis. Report with ICD-9-CM code 729.31.

camera oculi anterior Space in the eye located between the cornea and the lens that contains aqueous humor. The anterior chamber is bounded by the sclera and cornea in front and the ciliary body, iris, and pupillary portion of the lens in the back. *Synonym(s): anterior chamber, camera anterior bulbi.*

Cameron ulcer Gastric ulcer within a sliding hiatal hernia, usually associated with inflammation and chronic blood loss, but seldom causing perforation.

camisole Canvas jacket with extra long sleeves that fasten behind the back for restraining a violent person's arms. *Synonym(s): straightjacket.*

Campath Brand name chemotherapy drug used to treat chronic B-cell lymphocytic anemia by binding to CD52 and causing antibody-dependent destruction of leukemic cells. Supply is reported with HCPCS Level II code J9010. Campath contains alemtuzumab.

Campbell arthrodesis Extra-articular fusion of the ankle and subtalar joint, done to treat arthritic conditions, infection, or a failed prior surgery on the joint. Report CPT code 27870 for open ankle arthrodesis.

camptodactyly Congenital deformity in which a finger is bent and fixed in a permanent flexed position and

cannot be completely straightened or extended. Report this condition with ICD-9-CM code 755.59.

Camptosar Brand name DNA inhibitor used to treat metastatic cancer of the colon and rectum in 5FU and leucovorin therapy. Supply is reported with HCPCS Level II code J9206. Camptosar contains irinotecan.

campylobacteriosis Infection with the gram-negative, motile bacteria campylobacter, found normally occurring in the mouth and genitourinary and gastrointestinal (GI) tracts of humans. It is the most prevalent cause of diarrhea with GI symptoms usually beginning two to five days from exposure and lasting as long as a week. Infection comes from undercooked or poorly preserved chicken, unpasteurized milk, and contaminated drinking water, such as from streams and rivers contaminated with feces from cows and birds. It is generally not treated but antibiotics are given in severe cases. Campylobacteriosis is reported with ICD-9-CM code 008.46.

canaliculitis Inflammation of the lacrimal ducts.

canaloplasty Surgical repair or reconstruction of the external auditory canal. Canaloplasty is reported with CPT codes 69310 and 69320 and is often performed in conjunction with tympanoplasty; see 69631-69646.

Canavan disease Genetic disorder of the nervous system causing degeneration of the brain due to errors in development of the myelin sheath. Canavan disease is reported with ICD-9-CM code 330.0. Genetic testing for Canavan disease is reported with HCPCS Level II code S3851.

cancellous bone Bone found mostly in the midshaft of long bones that is spongy and porous with a lattice-like construction. Cancellous bone is often referenced in orthopedic operative notes as being harvested and used as a bone graft with no direct bearing on code selection.

cancellous bone graft Highly porous, spongy bone composed of a lattice-like or trabecular meshwork structure, found in the interior of bones and harvested primarily from the iliac crest or rib to be tapped into place as a bone filler.

cancellous graft Transplant of cancellous or spongy medullary bone found in the midshaft of long bones, as opposed to cortical bone, the outer bone tissue used to provide mechanical support. Cancellous bone is used to promote osteogenesis as new cells are laid down in the grafted area. Cancellous bone is often used in spinal arthrodesis, in which case separate grafting codes for spinal surgery only, including harvesting, are reported in addition to the arthrodesis. If the primary procedure includes a graft, do not report a separate code for obtaining or transplanting the graft.

Cancidas See caspofungin acetate.

cancrum oris Severely destructive lesion of the mouth from fusospirochetal infection, found primarily in debilitated and malnourished children. This lesion destroys buccal, labial, and facial tissue and can be fatal. Cancrum oris is reported with ICD-9-CM code 528.1. *Synonym(s): gangrenous stomatitis.*

candida Yeast-like fungi causing itching and white, cheesy vaginal discharge.

candidiasis Yeast infection caused by the fungus Candida albicans. It commonly occurs in the vagina, but affects any moist skin or mucus membrane. Report candidiasis with a code from ICD-9-CM category 112.

cannula Tube inserted into a blood vessel, duct, or body cavity to facilitate passage.

cannulated screw Surgical nail or screw with a hole through the middle. The hole allows the surgeon to direct the nail or screw over a guidewire. This is a term frequently encountered in operative notes for orthopedic or neurosurgical procedures using internal fixation but has no bearing on coding.

cannulation Insertion of a flexible length of hollow tubing into a blood vessel, duct, or body cavity, usually for extracorporeal circulation or chemotherapy infusion to a particular region of the body. *Synonym(s): cannulization.*

Canthopexy

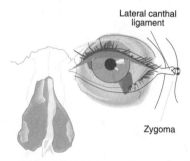

Lateral canthal ligament

Zygoma

Ligament and wire are passed through drilled hole and ligated to bone

canthopexy Procedure performed to stabilize the eyelid by reattaching the medial or lateral canthal ligament by placing a wire or suture through the nasal orbital or cheekbones. For medial canthopexy, report CPT code 21280. For lateral canthopexy, report 21282.

canthoplasty Procedure to restore the angle of the fissure between the eyelids at either side, most often meaning sectioning the lateral canthus to increase the lid margin and lengthen the fissure. Canthoplasty is reported with CPT code 67950.

canthorrhaphy Suturing of the palpebral fissure, the juncture between the eyelids, at either end of the eye. Report with CPT codes 67880-67882. *Synonym(s): tarsorrhaphy.*

canthotomy Horizontal incision at the canthus (junction of upper and lower eyelids) to divide the outer canthus and enlarge lid margin separation. This is reported with CPT code 67715 when it is not performed at the time of another related service.

canthus Angle formed at either end of the palpebral fissure, the junction of the upper and lower eyelids.

Cap *1)* Capitation. *2)* Contract maximum.

CAPD *1)* Continuous ambulatory peritoneal dialysis. Common form of dialysis done at home that uses the peritoneum, the natural lining of the abdomen, as the dialysis membrane. A special CD catheter is inserted into the abdomen and a fresh bag of dialysis solution is drained into the abdomen. After a dwell time of four to six hours or more, the solution, containing wastes, is drained out of the body. The process is repeated with a fresh bag of dialysis solution about four times a day. *NCD Reference: 230.13. 2)* Central auditory processing disorder. Inability to effectively utilize auditory information, especially when competing sounds are present.

capecitabine Oral chemotherapy for metastatic breast cancer and colorectal cancer. Supply of capecitabine is reported with HCPCS Level II codes J8520 and J8521. May be sold under the brand name Xeloda.

capillary Tiny, minute blood vessel that connects the arterioles (smallest arteries) and the venules (smallest veins) and acts as a semipermeable membrane between the blood and the tissue fluid.

capital epiphysis Ball or topmost portion of the femur that fits into the ball and socket joint in the hip. In a growing child, it is referred to as the capital epiphysis and is an anatomical landmark seen in operative reports and radiographic examinations. *Synonym(s): femoral head.*

capitation Contractual agreement whereby the provider is paid a fixed amount for treating enrolled patients regardless of utilization. *Synonym(s): cap.*

capitellum Rounded distal end of the humerus.

Caplan's syndrome Pulmonary condition in rheumatoid arthritis patients in which the lungs have multiple, spherical nodules or lesions throughout both lungs. Report this condition with ICD-9-CM code 714.81. *Synonym(s): rheumatoid pneumoconiosis.*

caps. Capsule.

CAPSO Cautery-assisted palatal stiffening operation. Procedure using heat to induce a midline scar of the palate to stiffen the upper palate and reduce snoring in

A-C

patients with obstructive sleep apnea. An unlisted code would be used to report this procedure.

capsule Structure made of cartilage, fibrous, membranous, or fatty tissue that encloses another structure or body part, such as a joint or the lens of the eye.

capsulectomy Surgical excision of a joint capsule or an area of fibrous scarring (capsular contraction) occurring with a breast prosthesis. CPT codes report this procedure by the anatomical structure involved.

capsulodesis Fixation or securing of a joint capsule to the neighboring structures to treat joint instability, most often done for carpal and metacarpophalangeal instability. CPT codes 25230 and 26516-26518 depict capsulodesis procedures of the hand and wrist.

capsulorrhaphy Suturing or repair of a joint capsule, most frequently done on the glenohumeral joint. CPT codes 23450-23466 and 29806 report this procedure done on the shoulder.

capsulorrhexis Procedure performed during cataract surgery to facilitate extraction of the lens nucleus by making a continuous circular tear in the anterior capsule.

capsulotomy Incision made into a capsule, such as the lens of the eye, the kidney, or a joint. CPT codes 25085, 26520-26525, 27036, 27435, and 28260-28272 depict a variety of joint capsulotomies in various anatomical areas.

Carb Carbohydrate.

Carbocaine Brand name agent used to produce regional, local, epidural, or caudal anesthesia. Supply is reported with HCPCS Level II code J0670.

carbohydrate-deficient glycoprotein syndrome Rare genetic disorder affecting the enzymes used in sugar synthesis, manifesting symptoms in infancy. Symptoms may include neurologic impairment, low blood sugar, gastrointestinal disturbances, and delayed development. CDGS is reported with ICD-9-CM code 271.8. *Synonym(s): CDGS.*

carboplatin Chemotherapy drug used to provide palliative treatment and in combination with cyclophosphamide for advanced ovarian cancer. Supply is reported with HCPCS Level II code J9045. May be sold under the brand names Paraplatin, Paraplatin AQ.

carboxyhemoglobinemia Carbon monoxide poisoning due to breathing vehicle exhaust or smoke from fire. Hemoglobin that normally carries oxygen changes to hemoglobin carrying carbon monoxide in the blood, causing tissue hypoxia, damage to the central nervous system (CNS), and death. Report this condition with ICD-9-CM code 986.

carbuncle Necrotic infection of the skin and subcutaneous tissues, occurring mainly in the neck and back, that produces pus and forms drainage cavities. Carbuncles arise from a collection of infected boils, usually from hair follicles infected by staphylococcus. Report this condition with a code from ICD-9-CM category 680. For incision and drainage of a carbuncle, report CPT codes 10060-10061. *Synonym(s): boil.*

carcinogen Any substance that can cause cancer. Epigenetic carcinogens do not damage the DNA, but cause changes in hormones, immunosuppression, or tissues, leading to cancer. Genotoxic carcinogens damage the DNA itself, causing cell alterations that lead to cancer.

carcinogenic thrombophlebitis syndrome Spontaneous development of thromboses in the upper and lower limbs because of visceral neoplasm. Report this disorder with ICD-9-CM code 453.1.

carcinoid syndrome Carcinoid tumors causing cyanotic flushing of the skin, diarrhea, watery stools, bronchoconstrictive attacks, hypotension, edema and ascites. Report this disorder with ICD-9-CM code 259.2. *Synonym(s): Bjorck-Thorson syndrome, Cassidy-Scholte syndrome, Hedinger's syndrome.*

carcinoid tumor Benign or malignant tumor that arises from neuroendocrine cells located throughout the body. The most common sites are the appendix, bronchi, rectum, small intestine, and stomach. Report carcinoid tumors with a code from ICD-9-CM category 209.

carcinoma Malignant growth of epithelial cells in the coverings and linings of organs and tissues. The cells tend to spread to other locations via the bloodstream or lymphatic channels.

carcinoma in situ Malignancy that arises from the cells of the vessel, gland, or organ of origin that remains confined to that site or has not invaded neighboring tissue. Carcinoma in situ codes are found in their own subchapter of neoplasms according to site.

carcinoma in situ of breast Malignant neoplasm that has not invaded tissue beyond the epithelium of the breast.

cardia Portion of the stomach next to and surrounding the cardiac esophageal opening.

cardiac arrest Sudden, unexpected cessation of cardiac action, including absence of heart sounds and/or blood pressure. Cardiac arrest is a major complication reported with ICD-9-CM code 427.5, which may accompany a more specific diagnosis, such as myocardial infarction, ventricular fibrillation, or asphyxia. Procedures associated with cardiac arrest include cardiopulmonary resuscitation, artificial ventilation, defibrillation, and cardiac massage.

cardiac contractility modulation Implantable, rechargeable cardiac device designed for the treatment of patients with moderate to severe heart failure.

A-C

Generating signals during the absolute refractory period that enhance the heart's strength and overall cardiac performance, the device may be implanted alone or concurrently with an AICD. Report implantation of a total system with ICD-9-CM procedure code 17.51 and implantation or replacement of the pulse generator only with 17.52. *Synonym(s): CCM.*

cardiac output Measurement of the volume of blood ejected by the heart ventricle that is usually measured by a catheter with an opening in the right atrium and pulmonary artery.

cardiac tamponade Interference with the venous return of blood to the heart due to an extensive accumulation of blood in the pericardium (pericardial effusion). Tamponade may occur as a complication of dissecting thoracic aneurysm, pericarditis, renal failure, acute myocardial infarction, chest trauma, or a malignancy. Treatment involves the emergent removal of the fluid. Report this condition with ICD-9-CM code 423.9. *Synonym(s): tamponade heart.*

cardiacos negros syndrome Cyanosis and hypertension resulting from sclerosis of the pulmonary arteries. Report this disorder with ICD-9-CM code 416.0. *Synonym(s): Arrilaga-Ayerza syndrome.*

cardialgia Pain that is localized in the area of the heart, reported with ICD-9-CM code 786.51. *Synonym(s): cardiodynia.*

cardiectomy Excision of the cardiac portion of the stomach.

cardio- Relating to the heart.

cardiochalasia Relaxation or ineffectiveness of the action of the stomach's cardiac orifice sphincter, causing gastroesophageal reflux in adults and infantile vomiting, reported with ICD-9-CM code 530.81.

CardioGenesis SoloGrip Brand name laser used in transmyocardial revascularization (TMR), reported with CPT codes 33140 and 33141. Laser energy is directed into the heart muscle through an incision in the chest, creating small channels in the heart muscle that restore the flow of blood and oxygen. TMR relieves severe angina in patients who are not candidates for bypass surgery.

cardiogenic shock Shock caused by an inadequate supply of oxygen to the body's tissues due to a malfunction of the pumping action of the heart.

cardiointegram Experimental, noninvasive analysis of electrical signals of the heart. Cardiointegram converts analog EKG signals to digital and performs a computer analysis that considers the time element. Report this procedure with HCPCS Level II code S9025. *Synonym(s): CIG. NCD Reference: 20.27.*

cardiomalacia Softening or degeneration of the heart's musculature, reported with ICD-9-CM code 429.1.

cardiomegaly Enlargement of the heart due to a thickened heart muscle or an enlarged heart chamber. Cardiomegaly is a result of the heart having to work harder than normal. Cardiomegaly as a result of high blood pressure is reported with ICD-9-CM code 402.90; idiopathic cases with 429.3; and congenital cardiomegaly is reported with 746.89.

cardiomyopathy General term used to describe a number of conditions of the heart muscle.

cardiopericarditis Inflammation of the heart and the pericardium.

cardiophobia Anxiety disorder manifested by repeated complaints of chest pain, pounding or racing heartbeats, and other somatic events combined with fear of experiencing a heart attack and death. Report this condition with ICD-9-CM code 300.29.

cardiophrenic angle Angle formed by the junction of the shadows of the diaphragm and the heart, seen in posteroanterior x-ray chest films.

cardioptosis Congenital condition in which the heart is displaced downward, reported with ICD-9-CM code 746.87.

cardiopulmonary bypass Venous blood is diverted to a heart-lung machine, which mechanically pumps and oxygenates the blood temporarily so the heart can be bypassed while an open procedure on the heart or coronary arteries is performed. During bypass, the lungs are deflated and immobile.

cardiopulmonary obesity syndrome Obesity, hypoventilation, somnolence, and erythrocytosis. Report this disorder with ICD-9-CM code 278.03. *Synonym(s): Pickwickian syndrome.*

cardiotomy Incision of the heart, the cardiac orifice, or the cardiac end of the stomach.

cardiovasorenal syndrome Abnormal accumulations of neutral glycolipids in histiocytes in blood vessel walls, cornea verticillata, paresthesia in extremities, cataracts, and angiokeratomas on the thighs, buttocks and genitalia. Report this disorder with ICD-9-CM code 272.7.

cardioversion Measured electric shock administered with a defibrillator chest paddle to the heart to convert the heartbeat to a regular rhythm. This procedure can be performed externally or internally. *Synonym(s): rhythm "shock."*

cardioverter-defibrillator Device that uses both low energy cardioversion or defibrillating shocks and antitachycardia pacing to treat ventricular tachycardia or ventricular fibrillation.

CardioWest Brand name temporary totally artificial heart. *NCD Reference: 20.9.*

care plan oversight services Physician's ongoing review and revision of a patient's care plan involving complex or multidisciplinary care modalities.

care unit Specific department or facility within a hospital or long-term care facility designed and staffed for treating a particular type of patient.

caries Localized section of tooth decay that begins on the tooth surface with destruction of the calcified enamel, allowing bacterial destruction to continue and form cavities or even reach the dentin and pulp; reported with a code from ICD-9-CM subcategory 521.0. *Synonym(s): cavity.*

carina Ridge at the junction of the trachea and the bronchi formed by a projection of the lowest tracheal cartilage separating the openings of the two bronchi.

carini's syndrome Scaling of skin accompanying other congenital syndromes. Report this disorder with ICD-9-CM code 757.1.

C-arm Portable x-ray fluoroscopy machine often used in surgery.

carmustine Chemotherapy drug used to treat Hodgkin's lymphoma, recurrent glioblastoma, and malignant melanomas. This drug interferes with enzyme reactions needed for DNA and RNA transcription, leading to cell death. Supply is reported with HCPCS Level II code J9050. May be sold under the brand name BCNU, Gliadel.

carneous mole Condition following a missed abortion in which the blood clots fuse and form an organized mass. This condition is reported with ICD-9-CM code 631.

Carnitor Therapeutic replacement for depleted levels of carnitine, a naturally occurring carrier molecule that delivers long chain fatty acids to mitochondria in the cells for energy production. Childhood deficiency is usually secondary to an inborn error of metabolism. Acquired deficiency in adults is of uncertain etiology, although organic acidemia and dialysis are primary contributors. Supply is reported with HCPCS Level II code J1955. Carnitor contains levocarnitine. *NCD Reference: 230.19.*

carotenemia Elevated blood carotene level as a result of excessive carotenoid ingestion or an inability to convert carotenoids to vitamin A. Characteristics often include yellow discoloration of the skin, especially the palms, soles, and the area behind the ears. Report this condition with ICD-9-CM code 278.3. *Synonym(s): hypercarotenemia.*

carotenosis Yellow discoloration of the skin, especially the area behind the ears, the palms, and the soles, that is usually a sign of carotenemia. Carotenosis is reported with ICD-9-CM code 278.3.

carotid bodies Small, oval nodules of highly neurovascular structure located at the fork of the carotid arteries. The carotid bodies monitor the oxygen content of the blood and help regulate respiration, blood pressure, and heart rate in response to changes in hydrogen and carbon dioxide levels.

carotid body syndrome Stimulation of an overactive carotid sinus, causing a marked drop in blood pressure, which, in turn, may stop the heart. Report this disorder with ICD-9-CM code 337.01. *Synonym(s): carotid sinus syndrome, Charcot-Weiss-Baker syndrome.*

carotid body tumor Benign growth that forms at the fork of the common carotid artery causing symptoms such as dizziness due to its effect on carotid body functions. *NCD Reference: 20.18.*

carotid sinus syndrome Stimulation of an overactive carotid sinus, causing a marked drop in blood pressure, which, in turn, may stop the heart. Report this disorder with ICD-9-CM code 337.01. *Synonym(s): carotid body syndrome, carotid sinus syncope, Charcot-Weiss-Baker syndrome.*

carotid-cavernous fistula Direct communication between the arterial flow from an injured carotid artery and the venous compartment of the cavernous sinus or the orbital veins, with subsequent drooping and swelling of the eyelid, and visual disturbances from the swollen veins pressing against ocular nerves. A bruit is usually present over the globe.

carpal bone One of eight bones that comprise the anatomic wrist arranged in two rows and held tightly together by ligaments. The eight carpal bones are the scaphoid (navicular) lunate (semilunar), triquetrum (triangular), pisiform, trapezium, trapezoid, capitate, and hamate.

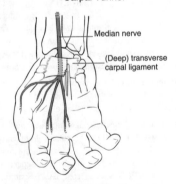

Carpal Tunnel

Median nerve

(Deep) transverse carpal ligament

carpal tunnel Anatomical landmark referring to the space in the wrist on the palmar side that houses the median nerve and all nine of the flexor tendons serving the fingers and thumb. The space is created by the bones of the wrist on either side and a thick ligament called the transverse carpal ligament.

carpal tunnel syndrome Swelling and inflammation in the tendons or bursa surrounding the median nerve caused by repetitive activity. The resulting compression on the nerve causes pain, numbness, and tingling especially to the palm, index, middle finger, and thumb. A brace and nonsteroidal anti-inflammatories are often used initially to treat the condition. This syndrome is reported with ICD-9-CM code 354.0. Open decompression for carpal tunnel syndrome is reported with CPT code 64721. Arthroscopic decompression is reported with CPT code 29848.

carpectomy Removal of one or more of the eight carpal bones of the wrist. Report CPT code 25210 for removal of one bone. In orthopedics, this term is used synonymously to describe the excision and removal of all of the carpal bones in the proximal row, reported with CPT code 25215. This is usually performed for severe arthritis or contracture.

Carpenter's syndrome Rare congenital craniofacial condition of unknown causes manifested by a tower-shaped skull, additional or fused digits, a reduction in height, mental disorders, speech difficulty, and obesity. An asymmetrical skull is often present because of craniosynostosis. This syndrome is reported with ICD-9-CM code 759.89.

carpo- Relating to the wrist.

carpoptosis Inability to extend the hand, which droops permanently at the wrist, due to extensor muscle paralysis. Report this condition with ICD-9-CM code 736.05. **Synonym(s):** hand drop, wrist drop.

Carpue's operation Repair of the nose by folding a flap from the forehead and pedicle at the root of the nose around the area to be repaired. Carpue's operation is reported with CPT code 15731.

carrier Person who generally appears in good health, but who harbors organisms that can infect and cause disease in others. Carriers are reported with a code from ICD-9-CM category V02, with a fourth digit designating the type of infection. **CMS c.** Organization that contracts with CMS to process Medicare claims under Part B, the supplemental medical insurance program for professional services. **insurance c.** Insurer or health plan that may underwrite, administer, or sell a range of health benefit programs.

carrier integrity committee Carriers are required to have a CAC to review and participate in the development of local medical review policies (LMRP). CAC functions are threefold. It provides a formal mechanism for physicians in the state to be informed of and participate in the development of an LMRP in an advisory capacity; a mechanism to discuss and improve administrative policies that are within carrier discretion; and a forum

for information exchange between carriers and physicians. **Synonym(s):** CAC.

carrion's disease Acute form of bartonellosis, an infectious, bacterial disease with sudden onset that is transmitted by sandflies, and usually has a short course manifested by hemolytic anemia and fever. Report this condition with ICD-9-CM code 088.0. **Synonym(s):** Oroya fever.

CART CMS Abstraction and Reporting Tool.

Carticel Brand name for autologous cultured chondrocytes. Chondrocytes are harvested and sent for tissue culture under patented methodology to produce more of the patient's own cells. Cultured cells are returned and used to repair a damaged joint, particularly the knee. Supply is reported with HCPCS Level II code J7330.

cartilage Variety of fibrous connective tissue that is inherently nonvascular. Usually found in the joints, cartilage helps joints move and provides a cushion to absorb jolts and shocks. It does not show up on x-ray, making diagnosis of chondral injuries difficult. Chondropathy is reported with a code from ICD-9-CM category 732.

carve-out Medical benefits for a specific type of care considered covered by separate guidelines or not covered by the payer.

CAS Computer-assisted surgery. Adjunct to surgical procedures in which imaging, markers, reference frames, and intraoperative sensing are utilized along with a computer workstation. CAS affords improved visualization and enhanced navigational techniques via minimally invasive surgical approaches. Report CAS with a procedure code from ICD-9-CM subcategory 00.3.

cascade stomach Abnormal form of hourglass stomach in which the upper posterior wall pushes forward, causing the upper part of the stomach to fill until it reaches a certain volume, at which time it spills into the antrum. Report this condition with ICD-9-CM code 537.6.

case Condition of having an illness or problem. **c. management** Ongoing review of cases by professionals to ensure the most appropriate utilization of services. **c. manager** Clinical professional (e.g., nurse, doctor, or social worker) who works with patients, health care providers, physicians, and insurers to determine and coordinate a plan of medically necessary and appropriate health care. **c. mix index** Sum of all DRG relative weights, divided by the number of Medicare cases. A low CMI may denote DRG assignments that do not adequately reflect the resources used to treat Medicare patients.

case management Ongoing review of cases by professionals to assure the most appropriate utilization of services

A-C

case management services Physician case management is a process of involving direct patient care as well as coordinating and controlling access to the patient or initiating and/or supervising other necessary health care services.

case manager Medical professional (usually a nurse or social worker) who reviews cases every few days to determine necessity of care and to advise providers on payers' utilization restrictions. Certifies ongoing care.

case mix Categories of patients (type and volume) treated by a hospital that represents the hospital's case load.

case mix index Sum of all DRG relative weights for cases over a given period of time, divided by the number of Medicare cases.

cash deductible Dollar amount assumed by the hospital to be applied to the patient's deductible for a particular insurance benefit program. The Medicare cash deductible is the amount the patient must pay each benefit period for inpatient hospital (Part A) services. Under Part B, it is an annual deductible amount that the patient is responsible for paying before Medicare payment can be made.

caspofungin acetate Antifungal/antibiotic used to treat aspergillosis in patients who are intolerant of other drugs, such as amphotericin B. It prevents formation of fungi by inhibiting the synthesis of cell walls in susceptible filamentous fungi. Supply is reported with HCPCS Level II code J0637.

Cassi Brand name rotational core biopsy device for percutaneous needle breast biopsy. Biopsy using the Cassi device is reported using CPT code 19103. Imaging guidance is reported separately.

Cassidy (-Scholte) syndrome Carcinoid tumors that cause cyanotic flushing of the skin, diarrheal watery stools, bronchoconstrictive attacks, hypotension, edema, and ascites. Report this disorder with ICD-9-CM code 259.2. *Synonym(s): Bjorck-Thorson syndrome, Hedinger's syndrome.*

cast *1)* Rigid encasement or dressing molded to the body from a substance that hardens upon drying to hold a body part immobile during the healing period; a model or reproduction made from an impression or mold. Generally, the supply of a cast is included in the codes describing the reduction. *2)* In dentistry and some other specialties, model or reproduction made from taking an impression or mold.

Castellani's bronchitis Chronic bronchitis occurring with the coughing up of blood, caused by a spirochetal infection. Report this condition with ICD-9-CM code 104.8. *Synonym(s): bronchopulmonary spirochetosis, bronchospirochetosis, hemorrhagic bronchitis.*

casting Material used for encasing a body part to immobilize it for injury repair; usually made from plaster or fiberglass.

casting process Creation of a model of teeth and adjoining tissues used to determine how relationships between structures will be affected by dental restoration or appliances. The model may be made of plaster or any other substance.

casting tape Material used for molding casts, usually made from fiberglass, but can be composed of plaster strips.

CAT Computerized axial tomography.

cata- Down from, down, according to.

catagonic stupor Psychomotor disturbances often alternating between extremes such as hyperkinesis or excitement and stupor or automatic obedience and negativism. May be accompanied by depression, hypomania, or submission to physical constraints.

Catalepsy schizophrenia Psychomotor disturbances often alternating between extremes such as hyperkinesis or excitement and stupor or automatic obedience and negativism. May be accompanied by depression, hypomania, or submission to physical constraints.

catamenial Related to menstruation.

catamnesis History or follow-up of a patient after the onset of medical or mental illness or after discharge from the hospital.

cataphasia Meaningless repetition of the same words or phrases like stereotypical chatter. Cataphasia is often seen in cases of schizophrenia. Report this disorder with ICD-9-CM code 315.35. *Synonym(s): verbigeration.*

cataplexy Sudden episode of muscle weakness triggered by emotions. The patient's knees may buckle and give way, the head drop, or the jaw become slack upon laughing, anger, or surprise. In severe cases, the patient may fall and become completely paralyzed for a brief period. Classified to category 347 of ICD-9-CM, code choice is determined by the presence of cataplexy with narcolepsy.

Catapres See clonidine HCl.

cataract Clouding or opacities of the lens that stop clear images from forming on the retina, causing vision impairment or blindness. The classification and coding of cataracts are dependent upon size, shape, location, and etiology.

cataract extraction Most common surgical procedure performed on adults. Most ophthalmologists perform cataract surgery in an ambulatory surgical setting. Anterior chamber lenses are inserted in conjunction with intracapsular cataract extraction and posterior chamber lenses are inserted in conjunction with extracapsular cataract extraction. *NCD References: 10.1, 80.10.*

A-C

catastrophic case management Method of reviewing ongoing cases in which the patient sustains catastrophic or extremely costly medical problems. *Synonym(s): large case management.*

catastrophic limits Maximum amount of certain covered charges patients have to pay out of pocket during the year. Separate limits are usually applied on a per person and per family basis.

catastrophic stress Acute transient disorders of any severity and nature of emotions, consciousness, and psychomotor states (singly or in combination) that occur in individuals, without any apparent pre-existing mental disorder, in response to exceptional physical or mental stress, such as natural catastrophe or battle, and which usually subside within hours or days.

catatonia (schizophrenic) See Catalepsy schizophrenia.

catatonic excitation Psychomotor disturbances often alternating between extremes such as hyperkinesis or excitement and stupor or automatic obedience and negativism. May be accompanied by depression, hypomania, or submission to physical constraints.

CATCH 22 syndrome Cardiac defects, abnormal facies, thymic hypoplasia, cleft palate, and hypocalcemia in a patient with a deletion on chromosome 22. This syndrome is reported with ICD-9-CM code 759.89. *Synonym(s): 22q11.2 deletion syndrome, DiGeorge sequence, Shprintzen syndrome, VCFS, Velo-cardio-facial syndrome.*

catchment area Geographical area from which a health care organization draws its members.

cat-cry syndrome Microcephaly, antimongoloid palpebral fissures, epicanthal folds, micrognathia, strabismus, mental and physical retardation, and a cat-like whine. Report this disorder with ICD-9-CM code 758.31. *Synonym(s): cri-du-chat syndrome.*

Category III codes Alphanumeric codes (four digits followed by the letter T) intended to permit specific data collection for new services or procedures. The use of these codes allows identification of new and emerging technology, services, and procedures. Codes released on January 1 are effective July 1, allowing six months for implementation. Codes released on July 1 are effective January 1. If available, a Category III code must be reported instead of a Category I unlisted code.

cath Catheterize.

catheter Flexible tube inserted into an area of the body for introducing or withdrawing fluid.

catheterization Use or insertion of a tubular device into a duct, blood vessel, hollow organ, or body cavity for injecting or withdrawing fluids for diagnostic or therapeutic purposes. *NCD Reference: 20.25.*

Cauda Equina

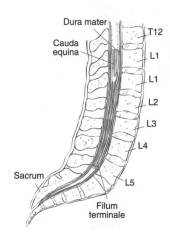

cauda equina Spinal roots occupying the lower end of the vertebral canal and descending from the distal end of the spinal cord, named for their appearance resembling that of the tail of a horse. *c.e. syndrome* Compression of the spinal nerve roots presenting with pain and tingling radiating down the buttocks, back of the thigh, calf, and into the foot in a sciatic manner with aching in the bladder, perineum, and sacrum. Loss of bowel and bladder control may also occur. This syndrome is reported with a code from ICD-9-CM subcategory 344.6.

caudad Anatomic point of reference frequently seen in radiology and operative reports that refers to a point on the body toward the back or lower end of the trunk. *Synonym(s): caudal.*

caudal anesthesia Regional loss of feeling or sensation produced by injection of a local anesthetic into the caudal or sacral canal, where the vertebral canal continues through the sacrum. *Synonym(s): epidural block, saddle block.*

cauliflower ear Condition in which infection or trauma has destroyed the underlying cartilage of the outer ear, resulting in the ear being misshapen. It is often seen in those who have repeated trauma to the ear, such as boxers or wrestlers. Cauliflower ear is reported with ICD-9-CM code 738.7.

causal Reason for the condition; the cause, or cause and effect.

causalgia Condition due to an injury of a peripheral nerve causing burning pain and possible trophic skin changes.

cauterization Tissue destruction by means of a hot instrument, an electric current, or a caustic chemical.

cauterize Heat or chemicals used to burn or cut.

cautery Destruction or burning of tissue by means of a hot instrument, an electric current, or a caustic chemical, such as silver nitrate.

Caverject See alprostadil.

cavernosography Diagnostic radiology study to evaluate erectile dysfunction in which a drug that dilates the blood vessels is injected into the corpus cavernosa. A constricting rubber band is placed around the penis and a contrast medium is injected into the body of the penis. The band is removed and x-rays are taken to demonstrate the function and integrity of the corpora cavernosa and blood flow of the penis. Report this procedure with CPT code 54230. Radiological supervision and interpretation is reported with 74445.

cavernosometry Evaluation of erectile dysfunction in which vasoactive drugs are injected into the corpora cavernosa. A rubber band is then placed around the base of the penis and the intracavernous pressure is measured using instrumentation. The physician evaluates the penis for leakage between the diastolic and the systolic pressures. A swift rate of decay between the two indicates arterial and/or venous insufficiency of the penis. This procedure is reported with CPT code 54231.

cavernous sinus One of two venous spaces between two folds of the dura on either side of the sphenoid bone, containing the veins that collect the venous blood from the superior ophthalmic vein and the sphenoparietal sinus. A length of the internal carotid artery is contained within the cavernous sinus, in addition to several of the cranial nerves including III (oculomotor), IV (trochlear), VI (abducens) and the first and the second branches of V (trigeminal).

cavity Tooth decay.

cavus foot Higher than normal longitudinal arch in the foot, usually associated with other deformities of the leg and/or foot. This can be a congenital or acquired problem reported with ICD-9-CM code 736.73 or 754.71, respectively. *Synonym(s): talipes cavus.*

CB HCPCS Level II modifier, for use with CPT or HCPCS Level II codes, that identifies when a service is ordered by a renal dialysis facility (RDF) physician as part of the end stage renal disease (ESRD) beneficiary's dialysis benefit, but is not part of the composite rate and is separately reimbursable. The patient must be entitled to ERSD coverage and must be admitted to a Medicare Part A stay.

CBC Complete blood count. Blood test to check the number of red blood cells, white blood cells, and platelets in a sample of blood. Report a CBC with CPT codes 85025-85027. *NCD Reference: 190.15.*

CBGCD Closed-loop blood glucose control device. Bedside apparatus designed for short-term management of patients with Type 1 diabetes mellitus, primarily used for stabilization during periods of stress when blood sugar levels fluctuate extensively. Specialized training and continuous observation is required for its use. *NCD Reference: 40.3.*

CBN Chronic benign neutropenia. A common form of neutropenia in infants and children in which there is a decrease in the number of neutrophils in the blood, and frequent infections are common.

CBO Congressional Budget Office or Cost Budget Office.

CBR Complete bedrest.

CBSA Core-based statistical area, as designated by CMS.

CC *1)* Complication or comorbid condition. *2)* Chief complaint. *3)* Cubic centimeter. *4)* HCPCS Level II modifier, for use with CPT or HCPCS Level II codes, indicating that the carrier changed the procedure code submitted either for administrative reasons or because an incorrect code was originally filed.

CCI Correct coding initiative. Official list of codes from the Centers for Medicare and Medicaid Services' (CMS) National Correct Coding Policy Manual for Part B Medicare Carriers that identifies services considered an integral part of a comprehensive code or mutually exclusive of it. *Synonym(s): national correct coding initiative.*

CCM Cardiac contractility modulation.

C-collar Cervical collar.

CCP Cyclic citrullinated peptide. Serum marker for rheumatoid arthritis. An antibody test for CCP is reported with CPT code 86200. Rheumatoid arthritis is reported with a code from ICD-9 category 714.

CCPD Continuous cycler-assisted peritoneal dialysis. Dialysis that utilizes a mechanized cycler to perform three to five exchanges at night to filter the blood while the patient is sleeping. After awakening, the patient begins another exchange with a daylong dwell time.

CCR Cost-to-charge ratio.

CCU Coronary care unit. Facility dedicated to patients suffering from heart attack, stroke, or other serious cardiopulmonary problems.

CDC Centers for Disease Control and Prevention.

CDGS Carbohydrate-deficient glycoprotein syndrome. Inherited metabolic disorder characterized by cardiac, dysmorphic, endocrine, gastrointestinal, hematologic, hepatic, and other body system disorders or disturbances. CDGS is caused by an inability of cells to produce glycoproteins integral to the transport of proteins in the body. CDGS is reported with ICD-9-CM code 271.8.

CDH Congenital dislocation of hip.

CDI Clinical documentation improvement. Program tasked with the generation of more specific and complete chart documentation in order to assure the proper use of resources, correct assessment of the patient's severity of illness, and compliance with regulatory requirements.

CDP Complex decongestive physiotherapy. Massage and manipulation of the affected tissue as a treatment for chronic intractable lymphedema. Lymphedema is reported with ICD-9-CM code 457.1 when an acquired chronic condition; postmastectomy lymphedema is reported with 457.0; and hereditary edema of the legs is reported with 757.0. *Synonym(s): CLT, complex lymphedema therapy.*

CDT Current Dental Terminology. Medical code set, maintained and copyrighted by the American Dental Association, that has been selected for use in the HIPAA transactions.

CE *1)* Cardiac enlargement. *2)* Covered entity. Under HIPAA, a health plan, a health care clearinghouse, or a health care provider who transmits any health information in electronic form in connection with a HIPAA transaction.

CEA Carcinoembryonic antigen. Elevated CEA is reported with ICD-9-CM code 795.81. *NCD Reference: 190.26.*

cec(o)- Having to do with the cecum.

CEDIA Cloned enzyme donor immunoassay test to measure the concentration of sirolimus in whole blood. Sirolimus is an immunosuppressant used to prevent organ rejection in patients receiving kidney transplant.

CEFACT See United Nations Centre for Facilitation of Procedures and Practices for Administration, Commerce, and Transport (UN/CEFACT).

Cefadyl See cephapirin sodium.

cefazolin sodium First generation cephalosporin antibiotic used as a preoperative prophylaxis and to treat a broad spectrum of infections from microorganisms. Supply is reported with HCPCS Level II code J0690. May be sold under the brand names Ancef, Kefzol.

cefepime HCl First generation cephalosporin antibiotic used as a preoperative prophylaxis and to treat a broad spectrum of infections from microorganisms. Supply is reported with HCPCS Level II code J0692. May be sold under the brand name Maxipime.

Cefizox See ceftizoxime sodium.

cefotaxime sodium Third generation cephalosporin antibiotic used to treat a broad spectrum of infections from microorganisms, especially skin infections and gonococcal infections. Supply is reported with HCPCS Level II code J0698. May be sold under the brand name Claforan.

cefoxitin sodium Second generation cephalosporin antibiotic used to treat a broad spectrum of infections from microorganisms, especially serious urinary tract and respiratory infections. Cefoxitin sodium is also used preoperatively as a prophylaxis. Supply is reported with HCPCS Level II code J0694. May be sold under the brand name Mefoxin.

ceftazidime Third generation cephalosporin antibiotic used as a preoperative prophylaxis and to treat a broad spectrum of infections from microorganisms, especially serious urinary tract and respiratory infections. Supply is reported with HCPCS Level II code J0713. May be sold under the brand name Fortaz, Tazidime.

ceftizoxime sodium Third generation cephalosporin antibiotic used to treat a broad spectrum of infections from microorganisms, especially serious urinary tract and respiratory infections and acute bacterial otitis media. Supply is reported with HCPCS Level II code J0715. May be sold under the brand name Cefizox, Ceftizoxime.

ceftriaxone sodium Third generation cephalosporin antibiotic used to treat a broad spectrum of infections from microorganisms, particularly uncomplicated gonococcal vulvovaginitis, meningitis, chronic otitis media in children, and sexually transmitted epididymitis. This antibiotic is also given status post sexual assault and as a preoperative prophylaxis. Supply is reported with HCPCS Level II code J0696. May be sold under the brand name Rocephin.

cefuroxime sodium Second generation cephalosporin antibiotic used to treat a broad spectrum of infections from microorganisms, particularly upper respiratory and urinary tract infections, otitis media, early Lyme disease, and gonorrhea. Supply is reported with HCPCS Level II code J0697. May be sold under the brand names Kefurox, Zinacef.

celiac plexus *1)* Cluster of nerve ganglions functioning as the largest autonomic nerve center in the abdomen, controlling activities such as intestinal contraction and adrenal secretion. *2)* Located at the origin of the celiac trunk, the superior mesenteric and renal arteries on either side and front of the aorta. *Synonym(s): solar plexus.*

celiotomy Incision into the abdominal cavity.

cellulitis Sudden, severe, suppurative inflammation and edema in subcutaneous tissue or muscle, most often caused by bacterial infection secondary to a cutaneous lesion. Progression of the inflammation may lead to abscess and tissue death, or even systemic infection-like bacteremia. Cellulitis and abscesses are reported by the affected site with a code from ICD-9-CM categories 681 and 682.

celo- *1)* Tumor or hernia. *2)* Cavity.

A-C

A-C

cement Any substance that solidly bonds two objects or surfaces together.

cement line Outer circle of an osteon, the basic building block of compact bone seen at the microscopic level, directed along the long axis of a bone. The cement line surrounds the concentric layers of lamellae around each osteon, separating it from interstitial bone, and studied for its ability to absorb shock and prevent micro fractures from spreading. It is an anatomic term, most likely seen in a pathology report, with no bearing on coding. *Synonym(s): tide-line.*

cementum Hard connective tissue that covers a tooth root, lines the apex of the root canal, and attaches to the periodontal ligament.

CEN European Center for Standardization, or Comite Europeen de Normalisation.

Cenacort A-40 Synthetic corticosteroid used as an antiinflammatory or immunosuppressive agent to treat a wide variety of disorders, including inflammatory conditions, certain forms of arthritis, gout, and certain respiratory conditions. Supply is reported with HCPCS Level II code J3301. Cenacort A-40 contains triamcinolone acetonide.

census In medical reimbursement, number and demographics of patients or members

Center for Healthcare Information Management Health information technology industry association. *Synonym(s): CHIM.*

Centers for Disease Control and Prevention Organization that maintains several code sets included in the HIPAA standards, including the ICD-9-CM codes. The ICD-9-CM codes are created by the World Health Organization. The clinical modifications that occur in the United States are made by the CM committee. The CDC participates in the committee. *Synonym(s): CDC.*

Centers for Medicare and Medicaid Services Federal agency that oversees the administration of the public health programs such as Medicare, Medicaid, and State Children's Insurance Program.

-centesis Puncture, as with a needle, trocar, or aspirator; often done for withdrawing fluid from a cavity.

centesis Puncture, as with a needle, trocar, or aspirator, often done for withdrawing fluid from a cavity.

centigray (cGy) Measurement of the amount of radiation dose absorbed by the body (1 cGy = 1 rad). Associated with CPT codes in the 77261-77470 range.

centimeter Metric length measurement equal to 0.3937 inches.

central axis Midline of any given body section around which the specified body parts are organized or rotate;

the midpoint of directly opposing beams in radiation treatment.

central fracture Acetabular fracture of the hip joint that is centrally displaced through the inner wall of the acetabulum to the pelvis.

central slip Portion of the extensor digitorum communis tendon that inserts into the back of the middle phalanx and acts to straighten the finger. Repair of the central slip is specific to boutonniere deformity correction, reported with CPT codes 26426-26428.

central venous access device Catheter or other device introduced through a large vein, such as the subclavian or femoral vein, terminating in the superior or inferior vena cava or the right atrium and used to measure venous pressure or administer medication or fluids. Report with CPT codes 36560-36566, 36570-36578, 36589-36591, and 36593-36596. *Synonym(s): CAVD.*

central venous catheter Catheter positioned in the superior vena cava or right atrium and introduced through a large vein, such as the jugular or subclavian, and used to measure venous pressure or administer fluids or medication.

centrifuge Machine used to simulate gravitational effects or centrifugal force to separate substances of different densities.

centrilobular emphysema Most common type of emphysema in smokers, in which the condition begins in the respiratory bronchioles and spreads peripherally. It is classified to ICD-9-CM code 492.8.

-cephal Relating to the head.

cephalad Toward the head.

cephapirin sodium First generation cephalosporin antibiotic used as a preoperative prophylaxis and to treat a broad spectrum of infections from microorganisms. Supply is reported with HCPCS Level II code J0710. May be sold under the brand name Cefadyl.

cerclage Looping or encircling an organ or tissue with wire or ligature for positional support. *obstetric c.* Surgical procedure that encircles an incompetent cervix with heavy suture material or wire for support in an attempt to retain a pregnancy and prevent preterm delivery. Cerclage is usually performed between 12 and 16 weeks gestation and often employed in patients with a history of spontaneous abortion in otherwise normal pregnancies. The ligature is generally removed at 36 to 38 weeks. This procedure is reported with ICD-9-CM procedure code 67.51 or 67.59 and CPT code 59320 or 59325.

cerebellar cyst Cyst that develops in the white matter of the cerebellum and may be associated with a malignant tumor. Report cerebellar cyst with ICD-9-CM code 348.0.

cerebellomedullary malformation syndrome Displacement of the caudal spinal cord due to tethering with or without spina bifida and meningomyelocele. Report this disorder with a code from ICD-9-CM range 741.00-741.03.

cerebellopontine angle tumor Tumor arising in the area where the cerebellum, pons, and medulla meet.

cerebellum Portion of the brain in the rear cranial fossa behind the brain stem responsible for movement coordination.

cerebral angiography Injection of contrast medium (dye) into an artery, x-raying the blood vessel system of the brain.

cerebral palsy Brain damage occurring before, during, or shortly after birth that impedes muscle control and tone.

cerebrohepatorenal syndrome Rare autosomal recessive disorder presenting with enlarged liver, high levels of copper and iron in the blood, polycystic kidneys, jaundice, lack of muscle tone, and abnormal craniofacial characteristics. Results in death in early infancy. Report this syndrome with ICD-9-CM code 759.89. *Synonym(s): Zellweger syndrome.*

cerebrospinal fluid Thin, clear fluid circulating in the cranial cavity and spinal column that bathes the brain and spinal cord.

cerebrovascular accident Disruption in blood flow to the brain caused by an embolism, thrombosis, or other occlusion, resulting in a lack of perfusion and infarction of brain tissue. Current CVAs are reported with codes from the 434 rubric of ICD-9-CM with a fifth digit of 1 to indicate that cerebral infarction has occurred. An impending CVA is reported as an unspecified transient ischemic attack (TIA), 435.9, in which intermittent ischemia of the brain tissue occurs. When a cerebrovascular accident occurs postoperatively, report 997.02. Sequelae or late effects of CVA can include paralysis, weakness, speech problems, and aphasia, and are reported within the 438 category reserved for late effects of cerebrovascular disease. A healed or old cerebral infarction is coded to V12.59, a personal history of circulatory system disease. *Synonym(s): CVA, stroke.*

cerebrum Primary portion of the brain in the upper part of the cranium that is the largest part of the central nervous system. It is divided into two hemispheres connected by the corpus callosum with the hemispheres divided into the frontal, parietal, temporal, occipital, and insular lobes. The functions of the cerebrum include intelligence, personality, motor function, planning and organization, and interpretation of sensory input.

Cerebryx See fosphenytoin sodium.

Ceredase See alglucerase.

ceroid lipofuscinosis Inherited disorder in which the body stores excessive amounts of lipofuscin, the pigment that remains after damaged cells are broken down and digested, resulting in progressive nervous tissue damage. This term actually denotes a group of genetic lipidoses, named for the type by age, all characterized by continual neurodegeneration manifesting in muscle incoordination, vision loss, retardation, seizures, and fatality. Report this disorder with ICD-9-CM code 330.1. *Synonym(s): amaurotic familial idiocy, neuronal ceroid lipofuscinosis.*

Cerovive Brand name neurovascular protectant for treatment of stroke. Infusion of Cerovive is reported with a CPT code from range 96365-96368 or ICD-9-CM procedure code 99.75. *Synonym(s): NXY-059.*

CERT Comprehensive Error Rate Testing. Program to measure and improve the quality and accuracy of Medicare claims submission, processing, and payment. The program calculates the error rates for all Medicare Administrative Contractors (MAC) and, until the transition to MACs is complete, the CERT program also reports on carriers and fiscal intermediaries (FI).

certificate of authority State license to operate as an HMO.

Certificate of Coverage Benefits included in an individual's health plan. State law requires all insured individuals and employers to receive a COC from the health plan providing coverage. *Synonym(s): COC.*

Certificate of Medical Necessity Form required by Medicare to establish the medical necessity of certain DMEPOS. It is completed by both the physician and the supplier, detailing the medical diagnosis and other information specific to the device ordered. *Synonym(s): CMN.*

certification Approval by a payer's case manager to continue care for a given number of days or visits.

certified nurse midwife Registered nurse who has successfully completed a program of study and clinical experience or has been certified by a recognized organization for the care of pregnant or delivering patients.

certified registered nurse anesthetist Nurse trained and specializing in the administration of anesthesia. *Synonym(s): CRNA.*

Cerubidine See daunorubicin hydrochloride.

cerumen Wax-like substance secreted by the ceruminous glands in the external ear canal. If it becomes firm and blocks the ear canal it may interfere with hearing and require removal. Report impacted cerumen with ICD-9-CM code 380.4. *Synonym(s): earwax.*

Cervarix Brand name human papillomavirus (HPV) vaccine. Supply of the vaccine is reported with CPT code 90649 and administration with 90471.

A-C

cervical Relation to the cervical spine or to the cervix. *c. compression syndrome* Degenerative disorder of the cervical spinal cord. Report this disorder with ICD-9-CM code 721.1. *Synonym(s): anterior spinal artery compression, cervical spondylosis, vertebral artery compression.* *c. smear* Sample of secretions and superficial cells collected from the cervix and prepared for microscopic cytopathology testing by smearing the material across a glass slide in order to screen for cancer cells. *Synonym(s): PAP smear.* *c. sympathetic syndrome* Irritation of nerve roots emanating from the posterior cervical spinal cord. Report this disorder with ICD-9-CM code 723.2. *Synonym(s): cervicocranial syndrome.*

cervical cap Contraceptive device similar in form and function to the diaphragm but that can be left in place for 48 hours.

cervical diaphragm Flexible, dome-shaped rubber cap that fits over the cervix and acts as a barrier to sperm. It is used in conjunction with spermicidal cream or jelly and generally left in place for eight hours after coitus.

cervical ectropion Eversion or turning outward of the cervical canal with epithelium extending further out of the external os of the cervix.

cervical intraepithelial neoplasia Classification system used to report abnormalities in the epithelial cells of the cervix uteri:

CIN I: Cervical intraepithelial neoplasia I; low-grade abnormality; mild dysplasia.

CIN II: Cervical intraepithelial neoplasia II; high-grade abnormality; moderate dysplasia.

CIN III: Cervical intraepithelial neoplasia III; carcinoma in situ; severe dysplasia.

cervicalgia Pain localized to the cervical region, generally referring to the posterior or lateral regions of the neck. Cervicalgia is reported with ICD-9-CM code 723.1. *Synonym(s): cervicodynia.*

cervico- Relating to the neck or neck of an organ.

cervicobrachial syndrome Neuropathy of the brachial plexus causing pain leading from the neck and radiating down the arm.

cervicodorsal outlet syndrome Pain or anesthesias affecting the neck and the upper back. Report this disorder with ICD-9-CM code 353.2.

cervicodynia Pain localized to the cervical spine, generally referring to the posterior or lateral regions of the neck. Cervicodynia is reported with ICD-9-CM code 723.1. *Synonym(s): cervicalgia.*

cervicography System of cervical cancer screening that uses a static photographic image of the ectocervix after application of acetic acid, taken with a specially designed camera for evaluation purposes, and providing photo documentation. Cervicography is considered investigational.

cervicoplasty Plastic repair, reconstruction, or revision of the neck.

cervicothoracic Transition between the neck and the thorax.

Cesamet Brand name synthetic version of THC, the active ingredient in marijuana. Cesamet is prescribed in capsules to treat nausea that may accompany chemotherapy.

Cesarean Section

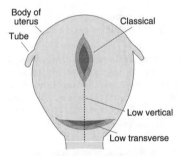

Cesarean section is delivery through incisions in the anterior abdominal and uterine walls. Low transverse is preferred to decrease chance of uterine rupture during future pregnancies

cesarean section Delivery of fetus by incision. *classical c.* Delivery of the fetus by an incision made in the upper part of the uterus, or corpus uteri, via an abdominal peritoneal approach. This type of delivery is performed when a vaginal delivery is not possible or advisable and is reported with ICD-9-CM procedure code 74.0. *low cervical c.* Delivery of the fetus by an incision in the lower segment of the uterus, either through a transperitoneal incision or extraperitoneally with the peritoneal fold being displaced upwards. Low cervical cesarean is reported with 74.1. *Synonym(s): corporeal cesarean section, fundal cesarean section, lower uterine segment cesarean section, transverse cesarean section.*

cesium teletherapy Form of radiation therapy to eradicate cancer cells, often delivered through intracavitary placement. It is the most electropositive and alkaline metallic element, but far less toxic than radium.

Cesium-137 Radioactive isotope used in brachytherapy, generally in the form of needles or tubes.

Céstan (-Raymond) syndrome Quadriplegia, anesthesia, and nystagmus caused by obstruction of twigs of the basilar artery and lesions in the pontine region. Report this disorder with a code from ICD-9-CM range 433.80-433.81.

Céstan's syndrome Paraplegia and anesthesia over part of the body caused by lesions in the brain or spinal cord. Report this disorder with ICD-9-CM code 344.89. *Synonym(s): Avellis syndrome, Babinski-Nageotte syndrome, Benedikt's syndrome, Brown-Sequard syndrome, Céstan-Chenais syndrome, Foville's syndrome, Gubler-Millard syndrome, Jackson's syndrome, Weber-Leyden syndrome.*

Céstan-Chenais syndrome Paraplegia and anesthesia over part of the body caused by lesions in the brain or spinal cord. Report this disorder with ICD-9-CM code 344.89. *Synonym(s): Avellis syndrome, Babinski-Nageotte syndrome, Benedikt's syndrome, Brown-Sequard syndrome, Céstan's syndrome, Foville's syndrome, Gubler-Millard syndrome, Jackson's syndrome, Weber-Leyden syndrome.*

cetuximab Monoclonal antibody for treatment of metastatic colorectal cancer or squamous cell carcinoma of the head and neck. Cetuximab is administered by infusion, reported with CPT code 96409, 96411, 96413, 96415, or 96417 or inpatient ICD-9-CM code 99.28. May be sold under the brand name Erbitux.

CF Cystic fibrosis. Genetic disorder affecting the respiratory, digestive, and reproductive systems in infants to young adults by disturbing exocrine gland function and causing chronic pulmonary disease with excess mucous production and pancreatic deficiency. CF results in early death, although life expectancy has been increasing. CF should be sequenced first with a code from ICD-9-CM subcategory 277.0. Complications arising from CF are reported secondarily.

CFR Code of Federal Regulations.

CGF Congenital generalized fibromatosis, reported with ICD-9-CM code 759.89.

CGM Continuous glucose monitoring, reported with CPT codes 95250-95251.

CGMS Continuous glucose monitoring system. Equipment required to provide 72-hour monitoring of a patient's blood sugars via a subcutaneous sensor. A rented device is reported with HCPCS Level II code S1031 and a purchased device with S1030.

CH Cholesterol.

Chadwick's sign Dark blue or deep purple-red discoloration of the cervix and vagina, which is a sign of pregnancy.

chain of trust Pattern of agreements that extend protection of health care data. Each covered entity that shares health care data with a second entity must require the second entity to provide protections comparable to those provided by the covered entity. The second entity, in turn, must require any other entities with which it shares the data to satisfy the same requirements.

chalasia Relaxation of a bodily opening or the sphincter action of a bodily orifice.

chalazion Small mass in the eyelid that results in chronic inflammation.

chalcosis Copper deposits in tissue. In the eye, chalcosis corneae, deposits of copper cause a colored ring in the deep layers, reported with ICD-9-CM code 371.15. Chalcosis of the globe is reported with ICD-9-CM code 360.24.

chalk stick fracture Fracture seen in cases of established ankylosing spondylitis, a rheumatoid arthritic condition causing fusion of the spine. These fractures occur at the cervicothoracic and thoracolumbar junctions. They are normally transverse, traveling from front to back, and often pass through the ossified disk.

CHAMPUS Civilian Health and Medical Program of the Uniformed Services. See Tricare.

CHAMPVA Civilian Health and Medical Program of the Veteran's Administration.

Chance fracture Unstable distraction fracture of the vertebrae that extends from the spinous processes to the front of the vertebral body. These occur most often in the lumbar spine and are associated with ecchymoses on the anterior abdomen and an open pedicle sign on radiographic exam (lucency on the medial aspect of spinal pedicles). A Chance fracture is coded to the appropriate fracture of the vertebra.

chancriform syndrome Symptoms resembling a syphilitic lesion. Report this disorder with ICD-9-CM code 114.1.

chandelier's sign Intense pain upon movement of the cervix during a manual pelvic examination, which may indicate pelvic inflammatory disease. *Synonym(s): cervical motion tenderness.*

Chandler's syndrome Predominant corneal edema and changes to the iris in an iridocorneal endothelial syndrome caused by a proliferation of the lining of the cornea. Secondary glaucoma is a risk in Chandler's syndrome. Do not confuse Chandler's syndrome with Chandler's disease, a disease of the hip bone. Chandler's syndrome is not indexed in ICD-9-CM. According to official coding guidelines, code selection is based upon presenting symptoms.

change of ownership Providers that undergo a change in their ownership structure are required to notify CMS concerning the identity of the old and new owners. They are also required to inform CMS on how they will organize the new entity and when the change will take place. A terminating cost report will be required from the seller owner in all CHOWs for certification purposes. *Synonym(s): CHOW.*

Chaput fracture Fracture of the ankle usually involving a fracture of the medial malleolus with a small avulsion

A-C

fracture pulling away the anterior portion of the tibia. Report the ICD-9-CM code that describes the fracture sites.

character neurosis Deeply ingrained maladaptive patterns of behavior generally recognizable by adolescence or earlier and continuing throughout most of adult life, although often becoming less obvious in middle or old age. The personality is abnormal either in the balance of its components, quality and expression, or in its total aspect.

Charcot's disease Progressive neurologic arthropathy in which chronic degeneration of joints in the weight-bearing areas with peripheral hypertrophy occurs as a complication of a neuropathy disorder, such as diabetic neuropathy or syringomyelia. Supporting structures relax from a loss of sensation resulting in chronic joint instability. This condition is reported with ICD-9-CM code 713.5 and requires the code for the underlying neuropathy to be listed first (e.g., diabetic 249.6x, 250.6x). *Synonym(s): Charcot's arthropathy, Charcot's joint, neurogenic arthropathy, neuropathic arthritis.*

Charcot's syndrome Degenerative disease of the motor neurons of the spinal tract and the motor cells of the brain that ends fatally within three years. This is not the same disease process referred to as Charcot's joint disease. Charcot's syndrome is reported with ICD-9-CM code 335.20. *Synonym(s): amyotrophic lateral sclerosis, Lou Gehrig's disease.*

Charcot-Marie-Tooth syndrome Pain across the shoulder and upper arm. Report this disorder with ICD-9-CM code 356.1.

Charcot-Weiss-Baker syndrome Stimulation of an overactive carotid sinus, causing a marked drop in blood pressure which, in turn, may stop the heart. Report this disorder with ICD-9-CM code 337.01. *Synonym(s): carotid sinus syndrome.*

CHARGE association Acronym for a recognizable pattern of birth defects that include coloboma (cleft or failure to close the eyeball), heart defects, atresia of the choanae (blockage of the back of the nasal passage), retardation (referring to various degrees of physical and developmental delay), genital and urinary difficulties (including underdevelopment of reproductive organs), and ear abnormalities (deformed pinna and/or hearing loss). The specific combination of features may vary widely among patients. The underlying cause is unknown. Report CHARGE with ICD-9-CM code 759.89.

chargemaster File, usually in an electronic billing system, where charge amounts are kept for all procedures, services, and supplies in a hospital for use with billing software in claims submission.

charges Dollar amount assigned to a service or procedure by a provider and reported to a payer.

Charite Brand name artificial lumbar disc for total spinal disc replacement. The natural disc is replaced with an artificial disc made of cobalt-chromium endplates and a high-density polyethylene pad. As a treatment for degenerative disc disease, ICD-9-CM diagnosis codes appropriate to the insertion of a Charite disc include 722.52 and 722.73. The procedure is reported with ICD-9-CM procedural code 84.65 for insertion or 84.68 for revision, or with CPT codes 22857 and 22862.

charleyhorse Colloquial name for a sudden, painful, leg cramp, likened to the kick of a horse. The cramp may occur in the thigh or the arch of the foot, but most often affects the calf muscle.

charts Compilation of documents maintained by the provider for each patient that includes treatment/progress notes, test orders and results, correspondence from other health care providers, and other documents pertinent to the patient's care.

chauffeur's fracture Fracture of the styloid process of the ulna, occurring as a result of avulsion, with fragments varying in size and usually nondisplaced. Report this fracture with ICD-9-CM code 813.43.

CHCT Caffeine halothane contracture test. Test to diagnose malignant hyperthermia susceptibility. It is performed on freshly biopsied muscle, which is exposed to caffeine and halothane separately. The strength of sustained muscle tension responses is evaluated to determine malignant hyperthermia susceptibility. Report CHCT with CPT code 89049.

CHD *1)* Congenital heart disease. *2)* Congestive heart disease.

Cheadle syndrome Anemia, spongy gums, weakness, induration of leg muscles, and mucocutaneous hemorrhages. Report this disorder with ICD-9-CM code 267. *Synonym(s): Cheadle-Barlow syndrome, Cheadle-Möller syndrome.*

Chealamide Brand name of edetate disodium, a chelating agent used in the treatment of hypercalcemia and arrhythmias induced by cardiac glycosides. Supply is reported with HCPCS Level II code J3520.

Chédiak-Higashi (-Steinbrinck) syndrome Hepatosplenomegaly, lymphadenopathy, anemia, thrombocytopenia and changes in the bones, cardiopulmonary system, skin, psychomotor skills, abnormalities of granulation, and nuclear structure of white cells open the patient to infection. Report this disorder with ICD-9-CM code 288.2. *Synonym(s): Chediak-Higashi syndrome, Dohle body syndrome, Hegglin syndrome, Jordan's syndrome, May syndrome.*

cheese washers' lung Form of hypersensitivity pneumonitis found in individuals who inhale penicillium spores in the process of washing moldy cheese casings.

Symptoms include weight loss, cough, and shortness of breath. Report this condition with ICD-9-CM code 495.8.

cheilectomy Chiseling off an irregular bony edge from a joint cavity that is interfering with the motion of the joint.

cheilitis Inflammation, pain, and swelling of the lips due to a variety of underlying factors. ICD-9-CM code 528.5 is the default for any unspecified type of cheilitis, as well as most infective, ulcerative cases, while radiation causes are reported with 692.72, 692.74, and 692.82.

cheilo- Relating to the lip or lips.

cheilodynia Lip pain, reported with ICD-9-CM code 528.5.

cheilophagia Condition in which one bites the lips, reported with ICD-9-CM code 528.9.

cheiloschisis Congenital fissure or separation of the upper lip due to failure of embryonic cells to fuse completely. Cheiloschisis can occur unilaterally or bilaterally and may accompany other abnormalities of the upper jaw, nose, or oral structures. Code assignment is dependent upon whether the cleft lip is unilateral or bilateral, complete or incomplete, and whether or not it is accompanied by a cleft palate. See ICD-9-CM category 749 for code assignment. Report repair of a cleft lip with CPT codes 40700-40761. **Synonym(s):** *cleft lip.*

cheiro- Relating to the hand.

cheiromegaly Condition in which the hands are abnormally large, reported with ICD-9-CM code 729.89. **Synonym(s):** *macrocheiria.*

chelate To bind or combine a metal into a complex, forming a ring within which the metal is firmly bound, removing its potential to bind elsewhere; agent or molecule that binds to a metal ion, forming a ring. Chelating agents are used in therapeutic treatment of metal poisoning.

chelating agent Synthetic amino acid used in the treatment of metal poisoning that binds a metallic ion firmly within the molecular ring of the chelating agent to facilitate removal of unwanted mineral deposits.

chemodenervation Chemical destruction of nerves. A substance, for example, Botox, is used to temporarily inhibit the transfer of chemicals at the presynaptic membrane, blocking the neuromuscular junctions.

chemoembolization Administration of chemotherapeutic agents directly to a tumor in combination with the percutaneous administration of an occlusive substance into a vessel to deprive the tumor of its blood supply. This ensures a prolonged level of therapy directed at the tumor. Chemoembolization is primarily being used for cancers of the liver and endocrine system. **Synonym(s):** *transcatheter arterial chemoembolization (TACE) of the liver.*

chemonucleolysis Process of injecting a chemolytic agent to dissolve the nucleus pulposus of a herniated intervertebral disk. **Synonym(s):** *discolysis.*

chemosis Swelling of the conjunctiva.

chemosurgery Application of chemical agents to destroy tissue, originally referring to the in situ chemical fixation of premalignant or malignant lesions to facilitate surgical excision. For Mohs micrographic technique, see CPT codes 17311-17315. If chemosurgery is performed on skin lesions, see 17004, 17110, 17270, and 17280.

chemotherapeutic Treatment for systemic or localized disease that employs a drug or chemical agent, usually designed to treat cancerous conditions.

Chemotherapy

Cannulization is accomplished for prolonged chemotherapy infusion

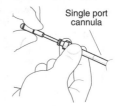

Single port cannula

chemotherapy Treatment of disease, especially cancerous conditions, using chemical agents. **NCD References:** *110.6, 110.17, 110.18.*

cherry picking In medical reimbursement, the practice of enrolling only healthy individuals and excluding those with existing problems.

cherubism Inherited childhood disorder manifested by loss of bone in the maxilla and mandible. The bone is replaced by excess fibrous tissue, resulting in a prominent lower face that resembles cherubs in Renaissance art. Report this condition with ICD-9-CM code 526.89.

chevron procedure Surgical treatment generally used for a large bunion deformity in which there is minimal angulation of the great toe, and involves a resection of the medial eminence of the first metatarsal. A "V" or chevron-shaped cut is made near the end of the bone, which allows the surgeon to slide the head of the bone laterally, or toward the little toe. Report this procedure with CPT code 28296. **Synonym(s):** *Austin procedure, Mitchell procedure.*

Cheyne-Stokes respiration Breathing pattern characterized by a period of apnea, followed by gradually increasing depth and frequency of respirations, occurring in cases of frontal lobe and diencephalic dysfunction. Report Cheyne-Stokes respiration with ICD-9-CM code 786.04.

CHF Congestive heart failure.

chgd Changed.

Chiari osteotomy Top of the femur is altered to correct a dislocated hip caused by congenital conditions or cerebral palsy. Plate and screws are often used.

Chiari's syndrome Thrombosis of the hepatic vein with enlargement of the liver and severe hypertension. Report this disorder with ICD-9-CM code 453.0.

Chiari-Frommel syndrome Unphysiological lactation and amenorrhea following pregnancy caused by hyperprolactinemia and a pituitary adenoma. Report this disorder with a code from ICD-9-CM range 676.60-676.64.

chiasmatic syndrome Impairment of vision, limitations of the field of vision, scotoma, headache, syncope, and vertigo. Report this disorder with ICD-9-CM code 368.41.

chickenpox Highly contagious infection by the varicella-zoster virus causing a rash of very pruritic pustules breaking out over the body and accompanied by fever. Complications may include pneumonia, cerebral edema, and bacterial skin infections. This disease is preventable with the varicella vaccination. Report chickenpox with a code from ICD-9-CM rubric 052.

chief complaint In medical documentation, the presenting problem bringing the patient to the health encounter.

Chiene test Measurement taken as part of a physical examination to determine if a fracture of the neck of the femur has occurred. A tape measure is simply used to measure around the femur. When there is a fracture of the neck, the affected side will measure larger as the shaft will have rotated outward.

chiggers Six-legged, red-colored larvae of a mite from the Trombiculidae family that attaches to the skin and whose bite results in wheals, causing an itchy rash and dermatitis. Treatment often consists of antihistamines and cortisone cream. Report chigger infestation with ICD-9-CM code 133.8.

chigoe disease Disease spread by the parasitic flea, Tunga penetrans, the pregnant female of which burrows into the host's skin, often the lower limbs and under nails, causing inflammation, swelling, and cyst formation that turns ulcerative. Gas gangrene, bacteremia, or tetanus may occur in cases of severe infestation, as well as spontaneous loss of a digit. Report this condition with ICD-9-CM code 134.1. *Synonym(s): burrowing flea disease, jigger disease, sand flea disease.*

Chilaiditi's syndrome Interposition of the colon between the liver and diaphragm. Report this disorder with ICD-9-CM code 751.4.

chilblains Unusual, localized inflammatory reaction manifested by redness and subcutaneous swelling after exposure to a cold and damp environment. The redness and swelling is accompanied by itching and a burning sensation and may take one to three weeks to heal. It often affects different areas such as legs and toes in women and hands and fingers in men, while children may have this response in the ears and face as well as the hands and feet. Report this condition with ICD-9-CM code 991.5. *Synonym(s): perniosis.*

childhood autism Syndrome beginning in the first 30 months of life affecting interaction with others, characterized by abnormal response to auditory and visual stimuli accompanied by difficulty understanding spoken language and limiting the ability to communicate or develop social skills.

childhood dementia-aphonia syndrome Dementia in which a child has impaired development of reciprocal social skills, verbal and nonverbal communication skills and has imaginative play. Report this disorder with a code from ICD-9-CM range 299.10-299.11.

childhood schizophrenia syndrome Schizophrenia occurring in childhood that exhibits itself with disturbances in thought (delusions, hallucinations), mood (blunted, flattened, inappropriate affect), sense of self, and may include strange, purposeless behavior, repetitious activity or inactivity. Report this disorder with a code from ICD-9-CM range 299.90-299.91.

childhood type schizophrenia Group of disorders in children characterized by distortions in the timing, rate, and sequence of many psychological functions involving language development and social relations in which the severe qualitative abnormalities are not normal for any stage of development.

chilo- Relating to the lip. *Synonym(s): cheilo-.*

CHIM Center for Healthcare Information Management.

CHIME College of Healthcare Information Management Executives.

CHIP Child Health Insurance Program.

chip fracture Fracture denoting a "chip" or corner broken from the growing end of a bone. Code to the bone, type, and end of bone involved.

chisel Instrument for cutting or planing bone.

chisel fracture Incomplete fracture of the intra-articular radial head usually resulting from falling on an outstretched hand.

CHL Conductive hearing loss. Dysfunction in sound-conducting structures of the external or middle ear, reported with ICD-9-CM codes 389.00-389.08.

chlamydia trachomatis Bacterium that causes a common venereal disease. Symptoms of chlamydia are usually mild or absent, however, serious complications may cause irreversible damage, including cystitis, pelvic inflammatory disease, and infertility in women and discharge from the penis, prostatitis, and infertility in men. Genital chlamydial infection can cause arthritis, skin lesions, and inflammation of the eye and urethra (Reiter's syndrome). Report this condition with ICD-9-CM codes 099.1, 099.3, 099.41, and 099.50-099.59.

chloasma Condition frequently seen in women who take birth control pills in which the skin develops brown patches with distinct edges. Primary sites include the cheekbones, forehead, and upper lip, but development may also occur on the nose, chin, and neck. This condition may also be seen in pregnant females, menopausal women, those with hormonal or ovarian disorders, or patients using the medication Dilantin. Chloasma is infrequently seen in men. Code assignment depends upon etiology and location. *Synonym(s): melasma.*

chlorambucil Antineoplastic drug used primarily to treat chronic lymphocytic leukemia. One of the alkylating-agent class, it is also indicated in the treatment of breast and ovarian cancer, Hodgkin's disease, and non-Hodgkin's lymphoma. Supply is reported with HCPCS Level II code S0172. May be sold under the brand name Leukeran.

chloramphenicol sodium succinate Bacteriostatic drug that inhibits bacterial protein synthesis used in the treatment of bacteremia and meningitis caused by Salmonella and Haemophilus influenzae. Supply is reported with HCPCS Level II code J0720. May be sold under the brand name Pentamycetin.

chlordiazepoxide HCl Antianxiety agent used to promote sleep and calmness, to treat alcohol withdrawal, and to lessen anxiety preoperatively. Supply is reported with HCPCS Level II code J1990. May be sold under the brand names Apo-Chlordiazepoxide, Librium, Novopoxide.

chloroleukemia Disorder manifested by numerous malignant tumors produced by bony infiltrates in myelogenous leukemia. The masses are most often found in the skull, but may occur in any part of the skeleton. The tumors appear green colored, due to pigment effects of myeloperoxidase. Report this condition with a code from ICD-9-CM category 205.3. *Synonym(s): Aran's cancer, Balfour's disease, chloroma, chloromyeloma, chlorosarcoma, granulocytic sarcoma, green cancer, Naegeli's disease.*

chloroma Disorder manifested by numerous malignant tumors produced by bony infiltrates in myelogenous leukemia. The masses are most often found in the skull, but may occur in any part of the skeleton. The tumors appear green colored, due to pigment effects of myeloperoxidase. Report this condition with a code from ICD-9-CM category 205.3. *Synonym(s): Aran's cancer, Balfour's disease, chloroleukemia, chloromyeloma, chlorosarcoma, granulocytic sarcoma, green cancer, Naegeli's disease.*

Chloromycetin sodium succinate See chloramphenicol sodium succinate.

chloromyeloma Disorder manifested by numerous malignant tumors produced by bony infiltrates in myelogenous leukemia. The masses are most often found in the skull, but may occur in any part of the skeleton. The tumors appear green colored, due to pigment effects of myeloperoxidase. Report this condition with a code from ICD-9-CM category 205.3. *Synonym(s): Aran's cancer, Balfour's disease, chloroleukemia, chloroma, chlorosarcoma, granulocytic sarcoma, green cancer, Naegeli's disease.*

chloroprocaine HCl Agent used to produce regional, local, epidural, or caudal anesthesia and often employed in dental procedures. Supply is reported with HCPCS Level II code J2400. May be sold under the brand name Nesacaine.

chloroquine HCl Antimalarial agent used to treat acute infectious attacks of malaria, as well as for the prevention of malaria from a variety of Plasmodium strains. May be sold under the brand name Aralen.

chlorosarcoma Disorder manifested by numerous malignant tumors produced by bony infiltrates in myelogenous leukemia. The masses are most often found in the skull, but may occur in any part of the skeleton. The tumors appear green colored, due to pigment effects of myeloperoxidase. Report this condition with a code from ICD-9-CM category 205.3. *Synonym(s): Aran's cancer, Balfour's disease, chloroleukemia, chloroma, chloromyeloma, granulocytic sarcoma, green cancer, Naegeli's disease.*

chlorothiazide sodium Diuretic used to treat edema and hypertension by inhibiting sodium reabsorption in the renal tubules. Supply is reported with HCPCS Level II code J1205. May be sold under the brand names Chlotride, Diurigen, Diuril.

chlorpromazine HCl Antipsychotic drug given to counteract psychoses in patients with schizophrenia and other manic psychotic conditions. Chlorpromazine is also used to treat nausea and vomiting at the time chemotherapy is administered, intractable hiccups, and tetanus. Supply is reported with HCPCS Level II codes Q0171, Q0172, and J3230. May be sold under the brand names Chlorpromanyl, Largactil, Novo-Chlorpromazine, Thorazine.

choanal atresia Congenital, membranous, or bony closure of one or both posterior nostrils due to failure of the embryonic bucconasal membrane to rupture and open up the nasal passageway. Choanal atresia is reported with ICD-9-CM code 748.0.

chocolate cyst of ovary Aberrant uterine tissue, or endometriosis, found on the ovaries, creating a cyst that is filled with blood. If small, they can sometimes be treated medically, but usually require surgical

A-C

intervention. Chocolate cysts are reported with ICD-9-CM code 617.1.

cholangitis Inflammation of the bile ducts.

chole- Relating to the gallbladder.

cholecystectomy Surgical removal of the gallbladder and its contents. Cholecystectomy may be performed by an open incision into the abdominal cavity or laparoscopically via instruments inserted through small incisions into the peritoneum for video-controlled imaging. *NCD Reference: 100.13.*

cholecystitis Inflammation of the gallbladder. Acute cholecystitis is most often the result of an obstruction at the outlet of the gallbladder, with consequent edema and congestion that can progress to serious cases of gangrene and perforation. Acute cholecystitis is reported with ICD-9-CM code 575.0. Chronic cholecystitis is a mild symptomatic inflammation of the gallbladder that continues over a long period and is reported with ICD-9-CM code 575.11. Acute and chronic forms may also occur together and are coded to 575.12.

choledochitis Inflammation of the common bile duct, reported with ICD-9-CM code 576.1 whether chronic, acute, secondary, primary, or recurrent. *Synonym(s): cholangitis.*

choledocholithiasis Presence of gallstones or calculi within the common bile duct. When the gallstones or other calculi are obstructing the bile duct, it is reported with ICD-9-CM code 574.51. If there is no obstruction of the bile duct with the stone, it is reported with 574.50. Calculus of the bile duct occurring with cholecystitis is not coded as two separate diagnoses. ICD-9-CM provides codes for this condition, with or without obstruction, in subcategory 574.3 for calculus of the bile duct with acute cholecystitis and subcategory 574.4 for calculus of the bile duct with chronic cholecystitis.

choledochotomy Surgical incision into the common bile duct for exploration or for the removal of stones, reported with CPT codes 47420 and 47425.

cholelithotomy Surgical incision into the gallbladder for the removal of gallstones.

cholera Acute infection of the entire bowel due to vibrio cholerae, a genus of gram-negative, anaerobic, rod-shaped, mobile bacteria divided into six serogroups. It presents with profuse diarrhea, cramps, and vomiting. The rice water diarrhea produced by the cholera enterotoxin results in severe dehydration, electrolyte imbalance, and death. It is spread through ingestion of food or water contaminated with feces of infected persons and is still prevalent in countries with poor socioeconomic conditions. Cholera is the acute infectious enteritis caused by this class of bacteria, reported with ICD-9-CM codes 001.0-001.9; suspected carrier, V02.0; exposure to or contact with, V01.0; and prophylactic

vaccination against, V03.0. Until recently cholera has only been diagnosed with bacterial stool culture or other advanced scientific method, rarely available in the prevalent area of disease. Recently a dipstick method (CPT code 87450) has become available for early detection. *Synonym(s): vibrio cholerae.*

cholestasis Blockage of the flow of bile from the liver or bile ducts, caused by a variety of underlying diseases. Symptoms may include itching, jaundice, and digestion difficulties. Treatment depends upon the underlying condition. Report cholestasis with ICD-9-CM code 576.8.

cholesteatoma Cyst-like mass of cell debris including cholesterol and epithelial cells found in the middle ear and mastoid (ICD-9-CM subcategory 385.3), external ear canal (380.21), and following mastoidectomy (383.32), resulting from trauma, improperly healed infections, and congenital enclosure of epidermal cells.

cholesterolemia Elevated levels of cholesterol in the blood that may be an inherited disorder or caused by certain environmental factors. Report this condition with ICD-9-CM code 272.0.

cholesterolosis of gallbladder Accumulation of cholesterol deposits within the tissues of the gallbladder. This condition is reported with ICD-9-CM code 575.6. *Synonym(s): strawberry gallbladder.*

choluria Condition in which bile is present in the urine, often causing discoloration. Report this condition with ICD-9-CM code 791.4.

chondr(o)- Relating to or denoting cartilage.

chondral Relating to cartilage.

chondralgia Perception of pain originating in cartilage experienced as pain in an affected joint.

chondritis Abnormal inflammatory response within cartilage that may be due to another disease process, injury, or direct infection and is coded to the affected site.

chondroblastoma Rare benign neoplasm typically found at the growth plate or epiphysis of a long bone in adolescents. Chondroblastoma is derived from immature cartilage cells, or chondroblasts, surrounded by a coarse matrix of eosinophils with calcifications arranged in a hexagonal pattern.

chondrocalcinosis Presence of calcium salt deposits within joint cartilage.

chondrodystrophy Abnormal development of cartilage, the primary cause of short limb dwarfism, reported with ICD-9-CM code 756.4.

chondroectodermal dysplasia Congenital disorder of inadequate enchondral bone formation, characterized by impaired development of hair, skin, teeth, and cartilage with polydactyly and cardial septal defects also present. This disorder is reported with ICD-9-CM code 756.55.

chondrolipoma Rare type of benign neoplasm of mesenchymal origin comprised of hyaline cartilage and adipose tissues found throughout the body but mainly in connective tissue of the skeletal system, breast, pharynx, and nasopharynx.

chondroma Benign tumor composed of bone and mature hyaline cartilage that may grow within the bone or cartilage tissue affected or on the surface of the affected tissue. Chondromas are most often seen in teenagers and young adults and are coded as a benign neoplasm of bone and articular cartilage within the 213 rubric of ICD-9-CM with the 4th digit denoting the involved bone(s).

chondromalacia Condition in which the articular cartilage softens, seen in various body sites but most often in the patella. Chondromalacia may be congenital or acquired, and code assignment is dependent upon the affected site.

chondromyoma Benign neoplasm of mesenchymal origin comprised of cartilage and muscle cells.

chondromyxoid fibroma Rare benign neoplasm of the cartilage comprised of fibrous, myxoid, and cartilaginous cells in varying quantities. It originates in the marrow of long bones, especially the tibia and the femur near the knee.

chondroplasty Surgical repair of cartilage.

chordee Ventral (downward) curvature of the penis due to a fibrous band along the corpus spongiosum seen congenitally with hypospadias, or a downward curvature seen on erection in disease conditions, causing a lack of distensibility in the tissues. Congenital chordee is reported with ICD-9-CM code 752.63. Acquired chordee is reported with ICD-9-CM on code 607.89, and that specified as gonococcal is reported with 098.2.

chorditis Condition in which the vocal cords are inflamed, most often as a result of overuse of the voice. Cancer may also be an underlying cause. Chorditis is reported with ICD-9-CM code 478.5.

chorea-athetosis-agitans syndrome Accumulation of copper in the brain, cornea, kidney, liver, and other tissues causing cirrhosis of the liver and deterioration in the basal ganglia of the brain. Report this disorder with ICD-9-CM code 275.1.

Chorex See chorionic gonadotropin.

chorionic gonadotropin Hormone normally produced by the placenta in pregnancy. This injectable hormone drug has the same action as luteinizing hormone manufactured in the pituitary gland and helps women to conceive. In men, it stimulates the testes to manufacture testosterone. Supply is reported with HCPCS Level II code J0725. May be sold under the brand names Chorex, Choron, Gonic, Novarel, Ovidrel, Pregnyl, Profasi.

chorionic villus sampling Aspiration of a placental sample through a catheter, under ultrasonic guidance. The specialized needle is placed transvaginally through the cervix or transabdominally into the uterine cavity. This sampling is performed to provide a rich source of fetal genetic information to help diagnose defects. The transabdominal approach can be performed throughout pregnancy. The other approaches are usually done between nine and 12 weeks of gestation. CPT code 59015 reports the procedure and 76945 reports the guidance, radiological supervision and interpretation. This procedure is excluded from the maternity care global package. *Synonym(s): CVS.*

chorioretinitis Inflammation of the retina extending to the choroid (middle vascular layer of the eyeball).

choroid Thin, nourishing vascular layer of the eye that supplies blood to the retina, arteries, and nerves to structures in the anterior part of the eye.

choroideremia Hereditary choroid degeneration occurring in the first 10 years of life and affecting males and females differently due to its X-linked transmission. In males, it causes night blindness, then a constricted visual field, ultimately ending in blindness as the retina atrophies. In females, the disease is less debilitating and is not progressive, usually consisting of a retinopathy with normal vision. Report choroideremia with ICD-9-CM on code 363.55.

Choron 10 See chorionic gonadotropin.

chr. Chronic.

Christian's syndrome Multiple-system defects of the membranous bones, exophthalmos, diabetes insipidus, soft tissues, and bone involvement. Report this disorder with ICD-9-CM code 277.89.

Christmas disease Second most common form of hemophilia, a hereditary blood disorder in which the clotting properties are affected. Christmas disease almost always occurs in males, caused by a coagulation factor IX deficiency. Symptoms include prolonged or spontaneous bleeding, ecchymosis, hematuria, and muscular and joint pain and swelling. Report this disorder with ICD-9-CM code 286.1. *Synonym(s): hemophilia B.*

Christmas factor assay Blood test that measures the activity for factor IX, a plasma thromboplastin component, one of the substances involved in the intrinsic pathway of coagulation or blood clotting. This test is performed on people with bleeding problems as a deficiency in this factor causes hemophilia B. *Synonym(s): factor IX assay, PTC assay.*

chrom(o)- Term denoting color.

chromatopsia Skewed perception of color or visual disorder in which objects with color appear to have unnatural hues. Objects lacking color appear as tinged with color. Drugs, cataract extraction, optic center damage, or blinding light may bring this on. The specific types of chromatopsia are named for the colors seen. Report chromatopsia with ICD-9-CM code 368.59.

chromhidrosis Rare condition in which a person secretes sweat that is colored, reported with ICD-9-CM code 705.89.

chromomycosis Chronic fungal skin infection that usually originates at the site of a puncture wound in a leg or foot, although other areas of the body may be involved. Manifestations include nodules resembling warts that have brownish bodies seen microscopically. Ulcerations may or may not be present. Report this condition with ICD-9-CM code 117.2. **Synonym(s):** *chromoblastomycosis.*

chromosome 4 short arm deletion

syndrome Microcephaly, antimongoloid palpebral fissures, epicanthal folds, micrognathia, strabismus, mental and physical retardation, and a cat-like whine. Report this disorder with ICD-9-CM code 758.39.

chromotubation Injection of a medication or saline solution into the uterine cavity and fallopian tubes to verify patency of the tubes.

chronic Persistent, continuing, or recurring.

chronic alcoholic brain syndrome Nonhallucinatory dementias occurring in association with alcoholism but not characterized by the features of either alcohol withdrawal delirium (delirium tremens) or alcohol amnestic syndrome (Korsakoff's alcoholic psychosis).

chronic alcoholic syndrome Numerous symptoms caused by constant, long-time ingestion of alcohol affecting the nervous and gastrointestinal systems. Report this disorder with ICD-9-CM code 291.2.

chronic duodenal ileus Persistent obstruction in the first portion of the small intestine between the pylorus and the jejunum. This condition is reported with ICD-9-CM code 537.2.

chronic fatigue syndrome Persistent fatigue that significantly reduces daily activity with chronic sore throat, mild fever, muscle weakness, myalgia, headaches, and neurological problems. Report this disorder with ICD-9-CM code 780.71.

chronic granulocytic leukemia Chronic form of myelogenous leukemia, most often associated with a chromosome abnormality, and manifesting between ages 25 and 60. The cell type involved is seen as abnormal, excessive unchecked growth of granulocytes in the bone marrow, causing hepatosplenomegaly, anemia, and malaise. Report this condition with ICD-9-CM codes

205.10-205.12. **Synonym(s):** *chronic myelocytic leukemia, chronic myeloid leukemia, CML.*

chronic interstitial cystitis Persistently inflamed lesion of the bladder wall, usually accompanied by urinary frequency, pain, nocturia, and a distended bladder. **Synonym(s):** *Hunner's ulcer, panmural fibrosis of the bladder, submucous cystitis.*

chronic inversion of uterus Persistent abnormality in which the uterus turns inside out.

chronic kidney disease Decreased renal efficiencies resulting in reduced ability of the kidney to filter waste. The National Kidney Foundation's classification includes five clinical stages, based on the glomerular filtration rate (GFR). The stages of CKD are as follows: stage 1 (ICD-9-CM code 585.1), some kidney damage with normal or slightly increased GFR (>90); stage 2 (585.2), mild kidney damage with a GFR value of 60 to 89; stage 3 (585.3), moderate kidney damage with a GFR value of 30 to 59; stage 4 (585.4), severe kidney damage and a GFR value of 15 to 29; and stage 5 (585.5), severe kidney damage that has progressed to a GFR value of less than 15. Dialysis or transplantation is required at stage 5. **Synonym(s):** *CKD.*

chronic mesenteric syndrome Complete or partial block of the superior mesenteric artery with symptoms of vomiting, pain, blood in the stool, and distended abdomen resulting in bowel infarction. Report this disorder with ICD-9-CM code 557.1. **Synonym(s):** *Wilkie's syndrome.*

chronic pain management services Distinct services frequently performed by anesthesiologists who have additional training in pain management procedures. Pain management services include initial and subsequent evaluation and management (E/M) services, trigger point injections, spine and spinal cord injections, and nerve blocks.

chronic passive congestion of liver Abnormal accumulation of blood in liver tissue due to an obstruction that prevents the passage of blood out of the organ. This condition is reported with ICD-9-CM code 573.0.

chronic subinvolution of uterus Persistent uterine enlargement occurring after childbirth, typically accompanied by excessive, prolonged menstruation.

Chronicle Brand name implantable monitor for continuous hemodynamic monitoring in patients with class III to class IV heart failure. Placement of a Chronicle device would be reported with unlisted CPT code 33999 or inpatient ICD-9-CM codes 37.79 and 89.63. The Chronicle system consists of an external data storage system and internally, a single lead with a pressure sensor tip and a wireless antenna system that allows continuous transmission of data on the heart rate, right ventricular diastolic and systolic pressure, physical activity, and body temperature to the storage system. The lead is inserted transvenously.

Chrysalin   Brand name synthetic thrombin receptor-activating peptide injected directly into the fracture site for acceleration of fracture repair. It is still in clinical trials. In the facility, ICD-9-CM procedural code 99.29 would be used as a secondary code to report the injection during fracture reduction. To report injection of Chrysalin using CPT, report an unlisted procedure of the corresponding anatomy. To report the supply of Chrysalin, report an unlisted HCPCS Level II J code.

church plan   Health plan established by and offered to employees of a church or other religious organization.

Churg-Strauss syndrome   Form of systemic inflammation and cell death of vessels with prominent lung involvement, manifested by severe asthma, among other respiratory disorders. Report this disorder with ICD-9-CM code 446.4.

churning   *1)* Performance-based reimbursement system emphasizing provider productivity. *2)* When a provider sees a patient more than medically necessary with the intent of generating more revenue.

Chvostek's sign   Physical predictor of neuromuscular excitability related to hypocalcemia that is elicited by tapping the cheek in front of the ear and just underneath the zygoma to see if the ipsilateral facial muscles twitch or spasm.

chyle   Milky fluid produced during digestion composed of lymph and triglyceride fats that mix with blood in the veins through the thoracic duct.

chylothorax   Type of pleural effusion; an accumulation of fluid in the pleural space, between the lungs and the chest wall, made up of chyle-like fluid from a leakage of chyle from the thoracic duct or from a chronic infection, such as tuberculosis. Report ICD-9-CM code 457.8 for non-filarial chylothorax and 125.9 for filarial chylothorax.

chylous   Pertaining to chyle, a white or yellowish fluid transferred into the lymphatic system from the intestines as a part of the digestion process.

chyme   Thick liquid substance consisting of partially digested food, water, enzymes, and digestive juices. Chyme forms in the stomach in the early phase of digestion and then progresses to the small intestines.

CI   *1)* Cardiac index. Heart measurement based on the volume of blood the left ventricle ejects into circulation in one minute, measured in liters per minute. The blood volume is divided by the body surface area of the patient to determine the cardiac index. *2)* Chloride. *3)* Confidence interval.

CIC   Completely in the canal (hearing aid).

cicatricial   Of or relating to scarring. *c. entropion* Scarring that results in inversion of the eyelid, causing

the lid margin to rest against and irritate the eyeball. *c. lagophthalmos* Scarring that results in an eye that cannot be completely closed. *c. pemphigoid* Autoimmune disease causing blisters on the skin, often accompanied by itching and/or burning and resulting in scarring.

cicatrix   New tissue formed in the healing of a wound, not limited to skin or external structures. Correct diagnosis code assignment is dependent upon the anatomical location of the scar. *Synonym(s): scar.*

cidofovir   Drug used to treat cytomegaloviral retinitis in AIDS patients by selectively inhibiting viral DNA synthesis and reproduction. Supply is reported with HCPCS Level II code J0740. May be sold under the brand name Vistide.

CIDP   Chronic inflammatory demyelinating polyradiculoneuropathy. Chronically progressive bilateral sensorimotor disorder, reported with ICD-9-CM code 357.81.

CIG   Cardiointegram. Experimental, noninvasive analysis of electrical signals of the heart reported with HCPCS Level II code S9025. CIG converts analog EKG signals to digital and performs a computer analysis that considers the time element. *NCD Reference: 20.27.*

cilastatin sodium imipenem   Combination injectable antibiotic used to treat a number of bacterial infections, including bacteremia and septicemia, bone and joint infections, diabetic foot ulcers, endocarditis, respiratory tract and gynecologic infections, and urinary tract infections. Supply is reported with HCPCS Level II code J0743. May be sold under brand name Primaxin IV and IM.

ciliary   Pertaining to the eyelid, eyelashes, or specific structures of the eyeball. *c. block* Increase in intraocular pressure that is accompanied by a shallow anterior chamber and forward displacement of the iris and lens. *c. body* Structure of the eye that produces the aqueous humor within the anterior chamber that nourishes the lens and cornea. The ciliary body is part of the uvea and connects anteriorly to the root of the iris and posteriorly to the choroid at the ora serrata retinae. It is divided into the pars plana and the pars plicata.

CIM   Coverage Issues Manual. Revised and renamed the National Coverage Determination Manual in the CMS manual system, CIM contained national coverage decisions and specific medical items, services, treatment procedures, or technologies paid for under the Medicare program.

cimetidine HCl   Antiulcer drug that decreases gastric acid secretion by inhibiting the action of histamine at H2 receptor sites. It is used to treat gastric and duodenal ulcers, GERD, heartburn, pathologic hypersecretory conditions, and as a preventive measure against upper gastrointestinal bleeding in critically ill patients. Supply

A-C

is reported with HCPCS Level II code S0023. May be sold under the brand name Tagamet.

Cimino type arteriovenous anastomosis Direct anastomosis of a vein to an artery, usually at the wrist of the nondominant hand. Using only a moderate amount of arterial and venous dissection, a portion of the vein is sutured in an end-to-side fashion to the adjacent artery, allowing blood to flow both down the artery and into the vein. The increased blood flow through the vein is used for hemodialysis. This type of direct AV anastomosis is reported with CPT code 36821.

CIN Cervical intraepithelial neoplasia. Classification following cervical biopsy to rank abnormalities in the epithelial cells of the cervix uteri. CIN I: low-grade abnormality; mild dysplasia, is reported with ICD-9-CM code 622.11 CIN II: high-grade abnormality; moderate dysplasia is reported with 622.12 CIN III: carcinoma in situ; severe dysplasia is reported with 233.1. Note that cervical Pap smear results are reported with codes from ICD-9-CM range 795.00-795.09. An abnormal Pap result can lead to a cervical biopsy and a CIN designation. CIN is commonly seen in patients with high-risk human papilloma virus (HPV) infection. If HPV is present, report it secondarily with 079.4.

CIN I Cervical intraepithelial neoplasia I; low-grade abnormality; mild dysplasia

CIN II Cervical intraepithelial neoplasia II; high-grade abnormality; moderate dysplasia

CIN III Cervical intraepithelial neoplasia III; carcinoma in situ; severe dysplasia

cine Movement usually related to motion pictures.

cineplastic amputation Amputation in which muscles and tendons of the remaining portion of the extremity are arranged so that they may be utilized for motor functions. Following this type of amputation, a specially constructed prosthetic device allows the individual to execute more complex movements because the muscles and tendons are able to communicate independent movements to the device.

cineradiography High-speed x-ray images taken in exposure ranges of nanoseconds to milliseconds to capture a series of moving images of an organ or organ system in motion, such as the vocal cords or heart. Cineradiography may be included as part of a procedure or reported alone with CPT code 76120. When it is performed in addition to a routine examination, it should be reported separately using 76125. *Synonym(s):* cinefluorography, cinematography, cinematoradiography, cineroentgenofluorography, cineroentgenography.

cingulotomy Creation of small lesions burned into the cingulate gyrus, the section of the brain connecting the limbic region to the frontal lobes. The lesions are made using stereotactic introduction of electrodes or the use

of gamma knife surgery to focus beams of radiation, resulting in lesions where the beams converge. Candidates for the procedure include those with medically intractable obsessive-compulsive disorder, refractive depression, chronic pain syndromes, and addictive disorders. When the procedure is performed for a psychiatric disease, it may be considered as experimental or investigational. *NCD Reference: 160.4.*

ciprofloxacin Broad-spectrum antibiotic administered by slow infusion into a vein that is used to treat a wide variety of bacterial infections, including those of the genitourinary tract, lungs, GI tract, skin, and bone. Supply is reported with HCPCS Level II code J0744. May be sold under the brand name Cipro.

circadian Relating to a cyclic, 24-hour period.

circle of Willis Arterial vessels forming a circle at the base of the cranial cavity. Included in the circle of Willis are the anterior cerebral, anterior communicating, internal carotid, posterior cerebral, and posterior communicating arteries. The circle creates redundancies in the blood supply to the brain that enable cerebral circulation to continue if one of the vessels becomes occluded.

circular amputation One of the original methods of amputation performed by making a circular incision in the skin and dissecting down through the muscles and bone leaving a little skin and muscle to fold over the stump.

circum- Encircling or around.

circumcise Circular cutting around the genitals to remove the prepuce or foreskin.

circumduction maneuver Circular maneuver performed to evaluate range of motion, particularly of the thumb, but may be done on any area where a group of joints are placed through a rotational motion.

circumferential Pertaining to the perimeter of an object or body.

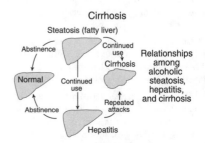

Cirrhosis

Steatosis (fatty liver)

Abstinence — Continued use — Cirrhosis

Normal — Continued use

Abstinence — Repeated attacks

Hepatitis

Relationships among alcoholic steatosis, hepatitis, and cirrhosis

cirrhosis Disease of the liver that has the characteristics of intertwining band of fibrous tissue that divides the parenchyma into micro- and macronodular areas. *alcoholic c.* Chronic disease of the liver that characteristically produces progressive fibrosis and nodules following initial enlargement with fatty infiltration of liver cells and inflammation caused by the poisoning from chronic alcohol consumption and its concomitant nutritional deficiency. Also called Laennec's cirrhosis, this alcoholic form of the liver disease is reported with ICD-9-CM code 571.2. **c. of liver** Chronic disease of the liver that characteristically produces intertwining bands of fibrotic tissue that change the normal structure of the lobes of the liver and destroys normal cells, which then regenerate into nodules and cause the liver to stop functioning over time. This form of cirrhosis is not alcohol related and is reported with 571.5.

CIS Carcinoma in situ.

cisplatin Antineoplastic drug used to treat advanced bladder cancer, head and neck cancer, non-small-cell cancer of the lung, osteogenic sarcoma, advanced esophageal cancer, and as an adjunct therapy in metastatic ovarian and testicular cancers. This drug has a high rate of cumulative renal toxicity and may even cause hearing loss. Supply is reported with HCPCS Level II code J9060. May be sold under the brand name Platinol AQ.

Cisterna Chyli

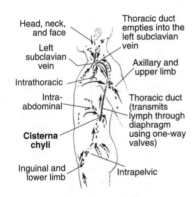

Head, neck, and face
Left subclavian vein
Intrathoracic
Intra-abdominal
Cisterna chyli
Inguinal and lower limb

Thoracic duct empties into the left subclavian vein
Axillary and upper limb
Thoracic duct (transmits lymph through diaphragm using one-way valves)
Intrapelvic

Nodes generally accompany large blood vessels

cisterna chyli Reservoir or dilation of the lymphatic system where the thoracic duct has its origin located in the center of the abdomen. Lymphatic fluid travels upward from the cisterna chyli through the thoracic duct into the diaphragm.

citrullinemia Rare genetic disorder in which there is a shortage or absence of argininosuccinate synthetase, one of six enzymes that function to break down and remove nitrogen from the body. The lack of this enzyme causes hyperammonemia, or excessive accumulation of nitrogen in the blood. Manifestations include vomiting,

anorexia, lethargy, and coma. Report this disorder with ICD-9-CM code 270.6.

CIU Chronic idiopathic urticaria. Wheals and swelling of the skin that persist for more than six weeks, of unknown etiology. CIU may continue for a few months or for years, and is reported with ICD-9-CM code 708.1.

civil monetary penalty Fine imposed on providers or suppliers by the DOJ for prohibited conduct in federal health care benefit programs, Medicare, and Medicaid. The monetary penalty may be up to $10,000 or three times the amount claimed, whichever is greater.

Civilian Health and Medical Program of the Uniformed Services Federal program that covered the health benefits for families of all uniformed service employees. The program has been replaced by TRICARE. *Synonym(s): CHAMPUS.*

Civilian Health and Medical Program of the Veteran's Administration Program similar to TRICARE under which the insured must be a disabled veteran's spouse or dependent or a survivor of someone who died of service-related causes. *Synonym(s): CHAMPVA.*

CJD Creutzfeldt-Jakob disease. Progressive destruction of the pyramidal and extrapyramidal systems with progressive dementia, wasting of muscles, tremor, and other symptoms leading to death. Report the various forms of this disorder with a code from ICD-9-CM subcategory 046.1.

CK Conductive keratoplasty. Surgery to correct vision by applying radiofrequencies generating heat to reshape the cornea. CK treats presbyopia, a form of far-sightedness associated with reduced accommodation seen in aging. Presbyopia is reported with ICD-9-CM code 367.4. It can also be used to treat hyperopia and normal farsightedness. CK is not covered by most insurance companies.

CKD Chronic kidney disease. Decreased renal efficiencies resulting in reduced ability of the kidney to filter waste. The National Kidney Foundation's classification includes five clinical stages, based on the glomerular filtration rate (GFR). The stages of CKD are as follows: stage 1 (ICD-9-CM code 585.1), some kidney damage with normal or slightly increased GFR (>90); stage 2 (585.2), mild kidney damage with a GFR value of 60 to 89; stage 3 (585.3), moderate kidney damage with a GFR value of 30 to 59; stage 4 (585.4), severe kidney damage and a GFR value of 15 to 29; and stage 5 (585.5), severe kidney damage that has progressed to a GFR value of less than 15. Dialysis or transplantation is required at stage 5.

cl liqs Clear liquids.

CLA Certified laboratory assistant.

cladosporiosis epidermica Minor fungal infection caused by cladosporium mansoni or Exophiala werneckii, producing lesions that most commonly appear on the hands and rarely on other areas. The lesions look like the characteristic dark ink or dye stain that occurs when silver nitrate is spilled on the skin. Report this condition with ICD-9-CM code 111.1. **Synonym(s):** *keratomycosis nigricans, microsporosis nigra, pityriasis nigra, tinea nigra, tinea palmaris nigra.*

cladribine Antimetabolite class of antineoplastic drug used in the treatment of hairy cell leukemia or other cancers. Supply is reported with HCPCS Level II code J9065. May be sold under the brand names Leustatin, Leustat.

Claforan See cefotaxime sodium.

claim Statement of services rendered requesting payment from an insurance company or a government entity. *c. adjustment reason code* National administrative code set that identifies the reasons for any differences, or adjustments, between the original provider charge for a claim or service and the payer's payment for it. This code set is used in the X12 835 Claim Payment & Remittance Advice and the X12 837 Claim Transactions and is maintained by the Health Care Code Maintenance Committee. *c. attachment* Any of a variety of hard copy forms or electronic records needed to process a claim in addition to the claim itself. *c. denial* Denial of an entire claim. The provider cannot resubmit the claim but can appeal the claim denial. *c. lag* Time incurred between the date of a claim and its submission or payment. *c. manual* Administrative guidelines used by claims processors to adjudicate claims according to company policy and procedure. *c. manager* Payer's manager who oversees the employee who processes routine claims. *c. rejection* Rejection of the entire claim. The provider may correct and resubmit the claim but cannot appeal the claim. *c. review* Examination of a submitted demand for payment by a Medicare contractor, insurer, or other group to determine payment liability, eligibility, or reasonableness or necessity of care provided. *c. reviewer* Payer employee who reviews claims like an auditor, looking at coding, prior authority, contract violations, etc. *c. status codes* National administrative code set that identifies the status of health care claims. This code set is used in the X12 277 Claim Status Notification transaction and is maintained by the Health Care Code Maintenance Committee.

claim adjustment reason codes National administrative code set that identifies reasons for any differences or adjustments between the original provider charge for a claim or service and the payer's payment. This code set is used in the X12 835 claim payment and remittance advice and the X12 837 claim transactions, and is maintained by the Health Care Code Maintenance Committee. **Synonym(s):** *CARC.*

claim attachment Any of a variety of hard copy documents or electronic records needed to process a claim in addition to the claim itself.

claim lag Time incurred between the date of a claim and its submission for payment. *c. manual* Administrative guidelines used by claims processors to adjudicate claims according to company policy and procedure.

claim manual Administrative guidelines used by claims processors to adjudicate claims according to company policy and procedure.

claim rejection Rejection of the entire claim. The provider may correct and resubmit the claim but cannot appeal the claim.

claim status category codes National administrative code set that indicates the general category of the status of health care claims. This code set is used in the X12 277 Claim Status Notification transaction, and is maintained by the Health Care Code Maintenance Committee.

claim status codes National administrative code set that identifies the status of health care claims. This code set is used in the X12 277 claim status notification transaction and is maintained by the Health Care Code Maintenance Committee.

claims review Examination of a submitted demand for payment by a Medicare contractor, insurer, or other group to determine payment liability, eligibility, reasonableness, or necessity of care provided.

clamp Tool used to grip, compress, join, or fasten body parts.

Clarke-Hadfield syndrome Obstructions of mucosal passageways, poor growth, chronic bronchitis, recurrent pneumonia, emphysema, clubbing of fingers, salt depletion, and abnormal secretions of exocrine glands. Report this disorder with ICD-9-CM code 577.8. **Synonym(s):** *Burke's syndrome.*

classification of surgical wounds Surgical wounds fall into four categories that determine treatment methods and outcomes:

clean wound: No inflammation or contamination; treatment performed with no break in sterile technique; no alimentary, respiratory, or genitourinary tracts involved in the surgery. Infection rate: up to 5 percent.

clean-contaminated wound: No inflammation; treatment performed with minor break in surgical technique; no unusual contamination resulting when alimentary, respiratory, genitourinary, or oropharyngeal cavity is entered. Infection rate: up to 11 percent.

contaminated wound: Less than four hours old with acute, nonpurulent inflammation; treatment performed with major break in surgical technique; gross contamination resulting from the gastrointestinal tract. Infection rate: up to 20 percent.

dirty and infected wound: More than four hours old with existing infection, inflammation, abscess, and nonsterile conditions due to perforated viscus, fecal contamination, necrotic tissue, or foreign body. Infection rate: up to 40 percent.

clastothrix Condition in which small, white nodules appear in the hair shafts where the hair shaft cortex has broken and split apart, causing the hair to break off, usually after growing only an inch or two. Report clastothrix with ICD-9-CM code 704.2. ***Synonym(s): bamboo hair, trichoclasia, trichorrhexis nodosa.***

Claude Bernard-Horner syndrome Disorder following a heart attack with pain and stiffness in the shoulder, and swelling and pain in the hand. Report this disorder with ICD-9-CM code 337.9. ***Synonym(s): Reilly's syndrome, Steinbrocker's syndrome.***

claudication Lameness, pain, and weakness occurring in the arms or legs during exercise due to muscles not receiving the needed oxygen and nutrients.

claustrophobia Anxiety disorder that involves an irrational fear of closed spaces, reported with ICD-9-CM code 300.29.

clavicotomy Dividing or cutting the collarbone of the fetus in order to aid in delivery, reported with ICD-9-CM procedure code 73.8. For CPT coding purposes, an unlisted code must be used, as there is no code supplied specifically for this procedure.

clavus Conical thickening or localized overgrowth of hyperkeratotic tissue of the epidermal layer of the foot or toes due to chronic irritation, friction, or pressure, reported with ICD-9-CM code 700. ***Synonym(s): callus, clavus mollis, Heloma molle, soft corn.***

claw hand deformity Abnormal positioning of the hand and fingers usually associated with ulnar nerve palsy, in which the metacarpal phalangeal joints are hyperextended with concomitant flexion of the proximal and distal interphalangeal joints. Acquired claw hand is reported with ICD-9-CM code 736.06 and congenital with 755.59.

claw toes Abnormal positioning of the toes. Claw toes can be congenital (ICD-9-CM code 754.71) or acquired (735.5), in which the proximal metatarsophalangeal joints are hyperextended with flexed middle and distal phalangeal joints. ***Synonym(s): hammer toe.***

CLC Creative living center.

CLD *1)* Chronic liver disease. *2)* Chronic lung disease.

-cle Small or little. ***Synonym(s): -cule.***

clean claim Submitted bill for services rendered that passes all edits and does not require any further investigation.

clean wound Wound with no inflammation and procedure performed under sterile operating room conditions with no break in sterile technique. No alimentary, respiratory, oropharyngeal, or genitourinary tracts are involved in the surgery. Infection rate: up to 5 percent.

clean-contaminated wound Wound with no inflammation and procedure performed with minor break in surgical technique. No unusual contamination found in alimentary, respiratory, genitourinary, or oropharyngeal cavity entered. Infection rate: up to 11 percent.

CLEAR Clear lens extraction and replacement. CLEAR surgery represents the same surgery performed on cataract patients. The natural lens is replaced with an artificial one. However, in CLEAR, the patient has no lens defect (cataract), and the surgery is done to correct the patient's near- or far-sightedness, not to correct a cataract. CLEAR is usually not covered by medical insurance, since it is considered cosmetic, akin to LASIK or other vision-correction surgeries. ***Synonym(s): CLE.***

clearinghouse See health care clearinghouse.

Cleft Palate

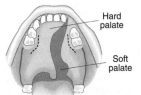

Cleft of alveolar ridge

cleft Fissure or abnormal separation from failure of parts to fuse during embryogenesis. ***c. hand*** Failure of the central ray of the metacarpals to fully develop, resulting in an extended separation between the fingers into the metacarpals or large fingers with absent middle fingers of the hand. Cleft hand is reported with ICD-9-CM code 755.58. ***c. lip*** Congenital fissure or separation of the upper lip due to failure of embryonic cells to fuse completely. A cleft lip can occur unilaterally or bilaterally and may accompany other abnormalities of the upper jaw, nose, or oral structures. Code assignment is dependent upon whether the cleft lip is unilateral or bilateral, complete or incomplete, and whether or not it is accompanied by a cleft palate. See ICD-9-CM category 749 for code assignment. For repair of a cleft lip, see CPT codes 40700-40761. ***c. palate*** Congenital fissure or separation in the roof of the mouth, allowing it to open into the nasal cavity, due to failure of the palatine processes to fuse completely. A cleft palate may appear as a complete separation of both the anterior bony hard palate and the posterior fleshy soft palate, or it may involve only one localized area. The deformity may be unilateral or bilateral and may be accompanied by a cleft lip. A cleft palate is reported with codes from ICD-9-CM rubric 749. See CPT codes 42200-42225 for repair.

cleido- Relating to the clavicle.

cleidocranial dysostosis Genetic disease most often characterized by the absence or hypoplastic development of the collarbone, an enlarged head, dental abnormalities, and underdeveloped pelvic bones. Cleidocranial dysostosis is reported with ICD-9-CM code 755.59. *Synonym(s): CCD, Cheuthauer-Marie-Sainton syndrome.*

cleidotomy Surgical separation of the fetus's clavicle in cases of difficult labor in order to allow the shoulders to pass through the birth canal. Report cleidotomy with ICD-9-CM procedure code 73.8.

Cleocin phosphate See clindamycin phosphate.

cleptomania Persistent, irrepressible impulse to steal objects that are not needed for personal use or financial gain, reported with ICD-9-CM code 312.32. *Synonym(s): kleptomania.*

Clerambault's syndrome Delusional belief that someone, often a person of high social status, is in love with the patient. Report this disorder with ICD-9-CM code 297.8.

clevidipine butyrate Intravenous medication indicated for the treatment of severe episodes of hypertension when oral antihypertensive administration is not an option. It metabolizes in the blood rather than the kidney or liver and does not accumulate in the body, making it suitable for patients with end-stage organ disease. May be sold under the brand name Cleviprex. Supply is reported with HCPCS Level II code C9248.

Cleviprex Intravenous medication indicated for the treatment of severe episodes of hypertension when oral antihypertensive administration is not an option. It metabolizes in the blood rather than the kidney or liver and does not accumulate in the body, making it suitable for patients with end-stage organ disease. Supply is reported with HCPCS Level II code C9248. *Synonym(s): clevidipine butyrate.*

CLIA Clinical Laboratory Improvement Amendments. Requirements set in 1988, CLIA imposes varying levels of federal regulations on clinical procedures. Few laboratories, including those in physician offices, are exempt. Adopted by Medicare and Medicaid, CLIA regulations redefine laboratory testing in regard to laboratory certification and accreditation, proficiency testing, quality assurance, personnel standards, and program administration.

Clifford's syndrome Placental dysfunction occurring in postmature fetuses. Report this disorder with ICD-9-CM code 766.22.

climacteric syndrome Chills, depression, hot flashes, headache, and irritability in menopausal women. Report this disorder with ICD-9-CM code 627.2.

clindamycin phosphate Anti-infective that kills sensitive strains of staph, strep, pneumococci, Clostridium perfringens, and other bacteria, both aerobic and anaerobic. It is used specifically for pelvic inflammatory disease, Pneumocystis carinii pneumonia, and as a prophylaxis against endocarditis prior to dental work. The injectable supply is reported with HCPCS Level II code S0077. May be sold under the brand names Cleocin Pediatric, Dalacin.

clinic Outpatient facility that provides scheduled diagnostic, curative, rehabilitative, and educational services for walk-in (ambulatory) patients.

clinical crown Part of the tooth that is not covered by any supporting structures such as the gums.

clinical documentation improvement Program tasked with the generation of more specific and complete chart documentation in order to assure the proper use of resources, correct assessment of the patient's severity of illness, and compliance with regulatory requirements. *Synonym(s): CDI.*

Clinical Laboratory Improvement Amendments Federal regulations imposed in 1988 to define laboratory certification and accreditation, proficiency testing, quality assurance, personnel standards, and program administration.

clinical manifestation Display or disclosure of signs and symptoms of an illness.

clinical service organization Health care organization developed by academic medical centers to integrate the medical school, the faculty practice plan, and the hospital plan. *Synonym(s): CSO.*

clinical social worker Individual who possesses a master's or doctor's degree in social work and, after obtaining the degree, has performed at least two years of supervised clinical social work. A clinical social worker must be licensed by the state or, in the case of states without licensure, must completed at least two years or 3,000 hours of post-master's degree supervised clinical social work practice under the supervision of a master's level social worker.

clinodactyly Congenital deviation of the little finger where it curves toward the ring finger. It can occur alone or with Down syndrome. This is usually not treated. *Synonym(s): bent finger.*

clitoridectomy Surgical removal of all or part of the clitoris. This procedure may also include removal of the labia and is considered a form of female circumcision. Clitoridectomy is practiced in other countries as part of a culturally determined ritual. Clitoridectomy status is reported with ICD-9-CM 629.20-629.23. **Synonym(s):** *clitoral amputation, clitorectomy, female genital mutilation.*

CLL Chronic lymphatic leukemia.

cloacal anomaly Congenital anomaly resulting from the failure of one common urinary, anal, and reproductive vaginal passage of the early embryonic stage to develop into the properly divided rectal and urogenital sections.

clonidine HCl Antihypertensive drug that lowers peripheral vascular resistance blood pressure and heart rate. This drug is used not only to treat essential and renal hypertension, but also as an adjunctive therapy for smoking cessation, alcohol and opiate dependence, pain relief in dysmenorrhea and cancer, and as a prophylactic against migraines. Supply is reported with HCPCS Level II code J0735 for injectable supply. May be sold under the brand names Catapress, Dixarit, Duraclon.

clonorchiasis Infectious disease of the biliary passages by infestation with the Chinese liver fluke Clonorchis sinensis. Infection of humans occurs by eating infected raw, dried, salted, or pickled fish. Inflammation of the biliary tract, portal fibrosis, cirrhosis of the liver, and carcinoma of the biliary duct may occur. Report this condition with ICD-9-CM code 121.1. **Synonym(s):** *clonorchiosis.*

clonus Recurring, regular contractions of a muscle when trying to maintain it in a stretched position, considered normal in newborns, but in others may signify multiple sclerosis, injury of the spinal cord, spastic paraparesis, or other CNS diseases. Report this condition with ICD-9-CM code 781.0.

Cloquet's canal Embryonic vestige of A. hyoidea.

Cloquet's node Highest deep inguinofemoral lymph node.

closed angle glaucoma Progressive optic nerve disease associated with high intraocular pressure that can lead to irreversible vision loss. The aqueous humor is the clear fluid filling the chambers of the eye that is continually drained and renewed, produced by the ciliary body and passing out through the pupil and trabecular meshwork. Angle closure glaucoma causes an increase in intraocular pressure due to an impairment of aqueous outflow caused by a narrowing or closing of the anterior chamber angle as the iris comes into contact with the trabecular meshwork. This type of glaucoma is identified in four stages: latent, intermittent, acute, and chronic. In the latent and intermittent phases, minor or transient attacks of varying severity, duration, and frequency occur in which intraocular pressure (IOP) rises with accompanying pain and edema. Acute angle closure glaucoma is a grave medical emergency as IOP rises, the cornea swells, and excruciating pain radiates through the eye. Visual acuity falls rapidly as the eye swells and

blindness may result if the IOP is not lowered. The chronic stage manifests as irreversible IOP increases from progressive damage and scar tissue closing the anterior angle. Closed angle glaucoma is reported with ICD-9-CM codes 365.20-365.24. **Synonym(s):** *angle closure glaucoma, narrow angle glaucoma, pupillary block glaucoma.*

closed claim Claim for which all apparent benefits have been paid.

closed dislocation Simple displacement of a body part without an open wound.

closed fracture Break in a bone without a concomitant opening in the skin. A closed fracture is coded when the type of fracture is not specified.

closed panel Arrangement in which a managed care organization contracts providers on an exclusive basis, restricting the providers from seeing patients enrolled in other payers' plans.

closed reduction Treatment of a fracture by manipulating it into proper alignment without opening the skin.

closed treatment Realignment of a fracture or dislocation without surgically opening the skin to reach the site. Treatment methods employed include with or without manipulation, and with or without traction.

clostridium perfringens/difficile Gram-positive, spore forming, obligate anaerobic bacteria from the family bacillaceae. Pathogenic species have the ability to produce deadly exotoxins or enzymes. C. perfringens is the most common cause of gas gangrene in humans. Toxin A from C. perfringens is associated with gas gangrene and necrotizing colitis while type C toxin causes enteritis necroticans. C. difficile is often encountered in patients on antibiotic therapy as it is normally found in the colon as part of the normal flora and it colonizes in the intestine as other beneficial bacteria die off and the balance is offset. C. difficile is found to produce Toxin A and B that cause enterocolitis. C. difficile is also a prevalent form of nosocomial or hospital-acquired infection. Diagnosis is usually made by identifying toxin in the stool or by enzyme immunoassay.

closure Repairing an incision or wound by suture or other means.

Clouston's syndrome Congenital thickened nails and sparse or absent scalp hair, often accompanied by keratoderma of the palms and soles. Report this disorder with ICD-9-CM code 757.31.

Clsd Closed.

CLT Complex lymphedema therapy. Massage and manipulation of the affected tissue as a treatment for chronic intractable lymphedema. Lymphedema is reported with ICD-9-CM code 457.1 when an acquired chronic condition; postmastectomy lymphedema is

A-C

reported with 457.0; and hereditary edema of the legs is reported with 757.0. **Synonym(s):** *CDP, complex decongestive physiotherapy.*

clubfoot Congenital or acquired anomaly of the foot with the heel elevated and rotated outwards and the toes pointing inward. Clubfoot is reported with a code from ICD-9-CM rubric 736 or 754. It may be treated with serial casting and stretching or surgery. **Synonym(s):** *congenital talipes equinovarus.*

clump kidney Urogenital abnormality present at birth in which the two kidneys never separated, but fused into a single entity and drain through a single ureter. **Synonym(s):** *cake kidney.*

clumsiness syndrome Disorders in which the main feature is a serious impairment in the development of motor coordination that is not explicable in terms of general intellectual retardation and is commonly associated with perceptual difficulties.

cluster headache Characteristic grouping or clustering of attacks in which headache periods can last for a number of weeks or months and then completely disappear for months or years. One of the least common types of headache, the cause is unknown. Men are affected more often than women, and the headaches are typically not associated with gastrointestinal upset or light sensitivity as experienced in migraines. Cluster headaches are reported with an ICD-9-CM code from range 339.00-339.02. **Synonym(s):** *histamine headache, Horton's neuralgia.*

clysis Fluids injected into the body.

cm Centimeter.

cm2 Square centimeters.

CMA Certified medical assistant.

CMC Carpometacarpal (joint). Joint in the hand where the carpal bones of the wrist meet the metacarpal bones of the hand.

CMCH Community mental health center.

CMG Cystometrogram. Graphic recording of urinary bladder pressure at various volumes, which is useful in differentiating bladder outlet obstruction from other voiding dysfunctions. A simple CMG utilizes a pressure catheter inserted into the bladder connected to a manometer line filled with fluid to measure pressure through the changes in the height of the water column. CMG is reported with CPT code 51725. A complex CMG utilizes calibrated electronic equipment with a microtipped pressure catheter and is reported with 51726.

CMHC Community mental health center.

CMI Case mix index. Sum of all DRG relative weights, divided by the number of Medicare cases. A low CMI may

denote DRG assignments that do not adequately reflect the resources used to treat Medicare patients.

CML Chronic myelogenous leukemia.

CMML Chronic myelomonocytic leukemia. CMML is reported with ICD-9-CM codes 205.10-205.12.

CMN Certificate of medical necessity.

CMP Competitive medical plan. Federal designation allowing plans to obtain eligibility to receive a Medicare risk contract without having to qualify as an HMO.

CMRI Cardiac magnetic resonance imaging.

CMS *1)* Centers for Medicare and Medicaid Services. Federal agency that administers the public health programs. *2)* Circulation motion sensation.

CMS manual system Web-based manuals organized by functional area that contain all program instructions in the National Coverage Determinations Manual, the Medicare Benefit Policy Manual, Pub 100, one-time notifications, and manual revision notices.

CMS manuals Official government manuals prepared by CMS that detail procedures for processing and paying Medicare claims, preparing reimbursement forms, and billing procedures. These manuals were converted to web-based manuals (referred to as IOM, or Internet-only manuals) on October 1, 2003. At the time of the conversion, the manuals were streamlined, updated, and consolidated. Manuals may be accessed at http://www.cms.gov/manuals.

CMS-1450 Universal form used to file institutional claims. **Synonym(s):** *UB-92.*

CMS-1500 Universal form used to file professional claims.

CMSA Consolidated Metropolitan Statistical Area, as designated by CMS.

CMT Certified medical transcriptionist.

CMV Cytomegalovirus.

cn Cranial nerves.

CNA Certified nursing assistant.

CNM Certified nurse midwife.

CNP Continuous negative airway pressure.

CNS Central nervous system.

co Cardiac output.

CO Fick Cardiac output measured by the direct O2 Fick method, which does not require insertion of a catheter into the right heart, but does require invasive mixed venous and peripheral arterial blood drawings and oxygen uptake measurements at the mouth, limiting its practical application. This method is more the theoretical standard than the applied method. The cardiac output is calculated as the quotient of oxygen uptake and the difference between the arterial and mixed venous oxygen content.

CO2   Carbon dioxide.

CO2 indirect Fick   Cardiac output measured noninvasively using the indirect Fick method, an equation using carbon dioxide output instead of oxygen uptake. This method uses carbon dioxide rebreathing techniques that require only indirect measurements of arterial and venous CO2 levels, estimated by respective partial pressures: Arterial CO2 partial pressure from %CO2 of end tidal air determined by sampling gas from a breathing bag, and mixed venous partial pressure determined by rebreathing a mixture of CO2 and measuring changes in %CO2 in bag breath by breath. This indirect method is used more often than the direct method since carbon dioxide output is easier to measure than oxygen uptake. Reported this test with ICD-9-CM procedure code 89.67.

CO2 laser   Carbon dioxide laser that emits an invisible beam and vaporizes water-rich tissue. The vapor is suctioned from the site.

COA   Certificate of authority. State license to operate as an HMO.

coagulation   Clot formation.

coagulation-fibrinolysis syndrome   Decrease of elements needed for coagulation of blood causing profuse bleeding. Report this disorder with ICD-9-CM code 286.6. *Synonym(s): coagulopathy.*

Coaguloop   Brand name resection electrode designed for use with a resectoscope for prostate operations, used in transurethral electrosurgical prostate resection, reported with CPT code 52601.

coal workers' lung   Coal dust deposits in the lung. Prolonged exposure to coal dust in mining causes the development of small sacs containing coal dust. This condition is reported with ICD-9-CM code 500. *Synonym(s): anthracosis, black lung, coal workers' pneumoconiosis, miners' asthma.*

Coaptite   Brand name permanent implant gel injected into the submucosal wall of the urethra to treat female urinary stress incontinence, reported with ICD-9-CM code 625.5, and intrinsic sphincter deficiency, reported with 599.82. Injection of Coaptite would be reported with CPT code 51715. Supply of the gel would be reported with HCPCS Level II code L8606.

coarctation of aorta   Localized deformation of the aortic media that causes a severe constriction of the vessel, resulting in high blood pressure in the arms and low pressure in the legs. This condition must be treated to prevent a cerebrovascular accident, endocarditis, congestive heart failure, or rupture of the aorta. ICD-9-CM subcategory 747.1 is reserved for coarctation

of the aorta and CPT codes 33840-33853 report procedures for this condition.

Coat's disease   Retinal vascular anomaly associated with lipid exudate, seen unilaterally in young boys, reported with ICD-9-CM code 362.12.

COB   Coordination of benefits. In health care contracting, method of integrating benefits payable when there is more than one group insurance plan so that the insured's benefits and the payment of insurance benefits from all sources do not exceed 100 percent of the allowed medical expenses.

Cobalt teletherapy   First form of radiation therapy used to eradicate cancer cells using gamma rays, which caused less damage to skin surfaces.

Cobalt unit   Teletherapy treatment machine that emits a constant beam of cobalt to a predetermined beam size for a specifically calculated amount of time.

Cobalt-60   Radioactive isotope.

cobex   See cyanocobalamin.

COBRA   Consolidated Omnibus Reconciliation Act. Federal law that allows and requires past employees to be covered under company health insurance plans for a set premium, allowing individuals to remain insured when their current plan or position has been terminated.

COC   Certificate of coverage.

coccidiosis   Infection by the protozoan Isospora hominis or I. belli, usually asymptomatic and found by testing stool sample, reported with ICD-9-CM code 007.2. *Synonym(s): isosporiasis.*

coccygectomy   Surgical excision of the coccyx or tailbone.

coccygodynia   Pain in the coccyx, or tailbone, that may occur spontaneously or as a result of injury. Treatment normally consists of antiinflammatory drugs or steroid injections, although surgical removal of the coccyx may be required. Report this condition with ICD-9-CM code 724.79.

cochlea   Bony, spiral-shaped structure forming part of the inner ear labyrinth that leads from the oval window.

cochlear implant   Hearing device used in profoundly deaf individuals, consisting of a battery-operated processor that converts sound waves into an electrical current, an internal and external coil system that transmits the electrical impulses, and an electrode array implanted in the cochlea that stimulates the fibers of the auditory nerve. Diagnostic analysis of cochlear implants is classified to CPT codes 92601-92604. Insertion of the device is reported with 69930. Device and supplies for cochlear implants are classified to HCPCS Level II codes L8614-L8619 and L8627-L8628. *NCD Reference: 50.3.*

A-C

A-C

Cockayne's syndrome Dwarfism with deafness, retinal atrophy, mental retardation, and photo sensitivity. Report this disorder with ICD-9-CM code 759.89.

Cockayne-Weber syndrome Dwarfism with a precociously senile appearance, pigmentary degeneration of the retina, optic atrophy, deafness, sensitivity to sunlight, and mental retardation. Report this disorder with ICD-9-CM code 757.39.

cock-up splint Splint designed to hold the wrist in a position of dorsi-flexion to relieve pain to the radial side of the wrist and forearm. Supply is reported with HCPCS Level II code L3908. Generic prefabricated splints are reported to non-Medicare payers with S8451.

coctolabile Capable of being destroyed or altered when boiled.

code set Under HIPAA, any set of codes used to encode data elements, such as tables of terms, medical concepts, medical diagnosis codes, or medical procedure codes. This includes both the codes and their descriptions.

code set maintaining organization Under HIPAA, an organization that creates and maintains the code sets adopted by the secretary for use in the transactions for which standards are adopted.

codeine phosphate Narcotic analgesic used to relieve mild to moderate pain in adults and treat nonproductive coughs. Supply is reported with HCPCS Level II code J0745. May be sold under the brand name Paveral.

coder Professional who translates documented, written diagnoses and procedures into numeric and alphanumeric codes.

Code-set maintaining organization Under HIPAA, organization that creates and maintains the code sets adopted by the secretary for use in the transactions for which standards are adopted.

Codimal-A Brand name of brompheniramine, an antihistamine used primarily to treat symptoms of allergy and the common cold. Supply is reported with HCPCS Level II code J0945.

coding conventions Each space, typeface, indentation, and punctuation mark determining how ICD-9-CM codes are interpreted. These conventions were developed to help match correct codes to the diagnoses documented.

coding guidelines Criteria that specify how procedure, diagnosis, or supply codes are to be translated and used in various situations. Coding guidelines are issued by the AHA, AMA, CMS, NCHVS, and various other groups. Guidelines may vary by payer, type of coding system, and intended use.

coding rules Official rules and coding conventions used for diagnosis and procedure coding.

coding specificity Codes must be assigned the most specific available; i.e., a three-digit disease code is

assigned only when there are no four-digit codes within that category, a four-digit code is assigned only when there is no fifth-digit subclassification within that category, or a fifth digit is assigned for any category for which a fifth-digit subclassification is provided.

Codman sign Sign that is tested for in a simple maneuver to determine if rupture of the supraspinatus tendon has occurred. The arm is supported and moved away from the body without pain. The sign is positive if, when the support is removed, the deltoid muscle contracts and causes pain.

Codman triangle Triangular area of new subperiosteal bone usually found at the advancing edge of a tumor or abscess, seen on radiographic examination as it lifts the periosteum away from the bone. This is associated with osteosarcoma, Ewing's sarcoma, and subperiosteal abscesses, but has no direct bearing on code selection from a positive finding.

coenurosis Infestation by the tapeworm larvae of the genus Coenurus, found rarely in humans, almost always forming cysts in the central nervous system that block cerebrospinal fluid and cause increased intracranial pressure. Surgical removal of the cysts is often required. Report this condition with ICD-9-CM code 123.8.

Coffin-Lowry syndrome Genetic disorder characterized by craniofacial and skeletal abnormalities, mental retardation, short stature, and hypotonia (skeletal muscle weakness). Report this disorder with ICD-9-CM code 759.89.

Cogan's sign Twitching lid in a patient with myasthenia when the patient is instructed to look down for several seconds, then quickly look up.

Cogan's syndrome Abrupt onset of interstitial keratitis, tinnitus, and vertigo followed by deafness. Report this disorder with ICD-9-CM code 370.52.

Cogan-Reese syndrome Unilateral iris nevus with atrophy and corneal endotheliopathy and edema in an iridocorneal endothelial syndrome. Do not confuse Cogan-Reese syndrome with Cogan's syndrome, which is indexed in ICD-9-CM. Cogan-Reese syndrome is not indexed. To report it this syndrome, first code the nevus, reported with ICD-9-CM code 224.0. Report other presenting manifestations as well. Secondary glaucoma is a risk in Cogan-Reese syndrome.

Cogentin See benztropine mesylate.

cognitive Being aware by drawing from knowledge, such as judgment, reason, perception, and memory.

COH Controlled ovarian hyperstimulation. Use of fertility drugs to stimulate development of egg follicles.

coinsurance Limitation of the amount payable by the payer to the provider or member for care in traditional plans or in parts of managed care plans. Most traditional plans pay 80 percent of care costs resulting in 20 percent coinsurance or cost share by the patient.

coinsurance days Under Medicare hospital benefits, each day of hospitalization over 60 days, up to the 90th day, for which a coinsurance payment of one-fourth of the inpatient hospital's deductible must be made, along with a payment equal to one-half of the deductible for covered days after the 90th day not to exceed 150 days.

colchicine Drug used to prevent acute attacks of gout and gouty arthritis when used as a preventive or maintenance therapy. Supply is reported with HCPCS Level II code J0760. May be sold under the brand name Colgout.

COLD Chronic obstructive lung disease.

cold injury (newborn) syndrome Birth injury resulting from hypothermia. Report this disorder with ICD-9-CM code 778.2.

colectomy Excision of a segment or all of the colon.

colistimethate sodium Potent antibiotic used to treat Enterobacter aerogenes, Escherichia coli, Klebsiella pneumoniae, and Pseudomonas aeruginosa infections. Supply is reported with HCPCS Level II code J0770. May be sold under the brand name Coly-mycin M.

colitis Inflammation of the colon, caused by any number of infections, external influences such as laxatives or radiation, and antibiotics. Diagnosis codes are selected by cause or type.

collagen Protein based substance of strength and flexibility that is the major component of connective tissue, found in cartilage, bone, tendons, and skin. Collagen is often injected to improve the appearance of skin. Collagen injections may be used to decrease deep facial wrinkles, creases, and furrows or to fill out ôsunkenô cheeks or other skin depressions. For collagen injections, see CPT codes 11950-11954. Collagen is also used in wound dressing pads and as wound filler, reported with HCPCS Level II codes A6010-A6024.

collapsed lung Condition in which all or part of a lung remains airless and cannot completely expand and fill with air. Report this condition with ICD-9-CM code 518.0. *Synonym(s): atelectasis, pulmonary collapse.*

collar Device that encircles the neck to immobilize it, provide support, and/or severely limit its mobility.

collateral circulation Series of secondary blood vessels that form to provide blood supply to an area where the main artery is damaged or occluded. They generate spontaneously and are often responsible for saving an organ or limb. This is a term seen in operative notes and angiograms with no specific bearing on code selection.

College of Healthcare Information Management Executives Professional organization for health care chief information officers (CIOs). *Synonym(s): CHIME.*

Colles' Fracture

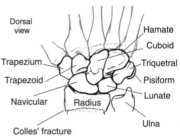

Colles' fracture

Colles' fracture Fracture of the radius at the wrist in which the distal fragment is pushed posteriorly. The dorsal angulation of the fragment results in the wrist cocking up.

Collet (-Sicard) syndrome Unilateral lesions of the ninth, tenth, eleventh, and twelfth cranial nerves producing paralysis of the vagal, glossal, and other nerves and the tongue on the same side. Report this disorder with ICD-9-CM code 352.6.

Coloboma

A congenital keyhole pupil is also called a coloboma of the iris

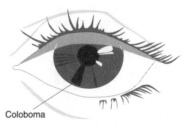

Coloboma

coloboma Defective or absent section of ocular tissue that may present as mild cupping or a small pit in the ocular disc due to extensive defects in the iris, ciliary body, choroids, and retina. *c. lentis* Cleft defect on the outer margin of the lens. *c. of the ciliary body* Common congenital defect of the ciliary body often appearing in trisomy 13 and seen as a white lesion with differing pigment around it. *c. of the iris* Keyhole-shaped defect within the lower, nasal quadrant of the eye. *choroidal c.* Fissure in the choroids that causes a scotoma on the retina. *complete c.* Typical type of coloboma seen extending from the margin of the pupil to the outer, posterior pole and involves the iris, ciliary body, choroid, retina, and the optic disc.

colonoscopy Visual inspection of the colon using a fiberoptic scope.

colorectal cancer screening test One of the following procedures performed for the purpose of detecting colorectal cancer: screening barium enema (HCPCS Level II code G0106, G0120, or G0122), screening fecal-occult blood test (CPT code 82270 or HCPCS Level II code G0328), screening flexible sigmoidoscopy (HCPCS Level II code G0104), screening colonography (CPT code 74263), and screening colonoscopy (HCPCS Level II code G0105 on a high-risk individual or G0121 for an individual not meeting criteria for high risk).

colostomy Artificial surgical opening anywhere along the length of the colon to the skin surface for the diversion of feces.

colpalgia Pain in the vagina.

colpocentesis Aspiration of fluid from the retrouterine cul-de-sac by puncture of the vaginal vault near the midline between the uterosacral ligaments. Report this procedure with CPT code 57020. *Synonym(s): culdocentesis.*

colpocleisis Surgical procedure in which the vaginal canal is closed in order to prevent uterine prolapse. Report colpocleisis with ICD-9-CM procedure code 70.8 and CPT code 57120.

colpopexy Suturing a prolapsed vagina to its surrounding structures for vaginal fixation.

colporrhaphy Plastic repair or reconstruction of the vagina by suturing the vaginal wall and surrounding fibrous tissue.

colporrhexis Laceration of the vaginal wall or sulcus occurring in childbirth without mention of perineal laceration. Reported this condition with a code from ICD-9-CM subcategory 665.4.

Colposcopy

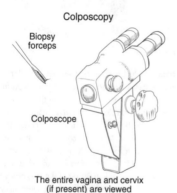

Biopsy forceps

Colposcope

The entire vagina and cervix
(if present) are viewed

colposcopy Procedure in which the physician views the cervix and vagina through a colposcope, which is a binocular microscope used for direct visualization of the vagina, ectocervix, and endocervix. Diagnostic vaginal/cervical colposcopy, not performed in conjunction with a surgical procedure, is reported with CPT code 57420 or 57452.

colpospasm Painful, involuntary contractions of the vagina, preventing intercourse. Colpospasm is reported with ICD-9-CM code 625.1, unless it stems from a psychogenic cause, reported with 306.51. *Synonym(s): vaginismus.*

colpotomy Incision into the vaginal wall for diagnostic or therapeutic purposes, reported with CPT code 57000 or 57010. *Synonym(s): Laroyenne operation.*

columella nasi Outer, distal margin of the nasal septum that divides the nostrils.

Coly-Mycin M See colistimethate sodium.

combat fatigue Brief, episodic, or recurrent disorders lasting less than six months after the onset of trauma.

Combidex Brand name molecular imaging agent for MRI for identifying lymph node metastases. Supply of Combidex is reported with HCPCS Level II code Q9953, or for outpatient facilities, C8903, C8905, C8906, or C8908. Injection of Combidex is bundled into the appropriate MRI with contrast code. Combidex contains ferumoxtran-10.

combined approach Periorbital and maxillary sinus approach performed together.

comedo necrosis Tissue death occurring within a gland, most commonly seen in the breast or prostate and associated with a malignancy. In comedo necrosis, a central luminal inflammation contains necrotic debris, and is usually indicative of a more invasive disease. There is no ICD-9-CM code specific to comedo necrosis; report the appropriate neoplasm code.

comedones Acne lesions that result from hair follicles becoming clogged with sebum, keratin, and/or bacteria. Comedones may be closed and appear as whiteheads or open and closer to the skin surface, appearing as blackheads. Comedones are reported with ICD-9-CM code 706.1. *Synonym(s): blackheads, whiteheads.*

comitant With, accompanying.

commemorative sign Any sign or indication of previous disease.

comment Public commentary on the merits or appropriateness of proposed or potential regulations provided in response to an NPRM, an NOI, or other federal regulatory notice.

commercial carriers For-profit insurance companies issuing health coverage.

commercial insurance carrier See commercial carriers.

commercial plan Health benefit coverage package offered by a commercial carrier.

comminuted Fracture type in which the bone is splintered or crushed.

comminuted fracture Any type of fracture in which the bone is splintered or crushed, resulting in multiple bone fragments.

commissure Juncture where two corresponding parts come together, especially referring to the union site of adjacent heart valve cusps.

commissure of lip Juncture where two corresponding parts come together, specifically the corner where the upper and lower lips meet.

commissurotomy Surgical division or disruption of any two parts that are joined to form a commissure in order to increase the opening. The procedure most often refers to opening the adherent leaflet bands of fibrous tissue in a stenosed mitral valve. Commissurotomy is referenced in CPT codes 33476 and 33478.

common carotid artery Artery that supplies the head and neck with oxygenated blood; it divides in the neck to form the external and internal carotid arteries.

common working file System of local databases containing total beneficiary histories developed by CMS to improve Medicare claims processing. Medicare fiscal intermediaries and carriers interact with these databases to obtain data on eligibility, utilization, Medicare secondary payer (MSP), and other detailed claims information. The CWF is authorized to deny payment on claims on a prepayment basis. There are nine CWF regionally based sectors. *Synonym(s): CWF.*

communicating hydrocephalus Excess cerebrospinal fluid in dilated brain cavities, caused by acquired, abnormal nonabsorption of fluid back into fluid pathways.

community mental health center Facility providing outpatient mental health day treatment, assessments, and education as appropriate to community members.

community mental health center, partial hospitalization services Services prescribed and supervised by a physician pursuant to an individualized, written plan of treatment that sets forth the diagnosis and the type, amount, frequency, and duration of care for a patient in a community mental health center. Services must be reasonable and necessary for the diagnosis or active treatment of the individual's condition and to prevent relapse or hospitalization. The items and services include the following: Individual and group therapy with physicians, psychologists, or other mental health professionals; Occupational therapy requiring the skills of a qualified occupational therapist; Services of social workers, trained psychiatric nurses, and other staff trained to work with psychiatric patients; Drugs and biologicals for therapeutic purposes that cannot be self-administered); Individualized activity therapies that are not primarily recreational or diversionary; Family counseling; Patient training and education; Diagnostic

services, and; Other items and services, excluding meals and transportation

community rating Methodology of state and federal governments that require qualified HMOs to request the same amount of money for each member in a plan.

comorbid condition Condition present on hospital admission that is not the primary reason for treating the patient, but one that effects the patient's care.

comorbidity Preexisting condition that causes an increase in length of stay by at least one day in approximately 75 percent of cases. Used in DRG reimbursement.

comparative performance report Report that provides an annual comparison of a physician's services and procedures with those of another physician in the same specialty and geographic area. *Synonym(s): CPR.*

compartment syndrome Compromised blood flow to the muscles and nerves within a closed anatomical space due to increased interstitial pressure buildup that has nowhere to go. Compartment syndrome is marked by pain, loss of sensation, and palpable tenseness in the compartment region. The resulting ischemia can cause necrosis and loss of myoneural function or even loss of the limb. Sometimes the compartment must be surgically opened by emergency fasciotomy to allow for release of the pressure and return of arterial blood flow. An interstitial tissue pressure measurement of 30 mm Hg is the threshold for concern and treatment with surgery. Compartment syndrome is classified according to whether it is traumatic or nontraumatic. Traumatic compartment syndrome is reported with a code from 958.9x and nontraumatic with a code from 729.7x.

Compa-Z Brand name of prochlorperazine, a drug used as an antiemetic and antipsychotic agent, primarily to control nausea and vomiting. Compa-Z is also indicated in the treatment of schizophrenia and migraine headaches. Supply is reported with HCPCS Level II code J0780.

Compazine See prochlorperazine.

compensation neurosis Type of neurosis in which features of secondary gain, such as a situation of financial advantage, are prominent.

compensators Customized treatment devices that are attached to the treatment port to manipulate the radiation dose.

competitive medical plan Federal designation allowing plans to obtain eligibility to receive a Medicare risk contract without having to qualify as an HMO. *Synonym(s): CMP.*

complete heart block Complete form of disruption or impairment in the conduction of electrical charges in which no impulses are conducted from the atria to the ventricles to maintain regular heartbeats, due to a block

A-C

in the conducting tissues. Complete heart block is reported with ICD-9-CM code 426.0. **Synonym(s):** *CHB, complete atrioventricular block, HB, third degree atrioventricular block, third degree heart block.*

complete past, family, and social history Comprehensive review of all elements of the patient's past, family, and social history. Two or three history areas are required depending on the category of E/M service.

complete procedure According to the AMA's CPT coding guidelines, a procedure performed by one physician who is responsible for all pre- and postinjection services, including administration of local anesthesia, placement of needle, injection of contrast materials, supervision of the study and interpretation of the study results. Hospitals should use the CPT codes for the complete procedure to bill for the technician's work and for the equipment, film, room, and clerical support.

complete system review Narrative of organ systems reviewed including systems related to the problems identified in the chief complaint and/or history of presenting illness plus a review of all other systems.

complex Composite or collection of related things, such as symptoms, anatomical parts, or surgical procedures.

complex diagnoses Specific diagnoses that affect DRG 124, Circulatory Disorders (except acute myocardial infarction) with Cardiac Catheterization.

complex problems Multiple system impairments that relate to functional limitation and physical disability.

complex repair Surgical closure of a wound requiring more than layered closure of the deeper subcutaneous tissue and fascia (i.e., debridement, scar excision, placement of stents or retention sutures, and sometimes site preparation or undermining that creates the defect requiring complex closure).

complexity Difficulty of clinical decision-making: low complexity follows well-known and established parameters and protocols; moderate complexity takes into account extra factors, such as comorbidities; high complexity relies on case-by-case analysis, without the assistance of established protocols.

complexus basalis choroideae Transparent inner layer of the choroid that comes in contact with the pigmented layer of the retina. **Synonym(s):** *basal lamina, Bruch's membrane, lamina basalis choroideae, vitreal lamina.*

compliance Satisfying official requirements. *c. audits* Internal or external monitoring and review of activities to ensure compliance with all laws, regulations, and guidelines related to health care. *c. committee* Individuals assigned to help the compliance officer teach and comply with all laws, regulations, and guidelines related to health care. *c. date* Under HIPAA, date by which a covered entity must comply with a standard, an

implementation specification, or a modification. This is usually 24 months after the effective date of the associated final rule for most entities but 36 months after the effective date for small health plans. For future changes in the standards, the compliance date would be at least 180 days after the effective date but can be longer for small health plans and for complex changes. *c. officer* Individual with authority, funding, and staff to perform all necessary compliance activities, including planning, implementing, and monitoring the compliance program. *c. plan* Plan of established methods to eliminate errors in coding, billing, and other issues through auditing and monitoring, training, or other corrective actions. Such a plan also provides an avenue for employees and others to report problems. *c. program* Set of written policies and procedures related to the delivery of services and developed and monitored internally to ensure that the facility/business is providing high-quality services, while at the same time eliminating waste, fraud, and abuse.

compliance date Under HIPAA, date by which a covered entity must comply with a standard, implementation specification, or modification. This is usually 24 months after the effective date of the associated final rule for most entities but 36 months after the effective date for small health plans. For future changes in the standards, the compliance date would be at least 180 days after the effective date but may be longer for small health plans and complex changes.

complicated fracture Open or closed fracture in which a bone fragment has injured a neighboring organ or adjacent tissue.

complication Condition arising after the beginning of observation and treatment that modifies the course of the patient's illness or the medical care required, or an undesired result or misadventure in medical care.

complication/comorbidity Diagnosis codes that increase the level of severity and potentially the payment in the inpatient DRG IPPS system.

component code In CCI, the code following the comprehensive code that cannot be charged to Medicare when the comprehensive code is charged.

component code, column II In the Corrective Coding Initiative (CCI) edits, the code following the column I code that cannot be charged when the more comprehensive code is charged.

component coding Coding a service that represents only a portion of the entire service provided, meant to standardize the reporting of interventional radiology services. Component coding allows a physician, regardless of specialty, to specifically identify and report those aspects of the service he or she provided, whether the procedural component, the radiological component, or both.

composite In dentistry, synthetic material such as acrylic resin and quartz particles used in tooth restoration.

composite graft Tissue taken from one body site of an individual to be transplanted to another site of the same individual. A composite graft includes more than one tissue type, such as the cartilage and skin mix taken together from the nose or ear. A composite graft is also multiple pieces of a patient's vein taken from distant sites and used in another limb as an arterial bypass graft conduit.

composite rate Prospective payment for outpatient maintenance dialysis services furnished to Medicare beneficiaries either in a facility or at home. All maintenance dialysis treatments furnished to Medicare beneficiaries in an approved end-stage renal disease (ESRD) facility are covered by this reimbursement system. The composite rate system is one of two methods of Medicare payment for maintenance dialysis services rendered in the beneficiary's home. The payment does not include physicians' professional services, separately billable laboratory services, and separately billable drugs.

compound *c. dislocation* Subluxation or displacement of a joint in which there is a break in the skin and the joint is exposed to the open air. *c. presentation* Malposition of the fetus before birth in which more than one part of the fetus enters the birth canal at the same time, commonly an extremity together with the head. This condition is reported with ICD-9-CM code 652.8 and the appropriate fifth digit for the episode of care. *Synonym(s): open dislocation.*

comprehensive code, column I In the Corrective Coding Initiative (CCI) edits, a column I, comprehensive code represents the major procedure or service when reported with another code.

comprehensive codes Code behind which component codes fall.

comprehensive outpatient rehabilitation facility Facility that provides services that include physician's services related to administrative functions; physical, occupational, speech and respiratory therapies; social and psychological services; and prosthetic and orthotic devices. A service is covered as a CORF service if it is also covered as an inpatient hospital service provided to a hospital patient. CORF services require a plan of treatment within a maximum of 60-day intervals for rereviews. *Synonym(s): CORF.*

comprehensive physical examination Under the 1995 guidelines, examination of at least eight organ systems or one comprehensive single-system examination. Under the 1997 guidelines, an examination of at least nine organ systems or body areas, which must include all bullet point elements within each of the nine systems/areas for the multisystem exam or examination

of all bullet point elements from one of the 10 single organ system exams.

compressed air disease Decompression sickness caused by rapid reduction in atmospheric pressure in deep-sea divers and caisson workers who return to normal air pressure environments too quickly or pilots flying at high altitudes. It causes joint pain, respiratory problems, neurologic symptoms, and skin lesions. Report this disease with ICD-9-CM code 993.3. *Synonym(s): bends, Caisson disease, diver's palsy, dysbarism.*

compression sleeve Fitted wrap that accelerates recovery in patients with vein disease, lymphedema, or diabetes. Compression sleeves increase circulation and decrease swelling and fluid buildup following surgery.

compulsive conduct disorder Great internal tension resulting from an impulse, drive, or temptation to perform some action that is harmful to the individual or to others that may provide short-term pleasure, gratification, or release and may be followed by regret, self-reproach, or guilt; can take the form of intermittent explosive disorder, isolated explosive disorder, kleptomania, pathological gambling, and pyromania.

compulsive neurosis Feeling of subjective compulsion to carry out an action, dwell on an idea, recall an experience, or ruminate on an abstract topic or to perform a quasi-ritual that may result in anxiety or inner struggle as the individual tries to cope with the behavior.

compulsive personality Feelings of personal insecurity, excessive doubt, and incompleteness leading to excessive conscientiousness, stubbornness, perfectionism, meticulous accuracy, and caution with persistent checking in an individual who may also have intrusive thoughts or impulses.

Computer-based Patient Record Institute Healthcare Open Systems and Trials Industry organization that promotes the use of health care information systems, including electronic health care records.

computerized corneal topography Digital imaging and analysis by computer of the shape of the corneal.

computerized patient record Computer application that allows all or most elements of a patient's medical record to be stored in a computerized database. *Synonym(s): CPR, electronic medical record, EMR.*

Comvax Brand name haemophilus influenzae type B and hepatitis B vaccine provided in a single-dose vial. Supply of Comvax is reported with CPT code 90748; administration is reported separately. The need for vaccination is reported with ICD-9-CM code V06.8.

CON Certificate of need.

conc Concentrate.

concentration camp syndrome Brief, episodic, or recurrent disorders lasting six months or more following the trauma.

concentric fading Transient blind spot within the visual field or an area of lost or diminished vision surrounded by more sensitive or normal vision. This condition is reported with ICD-9-CM code 368.12. *Synonym(s): scintillating scotoma, scotoma.*

concomitant Occurring at the same time, accompanying. *c. operations* Accompanying procedures that are completed during the same surgical session.

concomitant operations Accompanying procedures that are completed during the same surgical session.

concrescence In dentistry, condition in which the roots of two teeth are joined by a cementum deposit. Report this condition with ICD-9-CM code 520.2.

concretion Calculus or inorganic mass within an organ, tissue, or body cavity.

concurrent care Medical care provided by two or more physicians on the same day. If care is medically necessary, payers usually pay both physicians. Generally, payers expect the physicians to be of different specialties and caring for different conditions or different aspects of the same condition or disease process.

concurrent review Review of services to determine medical necessity and appropriateness of care and occurring at the same time as the services are being provided.

concussion syndrome Persistent personality disturbance following a blow to the head featuring affective instability, bursts of aggression, apathy and indifference, impaired social judgment, and suspiciousness or paranoid ideation. Report this disorder with ICD-9-CM code 310.2.

condition code Two-digit numeric code that is entered on the UB-04 claim form to indicate that a condition applies to the bill that affects processing and payment of the claim. Condition codes indicate whether coverage exists under another insurance, whether the injury or illness is related to employment, whether the bill is an outlier, or if medical necessity affects room assignment.

condition code category Broad sets of similar diseases that are clinically and cost similar under the CMS-HCC Model for capitated payments to managed care organizations.

conditional payment Medicare payment requested by the provider for a claim for which Medicare is the secondary payer, but the provider anticipates a lengthy processing delay (more than 120 days) by the primary payer due to third-party liability. Once payment is received from the true primary payer, a refund or request for reconsideration must be issued to Medicare within 60 days.

conduct disorders Socially inappropriate, abnormal, aggressive, destructive behavior, or delinquency in individuals of any age not related to life stressors but possibly associated with emotional disturbances without other psychiatric conditions. *mixed disturbance of c. and emotions* Emotional disturbance demonstrated by anxiety, misery, or obsessive manifestations resulting in undersocialized or socially disturbed conduct. *socialized c.* Acquired values or behavior of a peer group that the individual is loyal to and with whom he or she characteristically steals, is truant, stays out late at night, and is sexually promiscuous or engages in other socially delinquent practices. *undersocialized c. aggressive type* Persistent pattern of disrespect for the feelings and well-being of others, aggressive antisocial behavior, and failure to develop close and stable relationships with others as manifested by physical aggression, cruel behavior, hostility, verbal and physical abuse, stealing, vandalism, lying, and defiance of authority. *undersocialized c. unaggressive type* Lack of concern for the rights and feelings of others resulting from a failure to establish a normal degree of affection, empathy, or bond with others. May be manifested by self-protection with fear, timidity, whining, making demands, and throwing tantrums, or by exploitation and self-gain through lying and stealing without apparent guilt.

conduit Surgically created channel for the passage of fluids.

condyle Rounded end of a bone that forms an articulation.

condylectomy Excision of a condyle.

condyloma Infectious, tumor-like growth caused by the human papilloma virus, with a branching connective tissue core and epithelial covering that occurs on the skin and mucous membranes of the perianal region and external genitalia. Report condylomas with ICD-9-CM code 078.11. *Synonym(s): genital wart, venereal wart.*

cone In radiology, cylindrical attachment used to shape a radiation beam.

conformer Plastic or silicone shell usually inserted after eye surgery to help form the eye socket and support the eyelids.

confusional arousal State of waking from sleep, typically deep sleep, marked by mental disorientation to time, place, or people.

confusional state acute Short-lived organic, psychotic states, lasting hours or days and characterized by clouded consciousness, disorientation, fear, illusions, delusions, hallucinations (notably visual and tactile), restlessness, tremor, and sometimes fever.

confusional state epileptic Short-lived organic, psychotic states, triggered by an epileptic episode, lasting hours or days and characterized by clouded consciousness, disorientation, fear, illusions, delusions, hallucinations (notably visual and tactile), restlessness, tremor, and sometimes fever.

confusional state subacute Organic, psychotic states characterized by clouded consciousness, disorientation, fear, illusions, delusions, hallucinations of any kind (notably visual or tactile), restlessness, tremor, and sometimes fever. The symptoms, usually of a lesser degree than acute, last for several weeks or longer, during which time they may show marked fluctuations in intensity.

congenital Present at birth, occurring through heredity or an influence during gestation up to the moment of birth. *c. anomaly* Abnormality that is present at birth that may be the result of genetic factors, teratogens, or other conditions that affect the fetus in utero. The abnormalities may be readily apparent at birth or may remain undiscovered until some point after birth. *c. biliary atresia* Fatal infection affecting the biliary tree in which there is progressive sclerosing and destruction of the intrahepatic ducts. *c. glaucoma* High intraocular pressure accompanied by hazy corneas and abnormally large eyes (buphthalmos) in a newborn or within the first six months of life. *c. muscle hypoplasia syndrome* Dysplasia of the fingernails and toenails, hypoplasia of the patella, iliac horns, thickening of the glomerular lamina densa, and a flask-shaped femur. Report this disorder with ICD-9-CM code 756.89. *c. oculofacial paralysis syndrome* Unilateral lesions of the ninth, tenth, eleventh, and twelfth cranial nerves producing paralysis of the vagal, glossal, and other nerves and the tongue on the same side. Report this disorder with ICD-9-CM code 352.6. *Synonym(s): Collet-Sicard syndrome. c. spondylolisthesis* Abnormal forward displacement of the fifth lumbar vertebra on the first sacral vertebra.

congestive heart failure Condition caused by the heart's inability to adequately pump and circulate blood, resulting in fluid accumulation in the lungs and other tissues.

conical cornea Noninflammatory, bilateral bulging protrusion of the anterior cornea thins, which forms a cone-shaped dome, with the apex displaced downward toward the nose, resulting in astigmatism and blurred, distorted vision. Corneal transplant may be required in severe cases. Report this condition with ICD-9-CM codes 371.60-371.62, unless specified as congenital, in which case it is reported with 743.41. *Synonym(s): keratoconus.*

conization Excision of a cone-shaped piece of tissue.

conjoined twins Monozygotic (identical) twins connected at corresponding points due to incomplete late division. Joining occurs in varying degrees and may be superficial between well-developed individuals or the attachment of one incompletely developed twin in a parasitic conjoining with a fully developed individual. Classification depends upon the site at which they are joined: thoracopagus is joined at the chest; xiphopagus or omphalopagus is joined at the abdomen; pygopagus is joined at the buttocks; ischiopagus is joined at the ischium; and craniopagus is joined at the head. Report conjoined twins with ICD-9-CM code 759.4. When this condition causes fetopelvic disproportion, it is reported with a code from ICD-9-CM subcategory 678.1. Cesarean section is the usual method of delivery in these cases. *Synonym(s): Siamese twins.*

conjugated estrogen See estrogen.

conjunctiva Mucous membrane lining of the eyelids and covering of the exposed, anterior sclera.

conjunctival foreign body Foreign body that has become imbedded in the cornea but does not penetrate any deeper within the eye.

conjunctivodacryocystostomy Surgical connection of the lacrimal sac directly to the conjunctival sac.

conjunctivorhinostomy Correction of an obstruction of the lacrimal canal achieved by suturing the posterior flaps and removing any lacrimal obstruction, preserving the conjunctiva.

conjunctivourethrosynovial syndrome Symptom of Reiter's disease. Report this disorder with ICD-9-CM code 099.3.

Conn syndrome Headaches, nocturia, polyuria, fatigue, hypertension, hypokalemic alkalosis, potassium depletion, hypervolemia, and decreased renin activity, caused by a benign pituitary tumor. Report this disorder with ICD-9-CM code 255.12.

connective tissue Body tissue made from fibroblasts, collagen, and elastic fibrils that connects, supports, and holds together other tissues and cells and includes cartilage, collagenous, fibrous, elastic, and osseous tissue.

Conradi (-Hünermann) syndrome Asymmetric shortening of the limbs and scoliosis. Caused by both genetic and maternal medication sources. Report this disorder with ICD-9-CM code 756.59.

consanguinity State of being related by blood. Parental consanguinity is sometimes associated with medical implications, such as congenital malformations, and is reported with ICD-9-CM code V19.7. *Synonym(s): kinship.*

conscious sedation See moderate sedation.

consistency edits Screening system that identifies potential and actual errors on claims. Edits address clinical, coding, billing, and other data errors. For Medicare purposes, claims must pass edits for all Medicare-required fields on the UB-92 claim form in order to be paid correctly. Otherwise, the bill will be returned to the provider and payment will be delayed until the claim is completed properly.

consolidated billing HHAs Balanced Budget Act of 1997 requires consolidated billing for all home health services rendered under a home health plan of care. Payment for all items and services provided during a home health prospective payment system (HHPPS) episode will be made to a single HHA, the primary HHA for billing purposes. The type of services that are subject to the HH consolidated billing provisions are skilled nursing care; home health aide services; physical therapy; speech-language pathology; occupational therapy; medical social services; routine and nonroutine medical supplies; medical services provided by an intern or resident-in-training of a hospital under an approved teaching program in the case of an HHA that is affiliated or under common control with that hospital; and care for homebound beneficiaries involving equipment too cumbersome to take home.

consolidated billing SNF Section 4432(b) of the Balanced Budget Act of 1997 requires consolidated billing for skilled nursing facilities. The SNF must submit all Medicare claims for all services that its residents receive (both Part A and Part B), except for certain excluded services to the Medicare fiscal intermediary on the UB-92 claim form. The beneficiary's status as a SNF resident for consolidated billing ends when one of the following occurs: the beneficiary is admitted as an inpatient to a Medicare-participating hospital or a critical access hospital (CAH); the beneficiary receives services from a Medicare participating home health agency (HHA) under a plan of care; the beneficiary receives outpatient services from a Medicare-participating hospital or CAH, but only for services that are not furnished under the SNF's resident assessment or comprehensive care plan; or the beneficiary is formally discharged from the SNF. Consolidated billing applies to physical, occupational and speech therapy services, psychological services furnished by a clinical social worker, and services furnished incident to the professional services of a physician. Services excluded from consolidated billing include physician services, physician assistants, nurse practitioners, certified nurse-midwives, qualified psychologists, certified registered nurse anesthetists, home dialysis supplies and equipment, self-care home dialysis support services, institutional dialysis services and supplies, erythropoietin or EPO, hospice care, and, for 1998 only, the transportation costs of electrocardiogram equipment. This provision was effective on or after July 1, 1998. Also excluded from SNF consolidated billing are drugs incident to a radiology procedure or surgery, supplies including surgical dressings that are incident to a radiology procedure and surgery, anesthesia for surgery and radiology, and laboratory services for surgery.

Consolidated Omnibus Budget Reconciliation Act Federal law that allows and requires past employees to be covered under company health insurance plans for a set premium, allowing individuals to remain insured when their current plan or position has been terminated. *Synonym(s): COBRA.*

constipation Infrequent or incomplete and difficult bowel movements.

constriction Narrowed or squeezed portion of a tubular or luminal structure, such as a duct, vessel, or tube (e.g., esophagus). The narrowing can be a defect that is occurring naturally, or one that is surgically induced for therapeutic reasons.

constrictive pericarditis Inflammation and scarring occurring in the sac around the heart, leading to a rigid and thickened pericardium with loss of elasticity. Constrictive pericarditis prevents the ventricles from filling to the full extent and sometimes results in congestive heart failure. Report this condition with ICD-9-CM code 423.2.

consultation Advice or opinion regarding diagnosis and treatment or determination to accept transfer of care of a patient that is rendered by a medical professional at the request of the primary care provider. Consultations may also be requested by another appropriate source. A request for consultation must be documented in the medical record, as well as a written report of the findings of the consultation. Effective January 1, 2010, Medicare no longer recognizes CPT consultation codes 99241-99245 and 99251-99255; however, telehealth consultation services reported with HCPCS Level II codes G0425-G0427 are a paid service under the MPFS. *NCD References: 70.1, 70.2.*

Cont Continuous.

cont. Continue.

contact dermatitis Superficial skin inflammation characterized by epidermal edema and irritated vesicles occurring as a reaction to a substance coming in contact with the skin. Some of the most common irritants include poison ivy or oak, cosmetics, detergents, and solvents. Correct code assignment is dependent upon the causative agent. See ICD-9-CM category 692. *Synonym(s): allergic dermatitis, poison ivy, poison oak.*

Contak Renewal Brand name cardiac resynchronization therapy device.

contaminated wound Acute nonpurulent inflammation noted and procedure performed with major break in surgical technique. Open wound less than four hours old. Gross contamination from gastrointestinal tract. Infection rate: up to 20 percent.

contamination Introduction of organisms or foreign bodies and material into a wound.

continuing claim Bill for the same confinement or course of treatment for which a bill already has been submitted and for which further bills are expected to be submitted. This type of claim can be submitted once a month (every 30 days) or every 60 days by PPS hospitals.

continuity of coverage In health care contracting, transfer of benefits from one plan to another without a lapse in coverage.

continuous positive airway pressure

device Pressurized device used to maintain the patient's airway for spontaneous or mechanically aided breathing. Often used for patients with mild to moderate sleep apnea. *Synonym(s): CPAP device.*

continuous suture Running stitch with tension evenly distributed across the single strand to provide a leakproof closure line.

contour Act of shaping along desired lines.

contraceptive pill Generic designation for oral contraception. Most oral contraceptives today are a combination of an estrogen and progestin, such as norgestimate and estradiol. There are three main types of oral contraceptives: nonphasic, biphasic, and triphasic. Monophasic provide a fixed amount of estrogen throughout the cycle. Biphasic holds the estrogen level steady and varies the progestin content throughout the cycle. In triphasic products, both the estrogen and progestin levels are varied throughout the cycle. Estrogen suppresses the release of follicular stimulating hormone (FSH) from the anterior pituitary gland, which in turn inhibits ovulation. Progestin suppresses the release of luteinizing hormone (LH), making cervical mucosa more viscous and harder to penetrate. Supply for all oral contraceptives is reported with HCPCS Level II code S4993.

contractor Entity who enters into a contractual agreement with CMS to service a component of the Medicare program administration, for example, fiscal intermediaries, carriers, program safeguard coordinators.

contracture Shortening of muscle or connective tissue.

contralateral Located on, or affecting, the opposite side of the body, usually as it relates to a bilateral body part.

contrast material Radiopaque substance placed into the body to enable a system or body structure to be visualized, such as nonionic and low osmolar contrast media (LOCM), ionic and high osmolar contrast media (HOCM), barium, and gadolinium.

contusion Superficial injury (bruising) produced by impact without a break in the skin.

conus medullaris syndrome Cerebral spinal fluid of a yellowish hue signaling neoplastic or inflammatory obstruction. Report this disorder with ICD-9-CM code 336.8. *Synonym(s): Froin's syndrome.*

conventional dentures Dentures made and inserted after the teeth have been extracted and the gums have healed. The patient is edentulous while the denture is being made.

conversion In health care contracting, shifting a member under a group contract to an individual contract in accordance with contract terms and occurring with a change in employer benefits or when the covered person leaves the group.

conversion factor *1)* Dollar value for each relative value unit. When this dollar amount is multiplied by the total relative value units, it yields the reimbursement rate for the service. *2)* National multiplier that converts the geographically adjusted relative value units into Medicare fee schedule dollar amounts that applies to all services paid under the MFS.

conversion hysteria Restriction of the field of consciousness or disturbance of motor or sensory function resulting in symbolic or psychological advantage, primarily of a body part as manifested by paralysis, tremor, blindness, deafness, and seizures.

Cooke-Apert-Gallais syndrome Type I acrocephalosyndactyly with peak head and fusion of digits (specifically the second through fifth digits) and severe acne vulgaris of forearms. Report this disorder with ICD-9-CM code 255.2.

Cooley's anemia Most severe type of beta thalassemia due to deletions in both beta chain genes and noted from birth by skeletal deformations and mongoloid facial appearance. Complete absence of hemoglobin A produces hemolytic, hypochromic, microcytic anemia and necessitates recurrent blood transfusions. If left untreated, enlargement of the liver, spleen, and heart occurs, and bones can deteriorate. Accumulation of iron in the heart and other organs may result in heart failure. Report this condition with ICD-9-CM code 282.49. *Synonym(s): thalassemia major.*

coordinated care In health care contracting, system of health care delivery that influences utilization, quality of care, and cost of services. Managed care integrates financing and management with an employed or contracted organized provider network that delivers services to an enrolled population.

coordination disorder Disorders in which the main feature is a serious impairment in the development of motor coordination that is not explicable in terms of general intellectual retardation and is commonly associated with perceptual difficulties.

coordination of benefits Agreement that prevents duplicate payment for services when the member is covered by two or more sources. The agreement dictates which organization is primarily and secondarily responsible for payment. *Synonym(s): COB.*

Coordination of Benefits Agreement Program that establishes a national standard contract between CMS and other health insurance organizations that defines the criteria for transmitting enrollee eligibility data and Medicare adjudicated claim data. CMS has transferred the claims crossover functions from individual Medicare contractors to a national claims crossover contractor, the Coordination of Benefits Contractor (COBC). This consolidation allows for the establishment of unique identifiers (COBA IDs) to be associated with each contract and create a national repository for COBA information. **Synonym(s):** COBA.

Coordination of Benefits Contractor Contractor who consolidates activities that support the collection, management, and reporting of other insurance coverage for Medicare beneficiaries. The purposes of the COB program are to identify the health benefits available to a Medicare beneficiary and to coordinate the payment process to prevent mistaken payment of Medicare benefits. The COBC does not process claims, nor does it handle any mistaken payment recoveries or claims -specific inquiries. The Medicare intermediaries and carriers are responsible for processing claims submitted for primary or secondary payment. **Synonym(s):** COBC.

coordination of care Care provided concurrently with counseling that includes treatment instructions to the patient or caregiver; special accommodations for home, work, school, vacation, or other locations; coordination with other providers and agencies; and living arrangements.

Copaxone See glatiramer acetate.

copayment Cost-sharing arrangement in which a covered person pays a specified portion of allowed charges. In relation to Medicare, the copayment designates the specific dollar amount that the patient must pay and coinsurance designates the percentage of allowed charges.

COPD Chronic obstructive pulmonary disease.

coping Thin covering that is placed over a tooth before attaching a crown or overdenture.

copper intrauterine contraceptive device Small device placed inside the uterus with vertical and horizontal arms containing copper, which is slowly released into the uterine cavity. Copper stops sperm from making their way up through the uterus into the tubes, thereby reducing the ability of sperm to fertilize an egg. Copper also prevents a fertilized egg from successfully implanting in the lining of the uterus if fertilization has occurred. This IUD is reportedly 99 percent effective. Supply is reported with HCPCS code J7300. Insertion of the IUD is reported with CPT code 58300; removal with 58301. May be sold under the brand name Gravigard.

coprolith Hard, intestinal concretion of fecal matter that may lead to impaction or appendicitis. Report

coprolith with ICD-9-CM code 560.32. **Synonym(s):** *fecalith, stercolith.*

coprophilia Psychosexual disorder in which one becomes aroused when focusing on feces, often seen in conjunction with such practices as bondage and discipline, sadomasochism, or infantilism. This disorder is reported with ICD-9-CM code 302.89. **Synonym(s):** *fecophilia.*

cor biloculare Congenital anomaly in which the heart is two-chambered, lacking both an atrial and a ventricular septum. Few newborns with this condition live to the first year. Cor biloculare is reported with ICD-9-CM code 745.7.

cor pulmonale Heart-lung disease appearing in identifiable forms as chronic or acute. The chronic form of this heart-lung disease is marked by dilation and hypertrophy failure of the right ventricle due to a disease that has affected the function of the lungs, excluding congenital or left heart diseases. The acute form is an overload of the right ventricle from a rapid onset of pulmonary hypertension, usually arising from a pulmonary embolism. Acute cor pulmonale is reported with ICD-9-CM code 415.0 while chronic cor pulmonale, also called chronic cardiopulmonary disease, is reported with 416.9.

cor triatriatum Congenital heart defect resulting in pulmonary venous obstruction due to failure in the embryonic development of the common pulmonary vein. A fibrous septum, like a diaphragm, divides the left atrium with the upper, back portion receiving the pulmonary venous return and the lower, front part of the chamber open between the mitral orifice and the left atrial appendage, resulting in three atrial chambers. This anomaly is reported with ICD-9-CM code 746.82.

CORB Cardiac output measured by noninvasive, rebreathing method of inert foreign gas within a closed system that continuously analyzes the gas concentrations using an infrared photoacoustic gas analyzing computer system. The system stores the retrieved gas concentration data and the software calculates the cardiac output from the rate of uptake into the blood.

Corbus' disease Infection thought to be due to a spirochetal infection in which there is rapid erosion and destruction of the glans penis and sometimes the entire external genitalia. Report this disease with ICD-9-CM code 607.1. **Synonym(s):** *balanoposthomycosis, gangrenous balanitis.*

Cordis Checkmate Brand name radiation delivery system designed to treat restenosis sites in the coronary artery. A delivery catheter is placed in the coronary artery at the site of the blockage through which radioactive ribbons are inserted, and then returned to the storage container after treatment.

corditis Condition in which the spermatic cord is inflamed and irritated. Report corditis with ICD-9-CM code 608.4, with an additional code to identify the causative organism if known.

cordocentesis Aspiration of a sample of fetal blood from the umbilical vein under ultrasonic guidance. The specialized amniocentesis needle is placed into the cavity of the pregnant uterus and into the umbilical vessels. This procedure is done in the second or third trimester and is used for rapid chromosome analysis for fetal genetic information to help diagnose defects. ICD-9-CM procedure code 75.33 reports fetal blood sampling and biopsy. CPT code 59012 reports cordocentesis by any method and 76941 reports the radiological interpretation and supervision during the procedure. This procedure is excluded from the maternity care global package. *Synonym(s): percutaneous umbilical blood sampling, PUBS.*

cordotomy Surgical interruption of the spinal cord, usually for the relief of intractable pain.

core biopsy Large-bore biopsy needle is inserted into a mass and a core of tissue is removed for diagnostic study.

core buildup Replacement of all or a portion of the tooth's crown in order to provide a base for the retention of a crown that has been indirectly fabricated.

core needle biopsy Large-bore biopsy needle inserted into a mass and a core of tissue is removed for diagnostic study.

corectopia Condition in which the pupil is abnormally positioned, sometimes associated with forms of myopia or ectopia. Report this disorder with ICD-9-CM code 743.46.

CORF Comprehensive outpatient rehabilitation facility. Facility that provides services that include physician's services related to administrative functions; physical, occupational, speech and respiratory therapies; social and psychological services; and prosthetic and orthotic devices. A service is covered as a CORF service if it is also covered as an inpatient hospital service provided to a hospital patient. CORF services require a plan of treatment within a maximum of 60-day intervals for rereviews.

corgonject-5 See chorionic gonadotropin.

cornea Five-layered, transparent structure that forms the anterior or front part of the sclera of the eye.

corneal abscess Pocket of pus and inflammation on the cornea.

corneal ectasia Congenital or acquired condition in which the cornea of the eye bulges or protrudes abnormally, being thin and scarred. If specified as congenital, report ICD-9-CM code 743.41, otherwise report 371.71. *Synonym(s): keratectasia.*

corneal endothelium Lining of the cornea's inner surface that constantly produces fluid to keep the cornea clear.

corneal limbus Juncture of the cornea and the sclera identified on the eye's surface by a slight indentation known as the sulcus sclerae. *Synonym(s): corneoscleral junction.*

corneal stroma Middle layer that forms 90 percent of the cornea. *Synonym(s): substantia propria of cornea.*

corneal ulcer Necrosis of corneal tissue caused by bacteria, fungus, virus, or amoeba, resulting in pain, photophobia, and lacrimation.

Cornelia de Lange's syndrome Mental retardation, eyebrows across bridge of nose, hairline well down on forehead, uptilted tip of nose with depressed bridge of nose, and small head with low-set ears. Report this disorder with a code from ICD-9-CM category 759.8.

cornua Paired superior lateral extremities of the uterus that mark the entrance to the uterine tube.

coronal Relating to the top of a tooth or the crown of the head.

coronal incision *1)* Incision across the crown of the head, starting over one ear and extending over the crown to the other ear. *2)* Incision made at the crown (head/top) of an anatomical structure, such as a coronal incision of the urethra, thumb, or penis.

coronary atherosclerosis Chronic condition marked by thickening and loss of elasticity of the coronary artery, caused by deposits of plaque containing cholesterol, lipoid material, and lipophages. Report coronary atherosclerosis with a code from ICD-9-CM subcategory 414.0.

coronary care unit Facility dedicated to patients suffering from heart attack, stroke, or other serious cardiopulmonary problems. *Synonym(s): CCU.*

coronary ostia One or both of the two openings in the aortic sinuses that mark the origins of the left and right coronary arteries.

coronoidectomy Procedure in which a diseased or fractured coronoid process of the mandible is removed. Coronoidectomy is reported with ICD-9-CM procedure code 76.31 and CPT code 21070.

corpectomy Removal of the body of a bone, such as a vertebra.

corporate integrity agreement Agreement between the government and a provider who has entered into a settlement with the government due to a health care fraud and abuse investigation. Providers must agree to follow the corporate integrity agreement, which is essentially a government-mandated compliance program.

A-C

corpus callosum Mass of thick fibers in the white matter of the brain that connects the right and left hemisphere. *Synonym(s): commissural magna cerebri.*

corpus luteum Yellowish mass of endocrine tissue in the ovary that secretes progesterone, formed by a mature follicle that has released its ovum. The corpus luteum dissolves after about 10 days if there is no fertilization but persists for several months if the ovum is impregnated. *c. l. cyst* Common type of ovarian cyst that occurs when the corpus luteum fails to dissolve after the ovum is released and not fertilized. The cyst normally goes away in a few weeks but may enlarge to more than 10 cm and require surgical intervention. Corpus luteum cysts are reported with ICD-9-CM code 620.1. *Synonym(s): corpus luteum hematoma, lutein cyst.*

corpus uteri Main body of the uterus, which is located above the isthmus and below the openings of the fallopian tubes.

correct Body part modification.

Correct Coding Council Develops coding methodologies based on established coding conventions to control improper coding that leads to inappropriate and increased payment of Part B claims.

correct coding initiative *1)* Official list of codes from the Centers for Medicare and Medicaid Services' (CMS) National Correct Coding Policy Manual for Part B Medicare Carriers that identifies services considered either an integral part of a comprehensive code or mutually exclusive of it. *2)* CCI edits are of two main types: comprehensive/component edits and mutually exclusive edits. Comprehensive/component edits are those that are applied to code combinations in which one of the codes is a component of the more comprehensive code; only the comprehensive code is paid. Mutually exclusive edits are those that are applied to code combinations in which one of the codes is considered either impossible to perform or improbable to be performed with the other code. *Synonym(s): CCI, NCCI.*

correct coding initiative edits CCI edits are of two main types. Comprehensive/component edits are applied to code combinations in which one of the codes is a component of the more comprehensive code. Only the comprehensive code is paid. Mutually exclusive edits are applied to code combinations in which one of the codes is considered impossible to perform or improbable to be performed with the other code. Current CCI edits have been incorporated in the Outpatient Code Editor except for anesthesiology edits.

CorRestore patch Brand name pericardial patch integral to anterior surgical ventricular endocardial restoration. This procedure is reported with CPT code 33548.

corridor deductible Fixed out-of-pocket amount the member must pay before benefits are available. *Synonym(s): deductible.*

cortical bone Thin, superficial layer of dense, compact bone that covers the cancellous bone and makes up most of the diaphysis (shaft) of the long bones, providing strength to the long bones of the body.

corticoadrenal insufficiency Underproduction of the adrenal hormones, aldosterone and cortisol, causing low blood pressure, weight loss, weakness, and anemia.

corticorelin ovine triflutate Injectable synthetic peptide salt used in a diagnostic test for ACTH-dependent Cushing's syndrome in order to distinguish between pituitary and ectopic sources of ACTH production. Supply is reported with HCPCS Level II code J0795. May be sold under the brand name ACTHREL.

corticotropin Adrenocorticotropic hormone (ACTH) used as a diagnostic aid to test adrenocortical function and related insufficiencies by stimulating the adrenal cortex to release its range of hormones. It is also used as an antiinflammatory or immunosuppressant. It is used in evocative testing found in CPT codes 80400-80406. May be sold under the brand names ACTH, Acthar.

Cortrosyn See corticotropin.

Corvert See ibutilide fumarate.

Cosmegen See dactinomycin.

cosmetic Superficial or external, having no medical necessity.

CosmoPlast Brand name injectable subcutaneous implant of human collagen used to correct major skin defects caused by acne scarring or aging. Injections are usually considered cosmetic.

COSOPT Brand name eye drop for the treatment of glaucoma. Glaucoma codes are found in ICD-9-CM category 365.

cost outliers Cases for which costs fall outside the norm. Costs may be higher or lower than is typical for the service provided.

cost report Annual report required of all institutions participating in the Medicare program. The report details the costs and charges the provider incurred in providing services to all patients and the Medicare (or Medicaid) payments received during a specified reporting period. Costs and reporting procedures are defined by the Medicare program.

Costen's syndrome Multiple symptoms including temporomandibular joint dysfunction, hearing difficulty, headache, vertigo, and burning sensations in the ear, nose, tongue, and throat. Underlying causes may include overclosure of the mandible, TMJ lesions, and stress. Report this condition with ICD-9-CM code 524.60.

Synonym(s): temporomandibular joint-pain dysfunction syndrome.

costochondral Pertaining to the ribs and the scapula.

costochondral junction syndrome Painful swelling of costal cartilages, especially of the second rib and interpreted as coronary artery disease. Report this disorder with ICD-9-CM code 733.6. *Synonym(s): Tietze's syndrome.*

costophrenic angle Angle at the junction between the rib and the diaphragmatic pleurae. *Synonym(s): costodiaphragmatic recess.*

costovertebral Site of rib and vertebra articulation.

costovertebral syndrome Arthritis of spine accompanying acromegaly, resembling rheumatoid arthritis and progressing to bony ankylosis with lipping of vertebral margins. Report this disorder with ICD-9-CM code 253.0.

costovertebral tenderness Pain and tenderness to the touch at the site of the kidney between the ribs and spine. Costovertebral tenderness is a finding that can indicate kidney disease and is reported with ICD-9-CM code 788.0 unless a more definitive diagnosis is made. *Synonym(s): kidney pain, renal colic.*

cosyntropin Hormone drug used to diagnose or treat adrenocortical hormone insufficiency and used in evocative testing found in CPT codes 80400-80406. The IV supply is reported with HCPCS Level II code J0833 or J0834.

COT *1)* Chain of trust. In health care contracting, pattern of agreements that extend protection of health care data. Each covered entity that shares health care data with a second entity must require the second entity to provide protections comparable to those provided by the covered entity. The second entity, in turn, must require any other entities with which it shares the data to satisfy the same requirements. *2)* Certified ophthalmic technician.

COTA Certified occupational therapy assistant.

Cotard's syndrome Paranoia marked by sensory disturbances, delusions of negation, and suicidal ideations. Report this disorder with ICD-9-CM code 297.1.

COTD Cardiac output thermodilution. Cardiac output measured by thermodilution method that requires heart catheterization and then injection of a thermal indicator, usually iced saline. A computer calculates the cardiac output using an equation that incorporates body temperature, injectate volume and temperature, time, and other calculated ratios over a denominator of the integral of the change in blood temperature during the cold injection, reflected by the area of the inscribed curve. Report COTD with ICD-9-CM procedure code 89.68 and CPT codes 93561-93562.

Cotte's operation Presacral neurectomy to relieve severe dysmenorrhea.

Cotting's operation Excisional treatment for ingrowing toenail.

Cotugno's disease Low back, buttock, and hip pain that radiates down the leg, sometimes accompanied by paresthesia and weakness, usually caused by a herniated disk in the lumbar spine or neuropathy affecting the sciatic nerve. Report this disease with ICD-9-CM code 724.3. *Synonym(s): sciatica.*

cotyloid cavity Cup-shaped socket in the hipbone into which the head of the femur fits, forming a ball-and-socket joint. *Synonym(s): acetabulum, cetabular bone, os acetabuli.*

counseling Discussion with a patient and/or family concerning one or more of the following areas: diagnostic results, impressions, and/or recommended diagnostic studies; prognosis; risks and benefits of management (treatment) options; instructions for management (treatment) and/or follow-up; importance of compliance with chosen management (treatment) options; risk factor reduction; and patient and family education. *E/M c.* Discussion with a patient and/or family concerning treatment, results of diagnostic services, recommended management options, prognosis, and education regarding disease process. *psychiatric c.* Interaction between provider and patient to understand, correct, or change communication, emotional, personality, or behavioral problems through various methodologies. Report a CPT code(s) from the Medicine section, under Psychiatry, 90801-90889.

Courvoisier's sign Indication of common bile duct obstruction with features including jaundice and an enlarged, painless gallbladder; based on the understanding that obstruction of the common bile duct caused by a stone rarely results in dilation of the gallbladder. An obstruction caused in some way other than a stone usually results in dilatation of the gallbladder.

couvercle Hematoma.

coverage Services paid for by the insurance policy, as well as the amount that will be paid for those services.

coverage analysis for laboratories Process by which changes are made to the coding component of the laboratory national coverage determinations (NCD). It is an abbreviated process, similar to the NCD process. The CAL process is used when changes are required to the covered or noncovered ICD-9-CM diagnosis codes or the coding guidance in the laboratory NCDs based on the narrative indications. A tracking sheet is posted opening a CAL and a 30-day public comment period follows. A decision memorandum announcing and explaining the decision is posted following the comment period. Changes

A-C

are implemented in the next available quarterly update of the laboratory edit module. *Synonym(s): CAL.*

coverage decision memorandum CMS prepares a decision memorandum before preparing the national coverage decision. The decision memorandum is posted on the CMS Web site. It tells interested parties that CMS concluded its analysis, describes the clinical position, which CMS intends to implement, and provides background on how CMS reached that stance. The decision outlined in the coverage decision memorandum will be implemented in a CMS-issued program instruction within 180 days of the end of the calendar quarter in which the memo was posted on the Web.

Coverage Issues Manual Revised and renamed the National Coverage Determination Manual in the CMS manual system, it contained national coverage decisions and specific medical items, services, treatment procedures, or technologies paid for under the Medicare program. This manual has been converted to the Medicare National Coverage Determinations Manual (NCD manual), Pub. 100-03. *Synonym(s): CIM.*

covered charges Charges for medical care and supplies that are medically necessary and met coverage and program guidelines.

covered days Days of inpatient care covered by the primary insurance benefits.

covered entity Under HIPAA, a health plan, a health care clearinghouse, or a health care provider who transmits any health information in electronic form in connection with a HIPAA transaction. *Synonym(s): CE.*

covered function Functions that make an entity a health plan, a health care provider, or a health care clearinghouse.

covered osteoporosis drug Injectable drug approved for treating post-menopausal osteoporosis provided to an individual that has suffered a bone fracture related to post-menopausal osteoporosis.

covered person Any person entitled to benefits under the policy, whether a member or dependent.

covered services Diagnostic or treatment services that are considered medically necessary and met coverage and program guidelines.

Cowden syndrome Inherited disorder characterized by hamartomas of stomach and gastrointestinal tract, breast, thyroid carcinoma, and brain. An increased incidence of malignant tumors of the breast, endometrial tissues, and thyroid gland is also described. Report this disorder with ICD-9-CM code 759.6. *Synonym(s): multiple hamartoma.*

coxa valga Hip joint deformity in which there is a lateral deviation.

coxa vara Hip joint deformity in which there is a medial deviation.

coxitis Inflammation in the hip joint. The condition may be transient or may be a degenerative process. Coxitis is reported with ICD-9-CM code 716.65.

coxsackie virus Heterogenous group of viruses associated with aseptic meningitis, myocarditis, pericarditis, and acute onset juvenile diabetes. Report this condition with ICD-9-CM code 079.2.

CP *1)* Cerebral palsy. Reported with a code from ICD-9-CM category 343. *2)* Clinical psychologist.

CPAP Continuous positive airway pressure. Respiratory modality used in the treatment of breathing difficulties or lung disease. Constantly pressurized air and oxygen are delivered to the lungs by a nasal cannula, facemask, or endotracheal tube, and may be administered with or without a ventilator. The lungs are kept partially inflated between breaths, making breathing less difficult. Report noninvasive CPAP with ICD-9-CM procedure code 93.90 and that delivered by endotracheal tube or tracheostomy with a code from category 96.7. Report the initiation and management of continuous positive airway pressure ventilation with CPT code 94660. *NCD Reference: 240.4.*

CPB Cardiopulmonary bypass.

CPD Cephalopelvic disproportion. Disparity between the size of the maternal pelvis and the fetal head that inhibits vaginal delivery. CPD is reported with a code from ICD-9-CM subcategory 653.4.

CPHA Commission on Professional and Hospital Activities.

CPI Consumer price index.

CPK Creatine phosphokinase.

CPM Continuous passive motion. Motorized therapy to improve range of motion in patients recovering from joint surgery, applied prior to the weight-bearing stage of recovery. The joint is conditioned but the muscles are not exercised in CPM.

CPR *1)* Comparative performance report. Report that provides an annual comparison of a physician's services and procedures with those of another physician in the same specialty and geographic area. *2)* Computerized patient record. Computer application that allows all or most elements of a patient's medical record to be stored in a computerized database. *3)* Cardiopulmonary resuscitation. Substitutionary action made for both the heart and lungs in sudden death cases by artificial respiration and external cardiac compression. Cardiopulmonary resuscitation in cardiac arrest is reported with CPT code 92950 and is reported separately from critical care service codes.

CPRI-HOST Computer-based Patient Record Institute-Healthcare Open Systems and Trials.

CPS Chronic pain syndrome. Localized chronic pain with duration of more than three months. CPS often has

A-C

psychosocial factors and responds poorly to treatment. CPS is reported with ICD-9-CM code 338.4.

CPT Current Procedural Terminology. Definitive procedural coding system developed by the American Medical Association that lists descriptive terms and identifying codes to provide a uniform language that describes medical, surgical, and diagnostic services for nationwide communication among physicians, patients, and third parties, used in outpatient reporting of services.

CPT codes Codes maintained and copyrighted by the AMA and selected for use under HIPAA for noninstitutional and nondental professional transactions.

CPT modifier Two-character code used to indicate that a service was altered in some way from the stated CPT or HCPCS Level II description, but not enough to change the basic definition of the service.

CPT-4 Current Procedural Terminology, Fourth Edition.

CQI Continuous quality improvement.

C-QUR Brand name polypropylene surgical mesh with bioabsorbable coating used in the surgical repair and reinforcement of soft tissue, including hernia repair. Use of C-QUR is reported in addition to the primary procedure with CPT code 49568 or 57267. Supply of the mesh can be reported with HCPCS Level II code C1781 for outpatient facilities.

CR *1)* Carrier replacement. *2)* Creatine. *3)* HCPCS Level II modifier used to denote services or supplies that are provided in disaster or catastrophe-related conditions.

cranial Relating to the cranium, or skull. *c. concha* Dome-shaped top portion of the skull, composed of the frontal and parietal bones and portions of the occipital and temporal bones. *Synonym(s): calvaria, skull cap. c. fossae* Three fossae (anterior, middle, and posterior) that form the floor of the cranial cavity (on the superior aspect of the base of the skull) and that provide a surface to support the various lobes of the brain. *c. halo* External fixation device for stabilizing the head and spine. It is applied around the skull and attached to frame pins inserted into the bone. *c. nerve* Twelve paired bundles of nerves connected to the brain that control ocular, auditory, and nasal senses; facial muscles; and oral and throat muscles.

craniectomy Surgical excision of a portion of the skull.

craniocleidodysostosis Inherited bone development disorder, characteristics of which include abnormalities of the head, face, and collarbones. Children with this disorder typically exhibit a square skull, dental abnormalities, a low nasal bridge, and the ability to bring the shoulders together. Report this condition with ICD-9-CM code 755.59.

craniofacial Relating to skull and facial bones.

craniofenestria Developmental defect of the top of the fetal skull in which there are areas where no bone develops. This abnormality is reported with ICD-9-CM code 756.0.

craniomegaly Enlarged cranium, often associated with hydrocephalus.

craniopagus Monozygotic (identical) twins who are joined at the head, sharing bones of the skull and occasionally parts of the brain. Report this abnormality with ICD-9-CM code 759.4.

craniopharyngioma Benign tumor located at the base of the skull in the area of the pituitary gland. Although benign, it can cause symptoms by exerting localized pressure on the brain or blocking the flow of spinal fluid with resulting hydrocephalus. This type of tumor represents 2 to 3 percent of all primary brain tumors, and 5 to 13 percent of brain tumors in children. *Synonym(s): ameloblastoma, pituitary adamantinoma, Rathke's (pouch) tumor, suprasellar cyst.*

craniorachischisis Congenital abnormality in which there is a fissure or slit in the vertebral column and skull, leaving the brain and spinal cord exposed. This abnormality is reported with ICD-9-CM code 740.1.

craniosynostosis Congenital condition in which one or more of the cranial sutures fuse prematurely, creating a deformed or aberrant head shape.

craniotomy Surgical incision made into the cranium or skull for a number of surgical reasons (e.g., decompression, implantation of electrode array, excision, etc.). A craniotomy code is selected based on the procedure performed.

craniovertebral syndrome Nerve root irritation emanating from posterior cervical spinal cord. Report this disorder with ICD-9-CM code 723.2.

CRAO Central retinal artery occlusion. Ocular stroke that presents with painless loss of vision in one eye, usually affecting the complete visual field. A medical emergency, CRAO can lead to permanent vision loss. CRAO is reported with ICD-9-CM code 362.35. *Synonym(s): central RAO.*

craterization Excision of a portion of bone creating a crater-like depression to facilitate drainage from infected areas of bone.

CRC Community rating by class.

creatinine clearance test Comparison of the creatinine level in the blood to that in the urine. The comparison is normally based on the results of a 24-hour urine sample and a blood sample taken at the end of the 24 hours. This test assesses kidney function. Abnormal results may be indicative of kidney disease, although they may also indicate congestive heart failure, dehydration, or shock. Report abnormal results with ICD-9-CM code 794.4.

A-C

credentialing *1)* Reviewing the medical degrees, licensure, malpractice, and any disciplinary record of medical providers for panel and quality assurance purposes and to grant hospital privileges. *2)* Coding certification.

crepitus Clinical symptom manifested by a crackling or crunching sound or feeling around the joints, often indicative of worn cartilage. Report this condition with a code from ICD-9-CM category 719.6.

Creutzfeldt-Jakob disease Progressive destruction of the pyramidal and extrapyramidal systems with progressive dementia, wasting of muscles, tremor, and other symptoms leading to death. Report the various forms of this disorder with a code from ICD-9-CM subcategory 046.1. *Synonym(s): CJD.*

crevicular Area between the tooth and the gingiva. *Synonym(s): sulcus.*

CRF Chronic renal failure. Slow progressive loss of the kidneys' abilities to filter waste from the blood and concentrate urine. It generally occurs over a number of years as a result of disease that produces slow loss of kidney function. The most common causes are diabetes and hypertension. It can range from mild to severe, and may progress to end stage renal disease. CRF alone is reported with ICD-9-CM code 585.9.

CRH Corticotropic releasing hormone.

crib death syndrome Unexpected death of healthy infant under 12 months old. Report this disorder with ICD-9-CM code 798.0. *Synonym(s): SIDS, sudden infant death.*

cricoid Circular cartilage around the trachea.

cri-du-chat syndrome Microcephaly, antimongoloid palpebral fissures, epicanthal folds, micrognathia, strabismus, mental and physical retardation, and a cat-like whine. Report this disorder with ICD-9-CM code 758.31. *Synonym(s): cat-cry syndrome.*

crigler massage Massage of the lacrimal sac in a neonate to resolve congenital nasolacrimal duct obstruction. This massage would be included as part of an E/M service.

crit. Hematocrit.

critical access hospital Freestanding hospital emergency department, not a prospective payment system facility. Provides limited inpatient care, as needed, to stabilize a patient before discharge or transfer to an essential access community hospital (EACH) for extensive treatment. Outpatient critical access hospital claims are billed under type of bill code 85X (FL 4) on the UB-92 claim form for facilities. *Synonym(s): CAH.*

critical care Treatment of critically ill patients in a variety of medical emergencies that requires the constant attendance of the physician (e.g., cardiac arrest, shock, bleeding, respiratory failure, postoperative complications, critically ill neonate).

CRM Cardiac rhythm management.

CRNA Certified registered nurse anesthetist. Nurse trained and specializing in the administration of anesthesia. Anesthesia services rendered by a CRNA must be reported with HCPCS Level II modifier QX, QY, or QZ.

crocodile tears syndrome Facial paralysis with dramatic lacrimation during eating prompted by lesion on the seventh cranial nerve, causing impulses to be misdirected from salivary glands to lacrimal glands. Report this disorder with ICD-9-CM code 351.8.

Crohn's disease Chronic inflammation of the gastrointestinal tract, most commonly affecting the intestines and the terminal ileum in particular. The cause is unknown and it tends to be recurrent after treatment and can result in obstruction and fistula or abscess formation. Crohn's disease is reported under ICD-9-CM rubric 555 by the site affected. *Synonym(s): regional enteritis.*

cromolyn sodium Drug that acts on the respiratory system by inhibiting the release of histamine and leukotrienes from most cells after exposure to antigens. It is used to treat persistent asthma and to prevent seasonal allergic rhinitis and exercise-induced bronchospasm. Supply is reported with HCPCS Level II code J7631 for the non-compounded inhalation solution and J7632 for the compounded product. May be sold under the brand name Nasal Chrom.

CROS Contralateral routing of signals.

cross match Test used to match the compatibility of a donor's blood or organ to the recipient.

Cross-over See Coordination of benefits.

CROSSSAIL Brand name coronary dilatation catheter used in percutaneous intraluminal balloon angioplasty as a treatment approach for blocked coronary arteries. The procedure is reported with CPT code 92982 for one vessel and 92984 for each additional vessel. If performed with atherectomy, 92995 would be reported, with 92996 for each additional vessel. Inpatient procedures would be reported with ICD-9-CM procedural codes 00.40-00.43 and 00.66.

crosswalk Cross-referencing of CPT codes with ICD-9-CM, anesthesia, dental, or HCPCS Level II codes. *Synonym(s): data mapping.*

croup Respiratory illness in children that causes a hoarse voice and a brassy, barking cough. Doctors sometimes call it croup laryngotracheitis because it usually involves inflammation of the larynx (voice box) and trachea (windpipe). Report this illness with ICD-9-CM code 464.20, 464.21, or 464.4. *Synonym(s): brassy cough.*

Crouzon's syndrome Rare congenital condition suspected to be related to gene alteration, appearing with craniosynostosis, underdeveloped midface, and prominent eyes. Other characteristics may include visual distance, loss of hearing, and obstruction of nasal airways. Crouzon's syndrome is reported with ICD-9-CM code 756.0. *Synonym(s): craniofacial dysotosis.*

CRP C-reactive protein. Protein produced in the liver during episodes of acute inflammation. A blood test for CRP may be performed to test for inflammatory processes like lupus, rheumatoid arthritis, or vasculitis. The test may be performed serially to determine the efficacy of antiinflammatory therapy. CRP tests are reported with CPT codes 86140 and 86141.

CRPS Complex regional pain syndrome. Chronic pain following injury to a peripheral nerve. The level of pain is much more severe than appropriate to the injury. CRPS is reported with ICD-9-CM code 338.0. *Synonym(s): causalgia, reflex sympathetic dystrophy.*

CRST syndrome Induration and thickening of the skin with circulatory and organ changes in the face and hands. The name is an acronym for calcinosis, usually of the fingers, Raynaud's, sclerodactyly (hardened skin and bone deformity of the fingers), and telangiectasia (microvascular red spotting of the skin). Esophageal involvement is termed CREST syndrome. Report this disorder with ICD-9-CM code 710.1.

CRT Certified respiratory therapist.

crural Relating to the leg.

crus *1)* Any body part resembling a leg. *2)* Lower part of the leg.

crushing compression syndrome Traumatic anuria (lack of urinary secretion due to renal failure or obstructed renal tract) following crushing. Report this disorder with ICD-9-CM code 958.5.

Cruveilhier-Baumgarten syndrome Cirrhosis of the liver with patent paraumbilical, varicose periumbilical, or umbilical veins. Report this disorder with ICD-9-CM code 571.5.

cryolathe Tool used for reshaping a button of corneal tissue.

cryosurgery Application of intense cold, usually produced using liquid nitrogen, to locally freeze diseased or unwanted tissue and induce tissue necrosis without causing harm to adjacent tissue. This method of tissue destruction is used in a variety of procedures. *NCD Reference: 230.9.*

cryotherapy Any surgical procedure that uses intense cold for treatment. *Synonym(s): cryosurgery. NCD Reference: 230.9.*

cryptomenorrhea Condition in which a woman experiences all the normal symptoms of menstruation without having any external bleeding; often a sign of an imperforate hymen. Report cryptomenorrhea with ICD-9-CM code 626.8.

cryptophthalmos Congenital anomaly in which there is uninterrupted extension of an eyelid continuing across the eyeball, reported with ICD-9-CM code 743.06.

cryptorchidism Undescended testicles, reported with ICD-9-CM code 752.51.

cryptorchism Congenital condition in which one or both testes fails to move into the scrotum as the male fetus develops, remaining in the inguinal canal or the abdominal cavity. Cryptorchism is reported with ICD-9-CM code 752.51. Surgical treatment is often necessary if the testes have not descended by one year of age.

cryptosporidiosis Infection by tiny coccidian protozoa usually seen in young farm animals and parasitic in the intestinal tract of many vertebrate animals. In humans, it causes self-limiting diarrhea that may require rehydration in the very young, pregnant, or very old. In immunosuppressed patients, the diarrhea becomes intractable. It is contracted via a fecal-oral transmission route from ingestion of unfiltered water, and mainly affects those who are immunocompromised or have had exposure to cattle. Cryptosporidiosis is reported with ICD-9-CM code 007.4.

cryptotia Rare congenital anomaly in which the top portion of the ear is covered by or buried in the scalp, reported with ICD-9-CM code 744.29.

Crystalens Brand name intraocular lens that is corrective for both near and far vision, used to replace the natural lens during or after cataract surgery. It is inserted only following extracapsular lens surgery, which is reported with CPT code 66984 if performed as a one-stage procedure (removal and replacement).

CS *1)* Central service. *2)* HCPCS Level II modifier denoting that an item or service was related in part or in whole to the 2010 Gulf oil spill.

CSE Convulsive status epilepticus. More than 30 minutes of continuous seizure or multiple sequential seizures without a return to consciousness in between. Treatment usually begins after five minutes of seizure, so the definition of CSE is evolving. Status epilepticus does not have bearing on the type of epilepsy coded; it simply is indicative of ongoing, active seizure.

CSF Cerebrospinal fluid.

CSO Clinical service organization. Health care organization developed by academic medical centers to integrate medical school, faculty practice plan, and hospital.

CST Certified surgical technologist.

CSW Clinical social worker.

CT *1)* Carpal tunnel syndrome. *2)* Corneal thickness. *3)* Computed tomography. *NCD Reference: 220.1.*

CTA Computed tomographic angiography.

CTLSO Cervical-thoracic-lumbar-sacral orthosis.

CTPN Central total parenteral nutrition. When a patient cannot tolerate enteral feeding (a tube into the stomach), nutrients are provided intravenously, through a central vein. CTPN has a high concentration of dextrose, irritating to smaller blood vessels, so a central line is required. CTPN is usually associated with long-term parenteral feeding.

CTR Capsular tension ring. Used in cataract surgery to provide additional support to the capsular bag surrounding the lens in patients with weakened or missing zonules. Documentation of CTR may establish the procedure as more complex than usual, possibly justification of the use of modifier 22.

CTZ Chemoreceptor trigger zone.

CU *1)* Chronic urticaria. Wheals and swelling of the skin that persist for more than six weeks, reported with a code from ICD-9-CM category 708. *2)* Cubic.

cube pessary Vaginal device inserted to treat uterine prolapse, procidentia, cystocele, or rectocele. Cube pessary is non-rubber. Supply is reported with HCPCS Level II code A4562.

Cubicin Brand name for daptomycin, an IV antibiotic approved for treatment of bacterial skin infections. Supply is reported with HCPCS Level II code J0878.

cubital tunnel syndrome Lesion of the ulnar nerve, affecting movement and feeling of hand. Report this disorder with ICD-9-CM code 354.2.

cubitus valgus Congenital or acquired condition in which the forearm deviates away from the midline on extension. Report ICD-9-CM code 755.59 if specified as congenital and 736.01 if acquired.

cubitus varus Congenital or acquired condition in which the forearm deviates inward toward the midline when extended. Report ICD-9-CM code 755.59 if specified as congenital and 736.02 if acquired.

Cuiffini-Pancoast syndrome Neoplasm of upper lobe of lung. Report this disorder with ICD-9-CM code 162.3.

cul-de-sac Blind pouch, or cavity, such as the pouch of Douglas (retro uterine) or the conjunctival fornix, which is the loose pocket of conjunctiva between the eyelid and the eyeball that permits the eyeball to rotate freely.

culdocentesis Aspiration of fluid from the retrouterine cul-de-sac by puncture of the vaginal vault near the midline between the uterosacral ligaments. Report culdocentesis with CPT code 57020. *Synonym(s): colpocentesis.*

culdotomy/colpotomy Incision through the vaginal wall into the cul-de-sac of Douglas (retro uterine pouch).

Cullen's sign Periumbilical discoloration due to cyanosis, indicating a subcutaneous intraperitoneal hemorrhage.

culture Growth of microorganisms in a medium conducive to their development.

culture shock Stress reaction associated with an individual's assimilation into a new culture vastly different from one in which he or she was raised.

CUPS Cancer of unknown primary site, reported with ICD-9-CM code 199.1.

curet Spoon-shaped instrument used to scrape out abnormal tissue from a cavity or bone.

curettage Removal of tissue by scraping.

curette Spoon-shaped instrument used to scrape out abnormal tissue from a cavity or bone.

Curling's ulcer Peptic ulcer seen secondary to severe skin burns.

Current Dental Terminology Medical code set, maintained and copyrighted by the American Dental Association, that has been selected for use in the HIPAA transactions. *Synonym(s): CDT.*

Current Medical Terminology Manual of preferred medical nomenclature published by the American Medical Association prior to Current Procedural Terminology (CPT). *Synonym(s): CMT.*

Current Procedural Terminology Definitive procedural coding system developed by the American Medical Association that lists descriptive terms and identifying codes to provide a uniform language that describes medical, surgical, and diagnostic services for nationwide communication among physicians, patients, and third parties. *Synonym(s): CPT.*

Current Procedural Terminology coding system Medical code set maintained and copyrighted by the AMA and selected for use under HIPAA for noninstitutional and nondental professional transactions.

Curschmann (-Batten) (-Steinert) syndrome Condition in which the peritoneal cover of the liver converts into a white mass resembling cake icing. Report this disorder with ICD-9-CM code 359.21. *Synonym(s): Batten-Steinert syndrome.*

Cushing's syndrome Abdominal striae, acne, hypertension, decreased carbohydrate tolerance, moon face, obesity, protein catabolism, and psychiatric disturbances resulting from increased adrenocortical secretion of cortisol caused by ACTH-dependent adrenocortical hyperplasia or tumor, or by effects of steroids. Report this disorder with ICD-9-CM code 255.0.

Cushing's ulcer Peptic ulcer seen secondary to head trauma.

cusp *1)* In cardiology, a leaflet or a closure device within the heart's valves. Surgical correction can repair or reinforce "floppy" or inadequate closure of the cusps. The mitral valve has two cusps and the tricuspid has three (as the name implies). Valves with a defect in closure allow backwash or regurgitation of blood back into the heart's chambers. Cusp or valvular defects can be acquired or congenital. Mitral, aortic, and tricuspid valve disorders not caused by rheumatic fever are coded to ICD-9-CM category 424. Congenital insufficiency of the aortic and mitral valves due to incomplete closure is reported with ICD-9-CM codes 746.4 and 746.6, respectively. Rheumatic valve insufficiencies are reported with 394.1, 395.1, and 397.0. *2)* In dentistry, the rounded or pointed portion of the surface of the tooth used for mastication.

custodial care Medical or nonmedical services that do not seek to cure, are provided during periods when the medical condition of the patient is not changing, and do not require continued administration by medical personnel. For example: assistance in the activities of daily living, such as bathing, feeding, and dressing.

custom fabricated Orthotic made from basic materials on an individual basis, by using actual measurements or positive molds of the patient.

custom fitted Premanufactured orthotics that can be adjusted to fit the patient by bending, trimming, or other minimal efforts.

customary charges Amount the hospital or skilled nursing facility is uniformly charging patients for specific services and accommodations.

customary, prevailing, and reasonable charge Basis for Medicare's reimbursement rates before the resource-based relative value scale (RBRVS) was implemented. CPR reimbursement rates were based on historical physician charges rather than relative values, which caused wide variation in Medicare payments among physicians and specialties.

cutaneocerebral angioma syndrome Formation of multiple angiomas in skin of head and scalp. Report this disorder with ICD-9-CM code 759.6. *Synonym(s): Kalischer's syndrome.*

cutaneous Relating to the skin. *c. appendico-vesicostomy* Treatment of urinary incontinence in which the appendix is used as a conduit between the bladder and the surface of the abdomen as an opening for urine. Report this procedure with ICD-9-CM procedure codes 57.21 and 57.88 or CPT code 50845. *Synonym(s): Mitrofanoff operation. c. nerve of thigh syndrome* Tingling, formication, itching, and other symptoms on lower part of the thigh. Caused by lateral femoral cutaneous nerve. Report this disorder with ICD-9-CM code 355.1.

cutback Reduction of the amount or type of insurance for a member who attains a specified age or condition (e.g., age 65, retirement).

cutdown Small, incised opening in the skin to expose a blood vessel, especially over a vein (venous cutdown) to allow venipuncture and permit a needle or cannula to be inserted for the withdrawal of blood or administration of fluids. Age is a factor in choosing the proper code for a cutdown procedure.

cutis laxa syndrome Congenital connective tissue disorder resulting from an abnormality in the production of collagen, which causes hyperelasticity of the skin, hypermobility of the joints, and fragility of the blood vessels, resulting in impaired wound healing. This syndrome is reported with ICD-9-CM code 756.83. If this condition is acquired, rather than congenital, report with ICD-9-CM code 701.8. *Synonym(s): cutis pendula syndrome, Ehlers-Danlos syndrome, elastic skin.*

CV Cardiovascular.

CVA Cerebrovascular accident. Disruption in blood flow to the brain caused by an embolism, thrombosis, or other occlusion, resulting in a lack of perfusion and infarction of brain tissue. Current CVAs are reported with codes from the 434 rubric of ICD-9-CM with a fifth digit of 1 to indicate that cerebral infarction has occurred. An impending CVA is reported as an unspecified transient ischemic attack (TIA), 435.9, in which intermittent ischemia of the brain tissue occurs. When a cerebrovascular accident occurs postoperatively, report 997.02. Sequelae or late effects of CVAs can include paralysis, weakness, speech problems, and aphasia, and are reported within the 438 category reserved for late effects of cerebrovascular disease. A healed or old cerebral infarction is coded to V12.59, a personal history of circulatory system disease. *Synonym(s): stroke.*

CVD *1)* Cardiovascular disease. *2)* Cerebrovascular disease.

CVI Chronic venous insufficiency.

CVL Central venous line.

CVMS Clean voided midstream urine.

CVP Central venous pressure.

CVS Chorionic villus sampling.

CVU Cerebrovascular unit.

CW Closed ward.

CWF Common working file. System of local databases containing total beneficiary histories developed by CMS to improve Medicare claims processing. Medicare fiscal intermediaries and carriers interact with these databases to obtain data on eligibility, utilization, Medicare secondary payer (MSP), and other detailed claims information. The CWF is authorized to deny payment on

A-C

claims on a prepayment basis. There are nine CWF regionally based sectors.

CXR Chest x-ray.

CXy Chest x-ray.

cyanocobalamin Vitamin B12 used to treat deficiency caused by a number of reasons such as inadequate diet, subtotal gastrectomy, or other conditions related to gastrointestinal disease and pernicious anemia. Report the injection supply with HCPCS Level II code J3420. May be sold under the brand names Anacoban, Bedoz, Crystamine, Crysti 1000, Cyanojet, Cyomin, Hydro-Cobex.

cyanosis Bluish discoloration due to an excessive amount of deoxygenated hemoglobin in the blood.

cycl(o)- Round or recurring. May refer to shape or to a sequence of events occurring at repeated intervals.

cyclic schizophrenia Pronounced affective manic or depressive features intermingled with schizophrenic features that tends toward remission without permanent defect, but which is prone to recur.

cyclodialysis Procedure used to separate the ciliary body from the sclera (a result of trauma or glaucoma surgery).

cyclophosphamide Antineoplastic drug that kills specific types of cancer by disrupting transcription of RNA. It is used against breast and ovarian cancers, leukemias, multiple myeloma, and Hodgkin's disease. Cyclophosphamide is also known to improve renal function in children with mild nephrotic syndrome. Supply is reported with HCPCS Level II codes J8530 and J9070. May be sold under the brand names Cycloblastin, Cytoxan, Endoaxan-Asta, Neosar, and Procytox.

cyclophotocoagulation Procedure done to prevent vision loss from glaucoma in which a neodymium: YAG laser is used to burn and destroy a portion of the ciliary body in order to decrease the amount of aqueous humor being produced in the eye. This procedure is only done when creating a drain for aqueous humor to reduce intraocular pressure would not be successful. Destroying portions of the ciliary body reduces the amount of fluid present in the eye. This treatment is reported with ICD-9-CM procedure code 12.73 and CPT codes 66710-66711.

cyclopia Single eye in the place where the root of the nose is normally located. The nose is either missing or consists of a tubular-shaped proboscis located above the eye. Cyclopia is reported with ICD-9-CM code 759.89.

cycloplegia Condition in which the ciliary muscle of the eye is paralyzed, causing paralysis of accommodation in which the eye's ability to automatically change focus when looking from one object to another is lost. Cycloplegia is reported with ICD-9-CM code 367.51.

cyclosporiasis Infection of the small intestine by the protozoa, Cyclospora cayetanensis, spread to humans through ingestion of contaminated food or water, causing watery diarrhea, frequent, explosive bowel movements, loss of weight and appetite, stomach cramps, nausea and vomiting, low grade fever, and muscle aches. Reported with ICD-9-CM code 007.5.

cyclosporine Immunomodulating drug used to prevent organ rejection after transplant and also prescribed for patients with rheumatoid arthritis who have failed to respond to methotrexate therapy. Supply for the oral form is reported with HCPCS Level II codes J7502 and J7515; parenteral is reported with J7516. May be sold under the brand name Gengraf, Neoral, Sandimmune.

cyclothymic personality Mood disorder manifested by fast and repeated alterations between hypomanic and depressed moods. Treatment consists of psychotherapy and/or medication. This condition is reported with ICD-9-CM code 301.13.

cyclotropia Deviation of the eye from the anteroposterior axis.

Cymbalta Brand name serotonin and norepinephrine reuptake inhibitor indicated for major depressive disorder. Also FDA-approved for the pain of diabetic peripheral neuropathy, it is administered in oral capsules. Report major depression with ICD-9-CM codes 296.20-296.36 and diabetic peripheral neuropathy with a code from ICD-9-CM subcategory 249.6 or 250.6 and 357.2 or 337.1. Cymbalta contains duloxetine hydrochloride.

cynorexia Condition of having an insatiable appetite, reported with ICD-9-CM code 783.6.

CYPHER Sirolimus-eluting stent Brand name drug-eluting coronary stent.

Cyriax syndrome Arthritis with degeneration of cartilage leading to collapse of the ears, nose, and tracheobronchial tree. Death may occur as the respiratory system is affected. Report this disorder with ICD-9-CM code 733.99. *Synonym(s): Davies-Colley syndrome, slipping rib.*

cyst Elevated encapsulated mass containing fluid, semisolid, or solid material with a membranous lining.

cyst(o)- Relating to the urinary bladder or a cyst.

cystectomy *1)* Excision or removal of the urinary bladder. *2)* Excision or removal of a cyst on any anatomical site.

cystic duct stump syndrome Recurrence of gall bladder pain following removal of the organ. Report this disorder with ICD-9-CM code 576.0.

cystic hygroma Large watery cyst of the lymphatic channel that frequently occurs in the neck and shoulder region.

cystic mastopathy Mammary dysplasia involving inflammation and the formation of fluid-filled nodular cysts in the breast tissue.

cystitis Inflammation of the urinary bladder. Symptoms include dysuria, frequency of urination, urgency, and hematuria. Underlying causes can include bacterial infections, trauma, or radiation. Cystitis is reported with a code from ICD-9-CM category 595.

cystitis cystica Inflammation of the bladder characterized by the formation of multiple cysts.

cysto Cystoscopy.

Cystocele

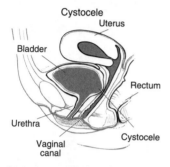

cystocele Herniation of the bladder into the vagina. *lateral c.* Most common form of hernia of the vagina in which a defect in the attachment of the supporting muscle tissue to the sides of the bladder and vagina (paravaginal defect) allows the bladder to protrude into the vaginal wall. When this defect occurs without uterine prolapse, it is reported with ICD-9-CM code 618.02. *midline c.* Form of hernia of the vagina in which a weakness in the midline supporting tissue between the bladder and vagina allows the bladder to protrude into the vaginal wall (central defect) with anterior disruption or bulging of the vagina. When this less common cystocele occurs without uterine prolapse, it is reported with 618.01.

Cystogram

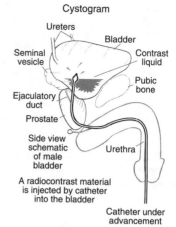

A radiocontrast material is injected by catheter into the bladder

cystogram X-ray of the bladder taken after the injection of opaque contrast solution. A delayed cystogram, where x-rays are taken for 30 minutes or longer, is useful in diagnosing cases of urinary reflux.

cystoid macular degeneration Retinal swelling and cyst formation in the macula.

cystometrogram Recorded measurement of bladder pressure from multiple volume amounts.

cystostomy Formation of an opening through the abdominal wall into the bladder.

cystotomy Surgical incision into the gallbladder or urinary bladder.

cytarabine Antimetabolite chemotherapy drug used primarily to treat acute leukemias, both lymphocytic and nonlymphocytic, and non-Hodgkin's lymphoma. Cytarabine liposome is indicated in the intrathecal treatment of lymphomatous meningitis. Report liposomal cytarabine with HCPCS Level II code J9098 and injectable supply with J9100. May be sold as brand name Cytosar.

-cyte Having to do with cells.

cyto- In relation to a cell.

cytogenetic studies Procedures in CPT that are related to the branch of genetics that studies cellular (cyto) structure and function as it relates to heredity (genetics). White blood cells, specifically T-lymphocytes, are the most commonly used specimen for chromosome analysis. *NCD Reference: 190.3.*

cytology Examination of cells for pathology, physiology, and chemistry content.

cytomegalovirus Herpes virus that infects directly through mucous membrane contact, tissue transplant, or blood transfusion, producing enlarged, infected cells containing inclusion bodies.

cytomegalovirus immune globulin Antibiotic glycoproteins effective in reducing the virulence of CMV disease in patients who are the recipient of a kidney from a seropositive donor and for general prophylaxis against CMV disease related to organ transplant. Supply is reported with HCPCS Level II code J0850. May be sold under the brand name CytoGam.

Cytosar See cytarabine.

Cytotec Brand name drug normally administered via vaginal suppository that induces contractions of the uterus and often used to facilitate expulsion of the products of conception after a second trimester missed abortion. It may also be used as a cervical ripening agent for the induction of labor, or to treat postpartum hemorrhage. Cytotec contains prostaglandin.

Cytovene See ganciclovir sodium.

Cytoxan See cyclophosphamide.

D *1)* Day. *2)* Diopter.

D codes HCPCS Level II alphanumeric codes, beginning with the letter D, used to report dental services.

D&C Dilation and curettage.

D.H.E. 45 See dihydroergotamine mesylate.

D/C *1)* Discharge. *2)* Discontinue.

D/R Dayroom.

D/W Dextrose in water.

D5W Dextrose, 5 percent in water. Sugars suspended in water administered by IV to keep an adult vein open, to provide a vehicle for mixing medications, or to provide hydration and carbohydrates for a patient. Supply of D5W is reported with HCPCS Level II codes J7060 and J7070.

da Vinci Surgical System Brand name robotic device used in performing various endoscopic, laparoscopic, and thoracoscopic surgical procedures. Tools, a light source, and a camera are inserted in the patient via small incisions. The physician guides the surgical tools from a video control console. Surgery performed with the da Vinci Surgical System is reported with the CPT code that represents the specific type of surgery. For example, a laparoscopic prostatectomy, reported with CPT code 55866, would still be reported with 55866 if the da Vinci Surgical System was employed during the surgical session. When assigning ICD-9-CM procedure codes, a code is assigned for the specific procedure, with an additional code assigned from subcategory 17.4 to indicate the type of robotic assistance employed.

dacarbazine Chemotherapy agent used primarily to treat metastatic malignant melanoma and Hodgkin's disease. Supply is reported with HCPCS Level II code J9130. May be sold under the brand name DTIC-Dome.

Daclizumab Brand name drug used as part of an immunosuppression regime with cyclosporin for renal transplant patients to prevent organ rejection. Supply is reported with HCPCS Level II code J7513. May be sold under the brand name Zenapax.

Dacogen Brand name hypomethylating agent under investigation for treatment of myelodysplastic syndrome. It is administered by injection. Supply of Dacogen is reported with unlisted HCPCS Level II code J9999. Myelodysplastic syndrome is reported with ICD-9-CM code 238.7. May be sold under the brand name decitabine.

dacry(o)- Pertaining to the lacrimal glands.

dacryadenoscirrhus Scirrhous carcinoma in the lacrimal gland.

dacryagogatresia Closure or perforation of the lacrimal duct.

dacryoadenalgia Pain in the lacrimal gland.

dacryoadenitis Inflammation of the lacrimal gland.

dacryoblennorrhea Discharge from the lacrimal gland.

dacryocanaliculitis Inflammation of the lacrimal duct.

dacryocystalgia Pain within the lacrimal sac.

dacryocystitis Lacrimal sac inflammation.

dacryocystoblennorrhea Discharge in the lacrimal sac, usually causing chronic inflammation.

dacryocystocele Hernia of the lacrimal sac.

dacryocystography Radiographic examination of the lacrimal system, or tear ducts. A catheter is introduced into the canaliculus and radiopaque dye is injected. Refer to CPT codes 68850, 70170, and 78660 for reporting the procedure.

dacryocystoptosis Displacement or prolapse of the lacrimal sac.

dacryocystorhinostomy Suturing the posterior flaps while the lacrimal obstruction is removed, preserving the conjunctiva. *Synonym(s): dacryorhinocystostomy.*

dacryocystostenosis Narrowing of the lacrimal sac.

dacryocystotome Instrument used for incising the lacrimal duct strictures. *Synonym(s): dacryocystitome.*

dacryohelcosis Ulcer of the lacrimal sac or lacrimal duct.

dacryohemorrhea Tears mixed with blood.

dacryolith Concretion or calculus of the lacrimal sac or duct.

dacryoma Swelling caused by obstruction in the lacrimal gland.

dacryops Distention of the lacrimal duct caused by its being overfilled with fluid.

dacryorhinocystostomy Suturing the posterior flaps while the lacrimal obstruction is removed, preserving the conjunctiva. *Synonym(s): dacryocystorhinostomy.*

dactinomycin Antibiotic with antineoplastic properties derived from Streptomyces parvulus that treats Wilms' tumor and rhabdomyosarcoma in childhood, other sarcomas such as Ewing's, Kaposi's, bone, and soft tissue sarcomas. Also metastatic, nonseminomatous testicular cancer. Supply is reported with HCPCS Level II code J9120.

-dactyl Relating to the fingers or toes.

DAE Distal acinar emphysema. Form of emphysema that occurs subpleurally and usually spares the rest of the lung. DAE is classified to ICD-9-CM code 492.8. *Synonym(s): paraseptal emphysema, subpleural emphysema.*

DAFO Dynamic ankle foot orthoses.

daily benefit Specified maximum benefit payable for room and board charges at a hospital.

D-F

Dalalone LA   See dexamethasone acetate.

Dalalone/Decadron phosphate/Decajet/Dexasone   See Dexamethasone (sodium phosphate)

Dalrymple's sign   Abnormal wideness in the palpebral fissure in thyrotoxicosis.

dalteparin sodium   Anticoagulant used to prevent blood clots from forming in the abdomen or hip for patients undergoing surgery and to decrease the risk of thrombus in patients with severely restricted mobility. It works by enhancing the inhibition of factor Xa and thrombin by antithrombin. It is also used for patients with unstable angina or non-Q wave myocardial infarction (MI). Supply is reported with HCPCS Level II code J1645. May be sold under the brand name Fragmin.

Dameshek's syndrome   One of the hemolytic anemias that share a common decreased rate of synthesis of hemoglobin polypeptide chains and classified according to chain involved. Report this disorder with an ICD-9-CM code from subcategory 282.4.

Damus-Kaye-Stansel procedure   Corrective procedure done for transposition of the great vessels, in which the pulmonary artery is cut just before it divides into the right and left branches and anastomosed to the side of the ascending aorta. This procedure is reported with CPT code 33606.

Dana rhizotomy   Posterior nerve roots of the spine are severed to relieve chronic pain or spasms.

Dana-Putnam syndrome   Numbness, tingling, weakness, a sore tongue, dyspnea, faintness, pallor of the skin and mucous membranes, anorexia, diarrhea, loss of weight, and fever. Strikes in the fifth decade. Report this disorder with ICD-9-CM code 281.0 and 336.2.

Danbolt (-Closs) syndrome   Zinc metabolism defect in young children with blisters, crusting, oozing eruptions, loss of hair, and diarrhea. Report this disorder with ICD-9-CM code 686.8. *Synonym(s): Brandt's syndrome.*

Dandy fever   Acute, self-limiting disease lasting up to a week, spread by the Aedes mosquito infected with one of four dengue virus serotypes of the Flavivirus genus. The disease is found in the tropics and subtropics and causes fever, headache, muscle and joint pain, generalized aches, prostration, rash, enlarged lymph nodes, and leukopenia. The muscle and joint pain experienced can be so severe the bones feel as if they are breaking. Report dandy fever with ICD-9-CM code 061. *Synonym(s): Aden fever, breakbone fever, dengue fever.*

Dandy ventriculocisternostomy   Operation in which an opening from the third ventricle to the interpeduncular cistern is established.

Dandy-Walker syndrome   Hydrocephalus with atresia of the foramina of Luschka and Magendie. Report this disorder with ICD-9-CM code 742.3.

Danlos' syndrome   Group of congenital connective tissue diseases with overly elastic skin, hyperextensive joints, and fragility of blood vessels and arteries. Report this disorder with ICD-9-CM code 756.83. *Synonym(s): Ehlers syndrome, Meekeren syndrome.*

Daptacel   Brand name pediatric diphtheria, tetanus, acellular pertussis vaccine provided in a single-dose vial. Supply of Daptacel is reported with CPT code 90700; administration is reported separately. The need for vaccination is reported with V06.1

darbepoetin alfa   Antianemic used to treat anemia related to chronic renal failure and recently used to treat anemia related to chemotherapy in patients who have non-myeloid malignancies. It increases red blood cell production and corrects hypoxia associated with the anemia by mimicking the effects of erythropoietin. Supply is reported with HCPCS Level II codes J0881 and J0882. May be sold under the brand name Aransep.

Darrach resection   Partial excision of the distal ulna. This resection was originally done by resecting 1 cm to 1.5 cm of the distal ulna, leaving a strip of bone on the ulnar side with ulnar styloid and associated ligaments attached to the carpus. However, it resulted in significant instability between the ulna and carpals. Recently, minimal resection of the ulna has proven more stable, sometimes performed to relieve rheumatoid arthritis. Report this procedure with CPT code 25240.

DAST   Drug abuse screening test. Report this assessment with intervention using HCPCS Level II codes G0396 and G0397.

data   Collection of factual information represented by numeric or alphanumeric characters. *d. condition* Description of the circumstances in which certain data are required. Under HIPAA, all of the data elements and code sets inherent to a transaction and not related to the format of the transaction. *d. council* Coordinating body within the Department of Health and Human Services that has high-level responsibility for overseeing the implementation of the A/S provisions of HIPAA. *d. dictionary* Document or system that characterizes the data content of a system. *d. elements* Smallest named unit of information in a transaction. Data elements are standardized throughout the transaction set (e.g., DTP03) and always consist of a date or time period. The information placed in the field depends on the loop that it occupies. For example, in loop 2300, DTP03 is the discharge hour. In loop 2400, it is the date of service. *d. mapping* Process of matching one set of data elements or individual code values to their closest equivalents in another set. This is sometimes called a crosswalk. *d. model* Conceptual model of the information needed to support a business function or process. *d. segment* Block or set of related data elements that contain related information (e.g., other diagnoses). A data segment may be one of two types: an information segment used to convey information about the provider, payer, or the services rendered; or a control segment that carries information necessary to the transmission and reception of the transaction.

data content Under HIPAA, all the data elements and code sets inherent in a transaction and not related to the format of the transaction.

Data Interchange Standards Association Body that provides administrative services to X12 and several other standards-related groups. *Synonym(s): DISA.*

database Electronic store of utilization information used by payers to pay claims, negotiate contracts, and track utilization and cost of services.

date of service Day the encounter or procedure is performed or the day a supply is issued. *Synonym(s): DOS.*

daunorubicin HCl Chemotherapy drug used to induce remission in acute nonlymphocytic leukemia and acute lymphocytic leukemia and is known to cause irreversible cardiomyopathy. Supply is reported with HCPCS Level II code J9150.

Daunoxome See liposomal daunorubicin citrate.

Daviel's operation Ocular lens is extracted through a corneal incision.

Davies-Colley syndrome Arthritis with degeneration of cartilage leading to collapse of the ears, nose, and tracheobronchial tree. Death may occur as the respiratory system is affected. Report this disorder with ICD-9-CM code 733.99. *Synonym(s): Cyriax's syndrome, slipping rib.*

DAW Dispense as written. Notation from a physician to a pharmacist requesting that the brand name medication be given in lieu of a generic medication.

Dawbarn sign Clinical sign tested for to help diagnose acute subacromial bursitis by palpating the shoulder while the arm is hanging at the side. In a positive exam, pain is elicited by palpating over the bursa. Pain goes away with abduction of the arm. Testing for this sign is part of the musculoskeletal evaluation and management (E/M) exam.

Dawson's fingers Condition seen in multiple sclerosis in which backflow of jugular blood damages the brain, resulting in finger-like lesions on the ventricles.

day test Test determines presence of blood in the feces.

days per thousand Standard unit of measurement of utilization determined by calculating the number of hospital days used in a year for each 1,000 covered lives. *Synonym(s): DPT.*

DBS Deep brain stimulation. Treatment for disabling neurological symptoms associated with diseases including Parkinson's. DBS requires three components: the implanted electrode, extension, and neurostimulator.

Electrical impulses are sent from the neurostimulator to the implant to block tremors. CPT codes for establishing DBS in a patient are 61867-61886. *NCD Reference: 160.24.*

DC *1)* Doctor of chiropractic medicine. *2)* Discontinue. *3)* Direct current.

DC'd *1)* Discharged. *2)* Discontinued.

DCC Data Content Committee.

DCCT Diabetes control and complications trial.

DCd *1)* Discharged. *2)* Discontinued.

DCI Duplicate coverage inquiry. Request made to insurance companies or medical providers to determine whether there is other medical coverage under another plan.

DCP Dynamic compression plate. Orthopedic plate used in open reduction internal fixation (ORIF) procedures for long bone fractures and for stabilization after osteotomy, designed to accommodate compression from muscles and weight bearing pressure. DCP has no direct bearing on code selection.

DCR Dacryocystorhinostomy.

DD *1)* Data dictionary. *2)* Down drain.

DDD Degenerative disc disease.

DDE Direct data entry.

DDH Developmental dysplasia of the hip. Inadequate development of the acetabulum that results in progressive and chronic problems such as subluxation and dislocation of the hip. DDH is reported with a code from ICD-9-CM subcategory 754.3, with a fifth digit identifying the presence of dislocation or subluxation and whether it is bilateral or unilateral. Report 755.63 for congenital hip dysplasia in the absence of dislocation.

DDST Denver developmental screening test.

DE Dose equivalent.

de Lange's syndrome Inherited deformity with impaired development, mental retardation, eyebrows growing across bridge of nose, hairline well down on forehead, uptilted tip of nose with depressed bridge of nose, and small head with low-set ears. Report this disorder with ICD-9-CM code 759.89.

de Quervain's disease Painful tenosynovitis with swelling and constriction secondary to inflammation resulting in stenosis of the first dorsal extensor compartment in the wrist. This disease is due to the narrowness of the common tendon sheath of both the abductor pollicis longus and the extensor pollicis brevis. Treatment can consist of rest, medication, and surgery. Report the diagnosis with ICD-9-CM code 727.04. If an incision into the extensor tendon sheath is made for relief of symptoms, report CPT code 25000.

D-F

de Toni-Fanconi (-Debré) syndrome Renal tubular malfunction, including cystinosis and osteomalacia and caused by inherited disorders or resulting from multiple myeloma or proximal epithelial growth. Report this disorder with ICD-9-CM code 270.0. *Synonym(s): Hart's syndrome.*

deactivate Provider or supplier is unable to use its billing number for claims processing. Upon taking this action, notify the applicant the contractor has done so and the reason.

DeBakey VAD Child Brand name miniaturized heart pump powered by electromagnetic energy, designed to help the left ventricle of the heart pump blood. It is intended for use in children 5 to 16 years of age awaiting heart transplant.

debility Nonspecific term denoting declining health, loss of strength, and feebleness. Report debility with ICD-9-CM code 799.3.

Debré syndrome Renal tubular malfunction, including cystinosis and osteomalacia and caused by inherited disorders or resulting from multiple myeloma or proximal epithelial growth. Report this disorder with ICD-9-CM code 270.0. *Synonym(s): Hart's syndrome.*

debride To remove all foreign objects and devitalized or infected tissue from a burn or wound to prevent infection and promote healing.

debridement Removal of dead or contaminated tissue and foreign matter from a wound.

Decadron LA See dexamethasone acetate.

decapitation Inadequate capitation.

Decavac Brand name tetanus, diphtheria, adsorbed vaccine, for patients older than 7, provided in a single-dose syringe. Supply is reported with CPT code 90714 or 90718, depending on whether the Decavac is preservative free. Administration is reported separately. Report ICD-9-CM code V06.5 for the need for vaccination secondary to injury codes if the patient presents with wounds that prompt the vaccination.

DeCC Dental Content Committee. Organization, hosted by the American Dental Association, that maintains the data content specifications for dental billing. The DeCC has a formal consultative role under HIPAA for all transactions affecting dental health care services.

decem Ten.

deciduoma malignum Malignant neoplasm of the placenta. *Synonym(s): choriocarcinoma, chorioepithelioma, placental deciduoma.*

deciduous tooth Any of 20 teeth that usually erupt between the ages of 6 and 24 months and are later shed as the permanent, adult teeth displace them. *Synonym(s): baby teeth, first set of teeth, primary teeth.*

decitabine Hypomethylating agent under investigation for treatment of myelodysplastic syndrome. It is administered by injection. Supply of decitabine is reported with unlisted HCPCS Level II code J9999. Myelodysplastic syndrome is reported with ICD-9-CM code 238.7. May be sold under the brand name Dacogen.

decompress To relieve pressure.

decompression Release of pressure.

decortication Removal of the cortical substance, the encapsulating or encasing material, of an organ, such as the kidneys or lungs.

decortication of lung Removal of a constricting membrane or layer of pleural tissue from a portion of the lung surface to allow for lung expansion.

decub. *1)* Decubitus ulcer. *2)* Lying down.

decubitus *1)* Ulcer often resulting from bedrest. *NCD Reference: 270.4. 2)* Patient's position in bed.

Decubitus Ulcer

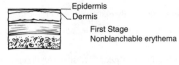
Epidermis
Dermis
First Stage
Nonblanchable erythema

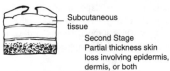
Subcutaneous tissue
Second Stage
Partial thickness skin loss involving epidermis, dermis, or both

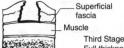
Superficial fascia
Muscle
Third Stage
Full thickness skin loss extending through subcutaneous tissue

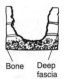
Fourth Stage
Full thickness skin loss extending to muscle and bone
Bone   Deep fascia

decubitus ulcer Progressively eroding skin lesion produced by inflamed necrotic tissue as it sloughs off. A decubitus ulcer is caused by continual pressure to a localized area, especially over bony areas, where blood circulation is cut off when a patient lies still for too long without changing position. It is classified to ICD-9-CM subcategory 707.0 with a fifth digit specifying the anatomical site. *Synonym(s): bedsore, pressure ulcer. NCD Reference: 270.4.*

deductible Predetermined dollar amount of covered billed charges that the patient must pay toward the cost of care.

deep dissection Cutting through the skin to the subcutaneous fat just above the fascial plane and deeper structures, including fascia, muscle, and related structures.

deep fascia Sheet of dense, fibrous tissue lying beneath the subcutaneous fat layer that lines extremities and the trunk and holds groups of muscles together.

def. Deficient, deficiency.

defect Imperfection, flaw, or absence.

defeminization syndrome Mature masculine somatic characteristics by prepubescent girl or woman, showing at birth or developing later as result of adrenocortical dysfunction. Report this disorder with ICD-9-CM code 255.2.

deferoxamine mesylate Chelating agent used to treat acute iron intoxication and iron overload often secondary to transfusion in cases of anemia. Supply is reported with HCPCS Level II code J0895. May be sold under the brand name Desferal.

defibrillation Arrest of cardiac arrhythmias (atrial or ventricular) with restoration of normal rhythm, usually by applying brief electroshock to the heart. *Synonym(s): cardioversion.*

defibrillator system System that includes a pulse generator and electrodes, implanted in the same manner as the pacemaker systems.

defibrination syndrome Dilution of fibrin by enzyme action. Report this disorder with ICD-9-CM code 286.6.

deficiency syndrome Any syndrome resulting from deficiencies in proteins, hormones, calories, trace minerals, vitamins, and other chemicals necessary for function or growth. Report this disorder with ICD-9-CM code 260.

deficit *1)* Amount by which funding is less than the required amount. *2)* Shortfall in funds.

definitive identification Identification of microorganisms using additional tests to specify the genus or species (e.g., slide cultures or biochemical panels).

deformity Irregularity or malformation of the body.

degarelix Injectable gonadotropin-releasing hormone (GnRH) receptor antagonist indicated for the treatment of patients with advanced prostate cancer. Degarelix may be sold under the brand name FIRMAGON. Report supply with HCPCS Level II code J9155.

degeneration Deterioration of an anatomic structure due to disease or other factors.

degenerative stenosis Narrowing of the neural foramina or the spinal canal that occurs as a result of the natural aging process and often manifests with numbness, pain, and tingling in the legs.

Degos' syndrome Malignant atrophic papulosis. Report this disorder with ICD-9-CM code 447.8.

Deheme cast Specialized cast applied to the hand to stabilize a fracture of the navicular bone, one of the carpal bones in the wrist. The cast incorporates the thumb and separately includes the index and middle fingers. Application is reported with CPT code 29085.

dehiscence Complication of healing in which the surgical wound ruptures or bursts open, superficially or through multiple layers. Report dehiscence with a code from ICD-9-CM subcategory 998.3.

dehydration Condition resulting from an excessive loss of water from the body.

Deiters' nucleus syndrome Ocular disturbances, deafness, nausea, thirst, anorexia, and symptoms traced to vagus centers resulting from lesion of Deiters' nucleus and its connections. Report this disorder with ICD-9-CM code 386.19. *Synonym(s): Bonnier syndrome.*

Déjérine sign Forcibly coughing, sneezing, or straining at stool to elicit radiating pain in a limb by aggravating symptoms of radiculitis, when positive. Done as a part of the evaluation and management (E/M) exam.

Dejerine-Roussy syndrome Hypersensitivity to pain as a result of damage to the thalamus. Pain and loss of sensation usually affects the face, arms, or legs and may be felt even in the absence of a stimulus. Dejerine-Roussy syndrome is reported with ICD-9-CM code 338.0. *Synonym(s): thalamic syndrome.*

Déjérine-Thomas syndrome Nerves between the striatum and pallidum are completely demyelinated. Report this disorder with ICD-9-CM code 333.0. *Synonym(s): Hallervorden-Spatz syndrome.*

del Delivery.

del Castillo's syndrome Cessation of menses not associated with pregnancy. Report this disorder with ICD-9-CM code 606.0.

Delatest See testosterone enanthate.

delayed graft Flap graft that is raised or incised from the skin but is not inset or attached immediately onto the prepared skin bed.

delegated official Individual who is delegated the legal authority by the authorized official of that provider or supplier to make changes and/or updates to the organization's status in the Medicare program (e.g., new practice locations, change of address, etc.) and to commit the provider or supplier to fully abide by the laws, regulations, and program instructions of Medicare.

D–F

deletion chromosomes syndrome General description of syndromes such as antimongolism and cat-cry in which chromosomes are missing rather than duplicated. Report this disorder with ICD-9-CM code 758.39.

Delhi boil Dry or urban cutaneous leishmaniasis, one form of Old World cutaneous leishmaniasis. This parasitic skin disease is caused by the protozoa Leishmania tropica, spread by the bite of sand flies, and occurring in large urban areas in the Middle East, especially Iran and Iraq, the Mediterranean, and India. Manifestation is mainly a single, large developing boil or furuncle type lesion that persists over a year. Lymphadenopathy may be present. Report this condition with ICD-9-CM code 085.1.

deligation Closure by tying up; sutures, ligatures.

delimiter Symbol used to separate and organize items of data; character used to group or separate words or values within printed material.

delirium Transient organic psychotic condition with a short course in which there is a rapidly developing onset of disorganization of higher mental processes manifested by some degree of impairment of information processing, impaired or abnormal attention, perception, memory, and thinking. Manifested by clouded consciousness, confusion, disorientation, delusions, illusions, and vivid hallucinations.

delirium acute Short-lived organic, psychotic states, lasting hours or days and characterized by clouded consciousness, disorientation, fear, illusions, delusions, hallucinations (notably visual and tactile), restlessness, tremor, and sometimes fever.

delirium subacute Organic, psychotic state characterized by clouded consciousness, disorientation, fear, illusions, delusions, hallucinations (notably visual and tactile), restlessness, tremor, and sometimes fever. The symptoms, lesser than those in an acute phase, last for several weeks or longer. During this time they may show marked fluctuations in intensity.

delirium tremens Acute or subacute organic psychotic states in alcoholics, characterized by clouded consciousness, disorientation, fear, illusions, delusions, hallucinations (notably visual and tactile), restlessness, tremor, and sometimes fever.

delivery Spontaneous delivery of an infant. *early onset d.* Spontaneous delivery of an infant after completion of 22 weeks of gestation but before completion of 37 weeks. Early onset of delivery is reported with a code from ICD-9-CM subcategory 644.2. *normal d.* Spontaneous vaginal delivery of a single live infant after completion of 38 to 42 weeks of gestation, with cephalic presentation, without instrumentation, and with no antepartum or postpartum conditions or complications. A normal delivery may also include the performance of an episiotomy, artificial rupture of membranes, or fetal

monitoring. Normal delivery is reported with ICD-9-CM code 650. The physician services for vaginal delivery are reported with CPT codes 59400-59430 and 59610-59612. *d. trauma* Perineal tears are classified by degree of tissue involvement, with or without an episiotomy: first-degree lacerations are superficial and involve vaginal mucosa and perineal skin in the fourchette; second-degree lacerations involve the pelvic floor and muscles; third-degree lacerations affect the anal sphincter; fourth-degree lacerations extend to the anal or rectal mucosa.

delmadinone Delatestadiol Combination estrogen and testosterone used to prevent breast fullness in new mothers after childbirth and for relief of menopausal symptoms such as sweating, hot flashes, chills, faintness, and dizziness. It is also used as an adjunct to chemotherapy. It acts by restoring normal estrogen level in tissues, stimulating cells that produce male sex characteristics, and replacing normal androgens that are lost in menopausal women. This class of drugs is exempt from consideration as a controlled substance anabolic steroid in most states. Supply is reported with HCPCS Level II code J0900. May be sold under the brand names Andro-Estro, Androgyn, EstraTestrin, Valertest.

Delorme pericardiectomy Method for excising a diseased pericardium constricting the ventricle.

delusional syndrome Organic disorder including hallucinations, beliefs about being followed, being poisoned, etc., and not meeting criteria for schizophrenia. If an adverse effect of drugs, report this disorder with ICD-9-CM code 292.11. Also report a code from 960-979 to identify the drug, and an E code to identify the circumstances of its use.

demand bills Bills submitted to the intermediary or carrier for medical review at the beneficiary's request because the beneficiary disputes the provider's opinion that the bill will not be paid by Medicare and wishes the bill to be submitted for a payment determination.

dementia Progressive decrease in intellectual functioning of sufficient severity to interfere with occupational or social performance, with impairment of memory and abstract thinking, the ability to learn new skills, problem solving, and judgment. May involve personality change or impairment in impulse control. *alcoholic d.* Nonhallucinatory dementias occurring in association with alcoholism but not characterized by the features of alcohol withdrawal delirium (delirium tremens) or alcohol amnestic syndrome (Korsakoff's alcoholic psychosis). *arteriosclerotic d.* Dementia attributable, because of physical signs (confirmed by examination of the central nervous system), to degenerative arterial disease of the brain. *multi-infarct d.* Dementia attributable, because of physical signs, to degenerative arterial disease of the brain caused by multiple infarctions (an ischemic condition causing local

D-F

tissue death). **presenile d.** Dementia occurring usually before the age of 65 in patients with the relatively rare forms of diffuse or lobar cerebral atrophy usually caused by an associated neurological condition. **repeated infarct d.** Dementia attributable, because of physical signs, to degenerative arterial disease of the brain caused by repeated infarctions. **senile d.** Dementia occurring usually after the age of 65 in which any cerebral pathology other than that of senile atrophic change can be reasonably excluded.

Demerol HCl Injectable narcotic analgesic used to prevent or relieve pain that is moderate to severe in intensity. Supply is reported with HCPCS Level II code J2175. Demerol HCl with promethazine HCl is reported with J2180.

demi- Half the amount.

dendritic keratitis Form of herpes simplex keratitis with symptoms of foreign body, lacrimation, and photophobia.

denervation Resection or removal of a nerve.

dengue fever Acute, self-limiting disease lasting up to a week, spread by the Aedes mosquito infected with one of four dengue virus serotypes of the Flavivirus genus. The disease is found in the tropics and subtropics and causes fever, headache, muscle and joint pain, generalized aches, prostration, rash, enlarged lymph nodes, and leukopenia. The muscle and joint pain experienced can be so severe the bones feel as if they are breaking. Report dengue fever with ICD-9-CM code 061. **Synonym(s):** Aden fever, breakbone fever, dandy fever.

denial Refusal by an insurance plan to pay for services, procedures, or supplies. A denial may be made due to coverage limitations, medical necessity issues, or failure to follow appropriate prior authorization or claim submission guidelines.

denileukin diftitox Type of molecular targeted therapy called a fusion protein made up of interleukin-2 (IL-2) that is fused, or combined, with fragments of inactive diphtheria toxin. The drug attaches to specific cancer cells with receptors for IL-2 and pushes the diphtheria toxin into the cell, killing it. It is used to treat recurrent mycosis fungoides.

Denonvillier's operation Correction of defective nasal ala using a triangular flap from the opposite side of the nose.

dens axis Peg-shaped projection of the second vertebra that ascends up from the vertebral body to articulate with the atlas, allowing the atlas and head to rotate. **Synonym(s):** odontoid process.

dental accretions Accumulation of foreign material on the tooth surface, usually plaque, tartar, or calculus. This condition is reported with ICD-9-CM code 523.6.

dental arch Curved structure of a line created by the buccal surfaces or the central grooves of all natural teeth and the residual ridge of missing natural teeth in the upper or lower jaw.

dental bridge Partial denture anchoring onto adjacent teeth on either side.

dental calculus Concretion of calcium, cholesterol, salts, or other substances that forms around the tooth supragingivally or subgingivally.

dental cast Reproduction or model of a section or the entire mandibular or maxillary arch made by pouring plaster or plastic into an impression.

dental cement Any substance used in the mouth that sets from a viscous to a hard form and functions as a restorative material, a bonding force for fabricated restorations and orthodontics, or protective filling for insulation.

dental complication Problem arising after observation and treatment in dental care has begun.

dental consultation Advice or an opinion rendered by a dentist or dental specialist who is not the treating doctor provided at the request of the providing dentist, physician, or other appropriate professional.

Dental Content Committee Organization, hosted by the American Dental Association, that maintains the data content specifications for dental billing. It has a formal consultative role under HIPAA for all transactions affecting dental health care services. **Synonym(s):** DeCC.

dental plaque Thin film composed of organic and inorganic deposits from food and epithelial cells that adheres to the tooth surface and is not readily removed, providing a medium for bacterial growth.

dental sealant Material that can be bonded to the surface of a tooth to cover pits, fissures, and imperfections and protects against debris and bacterial microorganisms.

dental splint Device that allows loose, transplanted, or injured oral structures to be immobilized and protected.

dentin Hard substance of the tooth found beneath the enamel on the crown and the cementum on the root that surrounds the living pulp tissue.

dentoalveolar structure Area of alveolar bone surrounding the teeth and adjacent tissue.

denture Manmade substitution of natural teeth and neighboring structures.

denture base Portion of the artificial substitute for natural teeth that makes contact with the soft tissue of the mouth and serves as the anchor for the artificial teeth.

dep. Dependent.

D-F

Department of Health and Human Services   Cabinet department that oversees the operating divisions of the federal government responsible for health and welfare. HHS oversees the Centers for Medicare and Medicaid Services, Food and Drug Administration, Public Health Service, and other such entities. *Synonym(s): DHHS, HHS.*

Department of Justice   Attorneys from DOJ and the United States Attorney's Office have, under the memorandum of understanding, the same direct access to contractor data and records as OIG and the Federal Bureau of Investigation (FBI). DOJ is responsible for prosecution of fraud and civil or criminal cases presented. *Synonym(s): DOJ.*

deployment   Placement or launching of an endovascular repair device, commonly a stent, an endograft, or endoprosthesis, out of its applicator or containment sheath to allow it to expand to fit snugly to the vessel wall. Placement of such a device may require more than one deployment attempt to seat the device in the correct position. The number of deployment attempts is not a factor in coding the placement. The code choice depends on the type of device, the vessel being repaired, and the method of insertion.

DepoCyt   Form of cytarabine indicated in the intrathecal treatment of lymphomatous meningitis. Kills selected cancer cells by inhibiting DNA synthesis. Supply is reported with HCPCS Level II code J9098.

Depo-Provera   See medroxyprogesterone acetate.

depressed fracture   Fracture of the skull where the bone is pushed or caving inward.

depressed skull fracture   Skull bones that are broken and driven inward from a forceful blow.

depression   Disproportionate depressive state with behavior disturbance that is usually the result of a distressing experience and may include preoccupation with the psychic trauma and anxiety.

depression anxiety   Disproportionate depression with behavior disturbance that is usually the result of a distressing experience and may include delusions or hallucinations, anxiety, and preoccupation with the psychic trauma that preceded the illness.

depression endogenous   Manic-depressive psychosis in which there is a widespread depressed mood of gloom and wretchedness with some degree of anxiety, reduced activity, or restlessness and agitation. There is a marked tendency to recurrence; in a few cases this may be at regular intervals.

depression monopolar   Manic-depressive psychosis in which there is a widespread depressed mood of gloom and wretchedness with some degree of anxiety, reduced activity, or restlessness and agitation. There is a marked

tendency to recurrence; in a few cases this may be at regular intervals.

depression neurotic   Disproportionate depression with behavior disturbance that is usually the result of a distressing experience and may include delusions or hallucinations, anxiety, and preoccupation with the psychic trauma that preceded the illness.

depression psychotic   Manic-depressive psychosis in which there is a widespread depressed mood of gloom and wretchedness with some degree of anxiety, reduced activity, or restlessness and agitation. There is a marked tendency to recurrence; in a few cases this may be at regular intervals.

depression psychotic reactive   Manic-depressive psychosis in which there is a widespread depressed mood of gloom and wretchedness with some degree of anxiety, reduced activity, or restlessness and agitation. There is a marked tendency to recurrence; in a few cases this may be at regular intervals.

depression reactive   Disproportionate depression with behavior disturbance that is usually the result of a distressing experience and may include delusions or hallucinations, anxiety, and preoccupation with the psychic trauma that preceded the illness.

depressive personality or character   Affective personality disorder characterized by lifelong predominance of a chronic nonpsychotic disturbance involving either intermittent or sustained periods of depressed mood marked by worry, pessimism, low output of energy, and a sense of futility.

depressive reaction   State of depression associated with an abnormal or maladaptive reaction with emotional or behavioral characteristics as a result of a life event or stressor that is usually temporary.

depressor   Tool used to push body tissue out of the way.

depth of field   Distance of focus in sight.

Dercum's syndrome   Deposits of painful symmetrical nodular or pendulous masses of fat in various body regions. Report this disorder with ICD-9-CM code 272.8. *Synonym(s): Ander's syndrome.*

derealization   Awareness of the disturbed perception of external objects or parts of one's own body as changed in their quality, unreal, remote, or automatized.

dermabrasion   Cosmetic procedure that smooths out flaws and disfigured skin and promotes the growth of a new layer of skin cells by removing the outer layer of skin by mechanical or chemical means such as fine sandpaper, wire brushes, and caustic substances. Dermabrasion is assigned a CPT code from range 15780-15783. *Synonym(s): dermaplaning, microdermabrasion.*

D-F

Dermagraft Brand name bioengineered dermal substitute that is derived from human fibroblast cells and cryopreserved for up to six months. It is used for treating chronic diabetic skin ulcers to restore the dermal bed and accelerate the wound healing process. Its application is reported with CPT codes 15360-15366. Supply is reported with HCPCS Level II code Q4106.

dermal melanocytoma Benign, usually solitary, dark blue to black neoplasm made up of melanocytes that presents as a somewhat firm, well defined, and rounded nodule. *Synonym(s): blue nevus, Jadassohn-Tièche nevus.*

dermatitis Inflammation of the skin.

dermatochalasis Acquired form of connective tissue disease in which decreased elastic tissue formation and abnormal elastin production result in loss of elasticity. In the eyelid, this is associated with aging, although it is seen after onset of puberty. This condition may be a cosmetic problem only or in more severe cases, may affect the visual field. Blepharoplasty is the usual treatment method.

dermatophytosis Superficial parasitic fungal infections occurring in the skin, hair, or nails that involve the corneal stratum, or outermost layer of cells, commonly referring to ringworm and athlete's foot. See ICD-9-CM category 110 for correct code assignment based upon anatomical site.

dermatoplasty Surgical replacement of lost or destroyed skin.

dermatosclerosis Systemic disease characterized by excess fibrotic collagen build-up, turning the skin thickened and hard. Fibrotic changes also occur in various organs and cause vascular abnormalities and affect more women than men. Report this condition with ICD-9-CM code 710.1.

dermatosis Any disease related to the skin.

dermis Skin layer found under the epidermis that contains a papillary upper layer and the deep reticular layer of collagen, vascular bed, and nerves.

dermis graft Skin graft that has been separated from the epidermal tissue and the underlying subcutaneous fat, used primarily as a substitute for fascia grafts in plastic surgery.

dermoid cyst Closed pouch or sac containing elements of teeth, hair, or skin.

dermolipoma Asymptomatic, congenital, benign tumor-like lesion or dermoid of the subconjunctiva. Report dermolipoma with ICD-9-CM code 224.9.

DeROM Brand name dynamic range of motion splint used in soft tissue contracture. Supply of DeROM splints is reported with HCPCS Level II codes appropriate to the site.

descriptor Text defining a code in a code set.

desensitization *1)* Administration of extracts of allergens periodically to build immunity in the patient. *2)* Application of medication to decrease the symptoms, usually pain, associated with a dental condition or disease.

desert fever Coccidioidomycosis, a fungal infection caused by inhaling dust particles containing the spores of coccidioides immitis. The primary form is an acute, self-limiting respiratory disease and presents like a cold or the flu. The progressive, chronic, secondary form is virulent presenting as a severe granulomatous disease that affects most body tissues that can be due to a reinfection or reactivation of the primary disease. Report coccidioidomycosis with ICD-9-CM category 114. *Synonym(s): California disease, coccidioidal granuloma, coccidioidosis, desert rheumatism, Posadas-Wernicke disease, Posadas' disease or mycoses, San Joaquin or San Joaquin Valley fever.*

desferal mesylate Pituitary hormone drug used to treat an unusual combination of problems. This drug both increases the permeability of the renal tubular epithelium and increases factor VIII activity. It is given to treat non-nephrogenic diabetes insipidus, temporary polyuria and polydipsia from pituitary edema, hemophilia A and von Willebrand's disease. It is also used to treat nocturnal enuresis in children older than age 6. Supply is reported with HCPCS Level II code J2597. May be sold under the brand names desmopressin acetate DDVAP, Stimate.

designated code set Medical code set or an administrative code set that the Department of Health and Human Services has designated for use in one or more of the HIPAA standards.

Designated Data Content Committee Organization that HHS designated for oversight of the business data content of one or more of the HIPAA-mandated transaction standards. *Synonym(s): Designated DCC.*

designated record set Group of records used, in whole or in part, by a covered entity to make decisions about an individual.

designated standard Standard that HHS designated for use under the authority provided by HIPAA.

-desis Binding or fusion.

desmo- Relating to ligaments.

desmoid tumor Nonencapsulated, fibromatous neoplasm that develops within muscular or tendinous bands of tissue, usually in the abdomen.

desmoplasia Development of collagen tissue at the point of a cancer cell's invasion as part of the invaded cell's defense mechanisms. Desmoplasia is a hallmark of invasion and malignancy.

D-F

D-F

Desmoteplase Brand name genetically engineered form of the clot-dissolving protein found in the saliva of the vampire bat in Phase III clinical trials as a therapeutic treatment for ischemic stroke. Infusion of Desmoteplase would be reported with CPT code 37195 or inpatient ICD-9-CM code 99.10. Desmoteplase contains rDSPA 1-a.

destination therapy Permanent support for advanced-stage heart failure patients who require permanent mechanical cardiac support and who are not candidates for heart transplantation. *NCD Reference: 20.9.*

destruction Ablation or eradication of a structure or tissue.

det. Let it be given.

detailed physical examination Under the 1995 guidelines, examination of two to seven organ systems, with at least one system documented in detail. Under the 1997 guidelines, an examination of at least six organ systems or body areas, including at least two bullet point elements for each system/area or at least 12 bullet point elements from at least two organ systems or body areas.

detail-level code Revenue code is defined on a detailed level by the code's fourth digit. The general classification is represented by a zero, and the detail-level codes are represented by the numbers 1 through 9, as applicable to the particular revenue code.

detection Search for presence of a tissue or material.

determination Decision made to pay in full, in part, or deny a claim.

detrusor sphincter dyssynergia Condition in which urinary outflow is obstructed because the bladder neck fails to relax or tightens when the detrusor muscle contracts during urination. This condition occurs more often in males than in females. This condition is reported with ICD-9-CM code 596.55. *Synonym(s): bladder neck dyssynergia.*

deuter- Secondary or second.

development letter request Request for additional information required by the Medicare fiscal intermediary to process a claim accurately that must be returned within 35 days of the date on the request.

developmental delay disorders Various disorders manifested by a delay in development based on that anticipated for a certain age level or period of development. Both biological and nonbiological factors may be involved. Originating before age 18, these impairments may continue indefinitely. *arithmetical disorder* Serious impairment in the development of arithmetical skills without obvious intellectual deficit and with adequate schooling. *articulation disorder* Delay in the development of normal word-sound production resulting in defects of articulation frequently identified by omissions or substitutions of consonants. *coordination disorder* Serious impairment in the development of motor coordination that is not explicable in terms of general intellectual retardation and is commonly associated with perceptual difficulties. *mixed developmental disorder* Delay in the development of a specific skill such as reading, arithmetic, speech, or coordination, frequently associated with lesser delays in other skills. *motor retardation disorder* Serious impairment in the development of motor coordination that is not explicable in terms of general intellectual retardation and is commonly associated with perceptual difficulties. *reading disorder* Serious impairment in the development of reading or spelling skills. May include speech, language, right-left identification, and motor problems or psychosocial factors without general intellectual retardation or with adequate schooling. *speech or language disorder* Serious impairment or delay in the development of speech or language (syntax or semantic) with frequent articular defect of consonant sound that is not explicable in terms of general intellectual retardation. *specific disorder* Non-neurologic disorder demonstrated by specific delay in development not explained by general intellectual retardation or inadequate schooling that may be related to biological maturation.

developmental dislocation Displacement of a body part occurring in the developmental phase of childhood.

devitalized Deprivation of vital necessities or of life itself.

DEXA Dual energy x-ray absorptiometry. Radiological technique for bone density measurement using a two-dimensional projection system in which two x-ray beams with different levels of energy are pulsed alternately and the results are given in two scores, reported as standard deviations from peak bone mass density. This procedure is reported with CPT codes 77080-77082. *Synonym(s): DXA. NCD Reference: 150.3.*

dexamethasone Potent antiinflammatory with a wide range of uses, most commonly used to treat any kind of allergic reaction by suppressing the immune reaction, but also used in treating cerebral edema, hyaline membrane disease in premature newborns, and in the prevention of chemotherapy-induced nausea and vomiting. It is also administered in the course of a dexamethasone suppression test to evaluate for Cushing's syndrome. Supply is reported with HCPCS Level II code J1100 for dexamethasone sodium phosphate, J1094 for dexamethasone acetate, and J7637 and J7638 for inhalation solution and J8540 for oral. May be sold under the brand names AK-Dex, Cortastat, Cortostat, Dalalone, Decadrol, Decadron, Decadron phosphate, Decaject, Dexacen, Dexacorten, DexaMeth, Dexamethasone Intensol, Dexasone, Dexone, Hexadrol,

Hexadrol phosphate, Mymethasone, Oradexon, Primethasone, Solurex.

Dexasone LA See dexamethasone acetate.

DexCom STS Continuous glucose monitoring system available by prescription. The system consists of a subcutaneous sensor that continuously measures glucose levels and transmits the information wirelessly to a handheld receiver. The monitoring system is intended for use as an adjunctive device to complement, not replace, information obtained from standard home glucose monitoring devices. Supply of a DexCom STS is reported with HCPCS Level II codes S1030 and S1031. Sensor placement and patient training is reported with CPT codes 95250 and 95251.

dexrazoxane HCl Chelating drug that acts as a cardioprotectant indicated for reducing the incidence and severity of cardiomyopathy associated with doxorubicin administration in women with metastatic breast cancer who will continue to receive doxorubicin therapy for tumor control. It is administered by rapid IV infusion or IV push about 30 minutes before doxorubicin. Supply is reported with HCPCS Level II code J1190. May be sold under the brand name Cardioprotective Zinecard.

dexter Right.

dextra Right.

dextran 40 Low-molecular weight dextran. Drug acting on fluid and electrolyte balance that has an osmotic effect on interstitial fluid, drawing it into the intravascular space to cause plasma volume expansion for fluid replacement, prevention of venous thrombosis, and as a hemodilutent in extracorporeal circulation. Supply is reported with HCPCS Level II code J7100.

dextran 75 High-molecular weight dextran. Drug acting on fluid and electrolyte balance that has an osmotic effect on interstitial fluid, drawing it into the intravascular space to cause plasma volume expansion for fluid replacement and used in emergencies to increase circulating blood volume and maintain blood pressure. Supply is reported with HCPCS Level II code J7110. May be sold under the brand names Gentran, Macrodex.

dextro- Meaning on or to the right.

dextrocardia Congenital condition in which the heart is located on the right side of the chest rather than in its normal position on the left. This reversal may occur alone, reported with ICD-9-CM code 746.87, or with situs inversus, in which all the internal organs are transposed, reported with code 759.3.

dextrose 5% and normal saline Intravenous solution used to keep patients hydrated and maintain body fluids and nutrition using physiologic (normal) saline combined with a little sugar (dextrose). It provides 170 calories per liter and can be used as a base mixture for adding other

medications. Supply is reported HCPCS Level II code J7042 or S5010.

dextrose 5% in lactated ringers Intravenous solution loosely resembling the electrolyte composition of normal blood serum and plasma. It is used to treat fluid losses from the lower gastrointestinal (GI) tract and burns and can be used as a base solution to mix in other medications. Supply is reported with HCPCS Level II code S5011.

dextrose 5% with potassium chloride Intravenous solution that helps maintain fluid and electrolyte balance by providing hypotonic water to the extracellular and intracellular spaces, as the dextrose is quickly metabolized with the addition of potassium chloride as a critical electrolyte. Supply is reported with HCPCS Level II code S5012.

dextrose 5%/45% normal saline w/potassium chloride & magnesium sulfate Intravenous fluid with an added mixture of electrolytes for treating preeclampsia or eclampsia in pregnant women. Supply is reported using HCPCS Level II codes S5013 and S5014.

DHEA Dehydroepiandrosterone.

DHHS Department of Health and Human Services. Cabinet department that oversees the operating divisions of the federal government responsible for health and welfare. HHS oversees the Centers for Medicare and Medicaid Services, Food and Drug Administration, Public Health Service, and other such entities.

DHS Dynamic hip screw. Sliding screw and plate used to repair hip fractures.

DHT Dihydrotestosterone.

Di Guglielmo's syndrome Condition characterized by large numbers of nucleated red cells appearing in the bone marrow and blood. Report this disorder with an ICD-9-CM code from subcategory 207.0.

diabetes mellitus Endocrine disease manifested by high blood glucose levels and resulting in the inability to successfully metabolize carbohydrates, proteins, and fats, due to defects in insulin production and secretion, insulin action, or both. Type I results from the autoimmune or other destruction of the pancreatic beta cells, which cease producing insulin. This type is commonly seen at a young age and requires regular insulin injections. Type II is caused by the body's inability to respond to insulin that is produced, called insulin resistance. The pancreas gradually loses the ability to produce insulin. Type II is usually seen in adulthood and can often be treated with diet, exercise, and oral medications. Type II may also require insulin, however, and is also diagnosed among juvenile patients. Diabetes mellitus is coded within the 250 rubric of ICD-9-CM. Coding diabetes as type I or type II is determined by the level of function of the pancreatic cells

D-F

and is not dependent on the patient's status as insulin dependent or non-insulin dependent. The age of onset is also not a determining factor in selecting the code. *Synonym(s): DM. **d. m. in newborn infant syndrome*** Newborn that has the inability to metabolize carbohydrates, proteins, and fats with insufficient secretion of insulin. Report this disorder with ICD-9-CM code 775.1. ***d. m. hypertension-nephrosis syndrome*** High blood pressure and kidney failure resulting from diabetes in which carbohydrate utilization is reduced and lipid and protein use are enhanced. Report this disorder with a code from ICD-9-CM subcategory 249.4 or 250.4 and 581.81. ***secondary d. m.*** Diabetic condition in which the underlying cause is something other than environmental conditions or genetics. Report this disorder with a code from ICD-9-CM category 249. *NCD References: 40.1, 70.2.1, 290.1.*

diabetes outpatient self-management training services Educational and training services furnished by a certified provider in an outpatient setting. The physician managing the individual's diabetic condition must certify that the services are needed under a comprehensive plan of care and provide the patient with the skills and knowledge necessary for therapeutic program compliance (including skills related to the self-administration of injectable drugs). The provider must meet applicable standards established by the National Diabetes Advisory or be recognized by an organization that represents individuals with diabetes as meeting standards for furnishing the services. *NCD Reference: 40.1.*

diabetes-dwarfism-obesity syndrome Endocrine dysfunction causing diabetes and affecting growth and weight. Report this disorder with ICD-9-CM code 258.1.

diabetes-nephrosis syndrome High blood pressure and kidney failure resulting from diabetes in which carbohydrate utilization is reduced and lipid and protein use are enhanced. Report this disorder with a code from ICD-9-CM subcategory 249.4 or 250.4, and 581.81.

diabetic Relating to diabetes. ***d. amyotrophy syndrome*** Muscular atrophy resulting from diabetes. Report this disorder with a code from ICD-9-CM subcategory 249.6 or 250.6, and 353.5. ***d. gastroparesis*** Neurological manifestation of diabetes often seen in the later stages that effects the process of emptying food from the stomach into the small bowel because of a degree of paralysis within the stomach muscles. It is coded first with a combination diabetes code from ICD-9-CM subcategory 249.6 or 250.6 and the code for gastroparalysis, 536.3. ***d. ketoacidosis*** Diabetic hyperglycemic crisis causing ketones to be present in body fluids. An odor of sweet apples on the breath and signs of dehydration are common. Diabetic ketoacidosis is reported with a code from ICD-9-CM subcategory 249.1 or 250.1.

diabetic nephropathy Commonly seen in later stages of diabetes mellitus when proteinuria can develop and lead to renal disease.

diagnosis Determination or confirmation of a condition, disease, or syndrome and its implications.

diagnosis code Alphanumeric code that describes the patient's medical condition, symptoms, or the reason for the encounter.

diagnosis related group Method CMS uses to pay hospitals for Medicare recipients based on a statistical system of classifying any inpatient stay into one of several hundred groups. It is a classification scheme whose patient types are defined by patients' diagnoses or procedures and, in some cases, by the patient's age or discharge status. Each DRG is intended to be medically meaningful and would ordinarily require approximately equal resource consumption as measured by length of stay and cost. *Synonym(s): DRG.*

diagnostic Examination or procedure to which the patient is subjected, or which is performed on materials derived from a hospital outpatient, to obtain information to aid in the assessment of a medical condition or the identification of a disease. Among these examinations and tests are diagnostic laboratory services such as hematology and chemistry, diagnostic x-rays, isotope studies, EKGs, pulmonary function studies, thyroid function tests, psychological tests, and other tests given to determine the nature and severity of an ailment or injury.

Diagnostic and Statistical Manual of Mental Disorders, Fourth Edition, Text Revision Manual used by mental health clinicians as the diagnosis coding system for substance abuse and mental health patients. *Synonym(s): DSM-IV-TR.*

diagnostic coding Claims submitted to Medicare require diagnostic codes from the International Classification of Diseases, Clinical Modification, Ninth Edition (ICD-9-CM). Claims for certain services, especially when local policy has been established, may be denied based on diagnosis, so correct code selection is important. In the next several years, the current system will be replaced by the clinically modified ICD-10. Information about the new system is available from the National Center of Health Statistics (NCHS), which is a department under the Centers for Disease Control (CDC).

diagnostic dental procedure Procedure performed to evaluate the patient's complaints or symptoms and help the dentist establish the nature of the patient's disease or condition so that definitive care can be provided.

diagnostic laboratory services Laboratory services that are required to diagnose a disease or injury, regardless of where the services are rendered. These services include certain mechanical or machine tests such as EKGs and EEGs. For Medicare purposes, these services are paid under a fee schedule.

diagnostic procedures Procedure performed on a patient to obtain information to assess the medical condition of the patient or to identify a disease and to determine the nature and severity of an illness or injury.

diagnostic reference patient Patient who is referred to the hospital for diagnostic services.

diagnostic services Examination or procedure performed on a patient to obtain information to assess the medical condition of the patient or to identify a disease and to determine the nature and severity of an illness or injury (e.g., diagnostic laboratory tests, x-rays, EKGs, pulmonary function tests, or psychological tests).

diagnostic x-ray services X-ray and other related services performed for diagnostic purposes, including portable x-ray services.

dialysis Artificial filtering of the blood to remove contaminating waste elements and restore normal balance. *NCD Reference: 230.7.*

diameter Straight line connecting two opposite points on the surface of a lesion, spheric, or cylindric body.

diamond burr Surgical drill used to make holes in bones.

Diamond-Blackfan syndrome Congenital anemia of infancy requiring a number of blood transfusions to maintain life. Report this disorder with ICD-9-CM code 284.01.

Diamond-Gardener syndrome Bruising occurring easily and large, involving surrounding tissues, resulting in pain, and spawning others. Assumed to be a form of autoimmune problem. Report this disorder with ICD-9-CM code 287.2.

diaper dermatitis Nonallergic skin irritation in infants in the area that has contact with the diaper. It can be caused by extended contact with feces, urine, soaps, and ointments, and by friction and the irritating effects of ammonia by-products in urine. The rash is often accompanied by secondary yeast or bacterial infection. Report this condition with ICD-9-CM code 691.0. *Synonym(s): ammonia dermatitis, diaper rash, Jacquet's dermatitis, Jacquet's erythema, napkin rash.*

diaper syndrome Infantile form of Fanconi's syndrome, in which there is a rounded face, almond-shaped eyes, strabismus, low forehead, hypogonadism, hypostomia, mental retardation, an insatiable appetite, but includes cystinosis. Report this disorder with ICD-9-CM code 270.0.

diaphragm *1)* Muscular wall separating the thorax and its structures from the abdomen. *2)* Flexible disk inserted into the vagina and against the cervix as a method of birth control.

diaphysectomy Surgical removal of a portion of the shaft of a long bone, often done to facilitate drainage from infected bone.

diaphysis Central shaft of a long bone.

diastasis Dislocation of two bones that do not have a true joint, such as the pubic symphysis.

Diastat See diazepam.

diastematomyelia Congenital defect often seen in spina bifida in which the spinal cord is split into halves by bone tissue, cartilage, or fibrous tissue resembling a spike, with each half surrounded by a dural sac. This defect is reported with ICD-9-CM code 742.51.

diastole Relaxation period of the heart muscle between the first and second heart sounds, during which the chambers, particularly the ventricles, are filling in between contractions.

diastolic Pertaining to the time in between ventricular contractions (systole), when ventricular filling occurs.

diathermy Applying heat to body tissues by various methods for therapeutic treatment or surgical purposes to coagulate and seal tissue. *NCD References: 150.5, 240.3.*

diazepam Antianxiety medication used prior to endoscopic procedures, cardioversion, or as a preoperative sedative. It is also used for acute alcohol withdrawal, muscle spasms, and seizure control. Supply is reported with HCPCS Level II code J3360. May be sold under the brand names Apo-Diazepam, Diastat, Diazemuts, Diazepam Intensol, Novo-Dipam, PMS-Diazepam, Valium, Vivol.

diazoxide Vasodilator and antihypertensive used in hypertensive crisis and hypoglycemia secondary to hyperinsulinemia. Direct relaxation of arteriolar smooth muscle and a decrease in peripheral vascular resistance result in lowered blood pressure. The inhibition of pancreatic release of insulin and the stimulation of catecholamine release result in an increased hepatic release of glucose. Supply is reported with HCPCS Level II code J1730. May be sold under the brand names Hyperstat IV, Proglycem.

DIC Disseminated intravascular coagulopathy.

DIC syndrome Disseminated intravascular coagulation syndrome caused by a decrease of elements needed for coagulation of blood causing profuse bleeding. Report this disorder with ICD-9-CM code 286.6.

dicephalus Congenital abnormality in which a fetus has two heads, reported with ICD-9-CM code 759.4.

DICOM Digital imaging and communications in medicine.

dicyclomine HCl Drug that acts on the autonomic nervous system that also has some local anesthetic properties, used to relieve gastrointestinal spasms

D-F

brought on by irritable bowel syndrome and infant colic in babies six months and older. Supply is reported with HCPCS Level II code J0500. May be sold under the brand names Bemote, Bentyl, Bentylol, Byclomine, Di-Spaz, Dibent, Diolamine, Formulex, GI antispasmodic Antispas, Lomine, Merbentyl, Or-Tyl, Spasmoban.

Didronel See etidronate disodium.

diencephalohypophyseal syndrome Problem with the thalamus or pituitary gland not otherwise specified. Report this disorder with ICD-9-CM code 253.8.

DIEP flap Deep inferior epigastric perforator flap. Reconstructive surgery in which skin and fat from the abdomen are transferred and anastomosed to feeding blood vessels in the armpit following mastectomy. Report a free DIEP flap with ICD-9-CM procedure code 85.74 or CPT codes 19364 and 19366. *NCD Reference: 140.2.*

dietetic neuritis Disease caused by a lack of vitamin B1 (thiamine) causing cardiac damage, polyneuritis, and edema. The disease is found mostly in areas where white, polished rice is the main staple of the diet. Report this disorder with ICD-9-CM code 265.0. *Synonym(s): beriberi, endemic polyneuritis, rice disease.*

Dieulafoy lesion Abnormally large submucosal artery protruding through a defect in the stomach mucosa or intestines that can cause massive and life-threatening hemorrhaging, reported with ICD-9-CM code 537.84 or 569.86. *Synonym(s): Dieulafoy's vascular malformation.*

DIF Direct immunofluorescence.

diffuse cystic mastopathy Condition in which benign cysts are scattered throughout the breast, thought to be associated with ovarian hormones. This condition is reported with ICD-9-CM code 610.1.

diffuse toxic goiter Diffuse thyroid enlargement seen mostly in women that stems from the autoimmune process. It is accompanied by the secretion of excessive thyroid hormone, goiter, and bulging eyes. *Synonym(s): Graves' disease.*

Diflucan See fluconazole.

DiGeorge's syndrome Hypoplasia or aphasia of the thymus and parathyroid gland with congenital heart defects, anomalies of the great vessels, esophageal atresia, seizures, and facial deformities. Report this disorder with ICD-9-CM code 279.11.

Dighton's syndrome Blue sclera, little growth, brittle bones, and deafness. Report this disorder with ICD-9-CM code 756.51. *Synonym(s): van der Hoeve's.*

Digibind See digoxin fab.

digital imaging and communications in medicine Standard for communicating images, such as x-rays, in a digitized form. This standard could become part of the HIPAA claim attachments standards. *Synonym(s): DICOM.*

digital subtraction angiography Diagnostic imaging technique that applies computer technology to fluoroscopy for the purpose of visualizing the same vascular structures observable with conventional angiography. *NCD Reference: 220.9.*

digoxin Antiarrhythmic that slows cardiac conduction through the SA and AV node and strengthens myocardial contractions, used to treat heart failure. Supply is reported with HCPCS Level II code J1160. May be sold under the brand names Digitek, Digoxin, Lanoxicaps, Lanoxin.

digoxin fab Antidote that counteracts life threatening digoxin toxicity by binding the digoxin molecules and preventing them from binding to cells in the heart. Supply is reported with HCPCS Level II code J1162. May be sold under the brand names Digibind, DigiFab.

dihydroergotamine mesylate Drug used for the treatment of migraines or cluster headaches by constricting blood vessels. Supply is reported with HCPCS Level II code J1110. May be sold under the brand name D.H.E. 45.

Dilantin See phenytoin sodium.

dilation Artificial increase in the diameter of an opening or lumen made by medication or by instrumentation.

dilution Concentration reduction of a mixture or solution by adding more fluid.

dim. Divide in half.

dimenhydrinate Antiemetic that exerts a depressant action on hyperstimulated labyrinthine functions and associated neural pathways, indicated for prevention and relief of motion sickness, vertigo due to Ménière's disease, and other labyrinthine disturbances. It is also used for treatment or prophylaxis against nausea and vomiting related to radiation, chemotherapy, or anesthetic administration. Supply is reported with HCPCS Level II code J1240.

dimercaprol Chelating agent used as a heavy metal antagonist in severe arsenic, gold, or mercury poisoning, and in acute encephalopathy associated with lead poisoning. Supply is reported with HCPCS Level II code J0470. May be sold under the brand name BAL in Oil.

dimethyl sulfoxide 50% Solution applied via a sterile straight cath directly into the urinary bladder, approved by the FDA for treatment of interstitial cystitis. Supply is reported with HCPCS Level II code J1212. May be sold under the names DMSO, Rmso 50.

dimple sign Finding on examination in which the skin is dimpled or furrowed over the area of a dislocation. In an anterior shoulder dislocation, the dimple is seen just below the acromion process in the deltoid.

D-F

diode probe Device placed on or in the body, used to measure the actual amount of radiation being delivered to a particular area.

diopter Power of the lens used to assist vision.

DIOS Distal intestinal obstruction syndrome. Previously known as meconium ileus equivalent (MIE), a condition specific to cystic fibrosis in which viscous mucous and feces bind the intestine to bring on colicky symptoms. DIOS is reported with ICD-9-CM code 277.01. *Synonym(s): MIE.*

diphenhydramine HCl Drug that competes with histamine for the H1 receptor sites and prevent the histamine response in allergic reactions, especially in smooth muscle such as the bronchial tubes and the blood vessels. It also has an effect on the medulla to relieve cough symptoms and is often used as a sedative or sleep aid due to the drowsiness incurred from the antihistamine side effects. Supply is reported with HCPCS Level II code J1200. May be sold under the brand name Benadryl.

diplegia Paralytic loss or impairment of motor function affecting like parts on both sides of the body (e.g., both arms or both legs).

diplegic infantile cerebral palsy Bilateral paralysis and delayed or abnormal motor development caused by trauma at birth or intrauterine pathology.

diplopia Double vision, reported as a symptom with ICD-9-CM code 368.2. If caused by an inability of the lens to focus, report 368.15.

dipsomania Chronic, progressive state of dependence upon alcohol that is both psychological and physical with periodic or continuous episodes impairing health and the ability to function emotionally, socially, and occupationally.

dipyridamole Drug used to prevent clotting in patients with thromboembolic disorders, artificial heart valves, or those patients at risk for developing thrombosis. It is also used to treat chronic angina pectoris in patients with coronary artery disease and as a pharmacologic inducing stress alternative to exercise myocardial perfusion imaging. Supply is reported with HCPCS Level II code J1245. May be sold under the brand name Adp-Dipyridamole, Novo-Dipradol, Perstantin, Perstantine.

direct claim payment Method where members deal directly with the payer rather than submitting claims through the employer.

direct contract model Plan that contracts directly with individual private practice physicians rather than through an intermediary.

direct costs Costs that are directly associated with a specific service, including items such as nonphysician labor, medical equipment, and medical supplies.

direct data entry Under HIPAA, direct entry of data that are immediately transmitted into a health plan's computer. *Synonym(s): DDE.*

direct laryngoscopy Endoscopic instrument, such as a flexible or rigid fiberoptic scope, inserted into the larynx for direct viewing capabilities of the voice box and vocal cords.

direct restoration In dentistry, restoration produced inside of the mouth.

direct supervision Situation in which the physician must be present in the office suite and immediately available to provide assistance and direction throughout a given procedure. The physician is not, however, required to be present in the room when the procedure is performed.

direct treatment relationship Relationship between an individual and a health care provider. The health care provider reports the diagnosis or the results associated with the treatment directly to the individual, rather than through another provider.

dirty and infected wound Existing infection and inflammation prior to surgery in a dirty traumatic wound more than four hours old, or an old abscess and/or existing surgical infection. In either case, abscess and nonsterile conditions were present. Wound older than four hours. Perforated viscus, fecal contamination, necrotic tissue, or foreign body may be present. Infection rate: up to 40 percent.

DISA Data Interchange Standards Association.

disabled beneficiary Person eligible for Medicare benefits because he or she is totally and permanently disabled. Individuals younger than 65 who have been entitled to disability benefits under the Social Security or the Railroad Retirement System for at least two years are classified as disabled for Medicare purposes.

disarticulation Removal of a limb through a joint.

discectomy Surgical excision of an intervertebral disk.

discharge Secretion, flow, or evacuation. *d. date* For medical facilities, date the patient is formally released, expires, or is transferred. In other situations, the date that medical care or treatment ended. *d. disposition* Description of the patient's status and destination at discharge (e.g., discharged to home) used for data and quality assurance purposes. *d. plan* Treatment plan by the provider for continued patient care after discharge that may include home care, the services of case managers or other health care providers, or transfer to another facility. *d. planning process* Plan applicable to services furnished by the hospital to individuals entitled to medical benefits. Upon the request of a patient's physician, the hospital must arrange for the development and initial implementation of a discharge plan for the patient. The discharge planning evaluation must be

D-F

included in the patient's medical record for use in establishing an appropriate discharge plan and the results of the evaluation must be discussed with the patient or the patient's representative. Plan guidelines and standards should address the following: patients who are likely to suffer adverse health consequences upon discharge in the absence of adequate discharge planning and patients, their physicians, and their representatives requesting a discharge plan; appropriate arrangements for post-hospital care made before discharge and to avoid unnecessary delays in discharge; and evaluation of a patient's likely need for appropriate post-hospital services, including hospice services and the availability of those services, including the availability of home health services. ***d. status*** Disposition of the patient at discharge (e.g., left against medical advice, discharged home, transferred to an acute care hospital, expired). ***d. transfer*** Discharge of a patient from one facility to another.

disciform senile macular degeneration   New vessel formation in the oxygen-deprived tissues feeding the retina. This neovascularization results in tiny, delicate vessels that break easily, causing leakage, hemorrhaging, swelling, and damage to surrounding tissue, and accounts for 10 percent of all cases of macular degeneration in the United States. Report this condition with ICD-9-CM code 362.52. ***Synonym(s):*** *exudative senile macular degeneration, neovascular macular degeneration, wet macular degeneration.*

discission   Recreating a clear optical opening in the field of vision by puncturing a cataractous lens capsule remnant.

disclosure   Release or divulgence of information by an entity to persons or organizations outside of that entity. ***d. history*** Under HIPAA, list of entities that have received personally identifiable health care information for uses unrelated to treatment and payment.

discography   Radiographic imaging of an intervertebral disk, done after the injection of a contrast agent. Discography is reported with CPT codes 62290-62291 for the injection procedure, with the radiological supervision and interpretation reported separately using 72285 or 72295.

DISH   Diffuse idiopathic skeletal hyperostosis. Excessive bone growth along the sides of the vertebrae, inflammation at ligament attachments, and bone spurs as a form of degenerative arthritis, usually seen in people older than age 50. It is more common among men than women. DISH with vertebral involvement is reported with ICD-9-CM code 721.8. Bone spurs are coded according to site. ***Synonym(s):*** *Forestier's disease.*

DISI   Dorsal intercalated segment instability. Best visualized on wrist radiograph, lateral view. A classic pattern of zig-zag collapse seen on a lateral view wrist radiograph due to a displaced scaphoid fracture, carpal instability, or scapholunate instability. The lunate may follow the triquetrum down toward the palm.

diskectomy   Surgical excision of an intervertebral disk. ***Synonym(s):*** *discectomy.*

dislocation   Displacement of a bone in relation to its neighboring tissue, especially a joint. ***Synonym(s):*** *luxation.*

disorganized schizophrenia   Solitary, disorganized schizophrenic state with prominent affective changes, delusions, hallucinations, and fleeting, fragmented, irresponsible, or unpredictable behavior that is manifested by purposeless giggling or self-satisfied, self-absorbed smiling, or by a lofty manner, grimaces, mannerisms, pranks, hypochondriacal complaints, and reiterated phrases.

disp   Disposition.

Di-Spaz   See dicyclomine HCl.

dispense as written   Notation from a physician to a pharmacist requesting that the brand name medication be given in lieu of a generic medication. ***Synonym(s):*** *DAW.*

disposition of patient   Description of the patient's status and destination at discharge (e.g., discharged to home) used for data and quality assurance purposes.

dissect   Cut apart or separate tissue for surgical purposes or for visual or microscopic study.

dissection   Separating by cutting tissue or body structures apart.

disseminated   Spread over an extensive area.

disseminated platelet thrombosis syndrome   Fatal disease with central nervous system involvement due to formation of fibrin or platelet thrombi in arterioles and capillaries in many organs. Report this disorder with ICD-9-CM code 446.6.

dissociative hysteria   Restriction of the field of consciousness or disturbance of motor or sensory function resulting in symbolic or psychological advantage, primarily selective amnesia. May be manifested by change of personality or wandering.

distal   Located farther away from a specified reference point.

distention   Enlarged or expanded due to pressure from inside.

Diuril sodium   See chlorothiazide sodium.

diver's palsy   Decompression sickness caused by rapid reduction in atmospheric pressure in deep-sea divers and caisson workers who return to normal air pressure environments too quickly or pilots flying at high altitudes. This disease causes joint pain, respiratory problems, neurologic symptoms, and skin lesions,

D-F

reported with ICD-9-CM code 993.3. **Synonym(s):** *bends, Caisson disease, compressed air disease, dysbarism.*

diversion   Rechanneling of body fluid through another conduit.

diverticulosis   Saclike pouches of the mucous membrane lining the intestine herniating through the muscular wall of the colon and occurring without inflammation, reported with ICD-9-CM code 562.10.

diverticulum   Pouch or sac in the walls of an organ or canal.

divestiture   Act of a provider s supplier selling off part or all of its assets, whether voluntarily or by court order. Whether or not a divestiture constitutes a change of ownership or CHOW for a provider depends on the structure of the transaction.

division   Separating into two or more parts.

Dix-Hallpike test   Clinical observation of eye movements (nystagmus) occurring during calculated movements of the patient's head and body. The Dix-Hallpike test is considered a component of evaluation and management and is not reported separately. **Synonym(s):** *Nylen-Barany test.*

Dizac   See diazepam.

dizygotic   Derived from two separate ova fertilized by two sperm, producing fraternal twins, from different zygotes with separate placentas, chorions, and amnions. **Synonym(s):** *fraternal twins.*

DJD   Degenerative joint disease.

DKA   Diabetic ketoacidosis.

DLI   Donor leukocyte infusion.

DM   Diabetes mellitus.

DMAA   Distal metatarsal articular angle. Angle between the cartilage that articulates with the big toe relative to the first metatarsal. DMAA is a factor in determining what type of corrective surgery will be performed. It will not affect code selection. **Synonym(s):** *PASA.*

DMARDS   Disease-modifying antirheumatic drugs. Category of drugs used to suppress symptoms in autoimmune disorders, including lupus, colitis, myasthenia gravis, rheumatoid arthritis, Crohn's disease, and idiopathic thrombocytopenic purpura. DMARDS include methotrexate, gold salts, chloroquine, minocycline, leflunomide, azathioprine, and sulfasalazine.

DMD   Duchenne muscular dystrophy.

DME   Durable medical equipment. Medical equipment that can withstand repeated use, is not disposable, is used to serve a medical purpose, is generally not useful to a person in the absence of a sickness or injury, and is appropriate for use in the home. Examples of durable medical equipment include hospital beds, wheelchairs, and oxygen equipment. **NCD Reference:** *280.1.*

DME MAC   Durable medical equipment Medicare administrative contractor. Entity where claims for specific DMEPOS must be submitted for processing and reimbursement (instead of the Medicare contractor).

DME PDAC   Durable Medical Equipment Pricing Data Analysis and Coding. Medicare contractor responsible for maintaining the durable medical equipment classification system (DMECS), including HCPCS coding determinations, and providing durable medical equipment, prosthetics, orthotics, and supplies (DMEPOS) allowables.

DMEPOS   Durable medical equipment, prosthetics, orthotics, and supplies.

DMERC   Durable medical equipment regional carrier.

DMPA   Depot medroxyprogesterone acetate.

DMST   Diabetes self-management training.

DNA   Deoxyribonucleic acid.

DNET   Desembryoplastic neuroepithelial tumor. Low-grade astrocytoma or brain tumor. DNETs are usually localized and slow growing.

DNP   Do not publish.

DNR   Do not resuscitate.

DNS

DNS is the acronym for
deviated nasal septum

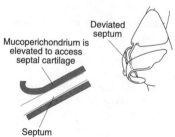

Deviated
septum

Mucoperichondrium is
elevated to access
septal cartilage

Septum

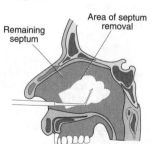

Area of septum
removal

Remaining
septum

D–F

DNS *1)* Deviated nasal septum, reported with ICD-9-CM code 470 if acquired or 754.0 if congenital. *2)* Deviated nasal septum. *3)* Dysplastic nevus syndrome. Syndrome involving high number of atypical melanocytic nevi, including a high number of moles on the patient's back. DNS puts the patient at high risk for developing melanoma. *Synonym(s): Atypical mole syndrome.*

DO Doctor of osteopathy.

DOA Dead on arrival.

Doan-Wiseman syndrome Inherited bronchiectasis and pancreatic insufficiency resulting in malnutrition, sinusitis, short stature, and bone abnormalities. Report this disorder with a code from ICD-9-CM category 288.0. *Synonym(s): Kostmann's syndrome, Schultz syndrome, Shwachman syndrome.*

DOB Date of birth.

dobutamine Drug used to increase cardiac output by directly stimulating beta 1 receptors to increase myocardial contractility and stroke volume. Often used supportively after cardiac surgery or in heart failure. Supply is reported with HCPCS Level II code J1250. May be sold under the brand name Dobutrex.

Dobutrex See dobutamine.

doc. Doctor.

docetaxel Antineoplastic used to treat locally advanced or metastatic breast cancer that has failed prior chemotherapy and non-small cell cancer of the lung for which platinum based chemotherapy has failed or which has not been treated with cisplatin. Supply is reported with HCPCS Level II code J9171. May be sold under the brand name Taxotere.

documentation Physician's written or transcribed notations about a patient encounter, including a detailed operative report or written notes about a routine encounter. Source documentation must be the treating provider's own account of the encounter and may be transcribed from dictation, dictated by the physician into voice recognition software, or be hand- or typewritten. A signature or authentication accompanies each entry.

DOE Dyspnea on exertion.

Döhle body syndrome Hepatosplenomegaly, lymphadenopathy, anemia, thrombocytopenia, changes in the bones, cardiopulmonary system, skin, and psychomotor skills. Granulation and nuclear structure of white cells opens patient to infection and results in death. Report this disorder with ICD-9-CM code 288.2. *Synonym(s): Chediak-Higashi syndrome, Hegglin syndrome, Jordan's syndrome, May syndrome.*

Dohle-Heller syndrome Inflammation of the aorta secondary to syphilis.

DOJ Department of Justice.

DOMS Delayed onset muscle soreness. Pain, fatigue, or stiffness beginning 24 to 48 hours and resolving within 96 hours after a physical workout.

Donohue's syndrome Slow physical and mental development, elfin facial features such as wide-set eyes and low-set ears, and severe endocrine disorders indicated by enlarged sexual organs. Rare and fatal. Report this disorder with ICD-9-CM code 259.8.

donor Person from whom tissues or organs are removed for transplantation.

Dooley nail Surgical nail, a modified version of the Smith-Peterson nail, with a groove located externally around the base, used to repair intracapsular hip fractures. It has no bearing on code selection.

doppler Ultrasonography used to augment two-dimensional images by registering velocity. When emitted sound waves reflect back off a moving object, the frequency of the reflected sound waves varies in relation to the speed of the moving object. This type of ultrasonography may be used in many different procedures and is not necessarily always coded. Some procedures are designed specifically using Doppler, such as fetal surveillance to determine the velocity of blood flow through the umbilical artery and some procedures may be enhanced by performing Doppler ultrasound in addition to the primary procedure, such as Doppler echocardiography.

DOR Diminished ovarian reserve. Fewer eggs remaining in the ovaries of a patient, usually a result of age. DOR reduces fertility and when associated with age is reported with ICD-9-CM code 628.8.

Dor procedure Therapeutic procedure to treat congestive heart failure by restoring the heart to a more normal size and shape. The ventricular muscle and chamber are resized with the aid of a plastic model, in hopes of improving heart function. This procedure is often performed with bypass or valve repair, which is reported separately. DOR procedure is reported with CPT code 33548. *Synonym(s): LV reconstruction, SAVER, SVR, TR3SVR.*

Doribax See doripenem.

doripenem Broad spectrum injectable antibiotic used to treat acute, complicated gram-positive and gram-negative bacterial infections, particularly those involving intraabdominal and urinary tract sites. May be sold under the brand name Doribax. Supply is reported with HCPCS Level II code J1267.

dornase alpha Inhaled treatment used to decrease the thickness of the mucous-based secretions that line the airways of cystic fibrosis patients. It is a genetically engineered form of deoxyribonuclease or DNAase. Supply is reported with HCPCS Level II code J7639. May be sold under the brand name Pulmozyme.

D-F

Dorsal

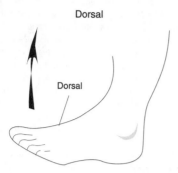

Dorsal

Dowager's Hump

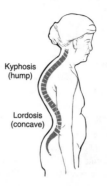

Kyphosis (hump)

Lordosis (concave)

dorsal Pertaining to the back or posterior aspect.

dorsi- Relating to the back. ***Synonym(s):*** *dorso-*.

dorsiflexion Position of being bent toward the extensor side of a limb.

dorsum Back side or back part of the body or individual anatomical structure.

DOS Date of service. In health care contracting, day the encounter or procedure is performed or the day a supply is issued.

dosimetry Component in the administration of radiation oncology therapy in which a radiation dose is calculated to a specific site, including implant or beam orientation and exposure, isodose strengths, tissue inhomogeneities, and volume. Dosimetry is reported in addition to the actual treatment delivery or management, with modifiers identifying technical and professional components. Report HCPCS code A4650 for the supply of each implantable radiation dosimeter.

double dipping Allowing one piece of information in the patient record to be counted as two data points in the calculation of an evaluation and management level for office visit coding. The practice is controversial, accepted by some payers and rejected by others.

double whammy syndrome Dislocation of eye ball. Report this disorder with ICD-9-CM code 360.81.

dowager's hump Finding on physical exam of inspection of the back in mature women with osteoporosis in which there is a rounded deformity of the upper back. Diagnosis must be made on radiograph or bone scan for osteoporosis. Finding dowager's hump alone does not drive diagnostic code selection.

Down syndrome One of the most common birth defects, due to an error in the formation of the 21st chromosome. Facial features common to Down syndrome patients include low set ears, skin folds in the inner eye corners, enlarged and protruding tongue, low nasal bridge, and upward-slanting eyes. Mental deficits are often present. Down syndrome is reported with ICD-9-CM code 758.0. ***Synonym(s):*** *Mongolism, Trisomy 21*.

downcode Reduction in the value and code on a claim when documentation does not support the level of service billed by a provider.

downcoding Reporting a lower-level code for a service so that an additional code may be used rather than using one higher-level and more comprehensive code.

doxercalciferol Drug that reduces the level of intact parathyroid hormone in patients with hyperparathyroidism secondary to long-term renal dialysis. Supply is reported with HCPCS Level II code J1270. May be sold under the brand name Hectorol.

Doxil See doxorubicin all lipid formulations.

doxorubicin Antineoplastic that kills cancer cells by interfering with DNA dependent RNA synthesis. It is used to treat bladder, breast, lung, ovarian, stomach, testicular, and thyroid cancers; Hodgkin's disease; acute lymphoblastic and myeloblastic leukemia; Wilma's tumor; neuroblastoma; lymphoma; and sarcoma. Supply is reported with HCPCS Level II code J9001. May be sold under the brand names Adriamycin, Adriamycin PFS, Adriamycin RDF, Rubex.

DPM *1)* Double-plated Molteno. Eponym for a shunt implant that mitigates glaucoma. Insertion of this shunt, which requires a two-quadrant dissection, is reported with CPT code 66180; revision with 66185; removal with 67120. **2)** Doctor of podiatric medicine.

DPNP Diabetic peripheral neuropathy pain, reported with the appropriate ICD-9-CM code from subcategory 249.6 or 250.6. and 357.2 or 337.1.

DPR Drug price review.

DPT **1)** Diphtheria-pertussis-tetanus. **2)** Days per thousand. Standard unit of measurement of utilization determined by calculating the number of hospital days used in a year for each 1,000 covered lives.

DPU Delayed pressure urticaria. Wheals and swelling occurring without other cause on skin that has been compressed during sitting, by clothes, or some other means. DPU is reported with ICD-9-CM code 708.8.

Dr Doctor.

DR **1)** Diagnostic radiology. **2)** Delivery room. **3)** Diurnalrhythm.

dr. Dram.

draft standard for trial use Archaic term for any X12 standard that has been approved since the most recent release of X12 American national standards. The current equivalent term is "X12 standard." **Synonym(s): DSTU.**

drain Device that creates a channel to allow fluid from a cavity, wound, or infected area to exit the body.

dramamine See dimenhydrinate.

Dramanate See dimenhydrinate.

Dramoject See dimenhydrinate.

drawer sign Clinical sign that checks for instability of knee ligaments. With the patient lying down, the hips are flexed 45 degrees and the knees are flexed 90 degrees with both feet flat on the exam table. The feet are held in position while firm pressure is placed on the lower leg just above the calf with both hands. The leg is pushed back (posterior drawer) then the knee is pulled forward (anterior drawer). If there is laxity in either direction, the test is positive.

DRE Digital rectal exam. The physician inserts a lubricated, gloved finger into the rectum to evaluate the back portion of the prostate for cancer and to check for other abnormalities. DRE is normally performed as a part of the annual physical and in conjunction with prostate specific antigen (PSA) testing. At times, women receive a DRE at their annual exam.

dressing Material applied to a wound or surgical site for protection, absorption, or drainage of the area.

Dressler's syndrome Fever, leukocytosis, chest pain, evidence of pericarditis, pleurisy, and pneumonia occurring days or weeks after a myocardial infarction. Report this disorder with ICD-9-CM code 411.0.

DRG Diagnosis related group. Method CMS uses to pay hospitals for Medicare recipients based on a statistical system of classifying any inpatient stay into one of several hundred groups. It is a classification scheme whose patient types are defined by patients' diagnoses or procedures and, in some cases, by the patient's age or discharge status. Each DRG is intended to be medically meaningful and would ordinarily require approximately equal resource consumption as measured by length of stay and cost. **d. grouper** Computer software that assigns diagnosis-related groups (DRGs) based on diagnoses and other criteria, such as the patient's age, sex, discharge status, and procedures performed. **d. payment rate** Payment rate a hospital receives for a Medicare patient assigned to a particular diagnosis-related group (DRG), reflecting the wage rates in the hospital's area and the cost associated with the DRG.

DRG grouper Computer software that assigns diagnosis-related groups (DRG) based on diagnoses and other criteria, such as the patient's sex, discharge status, and procedures performed.

drill Making a hole in a bone or hard tissue.

droperidol Antiemetic used in postoperative patients, as an adjunct to anesthesia, and as an antipsychotic. Supply is reported with HCPCS Level II Code J1790. May be sold under the brand name Inapsine.

drotrecogin alfa (activated) Anti-infective drug administered by intravenous infusion to adult patients with severe sepsis or systemic inflammatory response syndrome with associated acute organ dysfunction to reduce the risk of death.

DRS Duane's retraction syndrome. Unilateral disorder of eye abduction and/or adduction due to congenital errors in the formation of eye muscle. DRS can lead to amblyopic vision loss. Most patients are diagnosed before age 10. DRS is reported with ICD-9-CM code 378.71. **Synonym(s):** *retraction syndrome, Stilling-Turk-Duane syndrome.*

drug abuse Individual, for whom no other diagnosis is possible, who has come under medical care because of the maladaptive effect of a drug on which he is not dependent (see Drug dependence) and that he has taken on his own initiative to the detriment of his health or social functioning. **NCD References: 130.5, 130.6.**

drug dependence Psychic and physical dependence, resulting from taking a drug, characterized by behavioral and other responses that always include a compulsion to take a drug on a continuous or periodic basis to experience its psychic effects, and sometimes to avoid the discomfort of its absence. **NCD References: 130.5, 130.6.**

drug eluting stent Specialized device placed inside blood vessels for intraluminal support that is coated with a controlled time-release drug that enters the surrounding tissue and helps prevent or slow the growth of plaque or stenotic tissue.

drug formulary List of prescription medications preferred for use by a health plan and dispensed through participating pharmacies to covered persons.

drug psychoses Organic mental syndromes that are due to consumption of drugs (notably amphetamines, barbiturates, and opiate and LSD groups) and solvents.

drug withdrawal syndrome States associated with drug withdrawal ranging from severe, as specified for alcohol withdrawal delirium (delirium tremens), to less severe states characterized by one or more symptoms such as convulsions, tremor, anxiety, restlessness, gastrointestinal and muscular complaints, and mild disorientation and memory disturbance. *drug-induced hallucinosis* Hallucinatory states with auditory hallucinations, anxiety, or restlessness of more than a few days but not more than a few months' duration, associated with large or prolonged intake of drugs, notably of the amphetamine and LSD groups.

drug-induced organic delusional syndrome Paranoid states of more than a few days but not more than a few months' duration, associated with large or prolonged intake of drugs, notably of the amphetamine and LSD groups.

drug syndrome Number of physical symptoms resulting from long-time ingestion of, and dependence on, therapeutic and illicit drugs. Report this disorder with ICD-9-CM code 292.0.

drug utilization review Review to ensure prescribed medications are medically necessary and appropriate. *Synonym(s): DUR.*

drug-induced syndrome Description of symptoms, physiological and psychological, produced by drug abuse or dependence. Report this disorder with ICD-9-CM code 292.84.

drugs and biologicals Drugs and biologicals included - or approved for inclusion - in the United States Pharmacopoeia, the National Formulary, the United States Homeopathic Pharmacopoeia, in New Drugs or Accepted Dental Remedies, or approved by the pharmacy and drug therapeutics committee of the medical staff of the hospital. Also included are medically accepted and FDA approved drugs used in an anticancer chemotherapeutic regimen. The carrier determines medical acceptance based on supportive clinical evidence.

drum syndrome Sudden, severe infection of the middle ear with mucous. Report this disorder with ICD-9-CM code 381.02. *Synonym(s): Blue drum syndrome.*

drunkenness acute Current psychic and physical state resulting from alcohol ingestion, characterized by slurred speech.

drunkenness pathologic Physical state resulting from alcohol ingestion, affecting the psychological state, causing slurred speech.

drunkenness simple State of inebriation due to alcohol consumption without conspicuous neurological signs of intoxication.

drunkenness sleep Inability to fully arouse from the sleep state, characterized by failure to attain full consciousness after arousal due to alcohol consumption.

drusen White hyaline deposits on the retinal pigment epithelium, an early sign of macular degeneration in aging. Report ICD-9-CM code 362.57 for degenerative; 362.77 for hereditary; 377.21 of the optic disc.

Drusinoid macular degeneration Age-related, atrophic (dry, nonexudative) macular degeneration characterized by variable degrees of atrophy and progressive degeneration of the outer retina, retinal pigment epithelium, Bruch's membrane, and choriocapillaris. Report this degeneration with ICD-9-CM code 362.51. *Synonym(s): nonexudative macular degeneration.*

dry cutaneous leishmaniasis One of the forms of Old World cutaneous leishmaniasis. This parasitic skin disease caused by the protozoa Leishmania tropica is spread by the bite of sand flies and occurs in large urban areas in the Middle East, especially Iran and Iraq, the Mediterranean, and India. Manifestation is mainly a single, large developing boil or furuncle type lesion that persists over a year. Lymphadenopathy may be present. Report this condition with ICD-9-CM code 085.1. *Synonym(s): urban cutaneous leishmaniasis.*

dry eye syndrome Lacrimal glands are unable to provide enough moisture to cover the eye. Report this disorder with ICD-9-CM code 375.15.

dry skin syndrome Keratosis producing lesions appearing as dry skin. Report this disorder with ICD-9-CM code 701.1.

dry socket In dentistry, painful condition occurring when the blood clot disintegrates after tooth extraction, leaving the socket exposed to the air and infection; it may involve osteitis.

DSAP syndrome Skin disorder occurring on sun-exposed skin and characterized by numerous superficial, keratotic, brownish-red macules. Report this disorder with ICD-9-CM code 692.75. *Synonym(s): disseminated superficial actinic porokeratosis.*

Dsg Dressing.

DSH Disproportionate share hospital, as designated by CMS.

DSI Dysfunction of sensory integration. Inability of the brain to process sensory information correctly. A child with DSI will be hyposensitive or hypersensitive to

D-F

stimuli. Report DSI with ICD-9-CM code 299.8. **Synonym(s):** *SID.*

DSM-IV Diagnostic and Statistical Manual of Mental Disorders, Fourth Edition. Manual used by mental health workers as the diagnostic coding system for substance abuse and mental health patients

DSM-IV-TR Diagnostic and Statistical Manual of Mental Disorders, Fourth Edition, Text Revision. Manual used by mental health workers as the diagnosis coding system for substance abuse and mental health patients.

DSMO Designated Standard Maintenance Organization.

DSMT Diabetes self-management training. When the training subject is nutrition and when it has been certified by the American Diabetes Association, report HCPCS Level II codes G0108 and G0109. If the training is on another topic or if the nutritional training is not ADA approved, report CPT codes 97802-97804.

DSS Double simultaneous stimulation. Test in which both sides of the body are touched separately, then simultaneously. In a positive result, the patient can feel each side when stimulated separately, but doesn't distinguish touch on one side when both sides are touched simultaneously. It can be an indication of a dysfunction in the contralateral posterior parietal lobe. DSS would be included as part of the evaluation and management service.

DSTU Draft standard for trial use.

DT Delirium tremens.

DTI Diffusion tensor imaging. MRI technique to study white matter properties and fiber integrity within the brain.

DTIC-Dome See dacarbazine.

DTR Deep tendon reflexes.

dual chamber system System that includes a pulse generator with one electrode inserted into the atrium and one electrode inserted into the ventricle.

dual energy x-ray absorptiometry Radiological technique for bone density measurement using a two-dimensional projection system in which two x-ray beams with different levels of energy are pulsed alternately and the results are given in two scores, reported as standard deviations from peak bone mass density. This procedure is reported with CPT codes 77080-77082. **Synonym(s):** *DEXA, DXA.* **NCD Reference:** *150.3.*

dual option Offering of an HMO and traditional plan by one carrier.

dual photon absorptiometry Noninvasive radiological technique for bone density measurement using a small amount of radionuclide to measure the bone mass absorption efficiency of the dichromatic photon beam energy used. This provides a quantitative measurement of the bone mineral density of cortical bone in diseases like osteoporosis. This procedure is reported with CPT code 78351. **NCD Reference:** *150.3.*

dual-lead device Implantable cardiac device (pacemaker or implantable cardioverter-defibrillator [ICD]) in which pacing and sensing components are placed in only two chambers of the heart.

Duane's syndrome Simultaneous retraction of eye muscles causing an inability to abduct the affected eye with retraction of the globe. Report this disorder with ICD-9-CM code 378.71. **Synonym(s):** *Duane-Stilling-Turk syndrome, Still-Turk-Duane syndrome.*

Dubin-Johnson syndrome Nonhemolytic jaundice thought as a defect in concentrated bilirubin and other organs causing a brown granular pigment in the hepatic duct. Report this disorder with ICD-9-CM code 277.4. **Synonym(s):** *Dubin-Sprinz syndrome.*

Duchenne's syndrome Paralysis symptoms caused by medulla oblongata. Report this disorder with ICD-9-CM code 335.22.

ductogram X-ray of a mammary duct in the breast.

DUE Drug use evaluation.

Dührssen's incision Incision made into the cervix to aid in delivery of the fetal head, used when the head is in danger of becoming entrapped in a cervix that is not completely dilated. Dührssen's incision is reported with ICD-9-CM procedure code 73.93. In CPT, it would be included in the code used for delivery.

duloxetine hydrochloride Serotonin and norepinephrine reuptake inhibitor indicated for major depressive disorder. Also FDA-approved for the pain of diabetic peripheral neuropathy, it is administered in oral capsules. Report major depression with ICD-9-CM codes 296.20-296.36 and diabetic peripheral neuropathy with a code from ICD-9-CM subcategory 249.6 or 250.6, and 357.2 or 337.1. May be sold under the brand name Cymbalta.

dumping syndrome Emptying of contents of jejunum with nausea, sweating, weakness, palpitation, syncope, warmth, and diarrhea. Occurs after eating in patients who have had partial gastrectomy and gastrojejunostomy. Report this disorder with ICD-9-CM code 564.2.

Dunn arthrodesis Procedure in which the talus of the foot is fused.

duo Two.

duodecim. Twelve.

duodenum First portion of the small intestine connected to the stomach at the pylorus and extending to the jejunum.

Duplay's syndrome Inflammation of subacromial or subdeltoid bursa. Report this disorder with ICD-9-CM code 726.2.

duplex scan Noninvasive vascular diagnostic technique that uses ultrasonic scanning to identify the pattern and direction of blood flow within arteries or veins displayed in real time images. Duplex scanning combines B-mode two-dimensional pictures of the vessel structure with spectra and/or color flow Doppler mapping or imaging of the blood as it moves through the vessels.

duplicate coverage inquiry Request made to insurance companies or medical providers to determine whether there is other medical coverage under another plan. **Synonym(s):** DCI.

Dupré's syndrome Irritation of spinal cord and brain mimicking meningitis, but in which there is no swelling of membranes. Report this disorder with ICD-9-CM code 781.6.

Dupuy-Dutemp reconstruction Eyelid reconstruction involving the skin from the opposing lid.

Dupuytren's contracture Shortening of the palmar fascia resulting in flexion deformity of a finger.

DUR Drug utilization review. Review to assure prescribed medications are medically necessary and appropriate.

dur. dolor. While pain lasts.

dura mater Outermost, hard, fibrous layer or membrane that surrounds the brain and spinal cord.

durable medical equipment Medical equipment that can withstand repeated use, is not disposable, is used to serve a medical purpose, is generally not useful to a person in the absence of a sickness or injury, and is appropriate for use in the home. Examples of durable medical equipment include hospital beds, wheelchairs, and oxygen equipment. **Synonym(s):** DME, DMEPOS.

durable medical equipment regional carrier Medicare contractor that administers durable medical equipment (DME) benefits for a region. **Synonym(s):** DMERC.

durable medical equipment regional carrier advisory process Each DMERC is responsible for establishing workgroups in each region to discuss DME issues and concerns with physicians, clinicians, beneficiaries, suppliers, and manufacturers. The purpose of the DAP is to provide a formal mechanism to obtain input regarding regional medical review policy (RMRP) development and revision, a mechanism to discuss and improve administrative policies that are within the DMERCs discretion, and a forum for information exchange between the DMERCs, physicians, clinicians, beneficiaries, suppliers, and manufacturers. **Synonym(s):** DAP.

dural graft Patch placed to allow expansion and improve the flow of cerebrospinal fluid.

Duraloc Option Brand name ceramic hip replacement.

durasphere Urethral bulking material injected in an outpatient setting that acts like a kind of synthetic implant for treating urinary incontinence. Supply is reported with HCPCS Level II code L8606. The injection procedure is reported with CPT code 51715.

during labor syndrome Disorders of lung following vomiting and regurgitation by obstetric patients. Report this disorder with a code from ICD-9-CM range 668.00-668.04. **Synonym(s):** Mendelson's syndrome.

DuToit staple capsulorrhaphy Reattachment of the capsule of the shoulder and glenoid labrum to the glenoid lip using staples to anchor the avulsed capsule and glenoid labrum.

DVD Developmental verbal dyspraxia. Impaired ability to plan and follow through with motor tasks or sensory tasks. Patients with DVD may appear clumsy, inattentive, or immature due to the inability to adapt to environment. Report DVD with ICD-9-CM code 315.4.

DVM Doctor of Veterinary Medicine.

DVT Deep vein thrombosis.

dwell time Period of time that dialysis fluid remains in the abdomen in peritoneal dialysis. Typical dwell times are four to six hours.

Dwyer instrumentation Type of anterior spinal instrumentation to correct spinal deformities that consists of screws and a banding device.

Dwyer instrumentation technique Anterior procedure using rods and attachments to straighten the spine.

Dx Diagnosis.

Dyke-Young syndrome Anemia caused by exposure to trauma, poisons, and other causes. Report this disorder with ICD-9-CM code 283.9. **Synonym(s):** Hayem-Widal syndrome.

Dymelor Brand name oral medication exclusive to lowering blood glucose in Type II diabetics. Dymelor contains acetohexamide.

Dynalink Brand name biliary stent system.

dynamic Manifesting motion in response to force.

dynamic flexion device Highly specialized orthotic brace that allows for a controlled range of motion of a joint or joints during postoperative or post-traumatic convalescence.

dys- Painful, bad, disordered, difficult.

dysarthria Difficulty pronouncing words. If specified as being a late effect of cerebrovascular disease, report dysarthria with ICD-9-CM code 438.13; otherwise, report ICD-9-CM code 784.51.

D-F

dysbarism Decompression sickness caused by rapid reduction in atmospheric pressure in deep-sea divers and caisson workers who return to normal air pressure environments too quickly or pilots flying at high altitudes. This disease causes joint pain, respiratory problems, neurologic symptoms, and skin lesions, reported with ICD-9-CM code 993.3. *Synonym(s): bends, Caisson disease, compressed air disease, diver's palsy.*

dyscalculia Serious impairment in the development of arithmetical skills without obvious intellectual deficit and with adequate schooling.

dyschromia Abnormal pigmentation (coloring) of the hair or skin.

dysfunction Abnormal or impaired function of an organ, part, or system.

dysgenesis Defective development of an organ.

dyskinesia Impairment of voluntary movement.

dyskinesia of esophagus Difficult or impaired voluntary muscle movement of the esophagus.

dyslalia Delay in the development of normal word-sound production resulting in defects of articulation frequently identified by omissions or substitutions of consonants.

dyslexia Serious impairment of reading skills such as word blindness and strephosymbolia (letter or word reversal) that is not explicable in terms of general intellectual retardation or of inadequate schooling.

dysmenorrhea Painful menstruation that may be primary, or essential, due to prostaglandin production and the onset of menstruation; secondary due to uterine, tubal, or ovarian abnormality or disease; spasmodic arising uterine contractions; or obstructive due to some mechanical blockage or interference with the menstrual flow. All of these types are reported with ICD-9-CM code 625.3. Psychogenic dysmenorrhea, however, or that occurring secondary to anxiety or stress, is reported in the mental disorders chapter with 306.52. *Synonym(s): menorrhalgia, menstrual cramps.*

dysmetabolic syndrome Group of health risks that increase the likelihood of developing heart disease, stroke, and diabetes. Diagnosis of dysmetabolic syndrome is made if one has three or more of the following: waist measurement of 40 or more inches for men and 35 or more inches for women; blood pressure of 130/85 mm or higher; triglyceride level greater than 150 mg/dl; fasting blood sugar of more than 100 mg/dl; HDL level less than 40 mg/dl in men or less than 50 mg/dl in women. Report this condition with ICD-9-CM code 277.7, with additional codes to identify associated manifestations. *Synonym(s): insulin resistance syndrome, metabolic syndrome, syndrome X.*

dyspareunia Pain experienced during or after intercourse, commonly occurring in the clitoris, vagina, or labia. This condition is reported with ICD-9-CM code 625.0, unless the pain is specified as psychogenic or due to emotional causes, in which case it is reported with 302.76.

dyspepsia Epigastric discomfort after eating, due to impaired digestive function. *Synonym(s): indigestion.*

dysphagia Difficulty and pain upon swallowing. Common causes of dysphagia are esophagitis, Barrett's esophagus, or late effect of a stroke. Dysphagia is reported with a code from ICD-9-CM subcategory 787.2. Fifth-digit specificity is required and is determined by phase (oral, oropharyngeal, pharyngeal, pharyngoesophageal, other, or unspecified). If specified as a late effect of a cerebrovascular accident or stroke, ICD-9-CM code 438.82 should be coded first, followed by a code denoting the type of dysphagia. *NCD Reference: 170.3.*

dysphasia Speech impairment manifested by incoordination and the inability to arrange words in their proper order. If specified as a late effect of cerebrovascular disease, report dysphasia with ICD-9-CM code 438.12; otherwise, report 784.59.

dysplasia Abnormality or alteration in the size, shape, and organization of cells from their normal pattern of development. *cervical d.* Abnormal growth of epithelial cells on the surface of the cervix, classified in a continuum of changes from mild to moderate or severe dysplasia, and carcinoma in situ. The degree is identified by the type of change occurring within individual cells and the amount of extension into the epithelium. Cervical dysplasia is reported with a code from ICD-9-CM subcategory 622.1. Cervical intraepithelial neoplasia type I, or CIN I, is mild dysplasia; CIN II corresponds to moderate dysplasia, while CIN III is coded in the neoplasm chapter as carcinoma in situ. A definitive diagnosis from a biopsy sample, and not an abnormal Pap smear (795.00-795.09) is required for reporting these codes.

dysplastic nevi Moles that do not form properly and may progress to form a type of skin cancer called melanoma.

dyspnea Difficult or labored breathing. This symptom is reported with ICD-9-CM code 786.09. *Synonym(s): shortness of breath, SOB.*

dyspraxia syndrome Organic disorder affecting patient's ability to perform coordinated acts and not due to psychotic diagnosis. Report this disorder with ICD-9-CM code 315.4.

dysrhythmia Abnormality or disturbance in rhythm.

dyssocial personality Personality disorder characterized by disregard for social obligations, lack of feeling for others, and impetuous violence or callous unconcern and self-rationalization for behavior.

**dyssynergia cerebellaris myoclonica
syndrome** Disorder marked by myoclonus epilepsy and muscular tremors associated with disturbance of muscle tone and coordination. Report this disorder with ICD-9-CM code 334.2. *Synonym(s): Hunt's syndrome.*

dystonia Condition characterized by irregular elasticity of muscle tissue.

dystrophy of vulva Abnormal cell growth of the fleshy external female genitalia.

dysuria Pain upon urination. *psychogenic d.* Difficulty in passing urine due to psychic factors.

dz Disease.

E code ICD-9-CM diagnosis code that describes the circumstance that caused an injury, not the nature of the injury. E codes are used to classify external causes of injury, poisoning, or other adverse effects. An E code should not be used as a principal diagnosis because the intermediary will reject the claim.

E syndrome Congenital malformations in which extra chromosome is group E. Includes mental retardation, abnormal skull shape, malformed ears, small mandible, cardiac defects, short sternum, and other symptoms. Report this disorder with ICD-9-CM code 758.2. *Synonym(s): E3, Edward's, trisomy E.*

e.g. For example.

e.m.p. As directed.

E/M Evaluation and management services. Assessment, counseling, and other services provided to a patient and reported through CPT codes.

E/M codes Evaluation and management service codes.

E/M service components Key components in determining the correct level of E/M codes are history, examination, and medical decision-making.

E1 HCPCS Level II modifier for use with CPT or HCPCS Level II codes identifying a procedure or service specific to the upper left eyelid. The use of modifier E1 will not affect reimbursement, but its absence may cause payment delays.

E2 *1)* HCPCS Level II modifier for use with CPT or HCPCS Level II codes identifying a procedure or service specific to the lower left eyelid. The use of modifier E1 will not affect reimbursement, but its absence may cause payment delays. *2)* Estradiol. E2 levels may be monitored to track fertility in the female. Estradiol levels are measured in laboratory tests reported with CPT codes 80415 and 82670.

E3 HCPCS Level II modifier for use with CPT or HCPCS Level II codes identifying a procedure or service specific to the upper right eyelid. The use of modifier E3 will not affect reimbursement, but its absence may cause payment delays.

E4 HCPCS Level II modifier for use with CPT or HCPCS Level II codes identifying a procedure or service specific to the lower right eyelid. The use of modifier E4 will not affect reimbursement, but its absence may cause payment delays.

Ea Each.

EAC *1)* External auditory canal. *2)* Esophageal adenocarcinoma.

ead. Same.

Eagle-Barrett syndrome Congenital absence of lower rectus abdominis and lower and medial oblique muscles. Results in dilated ureters and bladder, dysplastic kidneys and hydronephrosis, commonly seen with undescended testicles. Report this disorder with ICD-9-CM code 756.71. *Synonym(s): prune belly.*

Eale's syndrome Retinal vasculitis marked by phlebitis, arteritis, and endarteritis. Report this disorder with ICD-9-CM code 362.18.

EAP Employee assistance program. Services designed to help employees, their family members, and employers find solutions for workplace and personal problems that affect morale, productivity, or financial issues such as workplace stress, family/marital concerns, legal or financial problems, elder care, child care, substance abuse, emotional/stress issues, and other daily living concerns.

early satiety Premature fullness that occurs when eating less than normal portions of food. This condition is reported with ICD-9-CM code 780.94.

EasyTrak Brand name cardiac lead system.

eating disorder Conspicuous disturbance in eating behavior such as anorexia, bulimia, pica, and psychogenic rumination.

Eaton-Lambert syndrome Progressive proximal muscle weakness resulting from antibodies directed against motor-nerve axon terminals. Report this disorder with ICD-9-CM code 199.1.

EB HCPCS Level II modifier for use with CPT or HCPCS Level II codes to denote that an erythropoietic-stimulating agent (ESA) was administered to treat anemia caused by anti-cancer radiotherapy.

Eberth's disease Infection caused by the Salmonella typhi bacteria, resulting in systemic toxic bacteremia with high fever, headache, a characteristic rose spot skin rash, abdominal pain, mesenteric lymphadenopathy, and leukopenia. Leads to an enlarged spleen, bradycardia, intestinal hemorrhage, and ultimately perforation of the intestine. It is transmitted by the ingestion of food or water contaminated from an infected person and is reported with ICD-9-CM code 002.0. Suspected carrier is reported using ICD-9-CM V02.1 and

D-F

typhoid vaccination with V03.1 or V06.2. **Synonym(s):** *typhoid fever.*

EBL   Estimated blood loss.

Ebstein's anomaly   Congenital malformation of the tricuspid valve in which leaflets attach to the right ventricle wall, causing the right ventricle and atrium to fuse, resulting in a small ventricle and large atrium. This anomaly causes right ventricle malfunction and complications such as heart failure and abnormal rhythm. Ebstein's anomaly is reported with ICD-9-CM code 746.2.

Ebstein's syndrome   Hypoplasia or atresia of the left ventricle and aorta or mitral valve with respiratory distress and extreme cyanosis. Cardiac failure and death often result in early infancy. Report this disorder with ICD-9-CM code 746.7. **Synonym(s):** *hypoplastic left heart.*

EBUS   Endobronchial ultrasound. Sound waves converted to picture form on screen to view the structure of the tracheobronchial wall by inserting a transducer or ultrasound probe within a flexible sheath, through a bronchoscope down the throat to the target area. Endobronchial ultrasound is often done during another primary therapeutic procedure and is reported as CPT add-on code 31620.

EBV   Epstein-Barr virus.

EC   *1)* Electronic commerce. Exchange of business information by electronic means. *2)* HCPCS Level II modifier for use with CPT or HCPCS Level II codes to denote that an erythropoietic-stimulating agent (ESA) was administered to treat anemia not caused by anti-cancer chemotherapy or radiotherapy.

ECCE   Extracapsular cataract extraction. Removal of natural lens with retention of posterior lens capsule in eye.

eccentric personality   Personality disorder characterized by oddities of behavior that do not conform to the clinical syndromes of personality disorders described elsewhere.

eccentro-osteochondrodysplasia   Inherited metabolic mucopolysaccharide disorder manifested by excess keratan sulfate excreted in the urine. Skeletal anomalies appear as genu valgum (knock knees), pectus carinatum (pigeon breast), short trunk and neck with flattened vertebrae, and broad-mouthed facial appearance with wide space between teeth. Secondary affects on the nervous system include gradual deafness and clouding of the cornea. Two biochemically distinct types exist that are clinically difficult to distinguish, as a result of a type A (N-acetylgalactosamine-6-sulfatase) enzyme deficiency or type B ([beta symbol]-galactosidase) enzyme deficiency. This disorder is reported with ICD-9-CM code 277.5. **Synonym(s):** *Morquio syndrome, mucopolysaccharidosis IV.*

ecchondroma   Abnormal development of excessive cartilage or dense connective tissue arising on a cartilaginous surface, such as the rib cage, ear, nose, intervertebral discs, or projecting from beneath the periosteal fibrous sheath covering a bone. Code assignment for ecchondroma depends upon the specific affected site, such as a benign neoplasm of bone. The general condition of ecchondrosis is coded as neoplasm of uncertain behavior of bone and cartilage, ICD-9-CM code 238.0. **Synonym(s):** *ecchondrosis.*

ecchymosis   Bruise.

eccrine   Sweat glands that are not necessarily associated with a hair follicle.

ECF   *1)* Extended care facility. *2)* Extracellular fluid.

ECG   Electrocardiogram. **NCD Reference:** *20.15.*

echinococcosis   Infection caused by larval forms of tapeworms of the genus *Echinococcus.*

echinococcus infection   Parasitic infection harbored in tissues, particularly the lungs, liver, and kidneys, caused by ingestion of tapeworm eggs found in contaminated food. The larvae form cysts within the infected tissue, causing allergic reactions and organ damage. Report *Echinococcus* infection with a code from ICD-9-CM category 122, according to the type and site of infection. **Synonym(s):** *hydatid cyst disease, hydatid disease, hydatidosis.*

echinostomiasis   Trematode infection from parasitic flukes ingested by eating certain types of fresh water snails or mussels. Infection is manifested by abdominal pain, profuse diarrhea, and even toxic anemia. Report this condition with ICD-9-CM code 121.8.

ECHO   *1)* Echocardiogram. *2)* Enterocytopathogenic human orphan virus.

echo-   Reverberating sound.

ECHO virus   Orphan enteric RNA virus, certain serotypes of which are associated with human disease, especially aseptic meningitis. Report this condition with ICD-9-CM code 079.1.

echography   Radiographic imaging that uses sound waves reflected off the different densities of anatomic structures to create images. **Synonym(s):** *ultrasonography.*

echolalia   Compulsive reiteration of another person's speech, often observed in catatonic schizophrenics, persons with Tourette's syndrome, or those with other neurologic disorders. Report echolalia with ICD-9-CM code 784.69. **Synonym(s):** *echophrasia.*

eclampsia   Tetany and toxemia producing seizure activity or coma in a pregnant patient who most often has presented with prior preeclampsia (i.e., hypertension, albuminuria, and edema). Eclampsia most commonly occurs during the third trimester or within the first 48

D-F

hours following birth, and is reported with a code from ICD-9-CM subcategory 642.6, unless it is superimposed on preexisting hypertension, then it is reported with a code from subcategory 642.7. **Synonym(s):** *eclamptic toxemia, toxemic convulsions.*

ECMO Extracorporeal membrane oxygenation.

ECochG Electric response audiometry in which a fine electrode is inserted through the tympanic membrane to record electrical potentials from the cochlea. This study is used to assess hearing loss in children who are unable to be tested by conventional audiometry or to evaluate endolymphatic hydrops, such as in Ménière's disease. **Synonym(s):** *electrocochleography.*

ECOG Electrocochleography. **Synonym(s):** *ECochG.*

ECT *1)* Electro-convulsive therapy. *2)* Emission computerized tomography.

ecto- External, outside.

ectocardia Rare congenital defect in which the heart and cardiac apex are displaced, inside or outside the thorax. There are many different types of ectocardia: dextrocardia in which the heart is located in the right half of the thorax with the apex pointing to the right; mesocardia in which the apex of the heart is located in direct midline of the thorax; abdominal heart in which the heart is found outside the thorax within the abdomen; and isolated levocardia in which the heart appears with congenital malformation in its usual location on the left but the other visceral organs are transposed in relation to the heart. Report ectocardia with ICD-9-CM code 746.87. **Synonym(s):** *exocardia.*

-ectomy Excision, removal.

ectopia cordis Form of ectocardia, a rare congenital defect in which the heart is located outside of the thoracic cavity due to developmental problems of the pericardium and sternum. This condition is reported with ICD-9-CM code 746.87.

ectopic ACTH syndrome Abdominal striae, acne, hypertension, decreased carbohydrate tolerance, moon face, obesity, protein catabolism, and psychiatric disturbances resulting from increased adrenocortical secretion of cortisol caused by ACTH-dependent adrenocortical hyperplasia or tumor, or administration of steroids. Report this disorder with ICD-9-CM code 255.0. **Synonym(s):** *Cushing's syndrome.*

ectopic beat Heartbeat that has its origin in an abnormal focus other than the sinoatrial (SA) node, such as an escape beat originating in the atrium when the SA node has not fired, or is not firing effectively. This is reported as other specified cardiac arrhythmias, ICD-9-CM code 427.89.

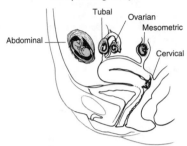

Ectopic Pregnancy

ectopic pregnancy Fertilized ovum that implants and develops outside the uterus. The ovum may implant itself in different sites, such as the fallopian tube, the ovary, the abdomen, or the cervix. The code is selected according to the site of the implantation. The most common site for ectopic implantation is the fallopian tube, reported with an ICD-9-CM code from subcategory 633.1 with a fifth digit denoting whether or not the tubal pregnancy coexists with an intrauterine pregnancy. Rupture of the tube due to the ectopic implantation is included. An ectopic pregnancy always requires medical intervention. **Synonym(s):** *abdominal pregnancy, fallopian pregnancy, intraperitoneal pregnancy, ovarian pregnancy, tubal pregnancy.*

ectro- Congenital absence of something.

ectrodactyly Congenital defect that involves the partial or complete absence of a finger or toe; reported with ICD-9-CM code 755.29 for absence of a finger, 755.39 for absence of a toe, and 755.4 for unspecified digit.

ectromelia Incomplete development or underdevelopment of one or more of the long bones in the upper or lower extremity, resulting in longitudinal deficiency. Ectromelia is reported as reduction deformities with ICD-9-CM subcategories 755.2 and 755.3.

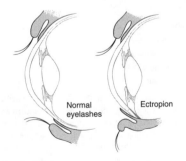

Ectropion

Normal eyelashes   Ectropion

D-F

ectropion *1)* Drooping of the lower eyelid away from the eye. *2)* Outward turning or eversion of the edge of the eyelid, exposing the palpebral conjunctiva and causing irritation. Ectropion is classified to ICD-9-CM subcategory 374.1, unless specific as congenital, 743.62. For repair of an ectropion, see CPT codes 67914-67917.

eculizumab Monoclonal antibody indicated for the treatment of paroxysmal nocturnal hemoglobinuria (PNH), a disease characterized by abnormal development of the red blood cells. Report the injectable supply with HCPCS Level II code J1300. *Synonym(s): Soliris.*

eczema Inflammatory form of dermatitis with red, itchy breakouts of exudative vesicles that leads to crusting and scaling that occurs as a reaction to internal or external agents. There are many causes of eczema, but the most common is a general allergic hypersensitivity reaction, known as atopic dermatitis or atopic eczema (ICD-9-CM code 691.8). Other eczematous conditions include infantile seborrheic dermatitis (cradle cap, 690.12) or contact with irritating substances (692.x). Eczema is coded in many different ICD-9-CM chapters based on the area affected, the cause, or type of eczema manifested.

eczema-thrombocytopenia syndrome Immunodeficiency shown by eczema, thrombocytopenia, and recurrent pyogenic infection with increased susceptibility to infection from encapsulated bacteria. Report this disorder with ICD-9-CM code 279.12.

ED *1)* Emergency department. *2)* Egg donation. *3)* Effective dose. *4)* HCPCS Level II modifier for use with CPT or HCPCS Level II codes to denote that, for three or more consecutive billing cycles (immediately prior to and including the current cycle), the patient's hematocrit level has exceeded 39 percent (or hemoglobin level has exceeded 13.0 g/dL).

EDC *1)* Estimated date of confinement. *2)* Expected date of confinement.

EdD Doctor of education.

Eddowes' syndrome Blue sclera, little growth, brittle and malformed bones, and malformed teeth. Report this disorder with ICD-9-CM code 756.51.

edema Swelling due to fluid accumulation in the intercellular spaces.

Eden-Hybinette procedure Anterior shoulder repair using an anterior bone block to augment the bony anterior glenoid lip.

edentulism Partial or complete absence of teeth due to a congenital defect involving the tooth bud, reported with ICD-9-CM code 520.0, or acquired as a result of caries, trauma, extraction, or periodontal disease, coded to causality within ICD-9-CM subcategory 525.1. The causal code is used in addition to a code for the class of edentulism: 525.40-525.44 (complete edentulism) or 525.50-525.54 (partial edentulism). *Synonym(s): adontia, anodontia, anodontism, edentia.*

edentulous Loss of all or some of the natural teeth.

edetate calcium disodium Chelating agent that forms a stable compound with lead used to treat lead poisoning with or without acute encephalopathy. Supply is reported with HCPCS Level II code J0600, not to be confused with J3520 for edetate disodium, also called Disodium EDTA, Endrate, or Diostate, which is used as a chelating agent for hypercalcemic crisis or Digoxin induced arrhythmias.

edetic acid Drug used to inhibit damage to the cornea by collagenase. Edetic acid is especially effective in alkali burns as it neutralizes soluble alkali, including lye. *Synonym(s): EDTA, ethylenediaminetetraacetic acid.*

Edex See alprostadil.

EDI Electronic data interchange. Transference of claims, certifications, quality assurance reviews, and utilization data via computer in X12 format. May refer to any electronic exchange of formatted data. *Synonym(s): EDI.* *e. translator* Software tool for accepting an EDI transmission and converting the data into another format, or for converting a non-EDI data file into an EDI format for transmission.

EDIFACT Electronic Data Interchange for Administration, Commerce, and Transport.

EDR Extreme drug resistance. Assay performed on cultured tumor samples to predict the outcome of chemotherapy. A screen to eliminate ineffective treatment courses, EDR is a multi-step procedure requiring multiple CPT codes including 87230, 88305, and 88358.

EDS Ehlers-Danlos syndrome. Group of hereditary connective tissue disorders with symptoms of skin elasticity, unstable joints, and slow-healing wounds. Bruising and skin wounds are also common. EDS is reported with ICD-9-CM code 756.83.

EDTA Drug used to inhibit damage to the cornea by collagenase. EDTA is especially effective in alkali burns as it neutralizes soluble alkali, including lye.

Edwards' syndrome Congenital malformations in which extra chromosome is group E. Includes mental retardation, abnormal skull shape, malformed ears, small mandible, cardiac defects, short sternum, and other symptoms. Report this disorder with ICD-9-CM code 758.2.

EE HCPCS Level II modifier for use with CPT or HCPCS Level II codes to denote that for three or more consecutive billing cycles (immediately prior to and including the current cycle) the patient's hematocrit level has not exceeded 39 percent (or hemoglobin level has not exceeded 13.0 g/dL).

EEG Electroencephalogram. *NCD References: 160.21, 160.22, 160.8, 160.9.*

EENT Eye, ear, nose, and throat.

effacement Shortening and thinning of the cervix during the early stages of labor. *Synonym(s): ripening.*

effective date Under HIPAA, the date that a final rule is effective, which is usually 60 days after it is published in the *Federal Register.*

efferent Moving or carrying away from.

efferent loop syndrome Distended efferent loop with illness and pain caused by acute or chronic obstruction of the duodenum and jejunum proximal to a gastrojejunostomy. Report this disorder with ICD-9-CM code 537.89. *Synonym(s): gastrojejunal loop obstruction.*

effusion Escape of fluid from within a body cavity.

EFT Electronic funds transfer.

EGA Estimated gestational age.

EGD Esophagus, stomach, and duodenum. *Synonym: esophagogastroduodenoscopy.*

EGFR Epidermal growth factor receptor. Aberrant EGFR is associated with advanced malignancies including breast, lung, ovarian, prostate, and squamous cell carcinoma of the head and neck.

egg Female gamete; an ovum. An ovum measures, on average, 145 micrometers in diameter.

Eggers procedure Hamstring muscles of the knee and thigh area are transferred to a new position on the femoral condyle.

eggshell nails Congenital or acquired condition in which the fingernails become thin and grow upward over the top of the finger. If congenital, report with ICD-9-CM code 757.5; if acquired, report 703.8.

EGHP Employer group health plan. Any health plan that is contributed to by an employer of 20 or more employees and that provides medical care directly or through other methods. The federal employee health benefits program, employee pay-all plans, multi-employer group health plans with at least one employer with 20 or more employees, and any health plan in which the beneficiary is enrolled because of his or her employment or his or her spouse's employment are all considered EGHPs.

EGIDs Eosinophilic gastrointestinal disorders. Disorders involving the accumulation of eosinophil in the tissues lining the gastrointestinal tract but without a known cause such as connective tissue disease, drug reactions, malignancy, or parasitic infection. Included are eosinophilic colitis, enteritis, esophagitis, gastritis, and gastroenteritis. Treatment may include diet limitation, use of a feeding tube, or steroid treatment.

EHBF Estimated hepatic blood flow.

Ehlers-Danlos syndrome Congenital connective tissue disorder, resulting from an abnormality in the production of collagen that causes hyperelasticity of the skin, hypermobility of the joints, and fragility of the blood vessels, resulting in impaired wound healing. This syndrome is reported with ICD-9-CM code 756.83. *Synonym(s): Cutis laxa syndrome, Cutis pendula syndrome.*

EHNAC Electronic Healthcare Network Accreditation Commission.

EHO Emerging healthcare organizations. Hospitals and other providers that are emerging or affiliating.

EHR Electronic health record.

ehrlichiosis Acute, bacterial febrile illness caused by infection from a tick bite. Symptoms range from mild to severe and include nausea, vomiting, diarrhea, headache, confusion, chills, myalgia, and malaise, with leukopenia and thrombocytopenia. Antibiotic treatment is sometimes required and death has been known to occur. Report this disease with a code from ICD-9-CM category 082.4.

EI Electrical impedance. In spectroscopy, low frequency electrical currents pass through tissue to create a computerized image of a cross section of that tissue.

EIN Employer identification number.

Eisenmenger's syndrome Pulmonary hypertension with congenital communication between two circulations so a right to left shunt results. Report this disorder with ICD-9-CM code 745.4.

EJ HCPCS Level II modifier, for use with CPT or HCPCS Level II codes, that identifies a subsequent claim or claims for a defined course of therapy, e.g., EPO, sodium hyaluronate, Infliximab. This modifier is reported for a single treatment in a defined course of multiple treatments and should not be used on the initial treatment.

ejection fraction Ratio of the volume of blood in the ventricles that is ejected during systole, determined by the stroke volume (the volume of blood ejected during a single contraction) to the end-diastolic volume. The normal range is between plus or minus 8 percent of 65. The ratio is an indicator of heart disease from ventricular dysfunction. Rest and exercise gated blood-pool scanning can be used for EF measurements, but it is now more frequently determined using SPECT myocardial perfusion imaging techniques or MR and CT imaging.

Ekbom's syndrome Indescribable uneasiness, restlessness, or twitching in the legs after going to bed. Often caused by poor circulation or antipsychotic medications, it can lead to insomnia. Report this syndrome with ICD-9-CM code 333.99. *Synonym(s): restless leg syndrome.*

EKG Electrocardiogram. Graphic recording of the changes in electrical voltage and polarity caused by the heart muscle's electrical excitation. The tracing follows atrial and ventricular activity over time, captured through

D-F

electrodes placed on the skin. An electrocardiogram is reported with CPT code 93000, 93005, or 93010. **Synonym(s):** *ECG.* **NCD Reference:** *20.15.*

Ekman's syndrome Blue sclera, little growth, brittle and malformed bones, and malformed teeth. Report this disorder with ICD-9-CM code 756.51.

Elaprase Enzyme replacement therapy administered by IV infusion and indicated for patients with Hunter syndrome or mucopolysaccharidosis II (MPSII), a rare lysosomal storage disorder that impairs the body's ability to break down mucopolysaccharides. By replacing the deficient enzyme, it assists in keeping the patient ambulatory, improving pulmonary function, and reducing organ size. Supply is reported with HCPCS Level II code J1743. **Synonym(s):** *idursulfase.*

elastic skin Congenital connective tissue disorder resulting from an abnormality in the production of collagen, which causes hyperelasticity of the skin, hypermobility of the joints, and fragility of the blood vessels, resulting in impaired wound healing. This syndrome is reported with ICD-9-CM code 756.83. If this condition is acquired, rather than congenital, report with ICD-9-CM code 701.8. **Synonym(s):** *cutis laxa syndrome, cutis pendula syndrome, Ehlers-Danlos syndrome.*

elastofibroma Rare, firm, noncancerous but unencapsulated connective tissue tumor composed of excessive sclerotic collagen and irregular elastic fibers that develop slowly. Found most often in older people in the subscapular area, it is associated with manual labor or fibrous reaction to trauma. Elastofibromas may be located elsewhere on the body. Treatment is usually by surgical excision. Code assignment depends upon site.

Elavil See amitriptyline.

ELBW Extremely low birth weight. Extreme immaturity referring to a newborn of less than 1,000 grams, usually born after 23 weeks gestation. These infants spend significant time in the newborn intensive care and are at high risk for long-term effects of prematurity. Extreme immaturity is reported with a code from ICD-9-CM subcategory 765.0 and a second code from subcategory 765.2 to report the completed weeks of gestation.

elderly primigravida Woman in her first pregnancy at an age beyond the norm, usually considered 35 years or older.

elective Optional, voluntary. *e. admission.* Admission made at the discretion of the patient and facility based on available resources.

elective mutism Pervasive and persistent refusal to speak in situations not attributable to a mental disorder, such as withdrawal in a specific stressful situation, shyness, or social withdrawal disorders.

electric feet syndrome Discomfort of feet and other extremities, excessive sweating, elevated skin

temperature, and riboflavin deficiency. Report this disorder with ICD-9-CM code 266.2. **Synonym(s):** *Gopalan's syndrome.*

electrical osteogenesis stimulation Special device applied externally to the skin with electrodes or implanted internally that creates a pulsing electromagnetic field around a damaged area to stimulate bone tissue into producing osteocytes and to promote neural regeneration, revascularization, epiphyseal growth, and ligament maturation.

electrocardiogram Recording of the electrical activity of the heart on a moving strip of paper that detects and records the electrical potential of the heart during contraction. **NCD Reference:** *20.15.*

electrocardiographic rhythm derived Analysis of data obtained from readings of the heart's electrical activation, including heart rate and rhythm, variability of heart rate, ST analysis, and T-wave alternans. Other data may also be assessed when warranted.

Electrocautery

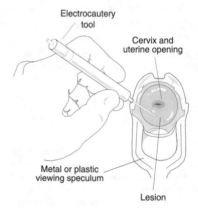

Electrocautery tool

Cervix and uterine opening

Metal or plastic viewing speculum

Lesion

electrocautery Division or cutting of tissue using high-frequency electrical current to produce heat, which destroys cells.

electrocorticography Electrodes are placed onto specific areas of the brain to record the brain's electrical activity while the cortex is irrigated to localize areas of seizure activity in patients with intractable epileptic seizures who are surgical candidates for excising the epileptic focus or a lobectomy.

electroculogram Method used to measure movement of the eye by placing electrodes around the eye. This test is helpful in determining rapid eye movement in sleep studies.

electrode Electric terminal specialized for a particular electrochemical reaction that acts as a medium between a body surface and another instrument, commonly termed a "lead." An electrode may carry a current of electrical activity from the body to a recording instrument, such as in electroencephalography or echocardiography, or it may conduct current into the body from a generator source, such as in pacemakers and cardioverter-defibrillators (AICDs). Placing leads on the skin surface as part of a graph recording is not reported separately. When electrodes are placed in the body as part of a permanent implantable device, the placement, replacement, or repositioning, and removal may have separately identifiable codes based on location, access route, and type of device.

electroejaculation Procedure that uses an electrovibratory device that stimulates ejaculation in order to collect semen for artificial insemination. This technique is most often used when a patient is paraplegic and wanting to reproduce. Electroejaculation is reported with CPT code 55870.

electroencephalography Testing involving amplification, recording, and analysis of the electrical activity of the brain.

electromechanical equipment Mechanical devices or systems that are electrically activated, as by a solenoid. May also include the use of computerized equipment for testing or training.

electromyogram Recording of nerve stimulation to determine if muscle weakness is present and if it is related to the muscles themselves or a problem with the nerves that supply the muscles.

electromyography Test that measures muscle response to nerve stimulation determining if muscle weakness is present and if it is related to the muscles themselves or a problem with the nerves that supply the muscles.

electron Negatively charged particle of an atom.

electronic Carrying of electrons. *e. claim* Claim submitted by a provider or electronic media claim (EMC) vendor via central processing unit (CPU) transmission, tape, diskette, direct data entry, direct wire, dial-in telephone, digital fax, or personal computer upload or download. Effective October 1, 1993, clean claims submitted to Medicare electronically are paid 13 days after the claim is received. *e. commerce* Exchange of business information by electronic means. *e. data interchange* Transference of claims, certifications, quality assurance reviews, and utilization data via computer in X12 format. May refer to any electronic exchange of formatted data. *e. media claim* Automated claims processing method that uses a data storage tool to transfer claims data to the payer. EMC has been replaced by electronic data interchange (EDI). *e. remittance advice* Any of several electronic formats for explaining the payments of health care claims.

electronic claim Claim submitted by a provider or an electronic media claim (EMC) vendor via central

processing unit (CPU) transmission, tape, diskette, direct data entry, direct wire, dial-in telephone, digital fax, or personal computer upload or download. Effective October 1, 1993, clean claims submitted to Medicare electronically are paid 13 days after the claim is received.

electronic data interchange Transference of claims, certifications, quality assurance reviews, and utilization data via computer in X12 format. May refer to any electronic exchange of formatted data.

electronic health record Electronic version of individual patients' health-related information that has the interoperability to be created, managed, and consulted by more than one health care organization's authorized staff and clinicians.

Electronic Healthcare Network Accreditation Commission Organization that tests transactions for consistency with the HIPAA requirements and that accredits health care clearinghouses. *Synonym(s): EHNAC.*

electronic media claim Automated claims processing method that uses a data storage tool to transfer claims data to the payer. EMC has been replaced by electronic data interchange (EDI).

electronic medical record Electronic version of individual patients' health-related information that can be created, managed, and consulted by single care organizations' authorized staff and clinicians.

electronic remittance advice Any of several electronic formats explaining the payments of health care claims.

electrophysiologic studies Electrical stimulation and monitoring to diagnose heart conduction abnormalities that predispose patients to bradyarrhythmias and to determine a patient's chance for developing ventricular and supraventricular tachyarrhythmias.

electrosurgery Use of electric currents to generate heat in performing surgery.

elephantiasis Obstructed lymphatic vessels that cause extreme swelling from fluid retention. The genitalia and legs are the most frequently involved areas. Elephantiasis is reported with ICD-9-CM code 457.1.

elevator Tool for lifting tissues or bone.

eligibility Individuals and services qualified for coverage under a specific health care plan.

eligibility for Part B Criteria hinge on an individual's being at least 65, a resident and citizen of the United States or an alien lawfully admitted for permanent residence who has resided in the United States continually for the five years preceding his/her application for enrollment for Part B benefits and is eligible for Medicare Part A benefits.

D-F

eligible professional Non-hospital based physician receiving Medicare and/or Medicaid reimbursement who is using a certified electronic health record.

Elliot's solution Intravenous solution used as a diluent for intrathecal methotrexate administration to treat meningeal leukemia or leukocytic lymphoma.

Ellison-Zollinger syndrome Peptic ulceration with gastric hypersecretion, tumor of the pancreatic islets, and hypoglycemia. Report this disorder with ICD-9-CM code 251.5. *Synonym(s): Zollinger-Ellison syndrome.*

Ellis-van Creveld syndrome Dwarfism with defective development of cardiac septum, skin, hair, and teeth. Report this disorder with ICD-9-CM code 756.55.

ELOS Estimated length of stay. Average number of days of hospitalization required for a given illness or procedure, based on prior histories of patients who have been hospitalized for the same illness or procedure.

Eloxatin Brand name pharmaceutical for treatment of advanced colorectal cancer. Eloxatin is infused with two other anti-cancer drugs, 5-FU and leucovorin. Supply of Eloxatin is reported with HCPCS Level II code J9263. Eloxatin contains oxaliplatin.

Elschnig bodies Transparent clusters resembling grapes resulting from the production of an excessive number of epithelial cells following cataract extraction. Report this condition with ICD-9-CM code 366.51. *Synonym(s): Elschnig pearls.*

Elspar See asparaginase.

elution Separation of one solid from another, usually by washing.

EM HCPCS Level II modifier, for use with CPT or HCPCS Level II codes, that identifies an emergency reserve supply (for end stage renal disease [ESRD] benefit only). Used only for supplies dispensed to patients on home dialysis and may be used for more than one item, but all supplies must be billed in the same month.

emaciation Condition of body tissue wasting, resulting in extreme thinness and depletion of subcutaneous fat. Underlying causes may include metabolic or malabsorptive disorders, eating disorders, or other physical or mental factors. Emaciation is reported with ICD-9-CM code 261. *Synonym(s): severe calorie deficiency severe malnutrition.*

emancipation disorder Adjustment reaction in adolescents or young adults following recent assumption of independence from parental control or supervision. Manifested by difficulty in making independent decisions, increased dependence on parental advice, and adoption of values deliberately oppositional to parents.

embolectomy Surgical excision of a blood clot or other foreign material that broke away from its original source and traveled in the blood stream, becoming lodged in a blood vessel and blocking circulation. Removal of an embolism is coded according to the vessel being accessed. *NCD Reference: 240.6.*

embolism Obstruction of a blood vessel resulting from a clot or foreign substance.

embolization Placement of a clotting agent, such as a coil, plastic particles, gel, foam, etc., into an area of hemorrhage to stop the bleeding or to block blood flow to a problem area, such as an aneurysm or a tumor. *NCD Reference: 20.28.*

embolus Any substance, such as air bubbles, cellular masses, calcium fragments, or blood clots, carried through the bloodstream that has become lodged in a vessel, resulting in an obstruction of circulation.

embryo Developing cells of a new organism that will become a fetus; the period defined from the fourth day after fertilization to the end of the eighth week.

embryonic fixation syndrome Eyebrow or upper or lower eyelid sags. Report this disorder with ICD-9-CM code 270.2. *Synonym(s): Mendes syndrome, van der Hoeve-Halbertsma-Waardenburg syndrome, Waardenburg-Klein syndrome.*

embryotomy Operation performed on a fetus in utero or within the birth canal to facilitate an otherwise impossible delivery. Embryotomy may consist of dismemberment, such as cutting the clavicle or removing a limb. Report embryotomy with ICD-9-CM procedure code 73.8.

EMC Electronic media claims. Automated claims processing method that uses a data storage tool to transfer claims data to the payer. EMC has been replaced by electronic data interchange (EDI).

emergency Serious medical condition or symptom (including severe pain) resulting from injury, sickness, or mental illness that arises suddenly and requires immediate care and treatment, generally received within 24 hours of onset, to avoid jeopardy to the life, limb, or health of a covered person. *E. admission* Admission in which the patient requires immediate medical or psychiatric attention because of life-threatening, severe, and potentially disabling conditions. *E. department* Organized hospital-based facility for the provision of unscheduled episodic services to patients who present for immediate medical attention. The facility must be available 24 hours a day. *E. outpatient* Patient admitted for diagnosis and treatment of a condition requiring immediate attention but who will not stay at that facility or be transferred to another.

emergent care Treatment for a medical condition or symptom (including severe pain) that arises suddenly and requires immediate care and treatment.

EMG Electromyogram.

EMI Electromagnetic interference. Disruption of an EKG in a clinical setting.

Eminase See anistreplase.

Emmet's operation Repair of the perineum and the cervix uteri.

emotional disturbances specific to childhood and adolescence Less well-differentiated, long-term emotional disorders characteristic of the childhood period not caused by stressors; can take the form of academic underachievement disorder, elective mutism, identity disorder, introverted disorder of childhood, misery and unhappiness disorder, oppositional disorder, overanxious disorder, and shyness disorder of childhood.

emphysema Pathological condition in which there is destructive enlargement of the air spaces in the lungs resulting in damage to the alveolar walls, commonly seen in long-term smokers. Emphysema is reported with ICD-9-CM code 492.8.

emphysematous bleb Formation of blisters or vesicles greater than 1.0 mm within an emphysematous lung, containing serum or blood, reported with ICD-9-CM code 492.0. *Synonym(s): giant bullous emphysema.*

employee assistance program Services designed to help employees, their family members, and employers find solutions for workplace and personal problems that affect morale, productivity, or financial issues such as workplace stress, family/marital concerns, legal or financial problems, elder care, child care, substance abuse, emotional/stress issues, and other daily living concerns. *Synonym(s): EAP.*

Employee Retirement Income Security Act of 1974 Law mandating reporting, disclosure of grievance and appeals requirements, and fiduciary standards for group life and health plans that are sponsored by private (but not public) employers. Also preempts state benefit mandates and premium tax laws for self-funded group health plans and allows these plans to be exempt from local or state reimbursement systems. *Synonym(s): Public Law 93-406.*

Employee Retirement Income Security Act of 1974 Law mandating reporting, disclosure of grievance and appeals requirements, and fiduciary standards for group life and health plans that are sponsored by private (but not public) employers. Also preempts state benefit mandates and premium tax laws for self-funded group health plans and allows these plans to be exempt from local or state reimbursement systems. *Synonym(s): ERISA.*

employer group health plan Any health plan that is contributed to by an employer of 20 or more employees and that provides medical care directly or through other methods. The federal employee health benefits program, employee pay-all plans, multi-employer group health plans with at least one employer with 20 or more employees, and any health plan in which the beneficiary is enrolled because of his or her employment or his or her spouse's employment are all considered EGHPs. *Synonym(s): EGHP.*

empty sella syndrome Sella turcica containing no pituitary gland caused by herniating arachnoid, radiotherapy, or surgery. Report this disorder with ICD-9-CM code 253.8.

empyectomy Removal of an accumulation of pus.

empyema Accumulation of pus within the respiratory, or pleural, cavity. This condition is reported with ICD-9-CM code 510.9 unless the infection communicates between the pleural cavity and another structure, and then it is coded as empyema with fistula, 510.0. *Synonym(s): purulent pleurisy.*

EMR Electronic medical record.

EMS Emergency medical service.

EMT Emergency medical technician.

EMTALA Emergency Medical Treatment and Active Labor Act.

EMT-P Paramedic.

en *1)* Clyster. *2)* Enema.

en bloc In total.

en bloc removal Take out as a whole or all in one mass.

enameloma Benign odontogenic growth containing enamel, dentin nucleus, or a small amount of dentin strand and pulp. Enamelomas may be located at the point where a multirooted tooth divides, at the tip of an enamel spur, or on the root surface. Report this condition with ICD-9-CM code 520.2. *Synonym(s): enamel drop, enamel pearl.*

Enbrel See etanercept.

encephal(o)- Pertaining to the brain.

encephalitis Inflammation of the brain, often caused by viral or bacterial infection. Code assignment requires more than one code and is dependent upon the specific infectious agent (herpes simplex, rubella, meningococcus), the type of underlying disease (viral, rickettsial, protozoal, other infectious disease), or whether it occurs postinfection, postimmunization, or from toxic poisoning.

encephalocele Congenital protrusion of brain tissue through a defect in the skull.

encephalocystocele Congenital abnormality in which a portion of the brain and meninges herniate through a defect in the skull known as a cranium bifidum. Report this condition with ICD-9-CM code 742.0. *Synonym(s): cephalocele, craniocele, encephalomeningocele, meningoencephalocele.*

encephalomyelitis Inflammatory disease, often viral in nature, that affects both the brain and spinal cord.

D-F

Code assignment is based upon type and underlying cause.

encephalomyeloneuropathy Illness that affects the brain, spinal cord, and peripheral nerves, reported with ICD-9-CM code 349.9.

encephalomyeloradiculitis Illness affecting the brain, spinal cord, and nerve roots of the spine, reported with ICD-9-CM code 357.0.

encerclage Wiring or banding fragments of fractured bone together along the shaft of a long bone, requiring an open approach and often done in tandem with intramedullary rod insertion.

enchondroma Benign neoplasm of the bone.

encoder Computer application that assists in the assignment of a diagnosis or procedure code and may also assign reimbursement categories and values.

encopresis Fecal incontinence from inability to control bowel movements. If traced to a psychological, not biological, cause, report with ICD-9-CM code 307.7. Unspecified encopresis without identified cause defaults to ICD-9-CM codes 787.60-787.63.

encounter Direct personal contact between a registered hospital outpatient (in a medical clinic or emergency department, for example) and a physician (or other person authorized by state law and hospital bylaws to order or furnish services) for the diagnosis and treatment of an illness or injury. Visits with more than one health professional that take place during the same session and at a single location within the hospital are considered a single visit.

encryption Transformation of ordinary text or data into a seemingly random and unintelligible string or sequence of characters. Once encrypted, data can securely be stored or transmitted over unsecured lines. The person receiving the encrypted data reverses the encryption process to restore the text to a readable form and to make it available for further processing. Only the person sending the text and the intended recipient have the key that allows them to encrypt and decrypt the data. **Synonym(s):** *encipherment.*

endarterectomy Removal of the thickened, endothelial lining of a diseased or damaged artery. Occlusion is often found in heavy or long-term tobacco users. Endarterectomy is performed on many different vessels, such as the carotids, the pulmonary artery, the common femoral, vertebral, and aortoiliac arteries and is coded accordingly.

endaural incision Incision within the ear.

endemic Within the normal incidence rate of infection or occurrence within a specific population.

endemic polyneuritis Disease caused by a lack of vitamin B1 (thiamine) causing cardiac damage, polyneuritis, and edema. The disease is found mostly in

areas where white, polished rice is the main staple of the diet. Report this disorder with ICD-9-CM code 265.0. **Synonym(s):** *beriberi, dietetic neuritis, rice disease.*

endo- Within, internal.

endocarditis Inflammatory disease of the interior lining of the heart chamber and heart valves, most commonly caused by bacteria. Risk factors include IV drug use, dental procedures, central venous catheters, and weakened or damaged heart valves. Code assignment is dependent upon site and causality.

Endocervical Curettage

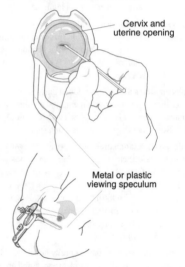

Cervix and uterine opening

Metal or plastic viewing speculum

endocervical canal Opening between the uterus and the vagina, through the cervix, lined with mucous membrane.

endocervicitis Inflammation of the cervix uteri mucous membranes, reported with ICD-9-CM code 616.0. When it occurs due to an IUD, report 996.65. For gonococcal endocervicitis, report 098.15 (acute) or 098.35 (chronic); for syphilitic cases, report 095.8; for trichomonal causes, report 131.09; and for tuberculous endocervicitis, report 016.7 with the appropriate fifth digit. **Synonym(s):** *endotrachelitis.*

endocervix Region of the cervix uteri that opens into the uterus or the mucous membrane lining the cervical canal.

EndoCinch Brand name device for suturing the esophagogastric junction during endoscopy as a treatment for gastrointestinal reflux disease (GERD).

endocrine-hypertensive syndrome Disorder of adrenal medullary tissue with hypertension, attacks of palpitation, headache, nausea, dyspnea, anxiety, pallor, and profuse sweating. Report this disorder with

ICD-9-CM code 255.3. **Synonym(s):** *Schroeder's syndrome, Slocumb's syndrome.*

endodontics Subspecialty of dentistry that deals primarily with the pulp of the tooth or the dentine complex.

endogenous depression Manic-depressive psychosis in which there is a widespread depressed mood of gloom and wretchedness with some degree of anxiety, reduced activity, or restlessness and agitation. There is a marked tendency to recurrence; in a few cases this may be at regular intervals.

endoleak Occurrence of blood-flow outside an endovascular graft that may be due to the graft, retrograde flow, disintegration, or tears.

endometrial carcinoma Cancer of the inner lining of the uterine wall.

endometrial cystic hyperplasia Abnormal cyst-forming overgrowth of the endometrium.

endometriosis Aberrant uterine mucosal tissue appearing in areas of the pelvic cavity outside of its normal location lining the uterus, and inflaming surrounding tissues. Predisposing factors may include heredity, previous uterine surgery, and associated conditions such as pelvic adhesions. Endometriosis can result in infertility and spontaneous abortion. Endometriosis is reported within ICD-9-CM rubric 617. *e. interna* Abnormal presence of endometrial glands and tissue within the myometrium, the smooth muscle walls of the uterus, causing hypertrophy of the myometrium. At menses, blood is trapped within the muscle of the uterus, causing pain and cramping. Report this condition with ICD-9-CM code 617.0. **Synonym(s):** *adenomyosis.*

endometrium Lining of the uterus, which thickens in preparation for fertilization. A fertilized ovum embeds into the thickened endometrium. When no fertilization takes place, the endometrial lining sheds during the process of menstruation.

endomyocardial Relating to the endocardium and the myocardium.

endophthalmitis Irritation, normally of an infectious origin, of the intraocular spaces or cavities and adjacent structures. Endophthalmitis that is not infectious in nature may be caused by a parasite, retained lens or fragment, embedded hairs, or a toxic substance. Report the various forms of endophthalmitis with codes from ICD-9-CM subcategories 360.0 and 360.1. **Synonym(s):** *endophthalmia.*

endoprosthesis Intravascular device in the form of a hollow stent placed within a duct or artery to provide passage through an obstructed area, such as in a bile duct, or to act as a replacement for damaged arterial walls, as in treating an aneurysm. **Synonym(s):** *EVP.*

endoscopy Visual inspection of the body using a fiberoptic scope. **NCD Reference:** *100.2.*

endosseous Within the bone.

endosteal implant Metal implants that are cylindrical or blade-like in structure, placed into the maxillary or mandibular bone. Metal posts that protrude through the mucosa into the mouth are attached to the implants so that artificial teeth or dentures can be attached to the roots to replace missing teeth. Report the surgical procedure with CPT code 21248 or 21249 and supply of the metal implants with HCPCS Level II code D6010.

Endotak Reliance Brand name cardiac lead system.

endotheliosis Rapid growth of epithelial cells that line the heart, blood, and lymph vessels, and serous cavities of the body. Endotheliosis is reported with ICD-9-CM code 287.8, whether it is identified as being infectional or hemorrhagic.

endotoxic shock Progression from septicemic infection to severe sepsis with shock, which carries a greater than 50 percent mortality rate. Septic shock presents with severe sepsis with low blood pressure, decreased urine output, and increased oxygen demands, followed by major organ failure, manifesting systemic inflammatory disease from bacterial toxins. Reporting septic shock correctly requires at least three codes to be assigned. Since septic shock is a systemic inflammatory response syndrome (SIRS) with organ dysfunction that has progressed from septicemic infection and not from trauma, the type of septicemia is identified first with a code from ICD-9-CM category 038, or the code for a specific systemic infection, such as systemic candidiasis, (ICD-9-CM code 112.5) to identify the type of bacteria, if known. The SIRS is coded secondarily with 995.92, followed by the additional code for septic shock, 785.52. When the specific organ failure is known, a fourth code is assigned. **Synonym(s):** *septic shock.*

endovascular therapy Intravascular catheters, scopes, stents, balloons, and other devices or methods used to treat vascular disease.

end-stage renal disease Chronic, advanced kidney disease requiring renal dialysis or a kidney transplant to prevent imminent death.

ENG Electronystagmogram.

eng. Engorged.

Engel-von Recklinghausen syndrome Osteitis with fibrous degeneration and formation of cysts with fibrous nodules on affected bones. Report this disorder with an ICD-9-CM code from subcategory 252.0. **Synonym(s):** *Jaffe-Lichtenstein-Uehlinger syndrome.*

Engerix-B Brand name hepatitis B vaccine provided in a single-dose vial or syringe. Supply of Engerix-B is reported with CPT codes 90743 and 90746. Administration of the vaccine is reported with HCPCS

D-F

Level II code G0010. Need for vaccination is reported with ICD-9-CM code V02.61.

ENOG Electroneuronography. Test to measure facial nerve integrity and diagnose facial paralysis disorders such as Bell's palsy. *Synonym(s): facial nerve function studies.*

enophthalmos Condition in which the eyeball recedes backwards into the eye socket. Underlying causes include atrophy, trauma, or surgery. Report this condition with ICD-9-CM codes 376.50-376.52.

enoxaparin sodium Anticoagulant used to prevent deep vein thrombosis (DVT) in patients following hip or knee replacement, abdominal surgery, or those at risk due to limited mobility. It also decreases ischemic complications of unstable angina and non-Q-wave myocardial infarction (MI) and can be used to treat patients who have already developed DVT with or without pulmonary embolism. Supply is reported with HCPCS Level II code J1650.May be sold under the brand name Lovenox.

enrollee In medical reimbursement, person who subscribes to a specific health plan.

enrollment Number of lives covered by the plan.

ENT Ear, nose, and throat.

enteraden Any gland found within the intestines.

enteral Pertaining to the intestines; enteral is often used in the context of nutrition management: formulas, jejunostomy tubes, nasogastric devices, etc.

enteral nutrition Feeding of a nutrient mixture directly into or just proximal to the upper end of the small bowel via a tube or through an existing stoma. Patients are usually able to absorb the nutrients. *NCD Reference: 180.2.*

enteralgia Intestinal pain, reported with ICD-9-CM codes 789.00-789.09. *Synonym(s): enterodynia.*

enterectomy Removal or resection of a portion of the intestine.

enteric-coated Pharmaceutical term denoting the specialized coating with which tablets or capsules are covered to prevent the contents from being released and absorbed until they reach the intestines.

enteritis Inflammation of the small intestine caused by any number of infections or external influences such as radiation. *Synonym(s): enterocolitis.*

entero- Relating to the intestines.

enteroarticular syndrome Association of arthritis, iridocyclitis, urethritis, and diarrhea. Report this disorder with ICD-9-CM code 099.3. *Synonym(s): Fiessinger-Leroy-Reiter syndrome.*

Enterobacter Gram negative, anaerobic bacteria found in the gastrointestinal (GI) tract of humans and animals. Strains of *Enterobacter* cause pneumonia and infections

of the urinary tract and bloodstream. Nosocomial (hospital-based) infections are often a result of *Enterobacter* contaminated medical devices and health care personnel.

enterobiasis Infection with pinworms, especially nematodes of the genus E. vermicularis, usually located in portions of the intestine. Symptoms include anal itching, restless sleep, decreased appetite, and lack of weight gain. Treatment is usually with oral medication. Report this condition with ICD-9-CM code 127.4.

enterobiliary Having to do with the small intestine and bile passages or biliary tract.

enterocele Intestinal herniation into the vaginal wall.

enterocystoma Congenital anomaly in which an intestinal cyst develops from a crease or pocket along the gastrointestinal (GI) tract, reported with ICD-9-CM code 751.5. *Synonym(s): enterocyst.*

enterogenous cyanosis Condition in which the intestines absorb nitrites or other toxic substances and the blood forms chemically altered types of hemoglobin. This results in cyanosis and other accompanying symptoms such as headache, nausea, dizziness, tachycardia, and dyspnea. Report this condition with ICD-9-CM code 289.7.

enterolith Any hard mass or concretion found within the intestines, not necessarily composed of fecal matter, that may cause obstruction. Report this condition with ICD-9-CM code 560.39. *Synonym(s): intestinal calculus.*

enterolysis Division of intestinal adhesions.

enteroptosis Condition in which the intestines are abnormally positioned downward in the abdominal cavity and often associated with displacement of other internal organs. Report this condition with ICD-9-CM code 569.89.

enterorrhagia Bleeding or hemorrhage within the gastrointestinal (GI) tract. If the underlying cause is identified, code the condition; if the cause is unidentified, code the intestinal hemorrhage with ICD-9-CM code 578.9.

enterospasm Frequent and painful contractions of the smooth muscles of the gastrointestinal (GI) tract, occurring on an irregular basis. This condition is reported with ICD-9-CM code 564.9, unless it is specified as psychogenic, in which case it is reported with 306.4.

enterostenosis Condition in which the intestine is uncharacteristically narrowed or strictured, reported with ICD-9-CM code 560.9, unless the stricture is noted to be congenital, in which case it is coded to 751.1 for the small intestine or 751.2 for the large intestine, rectum, and anal canal.

enterostomy Surgically created opening into the intestine through the abdominal wall.

D-F

enterovesical fistula Abnormal communication between the small intestine and the bladder.

enterovirus Genus of viruses inhabiting the intestinal tract and belonging to the family Picornaviridae. There are many different strains of non-polio enterovirus.

Enterra Brand name system for treating chronic nausea and vomiting associated with gastroparesis by using mild electrical impulses to stimulate the stomach.

Enteryx Brand name liquid polymer injected into the muscle of the lower esophageal sphincter through an endoscope to reduce the symptoms of gastrointestinal reflux disease (GERD). The injected material forms a spongy, permanent implant that supports the sphincter and keeps acid from backing up into the esophagus. The procedure, related to the use of Enteryx, is reported with CPT codes 43201 or 43236.

enthesopathy Disorders that occur at points where muscle tendons and ligaments attach to bones or joint capsules. Enthesopathy is reported with a code from ICD-9-CM category 726, dependent upon the location, or to 720.1 when affecting the spine.

Entropion

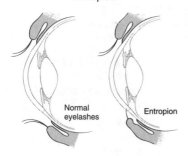

Normal eyelashes

Entropion

entropion Inversion of the eyelid, turning the edge in toward the eyeball and causing irritation from contact of the lashes with the surface of the eye. Entropion is classified to ICD-9-CM subcategory 374.0, unless specified as congenital (743.62). For repair of an entropion, see CPT codes 67921-67924. *Synonym(s): blepharelosis.*

enucleate Removal of a growth or organ cleanly so as to extract it in one piece.

enucleation Removal of a growth or organ cleanly so as to extract it in one piece. *eye e.* Surgical removal of the eye.

enuresis Urinary incontinence, without specification as to type. Different types of incontinence are reported with a code from ICD-9-CM subcategory 788.3 with any causal condition coded first. *Synonym(s): incontinence, nocturnal enuresis (bed wetting), postvoidal dribble, stress incontinence, urge incontinence. NCD Reference: 30.1.1.*

enzymopathy Condition in which enzymes are abnormally produced, deficient, or missing due to a genetic disorder. Report unspecified enzymopathy with ICD-9-CM code 277.9 and specified enzyme disorders with more specific codes from ICD-9-CM category 277.

EO Elbow orthosis.

EOB Explanation of benefits. Statement mailed to the member and provider explaining claim adjudication and payment.

EOG Electrooculography.

EOI Evidence of insurability.

EOM *1)* Extraocular muscles. Six orbital muscles (extrinsic) that move the eyeball. *2)* End of month.

EOMB Explanation of Medicare benefits. Explanation of Medicaid benefits. Explanation of member benefits. Typically sent to the provider and the patient, an explanation of how Medicare, Medicaid, or member benefits were paid, that is, the allowable amount paid, the coinsurance due to the provider or payable by the patient, or the reason why a claim may have been rejected or paid less or more than the original amount charged.

EOMI Extraocular motion intact.

EOP External occipital protuberance.

eosinopenia Reduced number of eosinophils (nucleated, granular leukocytes) in the blood. Report this condition with ICD-9-CM code 288.00.

eosinophilia Abnormally large accumulation or formation of eosinophils (nucleated, granular leukocytes) in the blood, characteristic of allergic states and infection. Report this condition with ICD-9-CM code 288.3.

eosinophilia myalgia syndrome Inflammatory, multisystemic fibrosis associated with ingesting elementary L-tryptophan. Symptoms include muscle aches and pains, weak limbs, sensory loss in distal areas, lack of reflexes, joint pain, cough, fever, fatigue, skin rashes, and elevated eosinophil (nucleated, granular leukocytes) counts greater than 1000/microliter. Report this disorder with ICD-9-CM code 710.5.

eosinophilic colitis Disorder involving the accumulation of eosinophil in the tissues lining the colon, but without a known cause such as connective tissue disease, drug reaction, malignancy, or parasitic infection. The resultant inflammation may cause extreme abdominal pain, diarrhea, or bloody stool, and may be misdiagnosed as Crohn's disease or irritable bowel. Report this disorder with ICD-9-CM code 558.42.

eosinophilic esophagitis Disorder involving the accumulation of eosinophil in the tissues lining the esophagus, resulting in severe inflammation. Affecting the ability to swallow, it may result in malnutrition and

D-F

possible failure to thrive in children. Report this disorder with ICD-9-CM code 530.13.

eosinophilic gastritis Disorder involving the accumulation of eosinophil in the tissues lining the stomach, but without a known cause such as connective tissue disease, drug reactions, malignancy, or parasitic infection. The resultant inflammation may cause severe abdominal pain and vomiting. Treatment may include diet limitation, use of a feeding tube, or steroid treatment. Report this disorder with a code from ICD-9-CM subcategory 535.7.

eosinophilic gastroenteritis Disorder involving the accumulation of eosinophil in the tissues lining the GI tract, but without a known cause such as connective tissue disease, drug reaction, malignancy, or parasitic infection. The resultant inflammation at multiple levels of the GI tract may cause severe abdominal pain and vomiting. Treatment may include diet limitation, use of a feeding tube, or steroid treatment. Report this disorder with ICD-9-CM code 558.41. **Synonym(s):** *eosinophilic enteritis.*

Eovist Brand name for gadoxetate disodium, an organ-specific intravenous MRI contrast agent used to detect and diagnose lesions in the liver. Supply is reported with HCPCS Level II code A9581.

EOY End of year.

EP *1)* Electrophysiologic. *2)* Eligible professional.

EPB Extensor pollicis brevis. Long extensor muscle of the thumb.

EPCA Early prostate cancer antigen. Tumor marker more specific than PSA used in identifying men at risk for prostate cancer. EPCA is currently in clinical trials.

EPF Endoscopic plantar fasciotomy. Treatment for plantar fasciitis in which a nick is made in the plantar fascia to relieve pain in the heel. Plantar fasciitis is reported with ICD-9-CM code 728.71. EPF is reported with CPT code 29893. If any bone is removed during the EPF, the EPF is bundled into the appropriate ostectomy code (e.g., 28119 or 28120).

epi- On, upon, in addition to.

epicardial electrode Stimulation device that is attached to or inserted into the heart muscle and connected to a generator.

Epicel Brand name cultured epidermal autograft that is a permanent skin replacement created from a culture of the patient's own skin cells. This technology is typically used in patients with deep burns over 30 percent or more of their bodies or in patients with congenital nevus. Application of Epicel is reported with CPT codes 15150-15157.

Epicondyle

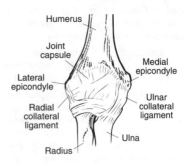

epicondyle Bony protrusion at the distal end of the humerus (elbow).

epidemic Outbreak of disease within a defined population that exceeds normal incidence rates.

epidemic pleurodynia Illness caused by infection with the coxsackie virus, affecting children and young adults. Symptoms include fever, abdominal pain, headache, and paroxysmal chest pain typically worsened by breathing or coughing. Report this illness with ICD-9-CM code 074.1. **Synonym(s):** *Bornholm disease.*

epidemic vomiting syndrome Nausea and vomiting attacking a group of people suddenly without prior illness or malaise. Headache, vomiting, abdominal pain, and giddiness end quickly. Report this disorder with ICD-9-CM code 078.82. **Synonym(s):** *winter's disease.*

epidermal Pertaining to or on the outer layer of skin.

Epidermis

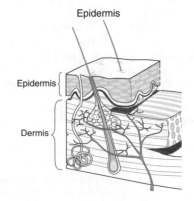

epidermis Outermost, nonvascular layer of skin that contains four to five differentiated layers depending on its body location: stratum corneum, lucidum, granulosum, spinosum, and basale. **Synonym(s):** *cuticle.*

epidermolysis bullosa Group of uncommon, inherited skin disorders manifested by frequently occurring painful blisters and open sores. Epidermolysis bullosa often

D-F

occurs as a result of minor trauma, due to the skin's abnormally fragile state. The eyes, tongue, and esophagus may be involved in the more severe forms of the disease, and scarring and musculoskeletal abnormalities may occur. Report this disorder with ICD-9-CM code 757.39. **Synonym(s):** *Köbner's disease.*

Epidex Brand name cultured epidermal autograft that is a permanent skin replacement created from the patient's own cells. This technology is typically used in patients with recalcitrant ulcers. Application of Epidex is reported with CPT codes 15150-15157.

Epididymis

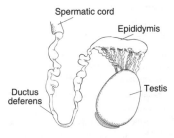

Spermatic cord

Epididymis

Testis

Ductus deferens

epididymis Coiled tube on the back of the testis that is the site of sperm maturation and storage and where spermatozoa are propelled into the vas deferens toward the ejaculatory duct by contraction of smooth muscle.

epididymitis Inflammation of the epididymis, which may be acute or chronic, and is generally caused by a bacterial infection. The most common etiology is a urinary tract infection, although it can also be caused by surgery, catheterization, congenital abnormalities, or sexually transmitted diseases. Nonvenereal and nontuberculous epididymitis is reported with a code from ICD-9-CM category 604, with an additional code to identify the causative organism. Other specified types are reported specifically within the infectious diseases chapter.

epididymo-orchitis Inflammation of the testes and epididymis.

epidural Anesthesia commonly used during labor and delivery achieved by the injection of anesthetic agent between the vertebral spines into the extradural space.

epidural block Anesthesia induced by injection of an anesthetic agent into the epidural space between the wall of the vertebral canal and dura mater. Most frequently used for normal spontaneous vaginal and cesarean deliveries. **Synonym(s):** *neuroaxial labor anesthesia.*

epidural space Area between the dura mater and the interior surface of the spinal canal, containing fat, veins, and arteries.

epigastric hernia Protrusion of a section of the intestine, omentum, or other structure through a fascial defect opening in the abdominal wall just above the umbilicus.

epiglottis Lid-like cartilaginous tissue that covers the entrance to the larynx and blocks food from entering the trachea.

epilation Depilation or removal of hair from the body by pulling the hair shaft out at the roots or employing electrical means to destroy the root. Electrolysis epilation is reported with CPT code 17380. **Synonym(s):** *electrolysis.*

epileptic confusional or twilight state Short-lived organic, psychotic states, caused by an epileptic episode, lasting hours or days, characterized by clouded consciousness, disorientation, fear, illusions, delusions, hallucinations of any kind, notably visual and tactile, restlessness, tremor, and sometimes fever.

epinephrine adrenalin Adrenergic drug with multiple effects and uses including vasopressor, cardiac stimulant, bronchodilator, local anesthetic, and topical antihemorrhagic. It is used to treat acute asthma attacks, bronchospasm, and to restore heart rhythm during cardiac arrest. Supply is reported with HCPCS Level II code J0171. May be sold under the brand names Adrenalin Chloride, ANA-Guard, AsthmaHaler Mist, Auto-injector, bronchodilator, Bronitin Mist, Bronkaid Mist, Bronkaid Mist Suspension, Bronkaid Mistometer, Adrenalin, Epi Pen, Epi Pen JR. Autoinjector, Medihaler-Epi, Primatene Mist, Primatene Mist Suspension, Sus-Phrine.

EpiPen Brand name automatic injector of epinephrine prescribed to adults or children with a history of anaphylaxis, for use in an allergic emergency.

epiphora Overflow of tears down the cheeks due to a stricture in the lacrimal passages. **Synonym(s):** *illacrimation.*

epiphysiodesis Surgical fusion of an epiphysis performed to prematurely stop further bone growth.

epiphysis End of a long bone.

epiphysitis of the calcaneus Inflammation of the calcaneus at the point of Achilles tendon insertion usually occurring in boys ages 8 to 14. Pain, tenderness, and localized swelling are present. Report this condition with ICD-9-CM code 732.5. **Synonym(s):** *calcaneal apophysitis, Sever's disease.*

epiploic Of or relating to the omentum, as in epiploic fat. **Synonym(s):** *omental.*

epirubicin HCl Cytotoxic drug used as a component of adjuvant therapy for patients with evidence of axillary node involvement following resection of primary breast cancer. Supply is reported with HCPCS Level II code J9178. May be sold under the brand name Ellence.

D-F

Epis. Episiotomy.

episiotomy Deliberate incision in the perineal tissue to facilitate delivery of the fetus and avoid traumatic tearing. In a midline or median episiotomy, the incision is made from the vagina straight down toward the anus. In a mediolateral episiotomy, the incision slants to one side. When episiotomy alone is performed, it is reported with ICD-9-CM procedure code 73.6, which includes the subsequent suturing for repair. In the CPT book, the episiotomy and its repair is included in the delivery code. If someone other than the attending physician repairs the episiotomy, report CPT code 59300. **Synonym(s):** *episioproctotomy, perineotomy.*

episode of care One or more health care services received during a period of relatively continuous care by a hospital or health care provider.

episode of payment Under HHPPS, a 60-day unit of payment.

Epispadias

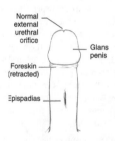

Normal external urethral orifice

Glans penis

Foreskin (retracted)

Epispadias

Dorsal view

epispadias *1)* Male anomaly in which the urethral opening is abnormally located on the dorsum of the penis, appearing as a groove with no upper urethral wall covering. *2)* Female anomaly with a slit in the upper wall of the urethra that may open toward or into the clitoris. Epispadias is reported with ICD-9-CM codes 752.62 and 753.8. This condition requires surgical correction.

epistaxis Nosebleed; hemorrhaging from the nose. If intervention is required, nasal packing or electrocautery are most common methods. Epistaxis is reported with ICD-9-CM code 784.7.

epithelial tissue Cells arranged in sheets that cover internal and external body surfaces that can absorb, protect, and/or secrete. Epithelial tissue includes the protective covering for external surfaces (skin), absorptive linings for internal surfaces such as the intestine, and secreting structures such as salivary or sweat glands.

epithelize Formation of epithelial cells over a surface.

Epley maneuver Therapy for benign positional paroxysmal vertigo. In the Epley maneuver, the clinician has the patient lie down and rotate his head to displace canaliths in the inner ear. The canaliths may be the source of dizziness in the patient. The Epley maneuver is reported with CPT code 95992.

EPO *1)* Epoetin alpha. *2)* Exclusive provider organization. In health care contracting, an organization similar to an HMO, but the member must remain within the provider network to receive benefits. EPOs are regulated under insurance statutes rather than HMO legislation.

EPO Exclusive provider organization. In health care contracting, an organization similar to an HMO, but the member must remain within the provider network to receive benefits. EPOs are regulated under insurance statutes rather than HMO legislation.

eponychium Thin layer of epidermis or skin found at the proximal portion and sides of the nail or the cuticle.

eponym Name of a drug, structure, disease, or procedure based on or derived from the name of a person. Example: Parkinson's disease.

epoprostenol Systemic prostaglandin that works to relax the pulmonary vasculature, used in cases of pulmonary hypertension. This takes the workload off the right side of the heart, which has to pump harder when the pressure is higher in the pulmonary vascular tree. Supply is reported with HCPCS Level II code J1325. May be sold under the brand name Flolan.

eposteal implant Dental implant receiving bone support by leaning on residual mandibular bone. **Synonym(s):** *subperiosteal dental implant.*

EPP Erythropoietic protoporphyria. Inherited disorder with a deficiency in ferrochelatase. Abnormally high levels of protoporphyrin IX in erythrocytes, feces, and plasma. Symptoms include erythema and edema, exacerbated by exposure to sunlight. EPP is reported with ICD-9-CM code 277.1.

e-prescribing Transmission of prescription or prescription-related information between the prescriber and the medication dispenser. For Medicare purposes, e-prescribing includes but is not limited to two-way transmission between the point of care and the dispenser.

EPS Electrophysiological study. Invasive diagnostic procedure that requires the intracardiac placing and repositioning of two or more electrode catheters, recording electrograms before and during pacing or electrical stimulation of multiple locations, and an analysis of the recorded information with a findings report. Electrophysiological studies are often performed with the induction of an arrhythmia by pacing in order to map out an induced tachycardia in its electrical path and site of origin, and then ablate the involved heart tissue. These procedures are reported separately unless it is specifically stated in combination with another code description. Intracardiac electrophysiological studies are found within their own subchapter of the medicine section of the CPT book, 93600-93662.

EPSDT Early and Periodic Screening, Diagnosis and Treatment Program. Preventive dental care.

epsom salts See magnesium salts.

Epstein's syndrome Nephrosis caused by chemical toxicity.

eptifibatide Antiplatelet drug that binds permanently to the IIb/IIIa glycoprotein receptor on platelets, inhibiting them from aggregating or sticking together to form a clot. This drug is used as medical intervention for acute coronary syndrome, unstable angina, and non-Q wave MI. Supply is reported with HCPCS Level II code J1327. May be sold under the brand name Integrilin.

ER Emergency room.

ER- Estrogen receptor negative status, reported with ICD-9-CM code V86.1.

ER+ Estrogen receptor positive status, reported with ICD-9-CM code V86.0.

ERA Electronic remittance advice. Any of several electronic formats for explaining the payments of health care claims.

Erb (-Oppenheim) -Goldflam syndrome Myoneural conduction-caused progressive muscular weakness beginning in face and throat. Report this disorder with ICD-9-CM code 358.00. *Synonym(s): Erb syndrome, Goldflam syndrome, Hoppe syndrome.*

Erbitux Brand name monoclonal antibody for treatment of metastatic colorectal cancer or squamous cell carcinoma of the head and neck. Erbitux is administered by infusion, reported with CPT codes 96409, 96411, 96413, 96415, or 96417 or inpatient ICD-9-CM code 99.28. Erbitux contains cetuximab.

ERC Endoscopic retrograde cholangiography.

ERCP Endoscopic retrograde cholangiopancreatography. Examination of the hepatobiliary system and gallbladder performed through a flexible fiberoptic endoscope. ERCP is reported with CPT codes 43260-43272. Radiologic supervision and interpretation is reported in addition to the procedure.

Erdheim's syndrome Spondylosis of the cervical spine in a patient with acromegaly, resembling rheumatoid arthritis and progressing to bony ankylosis with lipping of vertebral margins. Report this disorder with ICD-9-CM code 253.0.

Erecaid Brand name vacuum erection device to treat impotence. Supply of Erecaid is reported with HCPCS Level II code L7900.

ERG Electroretinogram.

ergonovine maleate Drug used to treat uterine hemorrhage secondary to uterine atony status post delivery of the placenta or abortion. It is also used as a diagnostic aid to test angina as it does cause the coronary arteries to constrict. Unlike other alkaloid ergots, this drug does not have an effect on migraines and is not indicated as such. Supply is reported with HCPCS Level II code J1330. May be sold under the brand name Ergotrate maleate.

Ergotrate maleate See ergonovine maleate.

ERISA Employee Retirement Income Security Act of 1974, Public Law 93-406. Mandates reporting, disclosure of grievance and appeals requirements, and fiduciary standards for private group life and health plans, and preempts state benefit mandates and premium tax laws for self-funded group health plans.

Erlacher-Blount syndrome Disease causing bowlegs in children. Report this disorder with ICD-9-CM code 732.4.

erlotinib Oral medication for the treatment of non-small cell lung cancer and pancreatic cancer.

erosion Eating away or gradual breaking down of the surface of a structure.

ertapenem sodium Parenteral antibiotic drug reserved for serious infections, such as intra-abdominal, skin, urinary tract, and pelvic inflammatory disease. Supply is reported with HCPCS Level II code J1335. May be sold under the brand name Invanz.

erupted tooth Tooth that protrudes through the gingival soft tissues.

erythema multiforme Complex of symptoms with a varied pattern of skin eruptions, such as macular, bullous, papular, nodose, or vesicular lesions on the neck, face, and legs. Gastritis and rheumatoid pain are also present as the first noticeable symptoms. This complex is secondary to a number of factors including infections, ingestants, physical agents, malignancy, and pregnancy. Erythema multiforme is reported with an ICD-9-CM code from range 695.10-695.19. *Synonym(s): scalded skin syndrome. e. m. exudativum* Type of erythema multiforme that begins with flu-like symptoms and produces severe mucocutaneous lesions affecting the mouth, nose, anal, and genital regions with formation of a grayish-white pseudomembrane, hemorrhagic crusting of the lips, ocular lesions, corneal opacities, even blindness. Other systemic lesions and visceral and thoracic organ involvement also occurs and can be fatal. This condition is reported with ICD-9-CM code 695.19. *e. m. of eye* Stevens-Johnson syndrome of the eye consisting of severe conjunctival inflammation with lesions and possible adhesion of eyelids and conjunctiva to the globe.

erythema nodosum Type of panniculitis or an inflammatory reaction of the deep dermis and

D-F

subcutaneous fat in women, usually a hypersensitivity response to infections, drugs, sarcoidosis, or specific enteropathies. Tender lesions pink to blue in color appear as nodules on the shins. The acute stage may have symptoms of fever, fatigue, and joint pain. This condition is classified to ICD-9-CM code 695.2.

erythrocyte fragmentation syndrome Fragmentation of red blood cells. Report this disorder with ICD-9-CM code 283.19. *Synonym(s): Lederer-Brill syndrome.*

eschar Leathery slough produced by burns.

escharotomy Surgical incision into the scab or crust resulting from a severe burn in order to relieve constriction and allow blood flow to the distal unburned tissue. This procedure is reported with CPT codes 16035 and 16036.

Escherichia coli Gram negative, anaerobic of the family Enterobacteriaceae found in the large intestine of warm-blooded animals, generally as a non-pathologic entity aiding in digestion. They become pathogenic when an opportunity to grow somewhere outside this relationship presents itself, such as ingestion of fecal contaminated food or water. The species coli (ICD-9-CM category 008) is the principle organism found in the human intestine and has both pathogenic and nonpathogenic strains. The enterotoxigenic form causes cholera-like illness while the enteroinvasive form causes dysentery by invading the epithelial cells of the human colon. Bloody stools are seen with the enterohemorrhagic strain. A relatively new strain of E. coli has been identified as E. coli O157:H7, found in undercooked beef and unpasteurized apple juice.

esophageal achalasia Failure of the smooth muscles at the esophagogastric junction to relax when swallowing, reported with ICD-9-CM code 530.0.

esophageal dyskinesia Difficulty swallowing due to impairment in the natural, voluntary movement of the esophagus. This condition is reported with ICD-9-CM code 530.5.

esophageal leukoplakia Thickening of the epithelium of the esophagus causing the appearance of white spots on the mucosa.

esophageal reflux Regurgitation of the gastric contents into the esophagus and possibly the pharynx. Report esophageal reflux with ICD-9-CM code 530.81.

esophageal varices Distended, tortuous varicose veins in the lower esophagus. Esophageal varices are frequently a cause of esophageal hemorrhaging and commonly a symptom of portal hypertension from chronic liver disease, especially alcoholic cirrhosis. This condition is reported with ICD-9-CM codes 456.0-456.21.

esophagismus Dispersed, involuntary esophageal spasms, often caused by increased activity of the

innervating vagus nerve. Report this condition with ICD-9-CM code 530.5. *Synonym(s): esophagism.*

esophagitis Inflammation of the esophagus.

esophagogastric fundoplasty See Nissen procedure.

esophagoscopy Internal visual inspection of the esophagus through the use of an endoscope placed down the throat. Esophagoscopy is reported with CPT codes 43200-43232.

esophagus Muscular tube that carries swallowed liquids and foods from the pharynx to the stomach.

esotropia Misalignment of the eye usually evidenced by the eye turning inward.

ESR Erythrocyte sedimentation rate.

ESRD End stage renal disease. Progression of chronic renal failure to lasting and irreparable kidney damage that requires dialysis or renal transplant for survival. ESRD is most often caused by diabetes, although hypertension is also a common cause. A diagnosis of ESRD alone is assigned ICD-9-CM code 585.6. Hypertensive renal disease or heart and renal disease specified as with renal failure is coded to the circulatory chapter in ICD-9-CM categories 403 and 404. ESRD-related physician services are reported with CPT range 90951-90970.

essential hypertension Elevated arterial blood pressure that occurs without an apparent organic cause. In the benign form, the blood pressure is mildly elevated. In the malignant form, the elevation is severe and may result in necrosis of the kidneys or retinas. Hemorrhage and death may occur, most often due to uremia or rupture of cerebral vessels. Report essential hypertension with a code from ICD-9-CM category 401.

essential modifiers Subterms listed below the ICD-9-CM main term and indented.

Essex-Lopresti fracture Comminuted fracture of the radial head due to longitudinal compression force, reported with ICD-9-CM code 813.05, and occurring with a distal dislocation of the radioulnar joint, reported with ICD-9-CM code 833.01.

Essure Brand name new product for female sterilization. Metal coils that occlude the fallopian tubes are inserted via a catheter threaded through the vagina and uterus into the fallopian tubes under radiologic guidance. No incision or general anesthesia is required.

EST Electroshock therapy.

established patient Patient who has received professional services in a face-to-face setting within the last three years from the same physician or another physician of the same specialty who belongs to the same group practice. If the patient is seen by a physician who is covering for another physician, the patient will be considered the same as if seen by the physician who is unavailable.

estimated length of stay Average number of days of hospitalization required for a given illness or procedure, based on prior histories of patients who have been hospitalized for the same illness or procedure. *Synonym(s): ELOS.*

estradiol Principal and most potent mammalian estrogen produced by the ovaries, which prepares the uterus for implantation after fertilization and is responsible for female reproductive organ maturation. Estradiol has been reproduced semisynthetically. *Synonym(s): E2.*

estriol Weak estrogen derived from estradiol that is produced in large quantities during pregnancy and detected in the urine. Estriol is believed to have some antineoplastic effects.

estrogen Group of estrus-stimulating hormones produced by the ovaries, possibly the adrenal cortex and testes, that have different functions in both sexes. They are the main female sex hormones (estradiol, estrone, and estriol) responsible for the maturation and development of female secondary sex characteristics and act on the reproductive organs to prepare for fertilization, implantation, and nourishment of the embryo. Estrogens also have nonreproductive actions such as minimizing calcium loss from bones by antagonizing the effects of parathyroid hormone and promoting blood clotting.

estrone Product of metabolism of estradiol, known to be less potent than estradiol but more so than estriol. This hormone is found circulating in human plasma and follicular fluid, and in human and horse urine in both males and pregnant females. This estrogen is reproduced synthetically to treat ovarian failure or removal, hypogonadism, atrophic vaginitis, menopausal symptoms, and advanced prostatic cancer. *Synonym(s): E1.*

estrone 5 See estrogen.

ESWL Extracorporeal shockwave lithotripsy. Destruction of calcified substances in the gallbladder or urinary system by means of directing shock waves at the calculus through a liquid medium to smash the concretion into small particles that can then be passed out of the body. ESWL is reported with CPT code 50590.

ESWT Extracorporeal shock wave therapy. ESWT devices generate pulses of high-pressure sound that travel through the skin. Soft tissue and bone subjected to these pulses of high-pressure energy heal stronger.

et And.

ET Endotracheal.

etanercept Drug used to treat moderate to severe rheumatoid arthritis (RA) and active polyarticular juvenile arthritis in patients who have not had relief from other

disease modifying RA drugs. It decreases the immune and inflammatory responses in these diseases triggered by tumor necrosis factor (TNF) by blocking TNF action. Supply is reported with HCPCS Level II code J1438. May be sold under the brand name Enbrel.

ETD Eustachian tube dysfunction.

ETG Episode treatment group.

Ethamolin See ethanolamine oleate.

ethanolamine oleate Drug used to treat esophageal varices either during or after hemorrhaging. It inflames the intimal lining of the vein, causing fibrosis and ultimately occlusion of the bleeding vessel. Supply is reported with HCPCS Level II code J1430. May be sold under the brand name Ethamolin.

Ethilon Brand name nylon suture used in wound repair. A nonabsorbable monofilament, its supply is incidental to the repair or procedure code.

ethmoid bone Cube-shaped bone located between the orbits.

ethmoid bulla Rounded projection from the ethmoid bone found in the space beneath the middle turbinate of the nose, enclosing an anterior ethmoid air cell.

ethmoidectomy Excision of all or a portion of the cube-shaped bone located between the orbits.

Ethyol See amifostine.

etidronate disodium Antihypercalcemic drug used for the treatment of symptomatic Paget's disease of bone and in the prevention and treatment of heterotopic ossification following total hip replacement as well as in the treatment of hypercalcemia that sometimes occurs in cancer patients. Supply is reported with HCPCS Level II code J1436. May be sold under the brand name Etidronate.

etiology Science and study of the causes of disease.

ETOH Alcohol.

etonogestrel implant Contraceptive implant consisting of a single rod that is inserted subcutaneously in the inner upper arm, where it slowly releases a progestogenic hormone. Supply of the implant system is reported with HCPCS Level II code J7307. *Synonym(s): Implanon.*

etoposide Chemotherapy drug used to treat testicular cancers, small cell cancer of the lung, and Kaposi's sarcoma secondary to AIDS. This plant alkaloid inhibits tumor growth by stopping cellular division. Supply is reported with HCPCS Level II codes J8560 and J9181. May be sold under the brand names Etopophos, Toposar, and Vespid (VP-16).

ETS Endoscopic thoracic sympathectomy. Surgery in which portions of the sympathetic nerve trunk are excised or destroyed, usually as a treatment for moderate to severe cases of sweaty palms (hyperhidrosis, ICD-9-CM code 705.21). ETS is reported with CPT code 32664.

D-F

eu- Well, healthy, good, normal.

Euflexxa Brand name high molecular weight glycosaminoglycan (GAG) that has viscous properties, most often used as a synovial fluid substitute injected directly into the knee for pain associated with osteoarthritis. It provides lubrication and shock absorption at the joint in the same manner as synovial fluid. Report the injection into the knee joint separately. Supply of the intra-articular injection is reported with HCPCS Level II code J7323. **Synonym(s):** *hyaluronic acid, sodium hyaluronate.*

Eulenburg's disease Uncommon, inherited disorder affecting the proximal muscles of the limbs, eyelids, and the tongue, manifested by failure of the muscles to relax after contracting (myotonia). The exacerbation is exposure to cold temperatures and aggravated by activity. Flaccid paresis may also occur on an irregular basis. This condition is not considered progressive. Report this disease with ICD-9-CM code 359.29. **Synonym(s):** *congenital paramyotonia.*

eunuchism Condition in which the testes or exterior genital organs of the male fail to develop or are removed, particularly in cases of castration prior to reaching puberty, resulting in the failure of secondary sex characteristics to develop, such as facial and body hair, deepening of the voice, and muscle mass development. Report this condition with ICD-9-CM code 257.2.

eustachian tube Internal channel between the tympanic cavity and the nasopharynx that equalizes internal pressure to the outside pressure and drains mucous production from the middle ear. **Synonym(s):** *auditory tube.*

euthyroid sick syndrome Transient alteration in thyroid hormone metabolism resulting in abnormally low levels of the thyroid hormone tri-iodothyronine in persons with systemic, non-thyroid illness or stress, and no symptoms of hypothyroidism. Report this condition with ICD-9-CM code 790.94.

evacuation Removal or purging of waste material.

evaluation Dynamic process in which the physical, occupational, sports, or other therapist makes clinical judgments based on data gathered during the examination.

evaluation Dynamic process in which the dentist makes clinical judgments based on data gathered during the examination.

evaluation and management Assessment, counseling, and other services provided to a patient reported through CPT codes.

evaluation and management codes Assessment and management of a patient's health care using CPT codes 99201-99499.

evaluation and management service components Key components of history, examination, and medical decision making that are key to selecting the correct E/M codes. Other non-key components include counseling, coordination of care, nature of presenting problem, and time.

Evans' syndrome Condition where number of platelets in circulating blood increases, causing bruising. Report this disorder with ICD-9-CM code 287.32.

EVAR Endovascular aortic repair. Deployment of a prosthetic stent via a catheter into the site of an abdominal aortic aneurysm (AAA). The stent provides a safe conduit for blood flow to relieve pressure on the aneurysm as the blood flows through the stent instead of continuing to bulge the sac formed by the aorta wall dilation. EVAR is reported with CPT codes 34800-34826.

event recorder Portable, ambulatory heart monitor worn by the patient that makes electrocardiographic recordings of the length and frequency of aberrant cardiac rhythm to help diagnose heart conditions and to assess pacemaker functioning or programming.

eventration Projection of the intestine through an abnormal opening in the abdominal wall; intestinal hernia.

Everbusch's operation Elevation of the levator muscle to correct ptosis of the upper eyelid.

evisceration Removal of contents of a cavity. *eye e* Removal of the contents of the eyeball, with the sclera being left intact. *organ e* Removal of internal organs. Although usually the result of trauma, evisceration may be surgically performed.

EVR Evoked visual response.

Ex *1)* Examination. *2)* Extended.

ExAblate Brand name high-focus ultrasound system requiring magnetic resonance guidance for ablation of uterine fibroid tumors. The fibroids are reported with a code from ICD-9-CM category 218, and the ablation, including ultrasound and magnetic resonance, is reported with CPT code 0071T or 0072T.

examination Comprehensive visual and tactile screening and specific testing leading to diagnosis or, as appropriate, to a referral to another practitioner.

Exanthema Skin rash appearing as a sign of a disease, such as measles. **Synonym(s):** *rash.*

exc Excise.

exchange Substitution of one thing for another.

Excimer laser Ultraviolet laser used in refractive surgery to remove corneal tissue.

excise Remove or cut out.

excision Surgical removal of an organ or tissue.

D-F

excluded services Services not covered by Medicare, including routine physical check-ups, eye exams, foot care, eyeglasses, hearing aids, immunizations not related to injury or immediate risk of infection, cosmetic surgery not related to an illness or injury, items and services not reasonable and necessary for diagnosing and treating an illness or injury, custodial care, personal comfort items, etc.

EXCLUDER Brand name, bifurcated endoprosthesis used to repair an abdominal aortic aneurysm where it branches into the two iliac arteries.

exclusions Services excluded from a plan's coverage by the employer or payer because of risk or cost.

exclusive provider organization Similar to an HMO, but the member must remain within the provider network to receive benefits. EPOs are regulated under insurance statutes rather than HMO legislation. *Synonym(s): EPO.*

exclusivity Sole right to provide a service or benefit, usually giving a provider or group the sole right to provide specific services without having to share the right with other providers or groups.

exemestane Antineoplastic used to treat estrogen dependent breast cancer in postmenopausal women who have progressed beyond Tamoxifen treatment. It permanently binds to aromatase, inhibiting the enzyme's ability to convert androgens to estrogens. Supply is reported with HCPCS Level II code S0156. May be sold under the brand name Aromasin. Report prophylactic use with ICD-9-CM code V07.52.

exenteration Surgical removal of the entire contents of a body cavity, such as the pelvis or orbit.

exfoliate Skin falling off in layers.

exfoliation Falling or sloughing off skin in layers. Report a code from ICD-9-CM subcategory 695.5 to identify percentages of skin exfoliation.

exhaustion delirium Acute transient disorders of any severity and nature of emotions, consciousness, and psychomotor states (singly or in combination) that occur in individuals, without any apparent pre-existing mental disorder, in response to exceptional physical or mental stress, such as natural catastrophe or battle. The symptoms usually subside within hours or days.

exhaustion syndrome Hypersomatic disorder. Report this disorder with ICD-9-CM code 300.5.

exhibitionism Sexual deviation in which the main sexual pleasure and gratification is derived from exposure of the genitals to a person of the opposite sex.

exo- Outside of, without.

exocervix Region of the cervix uteri that protrudes into the vagina.

exodontia Branch of dentistry related to the extraction or pulling of teeth.

exomphalos Congenital abnormality in which certain organs of the abdomen protrude or herniate into the umbilical cord, reported with ICD-9-CM code 756.79.

exophthalmos Abnormal bulging or protrusion of the eyeballs, seen in cases of hyperthyroidism, like Grave's disease and toxic diffuse goiter, or as a congenital condition.

exophytic Growing outward from the epithelium, usually describing a neoplasm. The term, ôexophyticô has no bearing on the status of the neoplasm's morphology (benign, malignant, etc.).

exostectomy Excision of a bony projection.

exostosis Abnormal formation of a benign bony growth.

exotropia Frequently occurring form of strabismus characterized by permanent or intermittent deviation of the visual axis when one eye turns outward while the other fixes upon an image, affecting one or both eyes. The various forms of exotropia are reported with codes from ICD-9-CM subcategories 378.1 and 378.2. *Synonym(s): Walleye.*

expanded problem focused physical examination Under the 1995 guidelines, examination of two to seven organ systems. Under the 1997 guidelines, examination of at least six bullet point elements in one or more organ systems from the general multisystem examination OR examination of at least six of the bullet point elements from one of the 10 single organ system exams.

expected outcomes Intended results of patient/client management, which indicate the changes in impairments, functional limitations, and disabilities and the changes in health, wellness, and fitness needs that are expected as the result of implementing the plan of care.

Exper Experimental.

experience rating In medical reimbursement, designation of a group's previous claims history to help determine premium rates.

explanation of benefits Statement mailed to the member and provider explaining claim adjudication and payment. *Synonym(s): EOB.*

explanation of Medicare benefits Medicare statement mailed to the member and provider explaining claim adjudication and payment. *Synonym(s): EOMB.*

exploration Examination for diagnostic purposes.

explosive personality disorder Instability of mood with uncontrollable outbursts of anger, hate, violence, or affection demonstrated by words or actions.

exposure In surgery, to display, reveal, or make accessible.

D-F

expression In surgery, the squeezing out of tissue.

exstrophy Congenital defect in the front of the bladder wall, associated with lack of closure of the pubic bone at the symphysis pubis.

exstrophy of bladder Congenital anomaly occurring when the bladder everts itself, or turns inside out, through an absent part of the lower abdominal and anterior bladder walls with incomplete closure of the pubic bone.

Ext External.

ext. Extremity.

extended care facility Institution that provides any type of long-term care. Usually refers to a skilled nursing facility, but may be used in reference to other types of long-term institutions.

extended care services Items and services provided to an inpatient of a skilled nursing facility, including nursing care, physical or occupational therapy, speech pathology, drugs and supplies, and medical social services.

extended history of present illness Detailed narrative of the presenting illness, including at least four elements: location, quality, severity, duration, timing, context, modifying factors, or associated signs and symptoms.

extended system review Narrative of two to nine organ systems reviewed directly related to the chief complaint or history of present illness plus a review of a limited number of additional, related systems.

extensive polyp Polyp that is thick at the base and firmly attached.

extensor Any muscle that extends a joint.

exteriorize In surgery, to expose an organ temporarily for observation.

external auditory canal/meatus External channel that leads from the opening in the external ear to the tympanic membrane (eardrum).

external carotid artery Major artery of the head and neck arising from the common carotid artery where it bifurcates into an internal and external branch.

external circulatory assist device Any mechanical device, such as anti shock trousers or air pressure cuffs, placed on the outside of the body to help increase myocardial perfusion, cardiac output, and peripheral circulation by applying counterpressure or synchronous compression to the muscles through rhythmic inflation and deflation with the patient's cardiac cycle. This therapeutic cardio-assist method is reported with CPT code 92971.

external electrical capacitor device External electrical stimulation device designed to promote bone healing. This device may also promote neural regeneration,

revascularization, epiphyseal growth, and ligament maturation.

external fixation
Rods and pins connected in a lattice to secure bone. There are several indications for external fixation:

acute fractures: External fixation may be required when a limb fracture is complicated by severe bony comminution, extensive soft tissue damage, or multiple trauma.

failure of previous treatment: External fixation may also be used after acute injury when there is delayed healing or nonunion of the fracture or when infection is present.

other uses include: Fixation in major pelvic disruption, joint fusion (arthrodesis), osteotomy, bone lengthening, or shortening procedures.

external os Uterine opening through the cervix and into the vagina.

external pulsating electromagnetic field External stimulation device designed to promote bone healing. This device may also promote neural regeneration, revascularization, epiphyseal growth, and ligament maturation.

external thrombosed hemorrhoid Reversed blood flow and clotted blood within a vein that extends beyond the anus.

extr. Extract.

extracoronal Portion of the tooth outside the corona or crown.

extracorporeal Located or taking place outside the body.

extracorporeal membrane oxygenation Procedure done for cardiopulmonary insufficiency that shunts the circulating venous blood through catheters inserted into the right atrium to the outside of the body where it is oxygenated, bypassing the lungs, then returned to the body through another cannula inserted in the femoral artery. Cannula insertion is reported with CPT code 36822, while the initial 24 hours of prolonged circulation is reported with 33960. *Synonym(s): ECMO.*

extract Condensed medication.

extraction Removal of a tooth and tooth fragments from the alveolus.

extradural Located outside of the dura mater.

extradural hemorrhage Bleeding or accumulation of blood within the skull but not invading the membrane covering the brain, or meninges, that may cause pressure against the brain.

extramural birth Infant born outside of a sterile environment.

extranasal approach Incision from outside of the nose to gain access into the sinus cavity.

extraocular muscles Six orbital muscles (extrinsic) that move the eyeball. *Synonym(s): EOM.*

extravasate Escape the confines. Most commonly used in reference to blood cells leaking outside the blood vessel into surrounding tissue.

extravasation Escape of fluid from a vessel into the surrounding tissue.

extrication collar Cervical collar with opening at the throat for patients who have a tracheotomy or tracheostomy.

exudate Fluid or other material, such as debris from cells, that has escaped blood vessel circulation and is deposited in or on tissues and usually occurs due to inflammation.

exudative eye cysts Protein or fatty fluid-filled sacs of the iris or ciliary body of unknown cause.

exudative macular degeneration Sharp central vision loss usually from the development of subretinal neovascularization (new blood vessels) and related exudative (leaking) maculopathy.

exudative retinopathy Destructive cholesterol-type deposits inflaming the retina in the posterior eye. *Synonym(s): Coats disease.*

exudative senile macular degeneration New vessel formation in the oxygen-deprived tissues feeding the retina. This neovascularization results in tiny, delicate vessels that break easily, causing leakage, hemorrhaging, swelling, and damage to surrounding tissue, and accounts for 10 percent of all cases of macular degeneration in the United States. Report this condition with ICD-9-CM code 362.52. *Synonym(s): disciform senile macular degeneration, neovascular macular degeneration, wet macular degeneration.*

EY HCPCS Level II modifier, for use with CPT or HCPCS Level II codes, that identifies that a physician or other licensed health care provider did not order an item or service. It does not override denial for services requiring an order from a physician or provider and cannot be used for procedures or services when an HHABN or ABN is required.

eye retraction syndrome Retraction of eye muscles with inability to abduct the affected eye with retraction of the globe. Report this disorder with ICD-9-CM code 378.71. *Synonym(s): Duane syndrome, Still-Turk-Duane syndrome.*

Eye

eye tarsus Inner framework of the eyelids that provides stiffness and shape.

eyelid-malar-mandible syndrome Malformations of derivatives of the first branchial arch, with palpebral fissures sloping outward and downward with notches in the outer third of the lower lids, defects of malar bones and zygoma, hypoplasia of the jawbone, high or cleft palate, low-set ears, unusual hair growth, and pits between mouth and ear. Report this disorder with ICD-9-CM code 756.0. *Synonym(s): Franceschetti's syndrome.*

Eyre-Brook capsulorrhaphy Reattachment of the capsule of the shoulder and glenoid labrum to the glenoid lip.

F *1)* Fahrenheit. *2)* Female. *3)* Firm. *4)* French.

f.m. Make a mixture.

F/U Follow-up.

FA *1)* Fractional anisotropy. In the medical record, diagnostic exploration via MRI of white matter of brain to identify flaws. In anisotropy, the image changes when the point of view changes, like the warp of velvet fabric. It is a useful technique when examining white matter via MRI. *2)* HCPCS Level II modifier indicating the left hand thumb and used in OPPS (outpatient hospital) billing.

fab fragment Immunoglobulin molecule fragment that is antigen binding with a light and heavy chain.

Faber's syndrome Central pallor in the red blood cells caused by lack of red cell hemoglobin in blood. Report this disorder with ICD-9-CM code 280.9. *Synonym(s): Hayem-Faber syndrome.*

Fabry (-Anderson) syndrome Neutral glycolipids in histiocytes in blood vessel walls, cornea verticillata, paresthesia in extremities, cataracts and angiokeratomas on the thighs, buttocks, and genitalia. Death comes from

D-F

cardiac, cerebrovascular and renal complications. Report this disorder with ICD-9-CM code 272.7.

face to face   Interaction between two parties, usually provider and patient, that occurs in the physical presence of each other.

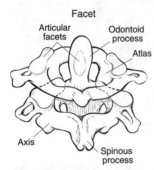

Facet

Articular facets   Odontoid process

Atlas

Axis

Spinous process

Posterior view of the first two vertebrae, the atlas (C-1) and the axis (C-2)

facet   Smooth surface area where the transverse and articular processes of certain vertebrae articulate with another vertebra. Each vertebra has two sets of facet joints, one on the left and one on the right. The superior articular facets face upward and the inferior articular facets face downward. **Synonym(s):** *apophyseal joints, zygapophyseal joints.*

facetectomy   Surgical excision of a vertebral articular facet, performed with laminectomy or laminotomy. This procedure is reported with CPT codes 63001-63048.

facial   Tooth surface that is facing the cheeks or lips.

facial diplegia syndrome   Unilateral lesions of the ninth, tenth, eleventh, and twelfth cranial nerves producing paralysis of the vagal, glossal, other nerves, and the tongue on the same side. Usually the result of injury. Report this disorder with ICD-9-CM code 352.6. **Synonym(s):** *Collet-Sicard syndrome.*

facial nerve   Seventh cranial nerve affecting hearing and vision, among other sensory abilities.

facial surface   In dentistry, tooth surface that is facing the cheeks or lips.

facility   Place of patient care, including inpatient and outpatient, acute or long term. *F. of payment* Contractual relationship that permits the payer to pay someone other than the member or provider.

facility component   Overhead related to the physical location, nursing and clerical staff, supplies including drugs and biologicals, special equipment, trained technicians, services of hospital ancillary departments, and all other services not performed by the physician

facility practice expense   One of the three components used to determine the relative value of physician services

paid under the resource-based relative value scale (RBRVS). Facility practice expense represents the physician's direct and indirect costs related to each service provided in a hospital, ambulatory surgery center (ASC), or skilled nursing facility (SNF).

facility services   Services that are furnished in connection with covered surgical procedures performed in an ASC or in a hospital on an outpatient basis.

factitious illness   Hysterical neurosis in which there are physical or psychological symptoms that are not real, genuine, or natural, which are produced by the individual and are under his or her voluntary control.

factitious illness physical symptom type   Presentation of physical symptoms that may be total fabrication, self-inflicted, an exaggeration or exacerbation of a pre-existing physical condition, or any combination or variation of these.

factitious illness psychological symptom type   Voluntary production of symptoms suggestive of a mental disorder with behavior that may mimic psychosis or the individual's idea of psychosis.

factor IX   Blood derivative of normal plasma that can be provided via recombinant DNA therapy to replace the patient's deficient clotting factor IX to treat Hemophilia B or Christmas disease. It is provided via IV infusion. Supply is reported with HCPCS Level II codes J7193, J7194, and J7195. May be sold under the brand names AlphaNine, Bebulin VH Immuno, Benefix, Konyne 80, Mononine, Profilnine SD, Proplex T.

factor VIIA   Recombinant form of activated factor VIII used to treat patients with Hemophilia A or B who have developed inhibitors to VIII or IX. Factor VIIA is successfully used in treating deficiencies without a means of replacing the missing clotting factor without massive plasma infusion. It is also used to treat bleeding from Warfarin therapy, trauma, and other acquired bleeding problems, and for other genetic platelet disorders. Supply is reported with HCPCS Level II code J7189. May be sold under the brand name NovoSeven.

factor VIII   Hereditary, sex-linked condition with missing antihemophilic globulin (AHG) (factor VIII). This condition causes abnormal coagulation characterized by increased bleeding; large bruises on the skin; bleeding in the mouth, nose, or gastrointestinal tract and hemorrhages into joints, resulting in swelling and impaired function. Report factor VIII disorders with ICD-9-CM code 286.0. Factor VIII deficiencies with vascular defect are reported with ICD-9-CM code 286.4. **Synonym(s):** *Helixate, Kogenate.*

fact-oriented V codes   Codes that do not describe a problem or a service; they simply state a fact. These generally do not serve as an outpatient primary or inpatient principal diagnosis.

Factrel   See gonadorelin HCl.

facultative anaerobe   Anaerobic bacteria that can grow in either oxygenated or non-oxygenated environments. Does not directly drive code selection, but does drive treatment decisions.

faculty practice plan   Group practice developed around a teaching program or medical school. *Synonym(s): FPP.*

failed attempted abortion   Induced medical abortion that does not eliminate the pregnancy, reported with a code from ICD-9-CM rubric 638.

failure   Inability to function.

fallopian tubes   Bilateral, paired tubes that extend from the uterus to the ovaries, through which an ovum released from the follicle travels to the uterus during ovulation. Thin projections that form a fringe around the ovarian end of the fallopian tube, called fimbria, collect the ova and deliver them into the tubes, where they are propelled toward the uterus by small hair-like projections called cilia. *Synonym(s): oviducts, uterine tube.*

Fallot's syndrome   Congenital cardiac defects with pulmonary stenosis, interventricular septal defect, dextroposeptum and venous as well as arterial blood, and right ventricular hypertrophy. Report this disorder with ICD-9-CM code 745.2. *Synonym(s): tetralogy of Fallot.*

Fallot's triad   Congenital anomaly of the heart involving pulmonary stenosis, atrial septal defect, and right ventricular hypertrophy, reported with ICD-9-CM code 746.09. *Synonym(s): trilogy of Fallot.*

False Claims Act   Governs civil actions for filing false claims. Liability under this act pertains to any person who knowingly presents or causes to be presented a false or fraudulent claim to the government for payment or approval.

familial acanthosis nigricans syndrome   Velvety acanthosis with gray, black, or brown pigmentation on axillae and other body folds. In adults, it results from internal carcinoma. In children, it results from obesity-producing endocrine disturbance. Report this disorder with ICD-9-CM code 701.2.

familial eczema-thrombocytopenia syndrome   Eczema, thrombocytopenia, and recurrent pyogenic infection with increased susceptibility to infection from encapsulated bacteria. Report this disorder with ICD-9-CM code 279.12. *Synonym(s): Aldrich syndrome, Wiskott-Aldrich syndrome.*

familial hepatitis   Rare, progressive, chronic disease caused by an inherited copper metabolism defect that results in the poisonous accumulation of copper in certain organs and tissues, such as the brain, kidneys, cornea, and liver. The disease causes cirrhosis, brain degeneration with progressive neurological dysfunction,

and pigmented Kayser-Fleischer corneal ring. Report this condition with ICD-9-CM code 275.1. *Synonym(s): hepatolenticular degeneration, Kinnier Wilson's disease, pseudosclerosis of Westphal, Westphal-Struempell disease, Wilson's disease.*

family history   Record of the health of family members, including the health status or cause of death of parents, siblings, and children, and specific diseases related to the patient's chief complaint, history of present illness, and/or review of systems.

famotidine   Antiulcer medication that prevents heartburn by decreasing the amount of stomach acid produced and inhibiting secretion by competing with histamine at the H2 receptor site on parietal cells. Supply is reported with HCPCS Level II code S0028. May be sold under the brand names Pepcid, Pepcid AC, Pepcid RPD, Pepcidine.

fanatic personality   Excessive self-reference and sensitiveness to setbacks or to what are taken to be humiliations and rebuffs, a tendency to distort experience by misconstruing the neutral or friendly actions of others as hostile or contemptuous, and a combative and tenacious sense of personal rights that may be manifested as jealousy or excessive self-importance, excessive sensitivity, or aggression.

Fanconi (-de Toni) (-Debré) syndrome   Renal tubular malfunction, including cystinosis and osteomalacia caused by inherited disorders, the result of multiple myeloma, or proximal epithelial growth. Report this disorder with ICD-9-CM code 270.0. *Synonym(s): Hart's syndrome.*

FAP   Familial adenomatous polyposis. Genetic predisposition to cancer of the large intestine and rectum. FAP patients usually begin developing polyps in their teens, and colon cancer in their third or fourth decade. Genetic testing for FAP is reported with HCPCS Level II codes S3833 and S3834.

FAQ   Frequently asked question.

FAR   Federal acquisition regulations. Regulations of the federal government's acquisition of services.

Farber (-Uzman) syndrome   Swollen joints, lymphadenopathy, subcutaneous nodules, and accumulation in lysosomes of affected cells of PAS-positive lipid consisting of ceramide. Begins soon after birth and caused by deficiency of ceramidase. Report this disorder with ICD-9-CM code 272.8.

farmer's lung   Hypersensitivity from exposure to moldy fermented hay causing inflammation of the lung air sacs. Symptoms can include cough, chills, fever, and tachycardia. Farmer's lung is reported with ICD-9-CM code 495.0.

Farnsworth-Munsell color test   Test evaluating depth perception.

D-F

Farr test   Antibody reacts to radioactive antigen and precipitates, leaving a free antigen in solution. Radio markers tag the suspected antigen.

FAS   Fetal alcohol syndrome.

fascia   Fibrous sheet or band of tissue that envelops organs, muscles, and groupings of muscles.

fasciectomy   Excision of fascia or strips of fascial tissue.

fasciocutaneous graft   Section of fascia with attached skin that is partially or fully removed from its donor site and transferred to a new recipient site.

fasciotomy   Incision or transection of fascial tissue.

Faslodex   See fulvestrant.

FAST   Functional assessment staging. Method for ranking cognitive abilities of geriatric patients as dementia progresses.

fat graft   Graft composed of fatty tissue completely freed from surrounding tissue that is used primarily to fill in depressions.

fatigue NEC syndrome   Hypersomatic disorder with no identifiable pathology. Report this disorder with ICD-9-CM code 300.5.

fatigue neurosis   Neurotic disorder characterized by fatigue, irritability, headache, depression, insomnia, difficulty in concentration, and lack of capacity for enjoyment (anhedonia).

FB   *1)* Foreign body. *2)* Finger breadths. *3)* HCPCS Level II modifier used to denote items that are provided without cost to the provider, supplier, or practitioner, or that full credit was received for a replaced device.

FBR   Foreign body removal.

FBS   Fasting blood sugar.

FC   HCPCS Level II modifier used to denote that partial credit was received for a replaced device.

FCE   Functional capacity evaluation.

FCR   Flexor carpi radialis. Radial flexor and abductor muscle of the wrist.

FDA   Food and Drug Administration. Federal agency responsible for protecting public health by substantiating the safety, efficacy, and security of human and veterinary drugs, biological products, medical devices, national food supply, cosmetics, and items that give off radiation.

FDG   2-(Flourine-18)-fluoro-2-dexoy-D-glucose.

FDG-PET   Positron emission with tomography with 18 fluorodeoxyglucose. *NCD References: 220.6.2-220.6.16.*

FDH syndrome   Focal dermal hypoplasia. Linear areas of dermal hyperplasia with soft yellow nodules of fat. Areas are widely distributed and resemble striae distensae. Report this disorder with ICD-9-CM code 757.39.

FDP   *1)* Flexor digitorum profundus tendon. Tendon originating in the proximal forearm and extending to index finger and wrist. A thickened FDP sheath, usually caused by age, illness, or injury, can fill the carpal canal and lead to impingement of the median nerve. *2)* Fibrin degradation products.

FDS   Functional dementia scale. Method for assessing functional disabilities in patients with dementia.

Fe   *1)* Female. *2)* Iron.

fecalith   Hard, intestinal concretion of fecal matter that may lead to impaction or appendicitis. Report this condition with ICD-9-CM code 560.32. *Synonym(s): coprolith, stercolith.*

fecophilia   Psychosexual disorder in which one becomes aroused when focusing on feces, often seen in conjunction with such practices as bondage and discipline, sadomasochism, or infantilism. This disorder is reported with ICD-9-CM code 302.89. *Synonym(s): coprophilia.*

federal acquisition regulations   Regulations of the federal government's acquisition of services.

Federal Bureau of Investigation   Along with the Office of Inspector General (OIG), the FBI investigates potential health care fraud. Under a special memorandum of understanding, the FBI has direct access to contractor data and other records to the same extent as the OIG. *Synonym(s): FBI.*

federal employee health benefits acquisition regulations (FEHBARS)   Federal regulations for acquisition of health services used by government agencies and subcontractors. *Synonym(s): FEHBARS.*

Federal Employee Health Benefits Program (FEHBP)   Provides health plans to federal workers. *Synonym(s): FEHBP.*

federal fiscal year in relation to the Medicare program   October 1 through September 30.

federal health care offense   Violation or conspiracy to violate any of the nine current statutes or four new health care crimes created under HIPAA.

Federal Register   Government publication listing changes in regulations and federally mandated standards, including coding standards such as HCPCS Level II and ICD-9-CM.

federally qualified HMO   HMO that meets CMS guidelines for Medicare reimbursement.

fee for service   *1)* Payment for services, usually physician services, on a service-by-service basis rather than an alternative payment system like capitation. Fee-for-service arrangements may be discounted or undiscounted rates. *2)* Situation in which the payer pays full charges for medical services. *Synonym(s): FFS.*

D-F

fee schedule List of codes and related services with pre-established billing amounts by a provider, or payment amounts by a payer that could be percentages of billed charges, flat rates, or maximum allowable amounts established by third-party payers. Medicare fee schedules apply to clinical laboratory, radiology, and durable medical equipment services.

feeble-minded Individuals with an IQ of 50-70 who can develop social and communication skills, have minimal retardation in sensorimotor areas, and often are not distinguished from normal children until a later age and can learn academic skills up to approximately the sixth-grade level. As adults they can usually achieve social and vocational skills adequate for minimum self-support but may need guidance and assistance when under social or economic stress. This is also known as a high grade defect.

FEF Frontal eye field. Area in the frontal lobe of the brain in which voluntary lateral eye movements originate. Following stroke, eyes look toward the side with the lesion; with seizure, the eyes look away from the affected side.

FEHB Federal Employee Health Benefits Program. Provides health plans to federal workers.

FEHBAR Federal Employee Health Benefits Acquisition Regulations. Federal regulations for acquisition of health services used by government agencies and subcontractors.

Feiba VH immuno See antiinhibitor coagulant complex.

Feil-Klippel syndrome Shorter than average neck and a low hairline. Caused by fewer than average cervical vertebrae or fusion of hemivertebrae into one bony mass. Report this disorder with ICD-9-CM code 756.16.

fellow Physician who has completed a basic residency program and is now in a formally organized and approved subspecialty program that may or may not be recognized as an approved residency program under Medicare for received GME funding.

felon Painful abscess on the palmar side of a distal fingertip, usually occurring after inoculation of a disease-causing microorganism, such as Staphylococcus aureus in the closed space of the terminal phalanx. Felon is reported with ICD-9-CM code 681.01. **Synonym(s):** *pulp abscess.*

Felty's syndrome Splenomegaly, leukopenia, arthritis, hypersplenism, anemia and other symptoms. Report this disorder with ICD-9-CM code 714.1.

Fem Female.

female stress incontinence Involuntary escape of urine at times of minor stress against the female bladder, such as coughing, sneezing, or laughing. *NCD Reference: 30.1.1.*

FemCap Brand name reusable contraceptive cervical barrier, sized to fit the patient, used in conjunction with a spermicide. Cervical cap supply is reported with HCPCS Level II code A4261.

femoral nerve Nerve that arises from the lumbar plexus that innervates the flexor (e.g., psoas major, rectus femoris, and sartorius) muscles and extensor (e.g., rectus femoris, vastus lateralis) muscles of the thigh.

fenestrate Pierce or perforate with one or more openings.

fenestration Presence of small openings from piercing or perforations.

fentanyl citrate Potent opioid analgesic used as an adjunct to anesthesia and to treat postoperative pain and break-through pain in cancer patients who have built a tolerance to other opioids. Supply is reported with HCPCS Level II code J3010. May be sold under the brand names Actiq, Fentanyl Duragesic, Fentanyl transmucosal, Sublimaze.

Fergusson speculum Device inserted into the vagina for viewing its walls and the cervix

-ferous Produces, causes, or brings about.

FERPA Family Educational Rights and Privacy Act.

ferrous fumarate/gluconate/sulfate Oral iron supplements used to treat iron deficiency, an essential ingredient in hemoglobin that carries oxygen on the red blood cells.

fertile eunuch syndrome Hypogonadism with gynecomastia, hypospadias, and postpubertal testicular atrophy, caused by an inherited defect of androgen receptors and insensitivity to testosterone. Report this disorder with ICD-9-CM code 257.2.

ferumoxtran-10 Molecular imaging agent for MRI for identifying lymph node metastases. Supply of ferumoxtran-10 is reported with HCPCS Level II code Q9953, or for outpatient facilities, C8903, C8905, C8906, or C8908. Injection of ferumoxtran-10 is bundled into the appropriate MRI with contrast code. May be sold as brand name Combidex.

FES Functional electrical stimulation. Method of stimulating nerves and muscles with electrical currents to activate function in prosthetic devices or to reduce wasting and bone loss by stimulating paralyzed limbs for stationary exercise.

FESS Functional endoscopic sinus surgery. Surgery to restore function to the patient's sinus, coded according to the site and the therapeutic procedure performed.

FET Frozen embryo transfer.

fetal alcohol syndrome Growth deficiency, craniofacial anomalies, and limb defects among offspring of mothers who are chronic alcoholics. Report this disorder with ICD-9-CM code 760.71.

D-F

fetal biophysical profile Monitoring by ultrasound the health of a term or near-term fetus by assessing fetal breathing movements, body movements, tone, and amniotic fluid volume. This profile is reported using CPT code 76819 if performed alone and 76818 if a nonstress test is included, which monitors the fetal heart rate for accelerations with the baby's movement. Fetal biophysical profiles are excluded from the maternity care global package. **Synonym(s):** *BPP.*

fetal contraction stress test Test performed to determine the ability of the fetus to tolerate the stress of normal labor and measure the ability of the placenta to provide sufficient oxygen to the fetus during contractions. The physician first applies external fetal monitors to the maternal abdominal wall. Uterine contractions are then induced by either a nipple stimulation protocol or intravenous administration of the hormone oxytocin, during which the fetal heart rate and uterine contractions are monitored and recorded. If the baby's heart rate slows in response to the stress rather than accelerating after a contraction, it may signify an inability to tolerate contractions well and can be an indication for a Cesarean delivery. This procedure is usually performed during the third trimester and is reported with ICD-9-CM procedure code 75.35 and CPT code 59020. Fetal contraction stress tests are excluded from the maternity care global package. **Synonym(s):** *CST oxytocin challenge.*

fetal nonstress test Noninvasive procedure in which the patient reports fetal movements as an external monitor records fetal heart rate changes. Electrodes that measure both the fetal heart rate as well as the ability of the uterus to contract are placed on the maternal abdomen over a conducting jelly and the accelerations of the fetal heart rate with normal movement are gauged. This test is reported using ICD-9-CM procedure code 75.34 and CPT code 59025, and is excluded from the maternity care global package. If a fetal biophysical profile is performed, the nonstress test is included in 76818 and 59025 would not be reported separately. **Synonym(s):** *fetal activity acceleration determinations, NST.*

Fetal Scalp Blood Sampling

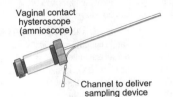

The physician removes a sample of fetal scalp blood

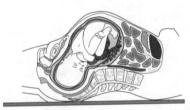

fetal scalp blood sampling Transvaginal procedure performed during active labor in order to assess fetal distress. The cervix must be dilated more than 2 cm with the fetal vertex low in the pelvis. The physician may need to break the amniotic sac and inserts an amnioscope through the vagina. The fetal scalp is cleansed and an incision is made in the scalp with a special narrow blade that penetrates no more than 2 mm. Blood is aspirated into a heparinized capillary tube. The incision is closely watched to ensure bleeding stops. This procedure tests the pH level of the blood and measures the oxygen to the baby's brain during labor and also measures clotting ability of the baby's blood by checking the platelet count. Fetal scalp blood sampling is reported with ICD-9-CM procedure code 75.33 and CPT code 59030. Fetal scalp blood sampling is excluded from the maternity care global package.

fetishism Sexual deviation in which nonliving objects are utilized as a preferred or exclusive method of stimulating erotic arousal.

fetoscopy Fetus and amnion are viewed through a thin, flexible instrument called a fetoscope, or amnioscope, inserted through a small abdominal access incision into the woman's uterus. Fetoscopy is performed under ultrasound guidance, and is useful in detecting some birth defects. Fetoscopy is reported with ICD-9-CM procedure code 75.31. An unlisted maternity care and delivery code, 59899, is used for CPT reporting. **Synonym(s):** *amnioscopy, laparoamnioscopy.*

fetus Unborn offspring past the embryonic stage that has developed major structures. It is the period defined from nine weeks after fertilization until birth.

FEV Forced expiratory volume.

fever Elevation of body temperature.

FFDM Full field digital mammography. Mammography in which a digital picture is produced rather than an x-ray.

FFL Flexible fiberoptic laryngoscopy, reported with CPT codes 31575-31579.

FFP Fresh frozen plasma.

FFR Fractional flow reserve.

FFS Fee for service. *1)* Payment for services, usually physician services, on a service-by-service basis rather than an alternative payment system like capitation. Fee-for-service arrangements may be discounted or undiscounted rates. *2)* Situation in which the payer pays full charges for medical services.

FGM Female genital mutilation. Female circumcision or castration, practiced as a culturally determined ritual in some countries. FGM patients may present with serious problems and concerns related to intercourse, childbirth, pelvic examinations, and pelvic infections. Code assignment is determined by the severity of the mutilation with a code from ICD-9-CM category 629.2.

FH Family history.

FHI Fuchs' heterochromic iridocyclitis.

FHR Fetal heart rate.

FHT Fetal heart tone.

FI Fiscal intermediary. Federally designated contractor that processes Medicare claims for Part A benefits and some Part B claims.

fibrillation Spontaneous contraction of individual muscle fibers. *atrial f.* Cardiac arrhythmia caused by small areas of muscle fibers becoming erratically and spontaneously activated through multiple circuits in uncoordinated phases of depolarization and repolarization. This causes the atria to quiver in a continuously erratic pattern instead of contracting in the regular rhythm. Atrial fibrillation can lead to ventricular arrhythmia and is distinguished from atrial flutter, in which the atrial contractions are rapid but regular. Atrial fibrillation is reported with ICD-9-CM code 427.31. *A fib. ventricular f.* Cardiac arrhythmia in which ventricular myocardial fibers are rapidly and repetitively excited from a random or ectopic focus of electrical impulse, causing the muscle fibers to contract in an erratic manner without corresponding contraction of the ventricles. Ventricular fibrillation is reported with 427.41. The condition requires immediate restoration of normal cardiac rhythm, often by electroshock through paddles placed on the chest. *Synonym(s): fib.*

fibrin Main fibrous composition of blood clots.

fibrin sheath Obstructive material or thrombus that forms around or within the lumen of an indwelling catheter or central venous access device. Pericatheter removal is reported with CPT code 36595 and intraluminal removal is reported with 36596.

fibro- Relating to fibers or fibrous tissue.

fibroadenoma Benign neoplasm of glandular epithelium frequently found in the breast.

fibroadenosis Fibrocystic breast disease in which nonneoplastic nodules composed of fibrous and glandular tissues develop in women of reproductive age, accounting for the most common cause of lumps found in the breast. Fibroadenosis is reported with ICD-9-CM code 610.2. *Synonym(s): chronic fibroadenosis, cystic fibroadenosis, diffuse fibroadenosis, periodic fibroadenosis, segmental fibroadenosis.*

fibrocutaneous tags Skin colored or light brown hyperplastic epidermal lesions that resemble a miniature polyp, usually occurring on the skin of the neck, upper chest, and axillae. *Synonym(s): acrochordon, cutaneous papilloma, skin tags.*

fibrosclerosis Hardening and induration with increased formation of fibrous connective tissue due to a disease process or inflammation.

fibrosis Formation of fibrous tissue as part of the restorative process.

fibrous tissue Connective tissues.

fibrous tuberosity Nodule or tubercle of the bone comprised of fibroblasts or connective tissue fibers.

Fick method Indirect method of measuring cardiac output based on pulmonary blood flow. The Fick principle states that the rate of oxygen consumed by the lungs when divided by the difference in oxygen concentration between the arterial and venous systems gives the rate of blood flow through the circulatory system, or cardiac output. Measuring cardiac output this way is accomplished by performing indicator dilution studies, done by different methods, in which a known quantity of a dye or radiolabeled tracer is injected and then monitored for concentration at one particular point over time. This type of study is reported with CPT codes 93561-93562. *Synonym(s): indicator dilution method.*

Fiedler's syndrome Isolated infection of heart muscle. Report this disorder with ICD-9-CM code 422.91.

field block Injection of a local anesthetic to manage pain from surgery for six to eight hours. This procedure is part of the surgical package and is not billable.

Fiessinger-Leroy (-Reiter) syndrome Association of arthritis, iridocyclitis, and urethritis, sometimes with diarrhea. While symptoms may recur, the arthritis is constant. Report this disorder with ICD-9-CM code 099.3. *Synonym(s): Fiessinger-Leroy-Reiter syndrome.*

D-F

Fiessinger-Rendu syndrome Necrolysis of the skin caused by toxins. Report this disorder with ICD-9-CM code 695.19.

fifth disease Infection with human parvovirus B19, mainly occurring in children. Symptoms include a low-grade fever, malaise, or a ôcoldö a few days before the appearance of a mild rash illness that presents as a ôslapped-cheekö rash on the face and a lacy red rash on the trunk and limbs. The condition usually resolves in seven to 10 days. Report this condition with ICD-9-CM code 057.0. *Synonym(s): megalerythema.*

FIGO Classification system of the International Federation of Gynecology and Obstetrics for cervical cancer, ranging from Stage I (confined to the uterus) to Stage IVB (distant metastasis).

filgrastim Biological response modifier that stimulates propagation and differentiation of hematopoietic cells, specifically neutrophils, to raise white blood cell levels. It is used to treat agranulocytosis; congenital, HIV related, or idiopathic neutropenia; and myelodysplasia. Supply is reported with HCPCS Level II codes J1440 and J1441. May be sold under the brand name Neupogen.

filiform Probe with woven-thread end.

filiform probe Slender instrument used for insertion and investigation within a body cavity, tract, or space, that has a woven-thread end.

filling In dentistry, restoration of lost tooth structure by utilizing substances such as metal, alloy, plastic, or porcelain.

filtered speech test Test most commonly used to identify central auditory dysfunction in which the patient is presented monosyllabic words that are low pass filtered, allowing only the parts of each word below a certain pitch to be presented. A score is given on the number of correct responses. This may be a subset of a standard battery of tests provided during a single encounter.

financial limitation Financial limitation on outpatient rehabilitation services for physical therapy, occupational therapy, and speech-language pathology claims. The limits apply to outpatient rehabilitation services provided by physicians, nurse practitioners, clinical nurse specialists, physician's assistants, physical therapists, occupational therapists, and speech-language pathologists. The limits apply in all settings that are paid under the Medicare physician fee schedule except the hospital outpatient setting.

fine needle aspiration 22- or 25-gauge needle attached to a syringe is inserted into a lesion/tissue and a few cells are aspirated for biopsy and diagnostic study. Aspiration is also used to remove fluid from a benign cyst. *Synonym(s): FNA.*

fine needle aspiration biopsy Insertion of a fine-gauge needle attached to a syringe into a tissue mass for the suctioned withdrawal of cells used for diagnostic study. *Synonym(s): FNA.*

Fineline 2 Brand name cardiac lead system.

finger-flicking One of a number of voluntary repetitive stereotypical movements that are not due to any psychiatric or neurological condition, manifested by head banging, head nodding and nystagmus, rocking, twirling, finger-flicking mannerisms, and eye poking. Common in cases of mental retardation with sensory impairment or with environmental monotony.

Finkelstein sign Clinical sign used to determine presence of de Quervain's disease. The thumb is placed in full opposition by bending it into the palm. Pain at this point suggests synovitis of the abductor pollicis longus tendon of the wrist. Then the wrist is passively flexed and deviated in the ulnar direction. Pain in the first dorsal extensor compartment is positive for de Quervain's disease.

Finsterer sign Slowed pulse in intraperitoneal bleeding.

FIPS Federal information processing standards. FIPS are developed when there are no existing voluntary standards to address federal requirements for the interoperability of computer systems. They are proposed and published in the *Federal Register*.

FIRMAGON See degarelix.

first arch syndrome Malformations of the first branchial arch with palpebral fissures sloping outward and downward with notches in the outer third of the lower lids, defects of malar bones and zygoma, hypoplasia of the jawbone, high or cleft palate, low-set ears, unusual hair growth, and pits between mouth and ear. Report this disorder with ICD-9-CM code 756.0. *Synonym(s): Franceschetti's syndrome.*

first order First vessel in the arterial or venous system that branches off the main vessel and supplies additional branches within the same vascular family; used for coding selective catheterization procedures.

first order selective Catheter placement into the first vessel that branches off the aorta; catheter placement into the first vessel that branches off the vessel into which percutaneous insertion was made.

first-degree burn Superficial partial-thickness burn in which only the epidermis or a portion of the dermis is involved, displaying redness but no blister formation. Burns that are the result of hot objects, flames, chemicals, or radiation are classified to ICD-9-CM categories 940-949. First-degree burns resulting from exposure to solar radiation (sunburn) are classified to 692.71.

fiscal intermediary Federally designated contractor that processes Medicare claims for Part A benefits and some Part B claims. *Synonym(s): FI.*

fiscal year Twelve-month period that an organization designates and uses to denote an accounting period or during which it plans to use funds. Fiscal years are referred to by the calendar year in which they end. The federal government's fiscal year runs from October 1 to September 30. *Synonym(s): FY.*

fish odor syndrome Rare disorder of trimethylamineuria metabolism that causes the patient to give off an odor of garbage or fish. Fish odor syndrome is reported with ICD-9-CM code 270.8.

Fisher scale Grade for evaluating nontraumatic subarachnoid hemorrhage by CT appearance. In grade 1, no blood is detected; in grade 2, diffuse blood is less than 1 mm thick; in grade 3, localized clots and vertical layers of blood up to 1 mm thickness; and grade 4 with intracerebral or intraventricular clots. Nontraumatic subarachnoid hemorrhage is reported with ICD-9-CM code 430.

Fisher's syndrome Paraplegia of limbs, flaccid paralysis, ophthalmoplegia, ataxia, and areflexia caused by disorder of immune system. Report this disorder with ICD-9-CM code 357.0. *Synonym(s): Guillain-Barre syndrome, Landry syndrome, Miller syndrome, Strohl syndrome.*

fissure Deep furrow, groove, or cleft in tissue structures.

fistula Abnormal tube-like passage between two body cavities or organs or from an organ to the outside surface.

fistulization Creation of a communication between two structures that were not previously connected.

fit Attack of acute symptoms.

Fitz's syndrome Acute infection of the pancreas with the formation of necrotic areas, bleeding in the gland, fever, leukocytosis, nausea, and pain. Report this disorder with ICD-9-CM code 577.0.

Fitz-Hugh and Curtis syndrome Peritonitis of the upper abdominal region in persons with a history of gonorrheal or other infections. Report this disorder with ICD-9-CM code 098.86.

FIX8 Brand name system for rigid fixation of the orbit during reconstructive surgery, treatment of orbital fractures and congenital anomalies, or for defects after surgery for the removal of tumors.

fixate Hold, secure, or fasten in position.

fixation Act or condition of being attached, secured, fastened, or held in position.

fixed Not able to be removed easily.

FL *1)* Fluid. *2)* Form locator. Area on the UB-92 claim form designated for specific billing or coding data. Every FL accepts a given number of characters, alphabetic or numeric and symbols or spaces. For Medicare billing purposes, FLs can be required, desirable, or optional, depending on the information.

flaccid hemiplegia Paralytic condition affecting one side of the body in which there is loss or impairment of motor function accompanied by lost muscle tone and tendon reflexes.

Flagyl IV RTU See metronidazole.

flail chest Instability of the chest wall resulting from a fracture of the sternum or ribs.

Flajani disease Enlargement of the thyroid gland seen mostly in women, stemming from an autoimmune process, and causing excessive secretion of thyroid hormone, goiter, and bulging eyes. The syndrome seen with hyperplasia of the thyroid and excessive hormone production consists of fatigue, nervousness, emotional lability and irritability, heat intolerance and increased sweating, weight loss, palpitations, and tremor of the hands and tongue. If there is no documentation of a thyrotoxic crisis or storm, report ICD-9-CM code 242.00; with thyrotoxic crisis or storm, report 242.01. *Synonym(s): Basedow syndrome, Begbie's disease, Graves' disease, Marsh's disease, Parry's disease, toxic diffuse goiter.*

flank Part of the body found between the posterior ribs and the uppermost crest of the ilium, or the lateral side of the hip, thigh, and buttock.

flap Mass of flesh and skin partially excised from its location but retaining its blood supply that is moved to another site to repair adjacent or distant defects. *F. rotation* Flap of skin is incised in a circular manner, leaving the existing blood flow to the skin intact, and then turned to cover the defect area or wound.

flat bones Bone of reduced thickness, usually curved in structure, comprised of only one or two layers of compact bone or spongy bone and marrow, such as the sternum, scapula, and ribs.

flat file File that consists of a series of fixed-length records that include some sort of record type code.

flexible fiberoptic bronchoscope Small, flexible endoscope with an external diameter between 3.0 and 6.0 mm composed of four channels: two light channels, one vision channel, and one open channel that accommodates biopsy forceps, cytology brush, suction tube, lavage tube, anesthetic, or oxygen. It is used to visualize the segmental and subsegmental bronchi. Flexible bronchoscopy may be performed with many different therapeutic procedures, in which case the diagnostic bronchoscopy is included.

flexion Act of bending or being bent.

Flexner-Wintersteiner rosette Flower-bud appearance of tissue under the microscope in retinoblastoma.

D–F

flexor   Muscle/tendon that bends or flexes a limb or part as opposed to extending it.

flexor digitorum profundus tendon   Tendon originating in the proximal forearm and extending to the index finger and wrist. A thickened FDP sheath, usually caused by age, illness, or injury, can fill the carpal canal and lead to impingement of the median nerve.

Flextend   Brand name cardiac lead system.

Flexzan   Brand name semi-occlusive polyurethane foam adhesive wound dressing used to protect and hydrate integumentary wounds as they heal. When the dressing is applied in the physician office, supply of the wound dressing is reported separately with HCPCS Level II codes A6209-A6214.

Flixene   Brand name vascular graft used in reconstruction and vascular access.

FLK   Funny looking kid.

Flolan   See epoprostenol.

floxuridine   Antimetabolite type of antineoplastic medication that interferes with the growth of cancer cells by inhibiting DNA and ultimately RNA synthesis. This drug is catabolized in the body to 5-Flurouracil and is primarily used to treat gastrointestinal adenocarcinoma with metastasis to the liver. *Synonym(s): FUDR.*

FLUARIX   Brand name influenza vaccine, indicated for patients 18 years and older, provided in a set of 10 single-dose syringes. Supply of FLUARIX is reported with CPT code 90656. Administration is reported with HCPCS Level II code G0008. Need for vaccination is reported with ICD-9-CM code V04.81.

fluconazole   Antifungal used most commonly to treat candidiasis. It is recommended for treatment of vaginal or oral candida albicans and for treatment of cryptococcal meningitis. It is also used as a prophylaxis against secondary fungal infections in patients who are immunocompromised, such as transplant and HIV patients. Supply is reported with HCPCS Level II code J1450. May be sold under the brand name Diflucan.

Fludara   See fludarabine phosphate.

fludarabine phosphate   Antineoplastic antimetabolite used to treat chronic B cell lymphocytic leukemia in patients who have not responded to at least one round of treatment with alkylating agents. Supply is reported with HCPCS Level II code J9185. May be sold under the brand name Fludara.

FluMist   Brand name influenza vaccine provided in a set of 10 single-dose sprayers. Supply of FluMist is reported with CPT code 90660. Administration is reported with HCPCS Level II code G0008. The need for immunization is reported with ICD-9-CM code V04.81.

flunisolide   Inhaled corticosteroid used to prevent an allergic response in asthma and allergic rhinitis, but is not for acute relief of asthma symptoms. It also helps patients dependent on systemic corticosteroid therapy to decrease their dosage by producing the desired effects with less systemic exposure. Supply is reported with HCPCS Level II code J7641. May be sold under the brand names Aerobid, Nasalide.

fluorescein stain   Fluorescein dye is instilled into the eye to stain local defects that are visible with cobalt blue illumination.

fluoride   Compound of the gaseous element fluorine that can be incorporated into bone and teeth and provides some protection in reducing dental decay.

fluoroscopy   Radiology technique that allows visual examination of part of the body or a function of an organ using a device that projects an x-ray image on a fluorescent screen.

fluorouracil   Antineoplastic antimetabolite used to treat various types of colorectal, breast, and pancreatic cancer, and to treat actinic keratosis and superficial basal cell cancer in topical form. Supply is reported with HCPCS Level II code J9190. May be sold under the brand names 5 Fluorouracil, 5 FU, Adrucil, Carac, Efudex, Fluoroplex.

fluphenazine   Antipsychotic medication of unknown action used to treat schizophrenia and other psychoses. It is generally taken in the smallest amounts necessary to manage the problem until therapeutic levels are reached, and then many patients are switched to the decanoate form in a long-acting injection. Supply is reported with HCPCS Level II code J2680. May be sold under the brand names Anatensol, Apo-Fluphenazine, Fluphenazine, Modecate, Moditen HCl, Permitil, Prolixin.

fluro   Fluoroscopy.

flush syndrome   Carcinoid tumors causing severe attacks of cyanotic flushing of the skin, diarrheal watery stools, bronchoconstrictive attacks, hypotension, edema, and ascites. Report this disorder with ICD-9-CM code 259.2. *Synonym(s): Bjorck-Thorson syndrome, Cassidy-Scholte syndrome, Hedinger's syndrome.*

Fluzone   Brand name influenza vaccine provided in a 10-dose vial or a single dose syringe (preservative free). Supply of Fluzone is reported with CPT codes 90655-90656 (preservative free) and 90657-90658. Administration is reported with HCPCS Level II code G0008. The need for immunization is reported with ICD-9-CM code V04.81.

Flynn procedure   Orthopaedic procedure performed as reduction, peg bone graft, and fixation for nonunion or delayed union of minimally displaced lateral condylar fractures in children.

FM   Face mask.

FMD   Fibromuscular dysplasia. Arterial disease of unknown etiology affecting the arteries, usually of women. It presents as a renal hypertension, thromboembolic stroke, dissection, or transient ischemic attack. FMD is reported with ICD-9-CM code 447.3 if renal artery and 447.8 for other than renal artery.

FME Full-mouth extraction.

FMG Fine mesh gauze.

FMP Final menstrual period.

FMPA Focused microwave phased array. Ablation technique for treating cancers in high-water content tissue, as in breast carcinoma. A subcutaneous transmitter emits microwaves to treat the tumor with heat. For FMPA of the breast, report CPT code 19499. Imaging guidance performed with this procedure is reported with 76942 and 76998.

FMR Focused medical review. The process of targeting and directing medical review efforts on Medicare claims where the greatest risk of inappropriate program payment exists. The goal is to reduce the number of noncovered claims or unnecessary services. CMS analyzes national data such as internal billing, utilization and payment data and provides its findings to the fiscal intermediary (FI). Local medical review policies are developed identifying aberrances, abuse, and overutilized services. Providers are responsible for knowing national Medicare coverage and billing guidelines and local medical review policies, and for determining whether the services provided to Medicare beneficiaries are covered by Medicare.

fMRI Functional magnetic resonance imaging. Technique to identify which part of the brain is activated by stimulus or activity; a type of brain mapping useful prior to brain surgery and in cases of epilepsy and mental disorders. fMRI is reported with CPT codes 70554 and 70555.

FNP Family nurse practitioner.

FO Finger orthosis.

FOBT Fecal occult blood test, reported with CPT codes 82270, 82272, and 82274. **NCD References:** *190.34, 210.3.*

focal length Distance between the object in focus and the lens.

FocalSeal-L Brand name liquid sealant painted on lung tissue to seal air leaks around sutures or staples following removal of lung tumors. FocalSeal-L is activated by light.

focused medical review Process of targeting and directing medical review efforts on Medicare claims where the greatest risk of inappropriate program payment exists. The goal is to reduce the number of noncovered claims or unnecessary services. CMS analyzes national data such as internal billing, utilization and payment data and provides its findings to the FI. Local medical review policies are developed identifying aberrances, abuse, and overutilized services. Providers are

responsible for knowing national Medicare coverage and billing guidelines and local medical review policies, and for determining whether the services provided to Medicare beneficiaries are covered by Medicare. *Synonym(s): FMR.*

FOD Free of disease.

Foix-Alajouanine syndrome Ophthalmoplegia, paresis of the sympathetic nerves, and neuroparalytic keratitis from compression of lateral wall of the cavernous sinus. Report this disorder with ICD-9-CM code 336.1.

Foldi technique Manual lymphatic drainage using gentle massage to reduce lymphedema. Lymphedema is reported with ICD-9-CM code 457.1 when an acquired chronic condition; postmastectomy lymphedema is reported with 457.0; and hereditary edema of the legs is reported with 757.0.

Foley catheter Temporary indwelling urethral catheter held in place in the bladder by an inflated balloon containing fluid or air.

Foley Y-pyeloplasty Y-shaped flap prepared from the renal pelvis of the kidney and advanced into the ureter to correct a defect.

Folie a deux Mainly delusional psychosis, usually chronic and often without florid features, that appears to have developed as a result of a close, if not dependent, relationship with another person who already has an established similar psychosis.

follicular cyst Common type of ovarian cyst related to the menstrual cycle that occurs when the follicle in which the ovum develops does not rupture and expel the egg. Follicular cysts normally disappear within two or three menstrual cycles and are usually benign. Follicular cysts are reported with ICD-9-CM code 620.0. *Synonym(s): cyst of graafian follicle.*

Follistim Brand name fertility drug administered by injection. Its active ingredient is follitropin beta. Supply is reported with HCPCS Level II code S0128.

following crush injury syndrome Traumatic anuria following crushing by a heavy object. Report this disorder with ICD-9-CM code 958.5.

following delivery syndrome Hepatorenal syndrome, cardiomyopathy, uterine hypertrophy, and other symptoms following childbirth. Report this disorder with an ICD-9-CM code from subcategory 674.8.

follow-up Visits or treatment following a procedure.

fomepizole Antidote for ethylene glycol (antifreeze) and methanol poisoning that inhibits alcohol dehydrogenase from catabolizing the alcohols into their metabolites, responsible for the toxic side effects. Fomepizole is usually administered via IV infusion in an emergency room or inpatient setting. Supply is reported with HCPCS Level II code J1451.May be sold under the brand name Antizol.

D-F

D-F

fomivirsen sodium Antiviral medication administered specifically for treatment of cytomegaloviral retinitis. Its mechanism of action is unique in that the nucleotide sequence in Fomivirsen is complimentary to the one on the mRNA of the virus and so takes its place and consequently inhibits the production of genes/proteins necessary for the virus to reproduce. It is administered directly into the vitreous humor. Supply is reported with HCPCS Level II code J1452. May be sold under the brand name Vitravene.

fondaparinux sodium Anticoagulant used for preventing deep vein thrombosis in patients undergoing surgical procedures for hip or knee replacement. Supply is reported with HCPCS Level II code J1652. May be sold under the brand name Arixtra.

Fong's syndrome Dysplasia of the fingernails and toenails, hypoplasia of patella, iliac horns, thickening of the glomerular lamina densa, and a flask-shaped femur. Report this disorder with ICD-9-CM code 756.89.

Fontan procedure Surgical bypass procedure that corrects tricuspid atresia and other selected congenital conditions by connecting the right atrium directly to the pulmonary artery by anastomosis or by inserting a closed prosthesis between the right atrium and the pulmonary artery and closing the interatrial communication. Fontan procedure is reported with CPT codes 33615 and 33617. *Synonym(s): ASD repair.*

fontanelle Membranous covering over cranial spaces in an infant skull that hasn't completely ossified and fused. *Synonym(s): soft spot.*

Food and Drug Administration Federal agency responsible for protecting public health by substantiating the safety, efficacy, and security of human and veterinary drugs, biological products, medical devices, national food supply, cosmetics, and items that give off radiation. *Synonym(s): FDA.*

foramen Natural opening or passage, especially one into or through a bone. *Synonym(s): foramina. f. magnum* Large opening in the base of the skull through which the spinal cord connects with the brain. *Synonym(s): great occipital foramen. f. magnum syndrome* Compression of brain from the space above. Report this disorder with ICD-9-CM code 348.4.

foramina Passage in the body that is naturally formed, usually through a bone.

foraminotomy Opening into the foramina, a passage in the body that is naturally formed, usually through a bone.

Forbes-Albright syndrome Persistent lactation and amenorrhea caused by pituitary tumor, marked by secretion of excessive amounts of prolactin. Report this disorder with ICD-9-CM code 253.1.

forceps Tool used for grasping or compressing tissue.

foreign body Any object or substance found in an organ and tissue that does not belong under normal circumstances.

Forestier's disease Excessive bone growth along the sides of the vertebrae, inflammation at ligament attachments, and bone spurs as a form of degenerative arthritis, usually seen in people older than age 50. It is more common among men than women. Forestier's disease with vertebral involvement is reported with ICD-9-CM code 721.8. Bone spurs are coded according to site. *Synonym(s): diffuse idiopathic skeletal hyperostosis, DISH.*

form locator Area on the UB-92 claim form designated for specific billing or coding data. Every FL accepts a given number of characters, alphabetic or numeric and symbols or spaces. For Medicare billing purposes, FLs can be required, desirable, or optional, depending on the information. *Synonym(s): FL.*

format Under HIPAA, data elements that provide or control the enveloping or hierarchical structure, or help identify data content of, a transaction. *Synonym(s): data-related concepts.*

formulary List of prescription medications preferred for use by the health plan and dispensed through participating pharmacies to covered persons.

fort. Strong (fortis).

Fortaz See ceftazidime.

foscarnet sodium Antiviral used to treat cytomegaloviral retinitis in patients with AIDS by blocking the pyrophosphate binding site on DNA polymerases and reverse transcriptase. Supply is reported with HCPCS Level II code J1455. May be sold under the brand name Foscavir.

Foscavir See foscarnet sodium.

fosphenytoin sodium Antiseizure medication used to treat status epilepticus, as a short-term substitute for Phenytoin, and to prevent or treat seizures in neurosurgery by stabilizing neuronal membranes. Supply is reported with HCPCS Level II codes Q2009 and S0078. May be sold under the brand name Cerebyx.

fossa Indentation or shallow depression.

fossa compression syndrome Compression of brain from the fossa underneath. Report this disorder with ICD-9-CM code 348.4.

Foster-Kennedy syndrome Meningioma of optic nerve with central scotoma and contralateral choked disk. Report this disorder with ICD-9-CM code 377.04. *Synonym(s): Gowers-Paton-Kennedy syndrome.*

Fournier's gangrene Necrotizing fasciitis of the scrotum, penis, or male perineum, caused by enteric, anaerobic, or gram-positive bacteria.

fourth and fifth digits Digits used in the ICD-9-CM coding system to provide more specific information about the diagnosis or procedure being coded. Certain ICD-9-CM codes require a fourth and fifth digit in order to be complete.

Foville's syndrome Paraplegia and anesthesia over part of the body caused by lesions in the brain or spinal cord. Report this disorder with ICD-9-CM code 344.89. *Synonym(s):* Avellis syndrome, Babinski-Nageotte syndrome, Benedikt's syndrome, Brown-Sequard syndrome, Cestan-Chenais syndrome, Cestan's syndrome, Gubler-Millard syndrome, Jackson's syndrome, Weber-Leyden syndrome.

Fowler's position Position assumed by patient when the head of the bed is raised 18 or 20 inches and the individual's knees are elevated.

FP *1)* Family planning. *2)* Family practitioner.

FPD Fixed partial denture.

FPL Flexor pollicis longus. Long flexor muscle of the thumb.

FPP Faculty practice plan. Group practice developed around a teaching program or medical school.

FQHC Federally qualified health center, as designated by CMS.

FR *1)* Federal Register. Government publication listing changes in regulations and federally mandated standards, including coding standards such as HCPCS Level II and ICD-9-CM. *2)* Family relationship.

fracture Break in bone or cartilage. *f. care* Packaged services for fracture management. Includes percutaneous pinning and open or closed treatment of the fracture, fixation, application and removal of the initial cast or splint, and normal, uncomplicated follow-up care. *f. types* There are three basic degrees of fracture: type I: a small crack in the bone without displacement; type II: a fracture in which the bone is slightly displaced; type III: a fracture in which there are more than three broken pieces of bone that cannot fit together.

fracture types There are three basic degrees of fracture: type I: a small crack in the bone without displacement; type II: a fracture in which the bone is slightly displaced; type III: a fracture in which there are more than three broken pieces of bone that cannot fit together.

fragile X syndrome Mental retardation, enlarged testes, big jaw, high forehead, and long ears in males. In females, fragile X presents mild retardation and heterozygous sexual structures. In some families, males have shown no symptoms but carry the gene. Report this disorder with ICD-9-CM code 759.83.

fragment Small piece broken off a larger whole; to divide into pieces.

Fragmin See dalteparin sodium.

Franceschetti's syndrome Malformations of derivatives of the first branchial arch, marked by palpebral fissures sloping outward and downward with notches in the outer third of the lower lids, defects of malar bones and zygoma, hypoplasia of the jawbone, high or cleft palate, low-set ears, unusual hair growth, and pits between mouth and ear. Report this disorder with ICD-9-CM code 756.0.

Fraser's syndrome Cryptophthalmus with ear malformations, cleft palate, laryngeal deformity, displacement of umbilicus and nipples, digital malformation, separation of symphysis pubis, maldeveloped kidneys, and masculine female genitals. Report this disorder with ICD-9-CM code 759.89.

FRAT Free radical assay test.

fraternal insurance Cooperative plan provided to members of an association or fraternal group.

fraud Intentional deception or misrepresentation that is known to be false and could result in an unauthorized benefit. Fraud arises from a false statement or misrepresentation that affects payments under the Medicare program. Examples include claiming costs for noncovered items and services disguised as covered items, incorrect reporting of diagnosis and procedures to maximize reimbursement, intentionally double billing for the same services, billing services that were not rendered, etc.

fraud alert CMS and the OIG periodically issue fraud alert statements that identify activities felt to pose legal and enforcement risks and urge incorporation of this information into existing compliance plans where appropriate.

fraud and abuse Method of obtaining unauthorized benefits. Fraud is an intentional deception, misrepresentation, or statement that is known to be false. Abuse is a practice that is inconsistent with accepted medical, business, or fiscal practices.

Fraud and Abuse Control Program Joint program between the DOJ and HHS that was established to coordinate federal, state, and local law enforcement efforts to control fraud and abuse.

Frazier-Spiller procedure Sensory root of the gasserian ganglion is compressed or decompressed to relieve trigeminal neuralgia.

FREDI Fallopian replacement of egg with delayed intrauterine insemination.

free flap Tissue that is completely detached from the donor site and transplanted to the recipient site, receiving its blood supply from capillary ingrowth at the recipient site.

free graft Unattached piece of skin and tissue moved to another part of the body and sutured into place to repair a defect.

D-F

free microvascular flap Tissue that is completely detached from the donor site following careful dissection and preservation of the blood vessels, then attached to the recipient site with the transferred blood vessels anastomosed to the vessels in the recipient bed.

Freeman-Sheldon syndrome Deviation of hands and face with protrusion of lips as in whistling, sunken eyes, and small nose. Report this disorder with ICD-9-CM code 759.89. *Synonym(s): whistling face syndrome.*

Freiberg's infraction Osteonecrosis of the metatarsal head, reported with ICD-9-CM code 732.5.

Frenulectomy

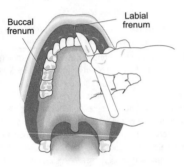

Physician excises the frenum
and underlying muscle

frenulectomy Excision of the labial, buccal, or lingual frenum, reported with CPT codes 40819, 41115, or HCPCS Level II code D7960. **penis f.** Incision of the frenulum, the membrane on the underside of the glans penis attaching it to the foreskin, to relieve tension. Reported with CPT code 54164. *Synonym(s): frenectomy.*

frenum Small, connected piece of skin or mucous membrane that serves to restrain, curb, or limit movement of the attached part.

frequency Number of times a given service is provided during a specified time period.

frequency-adjusted conversion factor Conversion factor obtained when converting a provider's fee schedule that is not based on the resource-based relative value scale to one that is based on it, using both current fees and frequencies. A frequency-adjusted conversion factor is more accurate than the more commonly used gross conversion factor because the income generated by each service provided is tied to the fee as well as the number of times the service is provided. Using a frequency-adjusted conversion factor allows development of an RBRVS fee schedule that generates the same amount of income that was generated under the non-RBRVS fee schedule.

Frey's syndrome Specific type of secondary focal hyperhidrosis caused by a lesion on the parotid gland that results in excessive sweating and redness in the auriculotemporal area of the cheek with eating. This syndrome is reported as secondary focal hyperhidrosis, which is ICD-9-CM code 705.22.

Frickman proctopexy To correct rectal prolapse, rectum is sutured to the anterior presacral fascia and attached to the sigmoid colon, which has been shortened to help suspend the rectum.

Friderichsen-Waterhouse syndrome Fulminating meningococcal septicemia in children below 10 years of age with vomiting, cyanosis, diarrhea, purpura, convulsions, circulatory collapse, meningitis, and hemorrhaging into the adrenal glands. Report this disorder with ICD-9-CM code 036.3.

Friedrich-Erb-Arnold syndrome Thickening of skin on extremities and face with clubbing of fingers and deformities in bone of the limb. Report this disorder with ICD-9-CM code 757.39.

frigidity Psychosexual dysfunction in which there is partial or complete failure to attain or maintain the lubrication-swelling response of sexual excitement until completion of the sexual act.

Fröhlich's syndrome Obesity and hypogonadism in adolescent boys. Dwarfism indicates hypothyroidism. Report this disorder with ICD-9-CM code 253.8. *Synonym(s): Babinski-Fröhlich syndrome, Launois-Cleret syndrome, Renon-Delille syndrome.*

Froin's syndrome Alteration in the cerebral spinal fluid resulting in a yellowish hue and indicative of neoplastic or inflammatory obstruction. Report this disorder with ICD-9-CM code 336.8.

Frommel-Chiari syndrome Hyperprolactinemia and a pituitary adenoma causing unphysiological lactation and amenorrhea following pregnancy. Report this disorder with a code from ICD-9-CM range 676.60-676.64.

frontal lobe syndrome Changes in behavior following damage to the frontal areas of the brain including reduction in self-control, foresight, creativity, spontaneity, emotional vivaciousness, and empathy. Report this disorder with ICD-9-CM code 310.0.

Frontal Sinusotomy

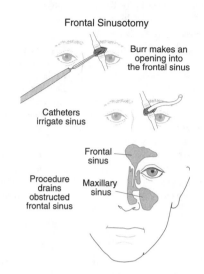

Burr makes an
opening into
the frontal sinus

Catheters
irrigate sinus

Frontal
sinus

Procedure   Maxillary
drains   sinus
obstructed
frontal sinus

frontal sinusotomy Surgical procedure in which the anterior wall of the frontal sinus is excised, the diseased tissue removed, and a permanent opening is created between the nasal cavity and the maxillary sinus in order to facilitate sinus drainage. Report this procedure with ICD-9-CM code 22.41 or CPT codes 31070-31087. *Synonym(s): Killian operation.*

Frost procedure Type of wedge excision utilizing an "L" shaped incision to remove the nail root and soft tissue usually performed on toe nails. Report this procedure with CPT code 11765.

frostbite Damage to skin, subcutaneous, and possibly deeper tissue caused by exposure to low temperatures, resulting in ischemia, thrombosis, even gangrene, and the loss of affected body parts.

frozen section Thin slice of frozen tissue removed for microscopic study with a special cutting instrument, often used to confirm the nature of tissue during a procedure.

frozen tissue Group of similar cells that have been frozen and thinly sliced according to specifications to preserve the tissue for diagnostic or histochemistry studies. Freezing methods include slow freeze or rapid freeze using sprays or carbon dioxide gas, solid carbon dioxide, or liquid nitrogen.

FSA Flexible spending account.

FSE Fetal scalp electrode.

FSF Frontal sinus fracture, reported with ICD-9-CM code 801.01.

FSH Follicle stimulating hormone. Gonadotropic hormone secreted by the anterior lobe of the pituitary gland. In women, it stimulates growth and maturation

of the ovum and its enclosing cells, the production of estrogen, and the endometrial changes that occur in the first phase of the menstrual cycle. In men, it stimulates the production of sperm.

ft Foot.

FTE Full time employee. Accounting equivalent of one full time employee that includes wages, benefits, and other costs.

FTND *1)* Fagerstrom Test for Nicotine Dependence. Survey assessing a smoking patient's dependence on nicotine. Tobacco dependence is reported with ICD-9-CM code 305.1. Do not report V15.82 History of tobacco use, if the patient still smokes. *2)* Full-term normal delivery.

FTQ Fagerstrom Tolerance Questionnaire. Survey assessing a smoking patient's dependence on nicotine. Tobacco dependence is reported with ICD-9-CM code 305.1. Do not report V15.82 History of tobacco use, if the patient still smokes.

FTSG Full thickness skin graft.

FTT Failure to thrive.

FUDR See floxuridine.

-fuge Drive out or expel.

Fukala's operation Lens is removed from the eye to treat near sightedness.

fulgurate Destruction by electric current.

fulguration Destruction of living tissue by using sparks from a high-frequency electric current.

full thickness skin graft Graft consisting of skin and subcutaneous tissue.

Fuller Albright's syndrome Patchy skin pigmentation, endocrine dysfunctions, and polyostotic fibrous dysplasia. Report this disorder with ICD-9-CM code 756.59. *Synonym(s): Albright's hereditary osteodystrophy syndrome, McCune-Albright syndrome.*

full-time employee Accounting equivalent of one full-time employee that includes wages, benefits, and other costs. *Synonym(s): FTE.*

fulvestrant Antineoplastic used to fight hormone receptor positive metastatic breast cancer. Supply is reported with HCPCS Level II code J9395. May be sold under the brand name Faslodex. Report prophylactic use with ICD-9-CM code V07.59.

function Special, normal, or proper action of any part or organ, including activities identified by an individual as essential to supporting physical and psychological well-being, as well as to creating a personal sense of meaningful living.

functional activities Activities that are goal directed and task specific.

functional activity training Teaching and practice of skills that will improve or enhance an individual's ability

D-F

to perform functional work-related activities, such as lifting and using an adaptive device.

functional capacity evaluation Evaluation based on procedures, questionnaires, and observation concerning the patient's ability to perform work from a physical, medical, behavioral, and ergonomic standpoint to determine whether the patient can safely return to work or other activity. *Synonym(s): FCE.*

functional dyspareunia Form of psychosexual dysfunction in which there is recurrent and persistent genital pain associated with coitus.

functional hemispherectomy Portions of one hemisphere of the brain not functioning normally or a nonfunctioning hemisphere are removed and the corpus callosum connecting the two hemispheres is split. This breaks the communications between the various lobes of the nonfunctioning hemisphere as well as the link between the two hemispheres, to prevent the spread of seizures to the functional side of the brain. This procedure is only used for those individuals with severe, uncontrollable, intractable seizures, failing all other treatments.

functional hyperinsulinism syndrome Hyperinsulinism due to organic endogenous factors with hypoglycemia, weakness, perspiration, jitteriness, tachycardia, mental confusion, and vision disturbances. Report this disorder with ICD-9-CM code 251.1. *Synonym(s): Harris' syndrome, organic hyperinsulinism.*

functional training Education and training of patients/clients in activities of daily living (ADL) and instrumental activities of daily living (IADL) that are intended to improve the ability to perform physical actions, tasks, or activities in an efficient, typically expected, or competent manner.

functional vaginismus Form of psychosexual dysfunction in which there is recurrent and persistent involuntary spasm of the musculature of the outer one-third of the vagina that interferes with sexual activity.

fund In a capitation contract, specific amount of money set aside and available to compensate the contracted entity.

fungal wet prep Diagnostic laboratory test used to detect a fungal or yeast infection of the skin. A scraping of the lesion is obtained, placed in a potassium hydroxide (KOH) solution, and examined under a microscope, where the fungus is visible if present. Report this test with CPT code 87220. *Synonym(s): KOH examination, potassium hydroxide examination.*

Fungizone See amphotericin B.

FUO Fever of unknown origin. Finding of fever on examination without apparent cause. FUO is reported with ICD-9-CM code 780.6.

furcation In dentistry, the area where roots separate in a multirooted tooth.

Furomide MD See furosemide.

furosemide Potent diuretic that inhibits sodium and chloride reabsorption in the kidneys to promote water and sodium excretion. It is indicated for the treatment of fluid overload and associated pulmonary edema, heart failure, and hypertension. Supply is reported with HCPCS Level II code J1940. May be sold under the brand names Apo-Furosemide, Furoside, Lasix, Lasix Special, Myrosemide, Novosemide, Uritol.

furuncle Inflamed, painful cyst or nodule on the skin caused by bacteria, often staphylococcus, entering along the hair follicle. It is classified to ICD-9-CM category 680. A fourth digit indicating the anatomical location should be assigned. *Synonym(s): boil.*

fusion Union of adjacent tissues, especially bone.

FVC Forced vital capacity.

fx Fracture.

fxBB Fracture, both bones.

FY Fiscal year. Twelve-month period that an organization designates and uses to denote an accounting period or during which it plans to use funds. Fiscal years are referred to by the calendar year in which they end. The federal government's fiscal year runs from October 1 to September 30.

G Gram.

G1 HCPCS Level II modifier, for use with CPT or HCPCS Level II codes, that identifies the most recent urea reduction ratio (URR) reading of less than 60. Medicare requires a URR to determine effectiveness of dialysis.

G2 HCPCS Level II modifier, for use with CPT or HCPCS Level II codes, that identifies the most recent urea reduction ratio (URR) reading of 60 to 64.9. Medicare requires a URR to determine effectiveness of dialysis.

G3 HCPCS Level II modifier, for use with CPT or HCPCS Level II codes, that identifies the most recent urea reduction ratio (URR) reading of 65 to 69.9. Medicare requires a URR to determine effectiveness of dialysis.

G4 HCPCS Level II modifier, for use with CPT or HCPCS Level II codes, that identifies the most recent urea reduction ratio (URR) reading of 70 to 74.9. Medicare requires a URR to determine effectiveness of dialysis.

G5 HCPCS Level II modifier, for use with CPT or HCPCS Level II codes, that identifies the most recent urea reduction ratio (URR) reading of 75 or greater. Medicare requires a URR to determine effectiveness of dialysis.

G6 HCPCS Level II modifier, for use with CPT or HCPCS Level II codes, that identifies an end stage renal disease (ESRD) patient for whom fewer than six dialysis sessions have been provided in a month. It should be appended to CPT code 90999 when submitted to Medicare.

G7 HCPCS Level II modifier, for use with CPT or HCPCS Level II codes, that identifies a pregnancy resulting from rape or incest or a pregnancy certified by the physician as life threatening. Appended to CPT procedure codes for abortion services.

G8 HCPCS modifier showing monitored anesthesia care for deep, complex, complicated, or markedly invasive surgical procedure.

G9 HCPCS modifier showing monitored anesthesia care of a patient with a severe cardiopulmonary condition.

GA *1)* HCPCS Level II modifier, for use with CPT or HCPCS Level II codes, that identifies that a waiver of liability statement is on file in the patient's records. This modifier indicates that there is a signed advanced beneficiary notice (ABN) retained in the physician's office. It has no effect on reimbursement, but potential liability determination is based on its use. *2)* Gastric analysis.

gadoxetate disodium Organ-specific intravenous MRI contrast agent used to detect and diagnose lesions in the liver. May be sold under the brand name Eovist. Supply is reported with HCPCS Level II code A9581.

Gafsa boil Dry or urban cutaneous leishmaniasis, one form of Old World cutaneous leishmaniasis. This parasitic skin disease is caused by the protozoa Leishmania tropica, spread by the bite of sand flies, and occurring in large urban areas in the Middle East, especially Iran and Iraq, the Mediterranean, and India. Manifestation is mainly a single, large developing boil or furuncle type lesion that persists over a year. Lymphadenopathy may be present. Report this condition with ICD-9-CM code 085.1.

Gaisböck's syndrome Associated with hypertension, but without hyposplenomegaly. Report this disorder with ICD-9-CM code 289.0.

gait Manner in which a person walks.

gait analysis Correlation of clinical findings and biomedical measures to determine the cause of a patient's postural and movement impairments when walking.

gait training Procedural intervention to restore normal stance, balance, arm and leg swing, speed, and sequence of muscle contractions for walking. May also include teaching the patient to use an assistive device.

galacto- Relating to milk.

galactocele Tumor or cyst-like enlargement of the milk-containing gland in the breast, reported with ICD-9-CM code 611.5. If occurring in pregnancy or the puerperium, report with a code from subcategory 676.8.

galactogram Following injection of a radiopaque dye into the ducts of the breast, radiographic pictures are taken of the milk-producing mammary ducts. *Synonym(s): ductogram.*

galactorrhea Rare condition in which breast milk is secreted in women who are not breast feeding, possibly indicative of a tumor or hormone imbalance. In obstetric cases, this is an excessive or persistent milk secretion, even in the absence of nursing. Galactorrhea is reported with ICD-9-CM code 611.6 unless occurring in an obstetric patient, in which case it is reported with an ICD-9-CM code from subcategory 676.6.

galactosemia Congenital disorder marked by the inability to metabolize galactose due to a missing enzyme.

galactosylceramide lipidosis Inherited disorder characterized by a deficiency of the enzyme galactosylceramidase, resulting in rapid destruction of cerebral myelin and globoid bodies in the brain's white matter. Infants develop seizures, deafness, blindness, paralysis, and mental deficiencies. Report this disorder with ICD-9-CM code 330.0. *Synonym(s): globoid cell leukodystrophy, Krabbe's leukodystrophy.*

Galeazzi fracture Break of the radius proximal to the wrist with a distal ulnar dislocation.

Galeazzi sign Evidence of congenital dislocation of the hip. The dislocated side is shorter when both thighs are flexed to 90 degrees, as demonstrated in infants. In older patients, a curvature of the spine is produced by the shortened leg.

G-I

Gallstone

Right and left bile ducts

Right hepatic artery

Cystic artery

Triangle of Calot

Common hepatic artery

Portal vein

Cystic duct

Gallstone in fundus

Common bile duct empties into Duodenum

gallstone Calculus composed of crystallized cholesterol or bile ionized calcium crystals. Once formed it can gradually grow to a size that completely blocks the gallbladder outlet into the biliary duct system, resulting in intense pain. In the absence of cholecystitis and obstruction, it is reported with ICD-9-CM code 574.20 *Synonym(s): biliary colic.* **g. ileus** Obstruction of the intestine by gallstone. This condition is reported with ICD-9-CM code 560.31.

gallstone ileus Obstruction of the intestine by gallstone.

GamaSTAN Brand name hepatitis A immune globulin provided in 2 ml and 10 ml vials. Supply of GamaSTAN is reported with unlisted CPT code 90399; administration is reported separately. Need for vaccination is reported with ICD-9-CM code V01.89.

gamekeeper's thumb Loosening of the ulnar collateral ligament of the thumb due to a chronic pattern of injury. The name comes from the practice of killing game by grasping the head of the animal between the thumb and index finger to break its neck. In chronic injury, the ulnar collateral ligament is stretched and damaged over time.

gamete Unfertilized male or female reproductive cell; an ovum or a spermatozoon.

Gamimune N See gamma globulin.

gamma globulin Serum immunoglobulins, glycoproteins that function as antibodies, are injected to provide passive immunity by increasing the amount of circulating antibodies. It is used to help prevent infections in patients exposed to certain pathogens and to boost immune systems in patients who suffer primary humoral immunodeficiency. Correct code assignment is dependent upon dosage. May be sold under the brand names BayGam, Carimune, Gamimune, Gammagard S/D, Gammar-P IV, IGIM, IGIV, Iveegam EN, Panglobulin, Polygam S/D, or Venoglobulin-S.

gamma knife Type of stereotactic radiosurgery that uses multiple cobalt sources and beams to deliver a precision treatment beam.

gamma ray Electromagnetic radiation emitted by a radioactive substance.

Gammagard Brand name injectable immune globulin derived from human plasma. Indicated for the treatment of patients with a primary immune deficiency disease. Supply is reported with HCPCS Level II code J1569.

Gammar P See gamma globulin.

Gamunex Brand name immune globulin indicated for the treatment of diseases that cause impaired antibody formation. It may also be administered to patients with idiopathic thrombocytopenia purpura (ITP) to quickly elevate platelet counts to prevent hemorrhage or to allow the patient to have surgery. Administered by intravenous infusion, the supply is reported with HCPCS Level II code J1561.

ganciclovir sodium Synthetic guanine derivative used to treat cytomegaloviral retinitis in immunocompromised patients. Supply is reported with HCPCS Level II code J1570. May be sold under the brand name Cytovene.

Ganglion

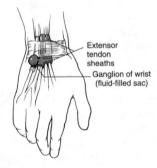

Extensor tendon sheaths

Ganglion of wrist (fluid-filled sac)

ganglion Fluid-filled, benign cyst appearing on a tendon sheath or aponeurosis, frequently found in the hand, wrist, or foot and connecting to an underlying joint. *gasserian g.* Large group of nerve cells at the root of the trigeminal nerve (cranial nerve V). *Synonym(s): trigeminal ganglion.* **geniculate g.** Group of nerve cell bodies of the facial nerve where the fibers turn sharply at the lateral end of the internal acoustic meatus.

gangrene Death of tissue, usually resulting from a loss of vascular supply, followed by a bacterial attack or onset of disease.

gangrenous balanitis Infection thought to be due to a spirochetal infection in which there is rapid erosion and destruction of the glans penis and sometimes the entire external genitalia. Gangrenous balanitis is reported with

G-I

ICD-9-CM code 607.1. **Synonym(s):** *balanoposthomycosis, Corbus' disease.*

ganirelix acetate Drug used in infertility treatment that blocks the release of luteinizing hormone (LH) and follicle stimulating hormone (FSH) early in the menstrual cycle, stopping premature surges in gonadotropin that can interfere with medically induced/supervised hyperstimulation of the ovaries. Supply is reported with HCPCS Level II code S0132. May be sold under the brand name Antagon.

Ganser's syndrome Psychotic-like condition, but without symptoms and signs of a traditional psychosis. Occurring in prisoners who feign insanity or who suffer head injury. Report this disorder with ICD-9-CM code 300.16. **Synonym(s):** *hysterical syndrome.*

GAO General accounting office.

GAP Gluteal artery perforator.

gap codes CPT codes that are not covered by Medicare and for this reason do not have relative values developed under the resource-based relative value scale (RBRVS).

Garamycin See gentamycin.

Gardasil Brand name human papillomavirus (HPV) vaccine. Supply of the vaccine is reported with CPT code 90649 and administration with 90471.

Gardner Wells tongs Immobilizing device used for cervical spine injuries. Two sharp metal pins are screwed into the superficial layer of the skull and then connected to traction devices for stabilization of the spine.

Gardner-Diamond syndrome Bruising occurring easily and large, involving surrounding tissues, resulting in pain, and spawning others. Assumed to be a form of autoimmune deficiency. Report this disorder with ICD-9-CM code 287.2.

gas tamponade Absorbable gas may be injected to force the retina against the choroid. Common gases include room air, short-acting sulfahexafluoride, intermediate-acting perfluoroethane, or long-acting perfluorooctane.

gastrectomy Surgical excision of all or part of the stomach, reported with CPT codes 43620-43634.

gastro- Relating to the stomach and abdominal region.

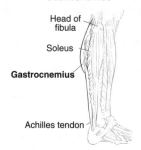

Gastrocnemius

Head of fibula

Soleus

Gastrocnemius

Achilles tendon

Medial head of gastrocnemius

Lateral head of gastrocnemius

Soleus

Achilles tendon

The gastrocnemius and soleus muscles share a common insertion as the Achilles tendon

The gastrocnemius muscle is surgically freed of its attachment to the soleus muscle and the Achilles tendon, with resultant lengthening of the muscle

gastrocnemius Large muscle of the back of the leg that flexes the foot and knee; the outermost portion of the muscle group that is commonly referred to as the calf muscle.

Gastrocrom See cromolyn sodium.

gastroduodenostomy Surgical creation of an opening from the stomach to the duodenum.

gastroesophageal laceration-hemorrhage syndrome Serious condition in which the mucosa of the esophagus or gastroesophageal junction is torn, usually preceded by vomiting. Although painless, it can be fatal.

gastroesophageal reflux disease Weakening of the lower esophageal sphincter allowing reflux of the stomach contents into the esophagus. One form is commonly defined as "heartburn." **Synonyms:** *GERD.*

gastrojejunal loop obstruction syndrome Distended afferent loop marked by illness and pain. Caused by acute or chronic obstruction of the duodenum and jejunum proximal to a gastrojejunostomy. Report this disorder with ICD-9-CM code 537.89. **Synonym(s):** *gastrojejunal loop obstruction.*

gastrojejunostomy Surgical creation of an opening from the stomach to the jejunum.

gastroparesis Delay in the emptying of food from the stomach into the small bowel due to a degree of paralysis in the muscles lining the stomach wall. This condition is reported with ICD-9-CM code 536.3.

gastroptosis Downward displacement of the stomach. This condition is reported with ICD-9-CM code 537.5.

gastrorrhaphy Repair or suturing of a perforation of the stomach or duodenum.

gastroschisis Congenital anomaly of the abdominal wall in which a fissure remains open, typically resulting in herniation of the small intestine and part of the large intestine.

gastrostomy Temporary or permanent artificial opening made in the stomach for gastrointestinal decompression or to provide nutrition when not maintained by other methods.

gatekeeper Primary care physician in a health care system in which a member's care must be provided by a primary care physician unless the physician refers the member to a specialist or approves the care provided by a specialist.

gatifloxacin Fluoroquinolone antibiotic that kills gram negative and gram positive susceptible bacteria, used to treat a long list of infections ranging from bronchitis to urinary tract infections. Supply is reported with HCPCS Level II code J1590. May be sold under the brand name Tequin.

Gaucher disease Genetic metabolic disorder in which fat deposits may accumulate in the spleen, liver, lungs, bone marrow, and brain, reported with ICD-9-CM code 272.7. Genetic testing for Gaucher disease is reported with HCPCS Level II code S3848.

gav. Gavage.

GAVE Gastric antral vascular ectasia. Dilated veins in the stomach that may resemble the markings on a watermelon. If bleeding is not present, report GAVE with ICD-9-CM code 537.82. If bleeding is present, report 537.83. *Synonym(s): watermelon stomach.*

Gayet-Wernicke's syndrome Thiamine deficiency, disturbances in ocular motility, pupillary alterations, nystagmus, ataxia with tremors, and coexisting organic toxic psychosis. Most often due to alcoholism. Report this disorder with ICD-9-CM code 265.1.

GB Gallbladder.

GBM Glioblastoma multiforme. High-grade astrocytoma or brain tumor. GBMs are usually aggressive and require intensive therapy.

GBS Group B Streptococcus, a bacterial infection reported with ICD-9-CM code 041.02; use 482.32 for GBS pneumonia.

GC HCPCS Level II modifier, for use with CPT or HCPCS Level II codes, that indicates a service that has been performed in part by a resident under the direction of a teaching physician. The teaching physician bills for the service and is certifying that he/she was present during the key portion(s) of the service and was immediately available during all other portions of the service.

GCA Giant cell arteritis. Inflammation of the lining of arteries, most commonly those in the temple. GCA is most commonly seen in aging patients. Risk comes from reduced blood flow in the artery due to swelling. Symptoms include headache, jaw pain, and blurred vision. Regardless of location, GCA is reported with ICD-9-CM code 446.5. *Synonym(s): granulomatous arteritis, Horton's disease, temporal arteritis.*

GCS Glasgow Coma Score. Assessment of trauma based on eye, verbal, and motor response in a coma patient. A score of 13 or higher correlates with mild brain injury in a coma patient; 9 to 12 is a moderate injury, and 8 or less is a severe brain injury.

G-CSF Filgrastim (granulocyte colony-stimulating factor).

GD HCPCS Level II modifier used to denote that units of service exceed the medically unlikely edit value and represents reasonable and necessary services.

GDD Glaucoma drainage device. Refers to an aqueous drainage shunt or tube placed to mitigate glaucoma. Insertion of the shunt is reported with CPT code 66180; revision with 66185; and removal with 67120.

GDM Gestational diabetes mellitus.

GDS Geriatric depression scale. Simple scale developed to diagnose depression in older persons, based on questions regarding how the patient views his or her current life. *Synonym(s): Brink-Yesavage, Yesavage-Brink.*

GE HCPCS Level II modifier, for use with CPT or HCPCS Level II codes, that indicates a service that has been performed by a resident without the presence of a teaching physician under the primary care exception.

Gee-Herter-Heubner syndrome Catarrhal dysentery. Malabsorption syndrome of all ages precipitated by gluten-containing foods. Children suffer growth retardation and irritability; adults suffer difficulty in breathing and clubbing of fingers. Wasting and fatigue in both adults and children Report this disorder with ICD-9-CM code 579.0.

Gehrung pessary Vaginal devise inserted to provide support to cystoceles or rectoceles and for uterine prolapse. Gehrung pessary is non-rubber. Supply is reported with HCPCS Level II code A4562.

Gélineau's syndrome Form of epilepsy where the patient abruptly falls asleep rather than suffering grand or petite mals. Report this disorder with an ICD-9-CM code from range 347.00-347.11. *Synonym(s): narcolepsy.*

Gellhorn pessary Vaginal device inserted to treat uterine prolapse or procidentia. Gellhorn pessary is non-rubber. Supply is reported with HCPCS Level II code A4562.

gemcitabine HCl Chemotherapeutic agent used to treat pancreatic and breast cancer. It is often given with cisplatin due to its synergistic effect in vitro. Supply is reported with HCPCS Level II code J9201. May be sold under the brand name Gemzar.

gemtuzumab ozogamicin Chemotherapy agent used to treat acute myeloid leukemia in patients who are not candidates for cytotoxic chemotherapy in the first relapse. Kills cancer cells by binding with an antigen on the cell membrane of immature leukemia cells and releasing the antibody complex in the cell, disrupting DNA strands. This drug is associated with many common and life-threatening side effects such as sepsis, hemorrhage, neutropenic fever, and leucopenia. Supply is reported with HCPCS Level II code J9300. May be sold under the brand name Mylotarg.

Gemzar See gemcitabine HCl.

general anesthesia State of unconsciousness produced by an anesthetic agent or agents, inducing amnesia by blocking the awareness center in the brain, and rendering the patient unable to control protective reflexes, such as breathing.

generalized convulsive epilepsy (tonic-clonic epilepsy) Abnormalities in the brain's electrical activity that cause convulsive seizures with tension of limbs (tonic) or rhythmic contractions (clonic).

-genic Production, causation, generation.

geniculate ganglion Part of the facial nerve where fibers turn sharply at the lateral end of the internal acoustic meatus.

geniculate ganglion syndrome Facial paralysis, otalgia, and herpes zoster caused by viral infection in seventh cranial nerve and geniculate ganglion. Report this disorder with ICD-9-CM code 053.11. *Synonym(s): Hunt's syndrome.*

geniculate ganglionitis Inflammation of nerve tissue at the bend in the facial nerve.

genioglossus Fan-shaped, extrinsic tongue muscle that forms the majority of the body of the tongue.

genioglossus advancement Surgical procedure where the base of the tongue is pulled forward, usually to increase airway size due to deformity or a sleep breathing disorder.

genioplasty Cosmetic surgery used to improve the appearance of a person's chin. *Synonym(s): mentoplasty.*

genitalia External organs related to reproduction.

genito- Relating to reproduction.

gentamicin sulfate Aminoglycoside antibiotic used to treat meningitis and serious infections secondary to sensitive strains of Pseudomonas aerugosa, E coli,

Proteus, Klebsiella, Serratia, Enterobacter, Citrobacter, and Staphylococcus. This is also used as a prophylaxis against endocarditis for gastrointestinal and genitourinary surgical procedures. Supply is reported with HCPCS Level II code J1580. May be sold under the brand names Cidomycin, Garamycin, Gentamycin Sulfate ADD-Vantage, Jenamicin.

Gentech See alteplase recombinant.

GentleLASE Brand name alexandrite laser with a long pulse and a cooling system for dermatologic procedures, treatment of vascular lesions, and hair removal.

genu recurvatum Congenital condition in which the knee is hyperextended so that the leg curves backward. This condition may occur either unilaterally or bilaterally and is reported with ICD-9-CM code 754.40. *Synonym(s): back knee.*

genu valgum Condition in which the thighs slant inward, causing the knees to be angled abnormally close together, leaving the space between the ankles wider than normal. If specified as congenital, report this condition with ICD-9-CM code 755.64, otherwise report 736.41. *Synonym(s): knock-knee.*

genu varum Condition in which the thighs and/or legs are bowed in an outward curve with an abnormally increased space between the knees. Report this condition with ICD-9-CM code 736.42 for acquired and 754.44 if congenital. *Synonym(s): bowleg, tibia vara.*

geographic practice cost indexes Cost indexes used to adjust for differences among geographic areas. Under the resource-based relative value scale, there are three GPCIs for each locality, one for work, practice expense, and malpractice. *Synonym(s): GPCI.*

geometric mean length of stay Statistically adjusted value for all cases for a given diagnosis-related group, allowing for the outliers, transfer cases, and negative outlier cases that would normally skew the data. The GMLOS is used to determine payment only for transfer cases (i.e., the per diem rate). *Synonym(s): GMLOS.*

geophagia Compulsive eating of dirt or gravel; reported with ICD-9-CM code 307.52.

GERD Gastroesophageal reflux disease. Disorder in which acidic gastric contents flow back into the esophagus as a chronic condition, causing pain, inflammation, and erosion of the esophagus. GERD is reported with ICD-9-CM code 530.81. The condition is commonly controlled with the use of acid pump inhibitors such as Nexium or Prilosec. *NCD Reference: 100.9.*

Gerhardt's syndrome Paralysis of vocal cords causing inspiratory dyspnea. Report this disorder with ICD-9-CM code 478.30.

Gerstmann's syndrome Right-left disorientation, finger agnosia, agraphia, and constructional apraxia, due to

G-I

lesion in the angular gyrus of the dominant hemisphere of the brain. Report this disorder with ICD-9-CM code 784.69.

Gerstmann-Straussler-Scheinker syndrome Rare, fatal neurodegenerative prion disease that is usually inherited. A slowly progressive condition, symptoms include difficulty speaking, unsteadiness, and worsening dementia. Report this disorder with ICD-9-CM code 046.71.

GES Gastric electric stimulation. Treatment for chronic nausea and vomiting associated with gastroparesis by using mild electrical impulses to stimulate the stomach.

gestational diabetes Glucose intolerance that develops in pregnant women who do not have a history of diabetes, most commonly developing in mid-pregnancy and resolving at delivery. It is treated primarily with diet but insulin may be required in some cases. Certain risk factors may predispose a woman to gestation diabetes, including being older than 25 years of age, obesity, a family history of diabetes, previous stillbirth, birth of a large infant, or one with a birth defect. This condition is reported with a code from ICD-9-CM subcategory 648.8.

GF HCPCS Level II modifier, for use with CPT or HCPCS Level II codes, that indicates nonphysician (e.g., nurse practitioner [NP], certified registered nurse anesthetist [CRNA], certified registered nurse [CRN], clinical nurse specialist [CNS], physician assistant [PA]) patient care services performed in a critical access hospital. Some Medicare carriers do not cover services of CRNAs with this modifier.

GFR Glomerular filtration rate.

GG HCPCS Level II modifier, for use with CPT or HCPCS Level II codes, that identifies the performance and payment of a screening mammogram and diagnostic mammogram on the same patient on the same day. It is required to be appended to the claim for the diagnostic mammogram. It is also required when a screening mammogram is converted to a diagnostic mammogram; the screening mammogram is not billed.

GH *1)* HCPCS Level II modifier, for use with CPT or HCPCS Level II codes, that identifies a diagnostic mammogram converted from screening mammogram on same day. *2)* Growth hormone.

GHAA Group Health Association of America. HMO trade organization.

GHP Group health plan.

GI Gastrointestinal.

Gianotti Crosti syndrome Papular acrodermatitis of childhood, usually benign. It is a self-limiting inflammatory response to Epstein-Barr, cytomegalovirus, or hepatitis B virus, manifest as a diverse exanthem. Report Gianotti Crosti syndrome with ICD-9-CM code

057.8 if the specific virus is undocumented or report the ICD-9-CM code for the specific virus if it is known.

giant cell tumor Common, usually benign tumor occurring most often in the hand.

giardiasis Infection by the flagellate protozoan Giardia lamblia causing gastrointestinal problems such as vomiting, chronic diarrhea, and weight loss in humans and other vertebrates. The cyst stage of the parasite is usually ingested through contaminated water. Once in the stomach, the cyst opens and the trophozoite moves into the small intestines and latches on. Report with ICD-9-CM code 007.1. Diagnosis is confirmed by running an enzyme immunoassay for G. lamblia, reported with CPT code 86674.

GID Gender identity disorder, reported with ICD-9-CM code 302.85 in adults and adolescents or 302.6 in children.

GIFT Gamete intrafallopian transfer.

gigantism Overgrowth of the short, flat bones. A chronic condition that is caused by overproduction of the pituitary growth hormone in which men can reach 80 inches in height. Gigantism is reported with ICD-9-CM code 253.0.

Gigli saw Saw made of thin, flexible wire with teeth along the edge used for cutting bones (e.g., craniotomy).

Gilbert's sign Increased urination during fasting, seen in patients with cirrhosis of the liver.

Gilbert's syndrome Benign elevation of unconjugated bilirubin with no liver damage or other deformities. Report this disorder with ICD-9-CM code 277.4.

Gilford (-Hutchinson) syndrome Precocious senility with death from coronary artery disease occurring before 10 years of age. Report this disorder with ICD-9-CM code 259.8. *Synonym(s): Hutchinson-Gilford syndrome.*

Gilles de la Tourette syndrome Familial neuropsychiatric disorder of variable expression that is characterized by multiple recurrent involuntary tics involving body movements (e.g., eye blinks, grimaces, or knee bends) and vocalizations (e.g., grunts, snorts, or utterance of inappropriate words). This syndrome often has one or more associated behavioral or psychiatric conditions (e.g., attention deficit disorder or obsessive-compulsive behavior) and is more common in males than females. It usually has an onset in childhood and often stabilizes or ameliorates in adulthood. Report this condition with ICD-9-CM code 307.23. *Synonym(s): TS.*

Gillespie's syndrome Congenital dysplasia of the eyes, teeth, and extremities. Report this disorder with ICD-9-CM code 759.89.

gingiva Soft tissues surrounding the crowns of unerupted teeth and necks of erupted teeth.

gingivectomy Surgical excision or trimming of overgrown gum tissue back to normal contours using a scalpel, electrocautery, or a laser. CPT code 41820 or HCPCS Level II code D4210 or D4211 is reported for each quadrant of the mouth in which gingivectomy is performed.

gingivitis Inflamed gingiva (oral mucosa) that surrounds the teeth. Most codes for gingivitis are found in category 523 of ICD-9-CM, and are chosen on the basis of whether the condition is chronic or acute, and whether it is caused by plaque. A few other specific forms of gingivitis cover conditions like herpetic gingivitis (054.2) or acute necrotizing ulcerative gingivitis (101).

gingivoplasty Repair or reconstruction of the gum tissue, altering the gingival contours by excising areas of gum tissue or making incisions through the gingiva to create a gingival flap. Gingivoplasty is reported with ICD-9-CM procedure code 24.2. CPT code 41872 is assigned for each quadrant in which gingivoplasty is performed.

GJ HCPCS Level II modifier, for use with CPT or HCPCS Level II codes, that identifies an ôopt outö physician or practitioner emergency or urgent service. For use with claims submitted to Medicare for services rendered by an opt-out provider who has not signed a contract with the Medicare patient requiring either emergent or urgent medical care.

GK HCPCS Level II modifier used to denote a reasonable and necessary item or service that is associated with modifier GA or GZ.

GL HCPCS Level II modifier used to denote a medically unnecessary upgrade that is provided instead of a non-upgraded item for no charge and with no advance beneficiary notice (ABN).

glabella Space between the eyebrows and above the nose, or the corresponding area on the frontal bone

gland Group of cells that secrete or excrete chemicals called hormones.

glanders Infection by actinobacillus, malleomyces, or pseudomonas mallei, which is usually seen in horses and transmitted to humans, causing inflammation of the mucous membranes and ulcers on the skin that break down into the deeper tissue layers and can ultimately affect tendons and bone. In the chronic form, as in farcy, the lymphatic system will also become involved. Report with ICD-9-CM code 024. *Synonym(s): farcy, Malleus.*

glandular plague Highly contagious, most common form of plague, caused by infection of Yersinia pestis. It is characterized by onset of fever, chills, headache, and swollen, tender, inflamed lymph glands called buboes, which develop intravascular coagulation, turning necrotic and gangrenous. Report this condition with ICD-9-CM

code 020.0. *Synonym(s): black death, bubonic plague, pestis bubonica.*

glans penis Distal end or head of the penis.

glatiramer acetate Biological response modifier that is thought to act on the immune processes that develop multiple sclerosis. It is a well-tolerated therapy that effectively reduces new brain lesions and the frequency of relapses in people with relapsing-remitting multiple sclerosis and is administered by subcutaneous injection. Supply is reported with HCPCS Level II code J1595. May be sold under the brand name Copaxone.

glaucoma Rise in intraocular pressure, restricting blood flow and decreasing vision.

glaucoma associated with pupillary block Functional defect of the pupil impeding aqueous flow and resulting in increased ocular pressure and decreased vision.

GLBA Gramm-Leach-Bliley Act.

GLC Gas liquid chromatography.

Gleason score Rating system assigned by a pathologist to characterize the aggressiveness of a malignancy. A score ranges from two to 10. The higher the number, the more aggressive the malignancy.

Gleevec See imatinab.

Glénard's syndrome Bloating, gas, pain, and fullness experienced in left upper abdominal quadrant with pain sometimes radiating up into left chest. Downward displacement of viscera may cause bulging of abdomen and other symptoms. Report this disorder with ICD-9-CM code 569.89.

Glenn procedure Creation of a shunt by anastomosing the superior vena cava to the pulmonary artery to increase perfusion to both lungs. Report CPT code 33766 for classical; 33767 for bidirectional procedure.

glenoid fossa Shallow depressed area on the lateral edge of the scapula that forms the junction with the head of the humerus. *Synonym(s): cavitas glenoidalis.*

glimepiride Oral medication exclusive to lowering blood glucose in Type II diabetics. May be sold as brand name Amaryl.

Glinski-Simmonds syndrome Wasting of pituitary gland as result of some other condition or affliction. Report this disorder with ICD-9-CM code 253.2.

glipizide Oral medication exclusive to lowering blood glucose in Type II diabetics. May be sold under the brand name Glucotrol.

GLM General linear modeling. Analysis to determine if functional magnetic resonance imaging correctly mapped an activity to the right part of the brain.

global surgery package Normal surgical procedure with no complications that includes all of the elements

G-I

needed to perform the procedure and includes routine follow-up care. **Synonym(s):** *follow-up days, FUD.*

globoid cell leukodystrophy Inherited disorder characterized by a deficiency of the enzyme galactosylceramidase, resulting in rapid destruction of cerebral myelin and globoid bodies in the brain's white matter. Infants develop seizures, deafness, blindness, paralysis, and mental deficiencies. Report this disorder with ICD-9-CM code 330.0. **Synonym(s):** *galactosylceramide lipidosis, Krabbe's leukodystrophy.*

glomerulonephritis Disease of the kidney with diffuse inflammation of the capillary loops of the glomeruli. It may be a complication of bacterial infection or immune disorders and can lead to renal failure and may be associated with hypertension or diabetes.

glossitis Inflammation and swelling of the tongue that may be associated with infection, adverse drug reactions, smoking, or injury. A severe case of glossitis may necessitate a tracheostomy to prevent asphyxia. This condition is reported with ICD-9-CM code 529.0.

glossodynia Tongue pain.

glossopharyngeal neuralgia Pain in the throat, tongue, or palate.

glossotomy Surgical cutting of the tongue.

glucagon Preparation of the hormone secreted by the islets of Langerhans cells of the pancreas in response to hypoglycemia that triggers the catabolism of glycogen in the liver to glucose for use by the body. Supply is reported with HCPCS Level II code J1610. May be sold under the brand name Glucagen.

Glucophage Brand name oral medication exclusive to lowering blood glucose in Type II diabetics. Glucophage contains metformin.

glucose tolerance test Timed test to detect diabetes consisting of hourly blood and urine tests after the patient has had a preparation containing a high level of glucose. **Synonym(s):** *GTT.*

Glucotrol Brand name oral medication exclusive to lowering blood glucose in Type II diabetics. Glucotrol contains glipizide.

glucuronyl transferase syndrome Benign elevation of unconjugated bilirubin with no liver damage or other deformities. Report this disorder with ICD-9-CM code 277.4.

glue ear syndrome Painless secretion of mucoid fluid in the middle ear, stopping up the eustachian tube and causing hearing loss. Report this disorder with ICD-9-CM code 381.20.

Gly. supp. Glycerin suppository.

glycopyrrolate Anticholinergic drug given prior to the induction of general anesthesia that blocks transmission of acetylcholine by postganglionic cholinergic nerves in smooth muscle. It reduces oral secretions and gastric acid, and inhibits vagal nerve stimulation that causes bradycardia and other cardiac arrhythmias. Administration in the process of prepping the patient is part of anesthesia induction. Supply is reported with HCPCS Level II code J7642 or J7643. May be sold under the brand name Robinul.

gm Gram.

GM HCPCS Level II modifier, for use with HCPCS Level II codes, that indicates that multiple patients were transported on one ambulance trip. The total number of patients transported should be listed.

GME Graduate medical education.

GMLOS Geometric mean length of stay. Statistically adjusted value for all cases for a given diagnosis-related group, allowing for the outliers, transfer cases, and negative outlier cases that would normally skew the data. The GMLOS is used to determine payment only for transfer cases (i.e., the per diem rate).

GMP Guanosine monophosphate.

GN HCPCS Level II modifier, for use with CPT or HCPCS Level II codes, that identifies services delivered under an outpatient speech language pathology plan of care

GNID Gram-negative intracellular diplocci.

GnRH Gonadotropin-releasing hormone.

goiter Abnormal enlargement of the thyroid gland commonly caused by a deficiency of dietary iodine, reported with ICD-9-CM code 240.9.

gold sodium thiomalate Gold salt antiarthritic used to treat rheumatoid arthritis. Supply is reported with HCPCS Level II code J1600. May be sold under the brand name Myochrysine.

Goldberg (-Maxwell) (-Morris) syndrome Male pseudohermaphroditism with an incompletely developed vagina, rudimentary uterus and fallopian tubes, scanty or absent axillary/pubic hair, and amenorrhea. Report this disorder with ICD-9-CM code 259.51. **Synonym(s):** *Goldberg-Maxwell syndrome, hairless women syndrome, Morris syndrome.*

Goldenhar's syndrome Congenital abnormality presenting with microtia of the ear, vertebral abnormality in the neck, and a growth of tissue over one eyeball. This syndrome is reported with ICD-9-CM code 756.0. **Synonym(s):** *oculoauriculovertebral dysplasia.*

Goldflam-Erb syndrome Progressive muscular weakness beginning in face and throat caused by a defect in myoneural conduction. Report this disorder with ICD-9-CM code 358.00. **Synonym(s):** *Erb syndrome, Goldflam syndrome, Hoppe syndrome.*

Goltz-Gorlin syndrome Irregular linear streaks of skin atrophy, skeletal malformations, papillomas of the lips and labia, and occasional alopecia. Report this disorder with ICD-9-CM code 757.39.

Gol-Vernet pyelotomy Calyces and renal pelvis of the kidney are explored.

gonadal dysgenesis Rare inherited disorder occurring in females that is characterized by the absence of an X chromosome and affects normal sexual development. It is evidenced by physical distinctions such as short stature, webbing of neck, absence of menses, retarded development of secondary sex characteristics, cortication of the aorta, and skeletal deformities.

gonadorelin HCl Medication used to test for suspected gonadotropin deficiency, regardless of its origin in the hypothalamus or the anterior pituitary, and also to check for residual gonadotropic function of the pituitary status post tumor removal. In CPT, the gonadotropin releasing hormone evocative test is reported with 80426. The drug and its administration are not included in the evocative test and should be reported separately. Supply is reported with HCPCS Level II code J1620. May be sold under the brand name Factrel.

Gonal-F Brand name fertility drug with the active ingredient follitropin alpha, administered by injection. Supply is reported with HCPCS Level II code S0126.

Gonin's operation Thermocautery of the fissure of a detached retina is performed through an incision in the sclera.

goniosynechiae Adhesion binding the front surface of the peripheral iris to the back surface of the cornea.

gono- Relating to the genitals, offspring, origination.

Goodpasture's syndrome Renal condition where nephritis progresses rapidly to death, leaving lungs showing extensive hemosiderosis or bleeding. Report this disorder with ICD-9-CM code 446.21.

Gopalan's syndrome Severe discomfort of the feet and other extremities associated with excessive sweating and elevated skin temperature; believed to be caused by a riboflavin deficiency. Report this disorder with ICD-9-CM code 266.2. *Synonym(s): burning feet syndrome.*

Gore Viabahn Brand name endoprosthesis.

Gorlin's sign Ability to touch the nose with the tongue, seen in patients with Ehlers-Danlos syndrome.

Gorlin-Chaudhry-Moss syndrome Congenital lesion of the basal cells. Report this disorder with ICD-9-CM code 759.89.

goserelin acetate implant Subcutaneous implant that decreases secretion of sex hormones by acting on the pituitary gland to decrease the release of follicle stimulating hormone and luteinizing hormone. It is used in the treatment of hormone sensitive prostate gland tumors and in cases of dysfunctional uterine bleeding to decrease endometrial tissue growth within the uterus.

Report CPT code 11980 for insertion. Supply is reported with HCPCS Level II code J9202. May be sold under brand name Zoladex. Report prophylactic use with ICD-9-CM code V07.59.

Gougerot (-Houwer) -Sjögren syndrome Complex of symptoms of unknown source in middle-aged women in which the following triad exists: keratoconjunctivitis sicca, zerostomia, and connective tissue disease (usually rheumatoid arthritis but sometimes systemic lupus erythematosus). Cause may be abnormal immune response. Report this disorder with ICD-9-CM code 710.2. *Synonym(s): sicca syndrome.*

Gougerot-Blum syndrome Purpuric skin eruption seen on the legs, thighs, and lower trunk of men 40 to 60 years of age and characterized by minute rust-colored papules that fuse into plaques. Report this disorder with ICD-9-CM code 709.1.

Gougerot-Carteaud syndrome Benign neoplasm producing finger-like projections from epithelial surface in girls nearing puberty. Papillas begin on back and between breasts, eventually spreading over the torso and throughout the body. Report this disorder with ICD-9-CM code 701.8.

Gouley's syndrome Restrictive pericarditis. Report this disorder with ICD-9-CM code 423.2.

government mandates Services mandated by state or federal law, such as the correct use of ICD-9-CM codes.

Gowers' syndrome Fall in blood pressure, slow pulse, and convulsions. Believed to be sudden stimulation of vagal nerve by receptors in heart, carotid sinus, or aortic arch. Report this disorder with ICD-9-CM code 780.2.

Gowers-Paton-Kennedy syndrome Meningioma of optic nerve with central scotoma and contralateral choked disk. Report this disorder with ICD-9-CM code 377.04. *Synonym(s): Foster-Kennedy syndrome, Gowers-Paton-Kennedy syndrome.*

GP General practitioner.

GPCI Geographic practice cost indexes. Cost indexes used to adjust for differences among geographic areas. Under the resource-based relative value scale, there are three GPCIs for each locality, one for work, practice expense, and malpractice.

GR HCPCS Level II modifier used to denote a service that was performed in whole or in part by a resident in a Department of Veterans' Affairs Medical Center or clinic. This modifier requires the resident to be supervised in accordance with VA policy.

gr. Grain.

graafian follicle Capsule surrounding a maturing egg cell within the ovary that is filled with fluid and acts to protect the egg as it develops.

G-I

grace days *1)* Days of an inpatient hospitalization that are billable to the patient because they occur after the hospital receives a quality improvement organization (QIO) denial notice. *2)* Number of days determined by the QIO to be necessary for the physician or family to make arrangements for discharge from the hospital.

grace period Set number of days past the due date of a premium payment during which medical coverage may not be canceled and the premium payment may be made, or after employment termination. It varies by health plan contract and state law but is generally 30 to 60 days.

Gradenigo's syndrome Localized meningitis in fifth and sixth cranial nerves, causing paralysis and pain in the temporal region. Report this disorder with ICD-9-CM code 383.02.

Graefe's operation Cataracts are corrected by removing the lens, lacerating the capsule, and performing an iridectomy via the sclera.

Graefe's sign Upper eyelid fails to follow the downward movement when the patient looks down.

graft Tissue implant from another part of the body or another person.

GraftJacket Brand name regenerative tissue matrix commonly used for lower extremity ulcers, particularly diabetic ulcers. Report supply with HCPCS Level II code Q4107. Injectable GraftJacket allograft is reported with Q4113.

graft-versus-host disease Acute or chronic complication of blood transfusion, bone marrow transplant, or any organ transplant in which white blood cells are present in the transplanted organ. Acute cases may result in skin disruption, diarrhea, hyperbilirubinemia, and an increase in susceptibility to infection. Chronic cases typically begin more than three months post-transplant. In addition to the symptoms noted above, dry eyes and mouth, loss of hair, and lung disorders may be present. Report this condition with a code from ICD-9-CM range 279.50-279.53.

-gram Drawn, written, and recorded.

gram-negative bacilli Bacteria having a cell wall made of a thin layer of peptidoglycan covered by an outer membrane of lipoprotein and lipopolysaccharide that lose their stain or are decolorized by alcohol in gram's staining method. They can be counterstained with a dye called safranin to make them visible again. This is a quick test that can be done to determine a course of treatment while other labs are pending and does not affect coding directly.

gram-positive bacilli Bacteria having a cell wall made of a thick layer of peptidoglycan with attached teichoic acids that retain and resist decolorization by alcohol in Gram's staining method. This is a quick test that can be

done to determine a course of treatment while other labs are pending and does not affect coding directly.

grand multiparity Condition of having had five or more pregnancies that resulted in viable fetuses.

granisetron HCl Antiemetic used to treat nausea and vomiting postoperatively or from cancer chemotherapy or radiation therapy. Supply is reported with HCPCS Level II code J1626 or Q0166. May be sold under the brand name Kytril.

granulation Formation of small, bead-like masses of cytoplasm or granules on the surface of healing wounds of an organ, membrane, or tissue.

granulation tissue Loose collection of fibroblasts, inflammatory cells, and new vessels in an edematous fleshy projection that forms at the base of open wounds over which new skin forms, unless excessive granulation tissue, or proud flesh, rises above the wound surface.

granulocytes Leukocytes, or white blood cells, that have granular cytoplasm.

granulocytic sarcoma Disorder manifested by numerous malignant tumors produced by bony infiltrates in myelogenous leukemia. The masses are most often found in the skull, but may occur in any part of the skeleton. The tumors appear green colored, due to pigment effects of myeloperoxidase. Report this disorder with a code from ICD-9-CM category 205.3. *Synonym(s): Aran's cancer, Balfour's disease, chloroleukemia, chloroma, chloromyeloma, chlorosarcoma, green cancer, Naegeli's disease.*

granuloma Abnormal, dense collections or cells forming a mass or nodule of chronically inflamed tissue with granulations that is usually associated with an infective process.

-graphic Written or drawn.

Grasset's phenomenon Inability to raise both legs at the same time, although the patient is able to raise either leg separately; a sign of incomplete organic hemiplegia.

grav Number of pregnancies.

Grave speculum Device inserted into the vagina for viewing its walls and the cervix.

Graves' disease Enlargement of the thyroid gland seen mostly in women, stemming from an autoimmune process, and causing excessive secretion of thyroid hormone, goiter, and bulging eyes. The syndrome seen with hyperplasia of the thyroid and excessive hormone production consists of fatigue, nervousness, emotional lability and irritability, heat intolerance and increased sweating, weight loss, palpitations, and tremor of the hands and tongue. If there is no documentation of a thyrotoxic crisis or storm, report ICD-9-CM code 242.00; with thyrotoxic crisis or storm, report 242.01.

Grawitz tumor Renal cell carcinoma, reported with ICD-9-CM code 189.0.

gray line Dividing line that demarcates the outer and inner margins of the eyelid, separating eyelid skin from conjunctival mucous membrane.

gray matter Gray nervous tissue, made up of demyelinated nerve fibers, supportive tissue, and nerve cell bodies.

gray syndrome Effects of chloramphenicol on the newborn, taken by mother during gestation. Report this disorder with ICD-9-CM code 779.4.

greater occipital nerve General sensory and motor nerve of the skin and scalp of the back of the head.

greater omentum Greater curvature of the stomach to the transverse colon.

green cancer Disorder manifested by numerous malignant tumors produced by bony infiltrates in myelogenous leukemia. The masses are most often found in the skull, but may occur in any part of the skeleton. The tumors appear green colored, due to pigment effects of myeloperoxidase. Report this disorder with a code from ICD-9-CM category 205.3. *Synonym(s): Aran's cancer, Balfour's disease, chloroleukemia, chloroma, chloromyeloma, chlorosarcoma, granulocytic sarcoma, Naegeli's disease.*

Greenfield filter Permanent umbrella-shaped filter implanted in the vena cava and designed to trap small clots of blood or plaque before they reach the lungs and cause pulmonary embolism. The filter is inserted intraluminally, usually through the femoral or jugular veins. Placement of a Greenfield filter is reported with CPT code 37620. Radiological supervision and interpretation of filter placement is reported with CPT code 75940.

Greig's syndrome Congenital anomaly involving multiple deformities of the hands and feet, macrocephaly, orbital hypertelorism, mild mental retardation, and a broad, flat nose. This syndrome is reported with ICD-9-CM code 756.0.

grey syndrome Effects of chloramphenicol on the newborn taken by mother during gestation. Report this disorder with ICD-9-CM code 779.4.

grice arthrodesis Bone graft is planted in the lateral part of the subtalar joint.

grief reaction Short-term depressive symptoms following a life event or stressor.

grievance Any issue or concern expressing dissatisfaction with products, services, operations, and/or protocol from a customer, state insurance department, or other party on behalf of a customer.

Gritti amputation Leg is amputated through the knee, and kneecap is used as the flap over the wound.

gross Macroscopic, as in gross pathology; the study of tissue changes without magnification by microscope.

gross conversion factor Conversion factor obtained when converting a fee schedule not based on the resource-based relative value scale to one that is, using only the current fee schedule without including frequencies. This calculation gives only a rough approximation of the conversion factor required to maintain income at the level currently generated using a non-RBRVS-based fee schedule. Since income is tied not only to the fee for each service but also to the frequency, a more accurate conversion factor is obtained when frequency is included.

gross stress reaction Acute transient disorders of any severity and nature of emotions, consciousness, and psychomotor states (singly or in combination) that occur in individuals, without any apparent pre-existing mental disorder, in response to exceptional physical or mental stress such as natural catastrophe or battle. The symptoms usually subside within hours or days.

group delinquency Acquisition of values or behavior of a peer group to which an individual is loyal and with whom the person characteristically steals, is truant, stays out late at night, is sexually promiscuous, or engages in other socially delinquent practices.

Group Health Association of America HMO trade organization. *Synonym(s): GHAA.*

group health plan Under HIPAA, employee welfare benefit plan that provides for medical care and either has 50 or more participants or is administered by another business entity.

group model HMO that contracts with a group of providers.

group practice Group of providers that shares facilities, resources, and staff, and who may represent a single unit in a managed care network.

group segment One or more related transaction sets. The group segment begins with the header and ends with the trailer. One complete transmission of a batch of institutional 837 claims is a group segment.

grouper Computer application that assigns diagnosis-related groups (DRGs).

GS HCPCS Level II modifier used to denote a 25 percent reduction of EPO or darbepoietin alfa from the previous month's dosage.

GSR Galvanic skin response.

GSS syndrome Gerstmann-Straussler-Scheinker syndrome, reported with ICD-9-CM code 046.71.

GSW Gunshot wound.

gt. Drop.

GTD Gestational trophoblastic disease. GTD can be any of four aberrant pregnancies: hydatidiform mole, invasive

G-I

mole, choriocarcinoma, or placental site trophoblastic tumor. Documentation stating GTD needs further clarification from the clinician. GTD is reported with ICD-9-CM code 181 if choriocarcinoma or placental site trophoblastic tumor; 630 if hydatidiform mole; or 236.1 if an invasive mole.

GTF Gunther Tulip filter. Retrievable, tulip-shaped filter implanted in the vena cava and designed to trap small clots of blood or plaque before they reach the lungs and cause pulmonary embolism. The filter is inserted intraluminally, usually through the femoral or jugular veins. Placement of a Gunther Tulip filter is reported with CPT code 37620. Radiological supervision and interpretation of filter placement is reported with CPT code 75940.

GTT Glucose tolerance test. Blood test to determine a fasting patient's ability to metabolize and store carbohydrates. The test is normally given orally, but may be performed using IV glucose solution. A blood test is administered before glucose administration and at intervals after administration. A GTT usually includes a series of three blood samples. In CPT, additional samples beyond three are reported in addition to the GTT code, 82951. If results are not normal, the patient may have simple hyperglycemia, impaired glucose tolerance, or diabetes mellitus. *Synonym(s): IVGTT, OGTT, oral GTT.*

gtt. Drops.

g-tube Gastrostomy tube. Feeding tube placed through the stomach wall to allow feeding or dosing of medication, or to vent gases or fluids. Percutaneous placement of a g-tube performed endoscopically is reported with CPT code 43246; nonendoscopic placement is reported with 49440. Open g-tube insertion is reported with codes from range 43830-43832.

Gu Guaiac.

GU Genitourinary.

guarantee of payment Provision that ensures that Medicare will pay for hospital inpatient services-even if benefits were exhausted before admission-assuming that the hospital acted in good faith in admitting the patient. The guarantee does not apply to patients not entitled to Medicare or to those whose entitlement has been terminated. All claims involving this provision must be accompanied by information substantiating the claim.

Gubler-Millard syndrome Paraplegia and anesthesia over half or part of the body caused by lesions in the brain or spinal cord. Report this disorder with ICD-9-CM code 344.89.

Guérin-Stern syndrome Congenital immobility of most joints, fixed in various postures, with little muscle development and growth. Report this disorder with ICD-9-CM code 754.89.

guidelines Information appearing at the beginning of each of the six major sections of the CPT book. They also may appear at the beginning of subsections and code ranges. The information contained in the guidelines provides definitions, explanations of terms, and factors relevant to the section.

guidewire Flexible metal instrument designed to lead another instrument in its proper course.

Guillain-Barré (-Strohl) syndrome Often follows viral infections and may be a disorder of immune system with paraplegia of limbs, flaccid paralysis, ophthalmoplegia, ataxia, and areflexia. Report this disorder with ICD-9-CM code 357.0.

guillotine Instrument used for severing tonsils from their attachments.

Gunn's syndrome Eyelids widen during chewing, sometimes with an elevation of the upper lid when the mouth is open and closing of the lid when the mouth is closed. Report this disorder with ICD-9-CM code 742.8. *Synonym(s): jaw-winking syndrome.*

Gunther Tulip filter Retrievable, tulip-shaped filter implanted in the vena cava and designed to trap small clots of blood or plaque before they reach the lungs and cause pulmonary embolism. The filter is inserted intraluminally usually through the femoral or jugular veins. Placement of a Gunther Tulip filter is reported with CPT code 37620. Radiological supervision and interpretation of filter placement is reported with CPT code 75940. *Synonym(s): GTF.*

Günther's syndrome Cutaneous photosensitivity leading to mutilating skin lesions, hemolytic anemia and splenomegaly, and greatly increased urinary excretion of uroporphyrin. Report this disorder with ICD-9-CM code 277.1.

gusset Triangular or diamond shaped patch that is placed for reinforcement or expansion.

gustatory sweating syndrome Localized sweating and flushing of cheek and ear in response to chewing. Report this disorder with ICD-9-CM code 350.8. *Synonym(s): Frey's syndrome.*

Guthrie test Bacterial inhibition assay measures serum phenylalanine; and is in widespread use for detection of phenylketonuria in newborn.

GV HCPCS Level II modifier, for use with CPT or HCPCS Level II codes, that identifies that the attending physician is not employed by the patient's hospice provider or paid under arrangement by the patient's hospice provider. Failure to append this modifier for services rendered to beneficiaries enrolled in hospice care will result in denial.

GVHD Graft-versus-host disease. Acute or chronic complication of blood transfusion, bone marrow transplant, or any organ transplant in which white blood cells are present in the transplanted organ. Acute cases

G-I

may result in skin disruption, diarrhea, hyperbilirubinemia, and an increase in susceptibility to infection. Chronic cases typically begin more than three months post-transplant. In addition to the symptoms noted above, dry eyes and mouth, loss of hair, and lung disorders may be present. Report this condition with a code from ICD-9-CM range 279.50-279.53.

GW HCPCS Level II modifier, for use with CPT or HCPCS Level II codes, that indicates that the service provided is not related to the hospice patient's terminal condition. This modifier is reported when medically necessary services are not part of the patient's hospice care. Failure to append this modifier to the codes for services rendered to beneficiaries enrolled in hospice care will result in denial.

GXT Graded exercise test. Another name for a stress test performed on a treadmill to evaluate cardiac function.

gyn Gynecology.

gyn- Relating to the female gender.

gynecomastia Condition in which the male mammary glands are abnormally large, reported with ICD-9-CM code 611.1. *Synonym(s): macromastia.*

Gynogen See estrogen.

H Hertel measurement.

h (hora) Hour.

H&P History and physical.

h.d. At bedtime.

H.O. House officer.

h.s. At bedtime.

H2O Water.

H2O2 Hydrogen peroxide.

H3O syndrome Rounded face, almond-shaped eyes, strabismus, low forehead, hypogonadism, hypostomia, mental retardation, and an insatiable appetite. Report this disorder with ICD-9-CM code 759.81.

HA *1)* Headache. *Synonym(s): cephalgia. 2)* Hearing aid.

HAA Hepatitis antigen.

HAAb Hepatitis antibody A.

HaAg Hepatitis antigen A.

HAART Highly active antiretroviral therapy. Protease inhibitors and reverse transcriptase inhibitors used in combination to effectively treat AIDS. The drugs work by disrupting HIV during different stages of its replication.

HAASC Hospital affiliated ambulatory surgical center.

habit spasm Tic disorder limited to three or less that starts in childhood and persists into adult life and rarely has a verbal component.

habitual aborter Spontaneous abortions or miscarriages in three or more successive pregnancies. In a currently non-pregnant female, the condition of habitual aborter is reported with ICD-9-CM code 629.9. In pregnancy, habitual abortion is reported with a code from subcategory 646.3.

Hadfield-Clarke syndrome Abnormal secretions of exocrine glands, obstructions of mucosal passageways, poor growth, chronic bronchitis, recurrent pneumonia, emphysema, clubbing of fingers, and salt depletion. Report this disorder with ICD-9-CM code 577.8. *Synonym(s): Burke's syndrome, Clarke-Hadfield syndrome, cystic fibrosis.*

haemophilus influenzae Gram negative, aerobic or facultatively anaerobic rod shaped or coccobacillus from the family Pasturellaceae causing pneumonia (ICD-9-CM code 482.2), meningitis (320.0), septicemia (038.41), and infections in other conditions coded elsewhere (041.2). *Synonym(s): Pfeiffer's bacillus.*

Haglund's deformity Retrocalcaneus bursitis concurrent to Achilles tendonitis with a bony growth at the back of the heel bone. The typical patient may have a history of wearing high-heeled shoes. Haglund's deformity may be treated with ice, compression, or cast walking boot; severe cases require surgical excision of the bony growth. Haglund's deformity is reported with ICD-9-CM code 726.73. Surgical excision of the exostosis is reported with CPT code 28119. *Synonym(s): pump bump.*

Haglund-Läwen-Fründ syndrome Traumatic separation of the cartilage of the patella with fissures. Report this disorder with ICD-9-CM code 717.89.

Hagner's disease Syndrome manifested by clubbed fingers and toes, enlarged extremities, pain in the joints, and vasomotor disturbance of the hands and feet. The periosteum of the radius and fibula is frequently inflamed, often due to underlying pulmonary problems such as lung cancer, tuberculosis, abscesses, emphysema, or cystic fibrosis. Conditions other than pulmonary disorders may also cause this syndrome. Report this disease with ICD-9-CM code 731.2. *Synonym(s): HPOA, hypertrophic pulmonary osteoarthropathy, Marie-Bamberger disease.*

HAI Hospital acquired infection.

hair follicle Tube-like opening in the epidermis where the hair shaft develops.

hairless women syndrome Male pseudohermaphroditism with incompletely developed vagina, rudimentary uterus and fallopian tubes, scanty or absent axillary/public hair, and amenorrhea. Report this disorder with ICD-9-CM code 259.51. *Synonym(s): Goldberg syndrome, Goldberg-Maxwell syndrome, Morris syndrome.*

Haldol See haloperidol.

G-I

Hallervorden-Spatz syndrome Nerves between the striatum and pallidum are completely demyelated. Report this disorder with ICD-9-CM code 333.0.

hallucinatory type syndrome Organic disorder in which the patient exhibits chronic hallucinations not occurring during the course of delirium. Report this disorder with ICD-9-CM code 293.82. *Synonym(s): hallucinosis.*

hallux malleus Deformity in which there is hammertoe of the great toe.

hallux rigidus Deformity in which there is severe flexion of the great toe causing pain and limited movement.

hallux valgus Deformity in which the great toe deviates toward the other toes and may even be positioned over or under the second toe.

hallux varus Deformity in which the great toe deviates away from the other toes.

halo Tool for stabilizing the head and spine.

haloperidol Antipsychotic drug that works on dopamine receptors in the brain. It is used primarily to treat psychotic disorders requiring long-term therapy and Tourette's syndrome. It is available in sustained release injection referred to as Decanoate or Lactate. Supply is reported with HCPCS Level II code J1630 (Haldol or haloperidol) or J1631 (Haldol Decanoate-50 or haloperidol decanoate). May be sold under the brand names Apo-Haloperidol, Haldol, Novo-Paridol, Paridol, PMS-Haloperidol, Serenace.

HALS Hand-assisted laparoscopic surgery.

Halsted mastectomy Radical mastectomy includes removal of the breast along with pectoral minor muscle.

Haltia-Santavuori disease Rare, infantile type of neuronal ceroid lipofuscinosis or amaurotic familial idiocy. It is an inherited disorder in which the body stores excessive amounts of lipofuscin, the pigment that remains after damaged cells are broken down and digested, resulting in progressive nervous tissue damage, vision loss, and fatality. Haltia-Santavuori manifests at about one year with myoclonic seizures, mental and motor deterioration, hypotonia, blindness, and death within five years. Report this disease with ICD-9-CM code 330.1.

Ham test Test checks for acidified serum.

hamartoma Benign tumor composed of an overgrowth of normally occurring mature cells and tissue from the presenting area.

Hamman's syndrome Pneumothorax or pneumopericardium resulting from presence of air or gas in the mediastinum beginning spontaneously or from trauma or disease. Sometimes induced to aid in diagnosis. Report this disorder with ICD-9-CM code 518.1.

Hamman-Rich syndrome Chronic inflammation, progressive fibrosis of the pulmonary alveolar walls, and progressive dyspnea leading to death by oxygen deprivation or right heart failure. Report this disorder with ICD-9-CM code 516.3.

hammertoe Deformity in which there is permanent flexion of the second or third toe joint causing a claw-like appearance.

hamstrings Designation given to three muscles of the thigh: the biceps femoris, semitendinosus, and semimembranosus muscles.

Hancock II Bioprosthesis Brand name aortic porcine valve.

hand drop Inability to extend the hand, which droops permanently at the wrist, due to extensor muscle paralysis. Report this condition with ICD-9-CM code 736.05. *Synonym(s): carpoptosis, wrist drop.*

hand-foot syndrome Sickle cell anemia. Report this disorder with ICD-9-CM code 282.61. *Synonym(s): Herrick's syndrome.*

Hand-Schüller-Christian syndrome Histiocytosis with an occasional accumulation of cholesterol, defects of the membranous bones, exophthalmos, diabetes insipidus, and multiple-system, soft tissue, and bone involvement. Report this disorder with ICD-9-CM code 277.89. *Synonym(s): Christian syndrome.*

hang-back technique Ophthalmic surgical method for performing bimedial rectus recession for correction of strabismus and exotropia. Two sets of sutures are placed in the muscle to be corrected in a patient under general anesthesia. One set is secured, and the second set is tucked behind the lids. Should the correction need to be modified once the patient is awakened, the suture is already in place.

hangover State of inebriation due to alcohol consumption without conspicuous neurological signs of intoxication.

Hanot-Chauffard (-Troisier) syndrome Hypertrophic cirrhosis with pigmentation and diabetes mellitus. Report this disorder with ICD-9-CM code 275.01.

HAPE High altitude pulmonary edema. Life-threatening condition of hypoxia-induced vasoconstriction of the pulmonary arterial vascular bed. HAPE is reported with ICD-9-CM code 993.2.

haptics Fixation portion of intraocular lenses, usually made of plastic and secured by loops, tension, or sutures.

hard palate Bony portion of the roof of the mouth.

Hare's syndrome Neoplasm of upper lobe of lung. Report this disorder with ICD-9-CM code 162.3. *Synonym(s): Ciuffini-Pancoast syndrome.*

harelip Congenital fissure or separation of the upper lip due to failure of embryonic cells to fuse completely. A cleft lip can occur unilaterally or bilaterally and may accompany other abnormalities of the upper jaw, nose, or oral structures. Code assignment is dependent upon whether the cleft lip is unilateral or bilateral, complete or incomplete, and whether or not it is accompanied by a cleft palate. See ICD-9-CM category 749 for code assignment. Repair of a cleft lip is reported with CPT codes 40700-40761. *Synonym(s): cheiloschisis, cleft lip.*

Harii procedure Complex repair of an injury that affects the dorsal skin, subcutaneous fat, including the nerves and blood vessels, and the covering immediately adjacent to the tendon.

Harkavy's syndrome Fever, conjunctival injection reddening of the oral cavity, ulcerative gingivitis, cervical lymph nodes, and skin eruptions that cover the hands and feet. Skin becomes puffy and sloughs off. Report this disorder with ICD-9-CM code 446.0. *Synonym(s): MCLS.*

harlequin fetus Congenital abnormality in which the fetal skin has thickened, armor-like plates of keratin resulting from an autosomal recessive keratinizing disorder, or the extreme form of congenital ichthyosis contraction anomalies of the eyes, ears, appendages, and mouth. Harlequin fetus is reported with ICD-9-CM code 757.1. Affected babies usually are stillborn or die within days of birth.

Harrington rod Device used in nonsegmental spinal instrumentation that affixes at the ends and may span several vertebral segments without attaching to the segments in between. Placed to correct spinal curvature problems and occasionally fractures. For insertion, report CPT code 22840; for removal, report 22850.

Harris' syndrome Hyperinsulinism due to organic endogenous factors, hypoglycemia, weakness, perspiration, jitteriness, tachycardia, mental confusion, and vision disturbances. Report this disorder with ICD-9-CM code 251.1.

Hart's syndrome Renal tubular malfunction, cytinosis, and osteomalacia caused by inherited disorders or the result of multiple myeloma or proximal epithelial growth. Report this disorder with ICD-9-CM code 270.0.

Hartley-Krause Gasserian ganglion is removed to relieve trigeminal neuralgia.

Hartmann's pouch *1)* The results of a procedure in which the lower end of the rectum is closed with sutures or staples and the proximal end of the colon is brought out as a descending colostomy. Report CPT code 44206 for a laparoscopic procedure or 44143 for an open procedure. *2)* A condition affecting the neck of the gallbladder, in which a sac-like projection forms. Hartmann's pouch is reported with ICD-9-CM code 575.8.

harvest Removal of cells or tissue from their native site to be used as a graft or transplant to another part of the donor's body or placed into another person. In ICD-9-CM diagnostic coding, harvest from a donor is classified to category V59, depending on the type of organ, cells, or tissue harvested. In CPT, see the appropriate anatomical site for organ harvest (e.g., conjunctiva, heart, lung, liver, kidney, etc.) or the type of harvested cells, such as stem cells from bone marrow or chondrocytes.

HAV Hepatitis A virus.

Havrix Brand name hepatitis A vaccine provided in a single-dose vial or syringe. Supply of Havrix is reported with CPT codes 90632 and 90633; administration is reported separately. Need for vaccination is reported with ICD-9-CM code V05.3.

hay fever Inflammation of the nasal lining from hypersensitive reactions to ambient particles in the air and flowering plants, causing nasal congestion, mucus secretion, and sneezing. Hay fever is reported with ICD-9-CM code 477.9. *Synonym(s): allergic rhinitis.*

Hayem-Faber syndrome Central pallor in red blood cells caused by lack of red cell hemoglobin in blood. Report this disorder with ICD-9-CM code 280.9. *Synonym(s): Faber syndrome.*

Hayem-Widal syndrome One of a group of anemic syndromes caused by exposures to trauma, poisons, and other causes that decreases the number of red blood cells. Report this disorder with ICD-9-CM code 283.9. *Synonym(s): Dyke-Young syndrome, Widal syndrome.*

HB *1)* Hepatitis B. *2)* HCPCS Level II modifier, for use with CPT or HCPCS Level II codes, that identifies a nongeriatric adult program. May be required for state Medicaid program.

HBcAg Hepatitis antigen B.

HBD Hydroxybutyric dehydrogenase.

Hbg Hemoglobin.

HBIG Hepatitis B immune globulin. Supply of HBIG is reported with CPT code 90371; administration is reported separately. The need for the injection is reported with ICD-9-CM code V01.89.

HBO Hyperbaric oxygen. *NCD Reference: 20.29.*

HbO2 Oxyhemoglobin.

HBP Hospital based physician.

HBsAb Hepatitis surface antibody B.

HBsAg Hepatitis antigen B.

HBV *1)* Hepatitis B virus. Report this disorder with codes from 070.20-070.23. 2) Hepatitis B vaccine.

HC HCPCS Level II modifier, for use with CPT or HCPCS Level II codes, that identifies a geriatric adult program. May be required for a state Medicaid program.

HCAHPS   Hospital Consumer Assessment of Healthcare Providers and Systems.

HCC   Hepatocellular carcinoma. Primary liver cancer.

HCC model   Hierarchical condition categories model. Centers for Medicare and Medicaid Services risk adjustment payment model for Medicare managed care organizations (MCOs) and other capitated programs. The CMS-HCC Model is a prospective payment system that uses a hierarchical diagnosis classification system as well as other demographic adjusters to predict costs and set the payment rates for managed care services.

HCG   Human chorionic gonadotropin. Hormone produced by the placenta early in pregnancy that can be detected in the blood and urine in certain pregnancy tests. *NCD Reference: 190.27.*

HCl   Hydrochloric acid.

HCM   Hypertrophic cardiomyopathy. Genetic disorder causing hypertrophy in any segment of the ventricle, carrying a risk of sudden death due to arrhythmia in children and adolescents. HCM is reported with ICD-9-CM code 746.84. *Synonym(s): ASH.*

HCP   Hereditary coproporphyria. Genetic hepatic porphyria causing nausea, fatigue, and, in some patients, photosensitivity of the skin. HCP is a deficiency in coproporphyrinogen oxidase, reported with ICD-9-CM code 277.1.

HCPCS   Healthcare Common Procedure Coding System. *HCPCS Level I:* Healthcare Common Procedure Coding System Level I. Numeric coding system used by physicians, facility outpatient departments, and ambulatory surgery centers (ASC) to code ambulatory, laboratory, radiology, and other diagnostic services for Medicare billing. This coding system contains only the American Medical Association's Physicians' Current Procedural Terminology (CPT) codes. The AMA updates codes annually. *HCPCS Level II:* Healthcare Common Procedure Coding System Level II. National coding system, developed by CMS, contains alphanumeric codes for physician and nonphysician services not included in the CPT coding system. HCPCS Level II covers such things as ambulance services, durable medical equipment, and orthotic and prosthetic devices. *HCPCS modifiers:* Two-character code (AA-ZZ) that identifies circumstances that alter or enhance the description of a service or supply. They are recognized by carriers nationally and are updated annually by CMS.

Hct   Hematocrit.

Hctz   Hydrochlorothiazide.

HCVD   Hypertensive cardiovascular disease.

HD   *1)* HCPCS Level II modifier, for use with CPT or HCPCS Level II codes, that identifies a pregnant/parenting women's program. May be required for a state Medicaid program. *2)* Hip disarticulation.

HDE   Humanitarian device exemption. Exemption granted by the FDA for devices treating rare medical conditions.

HDL   High-density lipoproteins.

HDM   House dust mite. Microscopic source of hypersensitivity reaction creating common allergic reactions of hay fever, asthma, or atopic dermatitis. Rhinitis due to HDM is reported with ICD-9-CM code 477.8.

HDS   Hasegawa Dementia Screening. Tool for evaluating dementia in the elderly.

HE   HCPCS Level II modifier, for use with CPT or HCPCS Level II codes, that identifies a mental health program. May be required for a state Medicaid program.

head-banging   Voluntary repetitive stereotypical movements not due to any psychiatric or neurological condition, manifested by head banging, head nodding and nystagmus, rocking, twirling, finger-flicking mannerisms, and eye-poking. Common in cases of mental retardation with sensory impairment or with environmental monotony.

header   Opening stream of data that tells the receiving party that a batch of institutional 837 claims is to follow.

Heaf test   Test checks for tuberculin antibodies.

Health and Human Services   Cabinet department that oversees the operating divisions of the federal government responsible for health and welfare. HHS oversees the Centers for Medicare and Medicaid Services, Food and Drug Administration, Public Health Service, and other such entities. *Synonym(s): DHHS, HHS.*

health care clearinghouse   Under HIPAA, entity that processes or facilitates the processing of information received from another entity in a nonstandard format or containing nonstandard data content into standard data elements or a standard transaction, or that receives a standard transaction from another entity and processes or facilitates the processing of that information into nonstandard format or nonstandard data content for a receiving entity.

Health Care Code Maintenance Committee   Organization administered by the Blue Cross and Blue Shield Association that maintains certain coding schemes used in the X12 transactions and elsewhere. These include the claim adjustment reason codes, the claim status category codes, and the claim status codes.

Health Care Financing Administration   Former name of the federal agency that oversees the administration of the public health programs (e.g., Medicare, Medicaid, State Children's Insurance Program), now known as the Centers for Medicare and Medicaid Services.

G-I

health care operations Specific set of activities related to an entity's covered functions.

health care provider Entity that administers diagnostic and therapeutic services.

Health Care Provider Taxonomy Committee Organization administered by the NUCC responsible for maintaining the provider taxonomy coding scheme used in the X12 transactions. The detailed code maintenance is done in coordination with X12N/TG2/WG15.

health care services Processes that contribute to the health and well-being of a patient. Services may be provided in a variety of health care settings including nursing, medical, surgical, or other health related services.

Health Industry Business Communications Council Council of health care industry associations that has developed a number of technical standards used within the health care industry. *Synonym(s): HIBCC.*

Health Informatics Standards Board Standards group accredited by the American National Standards Institute that has developed an inventory of candidate standards for consideration as possible HIPAA standards. *Synonym(s): HISB.*

health information Information, whether oral or recorded in any form or medium, that is created or received by a covered entity; relates to the past, present, or future physical or mental health or condition of an individual; the provision of health care to an individual; or for the past, present, or future payment for the provision of health care to an individual.

Health Insurance Association of America Industry association that represents the interests of commercial health care insurers. The HIAA participates in the maintenance of some code sets, including the HCPCS Level II codes. *Synonym(s): HIAA.*

health insurance claim number Number issued by the Social Security Administration to individuals or beneficiaries entitled to Medicare benefits. The HICN card provides the beneficiary information necessary for processing Medicare claims. *Synonym(s): HICN.*

Health Insurance Portability and Accountability Act of 1996 Federal law that allows persons to qualify immediately for comparable health insurance coverage when they change their employment relationships. Title II, subtitle F, of HIPAA gives the Department of Health and Human Services the authority to mandate the use of standards for the electronic exchange of health care data; to specify what medical and administrative code sets should be used within those standards; to require the use of national identification systems for health care patients, providers, payers (or plans), and employers (or sponsors); and to specify the types of measures required to protect the security and privacy of personally identifiable health care information. *Synonym(s): HIPAA, K2, Kassenbaum-Kennedy Bill, Kennedy-Kassenbaum Bill, Public Law 104-191.*

health insurance prospective payment system Procedure coding system used in the Medicare skilled nursing facility and home health, inpatient rehabilitation, and rural hospital swing beds prospective payment systems (PPS). *Synonym(s): HIPPS.*

health insurance purchasing cooperatives Purchasing pools that negotiate economic and equitable health insurance arrangements for employers and/or employees who voluntarily join. *Synonym(s): health plan purchasing cooperatives, HIPC.*

Health Level Seven Group accredited by the American National Standards Institute that defines standards for the cross-platform exchange of information within a health care organization. HL7 is responsible for specifying the Level Seven OSI standards for the health industry. The X12 275 transaction will probably incorporate the HL7 CRU message to transmit claim attachments as part of a future HIPAA claim attachments standard. The HL7 Attachment SIG is responsible for the HL7 portion of this standard. *Synonym(s): HL7.*

health maintenance organization Medical health insurance coverage that pays claims based on provider cost, per diem, or charge basis. Hospitals contract with an HMO to provide care at a contractually reduced price. HMO members pay a set monthly amount for coverage and are treated without additional cost, except for a copayment or deductible amount. Like all managed care organizations, HMOs use a variety of mechanisms to control costs, including utilization management, discounted provider fee schedules, and financial incentives. HMOs use primary care physicians as gatekeepers and emphasize preventive care. *Synonym(s): HMO.*

health plan Program that provides or pays the cost of health care services.

health plan ID System for uniquely identifying all organizations that pay for health care services. Formerly referred to as the payer ID. *Synonym(s): health plan ID, national payer ID, plan ID.*

health reimbursement account Health care coverage funded by the employer as an employee benefit, administered by a third-party administrator, and may include employee tax exempt contributions. *Synonym(s): HRA.*

health savings account Health care coverage plan with high deductible provided as part of a qualified trust that includes tax exempt employee contributions equal to the deductible up to a maximum level set by law. *Synonym(s): HSA.*

G-I

Healthcare Common Procedure Coding System Two levels of codes used by Medicare and other payers to describe procedures and supplies. Level I includes all of the codes listed in CPT, and Level II are alphanumeric supply and procedure codes. *Synonym(s):* HCPCS.

HCPCS Level I Numeric coding system used by physicians, facility outpatient departments, and ambulatory surgery centers (ASC) to code ambulatory, laboratory, radiology, and other diagnostic services for Medicare billing. This coding system contains only the American Medical Association's Physicians' Current Procedural Terminology (CPT) codes. The AMA updates codes annually. **HCPCS Level II** National coding system, developed by CMS, that contains alphanumeric codes for physician and nonphysician services not included in the CPT coding system. HCPCS Level II covers such things as ambulance services, durable medical equipment, and orthotic and prosthetic devices. **HCPCS modifiers** Alphanumeric code used to identify circumstances that alter or enhance the description of a service or supply reported to Medicare or other payers.

Healthcare Financial Management Association Organization promoting the improvement of the financial management of health-care-related organizations. The HFMA sponsors some HIPAA educational seminars. *Synonym(s):* HFMA.

Healthcare Information Management Systems Society Organization for health care information and management systems professionals. *Synonym(s):* HIMSS.

heart transplant complications Expected complications following a transplant include ECG changes, reduced cardiac output, arteritis, myocardial ischemia, and myocardial necrosis, as well as coronary artery atherosclerosis.

heartbeat Contraction of the heart muscles in a rhythmic pattern, circulating about 70 ml of blood and taking less than a second to complete. There are four phases to every heartbeat: 1) the atria relax and fill with blood from the main veins; 2) blood moves from the atria, through the tricuspid and mitral valves, into the ventricles; 3) the ventricles contract, forcing blood through the aortic and pulmonary valves into the main arteries; 4) the ventricles relax and the cycle begins again.

Heartsbreath Brand name noninvasive test for heart transplant rejection by evaluating the organic compounds in breath. This test is reported with CPT code 0085T.

heat exhaustion or prostration syndrome Salt depletion following exposure to sunlight and heat, causing heat exhaustion. Report this disorder with ICD-9-CM code 992.4.

hebephrenia Solitary, disorganized schizophrenic state with prominent affective changes, delusions, hallucinations, and fleeting, fragmented, irresponsible, or unpredictable behavior manifested by purposeless giggling or self-satisfied, self-absorbed smiling, or by a lofty manner, grimaces, mannerisms, pranks, hypochondriacal complaints, and reiterated phrases.

Heberden's syndrome Severe pain in the chest caused by ischemia of the heart prompted by coronary artery disease. Report this disorder with ICD-9-CM code 413.9. *Synonym(s):* angina pectoris.

HEDIC Healthcare EDI Coalition.

Hedinger's syndrome Carcinoid tumors causing severe attacks of cyanotic flushing of skin, diarrheal watery stools, bronchoconstrictive attacks, hypotension, edema, and ascites. Report this disorder with ICD-9-CM code 259.2. *Synonym(s):* Bjorck-Thorson syndrome, Cassidy-Scholte syndrome.

HEDIS Health plan employer data and information set. Series of standardized performance measures that allow for the comparison and measurement of performance among managed health care plans. HEDIS was developed by the National Committee for Quality Assurance to measure quality in key areas such as access to care, qualification of providers, preventative medicine, episodic illness, and chronic illness.

heel cup Plastic or rubber cup that fits into the back portion of the patient's shoe to provide protection, support, and stabilization.

HEENT Head, eyes, ears, nose, and throat.

Hegglin's syndrome Hepatosplenomegaly, lymphadenopathy, anemia, thrombocytopenia, and changes in the bones, cardiopulmonary system, skin, and psychomotor skills. Abnormalities of granulation and nuclear structure of white cells open patients to infection and result in death. Report this disorder with ICD-9-CM code 288.2. *Synonym(s):* Chediak-Higashi syndrome, Dohle body syndrome, Jordan's syndrome, May syndrome.

Heine's operation Ciliary body is destroyed to relieve glaucoma.

Heine-Medin disease Infection with any one of the three poliovirus organisms. Report this disease with a code from ICD-9-CM category 045. *Synonym(s):* Medin's disease.

Helicobacter pylori Bacteria found to be a causal agent in gastritis and pyloric ulcers, and has been known to be associated with gastric cancer. It is easily treatable with antibiotics. Tests for H. pylori include a simple breath test analysis, blood or stool sample analysis, or a combination of both, CPT codes 83009, 83013-83014, and 87338-87339. ICD-9-CM code 041.86 for H. pylori infection should be reported in addition to the code for the ulcer.

Helixate See factor VIII.

Heller myotomy Longitudinal division of the distal esophageal muscle down to the submucosal layer. Cardia muscle fibers may also be divided. This procedure is used to treat achalasia. Heller myotomy is reported with CPT code 43330 or 43331.

Heller's syndrome Dementia in which a child becomes mute with irritability, tantrums, and other behavioral disorders. Report this disorder with a code from ICD-9-CM range 299.10-299.11.

HELLP syndrome Hemolysis, elevated liver enzymes and low platelet count. Group of symptoms occurring in pregnancy, including hemolysis, elevated liver enzymes, and a low platelet count. These symptoms may occur simultaneously with preeclampsia or may be present prior to the patient becoming preeclamptic. HELLP is reported with a code from ICD-9-CM subcategory 642.5.

hem(ato)- Relating to blood.

hemangioma Benign neoplasm arising from vascular tissue or malformations of vascular structures. It is most commonly seen in children and infants as a tumor of newly formed blood vessels due to malformed fetal angioblastic tissues. *Synonym(s): lymphangioma, nevus flammeus, nevus vasculosus, port wine stain, strawberry nevus.*

hemarthrosis Occurrence of blood within a joint space.

hematemesis Vomiting of blood commonly caused by gastric or duodenal ulcers and treated with acid pump inhibitors such as Prilosec or Nexium. This condition is reported with ICD-9-CM code 578.0.

hematocele Effusion of blood into a body cavity.

hematoma Tumor-like collection of blood in some part of the body caused by a break in a blood vessel wall, usually as a result of trauma. A traumatic hematoma is coded according to the origin, nature, and site of the contusion injury (ICD-9-CM categories 920-924). Hematomas of the genital organs or the eyes are coded as diseases of those organs involved, while nontraumatic hematoma of the soft tissue or muscle is coded to 729.92. Hematomas of the skin and subcutaneous tissues are usually treated by incision and drainage or puncture aspiration.

hematometra Buildup of blood in the uterus, which causes uterine distention, reported with ICD-9-CM code 621.4.

hematopoietic progenitor cells Cells found in the bone marrow arising from stem cells that can differentiate into specialized cells for the formation of blood.

hematospermia Blood in the seminal fluid, often caused by inflammation of the prostate or seminal vesicles, or prostate cancer. In primary hematospermia, the presence of blood in the seminal fluid is the only symptom. In secondary hematospermia, an underlying cause of the bleeding is known or suspected but may be difficult to determine. Both are reported with ICD-9-CM code 608.82.

hematuria Blood in urine, which may present as gross visible blood or as the presence of red blood cells visible only under a microscope. Hematuria is reported with an ICD-9-CM code from range 599.70-599.72. Underlying conditions may include infections, neoplasms, radiation injury, calculi, kidney disease, genitourinary trauma, systemic disorders, and adverse effects of anticoagulant therapy. Hemoglobinuria (791.2) is excluded. Hematuria due to specified infectious diseases is coded to the disease within that chapter. *Synonym(s): hemuresis.*

hemi- Half.

hemiarthroplasty Partial prosthetic replacement of the joint structures of the humeral head in the arm, leaving the glenoid fossa intact.

hemibody Half the body. Commonly used in hemibody irradiation in which larger doses of irradiation are used to treat disseminated cancer or metastases.

hemiepiphyseal arrest Scraping or fusion of a growing bone to stop growth and even out unequal bone length.

hemilaminectomy Excision of a portion of the vertebral lamina.

hemin Enzyme inhibitor, derived from processed red blood cells, that is used to treat acute intermittent porphyria, a hereditary liver disturbance of porphyrin metabolism that manifests with attacks of abdominal pain, gastrointestinal problems, and neurologic disturbances. Supply is reported with HCPCS Level II code J1640. May be sold under the brand name Panhematin.

hemiphalangectomy Excision of part of the phalanx.

hemiplegia Paralysis of one side of the body. Many codes exist to report hemiplegia from various causes. If specified as a late effect of cerebrovascular disease, report with a code from ICD-9-CM subcategory 438.2.

hemisection In dentistry, surgical separation of a tooth that has multiple roots.

hemivertebra Congenital malformation of the spine in which there is incomplete development on one half of a vertebra, reported with ICD-9-CM code 756.14.

hemodialysis Cleansing of wastes and contaminating elements from the blood by virtue of different diffusion rates through a semipermeable membrane, which separates blood from a filtration solution that diffuses other elements out of the blood. The blood is slowly filtered extracorporeally through special dialysis equipment and returned to the body. Hemodialysis is reported with ICD-9-CM procedure code 39.95 or CPT codes 90935-90940. *Synonym(s): renal dialysis. NCD Reference: 130.8.*

Hemofil M See factor VIII.

hemofiltration Technique for treatment of end stage renal disease (ESRD) in which fluids, electrolytes, and toxic substances are removed from the blood by being filtered through hollow synthetic membranes. This procedure is generally performed in three weekly sessions, and imitates the course of filtration by normal kidneys. Hemofiltration is reported with ICD-9-CM procedure code 39.95 and CPT code 90945 or 90947. *Synonym(s): diafiltration.* **NCD Reference:** *110.15.*

hemoglobin Oxygen-carrying component of the red blood cell.

hemoglobinuria syndrome Acquired blood cell dysplasias in which there are many clones of stem cells producing red blood cells, platelets, and granulocytes. Report this disorder with ICD-9-CM code 283.2. *Synonym(s): Marchiafava-Micheli syndrome.*

hemolytic-uremic syndrome Enlargement of liver and spleen and many erythroblasts in circulation. Report this disorder with ICD-9-CM code 283.11.

hemoperfusion Process by which toxins or metabolites are removed from the blood through a dialysis membrane utilizing activated charcoal, enzymes, or resins. Hemoperfusion can be used in combination with renal dialysis and to treat drug overdose and aluminum toxicity. **NCD Reference:** *110.15.*

hemopericardium Presence of blood in the pericardial sac.

hemoperitoneum Effusion of blood into the peritoneal cavity, the space between the continuous membrane lining the abdominopelvic walls and encasing the visceral organs. Hemoperitoneum is reported with ICD-9-CM code 568.81 when it is not caused by any apparent traumatic injury to the abdominal area, with 868.03 when traumatic in nature but without an open wound into the cavity, and with 868.13 when there is an accompanying open wound into the cavity.

hemophilia A Abnormal coagulation characterized by increased bleeding; large skin bruises; bleeding in the mouth, nose, or gastrointestinal tract; and hemorrhages into joints, resulting in swelling and impaired function. This is a hereditary, sex-linked disease in which the patient is missing antihemophilic globulin (AHG) (factor VIII). Report hemophilia A with ICD-9-CM code 286.0.

hemophilia B Second most common form of hemophilia, a hereditary blood disorder in which the clotting properties are affected. Christmas disease almost always occurs in males, caused by a coagulation factor IX deficiency. Symptoms include prolonged or spontaneous bleeding, ecchymosis, hematuria, and muscular and joint pain and swelling. Report this disorder with ICD-9-CM code 286.1. *Synonym(s): Christmas disease.*

hemoptysis Coughing up or spitting out blood or blood-streaked sputum, reported with ICD-9-CM codes 786.30-786.39.

hemorrhage Internal or external bleeding with loss of significant amounts of blood. H. syndrome Fulminating meningococcal septicemia occurring in children below 10 years of age with vomiting, cyanosis, diarrhea, purpura, convulsions, circulatory collapse, meningitis, and hemorrhaging into adrenal glands. Report this disorder with ICD-9-CM code 036.3. *Synonym(s): Friderichsen-Waterhouse syndrome, Waterhouse syndrome.*

hemorrhage syndrome Fulminating meningococcal septicemia occurring in children below 10 years of age with vomiting, cyanosis, diarrhea, purpura, convulsions, circulatory collapse, meningitis, and hemorrhaging into adrenal glands. Report this disorder with ICD-9-CM code 036.3. *Synonym(s): Friderichsen-Waterhouse syndrome, Waterhouse syndrome.*

hemorrhagic bronchitis Chronic bronchitis occurring with the coughing up of blood, caused by a spirochetal infection. Report this condition with ICD-9-CM code 104.8. *Synonym(s): bronchopulmonary spirochetosis, bronchospirochetosis, Castellani's bronchitis.*

hemorrhagic detachment of retinal pigment epithelium Blood-filled blister causing localized detachment of the retina from the pigment epithelium.

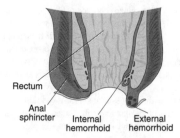

Hemorrhoid

Rectum

Anal sphincter   Internal hemorrhoid   External hemorrhoid

Varicose veins and hemorrhoids (varicose rectal veins) are often associated; internal hemorrhoids (also called piles) are varicosities of the tributaries of the superior rectal veins and are covered by mucous membranes; external hemorrhoids are of the inferior rectal veins and are covered by skin

hemorrhoid Dilated, varicose vein in the anal region caused by continually increased venous pressure. Hemorrhoids are reported under the ICD-9-CM rubric 455. *external thrombosed h.* Reversed blood flow and clotted blood within a vein that extends beyond the anus.

G-I

thrombosed h. Dilated, varicose vein in the anal region containing clotted blood within it.

hemostasis Interruption of blood flow or the cessation or arrest of bleeding.

hemostat Tool for clamping vessels and arresting hemorrhaging.

hemothorax Blood collecting in the pleural cavity.

Hench-Rosenberg syndrome Repeated episodes of arthritis and periarthritis marked by their complete disappearance after a few days or hours, usually affecting only one joint. There is no known cause. Report this disorder with a code from ICD-9-CM range 719.30-719.39.

Hendra virus Zoonotic virus of the family Paramyxoviridae, transmitted through animals in Australia. Hendra virus causes flu-like symptoms that may be mild or may progress to encephalitis. Fifty percent of clinically apparent cases die from Hendra virus, as no drug therapies are effective. There is no code specific to Hendra virus, nor is it indexed in ICD-9-CM. Report Hendra virus with ICD-9-CM other specified virus code 079.89, and also report any accompanying encephalitis.

Henoch-Schönlein syndrome Eruption of purpuric lesions with joint pain and swelling, colic, passage of bloody stools, and glomerulonephritis in young children. Report this disorder with ICD-9-CM code 287.0.

heparin sodium Anticoagulant that decreases the blood's clotting ability by accelerating the formation of antithrombin III-thrombin complex. This deactivates thrombin and prevents the conversion of fibrinogen to fibrin. Heparin has a wide variety of uses including keeping heparin locks unclogged and preventing deep vein thrombosis. Supply is reported with HCPCS Level II code J1642 for Hep lock flush or J1644 for regular heparin sodium. May be sold under the brand name Hep-Lock, Hepalean, Heparin Leo, Liquaemin sodium, Uniparin.

heparin-induced thrombocytopenia Life-threatening adverse effect of heparin therapy that is one of the three most common causes of iatrogenic thrombocytopenia. Initial indications include a drop in platelet count by 50 percent or more within five to 12 days of heparin therapy initiation. At least half of patients will experience arterial or venous thrombotic complications that may result in limb amputation, myocardial infarction, pulmonary emboli, or stroke. Report this disorder with ICD-9-CM code 289.84.

hepat(o)- Relating to the liver.

hepatic portal vein Blood vessel that delivers unoxygenated blood from the gastrointestinal tract, spleen, pancreas, and gallbladder to the liver.

hepatic vein thrombus Clotting of the hepatic vein. An enlarged liver, jaundice, ascites, and portal hypertension are the most common symptoms. Report this syndrome with ICD-9-CM code 453.0. *Synonym(s): Budd-Chiari syndrome.*

hepato- Relating to the liver.

hepatolenticular degeneration Rare, progressive, chronic disease caused by an inherited copper metabolism defect that results in the poisonous accumulation of copper in certain organs and tissues, such as the brain, kidneys, cornea, and liver. The disease causes cirrhosis, brain degeneration with progressive neurological dysfunction, and pigmented Kayser-Fleischer corneal ring. Report this condition with ICD-9-CM code 275.1. *Synonym(s): familial hepatitis, Kinnier Wilson's disease, pseudosclerosis of Westphal, Westphal-Struempell disease, Wilson's disease.*

hepatoma Tumor of the liver. *Synonym(s): hepatoblastoma, liver carcinoma.*

hepatorenal syndrome Liver and kidney failure characterized by cirrhosis with ascites or obstructive jaundice, oliguria, and low sodium values. This condition is reported with ICD-9-CM code 572.4.

hepatotomy Incision into the liver.

Herbst Cradle Brand name ankle foot orthosis for heel suspension to prevent ulcers. Also used for plantar flexion contractures, supply is reported with HCPCS Level II code L4396.

Herceptin Antineoplastic agent used to treat metastatic breast cancer. Supply is reported with HCPCS Level II code J9355. Herpeptin contains trastuzumab.

Hercules Nd:YAG Brand name laser system providing both pulsed and continuous laser energy for tissue ablation in numerous specialty applications, including ENT, gastroenterology, gynecology, thoracoscopy, and urology.

Hercules syndrome Type I acrocephalosyndactyly with peaked head, fusion of digits (specifically the second through fifth digits), and severe acne vulgaris of forearms. Report this disorder with ICD-9-CM code 255.2. *Synonym(s): Apert-Gallais syndrome, Cooke syndrome.*

Herculink Brand name biliary stent system.

hereditary cerebral leukodystrophy Inherited degenerative brain disease manifested by gradually advancing white matter sclerosis of the frontal lobes, mental deficits, and vasomotor disorders. Report this disease with ICD-9-CM code 330.0. *Synonym(s): aplasia axialis extracorticalis, Merzbacher-Pelizaeus disease, Pelizaeus-Merzbacher disease.*

hereditary hemorrhagic telangiectasia Post-pubescent appearing genetic disorder with small telangiectasia and dilated venules developing slowly on the skin and mucus

G-I

membranes of the lips, nasopharynx, and tongue with recurrent bleeding occurring. Report this disorder with ICD-9-CM code 448.0. **Synonym(s):** *Babington's disease, Rendu-Osler-Weber disease.*

Hernia

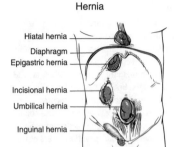

Hiatal hernia
Diaphragm
Epigastric hernia
Incisional hernia
Umbilical hernia
Inguinal hernia

hernia Protrusion of a body structure through tissue. *diaphragmatic h.* Protrusion of abdominal organs or structures into the thorax, mainly the stomach, through the esophageal opening within the diaphragm, creating a pouch in which food passing from the esophagus into the stomach gets caught and causes pain. Diaphragmatic is actually a broader classification of hernia that includes the different types of hiatal hernias, which for coding purposes are all reported as diaphragmatic with ICD-9-CM code 553.3, except when the condition is congenital, in which case, they are differentiated: diaphragmatic is coded as an anomaly of the diaphragm to 756.6 and hiatal is coded as 750.6 and classified as a congenital displacement of the stomach through the esophageal hiatus. *epigastric h.* Protrusion of a section of the intestine, omentum, or other structure through a fascial defect opening in the abdominal wall just above the umbilicus. Epigastric hernia is reported with ICD-9-CM code 553.29. *hiatal h.* The protrusion of an abdominal organ, usually the stomach, through the esophageal opening within the diaphragm and occurring in two types: the sliding hiatal hernia and the paraesophageal hernia, both reported as diaphragmatic with 553.3. *inguinal h.* Protrusion of an abdominal organ or tissue through the abdominal peritoneum into the inguinal canal, mainly occurring as a loop of intestine in the inguinal canal. Inguinal hernia is reported with a code from subcategory 550.9. *paraesophageal h.* Type of hiatal hernia in which a part or almost the entire stomach protrudes into the thorax lateral to the esophagus, leaving the gastroesophageal junction in place, reported as diaphragmatic with 553.3. *sliding hiatal h.* Type of hiatal hernia in which the upper stomach together with the gastroesophageal junction protrudes up into the mediastinum and is partially covered by a sac of peritoneum. It is coded as

diaphragmatic to 553.3. **Synonym(s):** *axial hiatal hernia, diaphragmatic hernia, esophageal sliding hiatal hernia, hiatal hernia, paraesophageal hernia, Spigelian hernia, Type I hiatal hernia, Type II hiatal hernia.*

herpes gestationis Rare skin disorder of unknown origin that appears on the abdomen in the second and third trimester as intensely itchy blisters that spread to other sites. Herpes gestationis is reported with a code from ICD-9-CM subcategory 646.8.

herpes simplex disciform keratitis Deep, localized area of corneal edema and haziness named for its disk shape.

herpes zoster keratoconjunctivitis Herpes zoster with involvement of the nasociliary nerve may affect the eye, and keratoconjunctivitis may lead to scarring or corneal hypoesthesia.

herpetic geniculate ganglionitis syndrome Facial paralysis, otalgia, and herpes zoster caused by viral infection in seventh cranial nerve and geniculate ganglion. Report this disorder with ICD-9-CM code 053.11. **Synonym(s):** *Hunt's syndrome.*

Herrick's syndrome Inherited blood disorder with sickle-shaped red blood cells that are hard and pointed, clogging blood flow. Report this disorder with ICD-9-CM code 282.61. **Synonym(s):** *sickle cell anemia.*

Herter(-Gee) syndrome Catarrhal dysentery. Inherited malabsorption syndrome of all ages precipitated by gluten-containing foods with wasting and fatigue. Children suffer growth retardation and irritability. Adults suffer difficulty in breathing and clubbing of fingers. Report this disorder with ICD-9-CM code 579.0. **Synonym(s):** *Heubner-Herter syndrome.*

heterograft Surgical graft of tissue from one animal species to a different animal species. A common type of heterograft is porcine (pig) tissue, used for temporary wound closure. Report a heterograft with CPT codes 15400-15431. **Synonym(s):** *xenograft.*

heterologous transplant Tissue from another species, such as porcine from a pig, that is grafted into a human recipient.

heterotopic transplant Tissue transplanted from a different anatomical site for usage as is natural for that tissue, for example, buccal mucosa to a conjunctival site.

Hexadrol phosphate See dexamethasone.

Heyd's syndrome Acute renal failure with disease of the biliary or liver tract. Cause is decreased renal blood flow, damaging both organs. Report this disorder with ICD-9-CM code 572.4.

HF HCPCS Level II modifier, for use with CPT or HCPCS Level II codes, that identifies a substance abuse program. May be required for a state Medicaid program.

HFMA Healthcare Financial Management Association. Organization promoting the improvement of the financial management of health-care-related organizations. The HFMA sponsors some HIPAA educational seminars.

HFO Hand-finger orthosis.

HG HCPCS Level II modifier, for use with CPT or HCPCS Level II codes, that identifies an opioid addiction treatment program. May be required for a state Medicaid program.

Hgb Hemoglobin.

HGH Human growth hormone.

HH *1)* HCPCS Level II modifier, for use with CPT or HCPCS Level II codes, that identifies an integrated mental health/substance abuse program. May be required for a state Medicaid program. *2)* Hard of hearing.

HHA Home health agency. Health care provider, licensed under state or local law, that provides skilled nursing and other therapeutic services. HHAs include visiting nurse associations and hospital-based home care programs. To participate in Medicare, an HHA must meet health and safety standards established by the U.S. Department of Health and Human Services (HHS). Home health services usually are provided in the patient's home, although some outpatient services performed in a hospital, SNF or rehabilitation center may be covered under home health if the equipment is required and cannot be used in the patient's home.

HHHO syndrome Rounded face, almond-shaped eyes, strabismus, low forehead, hypogonadism, hypotonia, mental retardation, and an insatiable appetite. Report this disorder with ICD-9-CM code 759.81. *Synonym(s): H3O syndrome.*

HHIC Hawaii Health Information Corporation.

HHNS Hyperosmolar hyperglycemic nonketotic syndrome. Elevated blood sugar with change in blood chemistry, but without the acidity related with the release of ketones. This is seen most typically in elderly patients with uncontrolled Type I or Type II diabetes and is most often precipitated by acute illness or infection. Report HHNS with an ICD-9-CM code from subcategory 249.2 or 250.2. *Synonym(s): hyperosmolar coma.*

HHS Health and Human Services. Cabinet department that oversees the operating divisions of the federal government responsible for health and welfare. HHS oversees the Centers for Medicare and Medicaid Services, Food and Drug Administration, Public Health Service, and other such entities. *Synonym(s): DHHS.*

HHT Hereditary hemorrhagic telangiectasia. Vascular disorder presenting with frequent nosebleeds and telangiectasis due to vascular system anomalies. HHT is reported with ICD-9-CM code 448.0.

HHV Human herpes virus.

HI HCPCS Level II modifier, for use with CPT or HCPCS Level II codes, that identifies an integrated mental health and mental retardation/ developmental disabilities program. May be required for a state Medicaid program.

HIAA *1)* Health Insurance Association of America. Trade organization for payers. *2)* Hydroxyindoleacetic acid.

hiatal hernia Protrusion of an abdominal organ, mainly the stomach, through the esophageal opening within the diaphragm.

Hib Hemophilus influenzae vaccine.

Hibb's fusion Intentional fracture of the spinous processes and pressing each tip downward to rest in the fractured area of the process below it.

HIBCC Health Industry Business Communications Council.

HibTITER Brand name haemophilus influenzae type B vaccine provided in a single-dose vial. Code selection for HibTITER is dependent upon the patient's immunization schedule. The number of doses specified does not necessarily have to be given; for children who start the Hib series late, fewer doses may be required. For children who start the schedule on time, CPT code 90648 would be reported. Administration is reported separately. Need for vaccination is reported with ICD-9-CM code V03.81.

HIC number Health insurance claim number or Medicare identification number.

Hickman catheter Central venous catheter used for long-term delivery of medications, such as antibiotics, nutritional substances, or chemotherapeutic agents.

hickory stick fracture Fracture unique to children seen as an incomplete, angulated fracture with a partial break. *Synonym(s): greenstick fracture, incomplete fracture, interperiosteal fracture, willow fracture.*

Hicks-Pitney test Thromboplastin generation test measures the efficiency of plasma in forming thromboplastin.

HICN Health insurance claim number. Number issued by the Social Security Administration to individuals or beneficiaries entitled to Medicare benefits. The HICN card provides the beneficiary information necessary for processing Medicare claims.

hidden penis Congenital condition in which a normal size penis is hidden by the foreskin or fat pad. This is reported with ICD-9-CM code 752.65.

hidradenitis Infection or inflammation of a sweat gland. It is classified to ICD-9-CM code 705.83, and is usually treated by incision and drainage.

HIE *1)* Hypoxic-ischemic encephalopathy, reported with a code from ICD-9-CM range 768.70-768.73. *2)* Health information exchange.

hierarchical condition category Groups included in the CMS-HCC Model. Categories of diseases that are

G-I

similar clinically and in cost, arranged to reflect severity rankings among related disease categories. A beneficiary is assigned to the condition category that reflects the most severe manifestation among related conditions. However, a case may be assigned to several non-related HCCs. **Synonym(s):** *HCC.*

hierarchy Ranking or ordering of information or people.

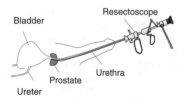

HIFU

HIFU is an acronym for
high intensity focused ultrasound

High intensity ultrasound
destroys prostate tissue

HIFU High-intensity focused ultrasound. Therapeutic ultrasound procedure in which high-intensity beams are focused on diseased tissue, which is then thermally coagulated. Indications may include benign prostatic hyperplasia, uterine fibroids, and certain cancers, particularly those of the prostate. **Synonym(s):** *acoustic ablation.*

high-grade defect Individuals with an IQ of 50-70 who can develop social and communication skills, have minimal retardation in sensorimotor areas, and often are not distinguished from normal children until a later age and can learn academic skills up to approximately the sixth-grade level. As adults they can usually achieve social and vocational skills adequate for minimum self-support but may need guidance and assistance when under social or economic stress. **Synonym(s):** *feeble minded.*

HIGHSAIL Brand name coronary dilatation catheter used in percutaneous intraluminal balloon angioplasty as a treatment approach for blocked coronary arteries. The procedure is reported with CPT code 92982 for one vessel and 92984 for each additional vessel. If performed with atherectomy, 92995 would be reported, with 92996 for each additional vessel. Inpatient procedures would be reported with ICD-9-CM procedural codes 00.40-00.43 and 00.66.

HI-LO High-low.

hilum Concave notch at the medial indentation of the kidney through which the ureter and renal vein exit and the renal artery enters the kidney.

HIM Health information management.

HIMSS Healthcare Information Management Systems Society. Organization for health care information and management systems professionals.

HIO Health information organization.

HIPAA Health Insurance Portability and Accountability Act of 1996. Federal law that allows persons to qualify immediately for comparable health insurance coverage when they change their employment relationships. Title II, subtitle F, of HIPAA gives the Department of Health and Human Services the authority to mandate the use of standards for the electronic exchange of health care data; to specify what medical and administrative code sets should be used within those standards; to require the use of national identification systems for health care patients, providers, payers (or plans), and employers (or sponsors); and to specify the types of measures required to protect the security and privacy of personally identifiable health care information. **Synonym(s):** *K2, Kassenbaum-Kennedy Bill, Kennedy-Kassenbaum Bill, Public Law 104-191.*

HIPAA data dictionary Data dictionary that defines and cross-references the contents of all X12 transactions included in the HIPAA mandate. It is maintained by X12N/TG3.

HIPC Health Information Policy Council.

hippotherapy Physical, occupational, and speech therapy treatment strategy using horses and horseback riding. Specific riding skills are not taught, but a foundation is established to improve neurological function and sensory processing. This foundation can be generalized to a wide range of daily activities. Hippotherapy is reported with HCPCS Level II code S8940. **Synonym(s):** *equestrian therapy.*

HIPPS Health insurance prospective payment system. Procedure coding system used in the Medicare skilled nursing facility and home health, inpatient rehabilitation, and rural hospital swing beds prospective payment systems (PPSs).

Hirschsprung's disease Congenital enlargement or dilation of the colon, with the absence of nerve cells in a segment of colon distally that causes the inability to defecate. This disease is reported with ICD-9-CM code 751.3. **Synonym(s):** *megacolon.*

hirsutism Excessive hair growth. In males, an excessive hair growth pattern usually occurs in androgen-stimulated locations, such as the face, chest, and areolae. In females, hair appears in locations where hair is usually absent. Hirsutism is frequently caused by abnormally high androgen levels, namely testosterone

G-I

or by hair follicles that have a greater sensitivity to normal androgen levels. Other diseases such as polycystic ovarian syndrome, adrenal hyperplasia, and Cushing syndrome can cause hirsutism. Hirsutism is reported with code ICD-9-CM code 704.1. *Synonym(s): hypertrichosis.*

HISB   Health Informatics Standards Board.

histiocytic necrotizing lymphadenitis   Benign lymphadenopathy syndrome manifested by swollen glands in the neck, fever, necrotizing lesions in the area around the thymus cortex, flu-like symptoms, and an increase in distinct types of histiocytes, monocytes, and immunoblasts. Predominantly occurring in females, this disease is sometimes considered a self-limiting form of systemic lupus erythematosus. Report this condition with ICD-9-CM code 289.3. *Synonym(s): Kikuchi disease, Kikuchi-Fujimoto disease, Kikuchi lymphadenitis, subacute necrotizing lymphadenitis.*

histiocytosis   Blood disease in which there is an abnormal multiplication of white blood cells.

histo-   Relating to tissue.

Histofreezer   Brand name cryosurgical device for the treatment of benign skin lesions including verruca vulgaris, verruca plantaris, HPV, acrochordon, molluscum contagiosum, seborrheic keratosis, verruca plana, actinic keratoses, and lentigo. The procedure is reported with CPT codes 17110 and 17111.

histology   Branch of science specializing in the microscopic study of tissues. There are four basic types of tissue. Epithelial (epi, upon or over) is found throughout the body and makes up the covering of external and internal surfaces. Connective tissue is the most widespread in the human body. It forms bones, cartilage, tendons, and ligaments. Muscle and nerve tissues are the remaining basic types and are further categorized.

history of present illness   Chronological account of signs and symptoms of the present condition.

histrelin acetate   Gonadotropin hormonal drug used to treat central precocious puberty of idiopathic or neurogenic origin occurring in girls younger than age 8 and in boys younger than age 9.5. Injectable supply is reported with HCPCS Level II code J1675; implant is reported with J9226. *Synonym(s): Supprelin.*

HIT   *1)* Heparin-induced thrombocytopenia. *2)* Home infusion therapy. *3)* Health information technology.

HITECH   Health information technology for economic and clinical health.

HIV   Human immunodeficiency virus. *NCD References: 190.9, 190.13, 190.14.*

HJ   HCPCS Level II modifier, for use with CPT or HCPCS Level II codes, that identifies an employee assistance program. May be required for a state Medicaid program.

HK   HCPCS Level II modifier, for use with CPT or HCPCS Level II codes, that identifies specialized mental health programs for high-risk populations. May be required for a state Medicaid program.

HKAFO   Hip-knee-ankle foot orthosis.

HL   HCPCS Level II modifier, for use with CPT or HCPCS Level II codes, that identifies services provided by an intern. May be required for a state Medicaid program.

HL7   Health Level Seven. Group accredited by the American National Standards Institute that defines standards for the cross-platform exchange of information within a health care organization. HL7 is responsible for specifying the Level Seven OSI standards for the health industry. The X12 275 transaction will probably incorporate the HL7 CRU message to transmit claim attachments as part of a future HIPAA claim attachments standard. The HL7 Attachment SIG is responsible for the HL7 portion of this standard.

HLA   Human leukocyte antigen.

HLV   Herpes-like virus.

HM   HCPCS Level II modifier, for use with CPT or HCPCS Level II codes, that identifies a service provided by an individual without a bachelor's degree.

HMD   Hyaline membrane disease.

HMES   Heat and moisture exchange system.

HMO   Health maintenance organization. Medical health insurance coverage that pays claims based on a provider cost, per diem, or charge basis. Hospitals contract with an HMO to provide care at a contractually reduced price. HMO members pay a set monthly amount for coverage and are treated without additional cost, except for a copayment or deductible amount, payable by the patient. Like all managed care organizations, HMOs use a variety of mechanisms to control costs, including utilization management, discounted provider fee schedules, and financial incentives. HMOs use primary care physicians as gatekeepers and tend to emphasize preventive care.

HMS   *1)* Hepatosplenomegaly. *2)* Haim-Munk syndrome. Rare syndrome of congenital calluses on soles and palms, frequent skin infections, overgrown nails, and degeneration of the gums and the bones surrounding the teeth. No specific code is indexed to HMS in ICD-9-CM. Coding guidelines indicate that if a syndrome is not indexed, its manifestations should each be coded separately.

HN   HCPCS Level II modifier, for use with CPT or HCPCS Level II codes, that identifies services provided by an individual with a bachelor's degree. May be required for a state Medicaid program.

HNAD   Hyperosmolar nonacidotic diabetes.

HNP Herniated nucleus pulposus. A fibrous extrusion of semifluid nucleus pulposus through a ruptured intervertebral disk, causing pain and disability.

HNPCC Hereditary nonpolyposis colorectal cancer. Inherited risk for multiple cancers primarily affecting the digestive tract, but also brain, skin, and urinary tract. Genetic testing for HNPCC is reported with HCPCS Level II code S3831. *Synonym(s): Lynch syndrome.*

HNS Hyperosmolar nonketotic syndrome. Elevated blood sugar with change in blood chemistry, but without the acidity related with the release of ketones. This is seen most typically in elderly patients with uncontrolled Type I or Type II diabetes and is most often precipitated by acute illness or infection. Report HNS with an ICD-9-CM code from subcategory 249.2 or 250.2. *Synonym(s): hyperosmolar coma.*

HO HCPCS Level II modifier, for use with CPT or HCPCS Level II codes, that identifies services provided by an individual with a master's degree. May be required for a state Medicaid program.

HOB Head of bed.

Hodgkin's disease Malignant disorder characterized by the presence of progressively swollen lymph nodes. Report with a code from the ICD-9-CM rubric 201.

Hoffa (-Kastert) syndrome Traumatic proliferation of fatty tissue on knee joint. Report this disorder with ICD-9-CM code 272.8.

Hoffman device External fixation device.

Hoffmann's syndrome Hypothyroidism beginning during infancy as a result of injury of the thyroid gland or presence of cretinism. Report this disorder with ICD-9-CM code 244.9 and 359.5.

Hoffmann-Bouveret syndrome Rapid action of the heart having sudden onset and cessation. Report this disorder with ICD-9-CM code 427.2.

HOH Hard of hearing.

hold harmless Contractual clause stating that if either party is held liable for malpractice, the other party is absolved.

Holländer-Simons syndrome Loss of subcutaneous fat of the upper torso, the arms, the neck, and face but with an increase in fat on and below the pelvis. Report this disorder with ICD-9-CM code 272.6.

Holmes' syndrome Cortical paralysis of visual fixation, optic ataxia, and disturbance of visual attention. Eye movements are normal. Report this disorder with ICD-9-CM code 368.16.

Holmes-Adie syndrome Pathological reaction in which the pupil does not react to changes in light and changes if focus is changed. Cause is certain tendon deficiency. Report this disorder with ICD-9-CM code 379.46.

holoprosencephaly Congenital abnormality in which the embryonic forebrain fails to adequately divide into the two lobes of the cerebral hemispheres, sometimes resulting in a single-lobed brain. Severe facial and skull abnormalities are often present, affecting the nose, eyes, and upper lip. This condition may be due to trisomy 13 or 18. This abnormality is reported with ICD-9-CM code 742.2 alone, with 758.1 when due to trisomy 13, and 758.2 when due to trisomy 18.

HoLRP Holmium laser resection of prostate. Thermal therapy using a laser to destroy tissue in benign prostatic hyperplasia.

Holten test Creatines are used to test renal efficiency.

Holter monitor Device worn by the patient for long-term continuous recording of electro-cardiographic signals on magnetic tape, replayed at rapid speed, for scanning and selection of significant but brief changes that might otherwise escape notice.

Holter monitor procedure Patient wears a portable instrument to chart long-term behavior of the heart.

hom(eo)/(o)- Indicates resemblance or likeness.

home environment assessment Determination of the patient's ability to interact within the home environment in the safest, most efficient manner and notation of anything that restrains or obstructs progress or access.

home health Palliative and therapeutic care and assistance in the activities of daily life to homebound Medicare and private plan members. *NCD References: 290.1, 290.2.*

home health agency Health care provider, licensed under state or local law, that provides skilled nursing and other therapeutic services. HHAs include visiting nurse associations and hospital-based home care programs. To participate in Medicare, an HHA must meet health and safety standards established by the U.S. Department of Health and Human Services (HHS). Home health services usually are provided in the patient's home, although some outpatient services performed in a hospital, SNF or rehabilitation center may be covered under home health if the equipment is required and cannot be used in the patient's home. *Synonym(s): HHA.*

home health services Services furnished to patients in their homes under the care of physicians. These services include part-time or intermittent skilled nursing care, physical therapy, medical social services, medical supplies, and some rehabilitation equipment. Home health supplies and services must be prescribed by a physician, and the beneficiary must be confined at home in order for Medicare to pay the benefits in full. *Synonym(s): HHS.*

homeo- Resemblance or likeness.

homogeneous Patients consuming similar types and amounts of hospital resources.

G-I

homogenous transplant Tissue or organ removed from a human donor and transplanted into another recipient.

homograft Graft from one individual to another of the same species. **Synonym(s):** *allogeneic graft, allograft.*

homonym One of two or more words spelled and pronounced alike but different in meaning.

homosexuality Exclusive or predominant sexual attraction for persons of the same sex with or without physical relationships.

Hoppe-Goldflam syndrome Progressive muscular weakness beginning in face and throat caused by a defect in myoneural conduction. Report this disorder with ICD-9-CM code 358.00. **Synonym(s):** *Erb syndrome, Goldflam syndrome, Hoppe syndrome.*

hor. decub. At bedtime.

hordeolum Acute localized infection of the gland of Zeis (external hordeolum) or Molt or of the meibomian glands (internal hordeolum) of the orbit.

HORF High output renal failure.

hormone Chemical substance produced by the body that has a regulatory effect on the function of its specific target organ(s).

Horner's syndrome Pain and stiffness in the shoulder, with puffy swelling and pain in the hand following a heart attack. Report this disorder with ICD-9-CM code 337.9. **Synonym(s):** *Claude Bernard-Homer syndrome, Reilly's syndrome, Steinbrocker's syndrome.*

horseshoe U-shaped device that stabilizes or immobilizes the patella when used with a knee orthosis.

horseshoe kidney Congenital anomaly in which the kidneys are fused together at the lower end during fetal development, resulting in one large, horseshoe shaped kidney, often associated with cardiovascular, central nervous system, or genitourinary anomalies. Reported with ICD-9-CM code 753.3.

hospice Organization that furnishes inpatient, outpatient, and home health care for the terminally ill. Hospices emphasize support and counseling services for terminally ill people and their families, pain relief, and symptom management. When the Medicare beneficiary chooses hospice benefits, all other Medicare benefits are discontinued, except physician services and treatment of conditions not related to the terminal illness.

hospice care Items and services provided to a terminally ill individual by a hospice program under a written plan established and periodically reviewed by the individual's attending physician and by the medical director: Nursing care provided by or under the supervision of a registered professional nurse; Physical or occupational therapy or speech-language pathology services; Medical social services under the direction of a physician; Services of a home health aide who has successfully completed a training program; Medical supplies (including drugs and biologicals) and the use of medical appliances; Physicians' services; Short-term inpatient care (including both respite care and procedures necessary for pain control and acute and chronic symptom management) in an inpatient facility on an intermittent basis and not consecutively over longer than five days; Counseling (including dietary counseling) with respect to care of the terminally ill individual and adjustment to his death; Any item or service which is specified in the plan and for which payment may be made.

hospice program Hospice program establishes the care and service plan and ensures that the services are available (as needed) on a 24-hour basis and also provides bereavement counseling for the immediate family of terminally ill individuals. The services may be delivered in an individual's home, on an outpatient basis, and on a short-term inpatient basis, directly or under arrangements made by the agency or organization. The Hospice agency is responsible for all services in an aggregate number of days of inpatient care provided in any 12-month period, as overseen by an interdisciplinary group of personnel that includes at least one physician, one registered professional nurse, and one social worker. A central clinical record must be maintained for each patient. According to federal law, an Hospice cannot discontinue its services with respect to a patient because of the inability of the patient to pay for care. Volunteers may provide care and services as long as the program maintains records on the cost savings and expansion of care and services achieved through volunteers.

hospital Institution that provides, under the supervision of physicians, diagnostic, therapeutic, and rehabilitation services for medical diagnosis, treatment, and care of patients. Hospitals receiving federal funds must maintain clinical records on all patients, provide 24-hour nursing services, and have a discharge planning process in place. The term "hospital" also includes religious nonmedical health care institutions and facilities of 50 beds or less located in rural areas.

hospital addiction syndrome Description of psychosomatic behavior with physical symptoms exhibited by some patients with histrionic personality disorder. Report this disorder with ICD-9-CM code 301.51. **Synonym(s):** *multiple operations syndrome, Münchhausen syndrome.*

hospital admission plan Used to facilitate admission to the hospital and to assure prompt payment to the hospital.

hospital hoboes Chronic form of factitious illness in which the individual demonstrates a plausible presentation of voluntarily produced physical symptomatology of such a degree that he or she is able to obtain and sustain multiple hospitalizations or courses of treatment. **Synonym(s):** *hospital addiction syndrome.*

hospital inpatient Person who is admitted to a hospital for bed occupancy for purposes of receiving inpatient hospital services. Generally, a patient is considered an inpatient if formally admitted as inpatient with the expectation that he or she will remain at least overnight and occupy a bed, even though it later develops that the patient can be discharged or transferred to another hospital and not actually use a hospital bed overnight.

hospital insurance Medicare Part A. **Synonym(s):** *HI.*

hospital issued notice of noncoverage Notice issued by a hospital to a beneficiary when the hospital determines that the care the beneficiary is receiving or is about to receive is not covered because it is not medically necessary, is not being delivered in the most appropriate setting, or is custodial in nature. The HINN may be given prior to admission, at admission, or at any point during the inpatient stay. **Synonym(s):** *HINN.*

hospital outpatient Person with known diagnoses that enters a hospital for a specific minor surgical procedure or other treatment that is expected to keep him or her in the hospital for only a few hours (less than 24), regardless of the hour the patient arrived at the hospital, whether the patient used a bed, or whether the patient remained in the hospital past midnight.

hospitalism Mild or transient adjustment reaction characterized by withdrawal seen in hospitalized patients. May be manifested by elective mutism in young children.

hot biopsy Using forceps technique, simultaneously excises and fulgurates polyps; avoids the bleeding associated with cold-forceps biopsy; and preserves the specimen for histologic examination (in contrast, a simple fulguration of the polyp destroys it).

Hover-T Bone attachment component used with SpineAssist surgery on the lumbar spine. Hover-T would be utilized in procedures reported with CPT code 22533, 22558, 22612, or 22630.

Howard test Both ureters are catheterized and urine is collected from each kidney to test renal function.

Howship's lacuna Pits in bone, the result of bone resorption by osteoclasts. Howship's lacuna is a normal finding and as such is not a coded diagnosis. **Synonym(s):** *absorption lacuna, resorption lacuna.*

HP HCPCS Level II modifier, for use with CPT or HCPCS Level II codes, that identifies services provided by an individual with a doctoral level degree. May be required for a state Medicaid program.

HPAG HIPAA Policy Advisory Group, a BCBSA subgroup.

HPF High power field. Magnification of a microscope during lab or pathology examination. It does not affect code selection.

HPG Human pituitary gonadotropin.

HPI History of present illness.

HPL Human placental lactogen. Placental hormone that breaks down maternal fats to provide nutrients to the fetus. HPL is measured in CPT chemistry code 83632, usually to assess the growth of the fetus.

H-plasty Adjacent tissue transfer or skin flap rearrangement approach resembling an ôHö with advancement flaps used for the closure of square or rounded defects, commonly used with injuries to the forehead. A series of CPT codes (14000-14350) are used to report this type of closure. These codes should not be reported when direct closure or rearrangement of traumatic wounds incidentally results in configurations like an H-plasty.

HPOA Hypertrophic pulmonary osteoarthropathy. Syndrome manifested by clubbed fingers and toes, enlarged extremities, pain in the joints, and vasomotor disturbance of the hands and feet. The periosteum of the radius and fibula is frequently inflamed, often due to underlying pulmonary problems such as lung cancer, tuberculosis, abscesses, emphysema, or cystic fibrosis. Conditions other than pulmonary disorders may also cause this syndrome. Report this disease with ICD-9-CM code 731.2. **Synonym(s):** *Hagner's disease, Marie-Bamberger disease.*

HPS *1)* Hanta virus pulmonary syndrome. *2)* Hot packs.

HPSA Health professional shortage area. Based on rural geographical areas that have a shortage of physicians, CMS provides incentive payments (also known as a bonus payment program) of 5 to 10 percent for physicians who furnish services in areas that are designated as HPSAs under the Public Health Service Act. There are three types of HPSAs: primary medical care, dental, and mental health. There is instruction on implementing this payment system in the Pub 100-4 (formerly the MCM).

HPV Human papilloma virus. Virus of several different species transmitted by direct or indirect contact and causing plantar and genital warts on skin and mucous membranes. HPV is most commonly associated with increased risk for cervical dysplasia and cancer in women. HPV infection is reported with ICD-9-CM code 079.4. Women with atypical cervical cells may be tested for exposure to HPV virus; positive findings for high-risk strains of HPV are reported with ICD-9-CM code 795.05.

HQ HCPCS Level II modifier, for use with CPT or HCPCS Level II codes, that identifies services performed in a group setting. May be required for a state Medicaid program.

G-I

HR *1)* HCPCS Level II modifier, for use with CPT or HCPCS Level II codes, that identifies services provided with a family/couple with the client present. May be required for a state Medicaid program. *2)* Harrington rod. *3)* Heart rate. *4)* Hour.

HRA Health reimbursement account.

HRT Hormone replacement therapy.

hrt. Heart.

HS *1)* HCPCS Level II modifier, for use with CPT or HCPCS Level II codes, that identifies services provided with a family/couple without the client present. May be required for a state Medicaid program. *2)* Heel stick.

HSA *1)* Health savings account. *2)* Health service agreement.

HSBG Heelstick blood gas.

HSG Hysterosalpingogram.

HSP Health service plan.

HSRV Hospital-specific relative value. Site specific weight added to DRG determination.

HSV Herpes simplex virus.

HT HCPCS Level II modifier, for use with CPT or HCPCS Level II codes, that identifies services provided by a multidisciplinary team. May be required for a state Medicaid program.

ht. Height.

HTA system Hydro Term Ablator System. Hysteroscopic device that performs endometrial ablation. The procedure is reported with CPT code 58563.

HTLV/III Human T-cell lymphotropic.

HTN Hypertension.

HU HCPCS Level II modifier, for use with CPT or HCPCS Level II codes, that identifies services or supplies that are funded by a child welfare agency. May be required for a state Medicaid program.

HUD Humanitarian use device. HUD is intended to benefit patients by treating or diagnosing a disease or condition that affects fewer than 4,000 individuals in the United States per year. HUDs are not held to the same FDA requirements as more widely used devices.

Huggins' orchiectomy Testes removed due to prostate cancer, among other diagnoses.

Hughes syndrome Autoimmune disorder associated with the development of arterial and venous thromboses. Hughes syndrome can be seen secondary to another disease, prominently lupus. It can also occur without an underlying disorder. It is reported with ICD-9-CM code 795.79. *Synonym(s): Antiphospholipid syndrome.*

human alpha 1 proteinase inhibitor Drug used to treat the genetic disorder of Alpha-1 antitrypsin deficiency, or AAT. This drug is a sterile, stable, lyophilized preparation of purified human Alpha 1-proteinase inhibitor. Prolastin is the common trade name. Supply is reported with HCPCS Level II code J0256. May be sold under the brand name Prolastin alpha 1-antitrypsin.

human antithrombin III Glycoprotein used to replace ATIII in patients with ATIII deficiency. It acts as an anticoagulant or antithrombolytic by inhibiting reactions in the coagulation cascade. Supply is reported with HCPCS Level II code J7197. May be sold under the brand name Atnativ, Thrombate III.

human papilloma virus Virus of several different species transmitted by direct or indirect contact and causing plantar and genital warts on skin and mucous membranes. HPV is most commonly associated with increased risk for cervical dysplasia and cancer in women. HPV infection is reported with ICD-9-CM code 079.4. Women with atypical cervical cells may be tested for exposure to HPV virus; positive findings for high-risk strains of HPV are reported with ICD-9-CM code 795.05.

Humate-P Mixture of Antihemophilic Factor (Factor VIII) and von Willebrand Factor (VWF) derived from human blood indicated in adult patients with hemophilia A. It is used in adult and pediatric patients for treatment of spontaneous and trauma-induced bleeding episodes in severe von Willebrand disease.

Humegon Injectable drug consisting of a mixture of follicle-stimulating hormone (FSH) and luteinizing hormone (LH), used to stimulate ovulation in instances when the ovaries are capable of producing a follicle but there is inadequate hormonal stimulation. This drug is also used to prompt the growth of multiple eggs for in vitro fertilization, as well as to stimulate sperm production in men who have inadequate hormonal stimulation but functioning testes. Supply is reported with HCPCS Level II code S0122.

Hummelshein operation Correction of strabismus by adjusting the eye muscles.

hungry bone syndrome Syndrome whose characteristics include hypocalcemia and sometimes hypophosphatemia and hypomagnesemia. Hungry bone syndrome commonly occurs following parathyroidectomy for primary or secondary hyperparathyroidism. Hypocalcemia may resolve in a number of weeks but in some cases may last for years. Report this disorder with ICD-9-CM code 275.5.

Hunt's syndrome Facial paralysis, otalgia, and herpes zoster caused by viral infection in seventh cranial nerve and geniculate ganglion. Report this disorder with ICD-9-CM code 053.11. *Synonym(s): Ramsey-Hunt syndrome.*

Hunter (-Hurler) syndrome Mucopolysaccharide sulfates affecting the eye, ear, skin, teeth, skeleton, joints, liver, spleen, cardiovascular system, respiratory system, and central nervous system. Report this disorder with ICD-9-CM code 277.5.

Hutchinson's sign Herpes zoster manifest on the tip of the nose, usually indicative of ocular involvement, due to the structure of the nasociliary nerve.

Hutchinson-Boeck syndrome Disorder with fibrosis, lymph nodes, skin, enlarged liver, eyes, enlarged spleen, phalangeal bones, parotid glands, and systemic granulomas composed of epithelioid and multinucleated giant cells. Report this disorder with ICD-9-CM code 135. *Synonym(s): Besnier-Boeck-Schaumann syndrome, Lofgren's syndrome, Schaumann's syndrome.*

Hutchinson-Gilford syndrome Precocious senility with death from coronary artery disease occurring before 16 years of age. Report this disorder with ICD-9-CM code 259.8. *Synonym(s): Gilford syndrome.*

HV HCPCS Level II modifier, for use with CPT or HCPCS Level II codes, that identifies services or supplies that are funded by a state addictions agency. May be required for a state Medicaid program.

HVA Homovanillic acid.

HW HCPCS Level II modifier, for use with CPT or HCPCS Level II codes, that identifies services or supplies that are funded by a state mental health agency. May be required for a state Medicaid program.

Hx History.

HX *1)* HCPCS Level II modifier, for use with CPT or HCPCS Level II codes, that identifies services or supplies that are funded by a county/local agency. *2)* History.

HY HCPCS Level II modifier, for use with CPT or HCPCS Level II codes, that identifies services or supplies that are funded by a juvenile justice agency. May be required for a state Medicaid program.

Hyalgan Brand name sodium hyaluronate indicated for the treatment of osteoarthritic knee pain. Administered by intraarticular injection, a treatment cycle typically consists of five injections given at weekly intervals. Supply of Hyalgan is reported with HCPCS Level II code J7321.

hyaluronic acid High molecular weight glycosaminoglycan (GAG) that has viscous properties, most often used as a synovial fluid substitute injected directly into the knee for pain associated with osteoarthritis. It provides lubrication and shock absorption at the joint in the same manner as synovial fluid. Report the injection into the knee joint separately. Supply of the intra-articular injection is reported with HCPCS Level II code J7321, J7323, J7324, or J7325. May be sold under the brand names Euflexxa, Hyalgan, Hyaluronan, Orthovisc, Supratz, or Synovisc. *Synonym(s): sodium hyaluronate.*

hyaluronidase Substance used for dispersing other medications through connective tissues. It changes the permeability of connective tissue to facilitate the absorption of injected fluids through the hydrolysis of hyaluronic acid. It is used in promoting absorption of radiographic substances and in anesthesia of the eye prior to surgery. May be sold under the brand name Vitrase. Report supply with HCPCS Level II codes J3470, J3471, J3472, and J3473.

Hybrid Capture 2 Brand name molecular technology used to perform a variety of laboratory tests, including an in vitro test for the detection of 13 high-risk types of human papilloma viruses (HPV) in cervical specimens from a Pap smear. HPV is associated with an increased risk for cervical dysplasia and cancer in women. Hybrid Capture 2 HPV DNA Pap Smear is reported with CPT code 88142 in combination with 87621.

hybrid entity Covered entity whose covered functions are not its primary functions.

hydatidiform mole Trophoblastic neoplasm that mimics pregnancy by proliferating from a pathologic ovum and resulting only in a mass of cysts resembling grapes, 80 percent of which are benign, but require surgical removal. Hydatidiform moles can be complete, in which there is no fetal tissue, or partial, in which fetal tissue is frequently present. Both are characterized by trophoblastic hyperplasia and proliferation of the chorionic villi, causing the grapelike appearance. If benign, it is reported with ICD-9-CM code 630; when malignant, it is reported with 236.1. *Synonym(s): cystic mole, hydatid mole, molar pregnancy, vesicular mole.*

hydralazine HCl Direct acting vasodilator used as an antihypertensive to manage severe essential hypertension, heart failure, and eclampsia or preeclampsia. Supply is reported with HCPCS Level II code J0360. May be sold under the brand names Alphapress, Apresoline, Novo-Hylazin.

hydro- Relating to fluid, water, or hydrogen.

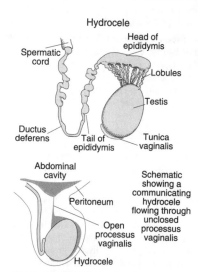

Hydrocele

Spermatic cord

Head of epididymis

Lobules

Testis

Ductus deferens

Tail of epididymis

Tunica vaginalis

Abdominal cavity

Peritoneum

Open processus vaginalis

Schematic showing a communicating hydrocele flowing through unclosed processus vaginalis

Hydrocele

The tunica vaginalis is a closed sac within the scrotum and is the lower remnant of the path taken by the testis as it descends from the abdomen just prior to birth. The testes, or testicles, are the male reproductive organs. Each produces sperm and male sex hormones

hydrocele Serous fluid that collects in the tunica vaginalis, the spermatic cord, or the canal of Nuck. Hydroceles may be congenital, due to a defect in the tunica vaginalis, or secondary, due to fluid accumulation, injury, infection, or radiotherapy. Secondary hydroceles are reported with a code from ICD-9-CM category 603. Congenital hydrocele is reported with ICD-9-CM code 778.6.

hydrocephalus Abnormal buildup of cerebrospinal fluid in the brain, causing dilation of the ventricles. Hydrocephalus is most often the result of obstructed cerebrospinal fluid pathways either congenital or acquired. The primary treatment method is to shunt the cerebrospinal fluid (CSF) to another body area. *Synonym(s): water on the brain.*

Hydrocol Brand name hydrocolloid wound dressing applied to protect a wound from infection that can be easily removed without disruption of the healing process. When the dressing is applied in the physician office, the supply of the wound dressing is reported separately with HCPCS Level II codes A6234-A6239.

hydromorphone Opioid analgesic used to control moderate to severe pain and cough by binding with opiate receptors to alter the central nervous system response to pain and suppressing the cough center in the medulla. Supply is reported with HCPCS Level II code S0092. May be sold under the brand name Dilaudid.

hydromyelia Dilation of the central canal of the spinal cord, in which there may be increased accumulation of cerebrospinal fluid that results in abnormal pressure on the spinal cord. Hydromyelia is reported with ICD-9-CM code 742.53. *Synonym(s): hydrorrhachis.*

hydronephrosis Distension of the kidney caused by an accumulation of urine that cannot flow out due to an obstruction that may be caused by conditions such as kidney stones or vesicoureteral reflux. Kidney infection and permanent damage may result. This condition is reported with ICD-9-CM code 591, which includes hydroureteronephrosis. *Synonym(s): hydrocalycosis, hydroureteronephrosis.*

hydrosalpinx Watery fluid within the fallopian tube that is commonly caused by a prior tubal infection in its last phase. Hydrosalpinx can be diagnosed by ultrasound, laparoscopy, or hysterosalpingogram. Hydrosalpinx is reported with ICD-9-CM code 614.1 as chronic salpingitis and oophoritis.

hydroureter Abnormal enlargement or distension of the ureter with water or urine caused by an obstruction. This condition is reported with ICD-9-CM code 593.5 unless specified as congenital, which is coded to 753.22.

hydroxyzine Antihistamine used for a variety of problems, known to relieve anxiety and itching from allergies. It is also used as a calming agent in pre and postoperative adjunctive sedative therapy or to relieve nausea and vomiting. Oral supply used as an approved antiemetic substitute for IV antiemetic therapy for cancer patients is reported with HCPCS Level II code Q0177 or Q0178. Report J3410 for an injection supply. May be sold under the brand names Anx, Apo-Hydroxyzine, Hydroxacen, Hyzine 50, Multipax, Neucalm, QYS, Vistacon-50, Vistaject-50, Vistaril.

hygroma Accumulation of serous fluid that resembles a cyst.

hylaform Injectable subcutaneous implant that temporarily reverses the effects of age or weight loss on the face. The effect lasts for about 12 weeks. After the initial treatment, follow-up treatments may be needed to achieve optimal skin smoothing. Injections are usually considered cosmetic.

hylan See hyaluronic acid.

hyoid bone Single, U-shaped bone palpable in the neck above the larynx and below the mandible (lower jaw) with various muscles attached but not articulating with any other bone.

hyoscyamine sulfate Acetylcholine inhibitor used to treat gastric ulcer disease as it decreases the secretion of stomach acid. It has an inhibitory affect on all postganglionic cholinergic nerves and muscles that respond to acetylcholine but lack cholinergic innervation including the cardiac muscle, AV node, SA node, all exocrine glands, and smooth muscles such as the intestines. It also decreases secretions in the trachea

G-I

and bronchi. Supply is reported with HCPCS Level II code J1980. May be sold under the brand name Levsin.

hyper- Excessive, above, exaggerated.

hyperabduction syndrome Malignant atrophic papulosis. Report this disorder with ICD-9-CM code 447.8.

hyperactive bowel syndrome Abdominal pain, watery stools, and gas. Report this disorder with ICD-9-CM code 564.1.

hyperaldosteronism Oversecretion of aldosterone causing electrolyte balance problems, fluid retention, and hypertension.

hyperaldosteronism with hypokalemic alkalosis syndrome Low or normal blood pressure, no edema, retarded growth, hypokalemic alkalosis, and elevated renin or angiotensin levels. Report this disorder with ICD-9-CM code 255.13. *Synonym(s): Bartter's syndrome.*

hyperalimentation Intake or ingestion of excessive amounts of food, reported with ICD-9-CM code 783.6. *Synonym(s): excessive eating, polyphagia.*

hypercalcemia Abnormally high levels of calcium in the blood, resulting in symptoms of muscle weakness, fatigue, nausea, depression, and constipation. Causes may include tumor or hyperthyroidism. Hypercalcemia is reported with ICD-9-CM code 275.42.

hypercalcemic syndrome Similar to hypoparathyroidism, Failure to respond to parathyroid hormone causing short stature, obesity, short metacarpals, and ectopic calcification. Report this disorder with ICD-9-CM code 275.42. *Synonym(s): Albright-Martin syndrome, Seabright-Bantam syndrome.*

hypercapnia Excess carbon dioxide in the blood.

hypercarotenemia Elevated blood carotene level as a result of excessive carotenoid ingestion or an inability to convert carotenoids to vitamin A. Characteristics often include yellow discoloration of the skin, especially the palms, soles, and the area behind the ears. Report this condition with ICD-9-CM code 278.3. *Synonym(s): carotenemia.*

hypercementosis Excess deposits of cementum on the tooth roots, reported with ICD-9-CM code 521.5.

hyperemesis gravidarum Persistent and severe nausea and vomiting in early pregnancy (before 22 completed weeks of gestation) that affects the management of the pregnancy. Mild hyperemesis gravidarum is reported with a code from ICD-9-CM subcategory 643.0. When it occurs with metabolic disturbances such as dehydration, carbohydrate depletion, or electrolyte disturbances, report it with a code from subcategory 643.1. *Synonym(s): HG.*

hyperestrogenism Excess secretion of estrogen by the ovaries. The most common diagnostic finding is ovaries containing many serous fluid filled follicular cysts. Hyperestrogenism is reported with ICD-9-CM code 256.0.

hyperglycemia Abnormally high blood sugar, usually greater than 140 mg/dl in a nonfasting, nondiabetic patient. Hyperglycemia in a diabetic patient is not easily quantified; levels will vary from patient to patient. Hyperglycemia is reported with ICD-9-CM code 790.29 when diabetes is not documented in the patient's medical record.

HyperHEP B Brand name hepatitis B immune globulin provided in a 1 ml or 5 ml vial or a 0.5 ml or 1 ml syringe. Supply of HyperHEP B is reported with CPT code 90371; administration is reported separately. The need for the injection is reported with ICD-9-CM code V01.89.

hyperhidrosis Condition of excessive perspiration beyond what the body requires for normal temperature control. This condition is classified as different types. Focal hyperhidrosis is coded differently than generalized hyperhidrosis. Primary focal hyperhidrosis is a rare disorder of the sweat glands localized to areas such as the axilla, face, palms, or soles and is reported with ICD-9-CM code 705.21. Secondary focal hyperhidrosis is usually the cause of a local condition or treatment, such as radiation, a lesion, or an injury, and is reported with ICD-9-CM 705.22. Generalized hyperhidrosis is a symptom of another underlying disease and includes secondary hyperhidrosis that is not localized, is reported with ICD-9-CM code 780.8.

hyperkinetic syndromes of childhood Disorders of short attention span and distractibility with impulsiveness, mood fluctuations, and aggression. In early childhood, characterized by disinhibited, poorly organized, and poorly regulated extreme overactivity; in adolescence, characterized by underactivity. *h. attention deficit disorder* Hyperkinetic syndrome with short attention span, distractibility, and overactivity without significant disturbance of conduct or delay in specific skills. *h. with developmental delay* Hyperkinetic syndrome associated with speech delay, clumsiness, reading difficulties, or other delays of specific skills. *h. conduct disorder* Hyperkinetic syndrome associated with marked conduct disturbance but not developmental delay. *hypersomnia h.* Hyperkinetic syndrome associated with difficulty in initiating arousal from sleep or maintaining wakefulness. *persistent h.* Chronic difficulty in initiating arousal from sleep or maintaining wakefulness associated with major or minor depressive mental disorders. *transient h.* Episodes of difficulty in arousing from sleep or maintaining wakefulness associated with acute or intermittent emotional reactions or conflicts.

hypermobility syndrome Movement of the joints beyond the normal range of motion.

G-I

hypernatremia Excessive amounts of sodium in the blood.

hyperosmolality Excessive electrolytes in the blood.

hyperostosis Abnormal overgrowth of bone.

hyperparathyroidism Abnormally high secretion of parathyroid hormones inducing hypercalcemia causing bone deterioration, reduced renal function, and kidney stones. Hyperparathyroidism may be primary, secondary, or tertiary and is coded respectively. The primary form is caused by a disorder of the glands that causes them to become overactive, 80 percent of the time due to a benign tumor or adenoma of the glands. The secondary form is caused by an increase in parathyroid hormone in response to another disease process, such as osteomalacia, vitamin D deficiency or malabsorption, or renal disease. The tertiary form is an adenomatous parathyroid gland developed from the secondary form due to renal impairment. These are reported with ICD-9-CM codes 252.01-252.08, with the secondary form due to renal causes reported in the genitourinary chapter, ICD-9-CM code 588.81.

hyperperfusion syndrome Potentially fatal, delayed, postoperative carotid endarterectomy complication occurring in approximately 0 to 3 percent of patients and characterized by throbbing headache, transient focal seizures, and intracerebral hemorrhage. Report this syndrome with ICD-9-CM code 997.01.

hyperphoria Upward deviation tendency occurring only when the eye is covered.

hyperplasia Abnormal proliferation in the number of normal cells in regular tissue arrangement.

hyperplasia of appendix Increase in the size and number of cells in the appendix.

HyperRAB Brand name rabies immune globulin provided in 2 ml and 10 ml vials. HyperRAB is administered to patients exposed to rabies. Supply of HyperRAB is reported with CPT codes 90375 and 90376; administration is reported separately. The need for treatment is reported with ICD-9-CM code V01.5.

hypersomnia Disorder identified by the need for excessive sleep.

hypersomnia-bulimia syndrome Hypersomnia associated with bulimia and occurring in males between 10 to 25 years of age. Ravenous appetite is followed by prolonged sleep, along with behavioral disturbances, impaired thought processes, and hallucinations. Report this disorder with ICD-9-CM code 349.89. *Synonym(s): Kleine-Levin syndrome, Parry-Romberg syndrome.*

Hyperstat IV See diazoxide.

hypersympathetic syndrome Pain and stiffness in the shoulder and swelling and pain in the hand following heart attack. Report this disorder with ICD-9-CM code

337.9. *Synonym(s): Claude Bernard-Homer syndrome, Reilly's syndrome, Steinbrocker's syndrome.*

HyperTED Brand name tetanus immune globulin provided in single-dose syringe for prophylaxis in cases where a patient has been exposed to tetanus. Supply of HyperTED is reported with HCPCS Level II code J1670 or CPT code 90389. Administration is reported separately.

hypertelorism Abnormally increased distance between the eyes reported as a congenital anomaly, ICD-9-CM code 756.0, except when it is specified as orbital, resulting from excessive spacing between the orbits in the skull, associated with disorders resulting in congenital craniofacial deformities and sometimes mental deficiency. In the latter case, it is coded to 376.41.

hypertension Abnormally increased pressure, usually referring to arterial pressure, exceeding an acceptable range.

Hyper-Tet See tetanus immune globulin.

hyperthermia Body temperature rising above 99 degrees Fahrenheit. This elevated temperature can be the result of illness or artificially created as a therapy. *NCD Reference: 110.1.*

hyperthyroidism Condition caused by the production of excessive quantities of thyroid hormones resulting in fibrillations, nervousness, weight loss, heat intolerance, excessive sweating, and weakness. This may stem from a goiter, malfunctioning thyroid gland, or the ingestion of a high dose of thyroid hormones in medication form or from iodine as a dietary supplement or contrast medium. Hyperparathyroidism is coded according to its cause in ICD-9-CM rubric 242. *Synonym(s): thyrotoxicosis.*

hypertonicity Excessive muscle tone and augmented resistance to normal muscle stretching.

hypertrophic Enlarged or overgrown from an increase in cell size of the affected tissue.

hypertrophy Overgrowth or enlargement of normal cells in tissue.

hypertrophy of breast Overgrowth of normal breast tissue.

hypertrophy of labia Overgrowth of the fleshy folds on either side of the vagina.

hypertrophy of nasal turbinates Overgrowth of bones within the nasal cavities.

hypertropia Misalignment of the eye when one eye turns upward or one eye is higher.

hyperviscosity syndrome Increase in macroglobulins in the blood, hyperviscosity, weakness, fatigue, bleeding disorders, and visual disturbances. Report this disorder with ICD-9-CM code 273.3.

G-I

hyphema Pooled blood in the anterior segment of the eye.

hypo Hypodermic injection.

hypo- Below, less than, under.

hypocalcemia Abnormally low levels of calcium in the blood, resulting in symptoms such as hyperactive deep tendon reflexes, muscle and abdominal cramping, and carpopedal spasm. This may be associated with diseases such as sepsis, pancreatitis, and acute renal failure. Hypocalcemia is reported with ICD-9-CM code 275.41.

hypochondriasis Excessive concern with one's health in general or the integrity and functioning of some part of one's body or, less frequently, one's mind. Usually associated with anxiety and depression.

hypoeosinophilia Reduced number of eosinophils (nucleated, granular leukocytes) in the blood. Report this condition with ICD-9-CM code 288.00. **Synonym(s):** *eosinopenia.*

hypoglycemia Abnormally low blood glucose level. Excessive insulin produced by the pancreas, sometimes associated with tumors, or an overdose of insulin to treat diabetes may be a cause. Hypoglycemia in a diabetic patient is reported with ICD-9-CM subcategory code 249.8 or 250.8. Hypoglycemia that is not occurring in a patient with diabetes mellitus is reported with 251.1. ***h. coma*** Loss of consciousness due to low blood sugar in a nondiabetic patient, commonly a blood sugar of less than 40 mg/dl as an iatrogenic reaction to treatment, reported with a code from ICD-9-CM subcategory 251.0. **Synonym(s):** *iatrogenic hyperinsulinism, non-diabetic insulin coma.* ***h. syndrome*** Hypoglycemia described as unspecified. Report this disorder with ICD-9-CM code 251.2. **Synonym(s):** *idiopathic familial hypoglycemia.*

hypomania Manic-depressive psychosis, circular type, in which the manic form is currently present.

hypomanic personality Affective personality disorder characterized by lifelong predominance of a chronic, nonpsychotic disturbance involving either intermittent or sustained periods of abnormally elevated mood (unshakable optimism and an enhanced zest for life and activity).

hyponatremia Decreased, deficient levels of sodium in the blood, reported with ICD-9-CM code 276.1.

hypoparathyroidism Abnormally low secretion of parathyroid hormones causing decreased levels of calcium and increased levels of phosphorus in the blood, muscle cramping, increased frequency of urination, and cataracts. This condition is reported with ICD-9-CM code 252.1.

hypoperfusion syndrome Respiratory distress in premature neonates associated with reduced amounts of lung surfactant. Frequently fatal. Report this disorder

with ICD-9-CM code 769. **Synonym(s):** *hyaline membrane syndrome.*

hypophyseal syndrome Relating to the pituitary. Report this disorder with ICD-9-CM code 253.8.

hypophysectomy Destruction of the pituitary gland.

hypophyseothalamic syndrome Relating to the pituitary and thalamus. Report this disorder with ICD-9-CM code 253.8.

hypopigmentation Abnormally diminished coloration.

hypopituitarism syndrome Decreasing production of pituitary hormones caused by lessening activity of the anterior lobe of the hypophysis. Report this disorder with ICD-9-CM code 253.2.

hypoplasia Condition in which there is underdevelopment of an organ or tissue.

hypoplastic left heart syndrome Hypoplasia or atresia of the left ventricle and aorta or mitral valve with respiratory distress and extreme cyanosis. Cardiac failure and death often result in early infancy. Report this disorder with ICD-9-CM code 746.7.

hypopnea Abnormal respiratory event lasting at least 10 seconds, with at least a 30 percent reduction in thoracoabdominal movement or airflow as compared to a baseline, and with at least a 4 percent oxygen desaturation.

hypopyon Accumulation of pus in the anterior chamber of the eye.

hyposmolality Deficiency of electrolytes in the blood.

hyposomnia Disorder of initiating or maintaining sleep.

Hypospadias

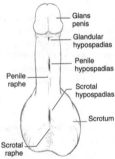

- Glans penis
- Glandular hypospadias
- Penile hypospadias
- Scrotal hypospadias
- Scrotum
- Penile raphe
- Scrotal raphe

Ventral View

hypospadias Fairly common birth defect in males in which the meatus, or urinary opening, is abnormally positioned on the underside of the penile shaft or in the perineum, requiring early surgical correction. Male hypospadias is reported with ICD-9-CM code 752.61. The equivalent defect in females is rare and consists of an opening of the urethra into the vagina. Female hypospadias is reported with ICD-9-CM code 753.8. Male repair reported with 54300-54352.

hypostasis Poor or insufficient circulation in a body part or organ resulting in vascular congestion within the area.

hypotension Decrease in blood pressure to below normal.

hypotensive anesthesia Anesthesia procedure in which the blood pressure is deliberately lowered to decrease blood loss during surgery. Use CPT add-on code 99135 with the appropriate anesthesia code.

hypothermia Therapeutic lack of heat or decrease in body temperature. *NCD Reference: 110.6.*

hypothermia with cardiac bypass Reduction of the body temperature using a bypass system to reduce the oxygen demands of tissue and to protect the myocardium during a procedure.

hypothermic anesthesia Anesthesia procedure that lowers the total body temperature during surgery. Use CPT add-on code 99116 with the appropriate anesthesia code.

hypothyroidism Underproduction of thyroid hormone causing a slow metabolic rate, fatigue, and lethargy. Hypothyroidism may result from surgical ablation of the gland, radiotherapy, iodine administration, or other iatrogenic cause, or from secondary reasons and is reported according to cause in ICD-9-CM rubric 244. When there is an underproduction of thyroid hormones from birth, it is reported with ICD-9-CM code 243.

hypotonia Diminished muscle tone and stretching resistance.

hypotonia-hypomentia-hypogonadism-obesity syndrome Rounded face, almond-shaped eyes, strabismus, low forehead, hypogonadism, hypotomia, mental retardation, and an insatiable appetite. Report this disorder with ICD-9-CM code 759.81. *Synonym(s): Prader-Willi syndrome.*

hypotrichosis of eyelid Less than normal or absent eyelashes.

hypovolemia Abnormal decrease in the total volume of blood circulating in the body. Hypovolemia differs from dehydration in that dehydration describes a reduction in total body waters without a reduction in body salts, while hypovolemia describes a decrease in the volume of blood. Report hypovolemia with ICD-9-CM code 276.52.

hypoxemia Inadequate oxygen in the blood.

hypoxia Organ or tissue receiving an oxygen supply that is below the necessary oxygen levels, even when there is adequate blood perfusion.

hyster(o)- Relating to either the womb or hysteria.

hysterectomy Surgical removal of the uterus. A complete hysterectomy may also include removal of tubes and ovaries.

hysteria Restrictions of the field of consciousness or disturbances of motor or sensory function that result in psychological advantage or have symbolic value. This is more commonly known as conversion disorder or dissociative disorder.

hysteria anxiety Neurotic states with abnormally intense dread of certain objects or specific situations that would not normally affect the patient.

hysteria psychosis Psychotic condition that is largely or entirely attributable to a recent life experience.

hysteria psychosis acute Affective psychosis with symptoms similar to manic-depressive psychosis, manic type, but apparently provoked by emotional stress.

hysterical personality Personality disorder characterized by shallow, labile affectivity, dependence on others, craving for appreciation and attention, suggestibility, and theatricality. There may be sexual immaturity and, under stress, hysterical symptoms (neurosis) may develop.

hysterosalpingography Radiographic pictures taken of the uterus and the fallopian tubes after the injection of a radiopaque dye.

Hysteroscopy

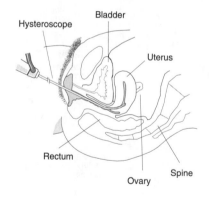

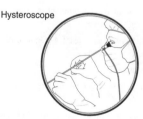

hysteroscopy Visualization and inspection of the uterus using a fiberoptic endoscope inserted through the vagina and cervical os into the uterine cavity. This may be done for diagnostic purposes alone or included with therapeutic procedures performed at the same time.

Hyzine-50 See hydroxyzine.

HZ HCPCS Level II modifier, for use with CPT or HCPCS Level II codes, that identifies services or supplies that are funded by a criminal justice agency. May be required for a state Medicaid program.

I&D Incision and drainage.

I&O Intake and output.

I-131 Iodine 131.

IA Intra-arterial.

-ia State of being, condition (abnormal).

IAB Intra-aortic balloon.

IABC Intra-aortic balloon counterpulsation.

IABP

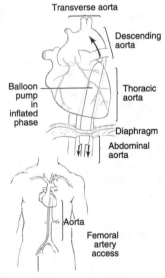

IABP is the acronym for intraaortic balloon pump

Transverse aorta

Descending aorta

Balloon pump in inflated phase

Thoracic aorta

Diaphragm

Abdominal aorta

Aorta

Femoral artery access

IABP Intra-aortic balloon pump or intra-arterial blood pressure.

IAIABC International Association of Industrial Accident Boards and Commissions.

-iasis Condition.

iatrogenic Adversely induced in the patient; caused by medical treatment.

iatrogenic pneumothorax Air trapped in the lining of the lung following surgery.

IBI Therapy Brand name device for cardiac ablation.

IBM Inclusion body myositis.

IBNR Incurred but not reported. Amount of money the payer's plan accrues to forestall unknown medical expenses.

IBS Irritable bowel syndrome.

ibutilide fumarate Cardiac antiarrhythmic given intravenously that works by slowing repolarizing the atria and ventricles, used to convert atrial fibrillation or flutter to normal rhythm. Supply is reported with HCPCS Level II code J1742. May be sold under the brand name Corvert.

IBW Ideal body weight.

IC Infant care.

ICAT Indirect Coomb's test.

ICBG

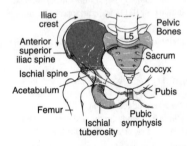

Iliac crest

Pelvic Bones

Anterior superior iliac spine

L5

Sacrum

Ischial spine

Coccyx

Acetabulum

Pubis

Femur

Ischial tuberosity

Pubic symphysis

ICBG is the acronym for iliac crest bone graft

ICBG is an autologous graft.
A piece of the iliac crest is removed

ICBG Iliac crest bone graft. Autologous donor graft common to reconstructive orthopedic surgery.

ICCE Intracapsular cataract extraction.

ICD *1)* Implantable cardioverter defibrillator. *2)* International Classification of Disease. Medical code set maintained by the World Health Organization (WHO). The primary purpose of ICD was to classify causes of death. *ICD-9-CM* International Classification of Diseases, Ninth Edition, Clinical Modification. Clinical modification of the international statistical coding system used to report, compile, and compare health care data, using numeric and alphanumeric codes to help plan, deliver, reimburse, and quantify medical care in the United States. Volumes 1 and 2 are a modification of the World Health Organization's ICD-9. Volume 3 was created in the United States and reports inpatient procedures and services. *ICD-10-CM* International Classification of Diseases, Tenth Edition, Clinical Modification. Diagnostic coding system developed to replace ICD-9-CM in the

United States. It is a clinical modification of the World Health Organization's ICD-10, already in use in much of the world, and used for mortality reporting in the United States. The implementation date for ICD-10-CM has not yet been set. **ICD-10-PCS** International Classification of Diseases, Tenth Edition, Procedural Coding System. Procedure coding system developed by 3M HIS under contract with CMS. This system is expected to replace ICD-9-CM Volume 3 for inpatient procedure reporting in the United States. The implementation date for ICD-10-PCS has not yet been set. **ICD-O** International Classification of Diseases, Oncology. First published in 1976, ICD-O provides a classification system for the morphology of neoplasms. The codes consist of five digits. The first four identify the histology of the neoplasm and the fifth identifies the neoplasm as benign, uncertain, carcinoma in situ, primary malignant, secondary malignant, or unknown whether primary or secondary. Abstracting ICD-O codes is a responsibility usually assigned to the cancer registry at facilities and some ambulatory care centers. *Synonym(s): morphology of neoplasms.*

ICD-10 International Classification of Diseases, Tenth Revision. Classification of diseases by alphanumeric code, used by the World Health Organization.

ICD-10-CM International Classification of Diseases, Tenth Edition, Clinical Modification. Diagnostic coding system developed to replace ICD-9-CM in the United States. It is a clinical modification of the World Health Organization's ICD-10, already in use in much of the world, and used for mortality reporting in the United States. The implementation date for ICD-10-CM is October 1, 2013.

ICD-10-PCS International Classification of Diseases, Tenth Revision, Procedure Coding System. Effective October 1, 2013, inpatient hospital services and surgical procedures must be coded using ICD-10-PCS. This code set will replace the current ICD-9-CM, Volume 3 for procedures.

ICD-9 Volume 3 was created in the United States and reports inpatient procedures and services.

ICD-9-CM International Classification of Diseases, Ninth Edition, Clinical Modification. Clinical modification of the international statistical coding system used to report, compile, and compare health care data, using numeric and alphanumeric (E codes and V codes) codes to help plan, deliver, reimburse, and quantify medical care in the United States.

ICE syndrome Iridocorneal endothelial syndrome. Primary proliferative endothelial degeneration as seen in progressive iris atrophy, Chandler syndrome, and Cogan-Reese syndrome. The iris is pulled in the direction of a peripheral anterior synechia. According to official coding guidelines, code selection is based upon presenting symptoms.

ICF *1)* International Classification of Functioning, Disability, and Health. World Health Organization coding system for reporting an individual's capacity to cope in situations that are the consequence of disease. The classification identifies functional limits set by the severity of the disease, without identifying the disease itself. Code examples include d550, to report the ability to open bottles and cans, use eating implements, and consume meals in a culturally accepted way; or the ability to walk, reported for different distances with codes in the d450 category of ICF. The United States has not adopted ICF for use. However, it is under investigation at the National Center for Health Statistics as a reporting mechanism for the future. *2)* Intermediate care facility. Health care facility that furnishes services to patients who do not require the degree of care provided by a hospital or skilled nursing facility or a step-down facility for patients who are leaving the hospital but who cannot be discharged to home because of continuing medical needs.

ICF syndrome Intravascular coagulation-fibrinolysis. Decrease of elements needed for coagulation of blood and profuse bleeding. Report this disorder with ICD-9-CM code 286.6.

ICH Intracranial/cerebral hemorrhage.

ICHI International Classification of Health Interventions. Basic coding system developed in Australia and distributed by the World Health Organization to other countries to report interventions and procedures for data collection purposes. It contains about 1,600 codes.

ICHT Intermittent combined hormone therapy or intracellular hyperthermia therapy.

ichthyosis congenita Congenital condition in which an excessive production of skin cells results in red, dry, scaly skin, reported with ICD-9-CM code 757.1.

ICM Implantable cardiovascular monitor.

ICN Internal control number. Unique, 15-digit identifying number the Medicare carrier assigns to every claim for control and inventory purposes that indicates the claim type, region, year, Julian date, batch number, and sequence.

ICP Intracranial pressure. *NCD Reference: 160.14.*

ICRS Intrastromal corneal ring segments. Rings implanted in the cornea to correct mild myopia. ICRS has also been approved to correct keratoconus, a corneal disease that causes distorted vision. The implant procedure is reported with CPT code 0099T.

ICS Intercostal space.

ICSH Interstitial cell stimulating hormone.

G-I

ICSI Intracytoplasmic sperm injection. Single spermatozoa injected into a mature egg in a laboratory using high-powered microscopy in order to achieve fertilization

icterus Increased bilirubin and accumulation of bile pigment in the skin and sclera, causing a yellow tint. This symptom is reported with ICD-9-CM code 782.4. *Synonym(s): jaundice.*

ICU Intensive care unit.

ID Infective dose.

ID card Wallet card carried by a plan member providing name, member and group numbers, effective dates, deductibles, and other information.

Id31 Radioactive iodine.

Idamycin See idarubicin HCl.

Idarubicin HCl Antibiotic that works as an antineoplastic, successfully treating a variety of leukemia and lymphoma conditions by having an inhibitory effect on DNA synthesis. Supply is reported with HCPCS Level II code J9211. May be sold under the brand names Idamycin, Idamycin PFS.

IDDM Insulin dependent diabetes mellitus. Diabetes requiring treatment with insulin injections to sustain the patient. Although IDDM is most often associated with type I diabetes, a severe form of diabetes in which the body manufactures no insulin, patients with type II diabetes may also be insulin dependent. Coding diabetes as type I or type II is determined by the level of function of the pancreatic cells and is not dependent on the patient's status as insulin dependent or non-insulin dependent. This terminology has been removed from the code set. Do not code diabetes based on the information of insulin dependence.

IDE Investigational device exemption. Status from the Food and Drug Administration allowing a company to sell or distribute devices for investigational purposes and clinical trials.

identification Recognition of body part or tissue.

identity disorder Emotional disorder caused by distress over the inability to reconcile aspects of the self into a relatively coherent and acceptable sense of self, not secondary to another mental disorder. May be manifested by intense subjective distress regarding uncertainty about various issues relating to identity, including long-term goals, career choice, friendship patterns, values, and loyalties.

IDET Intradiscal electrothermal therapy. A thin heating wire is threaded through a hollow needle into a painful disc, and heat is applied around the edge of the nucleus to close tears, shrink fibers, and cauterize nerve endings. This procedure may also be documented as intradiscal

electrothermal annuloplasty. Report IDET with CPT codes 22526 and 22527.

IDH Isocitric dehydrogenase.

idio- Distinct or individual characteristics.

idiopathic Having no known cause.

idiopathic cysts Fluid-filled sacs of the iris or ciliary body of unknown cause.

idiopathic nephrotic syndrome Affects the kidneys of a child with unknown cause. Report this disorder with ICD-9-CM code 581.9.

idiosyncratic alcohol intoxication Acute psychotic episodes induced by relatively small amounts of alcohol. These are regarded as individual idiosyncratic reactions to alcohol, not due to excessive consumption and without conspicuous neurological signs of intoxication.

idiot Individual with an IQ of less than 20 who have minimal capacity for sensorimotor functioning and need nursing care during the preschool period. May develop some further motor skills and may respond to minimal or limited training in self-help. During the adult years some motor and speech development may occur, and the individual may achieve very limited self-care and need nursing care.

IDK Internal derangement of the knee.

IDM Infant of diabetic mother. IDM syndrome is seen in a newborn infant of a diabetic or gestational diabetic mother exhibiting symptoms including macrosomia, hypoglycemia, and endocrine disturbances, and is reported with ICD-9-CM code 775.0. It is not necessary for the physician to document that these symptoms are due to the syndrome. If a normal infant is born to a diabetic mother but exhibits no signs of IDM syndrome, 775.0 should not be reported. Instead, assign V18.0 to identify a family history of diabetes.

IDN Integrated delivery network.

idursulfase Enzyme replacement therapy administered by IV infusion and indicated for patients with Hunter syndrome or mucopolysaccharidosis II (MPSII), a rare lysosomal storage disorder that impairs the body's ability to break down mucopolysaccharides. By replacing the deficient enzyme, it assists in keeping the patient ambulatory, improving pulmonary function, and reducing organ size. Supply is reported with HCPCS Level II code J1743. *Synonym(s): Elaprase.*

Ifex See ifosfamide.

ifosfamide Antineoplastic used to treat testicular, lung, breast, ovarian, gastric, pancreatic, uterine, and cervical cancers and a variety of leukemias and lymphomas. It works by creating crosslinked bonds in the cancer DNA, which interferes with RNA transcription. Supply is reported with HCPCS Level II code J9208. May be sold under the brand name Ifex.

G-I

IG *1)* Immunoglobulin. *2)* Implementation guide.

IgE Antibody class of immune globulin that binds to receptors on basophils and mast cells and is responsible for mediating immediate hypersensitivity (allergic) reactions.

IgG Most common and abundant antibody in blood and the only one to cross the placenta and endow the fetus with protection against infection.

IGS Implantable gastric stimulator. Placement, replacement, or removal of IGS electrodes designed for weight loss. IGS is reported with a CPT Category III code from range 0155T-0158T; electrodes for other indications are reported with CPT codes 43647-43648 and 43881-43882. For insertion, revision, or removal of the pulse generator, report CPT code 64590 or 64595. For electronic analysis and programming, see CPT codes 95980-95982.

IH Infectious hepatitis.

IHC Internet Healthcare Coalition.

IHSS Idiopathic hypertrophic sub-aortic stenosis. Obstruction in the left ventricular outflow tract due to overstretching or enlargement of the ventricular septum.

IHT Intermittent hormone therapy or induced hypothermic therapy.

II Cranial nerve in the inferior cranium. The optic nerve responsible for transmitting information from the retina to the brain. 2) Icteric index.

IIHI Individually identifiable health information.

III Cranial nerve at midbrain responsible for pupillary light reflex and some ocular muscle innervation.

IL-2 See aldesleukin.

ILC Interstitial laser coagulation.

ILD Interstitial lung disease.

ileo- Relating to the ileum (part of the small intestine).

ileocolostomy Surgical anastomosis that brings the end of the ileum to the colon.

ileostomy Artificial surgical opening that brings the end of the ileum out through the abdominal wall to the skin surface for the diversion of feces through a stoma. Ileostomy procedures are reported with CPT codes 44310-44316 for open approach and 44187 for a laparoscopic approach.

ileum Lower portion of the small intestine, from the jejunum to the cecum.

ileus Persistent obstruction of the intestines coded in different chapters in ICD-9-CM based on its type or cause, location, and whether it occurs in a newborn.

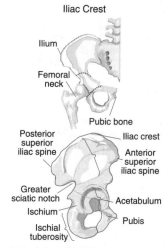

Iliac Crest

Lateral view of right hip and socket

iliac crest Edge of the iliac (hip bone).

ilio- Relating to the pelvis.

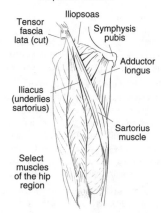

Illiopsoas Tendon

Select muscles of the hip region

iliopsoas tendon Fibrous tissue that connects muscle to bone in the pelvic region, common to the iliacus and psoas major.

ilium Part of the iliac bone. Superior part of the hip bone that expands.

illegally induced abortion Intentional termination of pregnancy that is performed outside the legal boundaries of state law or performed by someone or within a facility failing to meet qualification requirements. Illegally induced abortions are reported with an ICD-9-CM code from rubric 636, with fourth digits to indicate the presence or absence of complications and fifth digits to identify the stage of abortion (unspecified, incomplete, or complete). This category is only used for inpatient coding when a patient is admitted to the hospital to treat a complication of an illegal abortion performed outside the hospital, or to ensure that such an abortion is complete. *Synonym(s): criminal abortion, illegal abortion, self-induced abortion.*

ILP *1)* Interstitial laser photocoagulation. *2)* Isolated link perfusion.

ILR Implantable loop recorder. Cardiac monitor placed in subcutaneous tissue that continuously monitors the electrical activity of the heart and is activated by the patient using an external hand-held device to record a cardiac event as the patient experiences it happening. Electrocardiographic data of heart rates, rhythms, and events can be stored for long periods of time. *Synonym(s): patient activated cardiac event recorder.*

IM *1)* Infectious mononucleosis. *2)* Internal medicine. *3)* Intramuscular.

imaging Radiologic means of producing pictures for clinical study of the internal structures and functions of the body, such as x-ray, ultrasound, magnetic resonance, or positron emission tomography.

imatinib Antineoplastic used to treat acute or chronic blast crisis in chronic myeloid leukemia (CML); gastrointestinal stromal tumors with Kit positive (CD117) that are unresectable or metastatic in nature; and patients who are positive for the Philadelphia chromosome, status post stem cell transplant, and/or those who are resistant to interferon alpha therapy. Supply is reported with HCPCS Level II code S0088.

imbecile Individual with an IQ of 35 to 49 who can talk or learn to communicate and has fair motor development. He or she has poor social awareness and is unlikely to progress beyond the second-grade level in academic subjects. As an adult, the individual may achieve self-maintenance by performing unskilled or semi-skilled work under sheltered conditions with supervision and guidance when under mild social or economic stress.

imbricate Process of building a surface of overlapping layers of apposing material, such as tissue, for closing a wound or other opening in a body part.

imbrication Overlapping of tissues during closure.

IMC *1)* In my care. *2)* Intermediate care.

IME *1)* Independent medical evaluation. Examination carried out by an impartial health care provider, generally board certified, to resolve a dispute related to the nature and extent of an illness or injury. *2)* Indirect medical evaluation.

imiglucerase Analogue of the human enzyme beta-glucocerebrosidase produced by recombinant DNA therapy, and used for long-term enzyme replacement

therapy in type 1 Gaucher disease. Supply is reported with HCPCS Level II code J1786.

imipenem cilastatin sodium Broad spectrum beta-lactam antibiotic used for lower respiratory tract, skin, intra-abdominal, and gynecologic infections. Supply is reported with HCPCS Level II code J0743. May be sold under the brand name Primaxin.

Imitrex Neurological agent used to treat acute migraine attacks or cluster headaches. Supply is reported with HCPCS Level II code J3030. Imitrex contains sumatriptan succinate.

immediate denture Denture intended for placement immediately following removal of the remaining natural teeth.

immediate maternity Coverage provided for pregnancies that began prior to the date the member became insured.

immobility syndrome Paralysis of legs and lower part of body. Report this disorder with ICD-9-CM code 728.3.

immobilization To prevent the body or a body part from being capable of moving by holding it stable manually or with splints, casts, or strapping.

immobilizer Device used to restrain a part of the body, keeping the body part from moving.

immune globulin Serum immunoglobulins, glycoproteins that function as antibodies, are injected to provide passive immunity by increasing the amount of circulating antibodies. It is used to help prevent infections in patients exposed to certain pathogens and to boost immune systems in patients who suffer primary humoral immunodeficiency. Correct code assignment is dependent upon dosage. May be sold under the brand names Flebogamma, Gammagard, Gamunex, Hepagam B, Octagam, Privigen, and Vivaglobin.

immunoadsorption Chemical separation or removal of an antibody or antigen from a substance by using a homologous antigen or antibody to bind it respectively and then remove the specific antigen-antibody complex after aggregation has occurred.

immunoassay Method that uses binding between an antigen and antibody for determination of the presence of certain chemical substances. *NCD References: 190.28, 190.29, 190.30.*

immunologic deficiency syndrome Inherited immune deficiencies characterized by insufficient antibodies. Report this disorder with ICD-9-CM code 279.00. *Synonym(s): antibody deficiency.*

immunotherapy Therapeutic use of serum or gamma globulin.

IMO Integrated multiple option.

Imogam Rabies-HT Brand name, heat treated rabies immune globulin provided in 2 ml and 10 ml vials. Imogam Rabies-HT is administered to patients who have

G-I

been exposed to rabies. Supply of Imogam Rabies-HT is reported with CPT code 90376; administration is reported with 96372. The need for treatment is reported with ICD-9-CM code V01.5.

Imovax Brand name rabies vaccine provided in a single-dose vial. Imovax is administered to people who are at risk to being exposed to rabies, but have not been exposed. Supply of Imovax is reported with CPT code 90675 and administration is reported with 90471. The need for immunization is reported with ICD-9-CM code V04.5.

impacted tooth Tooth that is partially or totally unerupted that is unlikely to completely erupt because of its position to adjoining structures.

impaction State of being tightly wedged or lodged into or between something.

imperforate hymen Congenital condition in which the hymen completely covers the vaginal orifice, blocking the flow of menstrual blood. This condition requires surgery to remove the excess hymenal tissue and create a vaginal opening of normal size. Imperforate hymen is reported with ICD-9-CM code 752.42.

Implanon Brand name contraceptive implant consisting of a single rod that is inserted subcutaneously in the inner upper arm, where it slowly releases the hormone etonogestrel. Supply of the implant system is reported with HCPCS Level II code J7307. *Synonym(s): etonogestrel.*

implant Material or device inserted or placed within the body for therapeutic, reconstructive, or diagnostic purposes.

implantable cardiovascular monitor Implantable electronic device that stores cardiovascular physiologic data such as intracardiac pressure waveforms collected from internal sensors or data such as weight and blood pressure collected from external sensors. The information stored in these devices is used as an aid in managing patients with heart failure and other cardiac conditions that are non-rhythm related. The data may be transmitted via local telemetry or remotely to a surveillance technician or an internet-based file server. *Synonym(s): ICM.*

implantable cardioverter-defibrillator Implantable electronic cardiac device used to control rhythm abnormalities such as tachycardia, fibrillation, or bradycardia by producing high- or low-energy stimulation and pacemaker functions. It may also have the capability to provide the functions of an implantable loop recorder or implantable cardiovascular monitor. *Synonym(s): ICD.*

implantable loop recorder Implantable electronic cardiac device that constantly monitors and records electrocardiographic rhythm. It may be triggered by the patient when a symptomatic episode occurs or activated automatically by rapid or slow heart rates. This may be the sole purpose of the device or it may be a component of another cardiac device such as a pacemaker or implantable cardioverter-defibrillator. The data can be transmitted via local telemetry or remotely to a surveillance technician or an internet-based file server. *Synonym(s): ILR.*

implantable venous access device Catheter implanted for continuous access to the venous system for long-term parenteral feeding or for the administration of fluids or medications.

implantation cysts Defects caused by abnormal growth of epithelium following injury or surgery. *Synonym(s): epithelial downgrowth.*

implementation guide Document explaining the proper use of a standard for a specific business purpose. The X12N HIPAA IGs are the primary reference documents used by those implementing the associated transactions, and are incorporated into the HIPAA regulations by reference.

implementation specification Under HIPAA, specific instructions for implementing a standard.

impotence Psychosexual or organic dysfunction in which there is partial or complete failure to attain or maintain erection until completion of the sexual act. *NCD Reference: 230.4.*

impression Mold of a body part to be used as a pattern in making a replacement part, prosthesis, or stabilizing device for that area of the body.

impulse control disorder Great internal tension resulting from an impulse, drive, or temptation to perform some action that is harmful to the individual or to others. The action may provide short-term pleasure, gratification, or release but may be followed by regret, self-reproach, or guilt; can take the form of intermittent explosive disorder, isolated explosive disorder, kleptomania, pathological gambling, and pyromania.

IMRT Intensity modulated radiation therapy. External beam radiation therapy delivery using computer planning to specify the target dose and to modulate the radiation intensity, usually as a treatment for a malignancy. The delivery system approaches the patient from multiple angles, minimizing damage to normal tissue. The plan for IMRT is reported with CPT code 77301; the treatment itself is reported with 77418. Design and construction of multi-leaf collimator (MLC) devices for IMRT is reported with 77338. Compensator-based IMRT is reported with 0073T.

IMT Intima-media thickness. Measurement, for example, of the common carotid artery, the results of which may be an indicator of coronary artery disease. IMT testing is reported with CPT code 0126T.

Imuran See azathioprine.

G-I

IMV Intermittent mandatory ventilation.

in Inch.

in plan Services chosen from a network provider.

in situ Located in the natural position or contained within the origin site, not spread into neighboring tissue.

inadequate personality Personality disorder characterized by passive compliance with the wishes of elders and others and a weak, inadequate response to the demands of daily life. The individual may be intellectual or emotional with little capacity for enjoyment.

inappropriate secretion of antidiuretic hormone syndrome Low or normal blood pressure, no edema, and retarded growth found in children with hypokalemic alkalosis and elevated renin or angiotensin levels. Report this disorder with ICD-9-CM code 253.6. **Synonym(s):** *Schwartz-Bartter syndrome.*

Inapsine See droperidol.

inc. Incision.

inch Length measurement equal to 2.54 centimeters.

incident to Provision of a service concurrently with another service. For example, additional covered supplies and materials that are furnished after surgery typically are billed as "incident to" a physician's services and not as hospital services. This term is used specifically for revenue codes for pharmacy, supplies, and anesthesia furnished along with radiology and other diagnostic services.

incisal Biting edge of an incisor or a cuspid tooth.

incise To cut open or into.

incision Act of cutting into tissue or an organ.

incision and drainage Cutting open body tissue for the removal of tissue fluids or infected discharge from a wound or cavity. Incision and drainage of specified lesions or wounds is reported in the Integumentary chapter of CPT. **Synonym(s):** *I & D.*

inclusion body myositis Muscle disease characterized by chronic muscle inflammation and a gradual onset of muscle weakness. Both the proximal and distal muscles are affected, and the first obvious symptoms may be falling and tripping or, for some individuals, weakness in the fingers and wrists causing difficulty with buttoning, gripping, or pinching. Loss of muscle bulk (atrophy) in the muscles of the forearm or quadriceps muscles in the legs may be present. There is currently no cure and no standard course of treatment. Report inclusion body myositis with ICD-9-CM code 359.71. **Synonym(s):** *IBM.*

incompetence Inability of a valve or structure to perform its normal function.

incompetence Inability to perform normal functions.

incompetent cervix Narrow end of the uterus opening into the birth canal that abnormally dilates during the second trimester of the pregnancy and can lead to a miscarriage or premature delivery. This condition is reported with a code from ICD-9-CM subcategory 654.5.

incontestable clause Provision in a policy that prohibits the plan from disputing coverage for certain conditions after a specified period of time.

incontinence Inability to control urination or defecation. **NCD References:** *30.1.1, 230.10, 230.15, 230.18.*

incorrect code Reporting any code that does not accurately reflect the services documented.

incremental nursing charge Nursing care service charge that is assessed in addition to the room and board charge.

incubation Culture cultivation under controlled conditions.

incurred but not reported Amount of money the payer's plan accrues to forestall unknown medical expenses. **Synonym(s):** *IBNR.*

incus Second ossicle (bone) of the middle ear. **Synonym(s):** *anvil.*

IND Investigation of new drug.

indefinite delivery indefinite quantity Type of program safeguard contract that provides for program integrity and data analysis activities as defined in specific task orders. A program safeguard contractor (PSC) can perform one, some, all, or any subset of the work associated with the following payment safeguard functions: medical review, cost report audit, data analysis, provider education, and fraud detection and prevention. **Synonym(s):** *IDIQ.*

indemnification Type of hold-harmless clause that requires the responsible party in a liability claim to compensate the second party should the responsible party's actions result in liability to the second party.

indep Independent.

independent contractor Individual who performs full- or part-time work for which an IRS 1099 form is required.

independent medical evaluation Examination carried out by an impartial health care provider, generally board certified, to resolve a dispute related to the nature and extent of an illness or injury. **Synonym(s):** *IME.*

Indermil Brand name tissue adhesive. Use of tissue adhesive is usually bundled into the primary procedure. For Medicare claims, report HCPCS Level II code G0168 for wound closure as a primary procedure when tissue adhesive is the means of closure.

indexing Listing diseases and conditions according to classification system.

G-I

Indian tick fever Tick-borne rickettsioses caused by R. conorii found predominantly in the Mediterranean and India. Symptoms include rash, elevated temperature, headache, myalgia, and joint pain. This condition is reported with ICD-9-CM code 082.1. *Synonym(s): Marseilles fever, Mediterranean fever.*

Indian tick typhus Acute, febrile, rickettsial disease transmitted by tick bites and causing a primary lesion at the site of the bite, with rash, muscle and joint pain, headache, chills, fever, and sensitivity to light. It is commonly found in the Mediterranean and around the Black and Caspian Seas, having many names depending on the geographical region. This condition is reported with ICD-9-CM code 082.1. *Synonym(s): African tickbite fever, Boutonneuse fever, Kenya tick typhus, Marseilles fever, Mediterranean tick fever.*

indirect costs Practice costs not directly associated with the physician service being provided. Examples include general office supplies, rent, utilities, and other office overhead.

indirect laryngoscopy Viewing the larynx through a reflection in a strategically placed mirror as opposed to directly viewing it through the scope, reported with CPT codes 31505-31513.

indirect pulp cap In dentistry, insertion of a protective dressing to cover nearly exposed pulp.

indirect restoration In dentistry, restoration produced outside of the mouth.

indirect treatment relationship Relationship between an individual and a health care provider in which the health care provider delivers health care to the individual based on the orders of another health care provider.

individual practice association Organization made up of providers who, along with the rest of a group, contract with payers at a discounted fee-for-service or capitated rate. *Synonym(s): IPA.*

individual practice organization Organization made up of providers who, along with the rest of a group, contract with payers at a discounted fee-for-service or capitated rate. *Synonym(s): IPO.*

individually identifiable health information Information that is created or received by a health care provider, health plan, or health care clearinghouse that relates to an individual's physical or mental health, health care treatment, or payment for that treatment.

induced by drug syndrome Description of symptoms, physiological and psychological, produced by drug abuse or dependence. Report this disorder with ICD-9-CM code 292.11.

induced paranoid disorder Mainly delusional psychosis, usually chronic and often without florid features, that appears to have developed as a result of a close, if not dependent, relationship with another person who already has an established similar psychosis. *Synonym(s): folie a deux.*

inebriety State of inebriation due to alcohol consumption without conspicuous neurological signs of intoxication.

INF *1)* Inferior. *2)* Infusion.

Infanrix Brand name pediatric diphtheria, tetanus, acellular pertussis vaccine provided in a single-dose vial or syringe. Supply of Infanrix is reported with CPT code 90700; administration is reported separately. The need for vaccination is reported with ICD-9-CM code V06.1.

infant drug withdrawal of dependent mother syndrome Number of physical symptoms suffered by newborns whose drug-dependent mothers allowed drugs to cross the placenta. Report this disorder with ICD-9-CM code 779.5.

infantile autism Syndrome beginning in the first 30 months affecting interaction with others, characterized by abnormal response to auditory and visual stimuli accompanied by difficulty understanding spoken language and limiting the ability to communicate or develop social skills.

infantile nutritional atrophy Nutritional marasmus seen in children with severe calorie deficiency or malnutrition, characterized by hypoalbuminemia, tissue wasting, dehydration, and subcutaneous fat depletion. Report this condition with ICD-9-CM code 261.

infantilism syndrome Profound retardation of mental and physical development Report this disorder with ICD-9-CM code 253.3.

infarction Area of necrosis in tissue, due to ischemia from lack of circulation, usually from a thrombus or an embolus.

In-Fast Ultra Sling Brand name urethral sling for treatment of female stress incontinence and cystocele. The sling is inserted using a vaginal approach. Placement is reported with CPT code 57288.

infected postoperative seroma Infection within a tumor-like growth of serum following surgery.

infection Presence of microorganisms in body tissues that may result in cellular damage.

Infed See iron dextran.

Infergen See interferon.

inferior alveolar nerve Nerve that enters the mandible via the mandibular foramen and passes along the mandibular canal until it exits through the mental foramen and innervates the teeth of the mandible.

inferior vena cava syndrome Obstruction of the vena cava. Report this disorder with ICD-9-CM code 459.2.

infertility Inability or decreased ability to produce offspring. *female i.* Inability to conceive for at least one

G-I

year after regular intercourse in the absence of contraceptive measures. Infertility may be classified as primary, occurring in patients who have never conceived, or secondary, occurring in patients who have previously conceived. There are three basic types of infertility: functional, anatomic, and psychogenic. Functional infertility is due to impairment in hormonal interactions. Anatomic infertility can be the result of congenital malformation, scarring, or adhesions due to previous infection, atrophy, or surgery. Psychogenic infertility is caused by the effects of mental or emotional states on the body's functioning, such as a failure to ovulate due to stressors. Female infertility is reported with a code from ICD-9-CM category 628. **male i.** Inadequate amount of sperm production or an abnormality in the structure or motility of the sperm that makes it unable to reach or penetrate the egg. Contributing factors may include varicose veins in the spermatic cord, undescended testicles, radiation, chemotherapy, removal of one or both testicles, hypothalamic or pituitary disorder, or drug use. Male infertility is reported with a code from category 606.

INFH Ischemic necrosis of femoral head.

infibulation Total removal of the external female genitalia, including the clitoris, labia minora, and most or all of the labia majora. Both sides of the vulva are then sutured, eliminating the vaginal introitus except for a small opening to allow the passage of urine or menstrual blood. This procedure has often been practiced as a culturally determined ritual in other countries. The status of having undergone infibulation is reported as type III female genital mutilation with ICD-9-CM code 629.23.

inflammation Cytologic and chemical reactions that occur in affected blood vessels and adjacent tissues in response to injury or abnormal stimulation from a physical, chemical, or biologic agent.

inflammatory Pertaining to, characterized by, causing, or resulting from or affected by inflammation.

infliximab Antirheumatic drug used with methotrexate to prevent joint damage from rheumatoid arthritis. It is also used to phase Crohn's disease into remission and heal associated fistulas. Supply is reported with HCPCS Level II code J1745. May be sold under the brand name Remicade.

information model Conceptual model of the information needed to support a business function or process.

information services Internal administrators of the computer systems used by an organization or institution. *Synonym(s):* IS.

infra- Inferior to, beneath, under.

infraorbital nerve Maxillary branch of the trigeminal nerve. It transverses the infraorbital groove and emerges

on the face where it supplies sensation to the internal and external nasal areas, as well as the upper lip and lower eyelid.

infraorbital rim Edge around the inferior surface of the orbit.

infratentorial Located below or beneath the tentorium of the cerebellum, which is the dura mater supporting the occipital lobes and covering the cerebellum.

infundibulectomy Excision of the anterosuperior portion of the right ventricle of the heart.

infusate Therapeutic substance introduced through a vein.

infusion Introduction of a therapeutic fluid, other than blood, into the bloodstream.

infusion pump Device that delivers a measured amount of drug or intravenous solution through injection over a period of time. *NCD Reference:* 280.14.

inguinal Within the groin region.

INH Inhalation solution.

inhalation Act of drawing in by breathing.

inhalation anesthesia Anesthesia inducing a state of unconsciousness via the administration of gases or vapors through a mask or endotracheal tube. Agents used include Fluothane, Forane, nitrous oxide, Ethrane, or ether. To report general anesthesia provided by the physician performing the procedure, append modifier 47 to the procedure code.

inhibited female orgasm Form of psychosexual dysfunction in which there is recurrent and persistent inhibition of the female orgasm as manifested by a delay or absence of orgasm following a normal sexual excitement phase during sexual activity.

inhibited male orgasm Form of psychosexual dysfunction in which there is recurrent and persistent inhibition of the male orgasm as manifested by a delay or absence of the emission or ejaculation phases or, more usually, following an adequate phase of sexual excitement.

inhibited sexual desire Form of psychosexual dysfunction in which there is persistent inhibition of desire for engaging in a particular form of sexual activity.

inhibited sexual excitement Form of psychosexual dysfunction in which there is recurrent and persistent inhibition of sexual excitement during sexual activity, manifested by partial or complete failure to attain or maintain erection until completion of the sexual act (impotence) or partial or complete failure to attain or maintain the lubrication-swelling response of sexual excitement until completion of the sexual act (frigidity).

iniencephaly Rare neural tube defect in which there is marked retroflexion of the head and severe spinal defects. There is a disproportionately large head and the neck is generally absent. The spinal cord passes through the foramen magnum in an enlarged occipital bone with an absent vertebral bone layer and spinal processes, resulting in both a reduction in both the number and proper fusion of the vertebrae. Prognosis is poor. Iniencephaly is reported with ICD-9-CM code 740.2.

initial First stage in a series of events.

initial hospital care Admitting provider's evaluation and instructions for care, usually provided the day of admission to a facility. Note that only one initial care service can be reported per admission.

INJ Injection.

inject Introduction into body tissues.

injection Forcing a liquid substance into a body part such as a joint or muscle.

injury Harm or damage sustained by the body.

inlay Restoration made outside of the mouth to fit a prepared cavity and placed on the tooth.

innervate Supplying a stimulus or energy to nerve fibers connected to a part.

innervation Nerve distribution to a body part.

innominate Unnamed or nameless structure.

Innovar See droperidol and fentanyl citrate.

inpatient Time period in which a patient is housed in a hospital or facility offering medical, surgical, and/or psychiatric services, usually without interruption.

inpatient ancillary services Inpatient services other than accommodations or services included in "routine" for which separate charges are not submitted (i.e., routine nursing care).

inpatient hospitalization Period in which a patient is housed in a single hospital usually without interruption.

inpatient reimbursement Payment to hospital for the costs incurred to treat a patient.

inpatient services Items and services furnished to an inpatient, including room and board, nursing care and related services, diagnostic and therapeutic services, and medical and surgical services. An inpatient service requires the beneficiary to reside in a specific institutional setting during treatment.

INPH Idiopathic normal pressure hydrocephalus. Abnormal increase of cerebrospinal fluid in the brain's ventricles of unknown cause, most often diagnosed during the sixth or seventh decade of a patient's life. INPH is typically manifested by a triad of symptoms that includes dementia and progressive mental impairment, gait disturbance, and impaired bladder control. Diagnosis is determined through a combination of clinical signs and symptoms, diagnostic testing such as lumbar puncture, intracranial pressure monitoring or neuropsychological evaluations, and radiographic findings such as CT and/or MRI. Treatment may include surgical implantation of a ventriculoperitoneal (VP) shunt, which drains the excess cerebrospinal fluid into the abdomen where it can be absorbed. This allows the ventricles of the brain to return to their normal size. Report INPH with ICD-9-CM code 331.5.

inseminate Inject with semen.

insert To put into.

insert Surgical introduction or implant.

insertion Placement or implantation into a body part.

insight-oriented psychotherapy Development of insight or affective understanding and the use of behavior modification techniques, supportive interactions, cognitive discussion of reality, or any combination of the above to provide therapeutic change.

Insignia Ultra or Entra Brand name cardiac pacing system.

insoles Rubber or plastic orthotics that fit inside the shoes to correct a deformity or help aid in the healing of an injury.

insomnia Inability to sleep. *persistent i.* Chronic state of sleeplessness associated with chronic anxiety, major or minor depressive disorders, or psychoses. *transient i.* Episodes of sleeplessness associated with acute or intermittent emotional reactions or conflicts.

instill Instillation.

instillation Administering a liquid slowly over time, drop by drop.

institutional planning Overall plan and budget of a hospital, skilled nursing facility, comprehensive outpatient rehabilitation facility, or home health agency. Plans must be prepared and submitted to the state health agency. Plans must include an annual operating budget and a capital expenditures plan for at least a three-year period.

instrumentation Use of a tool for therapeutic reasons.

insufflation Blowing air or gas into a body cavity.

insulin resistance syndrome Group of health risks that increase the likelihood of developing heart disease, stroke, and diabetes. Diagnosis of insulin resistance syndrome is made if one has three or more of the following: waist measurement of 40 or more inches for men and 35 or more inches for women; blood pressure of 130/85 mm or higher; triglyceride level greater than 150 mg/dl; fasting blood sugar of more than 100 mg/dl; HDL level less than 40 mg/dl in men or less than 50 mg/dl in women. Report this condition with ICD-9-CM code 277.7, with additional codes to identify associated manifestations. *Synonym(s): dysmetabolic syndrome, metabolic syndrome, syndrome X.*

G-I

insurance fragmentation Breaking a single service into its multiple components, usually to increase total billing charges.

Intacs Brand name intrastromal corneal ring segments implanted in the cornea to correct mild myopia or keratoconus. The implant procedure is reported with CPT code 0099T.

Intal See cromolyn sodium.

INTEGRA Dermal Regeneration Brand name temporary wound dressing consisting of a polymer membrane of collagen and silicone used in treatment of surgically excised burns. When the dressing is applied in the physician office, supply of the wound dressing is reported separately. Application of INTEGRA is reported with CPT codes 15170-15176. Supply is reported with HCPCS Level II codes C9363, Q4104, Q4105, and Q4108. Report injectable INTEGRA with Q4114.

integrated delivery systems Health care delivery system that joins the various parts of the health care system, including facilities, physicians, and ancillary service providers, into a cohesive group to provide a complete network of health care services for a given patient population or geographic area.

integrated implant Implant attached to body parts to allow for transfer of motion from muscle to implant. In the eye, an integrated implant allows the muscles of the eye to transfer the motion from the muscle to the artificial eye via a peg system.

Integrelin See eptifibatide.

integument Covering.

integumentary Skin system covering the body that includes the epidermis, dermis, hair, nails, and glands. Procedures performed on the integumentary system are classified to CPT codes 10040-19499.

interactive psychotherapy Use of physical aids and nonverbal communication to overcome barriers to therapeutic interaction between a clinician and a patient who has not yet developed or has lost either the expressive language communication skills to explain his/her symptoms and response to treatment, or the receptive communication skills to understand the clinician if he or she were to use ordinary adult language for communication.

interarticular Between two joint surfaces.

intercarpal Between the carpal bones in the wrist.

interdental Gingival structures occupying the space between adjoining teeth.

interdisciplinary care Two or more health care professions working in a collaborative manner for the benefit of the patient.

interferometry Measuring minute distances or movements by the phenomena occurring when two rays of light or acoustics of sound interfere with each other.

interferon Naturally occurring glycoprotein found in the body, also created through recombinant genetic engineering. Interferons act in a host-specific manner to produce antiviral activity by inducing the transcription of the host's cellular genes that are coded for antiviral proteins, which in turn selectively inhibit the virus' synthesis of proteins and RNA. Alpha interferon is the drug of choice for treating hepatitis C. and is also used to treat hairy cell leukemia, condylomata acuminata, Kaposi's sarcoma, malignant melanoma, and other cancers. Beta interferon is used primarily to decrease the number of exacerbations in multiple sclerosis. Gamma interferon is used primarily to treat severe malignant osteopetrosis and chronic granulomatous disease. May be sold under the brand names Actimmune, Betaseron, Intron.

INTERGEL Brand name thick liquid made of sodium that separates and protects tissues as they heal, preventing adhesions. The gel is supplied in a single-use bottle and is applied prior to operative wound closure and absorbed over time by surrounding tissue. Check with your payer for reimbursement policies related to INTERGEL.

interim bill Bill that does not cover the complete hospital or skilled nursing facility stay. An interim bill is used when the hospital is expecting to submit a series of inpatient claims after a minimum confinement of 30 days. An interim claim may be submitted by a prospective payment system hospital every 60 days during the confinement or course of treatment.

intermediary Public or private agency or organization that has entered into an agreement with CMS to process Medicare claims under both Part A and Part B for institutional providers (e.g., hospitals, skilled nursing facilities (SNF), home health agencies (HHA), hospices, comprehensive outpatient rehabilitation facilities (CORF), outpatient physical therapy, occupational therapy, speech pathology providers, and end-stage renal disease (ESRD) facilities).

intermediate care facility Health care facility that furnishes services to patients who do not require the degree of care provided by a hospital or skilled nursing facility or a step-down facility for patients who are leaving the hospital but who cannot be discharged to home because of continuing medical needs. *Synonym(s): ICF.*

intermediate repair *1)* Surgical closure of a wound requiring closure of one or more of the deeper subcutaneous tissue and non-muscle fascia layers in addition to suturing the skin. *2)* Contaminated wounds with single layer closure that need extensive cleaning or foreign body removal.

G-I

intermittent bolus Intravenous procedure in which an agent or drug is administered intermittently by syringe into an intravenous catheter port.

intermittent explosive disorder Recurrent, uncontrollable episodes of sudden and significant loss of control of aggressive impulses that cannot be accounted for by any other mental disorder and that are disproportionate to any psychosocial stressors and result in assault or property destruction followed by genuine regret or self-reproach.

intern Medical school graduate who is in the first year of postgraduate training under the direction of a teaching physician and/or senior resident.

internal acoustic meatus Passage in the temporal bone through which the facial, intermediate, and vestibulocochlear nerves pass. *Synonym(s): internal auditory canal.*

internal carotid artery Major artery of the head and neck that helps supply blood to the brain.

internal control number Unique, 15-digit identifying number assigned by a Medicare carrier to every claim for control and inventory purposes that indicates the claim type, region, year, Julian date, batch number, and sequence. *Synonym(s): ICN.*

internal direct current stimulator Electrostimulation device placed directly into the surgical site designed to promote bone regeneration by encouraging cellular healing response in bone and ligaments.

internal fixation Wires, pins, screws, and plates placed through or within the fractured area to stabilize and immobilize the injury.

internal os Opening through the cervix into the uterus.

internal skeletal fixation Repair involving wires, pins, screws, and/or plates placed through or within the fractured area to stabilize and immobilize the injury.

International Association of Industrial Accident Boards and Commissions Trade association representing government agencies that administer workers' compensation programs. One of the association's standards is under consideration for use for the first-report-of-injury standard under HIPAA. *Synonym(s): IAIABC.*

International Classification of Disease Medical code set maintained by the World Health Organization (WHO). The primary purpose was to classify causes of death. A U.S. extension, ICD-9-CM, maintained by the National Center for Health Statistics within the Centers for Disease Control and Prevention, identifies morbidity factors, or diagnoses. The ICD-9-CM codes have been selected for use in the HIPAA transactions. *Synonym(s): ICD.*

International Classification of Diseases, Ninth Edition, Clinical Modification Clinical modification of the international statistical coding system used to report, compile, and compare health care data, using numeric and alphanumeric codes to help plan, deliver, reimburse, and quantify medical care in the United States. *Synonym(s): ICD-9-CM.*

International Classification of Diseases, Tenth Edition Classification of diseases by alphanumeric code, used by the World Health Organization but not yet adopted in the United States. *Synonym(s): ICD-10.*

International Classification of Diseases, Tenth Edition, Clinical Modification Clinical modification of ICD-10 developed for use in the United States. *Synonym(s): ICD-10-CM.*

International Classification of Diseases, Tenth Edition, Procedure Coding System Procedure coding system developed by 3M HIS under contract with the Centers for Medicare and Medicaid Services. *Synonym(s): ICD-10-PCS.*

International Organization for Standardization Organization that coordinates the development and adoption of numerous international standards. "ISO" is not an acronym, but the Greek word for "equal." *Synonym(s): ISO.*

internet-only manuals Internet-only manuals replace instructions previously contained in paper-based manuals. *Synonym(s): IOM.*

interposition Placement between objects.

interpretation Professional health care provider's review of data with a written or verbal opinion.

interrogation device evaluation Assessment of an implantable cardiac device (pacemaker, cardioverter-defibrillator, cardiovascular monitor, or loop recorder) in which collected data about the patient's heart rate and rhythm, battery and pulse generator function, and any leads or sensors present, are retrieved and evaluated. Determinations regarding device programming and appropriate treatment settings are made based on the findings. CPT provides required components for evaluation of the various types of devices.

interrupted suture Series of single stitches with tension isolated at each stitch, in which all stitches are not affected if one becomes loose, and the isolated sutures cannot act as a wick to transport an infection.

intersection syndrome Pain, swelling, and redness occurring at the intersection of the aductor pollicis longus and extensor pollicis brevis tendons on the wrist and forearm above the thumb, due to heavy and repetitive use of the wrist and thumb. It can be treated with antiinflammatory medications, rest, or splinting. Rarely, surgical release of the tendons is required.

G-I

Intersection syndrome is reported with ICD-9-CM code 727.05.

interspace Space between two similar objects.

InterStim Brand name implantable sacral nerve stimulator used as a treatment for managing urinary incontinence, urgency, overactive bladder, or urinary retention. The neurostimulator is implanted subcutaneously in the upper buttock or abdomen, and a lead is placed adjacent to the sacral nerve and attached to the neurostimulator. The patient controls urination with a hand-held programmer. In outpatient facilities, the supply of InterStim is reported with HCPCS Level II codes C1897, C1767 and C1787.

interstitial Within the small spaces or gaps occurring in tissue or organs.

interstitial fluid Extracellular fluid filtered through capillaries and drained as lymph that surrounds and bathes most tissue outside of blood or lymph vessels.

interstitial radiation Radioactive source placed into the tissue being treated.

interval history History documenting what has occurred in a given area since the last visit, usually associated with subsequent hospital, nursing home, rest home, and home visit services.

interventional radiology Performance of invasive procedures using imaging guidance.

interventional radiology component coding Coding allowing a physician, regardless of specialty, to specifically identify and report those aspects of the service provided, whether the procedural component, the radiological component, or both.

intervertebral disc Fibrocartilaginous cushion found between the vertebral bodies of the spine and composed of the annulus fibrosus, or the outer fibrous ring, surrounding a soft, central elastic area called the nucleus pulposus.

intestinal calculus Any hard mass or concretion found within the intestines, not necessarily composed of fecal matter, that may cause obstruction. Report this condition with ICD-9-CM code 560.39. *Synonym(s): enterolith.*

intestinal or peritoneal adhesions with obstruction Abnormal fibrous band growths joining separate tissues in the peritoneum or intestine, causing blockage.

intra Within.

intra-aortic Within the aorta.

intra-aortic balloon pump Internal cardiac assist device usually inserted through the femoral artery into the descending aorta, either percutaneously or by open approach, and connected to a drive console that monitors the patient's condition as the balloon is synchronously inflated and deflated to improve cardiac performance.

Insertion and removal codes differ by the approach used and are reported with CPT codes 33967-33974. *Synonym(s): IABP.*

intra-arterial Within an artery or arteries. *i. infusion pump* Implantable device consisting of a reservoir, or pump, that contains the drug to be administered. It is connected to a catheter that terminates in a specific artery. The pump delivers a measured amount of medication, such as a chemotherapeutic agent, directly into the arterial system through injection over a period of time. Initial placement, revision, and removal are reported separately using CPT codes 36260-36262. *Synonym(s): IAIP.*

intracavitary Within a body cavity.

intracoronal In dentistry, portion of the tooth inside the corona or crown.

intracranial Within the cranium (skull).

intractable Resistant to relief. *i. epilepsy* Seizure disorder that cannot be controlled with medication. Epilepsy is reported with a code from ICD-9-CM category 345, with fifth digit 1 indicating intractability. Intractability is a subjective clinical finding and should only be coded if specifically documented in the medical record. *i. migraine* Headache that cannot be controlled with medication. Migraines are reported with a code from ICD-9-CM category 346, with fifth digit 1 or 3 indicating intractability. Intractability is a subjective clinical finding and should only be coded if specifically documented in the medical record.

intralesional injection Medication delivered through a syringe and needle directly into a localized lesion. Report the first through seventh intralesional injections with CPT code 11900. If more than seven lesions are injected, report 11901. Intralesional chemotherapy administration is reported using 96405-96406.

intramedullary implants Nail, rod, or pin placed into the intramedullary canal at the fracture site. Intramedullary implants not only provide a method of aligning the fracture, they also act as a splint and may reduce fracture pain. Implants may be rigid or flexible. Rigid implants are preferred for prophylactic treatment of diseased bone, while flexible implants are preferred for traumatic injuries.

intramedullary nail Orthopaedic internal fixation device used to treat midshaft fractures in long bones, it is placed in the medullary canal of the bone and held in place with screws or cerclage. Reported as open reduction internal fixation by intramedullary nailing with appropriate CPT code by fracture site, e.g., for femur see 27506. *Synonym(s): Hansen-Street nail, Kuntscher nail, Lottes nail, Schnieder nail.*

intramural Within the wall of an organ.

intramural uterine leiomyoma Benign, smooth muscle tumor within the wall of the uterus.

intramuscular Within a muscle.

intranasal Within the nose.

intraocular lens Artificial lens implanted into the eye to replace a damaged natural lens or cataract. *Synonym(s): IOL.*

intraocular muscles Intrinsic muscles inside the eye.

intraosseous Within a bone.

intraparenchymal hematoma Tumor-like collection of blood located within the characteristic tissue cells of the brain.

intraperitoneal Within the cavity or space created by the double-layered sac that lines the abdominopelvic walls and forms a covering for the internal organs.

intrauterine copper contraceptive device Small plastic device in the shape of a T inserted into the uterus with a locator/extractor string that remains within the vagina. It contains a copper coil emitting a small amount of the metal, which creates a poor environment for sperm. This highly effective contraceptive device may be used for up to 10 years and works by preventing sperm from reaching the egg and by preventing implantation of a fertilized egg. Supply is reported with HCPCS Level II code J7300. Report insertion with CPT code 58300 and removal with 58301. May be sold under the brand names Copper T 380A and Paraguard T 380A.

intrauterine death Fetal death after 22 weeks of gestation. Report ICD-9-CM code 656.4X with the appropriate fifth digit (0, 1, or 3) to indicate the episode of care.

intrauterine synechiae Abnormal joining of tissues within the uterus.

intravascular Within a blood vessel.

intravenous Within a vein or veins.

intravenous anesthesia Anesthesia inducing a state of unconsciousness via the administration of IV anesthetics. Agents used include Pentothal, Ketamine, Ketalar, and Innovar. To report general or regional anesthesia provided by the physician performing the procedure, append modifier 47 to the procedure code.

intravenous pyelogram X-ray of the pelvis of the kidney and ureter after injection of a radiopaque contrast material. *Synonym(s): IVP.*

intravenous regional block Anesthesia of a local area of limb accomplished by applying a pneumatic tourniquet to the limb and injecting an anesthetic agent into the vein of the limb distal to the tourniquet.

intraventricular space Fluid-filled areas near the center of the brain that are within the ventricles.

intrinsic muscles of the foot These muscles are divided into two groups: dorsal and plantar. The dorsal group includes the extensor digitorum brevis; the plantar group includes the abductor hallucis, flexor digitorum brevis, abductor digiti minimi, quadratus plantae, lumbricals, flexor hallucis brevis, adductor hallucis, flexor digiti minimi brevis, and dorsal and plantar interossei.

introducer Instrument, such as a catheter, needle, or tube, through which another instrument or device is introduced into the body.

introduction Induction of an instrument, such as a catheter, needle, or endotracheal tube.

introitus Entrance into the vagina.

Intron A See interferon.

introverted disorder of childhood Emotional disturbance in children chiefly manifested by a lack of interest in social relationships and indifference to social praise or criticism.

introverted personality Profound defect in the ability to form social relationships and to respond to the usual forms of social reinforcements, often referred to as loners who do not appear distressed by their social distance and are not interested in greater social involvement.

intubate Insertion of a tube into a body canal or organ.

intubation Insertion of a tube into a hollow organ, canal, or cavity within the body.

intussusception Prolapse of one section of intestine into the lumen of an adjacent section of the bowel. This condition, which occurs mainly in children, causes pain, vomiting, and mucous passed from the rectum and requires surgical intervention. Intussusception is reported with ICD-9-CM code 560.0 or CPT code 44050..

inundation fever Acute infectious disease resembling typhus, caused by rickettsia bacteria and transmitted by the bite of infected larval mites, called chiggers. This disease occurs chiefly in Asia and the Pacific and is manifested by a specific telltale lesion or eschar at the site of the bite, fever, regional lymphadenopathy, and skin lesions and rashes. Report this disease with ICD-9-CM code 081.2. *Synonym(s): akamushi disease, island fever, Japanese flood fever, Japanese river fever, kedani fever, mite-borne typhus, Mossman fever, scrub typhus, shimamushi disease, tropical typhus, tsutsugamushi disease.*

invalid ICD-9-CM code Diagnosis code that is not specific because a digit is missing. Medicare and private payers will reject claims containing invalid ICD-9-CM codes.

InVance Brand name male urinary sling system to treat stress incontinence. Diagnosis is reported with ICD-9-CM code 788.32.

Invanz See ertapenem sodium.

G-I

invasive Insertion of an instrument, device, or foreign matter into the body or requiring puncture or incision of the skin.

Invega See paliperidone palmitate.

inversion Turning inward, inside out, or upside down.

inverted nipple Nipple that draws inward and does not protrude when compressed or cold, reported with ICD-9-CM code 611.79. If specified as congenital, report with 757.6 and if occurring in pregnancy, report with a code from subcategory 676.3.

involutional melancholia Manic-depressive psychosis in which there is a widespread depressed mood of gloom and wretchedness with some degree of anxiety, reduced activity, or restlessness and agitation. There is a marked tendency to recurrence; in a few cases this may be at regular intervals.

involutional paranoid state Paranoid psychosis in which there are conspicuous hallucinations, often in several modalities. May be associated with mild affective symptoms and well-preserved personality.

IOL Intraocular lens. Artificial lens replacing a natural one. *NCD Reference: 80.12.*

IOM Institute of Medicine.

iontophoresis Method of localized transdermal medication delivery using a low-level electrical current applied to a drug solution in a patch. The drug ions are propelled through the skin into underlying tissue. Iontophoresis is used to alleviate joint or muscle pain in sports medicine. It is also the method used for introducing pilocarpine in the sweat test for cystic fibrosis and as a treatment for hyperhidrosis. Application of iontophoresis patch for therapeutic drug delivery is reported with CPT code 97033; for cystic fibrosis diagnostic sweat test, see 89230.

IOP Intra-ocular pressure. High IOP is glaucoma.

IOPatch Brand name allograft for anterior and posterior eye segment patch grafting, used in a variety of procedures including glaucoma surgery, scleral buckle repair, eyelid reconstruction, and implant repair.

IP *1)* Interphalangeal. *2)* Intraperitoneal.

IPA Individual practice association. Organization made up of providers who, along with the rest of a group, contract with payers at a discounted fee-for-service or capitated rate.

IPD Intermittent peritoneal dialysis.

IPF *1)* Inpatient psychiatric facility. *2)* Interstitial pulmonary fibrosis. Fibrosis and scarring of the lungs as a result of an inflammatory reaction, commonly referred to as postinflammatory pulmonary fibrosis or interstitial pulmonary fibrosis. IPF is reported with ICD-9-CM code 515. *Synonym(s): cirrhosis of lung,*

fibrosis of lung, induration of lung, interstitial lung disease.

IPO Individual practice organization. Organization made up of providers who, along with the rest of a group, contract with payers at a discounted fee-for-service or capitated rate.

IPOL Brand name poliovirus vaccine provided in a single-dose or 10-dose vial. Supply of IPOL is reported with CPT code 90713; administration is reported separately. The need for vaccination is reported with ICD-9-CM code V04.0.

IPPB Intermittent positive pressure breathing. Therapeutic pulmonary procedure that provides short term inhalation therapy for the purpose of augmenting lung expansion, delivering aerosol medication, or assisting ventilation. IPPB is reported with CPT code 94640.

IPPS Inpatient short-term acute-care prospective payment system.

ipratropium bromide Acetylcholine agonist that inhibits reflexes stimulated by the vagus nerve, used in treating bronchospasm in COPD and to treat rhinorrhea occurring with allergies and colds. Supply is reported with HCPCS Level II code J7644. May be sold under the brand name Atrovent.

ipsilateral Located on, or affecting, the same side of the body, usually as it relates to a bilateral body part.

IPT Insulin potentiation therapy.

IPV *1)* Poliovirus vaccine, inactivated. Supply of IPV is reported with CPT code 90713 or 90698. Administration is reported separately. The need for vaccination is reported with ICD-9-CM code V04.0. *2)* Intrapulmonary percussive ventilator. *NCD Reference: 240.5.*

IQ Intelligence quotient.

IRB Institutional review board.

IRDS Idiopathic respiratory distress syndrome.

IRDS syndrome Infant reflex distress. Respiratory distress in premature neonates associated with reduced amounts of lung surfactant. Frequently fatal. Report this disorder with ICD-9-CM code 769. *Synonym(s): hyaline membrane syndrome.*

IRF Inpatient rehabilitation facility.

irid- Relating to the iris.

iridocyclitis Acute or chronic condition in which both the ciliary body and the iris are irritated and inflamed due to a variety of causes, such as another underlying disease, trauma, or immune or allergy reaction. Report iridocyclitis with a code from ICD-9-CM subcategories 364.0-364.3.

iridodialysis Tear at the base of the iris, separating it from the ciliary body.

iridolysis Tear at the base of the iris, separating it from the ciliary body.

iridoschisis Pathological condition causing the iris to split into two layers.

iridotomy Surgical incision into the iris.

irinotecan HCl First line chemotherapy drug used for metastatic colorectal cancer in combination with 5FU and leucovorin or in colorectal cancer progressing after 5-FU therapy. Supply is reported with HCPCS Level II code J9206. May be sold under the brand name Camptosar.

iris Pigmented membrane behind the cornea and in front of the lens that contracts and expands to enlarge or shrink the size of the pupil to regulate the light entering the eye.

iris pigment dispersion syndrome Lack of pigment in iris. Report this disorder with ICD-9-CM code 364.53.

iron dextran/sucrose Metallic element found in nature and an essential component in the formation of hemoglobin, which transports oxygen to the tissues. Iron dextran is a parenteral iron replacement used to treat iron deficiency anemia. Supply is reported with HCPCS Level II code J1750. Iron sucrose is also delivered parenterally to treat iron deficient patients on long-term hemodialysis, also receiving erythropoietin therapy. Supply is reported with HCPCS Level II code J1756.

irradiation Exposure to electromagnetic radiation from a source such as a light, laser, heat, or x-ray, usually for treatment of a disease.

irregular bones Bones of a shape that cannot be classified within long, short, or flat bones, such as the vertebrae, skull, and hipbones.

irrigate Washing out, lavage.

irrigation To wash out or cleanse a body cavity, wound, or tissue with water or other fluid.

IS Information services. Administrators of the computer systems used by payers and providers.

Isa Interchange control header segment. This is the HIPAA reference name for the data needed to contact the receiver and advise that a transmission of claims is being sent.

ISC Infant servo-control.

ischemia Deficiency in blood supply causing tissues to be deprived of oxygen, resulting from trauma, mechanical or functional constriction of blood vessels, or a physical obstruction.

ischial tuberosity Bony projection of the lower end of the ischium easily identified as the weight-bearing point in a sitting position.

ischio- Relating to the hip.

ischiopagus Monozygotic (identical) twins who are joined at the hip, reported with ICD-9-CM code 759.4.

ISD Intrinsic (urethral) sphincter deficiency. Malfunctioning of the urethral sphincter. There may be a posterior rotation and opening of the bladder neck and posterior urethra during straining that leads to intrinsic sphincteric damage. This condition is reported with ICD-9-CM code 599.82.

ISG Immune serum globulin.

Ishihara test Color blindness test using plates painted with dots depicting various figures.

ISHLT International Society for Heart and Lung Transplantation.

island fever Acute infectious disease resembling typhus, caused by rickettsia bacteria and transmitted by the bite of infected larval mites, called chiggers. This disease occurs chiefly in Asia and the Pacific and is manifested by a specific telltale lesion or eschar at the site of the bite, fever, regional lymphadenopathy, and skin lesions and rashes. Report this disease with ICD-9-CM code 081.2. *Synonym(s): akamushi disease, inundation fever, Japanese flood fever, Japanese river fever, kedani fever, mite-borne typhus, Mossman fever, scrub typhus, shimamushi disease, tropical typhus, tsutsugamushi disease.*

island pedicle Flap consisting of full-thickness skin and subcutaneous tissue that remains attached to its nutrient supply of blood vessels.

islet cell Islet of Langerhans, hormone producing pancreatic cells. *NCD Reference: 260.3.1. i. tumor* Benign tumor of the islets of Langerhans. This tumor may result in excessive hormonal production and is reported with ICD-9-CM code 211.7, with an additional code to identify functional activities or conditions. *Synonym(s): nesidioblastoma.*

ISMM In situ malignant melanoma. Melanoma on the outermost layers of epidermis. ISMM would be classified as an in situ carcinoma (172), rather than as a melanoma. *Synonym(s): Clark level I melanoma, ISM.*

ISO International Organization for Standardization.

iso- Equal.

isodose Equivalent dose of radiation delivered to two or more body areas.

isoetharine Adrenergic bronchodilator used to treat symptoms such as wheezing related to asthma, COPD, chronic bronchitis, and other lung diseases. Inhalant supply is reported with HCPCS Level II codes J7648 and J7649.

isograft Tissue or organ grafted between genetically identical persons, as from one identical twin to another. *Synonym(s): syngraft.*

G-I

isolated explosive disorder Disorder of impulse control in which there is a single discrete episode characterized by failure to resist an impulse that leads to a single, violent, externally directed act that has a catastrophic impact on others and for which the available information does not justify the diagnosis of another mental disorder.

isolated levocardia Form of ectocardia, a rare congenital defect in which the heart appears with malformation in its usual location on the left but the other visceral organs are transposed in relation to the heart. This condition is reported with ICD-9-CM code 746.87.

isolated phobia Fear of a discrete object or situation, such as animals, heights, or small spaces, that is neither fear of leaving the familiar setting of the home (agoraphobia) or of being observed by others in certain situations (social phobia).

isoproterenol Potent adrenergic used for dilating airways and stimulating the heart. It is prescribed to treat bronchospasm, heart block, ventricular arrhythmias, and shock, and used as a diagnostic aid in detecting mitral regurgitation and coronary artery disease. It relaxes smooth muscle in the bronchi by stimulating the beta 2-adrenergic receptors and acts on the beta 1-adrenergic receptors to stimulate the heart. Supply is reported with HCPCS Level II code J7658 or J7659.

Isosource Brand name enteral nutrition. Supply of Isosource is reported with HCPCS Level II code B4150 or B4152.

isotonic saline Salt solution used to irrigate or bathe tissue without causing water to be lost from cells by crossing the semipermeable membrane.

isotope Chemical element possessing the same atomic number (protons in the nucleus) as another, but with a different atomic weight (number of neutrons).

isthmusectomy Excision of the connecting tissue between two objections, usually in reference to the two thyroid lobes. This is not performed alone but in conjunction with a thyroid lobectomy or removal of a cyst or adenoma from the thyroid. These procedures are reported with CPT codes 60200-60225.

Isuprel See isoproterenol.

IT Intrathecal administration.

ITC In the canal, as seen in ENT documentation.

ITE In the ear, as seen in ENT documentation.

itemized statement Detailed statement of each item or service the patient received from the physician, hospital, or other health care supplier or professional. The BBA of 1997 gives Medicare beneficiaries the right to submit a written request for an itemized statement from their provider or supplier for any Medicare item or service.

Providers and suppliers are required to furnish the itemized statement within 30 days of the request or be subject to a civil monetary penalty of up to $100 for each offense. Recommended information to be included on the itemized statement includes date(s) of service, description of services provided, number of services provided, benefit days used, noncovered charges, deductible and coinsurance amounts, amount charged, beneficiary liability, total paid by Medicare, referring physician, provider/supplier submitting the claim, and the Medicare claim number.

-itis Inflammation.

ITP Idiopathic thrombocytopenic purpura, immune thrombocytopenic purpura. Disorder of coagulation due to a low number of platelets. Patients often have purple bruises due to bleeding in small blood vessels under the skin that looks like red or purple dots, called petechiae. ITP is reported with ICD-9-CM code 287.31.

itraconazole Antifungal used to treat a wide variety of fungal infections by interfering with fungal cell wall synthesis. It is especially useful in treating aspergillus and Blastomyces dermatides. Usually self administered by mouth but can be given by IV infusion. Injection supply is reported with HCPCS Level II code J1835.

Itsenko-Cushing syndrome Increased adrenocortical secretion of cortisol caused by ACTH-dependent adrenocortical hyperplasia or tumor with abdominal striae, acne, hypertension decreased carbohydrate tolerance, moon face, obesity, protein catabolism, and psychiatric disturbances. Report this disorder with ICD-9-CM code 255.0.

IU International units.

IUD Intrauterine device. Report encounters for IUD insertion with ICD-9-CM code V25.11; removal with V25.12; and replacement with V25.13.

IUGR Intrauterine growth restriction. Fetal size smaller than the gestational age would predict. IUGR is a significant factor in perinatal morbidity and mortality, and is reported with an ICD-9-CM code from subcategory 656.5 for the mother, or a code from subcategory 764.9 for the neonate.

IUI Intrauterine insemination, reported with CPT code 58322. The physician dilates the cervix and inserts a long plastic tube into the cavity of the uterus. Semen is then injected into the uterus by a syringe connected to the plastic tubing. *Synonym(s): artificial insemination.*

IV Cranial nerve on the brainstem responsible for motor control of the superior oblique muscle.

IVC *1)* Inferior vena cava. *2)* Intravenous cholangiogram.

IVC filter Filtering device placed into the inferior vena cava (IVC) to prevent venous emboli from the legs or pelvis from entering the pulmonary arteries. There are many different filters to choose from including the

G-I

Greenfield filter, DIL filter, Bird's nest filter, and the Vena
Tech LGM filter. Report the procedure with CPT code
37620; radiological supervision and interpretation for
the placement is reported with 75940.

IVC syndrome Intravascular coagulopathy. Decrease
of elements needed for coagulation of blood. Later stages
are marked by profuse bleeding. Report this disorder
with ICD-9-CM code 286.6.

IVEEGAM See gamma globulin.

Ivemark's syndrome Organs of left side of the body are
a mirror image of organs on right side. Splenic agenesis
and cardiac malformation are associated. Report this
disorder with ICD-9-CM code 759.0.

IVF In vitro fertilization.

IVH Intraventricular hemorrhage.

IVP Intravenous pyelogram. X-ray study of the renal
pelvis and ureter after injection of a radiopaque contrast
material in order to follow the normal flow of urine
through the tract (antegrade) and assess for function,
obstructions, or abnormalities. Contrast may be injected
through an existing nephrostomy or pyelostomy tube,
or an indwelling ureteral catheter (CPT code 50684).
Radiological supervision and interpretation during the
procedure is reported separately with 74425.

IVUS Intravascular ultrasound. Add-on service
performed during diagnostic evaluation or therapeutic
intervention on noncoronary vessels, reported with CPT
codes 37250 and 37251. Radiological supervision and
interpretation is reported separately with CPT codes
75945 and 75946. Facilities report IVUS with codes from
ICD-9-CM Volume 3 category 00.2.

Iwanoff cyst Cystic spaces on the periphery of the
retina that do not affect vision significantly, reported
with ICD-9-CM code 362.62. **Synonym(s):** *Blessig cyst.*

IX Cranial nerve on the surface of the rostral medulla
responsible for swallowing, posterior tongue taste
sensations, and carotid baroreception.

G-I

J code Subset of the HCPCS Level II alphanumeric code set used to identify certain drugs and other items.

J1 HCPCS Level II modifier used to denote a no-pay submission for a prescription number in a competitive acquisition program.

J2 HCPCS Level II modifier used to denote restocking of emergency drugs following an emergency.

J3 HCPCS Level II modifier used to denote that a prescribed drug is not available through a competitive acquisition program and will be reimbursed under the average sales price.

J4 HCPCS Level II modifier used to denote a DMEPOS item that is subject to the DMEPOS competitive bidding program and furnished by the hospital upon patient discharge.

Jaccoud's syndrome Chronic arthropathy that develops following a previous rheumatic fever infection, causing persistent arthritis with nodular fibrous changes in the joint capsules and tendons, but no bone loss. Malformation of the joints resembles rheumatoid arthritis. Hands are the most commonly affected anatomical site. Report this syndrome with ICD-9-CM code 714.4. *Synonym(s): Jaccoud's arthritis.*

Jace TRI /// BRACE Knee orthosis apparatus that may be utilized as a continuous passive motion brace, an immobilization brace for the postoperative period, or a rehabilitation brace.

Jackson's membrane Congenital intestinal abnormality in which the cecum, the first portion of the large intestine, is covered by a web of adhesions, like a sheet of peritoneum from the abdominal wall, causing bowel obstruction. This condition is reported with ICD-9-CM code 751.4. *Synonym(s): Jackson's veil.*

Jackson's syndrome Paraplegia and anesthesia over part of the body. Caused by lesions in the brain or spinal cord. Report this disorder with ICD-9-CM code 344.89. *Synonym(s): Avellis syndrome, Babinski-Nageotte syndrome, Benedikt's syndrome, Brown-Sequard syndrome, Cestan-Chenais syndrome, Cestan's syndrome, Foville's syndrome, Gubler-Millard syndrome, Weber-Leyden syndrome.*

Jacksonian epilepsy Focal motor seizures that occur unilaterally, causing a rapid succession of contraction and relaxation within the muscles of one group that travels to adjacent muscle groups in response to the progressive discharge of epileptic focal activity in the motor cortex on the opposite side. Alertness and awareness are not normally impaired during these attacks. Jacksonian epilepsy is reported with a code from ICD-9-CM subcategory 345.5. *Synonym(s): Bravais-Jacksonian epilepsy.*

Jacquet's dermatitis Nonallergic skin irritation in infants in the area that has contact with the diaper. It can be caused by extended contact with feces, urine, soaps, and ointments, and by friction and the irritating effects of ammonia by-products in urine. The rash is often accompanied by secondary yeast or bacterial infection. Report this condition with ICD-9-CM code 691.0. *Synonym(s): ammonia dermatitis, diaper dermatitis, diaper rash, Jacquet's erythema, napkin rash.*

Jadassohn-Lewandowski syndrome Abnormal thickness and elevation of nail plates with palmar and plantar hyperkeratosis. The tongue is white color. Report this disorder with ICD-9-CM code 757.5.

Jadassohn-Pellizzari disease Skin condition found predominantly in females between ages 20 and 40 in which circumscribed areas of round or oval flesh-toned lesions develop that become thin, atrophic, wrinkled, and pale protrusions with loss of elasticity. The lesions develop after an inflammatory outbreak. This condition is reported with ICD-9-CM code 701.3. *Synonym(s): Jadassohn's anetoderma.*

Jadassohn-Tièche nevus Benign, usually solitary, dark blue to black neoplasm made up of melanocytes that presents as a somewhat firm, well defined, and rounded nodule. *Synonym(s): blue nevus, dermal melanocytoma.*

Jaffe-Lichtenstein (-Uehlinger) syndrome Osteitis with fibrous degeneration and formation of cysts, along with fibrous nodules on affected bones due to misfunctioning parathyroid gland. Report this disorder with ICD-9-CM code 252.01. *Synonym(s): Engel-von Recklinghausen syndrome.*

Jahnke's syndrome Angioma in trigeminal nerve, homolateral meningeal angioma with intracranial calcification, and/or angioma of choroid. Report this disorder with ICD-9-CM code 759.6.

Jakob-Creutzfeldt disease Progressive dementia, wasting of muscles, tremor, and other symptoms. Communicable, rare spongiform encephalopathy occurring in middle life with progressive destruction of the pyramidal and extrapyramidal systems to death. Report this disorder with a code from ICD-9-CM subcategory 046.1.

Jaksch (-Hayem-Luzet) syndrome Anemic disorder among children younger than age 3 characterized by acute hemolytic anemia, infections, and gastrointestinal disorders. Report this disorder with ICD-9-CM code 285.8.

janiceps Form of craniopagus in which the heads of conjoined twins are fused with the faces looking in opposite directions. This condition is named after Janus, the two-faced Roman god, and is reported with ICD-9-CM code 759.4.

Jannetta decompression Microsurgery relieving pressure on the cranial nerves.

Jannetta procedure Microsurgical procedure done to relieve the pain caused by trigeminal neuralgia in which a tiny, nonabsorbable sponge is inserted to decompress the sensory root of the nerve by relieving the pressure put upon it by the surrounding blood vessels. Report this procedure with ICD-9-CM procedure code 04.41 or CPT code 61450. *Synonym(s): microvascular decompression, MVD.*

Jansky-Bielschowsky disease Late infantile type of neuronal ceroid lipofuscinosis or amaurotic familial idiocy. It is an inherited disorder in which the body stores excessive amounts of lipofuscin, the pigment that remains after damaged cells are broken down and digested, resulting in progressive nervous tissue damage, vision loss, and fatality. This disease is reported with ICD-9-CM code 330.1.

Japanese B type encephalitis Acute mosquito-borne, epidemic viral infection seen in southern and eastern Asia, affecting the central nervous system. Although frequently asymptomatic, patients may develop fever, chills, gastrointestinal symptoms, confusion, and agitation. In the most severe cases, meningoencephalomyelitis develops with cortical damage and spinal cord lesions forming like those occurring in polio, possibly becoming fatal. Report this condition with ICD-9-CM code 062.0. *Synonym(s): Russian autumnal encephalitis.*

Japanese flood fever Acute infectious disease resembling typhus, caused by rickettsia bacteria and transmitted by the bite of infected larval mites, called chiggers. This disease occurs chiefly in Asia and the Pacific and is manifested by a specific telltale lesion or eschar at the site of the bite, fever, regional lymphadenopathy, and skin lesions and rashes. Report this disease with ICD-9-CM code 081.2. *Synonym(s): akamushi disease, inundation fever, island fever, Japanese river fever, kedani fever, mite-borne typhus, Mossman fever, scrub typhus, shimamushi disease, tropical typhus, tsutsugamushi disease.*

Japanese river fever Acute infectious disease resembling typhus, caused by rickettsia bacteria and transmitted by the bite of infected larval mites, called chiggers. This disease occurs chiefly in Asia and the Pacific and is manifested by a specific telltale lesion or eschar at the site of the bite, fever, regional lymphadenopathy, and skin lesions and rashes. Report this disease with ICD-9-CM code 081.2. *Synonym(s): akamushi disease, inundation fever, island fever, Japanese flood fever, kedani fever, mite-borne typhus, Mossman fever, scrub typhus, shimamushi disease, tropical typhus, tsutsugamushi disease.*

Jatene procedure Corrective measure performed for transposition of the great vessels when there is subaortic stenosis and narrowing of the left aortic ventricular junction, requiring reconstruction of these sites as well

as surgical correction of the transposed aortic and pulmonary arteries. *Synonym(s): TGV repair.*

jaundice Increased bilirubin and deposits of bile pigment in the skin and sclera, causing a yellow tint. *Synonym(s): icterus.*

jaw-winking syndrome Eyelids widen during chewing, sometimes with an elevation of upper lid when mouth is open and closing of the lid when mouth is closed. Report this disorder with ICD-9-CM code 742.8.

JCAHO Joint Commission on Accreditation of Healthcare Organizations. Organization that accredits health care organizations. In the future, the JCAHO may play a role in certifying these organizations' compliance with the HIPAA A/S requirements. Previously known as the Joint Commission for the Accreditation of Hospitals.

JD Doctor of jurisprudence.

Jefferson's Fracture

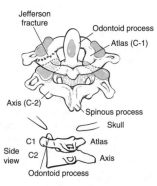

Jefferson's fracture Fracture of C1, usually the result of a diving accident or a heavy object falling onto the patient's head, reported with ICD-9-CM code 805.01 or a code from subcategory 806.0 if the fracture includes a spinal cord injury.

jejunal syndrome Emptying of contents of jejunum with nausea, sweating, weakness, palpitation, syncope, warmth, and diarrhea occurring after eating in patients who have had partial gastrectomy and gastrojejunostomy. Report this disorder with ICD-9-CM code 564.2. *Synonym(s): dumping syndrome.*

jejunitis Condition in which the upper portion of the small intestine between the duodenum and the ileum is inflamed and irritated. Report this condition with ICD-9-CM code 558.9.

jejuno- Relating to the jejunum (part of the small intestine).

jejunostomy Permanent, surgical opening into the jejunum, the part of the small intestine between the duodenum and ileum, through the abdominal wall, often used for placing a feeding tube.

jejunum Highly vascular upper two-fifths of the small intestine, extending from the duodenum to the ileum.

Jenamicin See gentamycin sulfate.

Jensen's disease Eye condition characterized by small areas of inflammation on the interior back portion of the eyeball (fundus) near the optic disc or papilla, found in young, healthy individuals. Report this condition with ICD-9-CM code 363.05. *Synonym(s): Jensen's retinitis, retinochoroiditis juxtapapillaris.*

Jericho boil Dry or urban cutaneous leishmaniasis, one form of Old World cutaneous leishmaniasis. This parasitic skin disease is caused by the protozoa Leishmania tropica, spread by the bite of sand flies, and occurring in large urban areas in the Middle East, especially Iran and Iraq, the Mediterranean, and India. Manifestation is mainly a single, large developing boil or furuncle type lesion that persists over a year. Lymphadenopathy may be present. Report this condition with ICD-9-CM code 085.1. *Synonym(s): Aleppo boil, Baghdad boil, Biskra boil, Delhi boil, Gafsa boil.*

Jervell-Lange-Nielsen syndrome Specific form of long QT syndrome, a potentially fatal condition precipitated by vigorous exertion, emotional upset, or startling moments due to an imbalance in the electrical timing mechanism that controls the pumping action of the heart's ventricles. This syndrome causes the patient to be susceptible to recurrent episodes of syncope, collapse, and possible ventricular fibrillation that can cause sudden death. Jervell-Lange Nielsen syndrome is characterized by the additional manifestation of neural deafness and is reported the same as long QT syndrome with ICD-9-CM code 426.82.

jet lag syndrome Imbalance of a normal sleep pattern rhythm resulting from airplane travel through a number of time zones. Leads to fatigue, irritability, and other constitutional disturbances. Report this disorder with ICD-9-CM code 307.45.

Jeune's syndrome Pelvis and phalanges are malformed, and cartilage of rib cage is unable to support breath action, leading to asphyxia. Report this disorder with ICD-9-CM code 756.4. *Synonym(s): asphyxiating thoracic dystrophy (ATD).*

JE-VAX Brand name Japanese encephalitis vaccine provided in a single-dose vial. Supply of JE-VAX is reported with CPT code 90735; administration is reported separately. The need for vaccination is reported with ICD-9-CM code V05.8.

Jevity Brand name enteral nutrition. Supply of Jevity is reported with HCPCS Level II code B4152.

JHITA Joint Healthcare Information Technology Alliance.

jigger disease Disease spread by the parasitic flea, Tunga penetrans, the pregnant female of which burrows into the host's skin, often the lower limbs and under nails, causing inflammation, swelling, and cyst formation that turns ulcerative. Gas gangrene, bacteremia, or tetanus may occur in cases of severe infestation, as well as spontaneous loss of a digit. Report this condition with ICD-9-CM code 134.1. *Synonym(s): burrowing flea disease, chigoe disease, sand flea disease.*

JNA Juvenile nasopharyngeal angiofibroma. Benign tumor in the nasopharynx in prepubescent and adolescent males. Symptoms of JNA include nasal obstruction, bleeding, and headache. Treatment may include radiation therapy, surgery, or hormone therapy. JNA is reported with ICD-9-CM code 210.7.

Job's syndrome Autosomal disorder of neutrophils with abnormal or absent chemotactic responses, eczema, and staphylococcal abscesses on the skin. Patients tend to be females with fair skin and red hair. Report this disorder with ICD-9-CM code 288.1.

jock itch Fungal infection of the groin (most common in men), reported with ICD-9-CM code 110.3. *Synonym(s): tinea cruris.*

jodbasedow phenomenon Iodine-induced hyperthyroidism, resulting from exposure to larger than normal amounts of iodine, such as contrast medium administration or diet supplement, resulting in thyrotoxicosis in a previously healthy person. Report this condition with a code from ICD-9-CM subcategory 242.8.

JODM Juvenile onset diabetes mellitus.

Johannsen procedure First stage of a two-phase surgical procedure in which the urethra is reconstructed. Report this procedure with ICD-9-CM procedure code 58.46 or CPT code 53400.

Johnson-Stevens disease Type of erythema multiforme that begins with flu-like symptoms and produces severe mucocutaneous lesions affecting the mouth, nose, anal, and genital regions with formation of a grayish-white pseudomembrane, hemorrhagic crusting of the lips, ocular lesions, corneal opacities, even blindness. Other systemic lesions and visceral and thoracic organ involvement also occurs and can be fatal. This condition is reported with ICD-9-CM code 695.13. *Synonym(s): Stevens-Johnson syndrome.*

joint Area of contact, or juncture, between two or more bones, often articulating with each other.

joint capsule Sac-like enclosure enveloping the synovial joint cavity with a fibrous membrane attached to the articular ends of the bones in the joint.

Joint Commission on Accreditation of Healthcare Organizations Organization that accredits health care organizations. In the future, the JCAHO may play a role in certifying these organizations' compliance with the HIPAA A/S requirements. Previously known as the Joint Commission for the Accreditation of Hospitals. *Synonym(s): JCAHO.*

Joint Healthcare Information Technology Alliance Health care industry association that represents the American Health Information Management Association, American Medical Informatics Association, Center for Healthcare Information Management, College of Healthcare Information Management Executives, and Healthcare Information Management Systems Society on legislative and regulatory issues affecting the use of health information technology. *Synonym(s): JHITA.*

joint replacement Insertion of new substitute material in place of damaged or diseased joint tissue to restore function and movement.

joint venture Business undertaking involving a one-time grouping of two or more entities. Although a joint venture is treated like a partnership for federal income tax purposes, it is different from the latter in that it does not involve a continuing relationship among the parties. Joint ventures are, in a sense, short-term partnerships.

Jones and Cantarow test Laboratory test to determine renal efficiency by testing collected urine for urea concentration. Report this procedure with CPT code 84540.

Jones Fracture

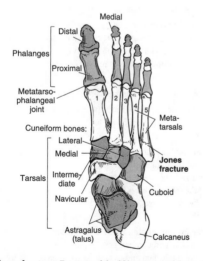

Jones fracture Fracture of the fifth metatarsal (base of the small toe) at the proximal end, next to the cuboid bone. Unlike dancer's fracture, in Jones fracture, the bone is not avulsed. This is a closed fracture treated with casting or a walking boot, so appropriate E/M and

radiology CPT codes apply. The fracture itself is reported with ICD-9-CM code 825.25. Jones fracture may become a chronic condition. In this case, surgery secures the fracture with a screw. A chronic Jones fracture would be reported as a nonunion of fracture, ICD-9-CM code 733.82

Joplin procedure Surgical operation on the foot in which bunions are corrected with tendon transplants. The extensor tendon of the big toe is cut to restore the toe to its correct alignment and then reattached to the head of the metatarsal bone. Other tendons may also be cut and reattached until correct anatomical alignment is achieved. Report this procedure with ICD-9-CM code 77.53 or CPT code 28294.

Jordan's syndrome Hepatosplenomegaly, lymphadenopathy, anemia, and thrombocytopenia with changes in the bones, cardiopulmonary system, skin, and psychomotor skills. Abnormalities of granulation and nuclear structure of white cells opens patient to infection and results in death. Report this disorder with ICD-9-CM code 288.2.

Joseph-Diamond-Blackfan syndrome Congenital anemia of infancy requiring a number of blood transfusions to maintain life. Report this disorder with ICD-9-CM code 284.0.

Joubert syndrome Rare genetic disorder, usually fatal in infancy, in which the middle part of the cerebellum remains partially or completely undeveloped, resulting in lack of coordination, breathing abnormalities, sleep apnea, aberrant movements of the eyes and tongue, decreased muscle tone, and mental retardation. Extra digits, cleft lip or palate, and seizures may also be present. Report this disorder with ICD-9-CM code 759.89.

JPA Juvenile pilocytic astrocytoma. Low-grade brain tumor. JPAs are usually localized and slow growing. They occur most often in children and young adults.

j-pouch Pouch or reservoir constructed from the last 18 inches of the small intestine and attached to the anus. Muscles surrounding the anus and anal canal enable people to control their bowel movements.

jugal bone Cheekbone or zygomatic bone.

jugular foramen Opening formed by the jugular notches on the temporal and occipital bones of the skull that serves as a pathway for the sigmoid sinus, the internal jugular vein, and nerves. J. syndrome Unilateral lesions of the ninth, tenth, eleventh, and twelfth cranial nerves producing paralysis of the vagal, glossal, and other nerves and the tongue on the same side resulting from injury. Report this disorder with ICD-9-CM code 352.6. *Synonym(s): Collet-Sicard syndrome.*

jugular vein Two pairs of veins on either side of the neck that open into the subclavian, sending blood from the head and neck to the heart.

jumpers' knee Form of patellar tendonitis in which partial rupture of the tendon connecting the kneecap to the tibia occurs, often affecting athletes who participate in sports focusing on jumping or throwing or resulting from overuse or injury. Inflammation or tissue degeneration sometimes follows. Report this condition with ICD-9-CM code 727.2.

jungle yellow fever Acute, rare, infectious, vector-borne viral disease contracted by humans bitten by mosquitoes infected with the flavivirus through animals, usually monkeys, in the setting of tropical rain forests in Africa and South America. Manifestations include fever, jaundice, possible kidney damage, and liver necrosis. Report this disease with ICD-9-CM code 060.0. *Synonym(s): sylvan yellow fever.*

juvenile kyphosis Increased curvature of the thoracic spine (kyphosis) usually occurring during growth spurts through adolescence and puberty. Most patients with Scheuermann's disease will have an increased roundback (e.g., hunch back or hump back), poor posture or slouching, and mild to moderate pain. Report this disease with ICD-9-CM code 732.0. *Synonym(s): Scheuermann's disease.*

juvenile retinoschisis Genetic, X-linked disease of the retina that mainly affects males, causing a tear or splitting in the nerve fiber layer of the retina, affecting the macula. Vision acuity loss is caused by the formation of tiny, spoke-like cysts that damage the nerve tissue. Peripheral vision loss is a result of the splitting of the inner layer of nerve cells from the outer layer of nerve cells. This condition is reported with ICD-9-CM code 362.73.

juxta- Next to, near.

JVD Jugular venous distention.

JVP Jugular venous pressure.

JW HCPCS Level II modifier, for use with CPT or HCPCS Level II codes, that identifies a drug amount discarded or not administered to any patient. This modifier is appended to codes for drugs where the dosage listed is greater than ordered and administered by the provider to indicate that the overage was discarded and not part of a multidose vial.

K Potassium.

K or K+ Symbol for potassium, the major electrolyte found in intracellular fluids. Potassium is an important facilitator of skeletal and cardiac muscle activity.

Kabikinase Brand name of streptokinase, an injectable enzyme used to break down and dissolve blood clots by stimulating extra plasmin production. This drug is primarily used to treat myocardial infarction, deep vein thrombosis, and pulmonary embolism. Supply is reported with HCPCS Level II code J2995.

Kabuki make-up syndrome Congenital or genetic disorder manifested by atypical facial features resembling the Kabuki makeup used in traditional Japanese theater. Other abnormalities include dwarfism and scoliosis, also accompanied by impaired intellect. This disorder is reported with ICD-9-CM code 759.89.

Kader operation Surgical procedure in which a temporary gastrostomy is constructed for the instillation of nutrients. Introduction of the feeding tube is via a valve-like flap that closes upon tube withdrawal. Report this procedure with ICD-9-CM procedure code 43.19 or a code from CPT range 43830-43832.

KAFO Knee-ankle-foot orthosis. External apparatus utilized to improve motor control, gait stabilization, and reduce pain. The device is attached to the leg in order to help correct flexible deformities and to halt the progression of fixed deformities.

Kahler (-Bozzolo) disease Rare form of cancer in which the bone marrow's plasma cells are produced at an increased rate, forming multiple bone marrow tumors and bone-destroying lesions that progress to other parts of the body in advanced stages. Symptoms involve bone pain, weakness, spontaneous fractures, anemia, fatigue, and hypercalcemia causing renal cast formation, nephropathy, and kidney failure. This condition is diagnosed by the presence of Bence-Jones protein in the urine. Report this condition with a code from ICD-9-CM subcategory 203.0. *Synonym(s): multiple myeloma, plasma cell myeloma.*

Kahler's syndrome Malignant neoplasm associated with anemia, hemorrhages, recurrent infections, and weakness that originates in bone marrow. Report this disorder with a code from ICD-9-CM range 203.00-203.02.

Kalginate See calcium gluconate.

Kalischer's syndrome Multiple angiomas in skin of head and scalp. Report this disorder with ICD-9-CM code 759.6.

Kallmann's syndrome Failure of sexual development resulting from inadequate secretion of pituitary gonadotropins. Associated with anosmia due to agenesis of the olfactory lobes in the brain, a product of X-linked inheritance. Report this disorder with ICD-9-CM code 253.4.

kanamycin sulfate Bactericidal aminoglycoside used as a bowel preparation prior to intestinal surgery to prevent infection and as an adjunctive therapy to treat hepatic coma. May be sold under the brand name Kantrex.

Kanavel's sign Indication of a tendon sheath infection in which there is a point of greatest tenderness in the palm, one inch proximal to the base of the little finger.

Kanner's syndrome Developmental disorder connected with neurophysiological factors, manifesting in early childhood with definitively impaired communication and social interaction marked by the inability to reciprocate in play, recognize other's feelings or existence, mimic or imitate, or seek comfort. Unusual activities and interests may be present, restricting others, as well as severe behavioral problems. Report this disorder with a code from ICD-9-CM subcategory 299.0. *Synonym(s): autism.*

Kantor's sign Threadlike pattern of contrast material through a filling defect seen in x-ray of the colon. *Synonym(s): string sign.*

Kantrex See kanamycin sulfate.

kaolinosis Occupational lung disease caused by inhaling particles of fine white clay known as kaolin. Report this condition with ICD-9-CM code 502. *Synonym(s): kaolin pneumoconiosis.*

Kaposi's sarcoma Malignant neoplasm caused by vascular proliferation of cutaneous tumors characterized by channels lined with endothelial tissue containing vascular spaced. These types of tumors usually remain confined to the skin and subcutaneous tissue, especially the legs, feet, and toes, but may spread to visceral organs as well. A herpes virus is said to cause the disease and it is most often associated with immunocompromised AIDS patients. Code by site in the 176 rubric of ICD-9-CM.

Kartagener's syndrome Reversal of the position or location of organs or viscera. Report this disorder with ICD-9-CM code 759.3.

karyo- Relating to the nucleus of a cell.

karyrrhexis Breakdown of cell matter during necrosis.

Kasabach-Merritt syndrome Small number of platelets in circulating blood, causing bruising. Report this disorder with ICD-9-CM code 287.39.

Kasai procedure Surgical procedure in which the jejunum is connected to the bile ducts and other portal structures of the liver and gallbladder. Report this procedure with ICD-9-CM procedure code 51.37 or CPT code 47701. *Synonym(s): portoenterostomy.*

Kaschin-Beck disease Endemic, chronic, and slowly progressing degenerative disease of the spine and peripheral joints believed to be caused by eating cereal grains infected with the fungus Fusarium sporotrichiella. This disease occurs mainly in children in Siberia, China, and Korea. Report this condition with a code from ICD-9-CM subcategory 716.0. *Synonym(s): Kashin-Bek, osteoarthritis deformans endemica.*

Kashin-Beck disease Debilitating, chronic, degenerative disease of the peripheral joints and spine, usually affecting children in endemic areas, that causes arthropathy, enlargement of joints, and eventual limb deformity. Afflicted persons have selenium deficiency and abnormal structure or function of lipids, RBC membranes, and cartilage.

Kast's syndrome Benign cartilaginous growths in bones with bleeding in viscera and skin. Report this disorder with ICD-9-CM code 756.4. *Synonym(s): Maffucci's syndrome.*

Katayama disease Acute, systemic illness caused by heavy infestation by the blood fluke Schistosoma japonicum. Manifestations include fever; chills; nausea and vomiting; cough; headache; itching; enlargement of the liver, spleen, and lymph nodes; and elevated levels of eosinophils, IgE, and IgG levels in the blood. Report this condition with ICD-9-CM code 120.2. *Synonym(s): Katayama fever.*

Kawasaki disease Syndrome of unknown origin causing fever; redness of the eyes, lips, and mucous membranes of the mouth; gingivitis; cervical lymphadenopathy, and a bright red raised rash in a glove-and-sock fashion over the hands and feet. The skin there becomes hard, swollen (edematous), and peels. This disease mainly affects children and is reported with ICD-9-CM code 446.1. *Synonym(s): MLNS, mucocutaneous lymph node syndrome.*

Kayser-Fleischer ring Condition found in Wilson's disease in which deposits of copper cause a pigmented ring around the cornea's outer border in the deep epithelial layers. Report this condition with ICD-9-CM codes 275.1 and 371.14.

Kaznelson's syndrome Congenital anemia of infancy and requiring a number of blood transfusions to maintain life. Report this disorder with ICD-9-CM code 284.01.

Kcal Kilocalorie.

KCL Potassium chloride.

Kearns-Sayre syndrome Condition manifested by chronic and progressive paralysis of one or more of the extraocular eye muscles and pigmentary retinal degeneration. Usually beginning before age 20, KSS produces progressive muscle weakness, deafness, dementia, and cataracts. Cardiac conduction abnormalities and cerebellar ataxia are also present. Report this condition with ICD-9-CM code 277.87. *Synonym(s): KSS, ophthalmoplegia plus.*

kedani fever Acute infectious disease resembling typhus, caused by rickettsia bacteria and transmitted by the bite of infected larval mites, called chiggers. This disease occurs chiefly in Asia and the Pacific and is manifested by a specific telltale lesion or eschar at the site of the bite, fever, regional lymphadenopathy, and skin lesions and rashes. Report this disease with ICD-9-CM code 081.2. **Synonym(s):** *akamushi disease, inundation fever, island fever, Japanese flood fever, Japanese river fever, mite-borne typhus, Mossman fever, scrub typhus, shimamushi disease, tropical typhus, tsutsugamushi disease.*

Keen laminectomy Removal of sections of the posterior branches of spinal nerves to affected muscles and spinal accessory nerves to correct torticollis.

Keen's sign Indication of a Pott's fibular fracture in which there is increased diameter of the leg at the malleoli.

Keflin Brand name for cephalothin sodium, an injectable systemic cephalosporin antibiotic used to treat bacterial infections. Supply is reported with HCPCS Level II code J1890.

Kefurox See cefuroxime sodium.

Kefzol See cefazolin sodium.

Kehr's sign Indication in some cases of splenic rupture in which there is severe left shoulder pain.

Keitzer test Sound is used to test the pressure of an external stream of urine.

Kelikian procedure Surgical procedure performed to correct a deformity of the foot when toes are missing and a large gap exists between the toes present. Osteotomies and bone alignments are performed to approximate the toes and eliminate the gap, producing an artificial syndactylism or webbing of the toes. Report this procedure with CPT code 28280.

Keller procedure Surgical correction of a bunion of the foot in which the median eminence and one-third of the base of the proximal phalanx are resected, followed by repair of the plantar plate and stabilization with a longitudinal K-wire. Report this procedure with ICD-9-CM code 77.59 and CPT code 28292.

Kellock sign Indication of pleural effusion in which there is increased vibration of the ribs when the examiner performs sharp percussion with the right hand while holding the left hand securely under the nipple on the thorax.

Kelly's syndrome Condition in middle-aged women with hypochronic anemia, cracks or fissures at the corners of the mouth, painful tongue, and dysphagia due to esophageal stenosis or webs. Report this disorder with ICD-9-CM code 280.8. **Synonym(s):** *Paterson-Brown-Kelly syndrome, Plummer-Vinson syndrome.*

keloid Progressive overgrowth of cutaneous scar tissue that is raised and irregular in shape, caused by excessive formation of collagen during connective tissue repair. This condition is reported with ICD-9-CM code 701.4. **Synonym(s):** *cheloid.*

Kenaject Synthetic corticosteroid used as an antiinflammatory or immunosuppressive agent to treat a wide variety of disorders, including inflammatory conditions, certain forms of arthritis, gout, and certain respiratory conditions. Supply is reported with HCPCS Level II code J3301. Kenaject contains triamcinolone acetonide.

Kenalog Synthetic corticosteroid used as an antiinflammatory or immunosuppressive agent to treat a wide variety of disorders, including inflammatory conditions, certain forms of arthritis, gout, and certain respiratory conditions. Supply is reported with HCPCS Level II code J3301. Kenalog contains triamcinolone acetonide.

Kenya tick typhus Acute, febrile, rickettsial disease transmitted by tick bites and causing a primary lesion at the site of the bite, with rash, muscle and joint pain, headache, chills, fever, and sensitivity to light. It is commonly found in the Mediterranean and around the Black and Caspian Seas, having many names depending on the geographical region. This condition is reported with ICD-9-CM code 082.1. **Synonym(s):** *African tickbite fever, Boutonneuse fever, Indian tick typhus, Marseilles fever, Mediterranean tick fever.*

Keppra Brand name for levetiracetam, an anticonvulsant used in combination with other medications to treat partial onset seizures, indicated for adult patients with a diagnosis of epilepsy. Supply of the injectable form is reported with HCPCS Level II code J1953 by facilities.

Keramos Brand name ceramic total hip replacement system.

keratectasia Congenital or acquired condition in which the cornea of the eye bulges or protrudes abnormally, being thin and scarred. If specified as congenital, report ICD-9-CM code 743.41, otherwise report 371.71. **Synonym(s):** *corneal ectasia.*

keratectomy Surgical removal of corneal tissue.

keratinocytes Largest population of epidermal cells in the skin. Keratinocytes acquire their name through their function as warehouses for keratin, the protein that provides a physical barrier in the most superficial dead cells of the skin.

keratitis Condition in which the cornea becomes inflamed and irritated. Etiology may be infection, injury, exposure to ultraviolet light, chemical or other external irritants, disease, or contact lens irritation. Symptoms include cloudy vision and painful, watering eyes.

kerato- Relating to the cornea or horny tissue.

keratoacanthoma Usually benign tumor of the skin that exhibits rapid growth into a dome-shaped nodule and then regresses and disappears, leaving localized scarring. Keratoacanthomas histologically resemble

J-N

squamous cell carcinoma and are associated with sunlight exposure, usually occurring on areas of exposed skin such as the face, neck, and back of the hands in light-skinned, middle-aged, or elderly adults. Report this condition with ICD-9-CM code 238.2. **multiple k.** Form of keratoacanthoma that erupts in adolescents and young adults in multiple tumors clinically identical to solitary keratoacanthomas, but also appearing on areas of skin not exposed to sunlight. Report this condition with ICD-9-CM code 238.2.

keratocele Bulging or herniation of Descemet's membrane, the cornea's innermost layer. Report this condition with ICD-9-CM code 371.72. **Synonym(s):** keratodermatocele.

keratoconjunctivitis Condition in which both the cornea and the conjunctiva are irritated and inflamed. Etiology may be infection, injury, exposure to ultraviolet light, chemical or other external irritants, disease, or contact lens irritation. Symptoms include cloudy vision and painful, watering eyes.

keratoconjunctivitis sicca Dryness of the cornea and conjunctiva caused by decreased tear secretion, causing irritation and burning. Can escalate to photophobia, ulceration, vascularization, and scarring as the corneal epithelium is eroded.

keratoconus Noninflammatory, bilateral bulging protrusion of the anterior cornea, which forms a cone-shaped dome, with the apex displaced downward toward the nose, resulting in astigmatism and blurred, distorted vision. Corneal transplant may be required in severe cases. Report this condition with ICD-9-CM codes 371.60-371.62, unless specified as congenital, in which case it is reported with 743.41. **Synonym(s):** conical cornea.

keratoderma Excessive growth of a horny, callous layer on the skin in three typical patterns: diffused over the palm and sole, focal with large keratin masses at points of friction, and punctate with tiny drops of keratin on the palmoplantar surface. If the condition is congenital, report ICD-9-CM code 757.39; if acquired, 701.1.

keratodermatocele Bulging or herniation of Descemet's membrane, the cornea's innermost layer. Report this condition with ICD-9-CM code 371.72. **Synonym(s):** keratocele.

keratoglobus Congenital or acquired condition in which the cornea has an abnormally large size, usually occurring bilaterally. Report this condition with ICD-9-CM code 371.70 or 743.22; if specified as congenital, report 743.41. **Synonym(s):** megalocornea.

keratolysis exfoliativa Congenital or acquired skin condition in which the palms and sometimes the soles develop blisters, followed by peeling of the outer layer of epidermis. Young adults are often affected during the summer months. If specified as congenital, report this condition with ICD-9-CM code 757.39, otherwise report 695.89. **Synonym(s):** peeling skin syndrome.

keratomalacia Ocular condition with symptoms of dryness of the eyes, poor night vision, corneal clouding, and softening. This condition is often caused by dietary or metabolic vitamin A deficiency and protein-calorie malnutrition. If specified as due to vitamin A deficiency, report ICD-9-CM code 264.4, otherwise report 371.45.

keratome Specialized surgical instrument or knife used for cutting into the cornea.

keratomileusis Ophthalmologic surgical procedure performed in order to improve visual acuity in which a partial-thickness central portion of the patient's cornea is removed, frozen, and reshaped on an electronic lathe. The revised cornea is then repositioned and secured with sutures. Report this procedure with ICD-9-CM procedure code 11.71 or CPT code 65760.

keratomycosis Corneal infection caused by a fungus. **Synonym(s):** mycotic keratitis.

keratomycosis nigricans Minor fungal infection caused by cladosporium mansoni or Exophiala werneckii, producing lesions that most commonly appear on the hands and rarely on other areas. The lesions look like the characteristic dark ink or dye stain that occurs when silver nitrate is spilled on the skin. Report this condition with ICD-9-CM code 111.1. **Synonym(s):** cladosporiosis epidermica, microsporosis nigra, pityriasis nigra, tinea nigra, tinea palmaris nigra.

keratopathy Disease or disorder of the cornea that is noninflammatory.

keratophakia Ophthalmologic surgical procedure performed in order to correct refractive error. A slice of donor corneal tissue is formed to the desired curvature and transplanted into the middle layer of the recipient's cornea, changing its curvature. Report this procedure with ICD-9-CM procedure code 11.72 or CPT code 65765.

keratoplasty Surgical transplant of all or a portion of the cornea, reported with CPT codes 65710-65756.

keratoprosthesis Surgical procedure in which the physician creates a new anterior chamber with a plastic optical implant that replaces a severely damaged cornea that cannot be repaired. Report this procedure with ICD-9-CM procedure code 11.73 or CPT code 65770.

keratosis Skin condition characterized by a wart-like or callus-type localized overgrowth, hardening, or thickening of the upper skin layer as a result of overproduction of the protein keratin.

keratosis pilaris Common skin condition characterized by small, discrete bumps around the hair follicles, especially on the back and sides of the upper arms and thighs. Report this condition with ICD-9-CM code 701.1; if congenital, report 757.39.

keratotomy Surgical incision of the cornea.

J-N

keraunoparalysis Temporary, short-lived paralysis resulting from the impact of being struck by lightning. Acute constriction of blood vessels and sensory disturbances of one or more extremities are also associated with this condition. Report keraunoparalysis with ICD-9-CM code 994.0. *Synonym(s): lightning paralysis.*

Kernig's sign Positive sign for meningitis. Severe stiffness in the hamstrings prevents legs from being straightened when the hip is flexed to 90 degrees. This test would be performed as part of an evaluation and management service. Codes for meningitis are selected according to causal agent.

Kestrone-5 See estrogen.

ketoacidosis Abnormal increase in the acidity of body fluids and tissues (acidosis) caused by the increased accumulation of ketone bodies, most often seen in Type 1 diabetes or excessive alcohol consumption. If ketoacidosis is specified as diabetic, report with a code from ICD-9-CM category 249.1 or 250.1; otherwise, report 276.2.

ketonuria Condition often seen in uncontrolled diabetes mellitus in which there are abnormally high levels of ketone bodies, a byproduct of cell breakdown, in the urine. Starvation, fasting, eating disorders, and dieting can also result in ketonuria. Symptoms may include increased thirst, urinary frequency, dehydration, nausea and vomiting, pupil dilation, confusion, and a fruity odor to the breath. Report ketonuria with ICD-9-CM code 791.6.

ketorolac tromethamine Nonsteroidal antiinflammatory used for short-term pain management. Supply is reported with HCPCS Level II code J1885. May be sold under the brand name Toradol.

key components Three components of history, examination, and medical decision making are considered the keys to selecting the correct level of E/M codes. In most cases, all three components must be addressed in the documentation. However, in established, subsequent, and follow-up categories, only two of the three must be met or exceeded for a given code.

key portion Part (or parts) of a service determined by the teaching physician to be the critical or key portion.

K-Feron See iron.

K-Flex Brand name of orphenadrine citrate, an injectable muscle relaxant used in the treatment of Parkinson's disease and muscle spasms. Supply is reported with HCPCS Level II code J2360.

kg Kilogram.

KG HCPCS Level II modifier for use with HCPCS Level II codes that identifies a durable medical equipment, prosthetics, orthotics, and supplies (DMEPOS) item that is subject to the DMEPOS competitive bidding program number 1.

KH HCPCS Level II modifier for use with HCPCS Level II codes that identifies a durable medical equipment, prosthetics, orthotics, and supplies (DMEPOS) item, initial claim, purchase or first month rental. Report with modifier RR for rented DME.

KI HCPCS Level II modifier for use with HCPCS Level II codes that identifies a durable medical equipment, prosthetics, orthotics, and supplies (DMEPOS) item, second- or third-month rental. Report with modifier RR for rented DME.

kickbacks Receiving payment (or other benefits) for making a referral.

kidney, ureter, bladder x-ray Radiographic pictures of the kidneys, ureters, and bladder to assess abnormalities.

Kienböck's disease Idiopathic, progressive osteochondrosis affecting the lunate bone of the wrist in which the bone undergoes osteonecrosis, or death of the bone tissue, due to a lack of blood supply. Symptoms may initially mimic those of a sprained wrist, but the lunate bone soon begins to collapse. Arthritis of the wrist develops. Advanced stages require surgical treatment. Report this condition with ICD-9-CM code 732.3 or 732.8. *Synonym(s): lunatomalacia.*

Kikuchi disease Benign lymphadenopathy syndrome manifested by swollen glands in the neck, fever, necrotizing lesions in the area around the thymus cortex, flu-like symptoms, and an increase in distinct types of histiocytes, monocytes, and immunoblasts. Predominantly occurring in females, this disease is sometimes considered a self-limiting form of systemic lupus erythematosus. Report this condition with ICD-9-CM code 289.3. *Synonym(s): histiocytic necrotizing lymphadenitis, Kikuchi-Fujimoto disease, Kikuchi lymphadenitis, subacute necrotizing lymphadenitis.*

Killian operation Surgical procedure in which the anterior wall of the frontal sinus is excised, the diseased tissue removed, and a permanent opening is created between the nasal cavity and the maxillary sinus in order to facilitate sinus drainage. Report this procedure with ICD-9-CM procedure code 22.41 or CPT codes 31070-31087. *Synonym(s): frontal sinusotomy.*

Kimmelstiel-Wilson syndrome High blood pressure and kidney failure resulting from a form of diabetes in which carbohydrate utilization is reduced and lipid and protein enhanced. Report this disorder with a code from ICD-9-CM subcategory 249.4 or 250.4, and 581.81.

Kimmerle's anomaly Small bridge of bone at C1, resulting from ossification of the atlanto-occipital membrane and thought to be a source of migraine headaches and potential disorders of the vertebral

J-N

arteries and cerebrum. Kimmerle's anomaly is reported with ICD-9-CM code 723.8 with secondary codes to describe symptoms. *Synonym(s): foramen arcual, ponticulus posticus.*

Kindercal TF Brand name pediatric enteral nutrition. Supply of Kindercal TF is reported with HCPCS Level II code B4150.

kinetics Motion or movement.

Kinnier Wilson's disease Rare, progressive, chronic disease caused by an inherited copper metabolism defect that results in the poisonous accumulation of copper in certain organs and tissues, such as the brain, kidneys, cornea, and liver. The disease causes cirrhosis, brain degeneration with progressive neurological dysfunction, and pigmented Kayser-Fleischer corneal ring. Report this condition with ICD-9-CM code 275.1. *Synonym(s): familial hepatitis, hepatolenticular degeneration, pseudosclerosis of Westphal, Westphal-Struempell disease, Wilson's disease.*

KJ *1)* HCPCS Level II modifier for use with HCPCS Level II codes that identifies a durable medical equipment, prosthetics, orthotics, and supplies (DMEPOS) item, parenteral enteral nutrition (PEN) pump or capped rental, months four to 15. Report with modifier RR for rented DME. *2)* Knee jerk.

KK HCPCS Level II modifier for use with HCPCS Level II codes that identifies a durable medical equipment, prosthetics, orthotics, and supplies (DMEPOS) item that is subject to the DMEPOS competitive bidding program number 2.

KL HCPCS Level II modifier for use with HCPCS Level II codes that identifies a durable medical equipment, prosthetics, orthotics, and supplies (DMEPOS) item that is delivered by mail.

Klauder's syndrome Necrolysis of skin caused by toxins. Report this disorder with ICD-9-CM code 695.19.

Klebcil See kanamycin sulfate.

Kleine-Levin syndrome Rare disorder causing excessive drowsiness and sleep. Symptoms may last for 20 hours a day, for days or weeks at a time. Onset is typically in adolescence and is more common in males. Kleine-Levin syndrome is reported with ICD-9-CM code 327.13. *Synonym(s): Critchley's syndrome, Kleine-Levin-Critchley syndrome.*

Klein-Waardenburg syndrome Eyebrow or upper or lower eyelid sags. Report this disorder with ICD-9-CM code 270.2. *Synonym(s): Mendes syndrome, van der Hoeve-Halbertsma-Waardenburg syndrome, Waardenburg-Klein syndrome.*

kleptomania Psychiatric disorder in which one experiences tension with an uncontrollable impulse to steal objects that are not needed, followed by pleasure or relief upon taking the object, without any precipitating factors of anger, delusions, vengeance, or hallucinations. Report this disorder with ICD-9-CM code 312.32.

Klinefelter's syndrome Male in development, but with seminal tube dysgenesis, gynecomastia, and urinary gonadotropins. Report this disorder with ICD-9-CM code 758.7. *Synonym(s): XXY syndrome.*

Klippel-Feil syndrome Shorter than average neck and a low hairline caused by fewer than average cervical vertebrae or fusion of hemivertebrae into one bony mass. Report this disorder with ICD-9-CM code 756.16.

Klippel-Trenaunay syndrome Rare congenital disorder characterized by large, benign cutaneous hemangiomas and port wine stains; excessive growth of the soft tissue and bone of the extremities, usually affecting one side; and varicose veins. This condition is classified to ICD-9-CM code 759.89.

Klumpke (-Déjérine) syndrome Atrophic paralysis of forearm and hand as result of birth trauma to brachial plexus. Report this disorder with ICD-9-CM code 767.6.

Klüver-Bucy (-Terzian) syndrome Bilateral temporal lobe ablation with psychic hyperreactivity to visual stimuli or blindness, increased oral and sexual activity, and depressed drive and emotional reactions. Report this disorder with ICD-9-CM code 310.0. *Synonym(s): lobectomy behavior syndrome.*

KM HCPCS Level II modifier, for use with CPT or HCPCS Level II codes, that identifies replacement of a facial prosthesis, including a new impression or moulage.

Knapp's operation Peripheral opening in the capsule is formed behind the iris to remedy a cataract.

knock-knee Condition in which the thighs slant inward, causing the knees to be angled abnormally close together, leaving the space between the ankles wider than normal. If specified as congenital, report this condition with ICD-9-CM code 755.64, otherwise report 736.41. *Synonym(s): genu valgum.*

KO *1)* HCPCS Level II modifier for use with HCPCS Level II codes that identifies a single drug unit dose formulation. May be used to report drugs used or supplied by DMERCs. *2)* Keep open. *3)* Knee orthosis.

Koate-HP See factor VIII.

Köbner's disease Group of uncommon, inherited skin disorders manifested by frequently occurring painful blisters and open sores. Köbner's disease often occurs as a result of minor trauma, due to the skin's abnormally fragile state. The eyes, tongue, and esophagus may be involved in the more severe forms of the disease, and scarring and musculoskeletal abnormalities may occur. Report this disorder with ICD-9-CM code 757.39. *Synonym(s): epidermolysis bullosa.*

Kocher maneuver Performed as a means of reducing anterior shoulder dislocations. The arm is abducted, rotated externally, then adducted and rotated internally;

J–N

reported as a closed reduction of anterior shoulder dislocation.

Koch-Weeks conjunctivitis Acute contagious inflammation and irritation of the conjunctiva that normally occurs in the spring or fall and is caused by a variant of the H. influenzae bacteria. Report this condition with ICD-9-CM code 372.03. **Synonym(s):** *pink eye.*

Kock Procedure

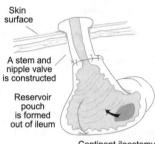

Skin surface

A stem and nipple valve is constructed

Reservoir pouch is formed out of ileum

Continent ileostomy
(44316)

A Kock style ileostomy involves the creation of a reservoir to hold waste material. A stem and nipple valve may also be constructed. The waste is drawn out by tube as needed

Kock procedure Surgical procedure in which the physician forms a reservoir of distal ileum (Kock pouch) and brings it through the abdominal wall onto the skin as a continent ileostomy. Report this procedure with ICD-9-CM procedure code 46.22 or CPT code 44316.

Kogenate See factor VIII.

KOH Potassium hydroxide. *K. examination.* Potassium hydroxide examination. Diagnostic laboratory test used to detect a fungal or yeast infection of the skin. A scraping of the lesion is obtained, placed in a potassium hydroxide solution, and examined under a microscope, where the fungus is visible if present. Report this test with CPT code 87220. **Synonym(s):** *fungal wet prep.*

Köhler-Pellegrini-Stieda syndrome Calcification of medial collateral ligament of the knee. Report this disorder with ICD-9-CM code 726.62.

koilonychia Congenital condition manifested by flattened, concave nails, reported with ICD-9-CM code 757.5.

Konakion Brand name for injectable phytonadione, a synthetic form of vitamin K. Primary indication is as an antidote for warfarin overdose, and is also used to control bleeding due to vitamin K deficiency. Supply is reported with HCPCS Level II code J3430.

König's syndrome Alternating constipation and diarrhea with pain meteorism and gurgling sounds in the right

iliac fossa. Report this disorder with ICD-9-CM code 564.89.

Konyne See factor IX.

Konyne 80 Brand name for one of the factor IX concentrates. Konyne 80 is normally prescribed to prevent or control bleeding episodes in hemophilia B, which causes factor IX deficiency.

Konyne-HT See factor IX.

Koop inguinal orchiopexy Undescended testicle is retrieved from the abdomen via an inguinal approach.

Koplik's spots Small, separate, raised bright red spots with bluish white centers appearing in the mouth on the inside of the cheeks that are a prodrome, or first indication, of measles infection. After the measles rash appears on the skin, these spots will lighten and disappear. Report this condition with ICD-9-CM code 055.9.

Korotkoff sounds Sounds heard during auscultatory determination of blood pressure. The sounds are produced by artery distension occurring suddenly upon release of the pneumatic cuff, which had first relaxed the artery walls.

Korsakoff (-Wernicke) syndrome Amnestic dementia in which the patient cannot remember short-term or long-term memories but is not delirious. Report this disorder with ICD-9-CM code 294.0.

Korsakoff's psychosis alcoholic Syndrome of prominent and lasting reduction of memory span, including striking loss of recent memory, disordered time appreciation, and confabulation, occurring in alcoholics as the sequel to an acute alcoholic psychosis or, more rarely, in the course of chronic alcoholism. It is usually accompanied by peripheral neuritis and may be associated with Wernicke's encephalopathy.

Korsakoff's psychosis nonalcoholic Syndrome of prominent and lasting reduction of memory span, including striking loss of recent memory, disordered time appreciation, and confabulation frequently caused by substance abuse and malnutrition. An amnestic syndrome may be present in early states of presenile and senile dementia, arteriosclerotic dementia, and in encephalitis and other inflammatory and degenerative diseases and certain temporal lobe tumors.

Korte-Ballance anastomosis Facial and hypoglossal nerves are joined.

Kostmann's syndrome Bronchiectasis and pancreatic insufficiency, resulting in malnutrition, sinusitis, short stature, and bone abnormalities. Report this disorder with ICD-9-CM code 288.01.

KP HCPCS Level II modifier for use with HCPCS Level II codes that identifies the first drug of a multiple drug unit dose formulation. May be used to report drugs used or supplied by DMERCs.

J-N

KQ HCPCS Level II modifier for use with HCPCS Level II codes that identifies the second or subsequent drug of a multiple drug unit dose formulation. May be used to report drugs used or supplied by DMERCs.

KR HCPCS Level II modifier for use with HCPCS Level II codes that identifies partial-month billing for a rental item. Report with modifier RR for rented DME.

Krabbe's leukodystrophy Inherited disorder characterized by a deficiency of the enzyme galactosylceramidase, resulting in rapid destruction of cerebral myelin and globoid bodies in the brain's white matter. Infants develop seizures, deafness, blindness, paralysis, and mental deficiencies. Report this disorder with ICD-9-CM code 330.0. *Synonym(s): galactosylceramide lipidosis, globoid cell leukodystrophy.*

Kraske Procedure

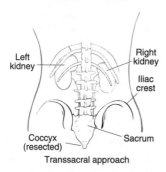

Left kidney

Right kidney

Iliac crest

Coccyx (resected)

Sacrum

Transsacral approach

Kraske procedure Surgical procedure in which a portion of the rectum is removed through a transsacral approach. Report this procedure with ICD-9-CM procedure code 48.64 or CPT code 45116.

kraurosis Condition in which the skin, mucous membrane, or body part becomes dry, shriveled, and atrophied. Underlying causes may include disease or disuse.

Krause decompression Gasserian ganglion is excised to relieve trigeminal neuralgia.

Krause operation Surgical procedure in which the physician releases pressure on the sensory root (gasserian ganglion) of the trigeminal nerve, which innervates the face, in order to relieve symptoms of trigeminal neuralgia. Report this procedure with ICD-9-CM procedure code 04.41 or CPT code 61450.

Krause's glands Accessory lacrimal glands.

Krimer's palatoplasty Physician sutures mucoperiosteal flaps from each side of the palatal cleft at the medial line.

Kroenlein procedure Lateral orbital decompression to relieve forward pressure on the eye when the orbital

contents have increased in size (e.g., Graves's disease, thyroid eye disease).

Krukenberg's spindle Condition in which the posterior surface of the cornea in both eyes contain a vertical, brown, spindle-shaped pigment. It is most often found in women age 20 or older who are nearsighted. Report this condition with ICD-9-CM code 371.13.

Krupin-Denver valve implant Eponym for an eye implant used to mitigate glaucoma. Insertion of the Krupin-Denver valve implant is reported with CPT code 66180; revision with 66185; and removal with 67120.

krypton laser Laser light energy that uses ionized krypton by electric current as the active source, has a radiation beam between the visible yellow-red spectrum, and is effective in photocoagulation of retinal bleeding, macular lesions, and vessel aberrations of the choroid.

KSPT Kaufman Speech Praxis Test. Language development test for children ages 24 to 71 months.

KSS Kearns-Sayre syndrome. Condition manifested by chronic and progressive paralysis of one or more of the extraocular eye muscles and pigmentary retinal degeneration. Usually beginning before age 20, KSS produces progressive muscle weakness, deafness, dementia, and cataracts. Cardiac conduction abnormalities and cerebellar ataxia are also present. Report this condition with ICD-9-CM code 277.87. *Synonym(s): ophthalmoplegia plus.*

KTS Klippel-Trenaunay syndrome.

KU HCPCS Level II modifier for use with HCPCS Level II codes that identifies a durable medical equipment, prosthetics, orthotics, and supplies (DMEPOS) item that is subject to the DMEPOS competitive bidding program number 3.

KUB Kidneys, ureters, bladder.

Kufs' disease Adult type of neuronal ceroid lipofuscinosis or amaurotic familial idiocy. It is an inherited disorder in which the body stores excessive amounts of lipofuscin, the pigment that remains after damaged cells are broken down and digested, resulting in progressive nervous tissue damage, vision loss, and fatality. Kufs' manifests around age 40 with excessive CNS lipofuscin storage causing neurological deterioration and a shorter life expectancy. Kufs' disease is the only form of neuronal ceroid lipofuscinosis in which blindness does not occur. Report this disease with ICD-9-CM code 330.1.

Kuhnt-Szymanowski Outdated method used to repair a lower eyelid that does not rest against the eyeball (ectropion).

Kunkel syndrome Chronic hepatitis with autoimmune manifestations. Report this disorder with ICD-9-CM code 571.49. *Synonym(s): lupoid hepatitis.*

J–N

Kussmaul breathing Rapid, labored breathing seen in patients with metabolic acidosis and most often associated with diabetic ketoacidosis. Diabetic ketoacidosis is reported with a code from ICD-9-CM subcategory 249.1 or 250.1. Known as air hunger, this respiratory compensation can also be seen in patients with renal failure, pneumonia, peritonitis, or severe hemorrhage. *Synonym(s): air hunger, Kussmaul-Kien respiration.*

KVO Keep vein open.

KW HCPCS Level II modifier for use with HCPCS Level II codes that identifies a durable medical equipment, prosthetics, orthotics, and supplies (DMEPOS) item that is subject to the DMEPOS competitive bidding program number 4.

kwashiokor Malnutrition syndrome, particularly of children, with increased carbohydrate intake and inadequate protein intake resulting in inhibited growth potential, anomalies in skin and hair pigmentation, edema, and liver disease.

K-wires Steel wires for skeletal fixation of fractured bones, inserted through soft tissue and bones. *Synonym(s): Kirschner wires.*

KX HCPCS Level II modifier for use with CPT or HCPCS Level II codes, that identifies when specific required documentation is on file. Used to indicate that the required documentation is on file at the DMERC suppliers. The documentation must be supplied if requested by the payer.

KY HCPCS Level II modifier for use with HCPCS Level II codes that identifies a durable medical equipment, prosthetics, orthotics, and supplies (DMEPOS) item that is subject to the DMEPOS competitive bidding program number 5.

kyphoscoliosis Combined posterior convexity and lateral curvature of the spine.

kyphosis Abnormal posterior convex curvature of the spine, usually in the thoracic region, resembling a hunchback.

Kytril See granisetron.

L *1)* Left vertebrae. *2)* Lumbar vertebrae.

L&A Light and accommodation.

L&W Living and well.

LA *1)* Long-acting. *2)* Left atrium.

LAA Left atrial appendage.

labial Around the lip or pertaining to a lip.

labial frenum Connecting fold of mucous membrane that joins the upper or lower lip to the gums at the inside midcenter.

labor Rhythmic, progressive contractions of the uterus that cause retraction and dilation of the cervix, resulting in the birth of a child.

laboratory results In the claims attachment proposed rule, clinic information as a result of biological, microbiological, serological, chemical, immuno-hematological, hematological, biophysical, cytological, pathology, or other examinations of materials from the human body.

labyrinth Another name for the inner ear because of its circular, maze-like series of canals, including the cochlea, semicircular canals, saccule, and utricle.

LAC Long arm cast.

laceration Tearing injury; a torn, ragged-edged wound.

lacosamide Generic injectable antiepileptic drug indicated for the treatment of partial-onset seizures. Approved for use as an add-on therapy in patients 17 years of age and older, lacosamide may also be sold under the brand name of Vimpat and is reported with HCPCS Level II code C9254.

lacrimal Tear-producing gland or ducts that provides lubrication and flushing of the eyes and nasal cavities. *l. punctum* Opening of the lacrimal papilla of the eyelid through which tears flow to the canaliculi to the lacrimal sac.

lacrimotome Knife for cutting the lacrimal sac or duct.

lacrimotomy Incision of the lacrimal sac or duct.

lactiferous duct Duct that drains the mammary glands of the breast.

lacuna Small anatomic cavity. A lacunar infarct of the brain describes an abnormal condition in which a small vessel in the brain is occluded. The condition is indexed to ICD-9-CM code 434.91. Urethral lacunae are naturally occurring pits in the mucous membrane of the urethra. Resorption lacunae are naturally occurring pits in bone. A visual lacuna refers to a defect in the visual field (scotoma) and is reported with a code from ICD-9-CM subcategory 368.4.

LAD Left anterior descending.

LADA Latent autoimmune diabetes in adults. Type I diabetes occurring in adults. Type I diabetes usually presents in children or very young adults; LADA presents as autoimmune disease in adults beyond their 20s. LADA is reported using ICD-9-CM fifth-digits 1 and 3 indicating Type I diabetes mellitus.

LAE Left atrial enlargement.

lag screw Screw with threads at the tip only; used for compression.

lag study Report used by plan managers to determine how long claims are pending and how much is paid out each month.

J-L

lagophthalmos Condition of the eye that prevents it from closing completely.

LAIS Lateral internal anal sphincterotomy. Usually performed as a treatment for anal fissure, LAIS involves cutting the internal sphincter muscle to relieve pressure. LAIS alone is reported with CPT code 46080; if performed concurrently with anal fissurectomy, report 46200. Acquired anal fissure is reported with ICD-9-CM code 565.0 and congenital with 751.5.

Lambert-Eaton syndrome Progressive proximal muscle weakness resulting from antibodies directed against motor-nerve axon terminals. Report this disorder with ICD-9-CM code 358.1.

Lambrinudi arthrodesis Triple fusion prevents the foot drop that may result from polio.

LAMC Large area metropolitan county, a CMS designation.

lamina Thin, flat plate or layer of membrane or other tissue; generally refers to the lamina of the vertebra.

lamina basalis choroideae Transparent inner layer of the choroid that comes in contact with the pigmented layer of the retina. *Synonym(s): basal lamina, Bruch's membrane, complexus basalis choroideae, vitreal lamina.*

laminectomy Removal or excision of the posterior arch of a vertebra to provide additional space for the nerves and widen the spinal canal.

laminoplasty Creating a gutter in the vertebral lamina, with one side acting like a hinge, and the other opening like a door to decompress a pinched spinal cord. The hinge is held in place with small bone struts and a bone graft may be fitted into the open door position with miniplates, wires, or suture. This procedure is reported with CPT codes 63050-63051.

laminotomy Surgical incision to divide the lamina, forming the posterior arch of a vertebra, to take pressure off nerve roots, sometimes caused by the rupture of a herniated vertebral disk.

lance Incise with a lancet.

lancet Pointed surgical knife.

Landboldt's operation Double pedicle or flap of eyelid skin is taken from the upper lid to form a lower eyelid.

Lane's operation Fecal production is halted by dividing the ileum near the cecum to close the distal portion of the colon. The proximal end of the colon is anastomosized with the upper part of the rectum or lower part of the sigmoid.

Langdon Down syndrome Congenital retardation with retarded growth, flat face with short nose, epicanthic skin folds, protruding lower lip, rounded ears, thickened tongue, pelvic dysplasia, broad hands and feet, stubby fingers, and absence of Moro reflex. Report this disorder with ICD-9-CM code 758.0.

Langer-Giedion syndrome Congenital defect characterized by a combination of mental retardation and deformities including peculiar faces with bulb-like nose, small head, little hair, redundant skin, multiple exostoses, and joint laxity. Report this syndrome with ICD-9-CM code 759.89. *Synonym(s): Ale-Calo syndrome.*

Lanoxin See digoxin.

lanugo Soft, fine hair that covers most of the fetus before birth. Persistent lanugo is the presence of this hair after birth, particularly on the limbs, trunk, or face, most commonly seen in premature births. Presence of lanugo is reported with ICD-9-CM code 757.4.

LAP Leucine aminopeptidase.

lap. *1)* Laparoscopy. *2)* Laparotomy.

laparo- *1)* Flank, loins. *2)* Operations through the abdominal wall.

laparoscope Endoscopic instrument placed through the peritoneum to visualize the abdominal cavity internally.

laparoscopic Minimally invasive procedure used for intraabdominal inspection; surgery that uses an endoscopic instrument inserted through small access incisions into the peritoneum for video-controlled imaging. *NCD Reference: 100.13.*

laparoscopy Direct visualization of the peritoneal cavity, outer fallopian tubes, uterus, and ovaries utilizing a laparoscope, a thin, flexible fiberoptic tube. Laparoscopy can be performed for diagnostic purposes alone or included as part of other surgical procedures accomplished by this approach.

laparotomy Incision through the flank or abdomen for therapeutic or diagnostic purposes. *Synonym(s): celiotomy.*

lapse Terminated policy.

Laroyenne operation Douglas pouch is punctured to evacuate pus and to facilitate drainage.

Larsen's syndrome Genetic, multi-system disorder presenting with multiple dislocations and other bony irregularities, as well as cylindrical fingers and a flattened face. Other symptoms include mental retardation, short stature, and cardiac abnormalities. This syndrome is reported with ICD-9-CM code 755.8.

laryng(o)- Relating to the larynx.

laryngeal nerves Superior and recurrent (inferior) laryngeal branches of the vagus nerve.

laryngo- Relating to the larynx.

laryngofissure Surgical opening into the larynx through the thyroid cartilage. *Synonym(s): median laryngotomy.*

laryngoscopy Examination of the larynx with an endoscope.

J–N

larynx Musculocartilaginous structure between the trachea and the pharynx that functions as the valve preventing food and other particles from entering the respiratory tract, as well as the voice mechanism. Also called the voicebox, the larynx is composed of three single cartilages: cricoid, epiglottis, and thyroid; and three paired cartilages: arytenoid, corniculate, and cuneiform.

Lasegue's sign Evidence at testing of sciatica. The knee is flexed and the thigh is brought up over hip, if flexion of the hip is painful when the knee is extended, the exam is positive for sciatica. Done as a part of an evaluation and management exam as a range of motion test.

LASEK Laser-assisted subepithelial keratomileusis. LASEK is not to be confused with LASIK, though each is reported with CPT code 65760. In LASEK, an excimer laser is used to shape the mid layers of cornea after the outer layers have been peeled back.

laser Concentrated light used to cut or seal tissue. *NCD Reference: 140.5.*

laser surgery Use of concentrated, sharply defined light beams to cut, cauterize, coagulate, seal, or vaporize tissue. The color and wavelength of the laser light is produced by its active medium, such as argon, CO2, potassium titanyl phosphate (KTP), Krypton, and Nd:YAG, which determines the type of tissues it can best treat. *NCD Reference: 140.5.*

LASIK Laser in situ keratomileusis.

Lasix See furosemide.

Lasègue sign Limitation of straight-leg raising; used in the diagnosis of a herniated lumbar disc.

Lasègue test Test for determining irritation of the nerve root. The physician elevates the supine patient's straight leg until there is ipsilateral extremity or back pain, or until the pain increases when the foot is bent backward.

LAT Lateral.

late charge In relation to facility billing, a charge posted to an account after the final bill has been produced.

late effect Abnormality, dysfunction, or other residual condition produced after the acute phase of an illness, injury, or disease is over. There is no time limit on when late effects can appear. The late effect may be apparent early, as with a stroke, or it can occur years later, as in arthritis following an injury. The code for the condition is sequenced first, and then the late effect code, unless the late effect code is combined with the manifestation in one code or the late effect is followed by the manifestation. *Synonym(s): sequela.*

latency Hidden, concealed, or dormant.

latent schizophrenia Eccentric or inconsequent behavior and anomalies of affect that give the impression of schizophrenia though no definite and characteristic schizophrenic anomalies, present or past, have been manifested.

lateral To/on the side.

lateral canthopexy Fixation or reattachment of the lateral canthal ligament.

lateral canthus Junction of the upper and lower eyelids away from the nose.

lateral extracavitary Lateral surgical approach that retracts muscles for access to the lateral and ventral vertebrae. Thoracic vertebrae may also include resection of the rib head and lumbar may include removal of the iliac crest.

lateral x-ray X-ray taken from the side.

lattice degeneration Retinal thinning with dense vitreous traction midway between the posterior and anterior eye.

laundering of monetary instruments Mixing funds obtained illegally with funds obtained legally. For example, depositing into a general account any payment from a fraudulent claim along with funds obtained from a legitimate claim may be interpreted as money laundering.

Launois' syndrome Pituitary secretions causing gigantism beginning before puberty with eosinophilic cell hyperplasia, eosinophilic adenoma, or chromophobe adenoma. Report this disorder with ICD-9-CM code 253.0. *Synonym(s): pituitary gigantism.*

Launois-Cléret syndrome Marked by obesity and hypogonadism in adolescent boys with dwarfism indicating hypothyroidism. Report this disorder with ICD-9-CM code 253.8.

LAUP Laser-assisted uvulopalatoplasty. Treatment for obstructive sleep apnea, reported with HCPCS Level II code S2080.

Laurence-Moon (-Bardet) -Biedl syndrome Retardation, pigmentary retinopathy, obesity, polydactyly, and hypogonadism. Report this disorder with ICD-9-CM code 759.89.

LAV Lymphadenopathy associated virus.

lavage Washing.

LAVH Laparoscopically assisted vaginal hysterectomy.

LAW Left atrial wall.

Lawford's syndrome Formation of multiple angiomas in skin of head and scalp. Report this disorder with ICD-9-CM code 759.6. *Synonym(s): Kalischer's syndrome.*

lazy eye Decreased or impaired vision in one or both eyes without detectable anatomic damage to the retina or visual pathways, brought on by disuse, often as a result of esotropia. Lazy eye is usually not correctable by eyeglasses or contact lenses. Report lazy eye with a

J-N

code from ICD-9-CM subcategory 368.0. *Synonym(s): amblyopia ex anopsia.*

LB *1)* Large bowel. *2)* Leg bag.

LBB Left branch bundle or left bundle branch. Part of the heart's electrical system carrying nerve impulses that cause the left ventricle to contract. If the impulses are blocked, the patient experiences left ventricular disease or cardiomyopathy.

LBBB Left bundle branch block.

LBD Lewy body disease. Degenerative dementia with progressive cognitive decline, Parkinson's like symptoms, and visual hallucinations. Lewy body dementia is reported with ICD-9-CM code 331.82 with a second code to identify with behavioral disturbance (294.11) or without behavioral disturbance (294.10).

LBP Lower back pain.

lbs Pounds.

LC HCPCS Level II modifier for use with CPT codes, that identifies the left circumflex coronary artery. Used to indicate the specific vessel involvement in a stent placement, balloon angioplasty, and/or atherectomy.

LCCA Left common carotid artery.

LCD Local coverage determination. Published decision by a fiscal intermediary or carrier regarding whether to cover a particular service or under what circumstances to cover it. The decision is valid only in the carrier's jurisdiction. LCDs replaced local medical review policies for CMS by year's end 2005.

LCH Langerhans cell histiocytosis. Pancreatic condition.

LCIS Lobular carcinoma in situ. Form of breast cancer, reported with ICD-9-CM code 233.0.

LCNB Large core needle biopsy.

LCSW Licensed clinical social worker.

LD *1)* HCPCS Level II modifier for use with CPT codes, that identifies the left anterior descending coronary artery. Used to indicate the specific vessel involvement in a stent placement, balloon angioplasty, and/or atherectomy. *2)* Lethal dose.

LDH Lactic dehydrogenase. Elevated LDH is associated with heart attack, liver and kidney disease, and some malignancies. LDH tests are reported with CPT codes 83615 and 83625. *Synonym(s): LD.*

LDL Low density lipoprotein.

LDS Lipodystrophy syndrome. Syndrome which involves the partial or total absence of fat and/or the abnormal deposition and distribution of fat in the body due to a disturbance of the lipid metabolism.

LDT Lymph drainage therapy. Massage using light touch to stimulate the lymphatic system. Lymphedema is reported with ICD-9-CM code 457.1 when an acquired chronic condition; postmastectomy lymphedema is

reported with 457.0; and hereditary edema of the legs is reported with 757.0.

LE *1)* Lower extremity. *2)* Lupus erythematosus.

Lea's Shield Brand name reusable contraceptive cervical barrier, sized to fit the patient, used in conjunction with a spermicide. Cervical cap supply is reported with HCPCS Level II code A4261.

leased employee Legal employment relationship established by a contract where an employer hires the services of an employee through another employer.

LEAT Least expensive alternative treatment. A limitation in a health care plan that allows benefits only for the least expensive treatment. *Synonym(s): LEAAT.*

leave of absence days Days during which a patient is discharged from the hospital temporarily. A patient may be placed on a leave of absence when readmission is expected for follow-up care or surgery and the patient does not require a hospital level of care during the interim period. Examples include situations in which surgery could not be scheduled immediately, a specific surgical team was not available, or further treatment is indicated following diagnostic tests but cannot begin immediately. Only one bill is prepared for a leave of absence, and one DRG payment is made. *Synonym(s): LOA.*

Lederer-Brill syndrome Anemic syndrome noted for fragmentation of red blood cells. Report this disorder with ICD-9-CM code 283.19.

LEEP Loop electrode excision procedure. Biopsy specimen or cone shaped wedge of cervical tissue is removed using a hot cautery wire loop with an electrical current running through it.

LeFort I type fracture Horizontal fracture of the maxilla in which a segment of the alveolar process containing teeth becomes detached.

J–N

LeFort Fracture

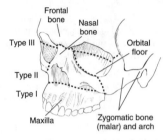

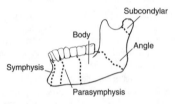

LeFort II type fracture Unilateral or bilateral fracture of the maxilla in which it is separated from the facial skeleton in a pyramid shape. The fracture can extend through the maxilla and hard palate, through the orbit floor, and into the nasal cavity.

LeFort III type fracture Fracture in which the entire maxilla, along with one or more other facial bones, is entirely separated from the craniofacial skeleton.

left heart Area of the heart consisting of the left atrium and left ventricle.

left heart failure Inability of the left ventricle to adequately pump blood, resulting in fluid accumulation in the lungs.

legal business name Name that is reported to the Internal Revenue Service (IRS).

legal counsel Individual who counsels other individuals on legal rights and obligations.

legally induced abortion Elective or therapeutic termination of pregnancy performed within legal parameters by a licensed physician or other qualified medical professionals. Report legally induced abortions with ICD-9-CM codes from rubric 635, with fourth digits to indicate the presence or absence of complications and fifth digits to identify the stage of abortion. *Synonym(s): elective abortion, induced or artificial abortion, termination of pregnancy, therapeutic abortion.* **NCD Reference:** *140.1.*

Legg-Calvé-Perthes syndrome Disease of children in growth centers, especially at top of femur, in which the epiphyses is replaced by new calcification. Report this disorder with ICD-9-CM code 732.1.

Legionnaire's disease Infection caused by the microorganism Legionella pneumophilia, transmitted by inhalation of the bacteria, not person to person. The bacteria reside and grow in damp, enclosed areas such as air conditioners, humidifiers, and shower heads. This is a kind of pneumonia with high fever, gastrointestinal pain, headache, muscle aches, and dry cough. This disease is reported with ICD-9-CM code 482.84.

leiomyoma Benign tumor consisting of smooth muscle in the uterus. Types of leiomyomas are classified according to the site of growth: intramural or interstitial leiomyomas are found in the wall of the uterus, subserous leiomyomas are beneath the serous membrane lining the uterus, and submucosal leiomyomas are beneath the inner lining of the uterus. Although often asymptomatic, these types of tumors can cause reproductive problems, pain and pressure, and abnormal menstruation. Leiomyomas are reported with a code from ICD-9-CM rubric 218. *Synonym(s): fibroid tumor, fibromyoma, myoma.*

Lekton Brand name absorbable metal stent used in the treatment of critical limb ischemia below the knee and coronary artery disease.

Lempert's fenestration Small window is drilled in the lateral semicircular canal and a skin flap is placed over the fistula to remedy otosclerosis.

length of stay Number of inpatient bed days for a single patient during a single admission. *Synonym(s): LOS.* **l. outliers** Cases in which length of stay falls outside the norm for a given diagnosis, procedure, or DRG. The length of stay may be longer or shorter than is typical.

lengthening Surgical procedure to lengthen a bone or tendon.

Lennox's syndrome Childhood epilepsy with slow brain waves. Report this disorder with a code from ICD-9-CM range 345.00-345.01.

lens Convex disc of the eye, behind the iris and in front of the vitreous body, that refracts light entering the globe.

lenticular syndrome Accumulation of copper in the brain, cornea, kidney, liver, and other tissues causing cirrhosis of the liver and deterioration in the basal ganglia of the brain. Report this disorder with ICD-9-CM code 275.1.

lepirudin Direct thrombin inhibitor used for anticoagulation in patients with heparin-induced thrombocytopenia and associated thromboembolic disease to prevent further thromboembolic complications. It is produced from a derivative of the medicinal leech Hirudo medicinalis via recombinant DNA synthesis. Supply is reported with HCPCS Level II code J1945. May be sold under the brand name Refludan.

Lepore hemoglobin syndrome Cardiac defects, coarse facial features, multiple lentigines, pulmonary stenosis, abnormalities of the genitalia, sensorineural deafness, and skeletal changes. Report this disorder with ICD-9-CM code 282.49.

Leriche sympathectomy Procedure involves sympathetic denervation.

Leriche's syndrome Syndrome caused by obstruction of the terminal aorta at its bifurcation, usually occurring in males, characterized by fatigue in the hips, thighs, or calves upon exercising, absence of pulsation in the femoral arteries, impotence, and often pallor and coldness of the lower limbs. This syndrome is reported with ICD-9-CM code 444.0.

Léri-Weill syndrome Dorsal dislocation of the distal ulna and carpal bones, bowing of the radius, and mesomelic dwarfism. Report this disorder with ICD-9-CM code 756.59.

Lermoyez's syndrome Vertigo, nausea, vomiting, tinnitus, and progressive deafness caused by endolymphatic hydrops. Report this disorder with ICD-9-CM code 386.00.

lesbianism Exclusive or predominant sexual attraction between women with or without physical relationship.

Lesch-Nyhan syndrome Physical and mental retardation, compulsive self-mutilation of the lips and fingers through biting, impaired renal function, choreoathetosis, spastic cerebral palsy, and purine synthesis and consequent hyperuricemia and uricaciduria. Report this disorder with ICD-9-CM code 277.2.

lesion Area of damaged tissue that has lost continuity or function, due to disease or trauma. Lesions may be located on internal structures such as the brain, nerves, or kidneys, or visible on the skin.

lesser omentum Liver to the lesser curvature of the stomach and duodenum.

Letterer-Siwe disease Rare, inherited, and progressive form of Langerhans cell histiocytosis characterized by skin lesions, bleeding tendency, anemia, and enlarged liver and spleen.

leucocoria Ocular symptom in which a pale, whitish mass is visible through the pupil behind the lens of the eye and is often indicative of retinoblastoma, reported with ICD-9-CM code 360.44. *Synonym(s): cat's eye reflex.*

leucovorin calcium Vitamin drug used to treat folic acid overdose, megaloblastic anemia caused by congenital enzyme deficiency, folate deficient megaloblastic anemia, and hematologic toxicity caused by pyrimethamine or trimethoprim. Also used as palliative treatment in advanced colorectal cancer. Supply is reported with HCPCS Level II code J0640. *Synonym(s): citrovorum factor, folinic acid.*

leukapheresis Isolation and removal of white blood cells from the circulating blood. Whole blood is drawn

out of one arm. It is then circulated through a separator, which performs anticoagulation with separation and collection of the white blood cells. The remainder of the blood is returned to the patient through the other arm. This is reported with CPT code 36511. *Synonym(s): lymphocytapheresis.*

leukemia Malignancy of the blood and blood-forming organs manifested by abnormal proliferation or development of leukocytes and their developmental precursors in the blood and bone marrow. Acute and chronic classifications in leukemia refer to the degree that the malignant cells have differentiated and not to the length of the disease itself. The predominant type of cell involved, whether myelogenous or lymphocytic, also determines classification.

leukocyte syndrome Bronchiectasis and pancreatic insufficiency, resulting in malnutrition, sinusitis, short stature, and bone abnormalities. Report this disorder with ICD-9-CM code 288.01.

leukoma Opacity of the cornea, dense and white in appearance. An adherent leukoma includes the cornea and a prolapsed, adherent iris.

leukonychia Congenital disorder manifested by white spots or streaks in the nails that may be associated with deafness, reported with ICD-9-CM code 757.5.

leukopenia Sudden and severe condition caused by a reduced number of white blood cells (WBC). The type of leukopenia is classified according to what kind of WBC is deficient (i.e., agranulocytosis for granulocytes or neutropenia for neutrophils). For coding purposes, these types are not reported with separate codes, but are reported with a single code, from ICD-9-CM category 288.0. When a drug or other specified cause brings on this condition, use an E code in addition to the code for the disease. *Synonym(s): agranulocytosis, aleukia, aleukocytosis, leukocytopenia, neutropenia.*

leukoplakia Thickened white patches or lesions appearing on a mucous membrane.

leukorrhea White mucousy vaginal discharge, reported with ICD-9-CM code 623.5 if not specified as infective. If specified as trichomonal, report with 131.00.

leuprolide acetate Brand name injectable drug that treats prostate and breast cancers, precocious puberty, uterine fibroid tumors, and endometriosis. In cases of infertility, it may be used to prepare the body for ovulation. Its active ingredient is leuprolide. Supply of Lupron is reported with HCPCS Level II code J9217 or J9218. A leuprolide implant (Viadur) is also available; placed under the skin of the upper, inner arm, it delivers medication continuously for 12 months and is reported with HCPCS Level II code J9219. May be sold under the brand names Epigard Lucrin, Lupron, or Lupron Depot. Report prophylactic use with ICD-9-CM code V07.59.

J-N

Lev's syndrome   Bundle branch block in patient with normal coronary arteries and myocardium resulting from calcification of the conducting system. Report this disorder with ICD-9-CM code 426.0. *Synonym(s): Rytand-Lipstitch syndrome.*

levalbuterol HCl   Bronchodilator used to treat patients with reversible obstructive airway disease. May be sold under the brand name Xopenex

Levaquin   See levofloxacin.

levator aponeurosis   Flat tendon attaching to the levator muscle of the eyelid that aids in opening and closing the eyelid.

level of specificity   Diagnosis coding specificity (i.e., a three-digit disease code is assigned only when there are no four-digit codes within that category, a four-digit code is assigned only when there is no fifth-digit subclassification within that category, or a fifth digit is assigned for any category for which a fifth-digit subclassification is provided).

levetiracetam   Anticonvulsant used in combination with other medications to treat partial onset seizures. It is indicated for adult patients with a diagnosis of epilepsy. May be sold under the brand name Keppra. Facilities report supply of the injectable form with HCPCS Level II code J1953.

Levi's syndrome   Dwarfism resulting from the absence of functional anterior pituitary gland. Report this disorder with ICD-9-CM code 253.3. *Synonym(s): Burnier syndrome, Lorain-Levi syndrome.*

levocarnitine   Therapeutic replacement for depleted levels of carnitine, a naturally occurring carrier molecule that delivers long chain fatty acids to mitochondria in the cells for energy production. Childhood deficiency is usually secondary to an inborn error of metabolism. Acquired deficiency in adults is of uncertain etiology, although organic acidemia and dialysis are primary contributors. Supply is reported with HCPCS Level II code J1955. Carnitor contains levocarnitine. *NCD Reference: 230.19.*

Levo-Dromoran   See levorphanol tartrate.

levofloxacin   Broad-spectrum quinolone antibiotic used to treat infections by preventing DNA replication and killing susceptible bacteria. Supply is reported with HCPCS Level II code J1956. May be sold under the brand name Levaquin.

levoleucovorin calcium   Folic acid derivative used to reduce the harmful side effects of anticancer medications such as methotrexate. Levoleucovorin calcium is also indicated to augment the effects of the anticancer drug fluorouracil in the treatment of advanced colorectal cancer. Supply is reported with HCPCS Level II code J0641.

levonorgestrel   Drug inhibiting ovulation and preventing sperm from penetrating cervical mucus. It is delivered subcutaneously in polysiloxone capsules. The capsules can be effective for up to five years, and provide a cumulative pregnancy rate of less than 2 percent. The capsules are not biodegradable, and therefore must be removed. Removal is more difficult than insertion of levonorgestrel capsules because fibrosis develops around the capsules. Normal hormonal activity and a return to fertility begins immediately upon removal.

levonorgestrel intrauterine device   T-shaped contraceptive device that gives off small doses of progesterone, a hormone that thickens cervical mucous and stops ovulation and is generally effective for up to five years. Supply is reported with HCPCS Level II code J7302. Insertion is reported with CPT code 58300 and removal with 58301. May be sold under the brand name Mirena.

levorphanol tartrate   Potent synthetic opioid similar to morphine used as a preoperative sedative or for postoperative pain management. Supply is reported with HCPCS Level II code J1960. May be sold under the brand name Levo-Dromoran.

Levsin   See hyoscyamine sulfate.

levulan Kerastick   See levonorgestrel intrauterine device.

LFH   Left femoral hernia.

LFT   Liver function test.

LGA   Large for gestational age. Excessive growth of a fetus that is more developed than is considered normal for the gestational age, measured in weeks and calculated from the first day of the mother's last menstrual period to the current date. The most common cause for LGA is maternal diabetes. If only LGA is documented, report with a code from ICD-9-CM subcategory 656.6. When it is documented as causing disproportion, report with a code from subcategory 653.5. When it causes obstructed labor, report a code from subcategory 660.1 in addition to the code from category 653.

LGHP   Large group health plan.

LGL   Large granular lymphoma.

LGV   Lymphogranuloma venereum. Rare, sexually transmitted disease causing painless genital ulcers, enlarged lymph nodes, and, in some cases, anal stricture. If untreated, it can lead to meningitis or encephalitis. LGV is reported with ICD-9-CM code 099.1.

LH   Luteinizing hormone. Gonadotropic hormone secreted by the pituitary gland. In women, it promotes ovulation, the release of the egg from the ovary, and sustains the luteal (second) phase of the menstrual cycle. It also promotes the secretion of progesterone. In men, it stimulates the development of testicular Leydig's cells.

J-N

LHC Left heart catheterization.

LHF Left heart failure.

LHR Leukocyte histamine release.

Li Lithium.

liability insurance Insurance, including self-insured plans, that provides payment based on legal liability for injuries, illness, or damage to property such as automobile, uninsured and underinsured motorist, homeowner's, malpractice, product liability, and general casualty insurance.

liability insurance Insurance that protects against claims for negligence or inappropriate action or inaction that resulted in injury to a person or damage to property.

Liberte stent Brand name coronary stent system.

Librium See chlordiazepoxide HCl.

LICA Left internal carotid artery.

lichen planus Inflammatory, pruritic disease of the skin, in acute or chronic form, sometimes involving the nails and oral and genital mucosa. It is manifested by violet, scaly papules with white puncta that may run together to form plaques, but usually resolves spontaneously.

Lichtheim's syndrome Numbness and tingling, weakness, a sore tongue, dyspnea, faintness, pallor of the skin and mucous membranes, anorexia, diarrhea, loss of weight, and fever. Most often strikes in the fifth decade. Report this disorder with ICD-9-CM code 281.0 and 336.2.

lid retraction "Pulled up" upper eyelid.

LIDO Lidocaine.

lidocaine HCl Antiarrhythmic that decreases the excitability of the ventricles of the heart to treat ventricular arrhythmias occurring as a result of myocardial infarction (MI), cardiac manipulation, or digoxin toxicity. Supply is reported with HCPCS Level II code J2001. May be sold under the brand names Lido-Pen autoinjector, Xylocaine, Xylocard.

LIDS Latex induced disease system.

lien- Relating to the spleen.

lifetime maximum Maximum amount an insurance plan pays on your behalf for covered services you receive while enrolled.

lifetime reserve days Sixty additional days that are granted only once in a lifetime allowed by Medicare hospital benefits (Part A) after a benefit period (90 days) has been exhausted.

ligament Band or sheet of fibrous tissue that connects the articular surfaces of bones or supports visceral organs.

ligate To tie off a blood vessel or duct with a suture or a soft, thin wire (ligature wire).

ligation Tying off a blood vessel or duct with a suture or a soft, thin wire.

lightning paralysis Temporary, short-lived paralysis resulting from the impact of being struck by lightning. Acute constriction of blood vessels and sensory disturbances of one or more extremities are also associated with this condition. Report lightning paralysis with ICD-9-CM code 994.0. *Synonym(s): keraunoparalysis.*

Lightwood's disease Metabolic acidosis that results from impaired renal function, marked by elevated urinary pH, hyperchloremic acidosis, bicarbonates in the urine, and a decrease in the expelling of ammonium and titratable acids. Lightwood's disease or syndrome is reported with ICD-9-CM code 588.89.

Lignac (-Fanconi) syndrome Metabolic disorder of kidney, involving failure to reabsorb water, minerals, and other substances as well as failure to transport. Report this disorder with ICD-9-CM code 270.0.

Likoff's syndrome Severe pain in the chest caused by ischemia of heart prompted by coronary artery disease. Report this disorder with ICD-9-CM code 413.9.

LIMA Left internal mammary artery.

limbal girdle of Vogt Concentric corneal opacity adjacent to the limbus, seen most commonly in women older than age 40.

limitation of liability Signed waiver a provider must obtain from the patient before performing a service that appears on a list of services Medicare classifies as medically unnecessary. The waiver notifies the patient in advance that the service may be denied coverage and that the patient is responsible for payment.

limited Bounded.

limiting charge Maximum amount a nonparticipating physician or provider can charge for services rendered to a Medicare patient.

limits In medical reimbursement, the ceiling for benefits payable under a plan.

Lincocin See lincomycin HCl.

lincomycin HCl Broad-spectrum macrolide antibiotic given to treat bacterial infection. Lincomycin HCl is successful against gram-positive bacteria, but has poor viability with oral dose, so is not used as often as erythromycin and clindamycin. Supply is reported with HCPCS Level II code J0210. May be sold under the brand name Lincocin.

line item Specific service or item detail of claim.

line item denial Fiscal intermediary's denial of a line item on a claim that may be otherwise processable. These

J-N

rejected line items cannot be corrected by the provider but can be appealed.

line item rejection Fiscal intermediary's rejection of a line item on a claim that may be otherwise processable for payment. These rejected line items may be corrected and resubmitted by the provider, but cannot be appealed.

line of business Different health plans offered by a larger insurer or insurance broker as a product line.

linear accelerator Device used to increase the energy of ions along a linear path. *mega voltage l.* High-energy radiation machine that creates and delivers fast moving subatomic particles to cancer sites.

lingua nigra Condition in which the papillae do not shed normally from the tongue, resulting in collections of debris, bacteria, and a dark fuzzy appearance. Report this condition with ICD-9-CM code 529.3. *Synonym(s): black hairy tongue.*

lingual Surface of the tooth closest to the tongue or relating to the tongue and its surrounding areas.

lingual nerve Nerve that is a branch of the mandibular nerve, which lies between the pterygoid muscle and the mandible. It supplies the mucous membrane of the floor of the mouth and the side of tongue.

linking codes To establish medical necessity, CPT and HCPCS Level II codes must be supported by the ICD-9-CM diagnosis and injury codes submitted on the claim form and supported by the documentation.

Linton ligation Radical subfascial ligation of the tributaries of the great saphenous vein, called perforator veins, connecting it to other veins of the lower leg. They are tied off to separate the communication of deep and superficial veins along the course of the leg. Linton ligation is reported with CPT code 37760.

Lioresal See baclofen.

LIP Lymphocytic interstitial pneumonia. Syndrome of fever, cough, and dyspnea, with bibasilar pulmonary infiltrates. LIP is reported with ICD-9-CM code 516.8.

lip(o)- Relating to fat.

lipectomy Surgical excision of fatty tissue. Lipectomy can be performed with or without suction-assistance. Correct code selection is dependent upon the anatomical site.

lipodystrophy Loss of fatty tissue in areas of the body due to a disturbance of metabolism. Lipodystrophy is reported with ICD-9-CM code 272.6.

lipofuscin Yellowish brown pigment found in muscle, liver, heart, and nerve cells after the breakdown and digestion of damaged cells, due to the oxidation of the lipids found in the membranes of cellular structures.

lipoma Benign tumor containing fat cells and the most common of soft tissue lesions, which are usually painless and asymptomatic, with the exception of an angiolipoma.

An angiolipoma has a proliferation of small vessels scattered throughout the fat and can be painful. See ICD-9-CM category 214 and assign the appropriate code based on anatomical site. This category includes angiolipoma. *Synonym(s): angiolipoma, fibrolipoma, hibernoma, myelolipoma, myxolipoma.*

liposomal daunorubicin citrate Cytotoxic, first-line drug for treatment of advanced HIV related Kaposi's sarcoma. Acts by inhibiting DNA synthesis to decrease tumor growth. The liposomal preparation is selective for solid tumors in situ. Supply is reported with HCPCS Level II code J9151. May be sold under the brand name DaunoXome.

liposuction Removal of fat deposits through suction.

liq. Solution (liquor).

Liquaemin sodium See heparin sodium.

Lisfranc injury Eponym describing a fracture-dislocation injury in the ball of the foot or distal to it, named for Napoleon's field surgeon who treated frostbite on the Russian front. The tarsometatarsal joint is also known as Lisfranc's joint.

LIT Leukocyte immune therapy.

lith(o)- Relating to a hard or calcified substance.

lithotripsy Destruction of calcified substances in the gallbladder or urinary system by smashing the concretion into small particles to be washed out. This may be done by surgical or noninvasive methods, such as ultrasound.

LITT Laser interstitial thermotherapy or laser-induced interstitial thermotherapy. Minimally invasive approach for treatment of soft tissue tumors, including those in the brain, breast, head and neck, liver, lung, and prostate in which a specially designed laser applicator is inserted, under guidance, into the targeted tumor to destroy tissue. Report LITT with procedure codes from ICD-9-CM subcategory 17.6.

little league elbow Injury consisting of tears and stretches to the muscles and ligaments of the elbow in addition to growth plate injury of the radius. It is caused by repetitively throwing a ball. This injury is reported with ICD-9-CM code 718.82. *Synonym(s): pitcher's elbow.*

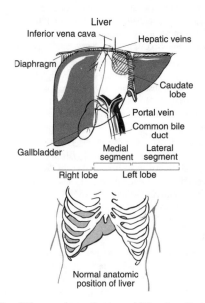

Liver
Inferior vena cava
Hepatic veins
Diaphragm
Caudate lobe
Portal vein
Common bile duct
Gallbladder
Medial segment
Lateral segment
Right lobe
Left lobe

Normal anatomic position of liver

liver-kidney syndrome Acute renal failure in patients with disease of biliary or liver tract. Cause seems to be decreased renal blood flow, damaging both organs. Report this disorder with ICD-9-CM code 572.4. *Synonym(s): Heyd's syndrome.*

lives Unit of measurement used by plans to determine the number of people covered. Calculated by multiplying the number of members by 2.5.

LKS Liver, kidneys, spleen.

LLB Long leg brace. Orthotic for the knee, ankle, and foot. *Synonym(s): KAFO.*

LLD Language-based learning disability.

LLETZ Large loop excision of transformation zone of cervix of uterus.

LLL Left lower lobe.

Lloyd's syndrome Endocrine dysfunction causing diabetes and affecting growth and weight. Report this disorder with ICD-9-CM code 258.1.

LLQ Left lower quadrant.

LLWC Long leg walking cast. A cast from the upper thigh to the toes.

LMA Laryngeal mask airway.

LMD Local medical doctor.

LMD 10% See dextran.

LML Left medio-lateral position.

LMM Lentigo malignant melanoma.

LMN Lower motor neuron.

LMP Last menstrual period.

LMRP Local medical review policy. Carrier-specific policy applied in the absence of a national coverage policy to make local Medicare medical coverage decisions, including the development of a draft policy based on a review of medical literature, an understanding of local practice, and the solicitation of comments from the medical community and Carrier Advisory Committee.

LMS Left mentum anterior position (chin).

LMT Left mentum transverse position.

LN+ Lymph node positive. Pathology finding that a malignancy has spread into the lymph node(s).

LNE Lymph node enlargement.

LNMP Last known menstrual period.

LNTX Long chain neurotoxin.

Lo Low.

Lo Dose syringe Brand name insulin syringe. Supply of a box of 100 is reported with HCPCS Level II code S8490 or A4206 x 100 for Medicare claims.

LOA Leave of absence days. Days during which a patient is discharged from the hospital temporarily. A patient may be placed on a leave of absence when readmission is expected for follow-up care or surgery and the patient does not require a hospital level of care during the interim period. Examples include situations in which surgery could not be scheduled immediately, a specific surgical team was not available, or further treatment is indicated following diagnostic tests but cannot begin immediately. Only one bill is prepared for a leave of absence, and one DRG payment is made.

LOAD Late onset Alzheimer's disease. Alzheimer's is reported with ICD-9-CM code 331.0 for the Alzheimer's and a code for the dementia: 294.10 without behavioral disturbance or 294.11 with behavioral disturbance. While no distinction is made between early and late onset Alzheimer's in ICD-9-CM, this distinction does affect coding in ICD-10-CM.

lobe (lung) (right) syndrome Incomplete expansion of right middle lobe of lung with chronic pneumonitis. Report this disorder with ICD-9-CM code 518.0. *Synonym(s): Brock syndrome.*

lobectomy Excision of a lobe of an organ such as the liver, thyroid, lung, or brain.

lobectomy behavior syndrome Bilateral temporal lobe ablation with psychic hyperreactivity to visual stimuli or blindness, increased oral and sexual activity, and depressed drive and emotional reactions. Report this disorder with ICD-9-CM code 310.0. *Synonym(s): Klüver-Bucy syndrome.*

lobotomy Psychosurgical procedure that involves cutting all of the nerve pathway fibers in a lobe of the brain, most often referring to the frontal lobes. This procedure is reported with CPT code 61490.

J–N

lobotomy syndrome Changes in behavior following damage to the frontal areas of the brain resulting in general diminution of self-control, concentration, memory, intellect, foresight, creativity, and spontaneity, which may be manifested as increased irritability, selfishness, restlessness, slowness, dullness, loss of drive and lack of concern for others. A considerable degree of recovery is possible and may continue over the course of several years. **Synonym(s):** *frontal lobe syndrome.*

LOC 1) Level of consciousness. 2) Loss of consciousness.

local allograft Graft taken directly from the patient through the same incision that is used for the definitive procedure.

local anesthesia Induced loss of feeling or sensation restricted to a certain area of the body, including topical, local tissue infiltration, field block, or nerve block methods.

local codes Generic term for code values that are defined for a state or other political subdivision, or for a specific payer. This term most commonly describes HCPCS Level III codes, but also applies to state-assigned institutional revenue codes, condition codes, occurrence codes, value codes, etc.

local coverage determination Statement of coverage and related usage specific to a Medicare contractor or designated geographic area.

local infiltration Local anesthesia procedure using injection of an anesthetic agent, such as lidocaine, into the skin and subcutaneous tissue of the area to be treated. This anesthesia is part of the global surgical package and is not billed separately.

local medical review policy Carrier-specific policy applied in the absence of a national coverage policy to make local Medicare medical coverage decisions, including the development of a draft policy based on a review of medical literature, an understanding of local practice, and the solicitation of comments from the medical community and Carrier Advisory Committee. **Synonym(s):** *LCDs, LMRP, local carrier decisions.*

localization Limitation to one area.

localize Identifying the site or location of a lesion or the process of confining within a limited area.

localized Limited to one area.

locked-in state or syndrome Brainstem infarction with consciousness, but the inability to move limbs or speak.

Löffler's syndrome Transient infiltrations of lungs by eosinophilia resulting in coughing, fever, and dyspnea. Report this disorder with ICD-9-CM code 518.3.

Löfgren's syndrome Involves fibrosis in lungs, lymph nodes, skin, liver, eyes, spleen, phalangeal bones, and parotid glands. Identified by systemic granulomas

composed of epithelioid and multinucleated giant cells. Report this disorder with ICD-9-CM code 135. **Synonym(s):** *Besnier-Boeck-Schaumann syndrome, Hutchinson-Boeck syndrome, Schaumann's syndrome.*

logical observation identifiers, names, and codes Set of universal names and codes that identify laboratory and clinical observations. These codes, which are maintained by the Regenstrief Institute, are expected to be used in the HIPAA claim attachments standard. **Synonym(s):** *LOINC.*

LOINC Logical observation identifiers names and codes. Universal code system for reporting laboratory and other clinical observations, maintained by the Regenstrief Institute. This coding system is HIPAA compliant. Laboratories can include LOINC codes in their outbound HL7 messages so their results can be integrated in clinical and research repositories.

LOM Limitation of motion.

lone star fever Tick-borne, rickettsial disease transmitted by the tick Amblyomma americanum, observed in soldiers who had been at Camp Bullis, Texas. Lone Star fever is marked by very low leukocyte count with neutropenia, headache, and constant lymphadenitis. Report this condition with ICD-9-CM code 082.8. **Synonym(s):** *Bullis fever.*

long arm 18 or 21 deletion syndrome Autosomal deletion causing a variety of symptoms. Report this disorder with ICD-9-CM code 758.39.

long bone Bone that has an extended longitudinal axis of the body or shaft, such as the humerus, tibia, and femur.

long face syndrome Vertical maxillary excess. Patients with long face syndrome develop more severe symptoms during orthodontic treatment, and may require a LeFort I procedure. Long face syndrome is reported with ICD-9-CM code 524.34 or a code from subcategory 524.9 to report an angle class defect.

long QT syndrome Potentially fatal condition precipitated by vigorous exertion, emotional upset, or startling moments due to an imbalance in the electrical timing mechanism that controls the pumping action of the heart's ventricles. This syndrome causes the patient to be susceptible to recurrent episodes of syncope, collapse, and possible ventricular fibrillation that can cause sudden death. Report this condition with ICD-9-CM code 426.82. **Synonym(s):** *prolonged QT interval syndrome, Romano-Ward syndrome.*

Longmire anastomosis Biliary obstruction is corrected with an intrahepatic cholangiojejunostomy and partial hepatectomy.

long-term care facility Nursing home or, more specifically, a facility offering extended, nonacute care

J-N

to a resident patient whose illness does not require acute care.

long-term care hospital Certified under Medicare as short-term acute care hospital with an average inpatient length of stay greater than 25 days. Provider number suffixes range from 2000-2299. LTCHs are paid under a per discharge PPS based on LTC-DRGs effective October 1, 2002. Under the PPS, the 25-day calculation is based only on the hospital's Medicare inpatients, counting total medically necessary days, not only covered days. The PPS will be phased in over five years with decreasing percentage of cost-based reimbursement and increasing percentage of prospective payment per discharge. *Synonym(s): LTCH.*

loop Set of related data. For example, all billing provider information is contained in loop 2000A.

Looser (-Debray) -Milkman syndrome Osteoporosis with frequent fractures striking middle-aged women. Report this disorder with ICD-9-CM code 268.2. *Synonym(s): milkman syndrome.*

LOP Left occipitoposterior. Referencing a fetal position in cephalic presentation, in which the occiput is directed toward the left.

LOPS Loss of protective sensation. Reduction in anatomic nerve function so the patient cannot sense minor trauma from heat, chemicals, or mechanical sources. This disorder is usually associated with the foot, and secondary to another disorder like diabetes or amyloidosis. Foot exams and educational training for patients with a diagnosis of LOPS are reported with HCPCS Level II codes G0245, G0246, and G0247.

Lorain-Levi syndrome Dwarfism resulting from absence of functional anterior pituitary gland. Report this disorder with ICD-9-CM code 253.3. *Synonym(s): Burnier syndrome, Levi syndrome.*

lorazepam Sedative hypnotic used to decrease anxiety, lessen seizures, treat nausea and vomiting, and as a preanesthesia sedative. Supply is reported with HCPCS Level II code J2060. May be sold under the brand name Apo-Lorazepam, Ativan, or Novolorazepam.

Lordosis

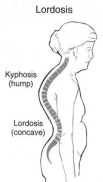

lordosis Congenital condition in which there is an exaggerated inward curvature of the lower back. This condition is reported with ICD-9-CM code 754.2.

Lorenz's operation Chronic dislocation of the hip is corrected by tying the head of the femur to the acetabulum to develop a socket.

LOS Length of stay. Number of inpatient bed days for a single patient during a single admission. *l. outliers* Cases in which length of stay falls outside the norm for a given diagnosis, procedure, or DRG. The length of stay may be longer or shorter than is typical.

loss ratio Ratio between the cost to deliver medical care and the amount of money taken in by the plan.

LOT Left occiput transverse position.

Louis-Bar syndrome Gonadal hypoplasia, insulin resistance and hyperglycemia, liver function problems, ataxia, nystagmus, and increased sensitivity to ionizing radiation. Report this disorder with ICD-9-CM code 334.8. *Synonym(s): Boder-Sedgwick syndrome.*

loupe Small magnifying lens used by clinicians to improve visualization during an examination. Use of a loupe does not qualify as an operating microscope and, thus, does not affect coding of the procedure.

Lovenox See enoxaparin sodium.

low utilization payment adjustment Under the home health prospective payment system, episode of four or less visits. They are paid under the national standardized per visit rates rather than a home health resource group (HHRG). *Synonym(s): LUPA.*

Lowe's syndrome Aminoaciduria, cataracts, mental retardation, hydrophthalmia, rickets, and reduced ammonia production by the kidney. Report this disorder with ICD-9-CM code 270.8. *Synonym(s): Lowe-Terrey-MacLachlan syndrome.*

lower radicular, newborn syndrome Damage of nerve root during birth. Report this disorder with ICD-9-CM code 767.4.

Lown (-Ganong)-Levine syndrome Electrocardiographic disorder indicated by a short P-R interval with normal duration of the QRS complex. Report this disorder with ICD-9-CM code 426.81.

Lowsley's operation Simple epispadias is corrected by closing the glandular cleft urethra, splitting the glans, and burying the repaired urethra deep into the soft tissue.

LOX Liquid oxygen.

LP Lumbar puncture.

LPF Low powered field. Magnification of a microscope during lab or pathology examination. It does not affect code selection.

LPM Liters per minute.

LPN Licensed practical nurse.

LR Lactated Ringer's.

LRD Living related donor.

LRSA Linezolid and methicillin resistant *Staphylococcus aureus*. Extremely rare *Staphylococcus aureus* that may include associated pneumonia and moderate organ dysfunction.

LS fusion Lumbar sacral fusion.

LSA Left sacrum anterior position.

LSB Left sternal border.

LSC Left subclavian.

LSD reaction Acute intoxication from lysergic acid diethylamide abuse, manifested by hallucinatory states lasting a few days or less.

LSO Lumbar sacral orthosis.

LT *1)* HCPCS Level II modifier for use with CPT or HCPCS Level II codes, that identifies procedures performed on the left side of the body. It does not indicate a bilateral procedure. Does not affect reimbursement, but failure to use when appropriate could result in delay or denial of the claim. *2)* Left.

LTC Long-term care.

LTC-DRG Inpatient long-term acute-care diagnosis-related group.

LTCH Long-term care hospital, a CMS designation.

LTK *1)* Laser thermal keratoplasty. *2)* Left total knee (replacement).

LTOT Long-term oxygen therapy.

Lucentis Brand name injectable drug used to treat subfoveal neovascularization due to age-related macular degeneration. Injection is reported with CPT code 67028, with modifier RT or LT appended to identify the eye treated. Supply is reported with HCPCS Level II code J2778. Lucentis contains ranibizumab.

Lucey-Driscoll syndrome Retention jaundice in newborn infants resulting from defective bilirubin conjugation, a product of a steroid in mother's blood being transferred to the infant. Report this disorder with ICD-9-CM code 774.30.

Ludwig's angina Infection of the subcutaneous connective tissue under the tongue, around the mouth floor. This condition is reported with ICD-9-CM code 528.3.

lul Left upper lobe.

LULA Laparoscopy under local anesthesia.

LUMA Brand name cervical imaging system that operates by shining a light on the cervix and analyzing how different areas respond to the light. LUMA creates a color map that helps the physician determine where to biopsy. LUMA is used after colposcopy and before a biopsy.

lumbago Low back pain.

lumbar plexus Network of spinal nerves from lumbar levels L1-L4 that supplies motor, sensory, and autonomic fibers to the lower extremity, as well as the gluteal and inguinal regions along with the sacral plexus.

lumbo- Relating to the loin region.

lumbosacral plexus lesions Acquired defect in tissue along the network of nerves in the lower back, causing corresponding motor and sensory dysfunction.

lumen Space inside an intestine, artery, vein, duct, or tube.

lunatomalacia Idiopathic, progressive osteochondrosis affecting the lunate bone of the wrist in which the bone undergoes osteonecrosis, or death of the bone tissue, due to a lack of blood supply. Symptoms may initially mimic those of a sprained wrist, but the lunate bone soon begins to collapse. Arthritis of the wrist develops. Advanced stages require surgical treatment. Report this condition with ICD-9-CM code 732.3 or 732.8. *Synonym(s): Kienböck's disease.*

lung syndrome Respiratory distress following surgery, shock or trauma, similar to but not caused by, adult respiratory distress system. Report this disorder with ICD-9-CM code 518.5.

LUPA Low utilization payment adjustment. Under the home health prospective payment system, episode of four or less visits. They are paid under the national standardized per visit rates rather than a home health resource group (HHRG).

Lupron Brand name injectable drug that treats prostate and breast cancers, precocious puberty, uterine fibroid tumors, and endometriosis. In cases of infertility, it may be used to prepare the body for ovulation. Its active ingredient is leuprolide. Supply of Lupron is reported with HCPCS Level II code J9217 or J9218. A leuprolide

J-N

implant (Viadur) is also available; placed under the skin of the upper, inner arm, it delivers medication continuously for 12 months and is reported with HCPCS Level II code J9219. Lupron contains leuprolide acetate.

LUQ Left upper quadrant.

Luschka proctectomy Technique used to resect the rectum.

LUSCS Lower uterine segment cesarean section. In LUSCS, the operative incision is across the lower part of the uterus. The type of incision does not impact code selection for cesarean birth. Report CPT code 59510 to also report ante- and postpartum care; 59514 for cesarean delivery only; or 59515 for cesarean delivery and postpartum care. For LUSCS after attempted vaginal delivery, see 59618, 59620, and 59622. *Synonym(s): LSCS.*

LUSS Liver ultrasound scan. Diagnostic ultrasound performed solely on the liver, reported with CPT code 76705.

Lutembacher's syndrome Atrial septal defect associated with mitral stenosis. Report this disorder with ICD-9-CM code 745.5.

LUTO Lower urinary tract obstruction.

Lutrepulse Brandname subcutaneous implant that decreases secretion of sex hormones by acting on the pituitary gland to decrease the release of follicle stimulating hormone and luteinizing hormone. It is used in the treatment of hormone sensitive prostate gland tumors and in cases of dysfunctional uterine bleeding to decrease endometrial tissue growth within the uterus. Report CPT code 11980 for insertion. Supply is reported with HCPCS Level II code J9202. Lutrepulse contains gonadorelin acetate.

LUTS Lower urinary tract symptoms.

LV Left ventricle.

LV reconstruction Left ventricle restoration. Treatment of congestive heart failure by restoring the heart to a more normal size and shape. The ventricular muscle and chamber are resized with the aid of a plastic model, in hopes of improving heart function. This procedure is often performed with bypass or valve repair, which is reported separately. LV reconstruction is reported with CPT code 33548. *Synonym(s): Dor procedure, SAVER, SVR, TR3SVR.*

LVAD Left ventricular assist device. Temporarily implanted device that helps the left ventricle of a damaged heart continue to pump an adequate supply of blood to meet the body's needs, generally used as a temporary measure while awaiting transplantation. *Synonym(s): VAD. NCD Reference: 20.9.*

LVEDP Left ventricular end diastolic pressure. Elevated LVEDP is a sign of congestive heart failure, and can be measured invasively by placing a catheter in the left ventricle (direct LVEDP) or in the pulmonary artery (indirect LVEDP). Another method to measure LVEDP involves measuring arterial pressure during the strain phase of the Valsalva maneuver using a Vericor device.

LVN 1) Licensed visiting nurse. 2) Licensed vocational nurse.

LVRS Lung volume reduction surgery. Treatment for patients with severe or end-stage emphysema. LVRS allows the remaining compressed lung to expand and thus improve respiratory function. The procedure is performed via video-assisted thoracoscopic or median sternotomy surgery. The procedure is reported with ICD-9-CM procedural code 32.22 for the facility and CPT code 32491 for physician services. CPT code 32491 reflects both unilateral and bilateral procedures; modifier 50 or 52 should not be used. HCPCS Level II codes G0302-G0305 identify preparation and post-discharge services for the patient undergoing LVRS. *Synonym(s): lung contouring, lung shaving, reduction pneumoplasty.*

Lyell's syndrome Life-threatening dermatological condition in which the epidermis (top layer of skin) detaches from the dermis (lower layers) all over the body, often as a result of medication reaction. Report this disorder with ICD-9-CM code 695.15. *Synonym(s): toxic epidermal necrolysis.*

lymph Clear, sometimes yellow fluid that flows through the tissues in the body, through the lymphatic system, and into the blood stream.

lymph nodes Bean-shaped structures along the lymphatic vessels that intercept and destroy foreign materials in the tissue and bloodstream.

lymphadenectomy Dissection of lymph nodes free from the vessels and removal for examination by frozen section in a separate procedure to detect early-stage metastases.

lymphadenitis Inflammation of the lymph nodes.

lymphangioma Benign, malformed lymph channels.

lymphangion Segment of lymphatic vessel between two lymphatic valves, acting to push the lymphatic fluid in one direction. *Synonym(s): angion.*

lymphangiotomy Incision into a lymphatic vessel, usually performed for cannulation before lymphangiography.

lymphangitis Inflammation of the lymph glands.

lymphatic fluid Clear, sometimes yellow fluid that flows through the tissues in the body, through the lymphatic system, and then into the blood stream.

J-N

Lymphatic System

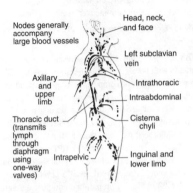

Nodes generally accompany large blood vessels

Head, neck, and face

Left subclavian vein

Axillary and upper limb

Intrathoracic

Intraabdominal

Thoracic duct (transmits lymph through diaphragm using one-way valves)

Cisterna chyli

Intrapelvic

Inguinal and lower limb

lymphatic system Lymph nodes, spleen, thymus gland, and bone marrow.

lymphedema Defect in which excessive lymph fluid accumulates in the tissues and causes the legs to swell, reported with ICD-9-CM code 757.0 when congenital and 457.1 when an acquired chronic condition. *Synonym(s): Nonne-Milroy's disease.*

lymphedema praecox Primary chronic lymphedema beginning at puberty, with swelling of the ankles and feet. It is hereditary. *Synonym(s): Meige syndrome, Milroy's disease.*

lymphedema tarda Primary chronic lymphedema presenting for the first time in a patient older than age 35.

lymphocele Cyst that contains lymph.

lymphocytes White blood cells formed in the body's lymph system.

lymphoma Tumors occurring in the lymphoid tissues (usually malignant).

lymphs Lymphocytes.

Lynch syndrome Hereditary nonpolyposis colorectal cancer, an inherited risk for multiple cancers primarily affecting the digestive tract, but also brain, skin, and urinary tract. Genetic testing for Lynch syndrome is reported with HCPCS Level II code S3831. *Synonym(s): HNPCC.*

Lysis of Intranasal Synechia

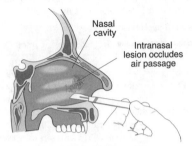

Nasal cavity

Intranasal lesion occludes air passage

Mucosal scar tissue is excised

lysis Destruction, breakdown, dissolution, or decomposition of cells or substances by a specific catalyzing agent.

-lysis Releasing, freeing, dissolution, loosening, or destruction.

lysis of adhesions Mobilization or release of an organ by dividing and freeing restricting adhesions.

lytes Electrolytes.

M *1)* Male. *2)* Manifest refraction.

M+CO See Medicare+Choice organization.

M. fiscal agent Organization responsible for administering claims for a state Medicaid program.

M1 Mitral first sound.

M2 Mitral second sound.

MA *1)* Master of arts degree. *2)* Medical assistant. *3)* Mental age.

MA1 Volume respirator.

MAAC Maximum allowable actual charge. Former provision of the Medicare program that applied to nonparticipating physicians before 1991, setting a limit on charges for physicians' professional services and most services provided incident to the professional services.

MAC *1)* Maximum allowable charge. Amount set by the insurer as the highest amount that can be charged for a particular medical service or by a pharmacy vendor. *2)* Monitored anesthesia care. No specific code is assigned to this service. MAC is reported with a regular anesthesia code and modifier QS. It is billed in the same manner as regular anesthesia based on time + base units times a conversion factor. *3)* Medicare administrative contractor. One of 15 jurisdictional organizations that contract with CMS to adjudicate professional claims under Part A and Part B, responsible for daily claims processing, utilization review, record maintenance, dissemination of information based on CMS regulations, and whether services are covered and payments are appropriate. Four of the jurisdictions will also include

J-N

home health services. There are four separate MAC jurisdictions for DME services.

MACE Major adverse cardiac event. Includes cardiac death, myocardial infarction, emergency coronary artery bypass graft surgery, and cerebrovascular accidents.

MacEwen hernia repair Hernia sack is used to construct a closing ring in this radical cure of a hernia.

MacLeod's syndrome Acquired unilateral hyperlucent lung with severe airway obstruction during expiration. Report this disorder with ICD-9-CM code 492.8. *Synonym(s): Swyer-James syndrome.*

macro- Oversized, large.

macrocephaly Congenital abnormality in which the head is abnormally large. It is differentiated from hydrocephalus in that the overgrowth is symmetrical and there is no increased intracranial pressure. Report this condition with ICD-9-CM code 756.0.

macrocheiria Condition in which the hands are abnormally large, reported with ICD-9-CM code 729.89. *Synonym(s): cheiromegaly.*

macrochilia Congenital hypertrophy of the lips, appearing abnormally large, reported with ICD-9-CM code 744.81.

macrocolon Congenital disorder in which the sigmoid colon is abnormally long, reported with ICD-9-CM code 751.3.

macrocornea Congenital condition in which the cornea is abnormally large. Report this condition with ICD-9-CM code 743.41; if associated with infantile glaucoma, report 743.22. *Synonym(s): megalocornea.*

macrocytosis Condition in which the blood contains abnormally large red blood cells (macrocytes). This abnormal finding is often a symptom of other disease processes, such as megaloblastic anemia. Report macrocytosis with ICD-9-CM code 289.89 if causative disease process is unknown.

macrodactylia Abnormal largeness of the fingers, reported with ICD-9-CM code 755.57, or of the toes, reported with 755.65. Repair of this condition is reported with CPT code 26590, once for each digit. *Synonym(s): dactylomegaly, macrodactylia, macrodactylism, macrodactyly, megalodactylia, megalodactylism, megalodactyly.*

macrodontia Unusually large teeth, reported with ICD-9-CM code 520.2. *Synonym(s): megadontism, megalodontia.*

macrogenia Increased jaw size, especially affecting the chin, which may involve the soft and/or bony tissue, reported with ICD-9-CM code 524.05.

macrogenitosomia praecox syndrome *1)* Excessive bodily development with unusual growth of sexual organs. *2)* A description of symptoms indicating

Donohue's and other syndromes. Report this disorder with ICD-9-CM code 259.8.

macroglobulinemia syndrome Earmarked by increase in macroglobulins in the blood. Has symptoms of hyperviscosity such as weakness, fatigue, bleeding disorders, and visual disturbances. Report this disorder with ICD-9-CM code 273.3. *Synonym(s): Waldenström's syndrome.*

macroglossia Congenital or acquired condition in which the tongue is abnormally large. If specified as congenital, report with ICD-9-CM code 750.15; if acquired, report 529.8.

macrognathia Condition in which the mandible and maxilla are distinctly overgrown, reported with a code from ICD-9-CM subcategory 524.0. If specified as alveolar, see subcategory 524.7.

macrogyria Congenital anomaly in which there is a modest decrease in the number of grooves and trenches on the surface of the brain (sulci), which sometimes results in increased size of the gyri, or convolutions, due to an increase in the brain matter. Report this condition with ICD-9-CM code 742.4.

macromastia Condition in which the breasts are abnormally large, reported with ICD-9-CM code 611.1. *Synonym(s): gynecomastia.*

macropsia Neurological condition in which one perceives objects as being larger than normal, reported with ICD-9-CM code 368.14.

macroscopic Of a size to be examined by the human eye.

macrosigmoid Congenital or acquired condition in which the sigmoid colon is abnormally large. If specified as congenital, report ICD-9-CM code 751.3; acquired, report 564.7.

macrosomia Abnormally large size, often in reference to a fetus or newborn. An infant with a birthweight greater than 4,500 grams (9.9 pounds) is reported with ICD-9-CM code 766.0. Many clinical definitions for macrosomia require a birthweight greater than 4,000 grams (8.8 pounds). For infants between 4,000 and 4,499 grams, report macrosomia with 766.1. Macrosomia in a fetus affecting the care of the mother is reported with a code from subcategory 656.6.

macrostomia Congenital abnormality in which one or both sides of the mouth are abnormally wide due to failure of the upper and lower jaw processes to unite properly during the first weeks of fetal development. Report this condition with ICD-9-CM code 744.83.

macrotia Abnormally large external ear, reported with ICD-9-CM code 744.22.

MACs Medicare administrative contractors.

macula Central region of the retina responsible for the sharpest vision, allowing for reading and color visualization.

maculae caeruleae Small spots produced by pubic lice, bluish in color and found on the trunk or thighs. Report this condition with ICD-9-CM code 132.1.

macular degeneration Age-related deterioration of the central portion of the retina (macula), causing blurring of central vision. There are two forms. The more advanced, wet macular degeneration, results from the formation of abnormal blood vessels behind the retina that grow under the macula. These fragile vessels leak blood and fluid and displace the macula from its normal position at the back of the eye. Central vision loss occurs quickly. Dry macular degeneration results from deterioration of the light-sensitive cells in the macula causing gradually blurring central vision. As macular degeneration progresses, central vision can be lost. Report wet macular degeneration with ICD-9-CM code 362.52; dry with 362.51. *Synonym(s): AMD, ARMD.*

macule Small, flat area of discolored skin that is not usually elevated and has no change in texture or thickness. Report this condition with ICD-9-CM code 709.8.

MAD Monoamine oxidase (inhibitor).

madarosis Condition in which one loses the eyelashes, reported with ICD-9-CM code 374.55. *Synonym(s): milphosis.*

Madelung's deformity Idiopathic progressive curvature of radius, a developmental defect of the wrist and forearm occurring in adolescence, usually in females. Madelung's deformity is reported with ICD-9-CM code 736.09. *Synonym(s): carpus curvus, Madelung's subluxation, manus valga.*

Madelung's disease Rare, idiopathic disorder often associated with hyperlipoproteinemia, manifested by masses of adipose tissue on the shoulders, neck, arms, and upper trunk. Surgical removal is often required. Report this condition with ICD-9-CM code 272.8.

Madlener Operation

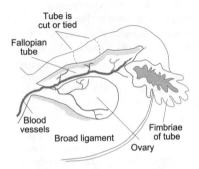

Madlener operation Sterilization method in which a clamp crushes the middle portion of the fallopian tube, which is then shut by suture. Report Madlener operation with ICD-9-CM procedure code 66.31 or CPT code 58600.

madura Fungal or bacterial infection, most often of the foot or leg, that is chronic, develops slowly, and is manifested by nodules that secrete pus with an oily consistency.

MAE Major arrhythmic event.

Maffucci's syndrome Benign, cartilaginous growths in bones with bleeding in viscera and skin. Report this disorder with ICD-9-CM code 756.4.

Magenblase syndrome Condition in which swallowed air accumulates in the stomach causing pain. Report this condition with ICD-9-CM code 306.4. *Synonym(s): stomach bubble syndrome.*

Magnan's sign Tactile hallucination often occurring in cocaine or amphetamine intoxication in which the subject feels as though there are bugs crawling over the skin. *Synonym(s): formication.*

magnesium sulfate/chloride Magnesium salt used as an anticonvulsant, electrolyte replacement, and a dietary supplement. Supply is reported with HCPCS Level II code J3475.

magnesium-deficiency syndrome Hyperexcitability of nerve and muscles due to decrease in concentration of extracellular ionized calcium, resulting in calcium and magnesium deficiency. Report this disorder with ICD-9-CM code 781.7.

magnetic resonance angiography Diagnostic technique utilizing magnetic fields and radio waves rather than radiation to produce detailed, cross-sectional images of internal body structures. CPT code assignment is dependent upon anatomical structure. *Synonym(s): MRA.*

magnetic resonance imaging Radiation-free, noninvasive technique that produces high quality, multiple plane images of the inside of the body by using the natural magnetic properties of the hydrogen atoms within the body that emit radiofrequency signals when exposed to radio waves in a strong magnetic field. *Synonym(s): MRI.*

Magnuson procedure Surgical procedure in which the subscapularis tendon is transferred to the greater tuberosity from the lesser tuberosity for treatment of recurrent anterior dislocations of the shoulder joint. Report Magnuson procedure with ICD-9-CM procedure code 81.82 or CPT code 23450.

Magnuson-Stack procedure Treatment for recurrent anterior dislocation of the shoulder that involves tightening and realigning the subscapularis tendon.

Magpi procedure Surgical procedure involving reconstruction of the meatus and glans, performed in order to correct hypospadias with chordee. Report this procedure with ICD-9-CM procedure code 58.45 or CPT code 54322.

MAHA Microangiopathic hemolytic anemia. Destruction and fragmentation of the red blood cells caused by stricture or blockage of the small blood vessels. Report this condition with ICD-9-CM code 283.19.

Mahler's sign Indication of thrombosis in which there is a continual elevation of the pulse rate but without concurrent temperature elevation.

Main en griffe Abnormal positioning of the hand and fingers usually associated with ulnar nerve palsy, in which the metacarpal phalangeal joints are hyperextended with concomitant flexion of the proximal and distal interphalangeal joints. If the condition is acquired, report ICD-9-CM code 736.06; congenital, report 755.59. *Synonym(s): claw hand deformity.*

Maisonneuve fracture Closed fracture of the proximal fibula due to external rotating force, reported with ICD-9-CM code 823.01. The fracture may be treated with casting alone, or may require two screws with two points of fixation.

Maisonneuve's sign Indication of a Colles' fracture in which the hand demonstrates marked hyperextensibility.

Majocchi's disease Dermatological condition in which there are circular skin lesions mainly on the lower extremities that consist of small telangiectases or tiny maroon spots containing blood hemosiderin deposits. Report this condition with ICD-9-CM code 709.1.

Majocchi's granuloma Uncommon type of fungal infection affecting the lower legs and the hairs of the lower legs. It is manifested by raised, soft granulomas that are red to blue in color and may occur in chains or may be scattered. After lasting for a number of months, the lesions are absorbed, resulting in depressed scars. Report this condition with ICD-9-CM code 110.6. *Synonym(s): MG.*

major complication/comorbidity Diagnosis codes that reflect the highest level of severity in the inpatient DRG IPPS system and have the potential to increase DRG reimbursement. *Synonym(s): MCC.*

major depressive disorder Manic-depressive psychosis in which there is a widespread depressed mood of gloom and wretchedness with some degree of anxiety, reduced activity, or restlessness and agitation. There is a marked tendency to recurrence; in a few cases this may be at regular intervals.

major diagnostic category Classification of diagnoses typically grouped by body system. Used in diagnostic-related group (DRG) reimbursement.

mal- Bad, poor, ill.

malabsorption Body's inability to absorb a substance or nutrient, usually occurring in the small intestine.

malabsorption syndrome Number of syndromes in which the body does not adequately absorb dietary constituents and loses nonabsorbed substances in the stool. Due to muscle, digestive, or lymphatic defect. Report this disorder with ICD-9-CM code 579.9.

malacia Abnormal softening of the tissues, most often found in a disease process.

malacoplakia vesicae Formation of soft, yellowish, raised patches on the mucous membranes of the urethra and bladder as a result of infection.

Maladie de Roger Congenital cardiac abnormality in which the interventricular septum contains a small defect. This defect is isolated and generally without symptoms. Report this condition with ICD-9-CM code 745.4. *Synonym(s): Roger's disease.*

malaise Generalized, nonspecific feeling of discomfort, distress, or uneasiness, sometimes indicative of an underlying disease process. Report this condition with ICD-9-CM code 780.79.

malar Buccal or zygomatic cheekbone area.

malaria Mosquito-borne parasitic infective disease manifested by cyclical chills, fever, and sweating.

malarial hemoglobinuria One of the most dangerous complications of malaria, having a high mortality rate, and occurring almost exclusively with infection from the parasite plasmodium falciparum. Symptoms include rapid pulse, high fever and chills, extreme prostration, rapidly developing anemia, and the passage of urine that is black or dark red in color. Report this condition with ICD-9-CM code 084.8. *Synonym(s): blackwater fever.*

Malassez's disease Testicular cyst, reported with ICD-9-CM code 608.89.

malassimilation Condition in which the body does not properly or adequately absorb nutrients after digestion. Report with malassimilation with ICD-9-CM code 579.9.

J-N

maldescent Common congenital condition in which the testes are incompletely or abnormally descended into the scrotum, often requiring surgical correction. Report this condition with ICD-9-CM code 752.51.

male infertility Inadequate amount of sperm production or an abnormality in the structure or motility of the sperm that makes it unable to reach or penetrate the egg. Contributing factors may include varicose veins in the spermatic cord, undescended testicles, radiation, chemotherapy, removal of one or both testicles, hypothalamic or pituitary disorder, or drug use. Male infertility is reported with a code from ICD-9-CM rubric 606.

male sling operation Procedure to correct male urinary incontinence by producing a mechanical obstruction in the urethra or bladder neck through the creation of a sling of fascia or synthetic material placed across the muscles surrounding the urethra. This puts pressure on the muscles, preventing passive leakage but still allows the patient to force urine.

male stress incontinence Involuntary escape of urine in men at times of minor stress against the bladder, such as coughing, sneezing, or laughing. *NCD Reference: 30.1.1.*

Malherbe tumor Benign follicular tumor containing features of the follicle matrix. Most often found in the head and neck area, these firm, button-like lesions are attached to the skin and underlying subcutaneous tissue. Report Malherbe tumor with a code from ICD-9-CM category 216. *Synonym(s): calcifying epithelioma, Malherbe, pilomatricoma, pilomatrixoma.*

malignant Any condition tending to progress toward death, specifically an invasive tumor with a loss of cellular differentiation that has the ability to spread or metastasize to other areas in the body.

malignant atrophic papulosis Endovasculitis of the skin, gastrointestinal tract, and possibly other organs, that typically occurs in men. Skin lesions appear in crops of erythematous papules with white centers and telangiectactic borders. These atrophy and leave scars. Usually fatal. *Synonym(s): Degas' syndrome.*

malignant carcinoid syndrome Carcinoid tumors causing cyanotic flushing of skin, diarrheal watery stools, bronchoconstrictive attacks, hypotension, edema, and ascites. Report this disorder with ICD-9-CM code 259.2. *Synonym(s): Bjorck-Thorson syndrome, Cassidy-Scholte syndrome, Hedinger's syndrome.*

malignant glaucoma Increase in intraocular pressure that is accompanied by a shallow anterior chamber and forward displacement of the iris and lens. This condition is reported with ICD-9-CM code 365.83

malignant melanoma Highly metastatic malignant neoplasm composed of melanocytes that occurs most often on the skin from a pre-existing mole or nevus, but may also occur in the mouth, esophagus, anal canal, or vagina.

malignant neoplasm Any cancerous tumor or lesion exhibiting uncontrolled tissue growth that can progressively invade other parts of the body with its disease-generating cells.

malignant pleural effusion Severe build-up of fluid in the pleural space from a disturbance of the normal processes that regulate fluid reabsorption. It is caused by an obstruction of the lymph that normally drains the parietal pleura or the transfer of a malignancy from a primary site to the lining of the lung, not to be confused with nonmalignant pleural effusion (ICD-9-CM code 511.9). Malignant pleural effusion is classified to 197.2.

malingerer Individual who intentionally, deliberately, and falsely claims or exaggerates symptoms of an illness or injury. Report this condition with ICD-9-CM code V65.2.

malingering Feigning of illness, as the result of intentional deceit or as the result of mental illness.

malleolus Rounded protuberances on each side of the ankle. The lateral malleolus is the fibula and the medial is the tibia.

mallet finger Congenital or acquired flexion deformity of the terminal interphalangeal joint that causes bowing of the fingertip and an inability to extend the fingertip.

malleus *1)* Outermost of the three bones of the middle ear, also called the hammer. *2)* Highly contagious bacterial disease often found in horses that may be passed on to humans, causing respiratory mucosal ulceration and nodular skin eruptions. Report this disease with ICD-9-CM code 024.

Mallory-Weiss syndrome Tear in the esophagus following several hours or days of vomiting, marked by vomiting of blood. Report this disorder with ICD-9-CM code 530.7.

malnutrition Nutritional insufficiency that may be due to inadequate dietary intake or a defect in the body's ability to absorb or utilize the food ingested.

malocclusion Condition in which the teeth are misaligned. Underlying causes may include accessory, impacted, or missing teeth; dentofacial abnormalities; thumb sucking; or sleeping positions.

Maloney dilator Flexible instrument with a tapered end used to dilate a stricture in the esophagus. When this type of dilator is used, it is considered unguided dilation reported with CPT code 43450.

malposition Congenital or acquired condition in which an organ or body part is in an abnormal or uncharacteristic position.

J-N

malpractice costs One of three components used to develop relative value units (RVUs) under the resource-based relative value scale. This portion represents the cost of professional liability insurance for each procedure.

malrotation Congenital abnormality in which all or a portion of an organ or system fails to rotate normally during development of the embryo.

Malta fever Infection in humans caused by the bacterium brucella, a gram negative, aerobic, coccobacilli microorganism, conveyed by contact with infected animals via infected meat and unpasteurized milk or cheese. Symptoms include fever, chills, sweating, weakness, fatigue, weight loss, aches, and abdominal pain. The various species or subclasses of brucellosis are based on the host animal: sheep, goat, cattle, pigs, or dogs. Malta fever is reported with a code from ICD-9-CM category 023. *Synonym(s): brucellosis, Cyprus fever, Mediterranean fever, rock fever, undulant fever.*

maltosuria Condition in which maltose, the essential structural unit of glycogen and starch, is found in the urine. Report this condition with ICD-9-CM code 271.3.

malt-worker's lung Extrinsic allergic alveolitis caused by inhalation of spores of aspergillus clavatus and aspergillus fumigatus from contaminated barley dust during the beer brewing process. It is classified to ICD-9-CM code 495.4.

malum coxae senilis Unilateral or bilateral osteoarthritis of the hips, usually affecting older persons. Report this condition with ICD-9-CM code 715.25.

malunion Fracture that has united in a faulty position due to inadequate reduction of the original fracture, insufficient holding of a previously well-reduced fracture, contracture of the soft tissues, or comminuted or osteoporotic bone causing a slow disintegration of the fracture. Report this condition with ICD-9-CM code 733.81.

mamillaplasty Surgical repair or reconstruction of the nipple and/or areola. Report this procedure with ICD-9-CM procedure code 85.87 or CPT code 19350 or 19355. *Synonym(s): theleplasty.*

mamillitis Irritation or inflammation of the nipple. Report this condition with ICD-9-CM code 611.0; when occurring in pregnancy report a code from ICD-9-CM subcategory 675.2. *Synonym(s): thelitis.*

mammaplasty Plastic or surgical repair of the breast.

mammary Concerning the breast.

mammary duct ectasia Condition characterized by dilated ducts of the mammary gland.

mammographic microcalcification Small white spots seen on mammography that consist of calcium salt deposits with cellular debris. They may be grouped in small clusters or spread all through the breasts and may be seen with malignant or benign conditions. Report this condition with ICD-9-CM code 793.81.

mammoplasia Condition in which there is further development of breast tissue, sometimes in response to certain drug therapies. Report this condition with ICD-9-CM code 611.1. *Synonym(s): mastoplasia.*

MammoReader Brand name computer-aided detection (CAD) system used by radiologists to read mammograms by highlighting suspicious tissue in the film and changing the mammogram into a digital read-out. The use of a MammoReader does not affect reimbursement.

mammotome Automated, vacuum-assisted biopsy needle used in breast biopsies of nonpalpable lesions; reported with CPT code 19103. Placement of a localization clip and imaging guidance is reported in addition to the biopsy code.

mammotomy Incision of the breast, often performed for exploration of suspicious tissue or for drainage of an abscess. Report this procedure with ICD-9-CM procedure code 85.0 or CPT code 19020. *Synonym(s): mastotomy.*

man. prim. First thing in the morning.

managed care organization Generic term for various health benefit plans that provide coverage for health care services in conjunction with management and review of services provided to ensure services are medically necessary and appropriate. *Synonym(s): MCO.*

managed health care *1)* Managing active cases to ensure care is the most appropriate, efficient, and effective. *2)* System of health care meant to manage overall cost. *3)* Method of health care whereby contracted physicians participate in managing health care costs.

management information system System incorporating hardware and software to facilitate claims management.

management services organization Organization that provides the strategic, financial, and operational plans required by physicians, physician groups, and ancillary service providers for a successful managed care venture. *Synonym(s): MSO.*

Manchester colporrhaphy Preservation of the uterus following prolapse by amputating the vaginal portion of the cervix, shortening the cardinal ligaments, and performing a colpoperineorrhaphy posteriorly.

mandated benefits Services mandated by state or federal law such as child abuse or rape, not necessarily covered by insurers.

mandated providers Providers of medical care, such as psychologists, optometrists, podiatrists, and chiropractors, whose licensed services must, under state or federal law, be included in coverage offered by a health plan.

J-N

mandatory assignment Although not in effect nationally, this alternative system stipulates that only those services for which the physician agrees to accept the Medicare payment as payment in full are fully reimbursable.

mandatory exclusion provisions Stipulations that any individual or entity that has been convicted of a health care felony that involves controlled substances, will be excluded from Medicare participation by the provider for 10 years for the first offense or permanently if convicted on two or more previous occasions.

mandible Lower jawbone giving structure to the floor of the oral cavity.

mandibular Having to do with the lower jaw.

mandibular canal Passage that carries vessels and nerves through the jaw and to the teeth.

mandibular dysostosis Inherited condition with dysostosis of the face, characterized by bilateral malformations, deformities of the outer and middle ear, and a usually smaller lower jaw. Report repair and reconstruction with CPT codes 21150-21151. *Synonym(s): Treacher Collins syndrome.*

mandibulofacial syndrome Malformations of derivatives of the first branchial arch, marked by palpebral fissures sloping outward and downward with notches in the outer third of the lower lids, defects of malar bones and zygoma, hypoplasia of the jawbone, high or cleft palate, low-set ears, unusual hair growth, and pits between mouth and ear. Report this disorder with ICD-9-CM code 756.0. *Synonym(s): Franceschetti's syndrome, mandibulofacial dysostosis syndrome.*

mania Manic-depressive psychosis characterized by states of elation or excitement out of keeping with the individual's circumstances and varying from enhanced liveliness (hypomania) to violent, almost uncontrollable, excitement. Aggression and anger, flight of ideas, distractibility, impaired judgment, and grandiose ideas are common.

manic depression syndrome Alternating major depressive and manic periods. Report this disorder with ICD-9-CM code 296.80. *Synonym(s): bipolar syndrome.*

manic disorder atypical Manic-depressive psychosis characterized by states of elation or excitement out of keeping with the individual's circumstances and varying from enhanced liveliness (hypomania) to violent, almost uncontrollable, excitement. Aggression and anger, flight of ideas, distractibility, impaired judgment, and grandiose ideas are common.

manic-depressive psychosis One of the affective psychotic states, including circular, manic, mixed, or atypical. *depressed type* Manic-depressive psychosis in which there is a widespread depressed mood of gloom and wretchedness with some degree of anxiety, reduced activity, or restlessness and agitation. There is a marked tendency to recurrence; in a few cases this may be at regular intervals. *manic type* Manic-depressive psychosis characterized by states of elation or excitement out of keeping with the individual's circumstances and varying from enhanced liveliness (hypomania) to violent, almost uncontrollable, excitement. Aggression and anger, flight of ideas, distractibility, impaired judgment, and grandiose ideas are common. *mixed type* Manic-depressive psychosis syndrome corresponding to both the manic and depressed types that cannot be classified more specifically.

manipulate Treatment by hand. *NCD Reference: 150.1.*

manipulation Skillful treatment by hand to reduce fractures and dislocations, or provide therapy through forceful passive movement of a joint or muscle beyond its active limit of motion. *NCD Reference: 150.1.*

Mankowsky's syndrome Symmetrical osteitis of limbs localized to phalanges and terminal epiphyses of the long bones of forearm and leg. Symptoms include kyphosis of spine and affection of joints. Report this disorder with ICD-9-CM code 731.2. *Synonym(s): Pierre Marie-Bamberger syndrome.*

Mannerfelt syndrome Rupture of flexor pollicis longus tendon from attrition caused by bony spur in carpal tunnel, most commonly due to rheumatoid arthritis. The rupture is reported with ICD-9-CM code 727.64. Code also the rheumatoid arthritis.

mannitol Diuretic used as a diagnostic agent in oliguria or renal dysfunction to determine glomerular filtration rate and to promote diuresis in the oliguric phase of renal failure to rid the patient of toxic chemicals and lower intracranial and intraocular pressure. Mannitol increases the osmolarity in the glomerular infiltrate, preventing tubular reabsorption of fluids, and promoting excretion of sodium and potassium. Supply is reported with HCPCS Level II code J2150. May be sold under brand name Osmitrol.

mannosidosis Inborn error of metabolism that results in a buildup of oligosaccharides, a type of short-chain sugar. Coarse facial appearance, upper respiratory problems, profound mental retardation, enlargement of the liver and spleen, and cataracts are often present in this disease. Two types of mannosidosis include infantile onset (type I) and juvenile-adult onset (type II). Both are reported with ICD-9-CM code 271.8.

manometric Pertaining to pressure, as measured in a meter.

manometry Pressure measurement of liquids and gases along the esophagus.

Manson's disease Intestinal infection by a parasitic worm Schistosoma mansoni. Symptoms may include diarrhea, melena, enlarged liver and spleen, and anemia.

Often asymptomatic during the early stages, later complications may include intestinal blockage or acute renal failure. Report this disease with ICD-9-CM code 120.1.

Manson's pyosis Infection most often caused by pus-producing bacteria and manifested by a severe localized inflammatory pustular response. Report this condition with ICD-9-CM code 684. **Synonym(s):** *pemphigus contagiosus.*

Mantoux test Skin test in which a small amount of liquid tuberculin, also known as purified protein derivative, is injected between the layers of the skin in order to determine if one has been infected with the bacteria that causes tuberculosis. **Synonym(s):** *PPD.*

manual transmittals Manual transmittals announce policy revisions. National coverage determinations are announced in transmittals for the *Medicare National Coverage Determinations Manual.* Changes to local medical review policy (LMRP) are announced in transmittals for the *Medicare Program Integrity Manual.*

MAP Mean arterial pressure.

maple bark disease Extrinsic allergic inflammation of the lungs' air sacs (alveoli) caused by inhalation of a fungus found in moldy maple bark. Report this condition with ICD-9-CM code 495.6.

maple syrup syndrome Anomaly in amino acid metabolism marked by urine and perspiration odor, hypertonicity, convulsions, coma, and death. Report this disorder with ICD-9-CM code 270.3.

mapping Multi-dimensional depiction of a tachycardia that identifies its site of origin and its electrical conduction pathway after tachycardia has been induced. The recording is made from multiple catheter sites within the heart, obtaining electrograms either simultaneously or sequentially. This is a separate procedure in addition to electrophysiological studies and is reported separately using CPT code 93609 or 93613.

Maquet procedure Surgical procedure performed for treatment of patellofemoral joint pain entailing anterior displacement of the tibial tubercle and insertion of a bony block. The result is decreased force on the patella as it crosses the femoral condyles and an alteration in its weight-bearing position. Report this procedure with ICD-9-CM procedure code 78.47 or CPT code 27418.

MAR Medication administration record.

Marable's syndrome Compression of celiac artery by median arcuate ligament in diaphragm. Report this disorder with ICD-9-CM code 447.4.

marasmus Protein-calorie malabsorption or malnutrition characterized by hypoalbuminemia, tissue wasting, dehydration, and subcutaneous fat depletion. Marasmus is reported with ICD-9-CM code 261. **Synonym(s):** *infantile atrophy, nutritional atrophy.*

marble bones Rare congenital condition in which the bones are excessively dense, resulting from a discrepancy in the formation and breakdown of bone. This disease manifests in various types and severity and can cause optic atrophy and deafness, hepatosplenomegaly, fractures, and depleted bone marrow and nerve foramina in the skull. This condition is reported with ICD-9-CM code 756.52. **Synonym(s):** *Albers-Schönberg disease, osteopetrosis.*

Marburg disease Animal-borne, viral hemorrhagic fever whose symptoms initially include fever, chills, and muscle aches, followed by a trunk rash, chest pain, sore throat, and GI symptoms. Symptoms increase in severity and may include jaundice, pancreatic inflammation, copious hemorrhaging, shock, and multi-system dysfunction. Report this condition with ICD-9-CM code 078.89.

Marcaine See bupivacaine HCl.

march foot Condition often associated with extreme foot strain in which the forefoot becomes painful and swollen due to fracture of one of the metatarsal bones. Report this condition with ICD-9-CM code 733.94.

march hemoglobinuria Condition occurring after extended or intense physical exercise in which hemoglobin is excreted in the urine. Report this condition with ICD-9-CM code 283.2.

Marchesani (-Weill) syndrome Short stature, heavy musculature, reduced joint mobility, myopic, glaucoma, and many other symptoms. Report this disorder with ICD-9-CM code 759.89.

Marchiafava (Bignami) disease Deterioration of the nerve fibers that connect the two hemispheres of the brain found most often in alcoholics. Symptoms include mental decline, dementia, and seizures. Report this disorder with ICD-9-CM code 341.8.

Marchiafava-Micheli syndrome Uncommon, acquired stem cell disorder in which the red blood cells undergo premature destruction, resulting in hemoglobin in the urine and a tendency to develop recurring blood clots. Some level of bone marrow dysfunction is also present. Report this condition with ICD-9-CM code 283.2. **Synonym(s):** *paroxysmal nocturnal hemoglobinuria, PNH.*

Marcus-Gunn syndrome Congenital anomaly of unknown causes characterized by the onset of rapid eyelid movement, producing a winking effect when the jaw moves. This syndrome is reported with ICD-9-CM code 742.8. **Synonym(s):** *jaw-winking syndrome.*

Marfan's sign Coating of the tongue with a red triangle at the tip. Often an indication of typhoid fever.

Marfan's syndrome Unusually long extremities, subluxation of the lens, dilation of the aorta, and other symptoms. Report this disorder with ICD-9-CM code 759.82.

J–N

margin Boundary, edge, or border, as of a surface or structure.

Marie's cerebellar ataxia Hereditary neurologic condition characterized by uncontrolled movements of the extraocular muscles, internal paralysis of the eye muscles, and optic wasting. Report this disorder with ICD-9-CM code 334.2. **Synonym(s):** *primary cerebellar degeneration.*

Marie's sign Indication of Graves' disease or other forms of hyperthyroidism manifested by body or extremity tremors.

Marie's syndrome Secondary to chronic conditions in lung and heart, localized to phalanges and terminal epiphyses of long bones of arm and leg, and accompanied by kyphosis. Caused by pituitary disorder. Report this disorder with ICD-9-CM code 253.0.

Marie-Bamberger disease Syndrome manifested by clubbed fingers and toes, enlarged extremities, pain in the joints, and vasomotor disturbance of the hands and feet. The periosteum of the radius and fibula is frequently inflamed, often due to underlying pulmonary problems such as lung cancer, tuberculosis, abscesses, emphysema, or cystic fibrosis. Conditions other than pulmonary disorders may also cause this syndrome. Report this disease with ICD-9-CM code 731.2. **Synonym(s):** *Hagner's disease, HPOA, hypertrophic pulmonary osteoarthropathy.*

Marie-Foix syndrome Ataxia, hemiparesis, and hemihyperesthesia for pain and temperature, seen following a stroke within the basilar artery's long circumferential branches or anterior inferior cerebellar artery, creating a lesion in the lateral pons.

Marie-Strumpell disease Rheumatic inflammation of the joints of the hips, spine, and pelvis most commonly affecting young men. This arthritic disease of the joints can lead to fusion and deformity of the spine. The cause is unknown. Report this condition with ICD-9-CM code 720.0. **Synonym(s):** *ankylosing spondylitis, rheumatoid spondylitis.*

Marinesco's sign Hand that is soft, edematous, cold, and bluish in color, caused by swelling and thickening of the subcutaneous tissues. Indication of fluid filed cyst within the spinal cord (syringomyelia). **Synonym(s):** *Marinesco's succulent hand, succulent hand.*

Marjolin's ulcer Malignancy rising from any site of chronic inflammation, as in a skin ulcer, usually in an extremity. Most Marjolin's ulcers develop from burn scars, but others may develop at the site of decubitus ulcers, osteomyelitis, or other non-healing wounds. Marjolin's ulcers are most typically squamous cell, but may be basal cell carcinoma, melanoma, or sarcoma. The ICD-9-CM code should be based on the type of malignancy and skin site.

Markus-Adie syndrome Paralysis of conjugate movement of eyes without paralysis of convergence. Caused by lesions of midbrain. Report this disorder with ICD-9-CM code 379.46.

Mar-Land pessary Vaginal device inserted to treat stress incontinence. Mar-Land pessary is non-rubber. Supply is reported with HCPCS Level II code A4562.

Marlex Brand name mesh reinforcement applied in herniorrhaphy.

Marlow's test Test for heterophoria (the eye's tendency to deviate) in which one eye is covered for a specific time. When the eye is uncovered, measurements for heterophoria are made.

Marmine See dimenhydrinate.

Maroteaux-Lamy syndrome Accumulation of mucopolysaccharide sulfates affecting eye, ear, skin, teeth, skeleton, joints, liver, spleen, cardiovascular system, respiratory system, and central nervous system. Report this disorder with ICD-9-CM code 277.5.

Marseilles fever Acute, febrile, rickettsial disease transmitted by tick bites and causing a primary lesion at the site of the bite, with rash, muscle and joint pain, headache, chills, fever, and sensitivity to light. It is commonly found in the Mediterranean and around the Black and Caspian Seas, having many names depending on the geographical region. This condition is reported with ICD-9-CM code 082.1. **Synonym(s):** *African tickbite fever, Boutonneuse fever, Indian tick typhus, Kenya tick typhus, Mediterranean tick fever.*

Marsh's disease Enlargement of the thyroid gland seen mostly in women, stemming from an autoimmune process, and causing excessive secretion of thyroid hormone, goiter, and bulging eyes. The syndrome seen with hyperplasia of the thyroid and excessive hormone production consists of fatigue, nervousness, emotional lability and irritability, heat intolerance and increased sweating, weight loss, palpitations, and tremor of the hands and tongue. If there is no documentation of a thyrotoxic crisis or storm, report ICD-9-CM code 242.00; with thyrotoxic crisis or storm, report 242.01. **Synonym(s):** *Basedow syndrome, Begbie's disease, Flajani disease, Graves' disease, Parry's disease, toxic diffuse goiter.*

Marshall-Marchetti-Krantz Surgical procedure to correct urinary stress incontinence in which the bladder is suspended by placing several sutures through the tissue surrounding the urethra and into the vaginal wall. The sutures are pulled tight so that the tissues are tacked up to the symphysis pubis and the urethra is moved forward. This procedure is normally reported with CPT codes 51840 and 51841. **Synonym(s):** *anterior vesicourethropexy.*

marsupial pouch Brand name belted pouch for use by ambulatory patients who have postsurgical drainage tubes.

marsupialization Creation of a pouch in surgical treatment of a cyst in which one wall is resected and the remaining cut edges are sutured to adjacent tissue creating an open pouch of the previously enclosed cyst.

Martin-Albright-Bantam disease Rare genetic disease in which there is sufficient amount of parathyroid hormone produced, but the body is unable to respond to it, due to a defective type of protein required for the hormone's signal transduction. This results in low blood calcium levels and high phosphate levels. Physical characteristics include a short physique, round face, obesity, and short hand bones. Report this disorder with ICD-9-CM code 275.49. **Synonym(s):** *Albright's hereditary osteodystrophy, Bantam-Albright-Martin disease, pseudohypoparathyroidism.*

Martorell-Fabré syndrome Progressive obliteration of the brachiocephalic trunk and the left subclavian and common carotid arteries above their source in the aortic arch causing ischemia, transient blindness, facial atrophy, and possibly other symptoms. Report this disorder with ICD-9-CM code 446.7. **Synonym(s):** *Marorell-Fabre syndrome, Raed-Harbitz syndrome, Takayasu-Onishi syndrome.*

masculinovoblastoma Benign neoplasm of the ovary that often results in different degrees of masculinization. Report this condition with ICD-9-CM code 220.

MASER Microwave amplification by stimulated emission of radiation.

masochism Sexual gratification derived from having pain, humiliation, or degradation threatened or inflicted on oneself, often in the form of whipping, beating, bondage, or acts of submission. Report this condition with ICD-9-CM code 302.83.

masochistic personality Personality disorder in which the individual appears to arrange life situations so as to be defeated and humiliated.

masons' lung Chronic respiratory disease caused by inhaling particles of stone dust or silica, often seen in stonemasons. Report this condition with ICD-9-CM code 502.

Massachusetts Health Data Consortium Organization that seeks to improve health care in New England through improved policy development, better technology planning and implementation, and more informed financial decision making. **Synonym(s):** *MHDC.*

massage Systematic and patterned stroking, kneading, and therapeutic friction applied to soft tissue by hand.

massive aspiration of newborn syndrome Intrauterine aspiration of amniotic fluid contaminated by meconium. Report this disorder with ICD-9-CM code 770.18.

MAST Military antishock trousers.

mast cells Cells found in the loose connective tissue of blood vessels and bronchioles responsible for acute hypersensitivity reactions, including anaphylactic shock. The IgE receptors on these cells bind with allergens causing cell degranulation and diffuse, widespread histamine release that results in airway constriction and vasodilation with decreased systemic blood pressure.

mastalgia Breast pain that may or may not be related to the menstrual cycle. Report this condition with ICD-9-CM code 611.71; if specified as psychogenic, add 307.89.

Modified Radical Mastectomy

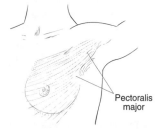

Pectoralis major

A modified radical mastectomy is performed where the pectoralis major muscle is preserved

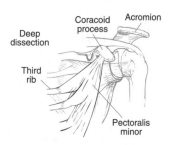

Coracoid process   Acromion

Deep dissection

Third rib

Pectoralis minor

mastectomy Surgical removal of one or both breasts. *modified radical m.* Large muscles of the chest that move the arm are preserved, reported with CPT code 19307. *partial m.* Removal of breast tissue with specific attention to surgical margins to remove a tumor or disease area, commonly referred to as a lumpectomy, tylectomy, quadrantectomy, or segmentectomy. Partial mastectomies are reported with 19300-19301. *radical m.* Lymph nodes of the axilla, some muscles of the chest wall, and sometimes the internal mammary nodes are removed, reported with 19305-19306. *simple m.* Only breast tissue, nipple, and a small portion of overlying skin are removed, reported with 19303. *subcutaneous m.* Breast tissue is removed via an incision under the breast with the skin and nipple left intact. It is performed primarily as a preventive measure for women who are

J-N

at a high risk of developing breast cancer. Subcutaneous mastectomy is reported with 19304. *Synonym(s): skin sparing mastectomy. NCD Reference: 140.2.*

Masterbrace 3   Knee orthosis formed of lightweight material. Bipivotal hinge devices enhance accommodation of the knee's natural motion. Supply is reported with HCPCS Level II code L2999.

Masters-Allen syndrome   Pelvic pain resulting from old laceration of broad ligament received during delivery. Report this disorder with ICD-9-CM code 620.6.

mastication   Process of chewing food to ready it for the digestive system.

mastitis   Inflammation of the breast. Acute mastitis is caused by a bacterial infection; chronic mastitis is caused by hormonal changes. Report acute mastitis with a code from ICD-9-CM category 610; chronic conditions with a code from category 611.

mastocytosis syndrome   Inherited disorder of skin (and sometimes other structures) in which pigmented lesions appear in linear, zebra stripe, and other configurations and are preceded by vesicles and bullae and followed by verrucal lesions. Report this disorder with ICD-9-CM code 757.33.

mastodynia   Pain, discomfort, or tenderness in the breast, often due to hormonal changes. Mastodynia is reported with ICD-9-CM code 611.71. If specified as psychogenic, code 307.89 is also reported. *Synonym(s): mastalgia.*

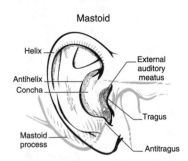

Mastoid

Helix
External auditory meatus
Antihelix
Concha
Tragus
Mastoid process
Antitragus

mastoid   Rounded process, or protrusion on the temporal bone behind the ear.

mastoidalgia   Pain or discomfort in the mastoid area, reported with ICD-9-CM code 388.70.

mastoidectomy   Surgical excision of a portion of the mastoid of the posterior temporal bone often performed in conjunction with other related procedures and not reported separately.

mastoiditis   Acute or chronic inflammation and irritation of the air space and air cells in the mastoid section of the temporal bone. Report mastoiditis with a code from ICD-9-CM category 383.

mastoidotomy   Surgical incision into the temporal bone's mastoid process or subperiosteum, often performed in conjunction with other procedures such as tympanoplasty. Report mastoidotomy with ICD-9-CM procedure code 20.21 or a code from CPT range 69635-69637.

mastopathy   Disease or disorder of the breast or lactiferous (mammary) glands.

mastopexy   Surgical procedure on the breast in which the nipple and areola are relocated to a higher position and the excess skin below the nipple and above the lower breast crease is excised. Report this procedure with ICD-9-CM procedure code 85.6 or CPT code 19316. *Synonym(s): breast lift.*

mastoplasia   Condition in which there is further development of breast tissue, sometimes in response to certain drug therapies. Report this condition with ICD-9-CM code 611.1. *Synonym(s): mammoplasia.*

mastotomy   Incision of the breast, often performed for exploration of suspicious tissue or for drainage of an abscess. Report this procedure with ICD-9-CM procedure code 85.0 or CPT code 19020. *Synonym(s): mammotomy.*

MAT   Multifocal atrial tachycardia, reported with ICD-9-CM code 427.89.

Matas' test   Test to determine collateral circulation in which a tourniquet is applied to the limb for a specified time. It is then removed and the extent of collateral circulation is ascertained by applying pressure to the main artery. *Synonym(s): tourniquet test.*

maternal hypotension syndrome   Significantly reduced blood pressure during pregnancy. Report this disorder with a code from ICD-9-CM range 669.20-669.24.

maternal obesity syndrome   Edema or excessive weight gain in pregnancy with no hypertension. Report this disorder with a code from ICD-9-CM range 646.10-646.14.

Matrix VSG   Brand name cardiac catheterization system.

Maverick   Brand name artificial implant for lumbar total disc replacement composed of a two-piece, metal-on-metal device with a posterior center of rotation ball-and-socket type joint between the endplates, inserted by anterior approach. Total disc replacement is currently being tested in clinical trials in the United States as an emerging technology, reported with CPT codes 22856 and 0092T.

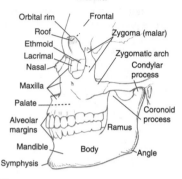

Maxilla

Orbital rim
Frontal
Roof
Zygoma (malar)
Ethmoid
Lacrimal
Zygomatic arch
Nasal
Condylar process
Maxilla
Palate
Coronoid process
Alveolar margins
Ramus
Mandible
Body
Angle
Symphysis

maxilla Pyramidally shaped bone forming the upper jaw, part of the eye orbit, nasal cavity, and palate and lodging the upper teeth.

maxillary Located between the eyes and the upper teeth.

maxillectomy Removal of all or a portion of a diseased maxilla. This procedure may also include removal of the eye and the orbital soft tissue for an en bloc resection. Report maxillectomy with a code from CPT range 31225-31230.

maximum allowable actual charge Former provision of the Medicare program that applied to nonparticipating physicians before January 1, 1991, and set a limit on charges for physicians' professional services and most services provided incident to the professional services. *Synonym(s): MAAC.*

maximum allowable charge Amount set by the insurer as the highest amount that can be charged for a particular medical service or by a pharmacy vendor. *Synonym(s): MAC.*

maximum defined data set Under HIPAA, required data elements for a particular standard based on a specific implementation specification. An entity creating a transaction is free to include whatever data any receiver might want or need. The recipient is free to ignore any portion of the data that are not needed to conduct its part of the associated business transaction, unless the inessential data are needed for coordination of benefits.

maximum out-of-pocket costs Limit on total number of copayments, deductibles, and coinsurance under a benefit contract.

Maxipime See cefepime HCl.

May (-Hegglin) syndrome Hepatosplenomegaly, lymphadenopathy, anemia, thrombocytopenia, along with changes in the bones, cardiopulmonary system, skin, and psychomotor skills. Abnormalities of granulation and nuclear structure of white cells open child to infection and result in death. Report this disorder

with ICD-9-CM code 288.2. *Synonym(s): Chediak-Higashi syndrome, Dohle body syndrome, Hegglin syndrome, Jordan's syndrome, May syndrome.*

Mayaro fever Mosquito-borne viral infection that manifests with headache, pain behind the eyes, muscle and joint pain, and gastrointestinal upset. Polyarthritis is a prominent aspect of this disease and may be severe. Report this condition with ICD-9-CM code 066.3.

Maydl colostomy Colon is drawn out through the wound and maintained in position by a glass rod until adhesions have formed.

Mayo hernia repair Surgical procedure in which the physician excises an umbilical hernia mass and overlaps the space with abdominal muscles. Report this procedure with ICD-9-CM procedure code 53.49 or a code from CPT range 49580-49587.

maze procedure Creation of multiple incisions in the left atria through the endocardium to obliterate aberrant atrial conduction pathways and allow a normal impulse to activate the atrium, thereby stopping atrial fibrillation or flutter. This procedure is reported with a code from CPT range 33254-33256.

MBC Maximum breathing capacity.

MBD Minimal brain dysfunction.

McArdle (-Schmid) (-Pearson) syndrome Glucose-6-phosphatase deficiency due to inherited defects of glycogen metabolism resulting in excess accumulation of glycogen in muscle, characterized by myopathies and hepatorenal effects. Report this disorder with ICD-9-CM code 271.0.

MCB *1)* Metastatic breast cancer. *2)* Male breast cancer.

McBride bunionectomy Repair of a thickened bulge at the base of the first toe. This procedure includes release of adductor hallucis, transverse metatarsal ligament, and lateral capsule, combined with excision of medial eminence and plication of the capsule medially. Report this procedure with CPT code 28292.

McBurney's sign Indication of appendicitis in which there is pain and tenderness at a site two-thirds the distance from the umbilicus to the anterior superior iliac spine.

McCall culdoplasty Vaginal suspension procedure for repair of uterine prolapse. This procedure suspends the vagina to the uterosacral ligaments and closes the cul-de-sac of Douglas, which treats an enterocele as well. It requires the normal attachment (uterosacral ligaments) be strong enough to be a firm support for the vaginal vault. Report CPT code 57283 for the procedure, along with any applicable codes for concurrent hysterectomy, anterior/posterior colporrhaphy, etc.

McCannel suture Securing the haptic loop of an intraocular lens to the iris by threading the suture

J-N

through the cornea without opening the eye, reported with CPT code 66682.

McCune-Albright syndrome Patchy skin pigmentation, endocrine dysfunctions, and polyostotic fibrous dysplasia. Report this disorder with ICD-9-CM code 756.59. *Synonym(s): Albright's hereditary osteodystrophy.*

MCD Macular corneal dystrophy.

McDonald operation Surgical procedure in which the opening of the cervix is decreased via pursestring sutures around the bottom of the cervix. Report this procedure with ICD-9-CM procedure code 67.59 or CPT code 57700. *Synonym(s): McDonald cerclage.*

McDonald procedure Polyester tape is placed around the cervix with a running stitch to assist in the prevention of pre-term delivery. Tape is removed at term for vaginal delivery.

McDonald's criteria Diagnostic criteria for multiple sclerosis. The neurologist examines the patient and MRIs to determine the number of brain and spinal lesions present.

MCE *1)* Medical care evaluation. *2)* Medicare code editor. Computer program used by Medicare fiscal intermediaries to identify coding inconsistencies in the information reported on an inpatient claim. In determining the appropriate DRG payment, the age, sex, discharge status, principal diagnosis, secondary diagnosis, and procedures performed are reviewed for accuracy and consistency with the other data reported on the claim. The MCE reviews codes, coverage, and clinical information.

mcg Microgram.

MCH Mean corpuscular hemoglobin.

MCHC Mean corpuscular hemoglobin concentration.

mCi Millicurie.

McIndoe vaginal construction Construction of an artificial vagina without using a graft.

MCKD Multicystic kidney disease.

MCL *1)* Modified chest lead. *2)* Midclavicular line.

MCLS Mucocutaneous lymph node syndrome. Syndrome of unknown origin causing fever; redness of the eyes, lips, and mucous membranes of the mouth; gingivitis; cervical lymphadenopathy, and a bright red raised rash in a glove-and-sock fashion over the hands and feet. The skin there becomes hard, swollen (edematous), and peels. This disease mainly affects children and is reported with ICD-9-CM code 446.1. *Synonym(s): Kawasaki disease.*

MCM Medicare Carriers Manual. Manual CMS provides to Medicare carriers containing instructions for processing and paying Medicare claims, preparing reimbursement forms, billing procedures, and adhering to Medicare regulations. This has been replaced by the Medicare manual system.

McMurray's test Test to determine a meniscus tear. The patient is placed supine with a flexed knee. While rotating the foot outward and extending the knee, a painful "click" suggests a medial meniscus tear. A lateral meniscus tear is indicated if the click takes place while the foot is being rotated inward.

MCO Managed care organization. Generic term for various health benefit plans that provide coverage for health care services in conjunction with management and review of services provided to ensure that services are medically necessary and appropriate.

MCP *1)* Metacarpophalangeal. *2)* Monthly capitation payment.

McQuarrie syndrome Hypoglycemia described as primary and unspecified, reactive, or spontaneous. Report this disorder with ICD-9-CM code 251.2.

MCR Modified community rating.

MCS Minimally conscious state. MCS differs from persistent vegetative state in that the patient may demonstrate self- or environmental awareness and have some response to stimuli. MCS is reported with ICD-9-CM code 780.01.

MCT Mediastinal chest tube.

MCTD Mixed connective tissue disease. Rare autoimmune disorder affecting mostly women with characteristics of lupus, scleroderma, and polymyositis. MCTD is reported with ICD-9-CM code 710.9.

MCV *1)* Major cardiovascular condition. Designation that allows for severity in determining a higher-paying diagnosis-related group for patients requiring a higher level of care. This designation was established by CMS for its 2006 fiscal year. *2)* Mean corpuscular volume.

MD *1)* Manic depression. *2)* Medical doctor. *3)* Muscular dystrophy. *4)* Myocardial disease.

MDC Major diagnostic category. Dividing all possible principal diagnoses into mutually exclusive categories. These broad classifications of ICD-9-CM diagnoses are typically grouped by organ system.

MDCT Multi-slice detector computed tomography. Noninvasive diagnostic imaging that can produce multiple, thin-slice, cross-section images simultaneously. *Synonym(s): multi-row detector CT, multi-slice CT.*

MDD Manic-depressive disorder.

MDH Medicare dependent hospital, a CMS designation. Major source of Medicare service in a locality.

MDR Multidrug resistance.

MDS *1)* Minimum data set. Contains a core set of screening, clinical, and functional status elements, including common definitions and coding categories that form the basis of a comprehensive patient assessment RUG-III classification system. The Medicare skilled nursing facility (SNF) prospective payment system (PPS) is based on the MDS. Under the PPS, SNFs are required to use the MDS 2.0 as the data source for classifying patients for case mix. All of the information necessary to classify a patient into one of the RUG-III categories is contained in the MDS 2.0. *2)* Myelodysplastic syndrome. Collection of disorders in which the bone marrow does not produce enough blood cells. MDS can be a precursor of leukemia, and is reported with ICD-9-CM codes 238.72-238.75.

MDUFMA Medical Device User Fee and Modernization Act of 2002. Federal law that classifies and sets standards for single use devices that may reenter the marketplace after undergoing sterilization and cleansing.

ME Medical examiner.

MEA Microwave endometrial ablation. Long slender tube inserted into the uterus to deliver microwave energy to destroy endometrial tissue and minimize excessive uterine bleeding. MEA is reported with CPT code 58563.

Mean's sign Indication of Graves' orbitopathy in which the upper eyelid springs upward more quickly than the eyeball does when a hand is placed level with the patient's eyes and then raised. *Synonym(s): Kocher's sign.*

meaningful use Sets of guidelines that must be followed as part of the HITECH act.

measles Highly contagious, acute airborne viral disease manifested by fever, small red spots, and flu-like symptoms. Measles is primarily a disease of childhood and is generally reported with a code from ICD-9-CM rubric 055. *Synonym(s): rubeola.*

measles, mumps, and rubella vaccine Combined subcutaneous vaccination for measles, mumps, and rubella. Report MMR with ICD-9-CM procedure code 99.48 or CPT code 90707. Also report the appropriate administration code. *Synonym(s): MMR.*

meatoplasty Surgery to enlarge or reconstruct a meatus (an opening, canal, or passageway in the body). Meatoplasty usually applies to the external auditory or urethral meatus.

meatus Opening or passage into the body.

meat-wrappers' asthma Occupational asthma caused by inhalation of irritants in the workplace, in this case fumes from hot-wire cuttings of PVC film and from the price labels that are heat activated. Report this condition with ICD-9-CM code 506.9.

Mec Meconium.

mechanical traction Use of tractive forces to produce a combination of distraction and gliding to relieve discomfort or increase tissue flexibility. *Synonym(s): passive mobilization.*

mechlorethamine HCl Alkylating antineoplastic used to treat a variety of lymphomas such as Hodgkin's disease and chronic myelocytic leukemia. It is also used to treat intracavitary effusions of malignant cells. This chemotherapeutic drug is administered via IV infusion or intracavitary instillation. Supply is reported with HCPCS Level II code J9230. May be sold under brand name Mustargen.

Meckel's diverticulum Abnormal remnant of embryonic digestive system development that leaves a sacculation or outpouching from the wall of the small intestine near the terminal part of the ileum made of acid-secreting tissue as in the stomach.

meconium First stool passed by a fetus, sometimes while still in the uterus. In this event, the meconium combines with the maternal amniotic fluid. Complications may occur if meconium is aspirated by the fetus while in utero or at the time of birth. *m. staining* Meconium passed in utero causing discoloration on the fetus' skin and nails, or on the umbilicus. This staining may be incidental or may be an indicator of significant fetal stress that could affect outcomes. Meconium staining is reported with ICD-9-CM code 779.84. *m. aspiration* Meconium in the trachea or seen on chest x-ray after birth. Aspiration of meconium is reported with codes from ICD-9-CM subcategory 770.1.

meconium aspiration syndrome Newborn respiratory complications resulting from the passage and subsequent aspiration of meconium (fetal intestinal waste material) prior to or during delivery.

MEd Master of education.

MED Minimal effective dose.

medial Middle or midline.

medial canthopexy Fixation or reattachment of the medial canthal ligament of the eye.

medial canthus Junction of the upper and lower eyelids near the nose.

median arcuate ligament syndrome Compression of celiac artery by median arcuate ligament in diaphragm. Report this disorder with ICD-9-CM code 447.4.

median nerve One of the five main nerves originating from the brachial plexus, the median nerve innervates the forearm and parts of the hand.

median sternotomy Standard incision for open chest cardiac surgeries, from above the bellybutton to just under the chin, down the center of the chest through the sternum into the thoracic cavity.

mediastinitis Acute or chronic inflammation and irritation of the cavity between the lungs, containing the heart, large vessels, trachea, esophagus, thymus, and

M-N

connective tissue. Report this condition with ICD-9-CM code 519.2.

mediastinoscope Endoscope used for direct, internal visualization of the mediastinum.

mediastinotomy Incision into the mediastinum for purposes of exploration, foreign body removal, drainage, or biopsy. Report this procedure with ICD-9-CM procedure code 34.1. Report a cervical approach with CPT code 39000 and a median or transthoracic approach with 39010.

mediastinum Collection of organs and tissues that separate the pleural sacs. Located between the sternum and spine above the diaphragm, it contains the heart and great vessels, trachea and bronchi, esophagus, thymus, lymph nodes, and nerves.

Medicaid Joint federal and state program that covers medical expenses for people with low incomes and limited resources who meet the criteria. The benefits for recipients vary from state to state.

Medicaid fiscal agent Organization responsible for administering claims for a state Medicaid program.

Medicaid state agency State agency responsible for overseeing the state's Medicaid program.

medical and other health services Any of the services provided to a patient to diagnose, treat, or maintain health status, including services of health care providers and professionals; rural, inpatient, outpatient, and diagnostic services; physical/occupational/speech/sports therapy; dialysis; immunization and vaccines; blood products; drugs; nutritional and diagnosis instruction; equipment; supplies; and ambulance services.

medical care evaluation Part of the quality assurance program that reviews the process of medical care. *Synonym(s): MCE.*

medical code sets Codes that characterize a medical condition or treatment. These code sets are usually maintained by professional societies and public health organizations.

medical consultation Advice or an opinion rendered by a physician at the request of the primary care provider.

medical decision making Consideration of the differential diagnoses, the amount and/or complexity of data reviewed and considered (medical records, test results, correspondence from previous treating physicians, etc.), current diagnostic studies ordered, and treatment or management options and risk (complications of the patient's condition, the potential for complications, continued morbidity, risk of mortality, any comorbidities associated with the patient's disease process).

medical doctor Allopathic, or traditional, physician. *Synonym(s): MD.*

medical documentation Patient care records, including operative notes; physical, occupational, and speech-language pathology notes; progress notes; physician certification and recertifications; and emergency room records; or the patient's medical record in its entirety. When Medicare coverage cannot be determined based on the information submitted on the claim, medical documentation may be requested. The Medicare Administrative Contractor (MAC) will deny a claim for lack of medical necessity if medical documentation is not received within the stated time frame defined by the MAC (usually within 35-45 days after the date of request).

medical loss ratio Ratio between the cost to deliver medical care and the amount of money taken in by the plan.

medical meaningfulness Patients in the same DRG can be expected to evoke a set of clinical responses that result in a similar pattern of resource use.

medical necessity Medically appropriate and necessary to meet basic health needs; consistent with the diagnosis or condition and rendered in a cost-effective manner; and consistent with national medical practice guidelines regarding type, frequency, and duration of treatment.

Medical Records Institute Organization that promotes the development and acceptance of electronic health care record systems. *Synonym(s): MRI.*

medical review Review by a Medicare fiscal intermediary, carrier and/or quality improvement organization (QIO) of services and items provided by physicians, other health care practitioners, and providers of health care services under Medicare. The review determines if the items and services are reasonable and necessary and meet Medicare coverage requirements, whether the quality meets professionally recognized standards of health care, and whether the services are medically appropriate in an inpatient, outpatient, or other setting as supported by documentation.

Medical staff-hospital organization (MeSH) Organization that forms a network from hospital and attending medical staff. *Synonym(s): MeSH.*

medically necessary Services or supplies that are warranted for the diagnosis or treatment of a medical condition; are used for diagnosis, direct care, and treatment of a medical condition; meet the standards of good medical practice in the local community; and are not solely for the convenience of the patient or the doctor.

Medicare Federally funded program authorized as part of the Social Security Act that provides for health care services for people age 65 or older, people with disabilities, and people with end-stage renal disease (ESRD).

Medicare administrative contractor Uniform type of Medicare administrative entity that will process both institutional and professional claims in specified geographic jurisdictions of the country. There will be 15 A/B MACs, four DME MACs, and four home health/hospice MACs. MACs will be phased in over the next few years with all jurisdictions operational by October 2011.

Medicare Benefit Policy Manual CMS Internet-only manual (Pub. 100-02) that consolidates general information that had been contained in various paper manuals. It outlines the different coverage components of Medicare benefits (e.g., inpatient hospital service, home health service).

Medicare carrier Organization that contracts with CMS to adjudicate professional claims under Part B, the supplemental medical insurance program. Medicare carriers are responsible for daily claims processing, utilization review, record maintenance, dissemination of information based on CMS regulations, and determining whether services are covered and payments are appropriate. This organization will be replaced by Medicare Administrative Contractors by 2011.

Medicare Carriers Manual Manual provided by the Centers for Medicare and Medicaid Services to Medicare carriers containing instructions for processing and paying Medicare claims, preparing reimbursement forms, billing procedures, and adhering to Medicare regulations. This has been replaced by the Medicare manual system. *Synonym(s): MCM.*

Medicare Claims Processing Manual CMS Internet-only manual (Pub. 100-04) that consolidated and replaced the paper hospital, intermediary, and carrier manuals. The manual outlines billing and processing instructions for all claim types.

Medicare code editor Computer program used by Medicare contractors to identify coding inconsistencies in the information reported on an inpatient claim. In determining the appropriate DRG payment, the age, sex, discharge status, principal diagnosis, secondary diagnosis, and procedures performed are reviewed for accuracy and consistency with the other data reported on the claim. The MCE reviews codes, coverage, and clinical information.

Medicare contractor Medicare Part A fiscal intermediary, Medicare Part B carrier, Medicare administrative contractor (MAC), or a Medicare durable medical equipment regional carrier (DMERC).

Medicare Coverage Advisory Committee Committee that advises CMS on whether specific medical items and services are reasonable and necessary under Medicare law. It performs this task via a careful review and discussion of specific clinical and scientific issues in an open and public forum. The MCAC is advisory in nature,

with the final decision on all issues resting with CMS. Accordingly, the advice rendered by the MCAC is most useful when it results from a process of full scientific inquiry and thoughtful discussion, in an open forum, with careful framing of recommendations and clear identification of the basis of those recommendations. The MCAC is used to supplement CMS's internal expertise and to ensure an unbiased and contemporary consideration of "state of the art" technology and science. Accordingly, MCAC members are valued for their background, education, and expertise in a wide variety of scientific, clinical, and other related fields. In composing the MCAC, CMS was diligent in pursuing ethnic, gender, geographic, and other diverse views, and to carefully screen each member to determine potential conflicts of interest. *Synonym(s): MCAC.*

Medicare durable medical equipment regional carrier Medicare contractor that administers durable medical equipment (DME) benefits for a region.

Medicare economic index Economic index used by Medicare to set limits on its fee schedule for physician reimbursement based on estimates of the costs of providing physician office services. The index also measures increases in earning levels in the general economy. *Synonym(s): MEI.*

Medicare Fee Schedule Fee schedule based upon physician work, expense, and malpractice designed to slow the rise in cost for services and standardize payment to physicians regardless of specialty or location of service with geographic adjustments.

Medicare focused (medical review) status report Management report that allows CMS to monitor the services being targeted for investigation and correction by carriers and the success of corrective actions being employed to address those areas. *Synonym(s): MFSR.*

Medicare identification number Generic term for any number that uniquely identifies the enrolling individual or organization. Some examples of Medicare identification numbers include the unique physician identification numbers (UPIN), provider identification numbers (PIN), online survey certification and reporting (OSCAR) numbers, and National Supplier Clearinghouse (NSC) numbers.

Medicare Integrity Program Provision of HIPAA that grants CMS the authority to enter into contracts with entities to promote the integrity of the Medicare program. This program was established, in part, to strengthen CMS's ability to deter fraud and abuse. There are basically two aspects of this program. One area deals with COB functions that ensure that Medicare is appropriately paying for services when any other type of insurance covers the beneficiary. The second large area of concern is the safeguard or monitoring and integrity of the data and payment of Medicare services.

Medicare National Coverage Determinations Manual CMS Internet-only manual (Pub. 100-03) that replaces the paper Coverage Issues Manual. The manual contains national coverage decisions and presents coverage criteria for specific medical items, supplies, procedures, or technologies. This manual is used by all Medicare contractors to determine if services, procedures, and supplies are covered and payable.

Medicare Part A Hospital insurance coverage that includes hospital, nursing home, hospice, home health, and other inpatient care. Claims are submitted to intermediaries for reimbursement.

Medicare Part A fiscal intermediary Medicare contractor that administers the Medicare Part A (institutional) benefits for a given region.

Medicare Part B Supplemental medical insurance that includes outpatient hospital care and physician and other qualified professional care. Claims from providers or suppliers other than a hospital are submitted to carriers for reimbursement. Hospital outpatient claims are submitted to their FI/MAC.

Medicare Part B carrier Medicare contractor that administers the Medicare Part B (professional) benefits for a given region.

Medicare physician fee schedule List of payments Medicare allows by procedure or service. Payments may vary through geographic adjustments. The MPFS is based on the resource-based relative value scale (RBRVS). A national total relative value unit (RVU) is given to each procedure (HCPCS Level I CPT, Level II national codes) by a physician. Each total RVU has three components: physician work, practice expense, and malpractice insurance.

Medicare Program Integrity Manual Pub. 100-08 manual that reflects the principles, values, and priorities for the Medicare Integrity Program. The primary principle of program integrity is to pay claims correctly. *Synonym(s): PIM.*

Medicare remittance advice remark codes National administrative code set for providing claim or service-level Medicare-related messages that cannot be expressed with a claim adjustment reason code. This code set is used in the X12 835 Claim Payment & Remittance Advice transaction, and is maintained by the Centers for Medicare and Medicaid Services.

Medicare secondary payer Specified circumstance when other third-party payers have the primary responsibility for payment of services and Medicare is the secondary payer. Medicare is secondary to workers' compensation, automobile, medical no-fault and liability insurance, EGHPs, LGHPs, and certain employer health plans covering aged and disabled beneficiaries. The MSP program prohibits Medicare payment for items or services if payment has been made or can reasonably be expected to be made by another payer, as described above.

Medicare secondary payer alert Medicare edit on inpatient and outpatient claims that may indicate that Medicare is the secondary payer. The Medicare Code Editor and Outpatient Code Editor use certain trauma diagnosis codes to identify claims involving accidents and other liability insurance for patients who may be covered under another insurance plan that would be primary over Medicare. The intermediary suspends these claims for further review and determination.

Medicare supplement Private insurance coverage that pays the Medicare deductible and copayments and may also pay the costs of services not covered by Medicare.

Medicare volume performance standard Standard set by Congress (or the Department of Health and Human Services by a default formula provided in the law) to determine how much growth is appropriate for Medicare Part B physician payments. This standard is based on factors such as inflation, the mix and age of the Medicare population, technological changes, inappropriate utilization, and inadequate beneficiary access to care. The MVPS is used to develop payments under the national Medicare fee schedule. *Synonym(s): MVPS.*

Medicare+Choice organization Created in 1997 as part of the Balanced Budget Act (BBA), which allows managed care plans, such as health maintenance organizations (HMOs) and preferred provider organizations (PPOs) to join the Medicare system.

medications Drugs and biologicals that an individual is already taking, that are ordered for the individual during the course of treatment, or that are ordered for an individual after treatment has been provided.

Medigap Individual health insurance offered by a private entity to those persons entitled to Medicare benefits and is specifically designed to supplement Medicare benefits. It fills in some of the gaps in Medicare coverage by providing payment for some of the charges, deductibles, coinsurance amounts, or other limitations imposed by Medicare.

Medigap policy Health insurance or other health benefit plan offered by a private company to those entitled to Medicare benefits. The policy covers charges not payable by Medicare because of deductibles, coinsurance amounts, or other Medicare-imposed limitations.

Medihaler ISO See isoproterenol.

Medin's disease Infection with any one of the three poliovirus organisms. Report this disease with a code from ICD-9-CM category 045. *Synonym(s): Heine-Medin disease.*

J-N

Mediskin Brand name wound dressing of porcine origin used primarily as a temporary dressing in burn cases. Its application is reported with CPT codes 15400 and 15401.

Mediterranean anemia Inherited blood disorder manifested by faulty hemoglobin production, resulting in decreased production and increased destruction of the red blood cells. Report this disorder with ICD-9-CM code 282.49. *Synonym(s): Cooley's anemia.*

Mediterranean tick fever Acute, febrile, rickettsial disease transmitted by tick bites and causing a primary lesion at the site of the bite, with rash, muscle and joint pain, headache, chills, fever, and sensitivity to light. It is commonly found in the Mediterranean and around the Black and Caspian Seas, having many names depending on the geographical region. This condition is reported with ICD-9-CM code 082.1. *Synonym(s): African tickbite fever, Boutonneuse fever, Indian tick typhus, Kenya tick typhus, Marseilles fever.*

MedPAC Medicare Payment Advisory Commission.

MedPAR Medicare provider analysis and review file.

Medralone Brand name for methylprednisolone acetate, an injectable steroid drug used to reduce swelling and to lower the body's immune reactions. Indications include hormonal, immunologic, and allergic disorders. Supply is reported with HCPCS Level II code J1030 or J1040.

Medrol Brand name for methylprednisolone, an oral corticosteroid drug used in multiple inflammatory diseases, including arthritis, asthma and allergies, adrenal insufficiency, disorders of the blood, dermatologic conditions, lupus, digestive diseases, and ophthalmic disorders. It acts to suppress inflammation and relieve symptoms. Supply is reported with HCPCS Level II code J7509.

medroxyprogesterone acetate Progestin replacement drug used as a contraceptive and to treat abnormal uterine bleeding, secondary amenorrhea, endometrial or renal cancer, and paraphilia in men. Supply is reported with HCPCS Level II code J1051 or J1055. May be sold under brand names Amen, Cycrin, Depo-Provera, Provera.

meds Medications.

med-surg Medical, surgical.

medulla Central or innermost portion of an organ or body structure.

medulloblastoma Malignant brain tumor that begins in the lower part of the brain and can spread to the spine or to other parts of the body. Report this condition with a code from ICD-9-CM category 191.

Meekeren-Ehlers-Danlos syndrome Group of congenital connective tissue diseases with overly elastic skin, hyperextensive joints, and fragility of blood vessels and arteries. Report this disorder with ICD-9-CM code 756.83. *Synonym(s): Danlos syndrome, Ehlers syndrome, Meekeren syndrome.*

Mefoxin See cefoxitin sodium.

MEG Magnetoencephalography. Measurement of the brain's magnetic fields that are produced by its electrical activity, utilizing a sensitive device known as a biomagnetometer. Used in patients with epilepsy to distinguish epileptiform spikes and in patients with brain tumors to locate eloquent cortex in preparation for surgery, this test is noninvasive. Report MEG with ICD-9-CM procedure code 89.15 or a code from CPT range 95965-95967.

megacolon Enlargement or dilation of the large intestines or the colon. *acquired m.* Enlargement or dilation of the large intestines, commonly caused by the use of drugs that slow intestinal motility, such as narcotic pain medications, or a disease process, such as ulcerative colitis. This condition is reported with ICD-9-CM code 564.7. *congenital m.* Congenital enlargement or dilation of the colon, with the absence of nerve cells in a segment of colon distally that causes the inability to defecate. This disease is reported with ICD-9-CM code 751.3.

megadontism Unusually large teeth, reported with ICD-9-CM code 520.2. *Synonym(s): macrodontia, megalodontia.*

megaduodenum Abnormal condition, most often as a result of motor function disorder, in which the duodenum is unusually large or dilated. Report megaduodenum with ICD-9-CM code 537.3.

megaesophagus Congenital or acquired condition in which the esophagogastric sphincter fails to relax with swallowing, causing the thoracic esophagus to lose its usual peristaltic movement and become dilated. If specified as congenital, report ICD-9-CM code 750.4; if acquired, report 530.0.

megalerythema Infection with human parvovirus B19, mainly occurring in children. Symptoms include a low-grade fever, malaise, or a ôcoldö a few days before the appearance of a mild rash illness that presents as a "slapped-cheek" rash on the face and a lacy red rash on the trunk and limbs. The condition usually resolves in seven to 10 days. Report this condition with ICD-9-CM code 057.0. *Synonym(s): fifth disease.*

megalocornea Congenital or acquired condition in which the cornea has an abnormally large size, usually occurring bilaterally. Report this condition with ICD-9-CM code 371.70 or 743.22; if specified as congenital, report 743.41. *Synonym(s): keratoglobus.*

megalocytic anemia Anemias of varied causes that are manifested by abnormally large red blood cells (macrocytes) that lack the normal central area of

J-N

paleness. Mean corpuscular volume and mean corpuscular hemoglobin are also increased. Report this condition with ICD-9-CM code 281.9.

megalodactylia Abnormal largeness of the fingers, reported with ICD-9-CM code 755.57, or of the toes, reported with 755.65. Repair of this condition is reported with CPT code 26590, once for each digit. *Synonym(s): dactylomegaly, macrodactylia, macrodactylism, macrodactyly, megalodactylism, megalodactyly.*

megalodontia Unusually large teeth, reported with ICD-9-CM code 520.2. *Synonym(s): macrodontia, megadontism.*

megalogastria Congenital condition in which the stomach is abnormally large, reported with ICD-9-CM code 750.7.

megalomania Psychological state manifested by delusions of grandeur, or the belief that one is more powerful or important than is actually the case. Report this condition with ICD-9-CM code 307.9.

megalophthalmos Congenital abnormality in which the eyes are unusually large, reported with ICD-9-CM code 743.8.

megalosplenia Congenital or acquired condition in which the spleen is abnormally enlarged. If no definitive cause is known, report ICD-9-CM code 789.2; if congenital, report 759.0. *Synonym(s): splenomegaly.*

megaloureter Congenital or acquired condition in which the ureter is dilated or distended. If specified as congenital, report ICD-9-CM code 753.22; acquired, report 593.89.

megarectum Idiopathic or acquired condition in which the rectum is abnormally dilated, reported with ICD-9-CM code 569.49.

megestrol acetate Synthetic oral hormone therapy that is similar to the female hormone progesterone. It is used primarily in the treatment of recurring breast cancer and may also be used to treat endometrial cancer, prostate cancer, hot flashes, and as an appetite stimulant. Supply is reported with HCPCS Level II code S0179. May be sold under brand name Megace. Report prophylactic use with ICD-9-CM code V07.59.

megrim Headaches that occur periodically on one or both sides of the head that may be associated with nausea and vomiting, sensitivity to light and sound, dizziness, distorted vision, and cognitive disturbances. Warning signs of an impending megrim, known as an aura, may or may not occur. These typically consist of visual sensations of flashing lights, zigzag lines, or temporary loss of vision. Report this condition with a code from ICD-9-CM category 346. *Synonym(s): migraine.*

MEI Medicare Economic Index, a CMS designation.

Meibomian gland Sebaceous gland located in the tarsal plates along the eyelid margins that produces the lipid

components found in tears. Chalazion is a cyst or enlargement of a meibomian gland due to inflammation. Warm compresses are the usual course of treatment to resolve a chalazion, but surgery may be required. Chalazion is reported with ICD-9-CM code 373.2; its excision is reported with a CPT code from series 67800-67808. If the meibomian gland is specified as infected, report with ICD-9-CM code 373.12. Meibomian gland can be the site of a neoplasm. If benign, the neoplasm is reported with ICD-9-CM code 216.1; if malignant, report 232.1 for carcinoma in situ, 173.1 for primary, or 198.2 for secondary site.

meibomianitis Inflammation of the meibomian glands, a group of oil-secreting (sebaceous) glands in the eyelids, resulting in a condition called hordeolum internum. Report this condition with ICD-9-CM code 373.12.

Meige syndrome Primary chronic lymphedema beginning at puberty, with swelling of the ankles and feet. *Synonym(s): lymphedema praecox, Millroy's disease.*

melan(o)- Dark or black in color.

melancholia Severe disturbance of mood or emotion that adversely affects the thinking process and that may be accompanied by delusions or hallucinations.

melancholia involutional Manic-depressive psychosis in which there is a widespread depressed mood of gloom and wretchedness with some degree of anxiety, reduced activity, or restlessness and agitation. There is a marked tendency to recurrence; in a few cases this may be at regular intervals.

melano- Dark or black in color.

melanoma Highly metastatic malignant neoplasm composed of melanocytes that occur most often on the skin from a preexisting mole or nevus but may also occur in the mouth, esophagus, anal canal, or vagina. Melanoma has four stages. Stage 0: cells are found only in the outer layer of skin cells and have not invaded deeper tissues. Stage I: Tumor is no more than 1 mm thick and the outer layer of skin may appear scraped or ulcerated; or the tumor is between 1 and 2 mm thick with no ulceration and no spread to nearby lymph nodes. Stage II: Tumor is at least 1 mm thick with ulceration or the lesion is more than 2 mm thick without ulceration and no spread to lymph nodes. Stage III: Cells have spread to one or more nearby lymph nodes or to tissues just outside the original lesion. Stage IV: Malignant cells have spread to other organs, lymph nodes, or areas of the skin distant from the original tumor.

melanoma of the choroid Most common primary malignancy of the inner eye.

melanoplakia Condition in which the tongue and mucous membranes of the mouth exhibit areas of pigmentation. Report this condition with ICD-9-CM code 528.9.

melanosis coli Gastrointestinal condition in which pigment-containing macrophages found within the lamina propria cause the colon's mucous membranes to assume a black or dark brown color. This pigment is not true melanin. Report this condition with ICD-9-CM code 569.89.

melanuresis Condition in which one excretes dark colored urine or in which standing urine becomes dark. Report this condition with ICD-9-CM code 791.9. *Synonym(s): melanuria.*

MELAS syndrome Mitochondrial myopathy, encephalopathy, lactic acidosis, stroke. Progressive neurodegenerative disorder typically manifested by features that encompass the name of the disorder. Diabetes and hearing loss may also be present. Report this syndrome with ICD-9-CM code 277.87.

melasma Condition frequently seen in women who take birth control pills in which the skin develops brown patches with distinct edges. Primary sites include the cheekbones, forehead, and upper lip, but development may also occur on the nose, chin, and neck. This condition may also be seen in pregnant females, menopausal women, those with hormonal or ovarian disorders, or patients using the medication Dilantin. Melasma is infrequently seen in men. Code assignment depends upon etiology and location. *Synonym(s): chloasma.*

Meleney's gangrene Gangrene of the skin and subcutaneous tissues that results in widespread tissue death and ulceration. Most often occurring after surgery, Meleney's gangrene is a result of a reaction between microaerophilic nonhemolytic streptococci and aerobic hemolytic staphylococci. This condition is reported with ICD-9-CM code 686.09. *Synonym(s): Meleney's ulcer.*

Meleney's ulcer Gangrene of the skin and subcutaneous tissues that results in widespread tissue death and ulceration. Most often occurring after surgery, Meleney's ulcer is a result of a reaction between microaerophilic nonhemolytic streptococci and aerobic hemolytic staphylococci. This condition is reported with ICD-9-CM code 686.09. *Synonym(s): Meleney's gangrene.*

melioidosis Infection by Burkholderia pseudomallei usually seen in rats and contagious for humans. Acute illness varies with symptoms ranging from local abscesses to benign pneumonia to fatal septicemia progression. Melioidosis is reported with ICD-9-CM code 025.

Melkersson (-Rosenthal) syndrome Facial paralysis with dramatic lacrimation during eating. Caused by lesion on seventh cranial nerve, prompting impulses to be misdirected from salivary glands to lacrimal glands. Report this disorder with ICD-9-CM code 351.8. *Synonym(s): crocodile tears.*

Meller's excision Removal of a tear sac obstructing the lacrimal passages.

melorheostosis Bone overgrowth affecting the long bones, manifested by the presence of streaks in the bones. Report with this condition with ICD-9-CM code 733.99.

meloschisis Rare congenital abnormality in which a facial cleft extends from the lip to the eye's inner canthus, usually separating the underlying bone. It may occur in conjunction with a cleft lip or palate, or with a lateral facial cleft. Report this abnormality with ICD-9-CM code 744.83. *Synonym(s): oblique facial cleft, prosopoanoschisis.*

melotia Developmental anomaly in which the ear is displaced onto the cheek, reported with ICD-9-CM code 744.29.

melphalan HCl Chemotherapeutic agent used to treat multiple myeloma and advanced ovarian cancer that is not surgically treatable. Supply is reported with HCPCS Level II code J8600 or J9245. May be sold under brand name Alkeran.

Meltzer's sign Indication of occlusion or tightening of the lower esophagus in which the normal second sound, usually heard on auscultation of the heart after swallowing, is absent.

member In medical reimbursement, subscriber of a health plan.

member Subscriber of a health plan.

member months In medical reimbursement, total of months each member was covered.

member months Total of months each member was covered.

member services In health care contracting, the payer department that works as a patient advocate to solve problems and may take claims appeals to a final committee after all other processes have been exhausted.

membranitis Potentially fatal inflammation affecting the chorion, fetal blood vessels, umbilical cord, and amnion. Report this condition with a code from ICD-9-CM category 658.4. If specified as affecting the fetus, report 762.7.

Memokath Brand name temporary prostatic urethral stent to replace a urinary catheter in patients who have undergone prostate seed implantation for the treatment of prostate cancer. The stent allows volitional urination and remains until swelling is reduced. Placement of the Memokath stent is reported with CPT code 53855.

memorandum of understanding Document describing the responsibilities that are to be assumed by two or more parties in their pursuit of some goal or goals. More specific information may be provided in an associated scope of work. *Synonym(s): MOU.*

J-N

MEN syndrome Multiple endocrine neoplasia syndromes. Men syndromes are a group of conditions in which several endocrine glands grow excessively (such as in adenomatous hyperplasia) and/or develop benign or malignant tumors. Tumors and hyperplasia associated with MEN often produce excess hormones, which impede normal physiology. There is no comprehensive cure known for MEN syndromes. Treatment is directed at the hyperplasia or tumors in each individual gland. Tumors are usually surgically removed and oral medications or hormonal injections are used to correct hormone imbalances. Three types of MEN syndromes (I, IIA, and IIB) have been identified; code selection is based on type. Report MEN syndrome with a code from ICD-9-CM subcategory 258.0.

Menactra Brand name meningococcal conjugate vaccine provided in a single-dose vial. Supply of Menactra is reported with CPT code 90734. Administration is reported separately.

menadione deficiency Vitamin K deficiency. Menadione, a fat-soluble vitamin, controls calcification of bones and is needed for the production of prothrombin and other blood clotting factors. Report this deficiency with ICD-9-CM code 269.0.

Mende's (ptosis-epicanthus) syndrome Eyebrow or upper or lower eyelid sags. Report this disorder with ICD-9-CM code 270.2. *Synonym(s): Mendes syndrome, van der Hoeve-Halbertsma-Waardenburg syndrome, Waardenburg-Klein syndrome.*

Mendelson's syndrome Pulmonary disorders caused by aspiration of matter into lung following vomiting or regurgitation during a medical procedure. Report this disorder with ICD-9-CM code 997.39.

Ménétrier's syndrome Giant hypertrophy of gastric mucosa. Report this disorder with a code from ICD-9-CM range 535.20-535.21.

meninges Tough membranous protectors of the central nervous system that cover the brain and spinal cord comprising three layers: the dura mater, arachnoid mater, and pia mater. The outer layer is the dura mater. The dura is tough and thick and restricts the movement of the brain within the skull, protecting it from stretched or broken blood vessels. The middle layer is the arachnoid, a delicate membrane separated from the pia mater by the subarachnoid space. The pia mater, or inner layer, lies closest to the brain, thinner over the cerebral cortex and thicker over the brain stem. Blood vessels enter the brain through the pia, covered for a short distance by a sheath of pia mater.

meningioma Slow growing benign vascular tumor originating in the meninges of the brain or spinal cord. They comprise 20 percent of all brain tumors and are found most frequently in middle-aged or elderly adults, mostly in women.

meningitis Inflammation of meningeal layers of the brain.

meningo- Relating to membranes covering the brain and spine.

Meningocele

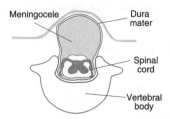

Meningocele — Dura mater — Spinal cord — Vertebral body

meningocele Herniation of the meninges through a defect in the skull or spine and most typically found in the sacral area. A simple meningocele is a protrusion of the meninges with the overlying skin intact and a mild bony deformity. Lateral meningoceles protrude through enlarged neural foramen, and can be asymptomatic. An anterior sacral meningocele is a herniation of the meninges through a focal erosion of the sacrum and coccyx, usually found in patients between ages 20 and 40.

meningococcic syndrome Acute fulminating meningococcal septicemia occurring in children below 10 years of age with vomiting, cyanosis, diarrhea, purpura, convulsions, circulatory collapse, meningitis, and hemorrhaging into adrenal glands. Report this disorder with ICD-9-CM code 036.3. *Synonym(s): Friderichsen-Waterhouse syndrome, Waterhouse syndrome.*

meningo-eruptive syndrome Enteric cytopathogenic human orphan (ECHO) virus. Common form of virus (which has many variations) is meningo-eruptive, with fever and aseptic meningitis. Report this disorder with ICD-9-CM code 047.1.

meniscocytosis Inherited type of anemia, occurring primarily in persons of African descent, that is chronic and often fatal, distinguished by crescent-shaped red blood cells, elevated temperature, leg ulcers, jaundice, and intermittent joint pain. Report this condition with ICD-9-CM code 282.60.

Meniscus Arrow Brand name fixation device for arthroscopic repair of bucket-handle tears of the meniscus.

Ménière's disease Distended, membranous labyrinth of the middle ear caused by a nonsuppurative disease with edema. This results in tinnitus or ringing in the ears, hearing loss from failure of nerve function, and dizziness or vertigo. This disease is reported with a code from ICD-9-CM subcategory 386.0. *Synonym(s):*

endolymphatic hydrops, labyrinth hydrops, Lermoyez's syndrome, Ménière's syndrome, recurrent aural vertigo. *NCD Reference: 50.7.*

Menkes' syndrome Congenital abnormality in copper absorption characterized by severe cerebral degeneration and arterial changes resulting in death in infancy. Report this disorder with ICD-9-CM code 759.89.

menolipsis Menstrual period ceases temporarily, reported with ICD-9-CM code 626.0.

menometrorrhagia Disproportionate amount of uterine bleeding during menstruation as well as at erratic intervals. This can be a sign of endometriosis, uterine fibroids, an imbalance of hormones, or malignancy. Menometrorrhagia is reported with ICD-9-CM code 626.2. *Synonym(s): menorrhagia.*

Menomune Brand name meningococcal polysaccharide vaccine provided in a single-dose vial. Supply of Menomune is reported with CPT code 90733. Administration is reported separately.

menopause Cessation of menstruation involving four physical stages: Premenopausal, in which periods may be irregular but without classic menopausal symptoms. Perimenopause, the onset of symptoms that indicate a drop in estrogen, such as erratic periods, hot flashes, and vaginal dryness lasting approximately four years, counting the first two years before and after the last period. Menopause, referring to the final menstrual period, marked once the female has had no periods for one year. Postmenopause, the phase in which a woman has been free of periods for at least one year. *premature m.* Complete and permanent cessation of ovarian function before the age of 40 from unknown causes and occurring naturally. Premature menopause is reported with ICD-9-CM code 256.31. *m. syndrome* Cessation of menstrual flow, usually midlife in most women, Symptoms are chills, depression, hot flashes, headache, and irritability Report this disorder with ICD-9-CM code 627.2.

menorrhagia Excessive or disproportionate amount of uterine bleeding during menstruation in which the period is regular but may be extended and is heavier than normal. This can cause anemia and may be indicative of underlying disorders such as endometriosis, uterine fibroids, hormonal imbalance, or malignancy, or it may be associated with premenopause. Menorrhagia is reported with ICD-9-CM codes 626.2 and 627.1.

menorrhalgia Painful menstruation that may be primary, or essential, due to prostaglandin production and the onset of menstruation; secondary due to uterine, tubal, or ovarian abnormality or disease; spasmodic arising uterine contractions; or obstructive due to some mechanical blockage or interference with the menstrual flow. All of these types are reported with ICD-9-CM code 625.3. Psychogenic dysmenorrhea, however, or that

occurring secondary to anxiety or stress, is reported in the mental disorders chapter with 306.52. *Synonym(s): dysmenorrhea, menstrual cramps.*

menoschesis Retention or suppression of the menses, reported with ICD-9-CM code 626.8.

menostaxis Excessive or disproportionate amount of uterine bleeding during menstruation in which the period is regular but may be extended and is heavier than normal. This can cause anemia and may be indicative of underlying disorders such as endometriosis, uterine fibroid, hormonal imbalance, or malignancy, or it may be associated with premenopause. This condition is reported with ICD-9-CM codes 626.2 and 627.1. *Synonym(s): menorrhagia.*

menotropins Injectable drug consisting of a mixture of follicle-stimulating hormone (FSH) and luteinizing hormone (LH), used to stimulate ovulation in instances when the ovaries are capable of producing a follicle but there is inadequate hormonal stimulation. This drug is also used to prompt the growth of multiple eggs for in vitro fertilization, as well as to stimulate sperm production in men who have inadequate hormonal stimulation but functioning testes. Supply is reported with HCPCS Level II code S0122. May be sold under brand names Humegon, Pergonal.

menstruation syndrome Monthly physiological and emotional distress during the several days preceding menses with symptoms of nervousness, fluid retention, weight gain, and depression. Report this disorder with ICD-9-CM code 625.4. *Synonym(s): PMS, premenstrual syndrome.*

mentagra Pus-containing rash appearing on the scalp or the bearded portion of the face, often caused by ringworm, acne, or impetigo. *Synonym(s): sycosis.*

mental health substance abuse Payer term for services rendered to members for emotional problems or chemical dependency.

mental or nervous Payer term for services rendered to members for emotional problems or chemical dependency.

mental retardation Condition of arrested or incomplete development of the mind, which is especially characterized by subnormality of intelligence, whether congenital or acquired, and is further defined according to tested or perceived intelligence and capabilities of learning and self care. *mild m. r.* Individuals with an IQ of 50 to 70 who can develop social and communication skills, have minimal retardation in sensorimotor areas, and often are not distinguished from normal children until a later age and can learn academic skills up to approximately the sixth-grade level. As adults they can usually achieve social and vocational skills adequate for minimal self-support but may need guidance and assistance when under social or economic stress.

moderate m. r. Individuals with an IQ of 35 to 49 who can talk or learn to communicate and have fair motor development. They have poor social awareness and are unlikely to progress beyond the second-grade level in academic subjects. As adults, they may achieve self-maintenance by performing unskilled or semi-skilled work under sheltered conditions with supervision and guidance when under mild social or economic stress. *profound m. r.* Individuals with an IQ of less than 20 who have minimal capacity for sensorimotor functioning and need nursing care during the preschool period. They may develop some further motor skills, and they may respond to minimal or limited training in self help. During the adult years some motor and speech development may occur, and they may achieve very limited self care and need nursing care. *severe m. r.* Individuals with an IQ of 20 to 34. They have poor motor development, minimal speech, and are generally unable to profit from training and self help during the preschool period. They can talk or learn to communicate, can be trained in elementary health habits, and may profit from systematic habit training. During the adult years they may contribute partially to self-maintenance under complete supervision.

Mentor Alpha I Brand name, multi-component penile implant device made from silicone and polyurethane rubber, with four implantable parts: two tubes or cylinders, a pump, and a reservoir container. When the pump is squeezed, fluid is sent from the reservoir into the tubes to facilitate erection. Placement of this device is reported with CPT code 54405.

Mepergan Brand name combination drug consisting of Demerol and Phenergan that combines pain relief with an antiemetic and is used as a preanesthetic or adjunct to anesthesia, usually administered by intramuscular injection to avoid arterial introduction through an IV. Supply is reported with HCPCS Level II code J2180. Mepergan contains meperidine and promethazine.

meperidine Injectable narcotic analgesic used to prevent or relieve pain that is moderate to severe in intensity. Supply is reported with HCPCS Level II code J2175. Meperidine with promethazine HCl is reported with J2180. May be sold under brand names Demerol HCl, Mepergan.

mEq Milliequivalent.

mEq/1 Milliequivalent per liter.

meralgia paresthetica Neurologic disorder due to constriction of the lateral femoral cutaneous nerve as it exits the pelvis, manifested by tingling, lack of sensation, and burning pain of the outer thigh. It is often associated with obesity, diabetes, pregnancy, or restrictive clothing. Report this disorder with ICD-9-CM code 355.1.

Mercedes-Benz sign Indication of gallstones wherein shadows resembling the Mercedes-Benz logo are evident on gallbladder x-rays. Even though gallstones may not be visible, this is indicative of gas-filled fissures inside the gallstones.

mercurialism Acute or chronic poisoning due to mercury or a mercury-containing compound. Report this condition with ICD-9-CM code 985.0. *Synonym(s): mercury poisoning.*

mercury poisoning Acute or chronic poisoning due to mercury or a mercury-containing compound. Report this condition with ICD-9-CM code 985.0. *Synonym(s): mercurialism.*

Merkel cell carcinoma Malignant cutaneous cancer predominantly found in elderly patients with sun exposure. Report this condition with ICD-9-CM codes 173.0-173.9. *Synonym(s): MCC, Merkel cell tumor.*

merocele Loop of the intestine herniated into the femoral canal. Report this condition with ICD-9-CM code 553.00. *Synonym(s): crural hernia, femorocele.*

Merogel Brand name nasal dressing and stent.

meromelia Congenital abnormality in which a portion of a limb is absent, reported with a code from ICD-9-CM range 755.20-755.4.

meropenem Injectable antibiotic used to treat certain bacterial infections. Supply is reported with HCPCS Level II code J2185. May be sold under brand name Merrem.

merosmia Sense of smell is partially lost, resulting in the inability to distinguish certain odors. Report this condition with ICD-9-CM code 781.1.

Merrem Injectable antibiotic used to treat certain bacterial infections. Supply is reported with HCPCS Level II code J2185. Merrem contains meropenem.

MERRF syndrome Myoclonus epilepsy associated with ragged-red fibers. Mitochondrial encephalomyopathy, a rare muscular disorder resulting from a defect in the portion of the cell structure that releases energy. This disorder causes brain and muscular dysfunction; microscopic tissue abnormalities are also present. Symptoms of MERRF include myoclonic seizures, incoordination, and lactic acidosis. Short stature, dementia, and speech, vision, and hearing abnormalities may also be present. Report this syndrome with ICD-9-CM code 277.87, with an additional code for associated abnormalities.

Meruvax II Brand name rubella vaccine provided in a single-dose vial. Supply of Meruvax II is reported with CPT code 90706; administration is reported separately. The need for vaccination is reported with ICD-9-CM code V04.3.

Merycism Regurgitation of food, without nausea, retching, or disgust followed by ejection or chewing with reswallowing. Frequently seen with failure to thrive or weight loss developing after a period of normal functioning. This condition may afflict any age group, but it is particularly found in the mentally retarded population.

Merzbacher-Pelizaeus disease Inherited degenerative brain disease manifested by gradually advancing white matter sclerosis of the frontal lobes, mental deficits, and vasomotor disorders. Report this disease with ICD-9-CM code 330.0. *Synonym(s): aplasia axialis extracorticalis, hereditary cerebral leukodystrophy, Pelizaeus-Merzbacher disease.*

mes(io)- *1)* Toward the middle. *2)* Secondary.

MESA Micro-epididymal sperm aspiration. Operation to retrieve sperm from the epididymis with a blocked vas deferens, carried out under general anesthetic. It would be reported with a CPT code for unlisted procedure.

mesenteric artery insufficiency syndrome Blocked superior mesenteric artery with vomiting, pain, blood in the stool, distended abdomen, and bowel infarction. Report this disorder with ICD-9-CM code 557.1. *Synonym(s): Wilkie's syndrome.*

mesenteric artery syndrome Complete or partial block of the superior mesenteric artery with symptoms of vomiting, pain, blood in the stool, and distended abdomen. Results in bowel infarction. Report this disorder with ICD-9-CM code 557.1. *Synonym(s): Wilkie's syndrome.*

mesentery Two layers of peritoneum that fold to surround the organs and attach to the abdominal wall.

mesh Synthetic fabric used as a prosthetic patch in hernia repair.

MeSH Medical staff-hospital organization.

mesial In dentistry, toward the dental arch's midline.

mesio- *1)* Toward the middle. *2)* Secondary.

mesiodens Small tooth that appears in addition to the regular number of teeth, consisting of a pointed crown and a short root between the central incisors of the maxilla. It may appear singly or in pairs, and may be erupted, impacted, or inverted. Report this condition with ICD-9-CM code 520.1. If specified as causing crowding, report 524.31.

mesna Detoxifying agent used to prevent hemorrhagic cystitis caused by the chemotherapeutic drug ifosfamide. Supply is reported with HCPCS Level II code J9209. Mesna contains sodium 2-mercaptoethane sulfonate.

Mesnex Detoxifying agent used to prevent hemorrhagic cystitis caused by the chemotherapeutic drug ifosfamide. Supply is reported with HCPCS Level II code J9209. Mesnex contains sodium 2-mercaptoethane sulfonate,

mesocardia Congenital abnormality in which the heart is centrally located in the middle of the thorax, reported with ICD-9-CM code 746.87.

MET Multiple employer trust. Group of employers that join together to purchase health insurance using a self-funded approach to lower costs by the broadening membership pool to prevent an adverse selection.

meta- Indicates a change.

metabolic syndrome Group of health risks that increase the likelihood of developing heart disease, stroke, and diabetes. Diagnosis of metabolic syndrome is made if one has three or more of the following: waist measurement of 40 or more inches for men and 35 or more inches for women; blood pressure of 130/85 mm or higher; triglyceride level greater than 150 mg/dl; fasting blood sugar of more than 100 mg/dl; HDL level less than 40 mg/dl in men or less than 50 mg/dl in women. Report this condition with ICD-9-CM code 277.7, with additional codes to identify associated manifestations. *Synonym(s): dysmetabolic syndrome, insulin resistance syndrome, syndrome X.*

metabolism Combination of processes occurring in any living organism to produce and maintain organized building blocks (anabolism) and to break down food substances into usable, available energy (catabolism).

metacarpal Five long bones of the hand that join with the carpal bones and with the proximal phalanges of the fingers.

metagonimiasis Intestinal disease caused by Metagonimus yokogawai, the smallest fluke that affects humans. Symptoms include abdominal pain and diarrhea. The eggs may migrate to other areas of the body, such as the brain and heart. Report this condition with ICD-9-CM code 121.5.

metamorphopsia Visual defect, most often of the retina, which causes objects to appear indistinct or unclear. Report this condition with ICD-9-CM code 368.14.

metaplasia Transformation of one type of mature differentiated cell type into another mature differentiated cell type. Examples include squamous metaplasia of the columnar epithelial cells of salivary gland ducts when stones are present and squamous metaplasia of the transitional epithelium of the bladder when stones are present.

Metaprel Bronchodilator administered by oral inhalation, used to treat asthma, bronchitis, or emphysema by relaxing the airway muscles in order to improve breathing. Supply is reported with HCPCS Level II code J7668 or J7669. Metaprel contains metaproterenol.

metaproterenol Bronchodilator administered by oral inhalation, used to treat asthma, bronchitis, or emphysema by relaxing the airway muscles in order to improve breathing. Supply is reported with HCPCS Level II code J7668 or J7669. May be sold under brand names Alupent, Metaprel.

metastasize Spread, invade, or extend to a new location.

J-N

metastatic carcinoid syndrome Carcinoid tumors that causes cyanotic flushing of skin, diarrheal watery stools, bronchoconstrictive attacks, hypotension, edema, and ascites. Report this disorder with ICD-9-CM code 259.2. *Synonym(s): Bjorck-Thorson syndrome, Cassidy-Scholte syndrome, Hedinger's syndrome.*

metastatic trophoblastic disease Invasive and invading cancerous tumor derived from a trophoblast, which is the layer of extraembryonic tissue that attaches the fertilized ovum to the uterine wall, supplies the embryo with nutrition, and gives rise to the chorion and amnion. Approximately 2 percent of hydatidiform moles become MTD. *Synonym(s): choriocarcinoma, chorioepithelioma, MTD.*

metatarsectomy Excision or resection of a metatarsal bone in the foot between the tarsal and phalangeal bones.

metatarsus One of the five long bones in the foot between the ankle bones and the phalanges, or toes.

meteorism Swelling from gas in the intestine or peritoneal cavity. *Synonym(s): tympanites.*

metformin Oral medication exclusive to lowering blood glucose in Type II diabetics. May be sold as brand name Glucophage.

methemoglobinemia Defect in the iron contained in the hemoglobin molecule, resulting in the inability of oxygen to be transported effectively to the body tissues. Report this disorder with ICD-9-CM code 289.7.

method I composite rate In health care contracting, the optional payment method for dialysis services. When the beneficiary elects method I, the dialysis facility assumes all responsibility for providing home dialysis equipment, supplies, and home support services. The facility is reimbursed under the composite rate system. The beneficiary pays the Medicare Part B deductible and coinsurance on the facility's composite rate.

method II dealing direct In health care contracting, the optional payment method for dialysis services. When the beneficiary elects method II, the beneficiary deals directly with a supplier of home dialysis equipment and supplies, not a dialysis facility. Each beneficiary has only one supplier. The beneficiary pays the Medicare Part B deductible and coinsurance. The Medicare carrier processes these claims. A dialysis facility cannot be paid for home dialysis equipment or supplies under this payment method. Such a facility receives method II payment for home dialysis support services only.

Methyldopate HCl Antihypertensive medication.

Metrodin Brand name fertility medication. Administered by injection, its active ingredient is urofollitropin. Supply is reported with HCPCS Level II code J3355.

metropathia hemorrhagica Abnormal condition in which an ongoing follicular phase of the menstrual cycle causes copious, excessive uterine bleeding that may be continuous. Report this condition with ICD-9-CM code 626.8.

metroperitonitis Uterine inflammation that involves the covering of the peritoneum or peritonitis as a result of infection after metritis. Metroperitonitis is reported with ICD-9-CM codes 614.5-614.7, unless it is postpartal, coded within subcategory 670.0.

metroplasty Surgical procedure performed to reshape or reconstruct the uterus and uterine cavity for correction of a double or septate uterus in order to improve the outcome of pregnancy. Metroplasty is reported with ICD-9-CM procedure code 69.49 and CPT code 58540.

metrorrhagia Prolonged, irregular uterine bleeding of an inconsistent amount occurring in frequent bouts.

metrostaxis Scant but continuous uterine bleeding, reported with ICD-9-CM code 626.6.

-metry Scientific measurement.

MEWA Multiple employer welfare association. Group of employers that join together to purchase health insurance using a self-funded approach to lower costs by the broadening membership pool to prevent an adverse selection.

Mexican hat sign Indication of a filling defect of the colon caused by a polyp attached to the inferior wall by a stalk-like base, resulting in a shadow on x-ray of the colon that resembles a large-brimmed Mexican hat.

Meyenburg-Altherr-Uehlinger syndrome Arthritis with degeneration of cartilage leading to collapse of ears, nose, and tracheobronchial tree. Death may occur as respiratory system is affected. Report this disorder with ICD-9-CM code 733.99.

Meyer-Schwickerath and Weyers syndrome Abnormally small nose with anteverted nostrils, dental anomalies, and missing phalanges of toes. Report this disorder with ICD-9-CM code 759.89. *Synonym(s): dysplasia oculodentodigitalis.*

MFD Minimum fatal dose.

MFS Medicare fee schedule. Fee schedule based upon physician work, expense, and malpractice designed to slow the rise in cost for services and standardize payment to physicians regardless of specialty or location of service with geographic adjustments. *Synonym(s): MPFS.*

MFT Muscle function test.

mg Milligram.

Mg Magnesium.

MGCRB Medicare Geographic Classification Review Board.

MGMA Medical Group Management Association.

mgs Milligrams.

MH/CD Mental health/chemical dependency.

MH/SA Mental health/substance abuse.

MHA Master of health administration.

MHC Mental health clinic.

MHDC Massachusetts Health Data Consortium.

MHDI Minnesota Health Data Institute.

MHT Megahertz.

MI *1)* Microwave imaging. In spectroscopy, microwaves passed through tissue create a computerized image of a cross section of that tissue. *2)* Myocardial infarct.

MIC Minimum inhibitory concentration. Measurement of bacterial sensitivity to an antibiotic, as seen in a test reported with CPT code 87186.

Micheli-Rietti syndrome Hemolytic anemias that share a common decreased rate of synthesis of one or more hemoglobin polypeptide chains and are classified according to the chain involved. Report this disorder with ICD-9-CM code 282.49.

Michotte's syndrome Malformation of spine in which kyphosis becomes so great nonadjacent vertebrae touch. Report this disorder with ICD-9-CM code 721.5. *Synonym(s): kissing spine.*

microangiopathic hemolytic anemia Thrombocytopenia with thrombi formation in the small arterioles and capillaries causing hemolytic anemia, purpura, azotemia, fever, and central nervous system disorders manifested by bizarre neurological effects. Report this condition with ICD-9-CM code 446.6. *Synonym(s): Baehr-Schiffrin disease, Moschcowitz disease, thrombotic microangiopathy, thrombotic thrombocytopenic purpura.*

microangiopathy Blood vessel disease in which the capillary walls thicken and weaken, resulting in bleeding, protein loss, and slowing of the blood flow. Peripheral microangiopathy often occurs as a complication of diabetes, reported with a code from ICD-9-CM subcategory 249.7 or 250.7 and an additional code, 443.81, to identify the manifestation. If the cause is unknown, report 443.9. Retinal microangiopathy is reported with 362.18.

microcephalus Extremely small brain or head.

microcephaly Congenital disorder in which the head circumference is more than two standard deviations below the mean for age, sex, race, and gestation and associated with a decreased life expectancy. This disorder is reported with ICD-9-CM code 742.1.

microcheilia Congenital condition of abnormally small lips; reported with ICD-9-CM code 744.82.

microcolon Uncommon congenital cause of intestinal obstruction thought to be a transient developmental delay and often related to maternal diabetes during the

pregnancy. Report this condition with ICD-9-CM code 751.5.

microcornea Congenital abnormality in which the corneal diameter is unusually small. This condition usually occurs bilaterally, and may be associated with other ocular anomalies. Report this condition with ICD-9-CM code 743.41.

microcurrent nerve stimulator Treatment of chronic, intractable pain by delivering low intensity electric currents via a device that is applied to the skin surface at the site of the pain. *Synonym(s): MNS.*

microdeletions Congenital abnormality in which there is loss of a minute portion of chromosome, detectable only by particular methods such as high-resolution chromosome banding, molecular chromosome analysis, or DNA testing. Microdeletions often result in disorders such as Angelman, DiGeorge, Prader-Willi, and Williams's syndromes. Report this abnormality with ICD-9-CM code 758.33, with additional codes to identify the associated conditions.

microdissection Dissection of tissue using a microscope.

microdontia Teeth are disproportionately small, reported with ICD-9-CM code 520.2.

MicroFlow Brand name phacoemulsification needle for use in ocular surgery.

microgastria Rare congenital abnormality in which the stomach is unusually small. This condition is often associated with other congenital abnormalities and frequently results in death or severe malnutrition. Report microgastria with ICD-9-CM code 750.7.

microgenia Abnormally small, underdeveloped mandible, characterized by an extremely small chin; reported with ICD-9-CM code 524.06.

microglossia Congenital anomaly of small tongue.

micrognathia Congenital hypoplasia or abnormal smallness of the maxilla or mandible, reported by site with ICD-9-CM code 524.03 or 524.04. The alveolar tissue of the upper or lower jaw may be incomplete or underdeveloped in micrognathia, coded to 524.73 and 524.74. *Synonym(s): micrognathism.*

micrognathia-glossoptosis syndrome Description of anomalies of face and skull. Report this disorder with ICD-9-CM code 756.0.

microgyria Congenital anomaly of the brain manifested by the growth of multiple minute convolutions, often causing mental retardation, reported with ICD-9-CM code 742.2.

microkeratome Surgical device used to cut a thin slice or create a thin flap from the surface of the cornea to a predetermined depth by a sharp blade affixed to the eye by a vacuum ring.

J–N

microneurovascular anastomosis Repair of lacerated or severed nerves, arteries, and veins using microscopic surgical technique.

microorganism Microscopic organisms, including bacteria, fungi, and protozoa.

micropenis Congenital abnormality in which testosterone fails to stimulate the gonadal tissues to develop, causing the penis to develop abnormally small. In a newborn, a penis less than 3/4 inches is considered a micropenis. This abnormality is reported with ICD-9-CM code 752.64. **Synonym(s):** *microphallus.*

microphthalmos Congenital anomaly of small eyeballs, assessed according to the level of debility, reported with ICD-9-CM codes 743.10-743.12.

microphthalmos syndrome Reduction in the size of the eye, opacities of the cornea and lens, and scarring of the retina. Report this disorder with ICD-9-CM code 759.89.

micropigmentation Permanent method of implanting pigment into the skin to add color for the treatment of vitiligo, skin grafts, or burn scars and for cosmetic purposes. Report this procedure with CPT codes 11920-11922. **Synonym(s):** *tattooing.*

microrepair Repair of tissue at a level that requires using a microscope.

microsporosis nigra Minor fungal infection caused by cladosporium mansoni or Exophiala werneckii, producing lesions that most commonly appear on the hands and rarely on other areas. The lesions look like the characteristic dark ink or dye stain that occurs when silver nitrate is spilled on the skin. Report this condition with ICD-9-CM code 111.1. **Synonym(s):** *cladosporiosis epidermica, keratomycosis nigricans, pityriasis nigra, tinea nigra, tinea palmaris nigra.*

microstomia Congenital condition of an abnormally small mouth; reported with ICD-9-CM code 744.84.

microsurgery Surgical procedures performed under magnification using a surgical microscope. CPT code 69990 is reported in addition to the appropriate procedure code when a surgical microscope is utilized and is not an inclusive component of the procedure. **Synonym(s):** *microrepair.*

microtia Congenital smallness of the external ear or pinna, sometimes associated with an absent or closed auditory canal that requires surgical intervention. Microtia is reported with ICD-9-CM code 744.23.

microvascular decompression Microsurgical procedure done to relieve the pain caused by trigeminal neuralgia in which a tiny, nonabsorbable sponge is inserted to decompress the sensory root of the nerve by relieving the pressure put upon it by the surrounding blood vessels. Report this procedure with ICD-9-CM procedure code 04.41 or CPT code 61450. **Synonym(s):** *Jannetta procedure, MVD.*

microvolt T-wave alternans Diagnostic test to evaluate electrical activity in the T-wave portion of the EKG; used to detect risk of sudden cardiac death and reported with CPT code 93025. **Synonym(s):** *MTWA.*

micturition Urination.

MIDAS Migraine disability assessment scale.

midbrain syndrome Infarction of postero-inferior thalamus causing transient hemiparesis, severe loss of superficial and deep sensation with crude pain in the hypalgic limbs, vasomotor, or trophic disturbances. Report this disorder with ICD-9-CM code 348.89.

middle cranial fossa Support for the temporal lobes of the brain comprising the greater wings of the sphenoid (anteriorly), the squamous portions of temporal bone (laterally), and the petrous portions of the temporal bones (posteriorly).

midlevel practitioners Professionals such as nurse practitioners, nurse midwives, physical therapists, physician assistants, and others who provide medical care but do so with physician input. **Synonym(s):** *MLP, nonphysician practitioners, NPP.*

MIE Meconium ileus equivalent. Condition specific to cystic fibrosis in which viscous mucous and feces bind the intestine and bring on colicky symptoms. MIE is reported with ICD-9-CM code 277.01. **Synonym(s):** *DIOS.*

Mieten's syndrome Affects multiple systems. Report this disorder with ICD-9-CM code 759.89.

MIF Migration inhibitory factor, reported with CPT code 86378.

migraine Headaches that occur periodically on one or both sides of the head that may be associated with nausea and vomiting, sensitivity to light and sound, dizziness, distorted vision, and cognitive disturbances. Warning signs of an impending migraine, known as an aura, may or may not occur. These typically consist of visual sensations of flashing lights, zigzag lines, or temporary loss of vision. Report this condition with a code from ICD-9-CM category 346. **Synonym(s):** *megrim.*

Mikity-Wilson syndrome Symptoms include hypercapnia and cyanosis of rapid onset during first month of life and frequently result in death. Rare pulmonary insufficiency in newborn babies, especially those with low birth weight. Report this disorder with ICD-9-CM code 770.7.

Mikulicz resection Procedure is done in stages and includes exteriorizing a section of intestine, usually the colon, resecting the exteriorized loop, and eliminating the fecal fistula by crushing the spur between the two barrels of the anastomosis. The fecal fistula is closed.

Mikulicz's syndrome Complex of lacrimal and salivary gland swelling, which may include enlargement

J-N

associated with other syndromes, such as Sjögren's. Report this disorder with ICD-9-CM code 527.1.

Miles' colectomy Lower sigmoid colon and rectum are removed for treatment of cancer. Physician removes the pelvic colon, mesocolon, and adjacent lymph nodes and establishes a permanent colostomy.

milia Tiny, round, white to yellow slightly elevated epidermal cysts containing keratin found on superficial skin in the hair follicles and sebaceous glands of all ages, even neonates. Milia are classified to ICD-9-CM code 706.2, unless it is the colloid form (709.3) or present on the eyelid (374.84). For removal of multiple milia, see CPT code 10040.

milk alkali syndrome Disorder of kidneys induced by ingestion of large amounts of alkali and calcium. While reversible in the early stages, it can lead to renal failure. Report this disorder with ICD-9-CM code 275.42. *Synonym(s): Burnett's (milk drinker's) syndrome.*

Milkman (-Looser-Debray) syndrome Osteoporosis striking middle-aged women with frequent fractures. Report this disorder with ICD-9-CM code 268.2.

Millard-Gubler syndrome Paraplegia and anesthesia over half or part of the body. Caused by lesions in brain or spinal cord. Report this disorder with ICD-9-CM code 344.89.

Millen-Read procedure Suprapubic approach is used in the procedure to remedy stress incontinence.

Miller Fisher's syndrome Often follows viral infections and may be a disorder of the immune system with symptoms of paraplegia of limbs, flaccid paralysis, ophthalmoplegia, ataxia, and areflexia. Report this disorder with ICD-9-CM code 357.0.

Milles' syndrome Formation of multiple angiomas in skin of head and scalp. Report this disorder with ICD-9-CM code 759.6. *Synonym(s): Kalischer's syndrome.*

Millner technique Technique for transurethral resection of prostate in which the initial resection attacks the bulk tissue of the lateral lobes without devascularization.

Milroy syndrome Lymphatic edema of the legs (and face and arms in severe cases) caused by obstruction of lymphatic ducts. Report this disorder with ICD-9-CM code 757.0.

min Minimum, minimal, minute.

Minerva cast Cast applied around the neck and trunk of the body, often following surgery on the neck or upper back area. Report the application of the cast with CPT code 29040.

Minerva jacket Spinal cast or brace that includes a sternal plate, dorsal plate, bonnet, and mandible piece attached to the superstructure of the sternal plate for cervical or high thoracic stability.

minimal brain dysfunction Disorders of short attention span and distractibility with impulsiveness, mood fluctuations, and aggression. In early childhood, characterized by uninhibited, poorly organized, and poorly regulated extreme overactivity; in adolescence characterized by underactivity. *Synonym(s): MBD.*

minimum data set Contains a core set of screening, clinical, and functional status elements, including common definitions and coding categories that form the basis of a comprehensive patient assessment. RUG-III classification system and the Medicare skilled nursing facility (SNF) prospective payment system (PPS) are based on the MDS. Under the PPS, SNFs are required to use the MDS 2.0 as the data source for classifying patients for case mix. All of the information necessary to classify a patient into one of the RUGs-III categories is contained in the MDS 2.0. *Synonym(s): MDS.*

minimum necessary Reasonable efforts a covered entity must make to limit the use, disclosure, or request of protected health information to the minimum necessary.

minimum scope of disclosure Principal that individually identifiable health information should be disclosed only to the extent needed to support the purpose of the disclosure.

Minkowski-Chauffard syndrome Hemolytic anemia with spherocytosis, fragility of erythrocytes, splenomegaly, and jaundice. Report this disorder with ICD-9-CM code 282.0.

Minnesota Health Data Institute Public-private partnership for improving the quality and efficiency of health care in Minnesota. MHDI includes the Minnesota Center for Healthcare Electronic Commerce (MCHEC), which supports the adoption of standards for electronic commerce and also supports the Minnesota EDI Healthcare Users Group (MEHUG). *Synonym(s): MHDI.*

Minnesota Multiphasic Personality Inventory Self-report personality assessment inventory consisting of multiple statements that depict feelings or actions with which the patient is asked to agree or disagree. This assessment is helpful in the identification of personal, social, or behavioral problems in psychiatric patients. Report administration and interpretation of this test with CPT codes 96101-96103. *Synonym(s): MMPI.*

minor procedure Self-limited procedure, usually with an assignment of 0 or 10 follow-up days by payers. A minor procedure may be considered by many payers to be part of the global package for a primary surgical service and cannot be billed separately from the primary procedure.

Minor's sign Indication of sciatica in which the patient rises from a seated position by supporting himself on the nonaffected side, placing a hand on the back,

J-N

bending the affected leg, and balancing on the healthy leg.

miosis Sustained abnormal contraction of the pupil less than 2 mm (that is not caused by miotics), reported with ICD-9-CM code 379.42.

miotic Agent that causes the pupil to contract.

miotic cysts Cysts causing restriction in the movement of the pupil.

MIP See Medicare Integrity Program.

Mircera Brand name injectable erythropoiesis-stimulating agent (ESA) indicated for the treatment of patients with anemia due to chronic renal failure. Mircera may be administered intravenously or subcutaneously. *Synonym(s): methoxy polyethylene glycol-epoetin beta.*

Mirena Brand name, hormone-eluting intrauterine device inserted through the cervix into the uterus by a clinician. Supply is reported with HCPCS Level II code J7302 and insertion is reported with CPT code 58300.

Mirizzi's syndrome Stone in cystic duct and chronic cystitis leading to spasms and scarring of connective tissue and obstruction of hepatic ducts. Report this disorder with ICD-9-CM code 576.2.

MIS *1)* Memory impairment screen. Short screening test to differentiate between normal forgetfulness and memory decline associated with Alzheimer's disease and other dementias. *2)* Management information system. Hardware and software facilitating claims management.

mis- Bad, improper.

misce. Miscellaneous.

miscoding Incorrect coding or using a code that does not apply to the procedure.

misery and unhappiness disorder Emotional disorder characteristic of childhood in which the main symptoms involve misery and unhappiness and may include eating and sleep disturbances.

misrepresented Deliberate false statement made, or caused to be made, that is material to entitlement or payment under the Medicare program.

missed abortion Retention of a dead fetus within the uterus in cases where fetal demise occurred before 22 weeks gestation. Abortion in this context refers to retained products of conception from the death of a normal fetus that does not follow spontaneous or induced abortion, or missed delivery. Indications are cessation of growth, hardening of the uterus, or a reduction in its size. Fetal electrocardiography or ultrasonography is used to confirm this diagnosis.

Mitchell procedure Correction of hallux valgus in which the metatarsal head is shifted laterally to a mild degree in order to correct the deformity. Report this

procedure with ICD-9-CM procedure code 77.51 or CPT code 28296.

mitral valve Valve with two cusps that is between the left atrium and left ventricle of the heart. *Synonym(s): bicuspid valve.*

Mitrofanoff operation Treatment of urinary incontinence in which the appendix is used as a conduit between the bladder and the surface of the abdomen as an opening for urine. Report this procedure with ICD-9-CM procedure codes 57.21 and 57.88 or CPT code 50845. *Synonym(s): cutaneous appendico-vesicostomy.*

mittelschmerz Pain related to ovulation. It typically occurs on one side of the lower abdomen depending upon which ovary is currently producing the ovum. This condition is reported with ICD-9-CM code 625.2. *Synonym(s): intermenstrual pain, midcycle pain, ovulation pain.*

mixed model HMO that includes both an open panel and closed panel option.

Mizuo's phenomenon Golden discoloration of the retina that reverts to normal after several hours of dark adaptation, as seen in various retinal disorders.

ml Milliliter.

ML Midline.

MLB test Monaural loudness balance test, reported with CPT code 92562.

MLC Midline catheter.

MLD Manual lymph drainage. Gentle massage of tissue to drain lymphatics and reduce lymphedema. Lymphedema is reported with ICD-9-CM code 457.1 when an acquired chronic condition; postmastectomy lymphedema is reported with 457.0; and hereditary edema of the legs is reported with 757.0.

MLM Manual lymphatic mapping. In lymphatic massage therapy, assessment of lymphatic circulation to determine drainage pathways. It is considered a component of lymphatic drainage therapy.

MLNS Mucocutaneous lymph node syndrome. Idiopathic disease affecting young children, involving the skin, mouth, and lymph nodes. Symptoms include a persistent fever; redness of the eyes, lips, and oral mucosa; gingival ulcers; swollen neck glands; and an edematous rash on the hands and feet with flaking from the fingers and toes. If left untreated, the disease can progress and affect the heart and blood vessels. Report this condition with ICD-9-CM code 446.1. *Synonym(s): Kawasaki disease.*

MLP Midlevel practitioners. Professionals such as nurse practitioners, nurse midwives, physical therapists, physician assistants, and others who provide medical care but do so with physician input.

MLT Medical laboratory technician.

MLV Modified live vaccine.

MM *1)* Malignant melanoma. *2)* Mucous membrane. *3)* Millimeter.

mmHg Millimeters of mercury.

M-mode One-dimensional procedure with movement of the trace to record amplitude and velocity of moving echo-producing structures.

MMPI Minnesota Multiphasic Personality Inventory. Self-report personality assessment inventory consisting of multiple statements that depict feelings or actions with which the patient is asked to agree or disagree. This assessment is helpful in the identification of personal, social, or behavioral problems in psychiatric patients. Report administration and interpretation of this test with CPT codes 96101-96103.

MMR Measles, mumps, and rubella. Combined subcutaneous vaccination for measles, mumps, and rubella. Report MMR with ICD-9-CM procedure code 99.48 or CPT code 90707. Also report the appropriate administration code. *Synonym(s): measles, mumps, and rubella vaccine.*

M-M-R II Brand name measles, mumps, rubella vaccine provided in a single-dose vial. Supply of M-M-R II is reported with CPT code 90707; administration is reported separately. The need for vaccination is reported with ICD-9-CM code V06.4.

MMRV Measles, mumps, rubella, and varicella, usually in reference to a vaccine. Supply of MMRV vaccine is reported with CPT code 90710; administration is reported separately. The need for vaccination is reported with ICD-9-CM code V06.4.

MNK Menkes syndrome. X-linked error of metabolism affecting the body's ability to absorb copper, leading to cerebral degeneration and death. MNK is reported with ICD-9-CM code 759.89. *Synonym(s): kinky hair disease, steely hair disease, copper transport disease.*

MNS Microcurrent nerve stimulator. Treatment of chronic, intractable pain by delivering low intensity electric currents via a device that is applied to the skin surface at the site of the pain.

MNT Medical nutrition therapy.

MoAbs Monoclonal antibodies.

mobile facility or portable unit Service that requires medical equipment be provided in a vehicle, OR the equipment for the service is transported to multiple locations within a geographic area. The most common types of mobile facilities/portable units are mobile independent diagnostic testing facilities, portable x-ray units, portable mammography units, and mobile clinics. Physical therapists and other medical practitioners (e.g., physicians, nurse practitioners, physician assistants) who perform services at multiple locations (i.e., house calls, assisted living facilities) are not considered to be mobile facilities or portable units.

mobilization Therapy that consists of small passive movements, usually applied as a series of gentle stretches in a smooth, rhythmic fashion to the individual vertebrae. The movements are applied at various locations on each of the affected vertebrae, and at various angles, directed at relieving restriction in movement at any particular level of the spine. Mobilization stretches stiff joints to restore range. It also relieves pain. For example, it is especially effective with arthritic joints. Report mobilization with CPT code 97140.

MOD Multiple organ dysfunction.

modality *1)* Form of imaging. These include x-ray, fluoroscopy, ultrasound, nuclear medicine, duplex Doppler, CT, and MRI. *2)* Any physical agent applied to produce therapeutic changes to biologic tissue; includes but is not limited to thermal, acoustic, light, mechanical, or electric energy.

moderate sedation Medically controlled state of depressed consciousness, with or without analgesia, while maintaining the patient's airway, protective reflexes, and ability to respond to stimulation or verbal commands.

modification Changing of tissues.

modifier Two-character code attached to a HCPCS code as a suffix to identify circumstances that alter or enhance the description of a service or supply.

modify or modification Under HIPAA, change adopted by the secretary, through regulation, to a standard or an implementation specification.

MODY Maturity-onset diabetes of the young. Type II diabetes occurring in children with a genetic predisposition for the defect. Type II diabetes usually occurs in adults; MODY presents in children but continues to be the diagnosis as the child matures into adulthood. MODY is reported using ICD-9-CM fifth-digits 0 and 2 indicating Type II diabetes mellitus.

Mohr's syndrome Cranial, facial, lingual, mandibular, digital, and palatal abnormalities. Report this disorder with ICD-9-CM code 759.89. *Synonym(s): oral-fascial-digital syndrome.*

Mohs micrographic surgery Special technique used to treat complex or ill-defined skin cancer and requires a single physician to provide two distinct services. The first service is surgical and involves the destruction of the lesion by a combination of chemosurgery and excision. The second service is that of a pathologist and includes mapping, color coding of specimens, microscopic examination of specimens, and complete histopathologic preparation.

molars Posterior teeth used for grinding.

J-N

mole Colored (pigmented) skin lesion. *Synonym(s): nevus.*

molluscum contagiosum Common, benign, viral skin infection, usually self-limiting, that appears as a gray or flesh-colored umbilicated lesion by itself or in groups, and later becomes white with an expulsable core containing the replication bodies. It is often transmitted sexually in adults, by autoinoculation, or close contact in children. For destruction of the lesions, see CPT codes 17110-17111. For destruction of penile molluscum contagiosum lesions, see 54050-54060. For destruction of vulvar molluscum contagiosum lesions, see 56501-56515.

Molteno valve/implant Eponym for an eye implant used to mitigate glaucoma. Insertion of the Molteno shunt is reported with CPT code 66180; revision with 66185; and removal with 67120.

MOM Milk of magnesia.

Monarch Subfascial Hammock Brand name urethral sling for treatment of female stress incontinence. The Monarch requires a transobturator approach, avoiding the space between the bladder, pubic bone, and abdominal wall.

monilethrix Rare congenital disorder in which the hair is dry, thin, and easily broken. The hair shaft resembles a string of beads and often breaks before reaching more than a few inches in length. Monilethrix is reported with ICD-9-CM code 757.4. *Synonym(s): nodose hair.*

monitored anesthesia care Sedation, with or without analgesia, used to achieve a medically controlled state of depressed consciousness while maintaining the patient's airway, protective reflexes, and ability to respond to stimulation or verbal commands. In dental conscious sedation, the patient is rendered free of fear, apprehension, and anxiety through the use of pharmacological agents.

monitoring Recording of events. compliance m. Keep track, regulate, or control the compliance process. patient m. Keep track, regulate, or control patient activities and record findings.

mono *1)* Monocyte. *2)* Mononucleosis.

monochromatism Complete color blindness or total inability to distinguish colors with all hues appearing as lighter or darker shades of grey. Monochromatism is reported with ICD-9-CM code 368.54. *Synonym(s): achromatism, achromatopsia.*

monocular Affecting one eye.

monocytic leukemia Malignancy of the blood forming tissues characterized by proliferation of monocytes and monoblasts. Report this condition with a code from ICD-9-CM category 206.

monofixation syndrome Strabismus of slight degree. Report this disorder with ICD-9-CM code 378.34.

mononeuritis Inflammation of one nerve.

mononeuritis multiplex Peripheral neuropathy involving isolated damage to at least two separate nerves.

monoplegia Loss or impairment of motor function in one arm or one leg.

Monorail stent Brand name coronary stent system.

monorchism Condition of having only one testis in the scrotum. This condition is reported with ICD-9-CM code 752.89 when congenital and V45.77 when acquired.

monosomy 9P-minus syndrome Rare congenital defect with a complex of disorders including mental retardation and muscle weakness, caused by a defect on the ninth chromosome. This syndrome is reported with ICD-9-CM code 759.89. *Synonym(s): Alfi's syndrome.*

monozygotic twins Identical twins arising from a single fertilized ovum that splits into two embryos at an early stage, resulting in two individuals with the same DNA. *Synonym(s): identical twins.*

Monteggia's fracture Break in the proximal half of the ulnar shaft accompanied by a dislocation of the radial head.

mood swings Mild disorders of mood (depression and anxiety or elation and excitement, alternating or occurring episodically) seen in affective psychosis.

Moore's syndrome Epilepsy with unilateral clonic movements starting in one group of muscles and spreading to adjacent groups, following the movement of the epilepsy through the contralateral motor cortex. Report this disorder with a code from ICD-9-CM range 345.50-345.51.

mor. dict. In the manner directed.

morbid obesity Accumulation of excess fat in the subcutaneous connective tissue with increased weight beyond the limits of skeletal requirements, defined as 125 percent or more over the ideal body weight. It is often associated with serious conditions that can become life threatening, such as diabetes, hypertension, and arteriosclerosis. Morbid obesity is reported with ICD-9-CM code 278.01. *NCD References: 40.5, 100.1, 100.11.*

morbidity Diseased condition or state.

morbidity rate In health care contracting, an actuarial term describing predicted medical expense rate.

morbidity rate Actuarial term describing predicted medical expense rate.

Morel-Moore syndrome Thickening of the inner table of the frontal bone related to obesity in women nearing menopause. Report this disorder with ICD-9-CM code

733.3. **Synonym(s):** *Morel-Morgagni syndrome, Stewart-Morel syndrome.*

Morgagni-Adams-Stokes syndrome   Heart block causing slow or absent pulse, vertigo, syncope, convulsions, and Cheyne-Stokes respiration. Report this disorder with ICD-9-CM code 426.9. **Synonym(s):** *Morgagni's disease syndrome, Spens syndrome, Stokes-Adams syndrome.*

Morquio (-Brailsford) (-Ulrich) syndrome   Accumulation of mucopolysaccharide sulfates affecting the eye, ear, skin, teeth, skeleton, joints, liver, spleen, cardiovascular system, respiratory system, and central nervous system. Report this disorder with ICD-9-CM code 277.5.

Morris syndrome   Male pseudohermaphroditism with incompletely developed vagina, rudimentary uterus and fallopian tubes, scanty or absent axillary/pubic hair, and amenorrhea. Report this disorder with ICD-9-CM code 259.51. **Synonym(s):** *Goldberg syndrome, Goldberg-Maxwell syndrome, hairless women syndrome.*

mortality   Condition of being mortal (subject to death).

mortality rate   Death rate often made explicit for a particular characteristic (e.g. gender, sex, or specific cause of death). Mortality rate contains three essential elements: the number of people in a population exposed to the risk of death (denominator), a time factor, and the number of deaths occurring in the exposed population during a certain time period (the numerator).

Morton's Neuroma

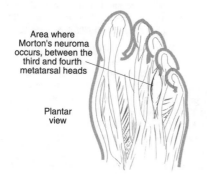

Area where Morton's neuroma occurs, between the third and fourth metatarsal heads

Plantar view

Morton's neuroma   Painful lesion of the plantar nerve. Report this disorder with ICD-9-CM code 355.6. Report injection of an anesthetic agent and/or steroid with CPT code 64455 and excision with 28080.

mosaicplasty   Multiple, small grafts composed of bone and cartilage placed to treat osteochondral defects of the knee. The grafts are cylindrical in shape and are placed in corresponding size holes made to the desired depth to fill the defect and allow for a more naturally shaped reconstruction. Graft may be harvested from the nonweight-bearing area of the patient's patellofemoral

area or an allograft from another donor and the arthroscopic mosaicplasty procedure is coded accordingly, see CPT codes 29866 and 29867.

Moschcowitz disease   Thrombocytopenia with thrombi formation in the small arterioles and capillaries causing hemolytic anemia, purpura, azotemia, fever, and central nervous system disorders manifested by bizarre neurological effects. Report this disease with ICD-9-CM code 446.6. **Synonym(s):** *Baehr-Schiffrin disease, microangiopathic hemolytic anemia, thrombotic microangiopathy, thrombotic thrombocytopenic purpura.*

Moschcowitz operation   Repair of a femoral hernia utilizing the inguinal approach, reported with CPT code 49555.

Mosenthal test   Urine test for kidney function that is taken while the patient prescribes to a general diet.

Mossman fever   Acute infectious disease resembling typhus, caused by rickettsia bacteria and transmitted by the bite of infected larval mites, called chiggers. This disease occurs chiefly in Asia and the Pacific and is manifested by a specific telltale lesion or eschar at the site of the bite, fever, regional lymphadenopathy, and skin lesions and rashes. Report this disease with ICD-9-CM code 081.2. **Synonym(s):** *akamushi disease, inundation fever, island fever, Japanese flood fever, Japanese river fever, kedani fever, mite-borne typhus, scrub typhus, shimamushi disease, tropical typhus, tsutsugamushi disease.*

most prevalent rate (charge)   Rate that applies to the greatest number of semiprivate or private beds in the institution.

most-favored-nation clauses   In health care contracting, contract provision requiring the provider to bill the third-party payer the lowest fee charged to any other person or entity.

motility   Capability of independent, spontaneous movement.

motor neuron disease   Group of disorders in which nerve cells (neurons) in the spinal cord and brain stem deteriorate and die. ALS is the most common motor neuron disease. This disease is reported with ICD-9-CM code 335.20.

motor tic disorders   Disorders of no known organic origin with quick, involuntary, apparently purposeless, and frequently repeated movements of the face or other body part that are not due to any neurological condition. May be manifested singly or simultaneously, alternately, or consecutively.

motor-verbal tic disorder   Rare disorder occurring in individuals of any level of intelligence in which facial tics and tic-like throat noises become more marked and more generalized. Later, whole words or short sentences (often

J-N

with obscene content) are cried out spasmodically and involuntarily. **Synonym(s):** *Gilles de la Tourette syndrome.*

MOU Memorandum of understanding.

moulage Model of an anatomical structure formed via a negative impression in wax or plaster.

Mounier-Kuhn syndrome Form of bronchiectasis where the bronchi is dilated with mucous and persistent cough. Report this disorder with a code from ICD-9-CM range 494.0-494.1. **Synonym(s):** *bronchiectasis.*

Moyamoya Rare, progressive vascular narrowing of the blood vessels causing a reduction of blood flow in the brain, thought to be caused by inherited anomalies. It usually presents in childhood. It is reported with ICD-9-CM code 437.5.

Moynihan test Radiological test determines hourglass stomach, a condition marked by the inability of the stomach muscles to contract, consequently resulting in digestive problems.

Mozobil See plerixafor.

MP Metacarpal phalangeal.

MPA Microscopic polyangiitis. Necrotizing vasculitis affecting small vessels, for example, in the kidneys and muscles. MPA is reported with ICD-9-CM code 446.0.

MPAP Mean pulmonary artery pressure. Arithmetic average of the pressure in the pulmonary artery during one heartbeat. This measurement is used in the evaluation of pulmonary hypertension.

MPD Maximum permissible dose.

MPFS Medicare physician fee schedule.

MPH Master of public health. Advanced degree.

MPNST Malignant peripheral nerve sheath tumor. Code according to nerve site. **Synonym(s):** *malignant schwannoma, neurofibrosarcoma.*

MPR Multifetal pregnancy reduction. Selective reduction, most often using potassium chloride injections, performed to eliminate one or more fetuses of a multiple pregnancy in an attempt to increase the viability of the remaining fetuses. Fetuses are usually eliminated in this procedure until only a twin or triplet pregnancy remains. Report this procedure with ICD-9-CM procedure code 75.0 or CPT code 59866. **Synonym(s):** *selective abortion.*

MR *1)* Medical review. *2)* Mitral regurgitation.

MRA Magnetic resonance angiography. Diagnostic technique utilizing magnetic fields and radio waves rather than radiation to produce detailed cross-sectional images of internal body structures. CPT code assignment is dependent upon anatomical structure. **NCD Reference:** *220.3.*

MRCP Magnetic resonance cholangiopancreatography. Technique for viewing the pancreatic and bile ducts and

gallbladder that requires no contrast imaging. MRCP is reported with HCPCS Level II code S8037 or CPT code 74181.

MRDD Mentally retarded/developmentally disabled.

MRG Murmurs, rubs, or gallops.

MRgFUS MR-guided, focused ultrasound system.

MRHFP Medicare Rural Hospital Flexibility Program, a CMS designation.

MRI *1)* Magnetic resonance imaging. Radiation-free, noninvasive technique that produces high quality, multiple plane images of the inside of the body by using the natural magnetic properties of the hydrogen atoms within the body that emit radiofrequency signals when exposed to radio waves in a strong magnetic field. **NCD Reference:** *220.2. 2)* Medical Records Institute.

MRM Modified radical mastectomy.

MRN *1)* Magnetic resonance neurography. *2)* Medical record number.

mRNA Messenger RNA.

MRND Modified radical neck dissection. Surgical treatment for head and neck cancers. There is no CPT code specific to MRND. Report the primary procedure first (e.g., a laryngectomy that is not a radical dissection [CPT code 31365]) and report secondarily the dissection of surrounding tissue with 38724.

MRS Magnetic resonance spectroscopy. Test that detects changes in chemicals that provide energy for heart contraction (phosphocreatine and adenosine triphosphate). Reductions in the ratio of the chemicals are indicative of reduced blood flow to the heart. MRS is reported with CPT code 76390. **NCD Reference:** *220.2.1.*

MRSA Methicillin resistant staphylococcus aureus. Bacterial infection resistant to treatment with all or most antibiotics. It is most commonly seen in inpatient situations. The infection with staphylococcus aureus is reported with ICD-9-CM code 041.12. Septicemia due to MRSA is reported with 038.12, and pneumonia due to MRSA is reported with 482.42. Report MRSA colonization with V02.54 and personal history with code V12.04.

MS *1)* Morphine sulfate. *2)* Multiple sclerosis. **NCD Reference:** *160.20. 3)* Mitral stenosis.

MSA *1)* Medical savings account. *2)* Metropolitan statistical area.

MS-DRG Medicare severity-adjusted diagnosis related group. Method CMS uses to pay hospitals for Medicare recipients based on a statistical system of classifying any inpatient stay into one of several hundred groups. It is a classification scheme whose patient types are defined by diagnoses or procedures and, in some cases, by the patient's discharge status. MS-DRGs are a modification of the prior DRG system that more accurately reflect the severity of a patient's illness and resources used.

MSHJ Medical staff hospital joint venture.

MSLT Multiple sleep latency test. Evaluation of excessive daytime sleepiness and narcolepsy in which the physiological parameters of a patient asleep in a lab setting are monitored for at least six hours. Report MSLT with ICD-9-CM procedure code 89.18 or CPT code 95805. This code applies to multiple sleep latency tests during periods of napping to assess sleepiness.

MSN Master of science in nursing.

MSO Management services organization. Organization that provides the strategic, financial, and operational plans required by physicians, physician groups, and ancillary service providers for a successful managed care venture.

MSP Medicare secondary payer. Specified circumstances when other third-party payers cover beneficiaries and Medicare is the secondary payer. Medicare is secondary to workers compensation, automobile, medical no-fault, and liability insurance. Medicare is also secondary to group health plans and certain group health plans covering aged and disabled beneficiaries. For end-stage renal disease beneficiaries, Medicare is the secondary payer during the first 30 months of the beneficiary's entitlement to ESRD benefits. MSP cases are identified by CMS through beneficiary questionnaires, provider identification of third-party coverage during the admissions process, data transfers with other state and federal agencies, and Common Working File edits. The MSP program prohibits Medicare payment for items or services if payment has been made or can reasonably be expected to be made by another payer, as described above.

MSP alert Medicare secondary payer alert. Medicare edit on inpatient and outpatient claims that may indicate that Medicare is the secondary payer.

MSS Medical social services.

MSSA Methicillin susceptible staphylococcus aureus, reported with ICD-9-CM code 041.11. Report MSSA septicemia or staphylococcus septicemia that is not otherwise specified with ICD-9-CM code 038.11, MSSA pneumonia with 482.41, and MSSA colonization with V02.53.

MSSU Midstream specimen urine.

MSW Master's in social work.

MT Medical technologist.

MTC Medullary thyroid carcinoma.

MTD Right eardrum.

MTM Metamucil.

MTP Metatarsophalangeal.

MTS Left eardrum.

MTWA Microvolt T-wave alternans. Diagnostic test to evaluate electrical activity in the T-wave portion of the EKG. MTWA is used to detect risk of sudden cardiac death and is reported with CPT code 93025. *NCD Reference: 20.30.*

MTX Methotrexate.

Mucha-Haberman syndrome Chronic dermatosis of unknown origin with scaling lesions that produce small pox-like scars. Recurrence of attacks are common, but disease is self-limiting. Report this disorder with ICD-9-CM code 696.2.

mucocele Serous fluid accumulation in the gallbladder, reported with ICD-9-CM code 575.3. *Synonym(s): hydrops of gallbladder.*

mucocutaneous leishmaniasis Form of leishmaniasis endemic in Mexico, Central America, and South America with sores limited to the skin and mucosa. Report this condition with ICD-9-CM code 085.5. *Synonym(s): American leishmaniasis.*

mucocutaneous lymph node syndrome Syndrome of unknown origin causing fever; redness of the eyes, lips, and mucous membranes of the mouth; gingivitis; cervical lymphadenopathy, and a bright red raised rash in a glove-and-sock fashion over the hands and feet. The skin there becomes hard, swollen (edematous), and peels. This disease mainly affects children and is reported with ICD-9-CM code 446.1. *Synonym(s): Kawasaki disease.*

mucopolysaccharidosis Progressive and chronic familial disease due to a deficiency of lysosomal enzymes and defects in the breakdown of sulfates, which are excreted and built up in tissues, affecting the central nervous system, the skeleton and joints, the liver, spleen, skin, teeth, and cardiovascular and respiratory systems.

mucosa Moist tissue lining the mouth (buccal mucosa), stomach (gastric mucosa), intestines, and respiratory tract.

Mucosperse Brand name cleaner that dissolves mucous and prevents blockage in ostomy appliances. Mucosperse is reported with HCPCS Level II code A4421.

mucous membranes Thin sheets of tissue that secrete mucous and absorb water, salt, and other solutes. Mucous membranes cover or line cavities or canals of the body that open to the outside, such as linings of the mouth, respiratory and genitourinary passages, and the digestive tube.

mucous polyp Outgrowth or projection of the mucous membrane tissue lining a body cavity.

MUGA scan Multiple gated acquisition scan. Noninvasive test that produces a moving image of the heart to assess the pumping function of the left ventricle. Technetium 99 is mixed with the patient's red blood cells, the cells are injected into the patient's bloodstream, and the patient is placed under a gamma camera so the ejection fraction of the left ventricle of the heart, an overall indicator of cardiac function, can be measured. MUGA scans identify the area of damage following a myocardial infarct or monitor the effects of chemotherapy upon the heart, as some drugs are toxic to heart muscle. *Synonym(s): RNV.*

Muir Torre syndrome Genetic syndrome that includes in situ sebaceous carcinoma, epithelioma or carcinoma, plus a visceral carcinoma in the absence of other precipitating factors like radiotherapy or AIDS. There is no single code in ICD-9-CM to describe this condition. Assign a code for each manifestation of the syndrome.

mulberry molars Berry-like molars seen in congenital syphilis. Report this condition with ICD-9-CM code 520.3. If due to congenital syphilis, see ICD-9-CM code 090.5.

Mullan set Brand name for trigeminal ganglion microcompression set using a balloon catheter for the treatment of trigeminal neuralgia.

Müller's sign Pulsation of the uvula accompanied by swelling of the palate and tonsils, seen in patients with aortic regurgitation or insufficiency.

multifetal pregnancy reduction Selective reduction, most often using potassium chloride injections, performed to eliminate one or more fetuses of a multiple pregnancy in an attempt to increase the viability of the remaining fetuses. Fetuses are usually eliminated in this procedure until only a twin or triplet pregnancy remains. Report this procedure with ICD-9-CM procedure code 75.0 or CPT code 59866. *Synonym(s): MPR, selective abortion.*

multigravida Female who has had two or more pregnancies. elderly m. Female in her second or more pregnancy who will be 35 years or older at her expected date of delivery. Multigravida is reported with a code from ICD-9-CM subcategory 659.6. Women in this category are considered to be at high risk during pregnancy. young m. Female in her second or more pregnancy who will be younger than age 16 at her expected date of delivery. Young multigravida is reported with a code from subcategory 659.8. Women in this category are considered to be at high risk during pregnancy.

multi-infarct dementia or psychosis Dementia attributable, because of physical signs (confirmed by examination of the central nervous system), to degenerative arterial disease of the brain.

Multi-Link Brand name coronary stent.

multip. Multipara.

multiparity Condition of having had two or more pregnancies that resulted in viable fetuses; producing more than one fetus or offspring in the same gestation.

multiplane external fixation device Stabilization device that uses more than one external fixation system to stabilize a fracture.

multiple birth Two or more infants delivered at the same time.

multiple employer group Group of employers who contract together to subscribe to a plan, broadening the risk pool and saving money. Different from a multiple employer trust.

multiple employer trust Group of employers that join together to purchase health insurance using a self-funded approach to lower costs by the broadening membership pool to prevent an adverse selection. *Synonym(s): MET.*

multiple employer welfare association Group of employers that join together to purchase health insurance using a self-funded approach to lower costs by the broadening membership pool to prevent an adverse selection. *Synonym(s): MEWA.*

multiple myeloma Rare form of cancer in which the bone marrow's plasma cells are produced at an increased rate, forming multiple bone marrow tumors and bone-destroying lesions that progress to other parts of the body in advanced stages. Symptoms involve bone pain, weakness, spontaneous fractures, anemia, fatigue, and hypercalcemia causing renal cast formation, nephropathy, and kidney failure. This condition is diagnosed by the presence of Bence-Jones protein in the urine. Report this condition with a code from ICD-9-CM subcategory 203.0. *Synonym(s): Kahler (-Bozzolo) disease, plasma cell myeloma.*

multiple operations syndrome Chronic form of factitious illness in which the individual demonstrates a plausible presentation of voluntarily produced physical symptomatology of such a degree that he or she is able to obtain and sustain multiple hospitalizations or courses of treatment. *Synonym(s): Munchhausen's syndrome.*

multiple personality Domination of the individual at any one time by one of two or more distinct, fully integrated, and complex personalities with memories, behavior patterns, and social friendships, that determine the nature of the individual's acts when uppermost in consciousness.

multiple sclerosis Chronic, demyelinating disease affecting the white matter of the spinal cord and brain. This disease may also be documented as disseminated or generalized multiple sclerosis. Report multiple sclerosis with ICD-9-CM code 340.

multiple-lead device Implantable cardiac device (pacemaker or implantable cardioverter-defibrillator

[ICD]) in which pacing and sensing components are placed in at least three chambers of the heart.

Mumpsvax   Brand name mumps vaccine provided in a single-dose vial. Supply of Mumpsvax is reported with CPT code 90704; administration is reported separately. The need for vaccination is reported with ICD-9-CM code V04.6.

Munchausen syndrome   Emotional condition in which patient exhibits physical, but psychosomatic, symptoms. Report this disorder with ICD-9-CM code 301.51. *Synonym(s): hospital addiction syndrome.*

Münchmeyer's syndrome   Diffuse progressive ossifying polymyositis. Report this disorder with ICD-9-CM code 728.11.

muscle deficiency syndrome   Absence of muscles of abdomen and genitourinary anomalies. Intestinal outlines are visible on patient's skin. Report this disorder with ICD-9-CM code 756.71. *Synonym(s): Eagle-Barrett syndrome, prune belly syndrome.*

muscle graft   Muscle taken from a donor site or person and inserted into a new site or person.

muscle tissue   Network of specialized cells for performing contraction to produce voluntary or involuntary movement of body parts, and skeletal, cardiac, or visceral muscles.

muscular tissue   Tissue consisting of cells that can contract and function automatically in the heart, voluntarily in the skeleton to allow movement, and rhythmically to move food in the digestive system.

musculature   Entire muscle tissue apparatus of the body or a specific part of the body.

Mustard procedure   Corrective measure for transposition of great vessels involves an intra-atrial baffle made of pericardial tissue or synthetic material. The baffle is secured between pulmonary veins and mitral valve and between mitral and tricuspid valves. The baffle directs systemic venous flow into the left ventricle and lungs and pulmonary venous flow into the right ventricle and aorta.

MVA   Motor vehicle accident or manual vacuum aspiration.

MVD   Microvascular decompression. Microsurgical procedure done to relieve the pain caused by trigeminal neuralgia in which a tiny, nonabsorbable sponge is inserted to decompress the sensory root of the nerve by relieving the pressure put upon it by the surrounding blood vessels. Report this procedure with ICD-9-CM procedure code 04.41 or CPT code 61450. *Synonym(s): Jannetta procedure.*

MVP   Mitral valve prolapse.

MVPS   Medicare volume performance standard. Standard set by Congress (or the Department of Health

and Human Services by a default formula provided in the law) to determine how much growth is appropriate for Medicare Part B physician payments. This standard is based on factors such as inflation, the mix and age of the Medicare population, technological changes, inappropriate utilization, and inadequate beneficiary access to care. The MVPS is used to develop payments under the national Medicare fee schedule.

MWS   Mickey-Wilson syndrome.

my-   Relating to muscle. *Synonym(s): myo-.*

myalgia   Pain in the muscles.

myasthenia gravis   Autoimmune neuromuscular disorder caused by antibodies to the acetylcholine receptors at the neuromuscular junction, interfering with proper binding of the neurotransmitter from the neuron to the target muscle, causing muscle weakness, fatigue, and exhaustion, without pain or atrophy.

myc-   Relating to fungus. *Synonym(s): myco-.*

mycotic keratitis   Corneal infection caused by a fungus. *Synonym(s): keratomycosis.*

mydriatic   Agent that contracts the iris, enlarging the pupil to allow better visualization or access to the eye.

myelo-   Relating to bone marrow or the spinal cord.

myelodysplasia   Defective formation of the spinal cord. Lesions may include spina bifida, meningocele, lipomyelomeningocele, or myelomeningocele.

myelodysplastic syndrome   Neoplasm of lymphatic and hematopoietic tissues, affecting the spinal cord. Report this disorder with ICD-9-CM code 238.72-238.75.

myelogram   Radiological images of the spinal cord after injection of contrast medium.

myelography   Introduction of radiographic contrast medium into the sac surrounding the spinal cord and nerves.

myelomeningocele   Congenital disorder in which the spinal cord and meninges herniate through a vertebral canal defect. If the birth of a child with myelomeningocele results in fetal disproportion, an ICD-9-CM code from subcategory 653.7 is reported. The condition of any age is reported as spina bifida with category 741 with fourth and fifth digits denoting with or without hydrecephalus and the spinal region. *Synonym(s): meningomyelocele, myelocystocele.*

myelopathy   Pathological or functional changes in the spinal cord, often resulting from nonspecific and noninflammatory lesions.

myelopore   Spinal column canal or opening.

myeloproliferative syndrome   Unusual proliferation of myelopoietic tissue. Report this disorder with ICD-9-CM code 238.72-238.75.

J–N

myelotomy Procedure performed to sever tracts in the spinal cord, a useful option for patients with intractable pain due to cancer and spasticity in spinal cord injuries.

myocardial ablation therapy Delivery of electrical energy, such as alternating radiofrequency current, to areas of the heart wall in order to selectively destroy cardiac muscle tissue and prevent arrhythmias.

myocardial infarction Obstruction of circulation to the heart, resulting in necrosis.

myocutaneous flap Skin, subcutaneous tissue, and intact muscle tissue that are transferred to a recipient site while retaining sufficient blood supply from its own vascular bed. CPT codes 15732-15738 report myocutaneous flap of the head and neck, trunk, and upper and lower extremities. CPT code 15756 identifies a free myocutaneous flap graft in which the blood vessels are attached to the new recipient bed with microvascular anastomosis.

myocutaneous flap graft Section of tissue containing muscle and attached skin is partially removed from its donor site so as to retain its own blood supply for transfer to a new recipient site.

myoelectrical Electric characteristics of muscle movement.

myofibrosis Muscle wasting and replacement of muscle tissue by fibrous tissue. Report myofibrosis with ICD-9-CM code 728.2.

myogenic ptosis Drooping of a muscle due to a defect.

myomectomy Excision of a benign lesion of the muscle.

myometrium Muscular middle layer of the uterine wall responsible for contractions associated with childbirth.

Myomo e-100 Noninvasive robotic tool worn as a portable upper arm brace. This robotic tool allows patients to initiate and control movement of affected limbs through the use of electrical muscle activity (EMG) signals, without the use of surgery or electrical stimulation. Myomo e-100 is indicated for individuals with upper extremity hemiparesis or hemiplegia secondary to stroke to assist in post-stroke motor recovery by engaging and reinforcing the neurological and motor pathways.

myoneural junction Neuromuscular junction.

myopathy Any disease process within muscle tissue.

myopia Defect in focusing in which the eye is overpowered and incoming distant light rays are focused in front of the retina because of a refractive or curvature defect in the lens. Myopia is reported with ICD-9-CM code 367.1 unless the condition is malignant or progressive. Malignant myopia is highly degenerative and complicated by serious disease of the choroid that leads to retinal detachment and blindness; reported with ICD-9-CM code 360.21. *Synonym(s): nearsightedness.*

myositis Inflammation of a muscle with voluntary movement.

myositis ossificans Inflammatory disease of muscles due to bony deposits or conversion of muscle tissue to bony tissue.

myotomy Surgical cutting of a muscle to gain access to underlying tissues or for therapeutic reasons.

myotonic chondrodystrophy Rare genetic disorder characterized by joint contractures, bone dysplasia, myotonic myopathy, and growth delays resulting in dwarfism. Treatment options for the various myotonic disorders may include anticonvulsant drugs, physical therapy, and other rehabilitative measures designed to improve muscle function. Report this disorder with ICD-9-CM code 359.23.

myotonic dystrophy Inherited multisystem disorder characterized by progressive degeneration and weakness of muscle and abnormal muscle contracture (myotonia). Myotonia is prominent in the hand muscles and ptosis is common even in mild cases. In severe cases, marked peripheral muscular weakness occurs, often with cataracts, premature balding, hatchet facies, cardiac arrhythmias, testicular atrophy, and endocrine disorders including diabetes mellitus. Mental retardation is common. This condition is reported with ICD-9-CM code 359.21. *Synonym(s): Steinert's disease.*

Myozyme Brand name drug used in treatment of Pompe's disease. Supply is reported with HCPCS Level II code J0220. *Synonym(s): alglucosidase alfa.*

myringotomy Incision in the eardrum done to prevent spontaneous rupture precipitated by fluid pressure build-up behind the tympanic membrane and to prevent stagnant infection and erosion of the ossicles. This incision is reported with CPT code 69420 and 69421 when general anesthesia is used. If a tube is inserted at the time of the incision, 69433 or 69436 is reported. *Synonym(s): tympanostomy, tympanotomy.*

mytonachol Cholinergic drug that stimulates receptors to increase muscle tone and contraction within the gastrointestinal tract and bladder. It is used to relieve urinary retention following surgery, childbirth, or due to atony of the bladder. Supply is reported with HCPCS Level II code J0520.

N Nitrogen.

N&V Nausea and vomiting.

N'ice Stretch Brand name night splint used as therapy for plantar fasciitis, Achilles tendonitis, plantar flexion contractures, and equinus and tight triceps surae. Supply is reported with HCPCS Level II code L4396.

n.p.o. Nothing by mouth.

N/T Not tender.

N0M0 Lymph node, zero; metastases, zero. Pathology finding on biopsy indicating malignancy has not spread.

N2O Nitrous oxide.

Na Natrium. Chemical symbol for sodium, the main positive ion in extracellular fluids.

NA Nurse assistant.

NAAT Nucleic acid amplification test. Laboratory test technique.

Nabi-HB Brand name hepatitis B immune globulin provided in a single-dose vial. Supply of Nabi-HB is reported with CPT code 90371; administration is reported separately. The need for the injection is reported with ICD-9-CM code V01.89.

nabilone Synthetic version of THC, the active ingredient in marijuana. Nabilone is prescribed in capsules to treat nausea that may accompany chemotherapy.

Naboth's cyst Retention cyst of endocervical cells common in adult women. If inflamed or infected, report ICD-9-CM code 616.0. *Synonym(s): nabothian cyst.*

NaCl Sodium chloride (salt).

NAD No acute distress.

Naegeli's disease Disorder manifested by numerous malignant tumors produced by bony infiltrates in myelogenous leukemia. The masses are most often found in the skull, but may occur in any part of the skeleton. The tumors appear green colored, due to pigment effects of myeloperoxidase. Report this disease with a code from ICD-9-CM category 205.3. *Synonym(s): Aran's cancer, Balfour's disease, chloroleukemia, chloroma, chloromyeloma, chlorosarcoma, granulocytic sarcoma, green cancer.*

nafcillin sodium Injectable penicillin antibiotic used in the treatment of various infections, including those of the urinary tract, respiratory tract, skin, bones, joints, blood, and heart valves. Supply is reported with HCPCS Level II code S0032. May be sold under brand names Nallpen, Unipen.

Naffziger operation Removal of the lateral and superior orbital walls to decompress the orbit in cases of severe malignant exophthalmos. Report this procedure with ICD-9-CM procedure code 16.09 or CPT code 61330.

Naffziger's syndrome Raynaud-like symptoms of vascular contractions caused by pressure of brachial plexus and subclavian artery against first thoracic rib. Report this disorder with ICD-9-CM code 353.0.

NAFLD Nonalcoholic fatty liver disease. Liver disease in individuals who drink little or no alcohol, manifested by a fatty liver without damage or inflammation. Diagnosis is confirmed by liver biopsy. Report this condition with ICD-9-CM code 571.8.

Naga sore Tropical, chronic skin ulcer, reported with ICD-9-CM code 707.9.

Nagel test Extended color vision examination involving an anomaloscope or equivalent, which is an instrument used to diagnose abnormalities of color perception in which one half of a field of color is matched by mixing two other colors. Report this test with CPT code 92283.

Nager-de Reynier syndrome Franceschetti's syndrome with limb deformities consisting of absence of the radius, radioulnar synostosis, and hypoplasia or absence of thumbs. Report this disorder with ICD-9-CM code 756.0.

NAHDO National Association of Health Data Organizations.

NAHMOR National Association of HMO Regulators.

NAIC National Association of Insurance Commissioners. Organization of state insurance regulators.

nail *1)* Thin, horny plate on the dorsal side of the phalanx of the distal toes and fingers. The nail root is the proximal end under the cuticle or skin fold. *2)* Metal, bone, or synthetic rod used as a surgical fastener.

nail bed Area of dermal layer beneath the nail.

nail fold Nail wall at the side and proximal end of the nail plate covered by a skin fold.

nail matrix Area of dermal layer beneath the nail and proximal skin. Nail bed is the portion of the matrix covered by the body of the nail.

nail-patella syndrome Dysplasia of the fingernails and toenails, hypoplasia of the patella, iliac horns, thickening of the glomerular lamina densa, and a flask-shaped femur. Report this disorder with ICD-9-CM code 756.89.

NAION Nonarteritic anterior ischemic optic neuropathy. Blood flow to the optic nerve is blocked, causing sudden vision loss. Report NAION with ICD-9-CM code 377.41.

nalbuphine HCl Synthetic injectable opiate analgesic used to relieve moderate to severe pain caused by acute or chronic medical conditions including cancer, colic, certain forms of headaches, and postoperative pain. It may also be used for labor and delivery analgesia. Supply is reported with HCPCS Level II code J2300. May be sold under brand name Nubain.

Nallpen Injectable penicillin antibiotic used in the treatment of various infections, including those of the urinary tract, respiratory tract, skin, bones, joints, blood, and heart valves. Supply is reported with HCPCS Level II code S0032. Nallpen contains nafcillin sodium.

naloxone HCl Injectable narcotic antagonist used to avoid or reverse the effects of opioids, including respiratory decline, sedation, and hypotension. Supply is reported with HCPCS Level II code J2310. May be sold under brand name Narcan.

NANDA North American Nursing Diagnoses Association.

Nandrobolic L.A. See nandrolone decanoate.

N-J

nandrolone decanoate Injectable anabolic steroid used to treat anemia due to chronic renal failure by increasing hemoglobin and red cell mass. It is also used in the treatment of osteoporosis. Supply is reported with HCPCS Level II code J2320. May be sold under brand names Anabolin LA 100, Andronolone-D 100, Deca-Durabolin, Decolone-50, Decolone-100, Hybolin Decanoate, Nandrobolic L.A., and Neo-Durabolic.

nanukayami Rodent-borne bacterial infection caused by Leptospira interrogans and manifested by fever and jaundice. Report this infection with ICD-9-CM code 100.89. *Synonym(s): autumn fever, seven-day fever.*

napkin rash Nonallergic skin irritation in infants in the area that has contact with the diaper. It can be caused by extended contact with feces, urine, soaps, and ointments, and by friction and the irritating effects of ammonia by-products in urine. The rash is often accompanied by secondary yeast or bacterial infection. Report this condition with ICD-9-CM code 691.0. *Synonym(s): ammonia dermatitis, diaper dermatitis, diaper rash, Jacquet's dermatitis, Jacquet's erythema.*

Narcan Injectable narcotic antagonist used to avoid or reverse the effects of opioids, including respiratory decline, sedation, and hypotension. Supply is reported with HCPCS Level II code J2310. Narcan contains naloxone HCl.

narcissistic personality Marked by an inflated sense of self-worth and indifference to the welfare of others. Achievement deficits and failure at meeting social responsibilities are justified and sustained by a boastful arrogance, expansive fantasies, facile rationalization, and frank prevarication.

narco- Indicates insensate condition or numbness.

narcolepsy Chronic neurological disorder caused by the brain's inability to regulate sleep-wake cycles normally. People with narcolepsy experience fleeting urges to sleep at various times throughout the day. People with this can fall asleep for periods lasting from a few seconds to several minutes and in some cases hours, if the urge becomes overwhelming. The major symptoms associated with narcolepsy include excessive daytime sleepiness (EDS); cataplexy (the sudden loss of voluntary muscle tone); vivid hallucinations during sleep onset or upon awakening; and brief episodes of total paralysis at the beginning or end of sleep.

narcosynthesis Psychiatric diagnostic or therapeutic procedure in which a hypnotic drug, known as sodium Amytal or amobarbital, is infused into the patient via an intravenous drip. This hypnotic sedative is used to diagnose dissociative disorders and to help treat trauma victims by accessing repressed memories, emotions, or events to facilitate healing, and is often used after other measures have failed and/or when gaining a definitive diagnosis is medically essential. Report narcosynthesis

with ICD-9-CM procedure code 94.21 or CPT code 90865. *Synonym(s): narcoanalysis.*

NARP syndrome Neuropathy-ataxia-retinitis pigmentosa syndrome. Inherited condition most often presenting in young adults and manifested by sensory-motor nerve disorders, cerebellar ataxia, and night blindness. Report this syndrome with ICD-9-CM code 277.87.

narrow angle glaucoma Progressive optic nerve disease associated with high intraocular pressure that can lead to irreversible vision loss. The aqueous humor is the clear fluid filling the chambers of the eye that is continually drained and renewed, produced by the ciliary body and passing out through the pupil and trabecular meshwork. Narrow angle glaucoma causes an increase in intraocular pressure due to an impairment of aqueous outflow caused by a narrowing or closing of the anterior chamber angle as the iris comes into contact with the trabecular meshwork. This type of glaucoma is identified in four stages: latent, intermittent, acute, and chronic. In the latent and intermittent phases, minor or transient attacks of varying severity, duration, and frequency occur in which intraocular pressure (IOP) rises with accompanying pain and edema. Acute angle closure glaucoma is a grave medical emergency as IOP rises, the cornea swells, and excruciating pain radiates through the eye. Visual acuity falls rapidly as the eye swells and blindness may result if the IOP is not lowered. The chronic stage manifests as irreversible IOP increases from progressive damage and scar tissue closing the anterior angle. This condition is reported with ICD-9-CM codes 365.20-365.24. *Synonym(s): angle closure glaucoma, closed angle glaucoma, pupillary block glaucoma.*

NAS Neonatal abstinence syndrome. Drug withdrawal symptoms seen in a newborn exposed to drugs from the mother in utero. NAS in the infant is reported with ICD-9-CM code 779.5.

Nasahist B Brand name for injectable brompheniramine maleate, an antihistamine used to treat hay fever, pruritic rashes, or allergic reactions to insect bites. Supply is reported with HCPCS Level II code J0945. Nasahist B contains brompheniramine maleate.

nasal polyp Fleshy outgrowth projecting from the mucous membrane of the nose or nasal sinus cavity that may obstruct ventilation or affect the sense of smell.

nasal septal prosthesis Use of an alloplastic button to close a nasal septal opening, reported with CPT code 30220 or HCPCS Level II code D5922. This procedure is performed as an option to surgical reconstruction of the septum such as grafting.

nasal septum Membrane made of cartilage, bone, and mucosa that partitions the two nostrils, or nasal cavities, down the middle.

nasal sinus Air-filled cavities in the cranial bones lined with mucous membrane and continuous with the nasal cavity, draining fluids through the nose.

NASH Nonalcoholic steatohepatitis. Liver disease occurring in individuals who drink little or no alcohol, manifested by a fatty, inflamed liver. Indications include elevated alanine aminotransferase (ALT) and aspartate aminotransferase (AST) and diagnosis is verified by liver biopsy. NASH can lead to cirrhosis. Report this condition with ICD-9-CM code 571.8.

NASMD National Association of State Medicaid Directors.

nasogastric tube Long, hollow, cylindrical catheter made of soft rubber or plastic that is inserted through the nose down into the stomach, and is used for feeding, instilling medication, or withdrawing gastric contents.

nasopharynx Membranous passage above the level of the soft palate.

NAT Nonaccidental trauma.

natal tooth Relatively rare condition in which one or more teeth are present at the time of birth, usually on the lower gum. Neonatal teeth are those that erupt in the first month following birth. Report this condition with ICD-9-CM code 520.6.

natalizumab Monoclonal antibody given in IV infusion as a treatment for relapsing forms of multiple sclerosis to reduce the frequency of clinical exacerbation. Report supply with HCPCS Level II code J2323. *Synonym(s): Tysabri.*

nateglinide Oral medication exclusive to lowering blood glucose in Type II diabetics. May be sold as brand name Starlix.

National Association of Health Data Organizations National organization for private, state and federal agencies to promote and improve health information and data systems in accordance with state and federal guidelines. *Synonym(s): NAHDO.*

National Association of Insurance Commissioners Organization of state insurance regulators. *Synonym(s): NAIC.*

National Association of State Medicaid Directors Association of state Medicaid directors. NASMD is affiliated with the American Public Health Human Services Association (APHSA). *Synonym(s): NASMD.*

National Center for Health Statistics Division of the Centers for Disease Control and Prevention that compiles statistical information used to guide actions and policies to improve the public health of U.S. citizens. The NCHS maintains the ICD-9-CM coding system. *Synonym(s): NCHS.*

National Committee for Quality Assurance Organization that accredits managed care plans, or HMOs. In the future, the NCQA may play a role in certifying these organizations' compliance with the HIPAA A/S requirements. *Synonym(s): NCQA.*

National Committee for Vital Health Statistics Federal advisory body within the Department of Health and Human Services that advises the secretary regarding potential changes to the HIPAA standards. *Synonym(s): NCVHS.*

National Committee on Health and Vital Statistics Statutory public advisory body to the Secretary of Health and Human Services in the area of health data and statistics.

National Committee on Vital and Health Statistics Federal advisory body within the Department of Health and Human Services that advises the secretary regarding potential changes to the HIPAA standards. *Synonym(s): NCVHS.*

National Council for Prescription Drug Programs Group accredited by the American National Standards Institute that maintains a number of standard formats for use by the retail pharmacy industry, some of which are included in the HIPAA mandates. *Synonym(s): NCPDP.*

national coverage analyses Documents that support the national coverage determination process. They include tracking sheets to inform the public of the issues under consideration and the status (i.e., pending, closed) of the review, information about and results of the Medicare Coverage Advisory Committee (MCAC) meetings, technology assessments, and the decision memorandums that announce CMS's intention to issue an NCD. These documents, along with the compilation of medical and scientific information currently available, any Food and Drug Administration (FDA) safety and efficacy data, clinical trial information, etc., provide the rationale behind the evidence-based NCDs. *Synonym(s): NCA.*

national coverage determination National policy statement granting, eliminating, or excluding Medicare coverage for a service, item, or test. NCDs state CMS policy regarding the circumstances under which the service, item, or test is considered reasonable and necessary or otherwise not covered for Medicare purposes. These polices apply nationwide. *Synonym(s): NCD.*

National Coverage Determination Manual Part of the Centers for Medicare and Medicaid Services manual system, it contains national coverage decisions and specific medical items, services, treatment procedures, or technologies paid for under the Medicare program and was revised from the Coverage Issues Manual (CIM). *Synonym(s): NCDM.*

J-N

national coverage policy Statement of Medicare coverage decisions that applies to all practitioners in states and regions. These policies indicate whether and under what circumstances procedures, services, and supplies are covered.

national coverage request Request from any party, including contractors, and CMS's internal staff, for CMS to consider an issue for a national coverage decision.

national drug codes Medical code set that identifies prescription drugs and some over-the-counter products and that has been selected for use in the HIPAA transactions. *Synonym(s): NDC.*

National Emphysema Treatment Trial Five-year randomized study of patients with severe emphysema that evaluates the safety and efficacy of lung volume reduction surgery. The three federal agencies involved within the Department of Health and Human Services include the National Heart, Lung, and Blood Institute; the Centers for Medicare and Medicaid Services; and the Agency for Healthcare Research and Quality. *Synonym(s): NETT.*

national employer ID System for uniquely identifying all sponsors of health care benefits.

National Health Care Survey Provides data related to the health care industry as a whole. Survey contents and sources are listed by individual survey titles, which include National Hospital Discharge Survey (NHDS), National Survey of Ambulatory Surgery (NSAS), National Ambulatory Medical Care Survey, National Hospital Ambulatory Medical Care Survey, National Nursing Home Survey (NNHS), National Nursing Home Survey Follow-up, National Home and Hospital Care Survey, National Health Provider Inventory.

National Health Information
Infrastructure Health-care-specific lane on the information superhighway, as described in the National Information Infrastructure (NII) initiative. Conceptually, this includes the HIPAA A/S initiatives. *Synonym(s): NHII.*

national patient ID System for uniquely identifying all recipients of health care services. *Synonym(s): health care ID, national individual identifier, NII.*

national payer ID System for uniquely identifying all organizations that pay for health care services. *Synonym(s): health plan ID, plan ID.*

national provider file Database envisioned for use in maintaining a national provider registry. *Synonym(s): NPF.*

national provider identifier Identification system developed by CMS to designate types of providers in the health care industry, including physicians, suppliers, home health agencies, and hospitals. *Synonym(s): NPI.*

national provider registry Organization envisioned for assigning national provider identifiers.

national provider system Administrative system envisioned for supporting a national provider identifier. *Synonym(s): NPS.*

national standard format Generically, this applies to any nationally standardized data format, but it is often used in a more limited way to designate the professional EMC NSF, a 320-byte flat file record format used to submit professional claims. *Synonym(s): NSF.*

National Supplier Clearinghouse Entity that approves providers and medical equipment vendors as "suppliers" under the Medicare program, issuing an identification number to approved applicants.

national supplier identification number Number with which providers or other health care professionals who disperse DMEPOS submit their claims. This number is obtained through an application to the National Supplier Clearinghouse, a centralized agency for DMEPOS suppliers.

National Uniform Billing Committee Organization, chaired and hosted by the American Hospital Association, that maintains the UB-92 hardcopy institutional billing form and the data element specifications for both the hardcopy form and the 192-byte UB-92 flat file EMC format. The NUBC has a formal consultative role under HIPAA for all transactions affecting institutional health care services. *Synonym(s): NUBC.*

National Uniform Claim Committee Organization, chaired and hosted by the American Medical Association, that maintains the CMS-1500 claim form and a set of data element specifications for professional claims submission via the CMS-1500 claim form, the Professional EMC NSF, and the X12 837. NUCC also maintains the provider taxonomy codes and has a formal consultative role under HIPAA for all transactions affecting nondental, noninstitutional professional health care services. *Synonym(s): NUCC.*

Natrecor Injectable cardiovascular agent used in the treatment of decompensated congestive heart failure. Supply is reported with HCPCS Level II code J2325. Natrecor contains nesiritide.

natrium Chemical symbol for sodium, the main positive ion in extracellular fluids. *Synonym(s): Na.*

natriuresis Excretion of salt in the urine.

Navelbine Brand name of vinorelbine tartrate, an injectable chemotherapeutic agent used to treat specific types of malignancies, including breast and non-small cell lung cancer. Supply is reported with HCPCS Level II code J9390. Navelbine contains vinorelbine tartrate.

NAW Nasoantral window. Creation of an opening to the maxillary, reported with CPT code 31256.

NB Newborn.

NBICU Newborn intensive care unit. Special care unit for premature and seriously ill infants. **Synonym(s):** *NICU.*

NBT Nitroblue tetrazolium.

NCA *1)* National coverage analyses. *2)* Neurocirculatory asthenia.

NCA closed When the decision memorandum is issued, the NCA is considered closed. However, the policy change is not effective until the manual transmittal is issued.

NCA decision memorandum Provides the reasons supporting an NCD and announces CMS's intent to issue an NCD. Prior to any new or modified policy taking effect, CMS must first issue a manual transmittal, CMS ruling, or *Federal Register* notice, giving specific directions to claims-processing contractors. That manual transmittal, or other issuance, which includes the effective date, is the actual NCD. If appropriate, the agency must also change billing and claims processing systems and issue related instructions to allow for payment. The NCD is published in the *Medicare National Coverage Determinations Manual.* Policy changes become effective as of the date listed in the transmittal that announces the *Medicare National Coverage Determinations Manual* revision.

NCA new National coverage analyses are considered new if CMS has received a coverage request or a current NCD is being edited. The "N" at the end of the tracking number (e.g., CAG-0000N) indicates a new NCA.

NCA pending National coverage analysis currently under review. The decision memorandum has not yet been issued. The subject may or may not be an existing NCD.

NCA reconsideration Formal reconsiderations can be requested if the requester presents documentation that meets either of the following criteria: additional medical material or scientific information that was not considered during the initial review; or arguments that the conclusion materially misinterpreted the existing evidence at the time the NCD was made. The "R" at the end of the tracking number (e.g., CAG-0000R) indicates reconsideration. Further reconsiderations are annotated with a number after the "R" (e.g., R2, R3, etc.).

NCAP Nasal continuous airway pressure.

NCCI National correct coding initiative. Official list of codes from the Centers for Medicare and Medicaid Services' (CMS) National Correct Coding Policy Manual for Part B Medicare Carriers that identifies services considered an integral part of a comprehensive code or mutually exclusive of it. **Synonym(s):** *CCI, correct coding initiative.*

NCD National coverage determinations. National policy statements granting, eliminating, or excluding Medicare coverage for a service, item, or test. NCDs state CMS policy regarding the circumstances under which the service, item, or test is considered reasonable and necessary or otherwise not covered for Medicare purposes. These polices apply nationwide.

NCHICA North Carolina Healthcare Information and Communications Alliance.

NCHS National Center for Health Statistics. Division of the Centers for Disease Control and Prevention that compiles statistical information used to guide actions and policies to improve the public health of U.S. citizens. The NCHS maintains the ICD-9-CM coding system.

NCHVS National Committee on Health and Vital Statistics.

NCI National Cancer Institute. *NCD Reference: 110.2.*

NCPDP National Council of Prescription Drug Programs.

NCPDP batch standard NCPDP standard designed for use by low-volume dispensers of pharmaceuticals, such as nursing homes. Use of version 1.1 of this standard has been mandated under HIPAA.

NCPDP telecommunication standard NCPDP standard designed for use by high-volume dispensers of pharmaceuticals, such as retail pharmacies. Use of version 5.1 of this standard has been mandated under HIPAA.

NCPR No cardiopulmonary resuscitation.

NCQA National Committee for Quality Assurance. Organization that accredits managed care plans, or HMOs. In the future, the NCQA may play a role in certifying these organizations' compliance with the HIPAA A/S requirements.

NCR No cardiac resuscitation.

NCS Nerve conduction study. Diagnostic testing performed to assess muscle or nerve damage. Nerves are stimulated with electric shocks along the course of the muscle. Sensors are utilized to measure and record nerve functions including conduction, amplitude, and latency/velocity. Report NCS with ICD-9-CM procedure code 89.15 or a code from CPT range 95900-95904.

NCV Nerve conduction velocity.

NCVHS National Center for Vital and Health Statistics. Federal advisory body within the Department of Health and Human Services that advises the secretary regarding potential changes to the HIPAA standards.

ND Doctor of naturopathy.

Nd:YAG laser Laser light energy that uses an yttrium, aluminum, and garnet crystal doped with neodymium ions as the active source, has a radiation beam nearing the infrared spectrum, and is effective in photocoagulation, photoablation, cataract extraction, and lysis of vitreous strands.

J–N

NDC National drug code.

Neapolitan fever Infection in humans caused by the bacterium brucella, a gram negative, aerobic, coccobacilli microorganism, conveyed by contact with infected animals via infected meat and unpasteurized milk or cheese. Symptoms include fever, chills, sweating, weakness, fatigue, weight loss, aches, and abdominal pain. The various species or sub-classes of Neapolitan fever are based on the host animal: sheep, goat, cattle, pigs, or dogs. Report this condition with a code from ICD-9-CM category 023. *Synonym(s): brucellosis, Cyprus fever, Malta fever, Mediterranean fever, rock fever, undulant fever.*

nearsightedness Defect in focusing in which the eye is overpowered and incoming distant light rays are focused in front of the retina because of a refractive or curvature defect in the lens. Nearsightedness is reported with ICD-9-CM code 367.1 unless the condition is malignant or progressive. Malignant nearsightedness is highly degenerative and complicated by serious disease of the choroid that leads to retinal detachment and blindness, reported with 360.21. *Synonym(s): myopia*

Nebcin Brand name for injectable tobramycin sulfate, an aminoglycoside antibiotic used to treat a wide variety of serious bacterial infections including septicemia, pneumonia, endocarditis, prostatitis, and pyelonephritis. Supply is reported with HCPCS Level II code J3260. Nebcin contains tobramycin sulfate.

Nebécourt's syndrome Dwarfism resulting from absence of functional anterior pituitary gland. Report this disorder with ICD-9-CM code 253.3. *Synonym(s): Burnier syndrome, Lorain-Levi syndrome.*

nebulization device Device used to vaporize liquid medication for the airborne delivery of the medication to the patient. The medication is absorbed into the body via the respiratory tract. Medications can also be administered with a nebulizer to fragment and mobilize thick, excess mucous in the respiratory tract; these medications are broadly termed mucolytics.

nebulizer Device pressurized by an oxygen tank for converting a liquid medication into a fine mist that can be inhaled.

Nebupent Inhalation solution used as a preventive treatment for pneumoocystis carinii pneumonia, a serious form of pneumonia commonly occurring in those with impaired immune systems. Supply is reported with HCPCS Level II code J2545. Nebupent contains pentamidine isethionate.

NEC *1)* Not elsewhere classifiable. Condition or diagnosis is not provided with its own specified code in ICD-9-CM, but included in a more broadly defined code for other specified conditions. *2)* Necrotizing enterocolitis.

necatoriasis Intestinal infection caused by the parasitic hookworm Necator americanus, reported with ICD-9-CM code 126.1.

neck sign Indication of meningitis wherein neck flexion often results in flexion of the hip and knee. *Synonym(s): Brudzinski's sign.*

NECMA New England county metropolitan areas.

necro- Indicates death or dead tissue.

necropsy Autopsy or postmortem examination performed in order to ascertain the cause of death or the changes caused by disease. Report necropsy with ICD-9-CM procedure code 89.8 or a code from CPT range 88000-88099.

necrosis Death of cells or tissue within a living organ or structure. Appropriate ICD-9-CM diagnosis code selection is dependent upon anatomical site.

necrospermia Dead or immobile sperm incapable of fertilizing an egg. This condition is reported with ICD-9-CM code 606.0.

necrotic Pathological condition of death occurring in a group of cells or tissues within a living part or organism.

necrotizing angiitis Inflamed blood vessels manifested by necrotic vascular tissue. Report this condition with ICD-9-CM code 446.0.

necrotizing enterocolitis Gastrointestinal disease seen primarily in premature infants. Most often occurring within the first two weeks of life, infection and inflammation cause injury to the bowel and disruption of the intestinal mucosa. Progression to serious complications, such as portal vein gas or perforation, may occur, necessitating emergent surgery. Report necrotizing enterocolitis with a code from ICD-9-CM subcategory 777.5.

NED No evidence of disease.

needle manometer technique Diagnostic procedure in which an interstitial fluid pressure monitoring device is inserted into a muscle compartment utilizing a needle manometer. This device monitors the escalation of pressure, which indicates developing compartment syndrome and tissue ischemia. Report this procedure with ICD-9-CM procedure code 89.39 and CPT code 20950.

neg. Negative.

negative pressure dressing Adjunctive therapy used to speed wound healing in skin grafts or large wounds. It has been shown to increase blood flow, decrease bacterial count, and increase formation of granulation tissues. A foam pad is placed on the defect and covered with an occlusive drape. A small tube that is non-collapsible is placed into the foam and attached to

J-N

a disposable pump that provides negative pressure up to -125 mmHg.

Negri bodies Characteristically shaped, sharply outlined inclusion bodies found in certain nerve cells, particularly in the hippocampus, that have been infected by the rabies virus. Report this condition with ICD-9-CM code 071.

Neill-Dingwall syndrome Small head and dwarfism. One of many syndromes affecting several body systems, but not elsewhere specified. Report this disorder with ICD-9-CM code 759.89.

Nembutal sodium solution Injectable short-acting barbiturate used primarily as a sedative hypnotic or anticonvulsant agent. Supply is reported with HCPCS Level II code J2515. *Synonym(s): pentobarbital sodium.*

neobladder Creation of a new urinary bladder utilizing a section of bowel following cystectomy. Report this procedure with ICD-9-CM procedure codes 57.79 and 56.51 or CPT code 51596.

Neocyten Brand name injectable muscle relaxant used to relieve the pain of muscle strains and spasms and also to alleviate the symptoms of Parkinson's disease. Supply is reported with HCPCS Level II code J2360. Neocyten contains orphenadrine citrate.

neodermis Artificial skin or skin substitute.

Neo-Durabolic See nandrolone decanoate.

neoformans cryptococcus infection Fungal infection caused by inhalation of dust containing the cryptococcus neoformans fungus, which is found in wild bird droppings. This infection may cause brain and spinal cord disease and those affected may experience headaches, dizzy spells, confusion, and drowsiness. Report this condition with ICD-9-CM code 117.5.

neonatal abstinence syndrome Drug withdrawal symptoms seen in a newborn exposed to drugs from the mother in utero. Neonatal abstinence syndrome in the infant is reported with ICD-9-CM code 779.5. *Synonym(s): NAS.*

neonatal period Period of an infant's life from birth to the age of 27 days, 23 hours, and 59 minutes.

neoplasm New abnormal growth, tumor.

Neoquess See dicyclomine HCl.

Neosar See cyclophosphamide.

neostigmine methylsulfate Injectable parasympathomimetic agent used to diagnose and treat acute exacerbations of myasthenia gravis. It is also used to reverse the effects of neuromuscular blocking agents, and to treat ileus and urinary retention. Supply is reported with HCPCS Level II code J2710. May be sold under brand name Prostigmin.

Neo-Synephrine Injectable synthetic sympathomimetic drug that works as a vasoconstrictor to shrink blood vessels. It is used to treat specific types of tachycardia and to prevent hypotension. Supply is reported with HCPCS Level II code J2370. Neo-Synephrine contains phenylephrine HCl.

neovascular macular degeneration New vessel formation in the oxygen-deprived tissues feeding the retina. This neovascularization results in tiny, delicate vessels that break easily, causing leakage, hemorrhaging, swelling, and damage to surrounding tissue, and accounts for 10 percent of all cases of macular degeneration in the United States. Report this condition with ICD-9-CM code 362.52. *Synonym(s): disciform senile macular degeneration, exudative senile macular degeneration, wet macular degeneration.*

neovascularization Formation of abnormal blood vessels in the eye, often found in diabetic retinopathy, central retinal vein obstruction, or macular degeneration. These blood vessels are fragile and tend to hemorrhage.

nephelometry Method of measuring the concentration of a suspension, such as that of albumin in body fluid, by using a specialized instrument (nephelometer) that assesses a solution's turbidity. Report nephelometry with CPT code 83883.

nephr- Relating to the kidney.

nephralgia Kidney pain, often experienced as a loin pain, reported with ICD-9-CM code 788.0.

nephrectomy Partial or total removal of the kidney that may be performed for indications such as irreparable kidney damage, renal cell carcinoma, trauma, congenital abnormalities, or transplant purposes.

nephritic syndrome Kidney condition resulting from damage to the glomeruli, characterized by proteinuria, hypoalbuminemia, hyperlipidemia, and massive edema. This can occur in multiple disease processes, including diabetic renal disease, and is often due to some form of glomerulonephritis. This syndrome is reported with codes from ICD-9-CM category 581.

nephritis Inflammation of the kidney, often due to infection, metabolic disorder, or an autoimmune process.

nephroblastoma Malignant tumor of the kidney, reported with ICD-9-CM code 189.0.

nephrocalcinosis Deposits in the kidneys formed by calcium phosphate and calcium oxylate, resulting in impaired kidney function. Report this condition with ICD-9-CM code 275.49.

nephrogenic diabetes insipidus Type of diabetes due to the kidneys failure to reabsorb filtered fluids. This diabetes is not responsive to vasopressin therapy, resulting in extreme thirst and frequent urination. This diabetes is reported with ICD-9-CM code 588.1. This may develop into chronic renal insufficiency.

nephrolithiasis Presence of a calculus, or stone, in the kidney, created when the urine becomes too concentrated

J-N

and forms crystals. This is a common condition, occurring more often in men than women and can cause urinary obstruction with severe pain, nausea and vomiting, and hematuria. Nephrolithiasis is reported with ICD-9-CM code 592.0; if congenital, see 753.3. *Synonym(s): renal calculus, renal stone, staghorn calculus.*

nephrolithotomy Removal of a kidney stone or calculus through an incision made directly into the kidney. The procedure is reported with CPT codes 50060-50075. Code selection is determined by factors such as whether the calculus fills other areas of the kidney, whether there are congenital abnormalities, or if there has been a previous surgery to remove a stone.

nephroma Tumor originating from renal tissue. Depending upon behavior, nephromas are reported with ICD-9-CM code 189.0 or a code from subcategory 236.9.

nephrons Functional units of the kidneys numbering more than one million in each kidney, making up the bulk of the organ's tissue. These are microscopic units that process blood and form urine by filtration, reabsorption, and secretion.

nephropexy Surgical fixation or suspension of a floating or mobile kidney. Nephropexy is reported with ICD-9-CM procedure code 55.7 or CPT codes 50400 and 50405.

nephroplasty Surgical repair of the kidney. Indications include fistula closure (CPT codes 50520-50526), correction of a horseshoe kidney (50540), correction of an obstruction or defect in the renal pelvis or ureteropelvic junction (50400-50405), or wound repair (50405).

nephroptosis Abnormal downward displacement or movement of the kidney; reported with ICD-9-CM code 593.0. *Synonym(s): floating kidney, mobile kidney, renal ptosis.*

nephropyosis Destruction of the kidney parenchyma wherein pus is produced and there is partial or total loss of kidney function. Report nephropyosis with ICD-9-CM code 590.2. *Synonym(s): pyonephrosis.*

nephrorrhagia Kidney hemorrhage, reported with ICD-9-CM code 593.81. *Synonym(s): renal hemorrhage.*

nephrorrhaphy Open surgical repair or suture of a wound or injury of the kidney. Nephrorrhaphy is reported with ICD-9-CM procedure code 55.81 and CPT code 50500.

nephrosclerosis Hardening of tissue in the kidney due to long-standing or poorly controlled hypertension that may result in renal failure and is often due to diabetes mellitus. *Synonym(s): arteriolar nephrosclerosis.*

nephrosis Nephrotic syndrome characterized by proteinuria more than 3.5 g/100 ml, hypoalbuminemia less than 3.0 g/100 ml, hyperlipemia (cholesterol greater than 300 mg/100ml), massive edema, and intercurrent infections. Nephrosis is usually due to some form of glomerulonephritis. It may progress to chronic renal failure. Report diagnosis codes from ICD-9-CM category 581, depending on the conditions. *Synonym(s): epimembranous nephritis, Epstein's syndrome, nephrotic syndrome.*

nephrosonephritis hemorrhagic Rodent-borne, febrile viral illness that occurs in epidemics. It is caused by the hantavirus and manifested by fever, loss of strength, vomiting, hemorrhaging, shock, and kidney failure. Report this condition with ICD-9-CM code 078.6. *Synonym(s): epidemic hemorrhagic fever.*

nephrostolithotomy Removal of a kidney stone through a percutaneous passageway created in the abdominal wall with a tube or stent inserted. This procedure is reported with CPT codes 50080-50081.

Nephrostomy Tube

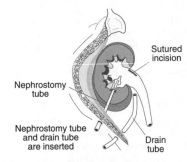

nephrostomy Placement of a stent, tube, or catheter that forms a passage from the exterior of the body into the renal pelvis or calyx, often for drainage of urine or an abscess, for exploration, or calculus extraction.

nephrotic Degeneration of renal epithelium.

nephrotomy Incision into the body of the kidney.

nerve block Regional anesthesia/analgesia administered by injection that prevents sensory nerve impulses from reaching the central nervous system.

nerve compression syndrome Pain in upper and posterior part of the shoulder radiating into neck and occiput, down the arm, and around the chest. Caused by abnormal positioning between the scapula and thorax, pain includes tingling in the fingers. Report this disorder with ICD-9-CM code 354.8.

nerve conduction study Diagnostic test performed to assess muscle or nerve damage. Nerves are stimulated with electric shocks along the course of the nerves. Sensors are utilized to measure and record nerve functions, including conduction, amplitude, and latency/velocity. Report NCS with ICD-9-CM procedure code 89.15 or a code from CPT range 95900-95904. *Synonym(s): NCS.*

nervous debility Neurotic disorder characterized by fatigue, irritability, headache, depression, insomnia, difficulty in concentration, and lack of capacity for enjoyment (anhedonia).

nervous tissue Highly specialized, organized cells for the function of the central peripheral nervous system, permitting information transfer between the brain and active tissue for both automatic and voluntary functions of skeletal, visceral, and cardiac muscle.

Nesacaine MPF See chloroprocaine HC1.

Nesbit technique Commonly performed technique for transurethral resection of the prostate that begins at the roof of the prostate and proceeds laterally along the capsule, allowing for control of major blood vessels.

nesidioblastoma Benign tumor of the islets of Langerhans (hormone-producing pancreatic cells). This tumor may result in excessive hormonal production and is reported with ICD-9-CM code 211.7, with an additional code to identify functional activities or conditions. *Synonym(s): islet cell tumor.*

nesiritide Injectable cardiovascular agent used in the treatment of decompensated congestive heart failure. Supply is reported with HCPCS Level II code J2325. May be sold under brand name Natrecor. *NCD Reference: 200.1.*

Netherton's syndrome Scaling of skin showing a peripheral double margin in and around the vagina. Report this disorder with ICD-9-CM code 757.1.

NETT National Emphysema Treatment Trial. Five-year randomized study of patients with severe emphysema that evaluates the safety and efficacy of lung volume reduction surgery. The three federal agencies involved within the Department of Health and Human Services include the National Heart, Lung, and Blood Institute; the Centers for Medicare and Medicaid Services; and the Agency for Healthcare Research and Quality.

nettle rash Red, itching rash that is often idiopathic, manifested by welts or swelling of the skin. Nettle rashes may be acute or chronic, reported with ICD-9-CM code 708.8.

Nettleship's disease Congenital condition in which cells accumulate in the dermis, characterized by persistent, small, reddish brown itchy macules and papules mostly on the trunk. The condition often goes away by puberty. Report this condition with ICD-9-CM code 757.33. *Synonym(s): mastocytoma, mastocytosis, urticaria pigmentosa.*

network model Plan that contracts with multiple groups of providers, or networks, to provide care.

Neulasta Injectable protein used to treat chemotherapy-induced neutropenia by stimulating production of white blood cells. Supply is reported with HCPCS Level II code J2505. Neulasta contains pegfilgrastim.

Neumann's disease Rare form of pemphigus bulgaris, a chronic dermatologic disease manifested by serous fluid-filled vesicles, bullae in the outermost layer of the skin, and persistent erosions. The lesions are predominantly on the face and within body folds. Bare areas heal with enlarged warty granulations. This condition is reported with ICD-9-CM code 694.4. *Synonym(s): pemphigus vegetans.*

Neumega Injectable synthetic hematopoietic stimulant used to prevent chemotherapy-induced thrombocytopenia. Supply is reported with HCPCS Level II code J2355. Neumega contains oprelvekin.

NeuraGen Nerve Guide Absorbable microporous collagen tube that provides an interface between a nerve and the tissue surrounding it. Designed to create a link across a nerve gap for axonal growth, it assists in rejoining severed peripheral nerves. Hospitals report the supply of each centimeter length with HCPCS Level II code C9352.

neuralgia Sharp, shooting pains extending along one or more nerve pathways. Underlying causes may include nerve injury, diabetes, or viral complications. Code assignment is dependent upon site and etiology.

neurapraxia Nerve injury, compression, or ischemia results in failure of nerve conduction. No structural change is present and there is normally a return of function. Code assignment is dependent upon affected nerve.

neurasthenia Mental disorder brought about by stress or anxiety. Manifestations are varied and may include weakness, exhaustion, chest pain, gastrointestinal complaints, palpitations, tachycardia, abnormal sensation of the hands and feet, hyperventilation, vertigo, syncope, or abnormal perspiration. Report neurasthenia with ICD-9-CM code 300.5 if all symptoms are present, 306.1 if only respiratory symptoms are present, or 306.4 if only gastrointestinal symptoms are present.

NeuraWrap Absorbable collagen implant that acts as a nerve protector by providing a non-constricting surrounding for injured peripheral nerves. Hospitals report the supply of each centimeter length with HCPCS Level II code C9353.

neuraxial anesthesia Regional anesthesia procedure in which an injection is given into the spine to relieve pain. It is used primarily in labor. *Synonym(s): epidural block, saddle block, spinal block.*

neurectasis Stretching of a nerve or nerve trunk, reported with ICD-9-CM procedure code 04.91 or CPT code 64999. *Synonym(s): neurotony.*

neurectomy Excision of all or a portion of a nerve. CPT code assignment is dependent upon specific nerve.

neuritis Inflammation of a nerve or group of nerves, often manifested by loss of function and reflexes, pain, and numbness or tingling. Code assignment depends upon site and underlying cause.

neurochorioretinitis Inflammation of the eye's middle layer (choroid), as well as the retina and optic nerve. Report this condition with ICD-9-CM code 363.20.

neurocutaneous syndrome Occurrence of nevi and skeletal deformities as result of gliosis and abiotrophy of central nervous system. Report this disorder with ICD-9-CM code 759.6.

neuroendoscopy Minimally-invasive technique involving the use of a specialized neuroendoscope to view inside the brain, spine, and peripheral nervous system through a small access hole just large enough to permit passage of the instrument. It may be used when treating conditions such as hydrocephalus, brain and spinal cord cysts, tumors, vascular lesions, nerve entrapments, and degenerative disease of the spine.

neurofibroma Tumor of peripheral nerves caused by abnormal proliferation of Schwann cells.

neurofibromatosis Autosomal dominant inherited condition with developmental changes in the nervous system, muscles, bones, and skin, producing coffee colored spots of pigmented skin (café au lait spots) and multiple soft tumor neurofibromas distributed over the entire body. Report this condition with ICD-9-CM code 237.71. *Synonym(s): von Recklinghausen's disease.*

neurofibrosarcoma Malignant tumor arising from the cells that surround peripheral nerves, most often affecting young and middle-aged adults. Most commonly found in the extremities, neurofibrosarcoma can spread extensively along nerve tissue. Metastasis to other parts of the body is rare, although lung metastasis sometimes occurs. *Synonym(s): peripheral nerve sheath tumor.*

Neuroform Brand name, microdelivery stent placed to prevent rupture of an intracranial aneurysm, formed by an abnormally weakened area in an artery wall.

neurogenic Originating in or related to the nervous system.

neurogenic bladder Dysfunctional bladder due to a central or peripheral nervous system lesion that may result in incontinence, residual urine retention, infection, stones, and renal failure.

neurolathyrism Neurodegenerative disease resulting in lower body paralysis. Neurolathyrism is caused by excessive consumption of the legume lathyrus sativus (Indian vetch), which produces a seed that contains a neurotoxic amino acid. Report this condition with ICD-9-CM code 988.2.

neurolemoma Tumor of a peripheral nerve sheath.

neuroleptic malignant syndrome Description of the effects of antipsychotic drugs on behavior and cognition. Report this disorder with ICD-9-CM code 333.92.

neurolipomatosis Numerous subcutaneous fat deposits that exert pressure on the nerves, resulting in sensitivity, pain, and burning or prickling sensations. Report this condition with ICD-9-CM code 272.8.

neurolysis Dissection of a nerve.

neurolytic Destruction of nerve tissue.

neuroma Any type of tumor growing from a nerve or comprised of nerve cells and fibers.

neuromuscular junction Nerve synapse at the meeting point between the terminal end of a nerve (motor neuron) and a muscle fiber.

neuromuscular reeducation Type of exercise that incorporates the concepts of motor control and motor learning to improve movement, balance, proprioceptive sense, kinesthetic sense, and perceptual motor skills.

neuromyopathy Disease or disorder affecting both the nerves and the muscles, particularly a muscular disease of nervous origin. Report this condition with a code from ICD-9-CM category 358.

neuron Nerve cell, the basic conduction unit of the nervous system, comprised of the cell body, dendrites, and the axon that terminates in branch-like projections, covered by a sheath, forming the nerve fiber. *Synonym(s): nerve cell.*

neuronal ceroid lipofuscinosis Inherited disorder in which the body stores excessive amounts of lipofuscin, the pigment that remains after damaged cells are broken down and digested, resulting in progressive nervous tissue damage. This term actually denotes a group of genetic lipidoses, named for the type by age, all characterized by continual neurodegeneration manifesting in muscle incoordination, vision loss, retardation, seizures, and fatality. Report this disorder with ICD-9-CM code 330.1. *Synonym(s): amaurotic familial idiocy, ceroid lipofuscinosis.*

neuropathy Abnormality, disease, or malfunction of the nerves.

neuroplasty Surgical release of adhesions around a nerve carried out to relieve pain and disability.

neuropsychological testing Evaluation of a patient's behavioral abilities wherein a physician or other health care professional administers a series of tests in thinking, reasoning, and judgment. Report CPT codes 96118-96120 for each hour of examination.

neuroretinitis Ophthalmologic condition in which the retina and the optic nerve are irritated and inflamed. If specified as syphilitic, report ICD-9-CM code 094.85, otherwise report 363.05.

neurorrhaphy Suturing cut ends of a severed nerve.

J-N

neurosis Mental disorder without any demonstrable organic basis in which the individual may have considerable insight and has unimpaired reality testing, in that he or she usually does not confuse his morbid subjective experiences and fantasies with external reality and usually remains within socially acceptable limits. Manifestations include excessive anxiety, hysterical symptoms, phobias, obsessional and compulsive symptoms, and depression.

neurosyphilis Syphilis of the central nervous system, reported with a code from ICD-9-CM subcategory 090.4 or category 094.

neurotic delinquency Emotional disturbance demonstrated by anxiety, misery, or obsessive manifestations resulting in undersocialized or socially disturbed conduct.

neurotic disorders Mental disorders without any demonstrable organic basis in which the individual may have considerable insight and has unimpaired reality testing, in that he or she usually does not confuse his morbid subjective experiences and fantasies with external reality and usually remains within socially acceptable limits. Manifestations include excessive anxiety, hysterical symptoms, phobias, obsessional and compulsive symptoms, and depression. *n. d. affecting occupation* Functional disorder of a group of muscles used chiefly in one's occupation, marked by the occurrence of spasm, paresis, or lack of coordination on attempt to repeat the habitual movements (e.g., writer's cramp). *anxiety state n. d.* Anxiety with physical and mental manifestations, not attributable to real danger and occurring diffusely, in attacks or as a persisting state. *n. d. compensation neurosis* Certain unconscious neurotic reactions focusing on secondary gain, such as a situational or financial advantage. *depersonalization n. d.* Awareness of the disturbed perception of external objects or parts of one's own body as unreal, remote, automatized, or changed in their quality. *n. d. with depression* Disproportionate depression with behavior disturbance that is usually the result of a distressing experience and may include delusions or hallucinations, anxiety, and preoccupation with the psychic trauma that preceded the illness. *hysteria n. d.* Restriction of the field of consciousness or disturbances of motor or sensory function that result in psychological advantage or symbolic value. *hysteria conversion type n. d.* Restriction of the field of consciousness or disturbance of motor or sensory function resulting in symbolic or psychological advantage, primarily of a body part as manifested by paralysis, tremor, blindness, deafness, and seizures. *hysteria dissociative type n. d.* Restriction of the field of consciousness or disturbance of motor or sensory function resulting in symbolic or psychological advantage, primarily of a body part as manifested by

selective amnesia, changes of personality, or a wandering state (fugue). *hysteria factitious illness n. d.* Restriction of the field of consciousness or disturbance of motor or sensory function resulting in symbolic or psychological advantage, primarily of a body part as manifested by physical or psychological symptoms that are not real, genuine, or natural, that are produced by the individual and are under his voluntary control. *neurasthenia n. d.* Neurotic disorder characterized by fatigue, irritability, headache, depression, insomnia, difficulty in concentration, and lack of capacity for enjoyment (anhedonia). *obsessive-compulsive n. d.* Feeling of subjective compulsion to carry out an action, dwell on an idea, recall an experience, ruminate on an abstract topic, or perform a quasi-ritual that may result in anxiety or inner struggle as the individual tries to cope with the behavior. *n. d. with phobia* Neurotic states with abnormally intense dread of certain objects or specific situations that would not normally affect the patient. *n. d. with somatization* Chronic, but fluctuating, neurotic disorder that begins early in life and is characterized by recurrent and multiple somatic complaints for which medical attention is sought but that are not apparently due to any physical illness.

neurotomy Dissection of a nerve.

neurotrophic keratoconjunctivitis Inflammation of the cornea and conjunctiva caused by a neurodefect.

Neurotube

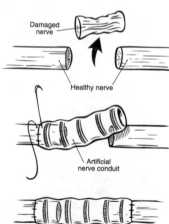

Damaged nerve

Healthy nerve

Artificial nerve conduit

A synthetic "bridge" is affixed to each end of a severed nerve with sutures
This procedure is performed using an operating microscope

Neurotube Brand name bioabsorbable nerve conduit used in peripheral nerve reconstruction. Its placement is reported with CPT code 64910.

neurovascular pedicle Section of skin and tissue retaining its nerves and veins that is partially excised from the donor location and grafted onto another site to repair adjacent or distant defects.

Neutrexin Injectable anti-infective agent used in conjunction with leucovorin to treat pneumoocystis carinii pneumonia in immunocompromised patients, such as those with cancer, AIDS, or who have undergone transplants. Supply is reported with HCPCS Level II code J3305. Newtrexin contains trimetrexate glucoronate.

nevus Benign, pigmented skin lesion that includes congenital lesions of the skin such as birthmarks, telangiectasias (permanent dilations of small blood vessels), vascular spider veins, hemangiomas, and moles. n. flammeus Port-wine stain. A cutaneous, vascular lesion appearing as flat, irregular, dark red to purple patches or marks present on the skin from birth that grow with the child, usually found on one side of the face and present with other developmental anomalies. They may eventually develop angiomatous growths over time and are sometimes removed by laser application. This condition is classified to ICD-9-CM code 757.32. *Synonym(s): strawberry nevus, vascular hamartomas.*

new patient Patient who is receiving face-to-face care from a provider or another physician of the same specialty who belongs to the same group practice for the first time in three years. For OPPS hospitals, a patient who has not been registered as an inpatient or outpatient, including off-campus provider based clinic or emergency department, within the past three years.

newborn admission Infant born in the facility.

newborn distress syndrome Intrauterine fetal aspiration of amniotic fluid contaminated by meconium. Report this disorder with ICD-9-CM code 770.6.

newborn hypertransfusion syndrome Polycythemia of newborn resulting from blood flow from mother. Report this disorder with ICD-9-CM code 776.4.

newborn idiopathic cardiorespiratory distress syndrome Respiratory distress in premature neonates associated with reduced amounts of lung surfactant. Frequently fatal. Report this disorder with ICD-9-CM code 769. *Synonym(s): hyaline membrane syndrome, respiratory distress syndrome.*

newborn inspissated bile syndrome Biliary obstruction in newborn resulting from plugging of outflow tract. Report this disorder with ICD-9-CM code 774.4.

newborn intensive care unit Special care unit for premature and seriously ill infants. *Synonym(s): NBICU, NICU.*

Nexavar Brand name oral pharmaceutical for treatment of advanced renal cell carcinoma in patients who have exhausted interferon-alpha or interleukin-2 based therapies. Nexavar blocks growth of the neoplasm by blocking growth of its vasculature. Renal cell carcinoma is reported with ICD-9-CM code 189.0. Nexavar contains sorafenib.

Nezelof syndrome Rare immunodeficiency disorder distinguished by severely deficient cellular immunity against opportunistic infections, making patients highly susceptible to life-threatening illnesses. Report this syndrome with ICD-9-CM code 279.13.

NF National formulary.

NFL Nerve fiber layer. Layer of the retina that is examined using a slit lamp, photography, or scanning laser polarimetry. NFL thickness can be a predictor of future field loss or disc changes caused by the presence of glaucoma. *Synonym(s): RNFL.*

NG Nasogastric.

NGU Nongonococcal urethritis. Infection of the urethra not attributed to gonococcus, typically seen in males. Though commonly considered a sexually transmitted disease, NGU can occur as a result of a urethral stricture or trauma or spreading of another urinary tract infection. If sexually transmitted, NGU is reported with a code from ICD-9-CM subcategory 099.4. If not sexually transmitted, report with 597.80. If occurring as a complication of pregnancy, childbirth, or the puerperium, report in addition to the appropriate code from subcategory 646.6 or 647.2. A discussion with clinicians regarding NGU is advised to ensure coding reflects intent of documentation.

NH Nursing home.

NHCS National Health Care Survey.

NHII National Health Information Infrastructure.

NHK Normal human keratinocytes.

NHL Non-Hodgkin's lymphoma.

niacin deficiency Disease caused by a deficiency of the B-complex vitamin niacin. Manifestations include diarrhea, nausea and vomiting, mouth ulcers, dermatitis, dementia, seizures, and ataxia. Death may occur. Report this disorder with ICD-9-CM code 265.2. *Synonym(s): pellagra.*

NIBP Non-invasive blood pressure. Blood pressure measurement taken with an external cuff or other noninvasive device.

NICE National Institute for Clinical Excellence.

NICO Neuralgia-inducing cavitational osteonecrosis. Facial pain due to chronic bone infection in the jaw or damage to nerve branches from chronic bone infection in the jaw. The jawbone infection is reported with ICD-9-CM code 526.4, and other manifestations are reported secondarily. *Synonym(s): alveolar cavitational osteopathosis, Ratner bone cavities, Robert's bone cavity, trigger point bone cavity.*

Nicolas-Durand-Favre disease Venereal disease caused by chlamydia trachomatis and manifested by inguinal lymphadenitis and weeping lesions. This disease is often found in tropical and subtropical climates. Report this disease with ICD-9-CM code 099.1.

NIDDM Noninsulin dependent diabetes mellitus. NIDDM is due to an insulin production or transport deficiency and is usually treated with oral medications or with diet and exercise. While the body manufactures insulin, it doesn't manufacture enough or is unable to release it effectively. This condition is reported with a code from ICD-9-CM rubric 250, unless it is associated with pregnancy, in which case it is reported with a code from category 648. If complications of diabetes are treated, report the complications secondarily to the diabetes code.

Niemann-Pick syndrome Accumulation of phospholipid in histiocytes in the bone marrow, liver, lymph nodes, and spleen, cerebral involvement, and red macular spots similar to Tay-Sachs disease. Most commonly found in Jewish infants. Report this disorder with ICD-9-CM code 272.7.

night blindness Impairment in the ability to see at night or in dim light. Night blindness is often a symptom of a variety of other medical conditions, such as vitamin A deficiency, retinitis pigmentosa, cystic fibrosis, diabetes, cataracts, or congenital disorders. Unless other medical conditions are indicated, report ICD-9-CM code 368.60 if stated as acquired or 368.61 if congenital. *Synonym(s): nyctalopia.*

night cramps Temporary nocturnal spasms of individual muscles or of entire muscle groups. Underlying causes may include dehydration, overexertion, ill-fitting shoes, or adverse affect of certain medications. Report this condition with ICD-9-CM code 729.82.

night sweats Profuse sweating occurring during sleep. Underlying causes may include menopause, andropause, HIV, tuberculosis, diabetes, sleep apnea, certain foods or drugs, or alcohol. Report this condition with ICD-9-CM code 780.8. *Synonym(s): nocturnal hyperhidrosis.*

night terrors Pathology of arousal from stage 4 sleep in which the individual experiences excessive terror and extreme panic (screaming, verbalizations), symptoms of autonomic activity, confusion, and poor recall of event.

nightmare Intense, terrifying dream that most commonly occurs during REM sleep at the end of the night or in the early morning hours. Underlying causes may be physiological, such as a high fever, or psychological, such as stress or trauma. Report this diagnosis with ICD-9-CM code 307.47.

Nightstick Fracture

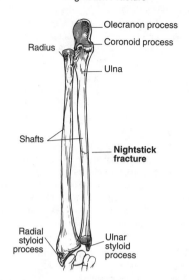

nightstick fracture Common closed fracture of the ulnar shaft, resulting from blunt forearm trauma and reported with ICD-9-CM code 813.22. In a nightstick fracture, there is no involvement of the radius and no dislocation, and the fracture itself is usually minimally displaced. The term is derived from the injury sustained if a person raises a forearm defensively against a baton or nightstick.

NIHL Noise induced hearing loss. Hearing loss due to exposure to loud noises or exposure to continuous noises. The hearing loss is the result of damage to sensitive hair cells of the inner ear and damage to the auditory nerve. NIHL is reported with ICD-9-CM code 388.12.

NINDS National Institute of Neurological Disorders and Stroke.

Nipah virus Zoonotic virus of the family Paramyxoviridae, transmitted through fruit bats in areas of the Pacific. Nipah virus causes flu-like symptoms that may be mild or may progress to encephalitis. Fifty percent of clinically apparent cases die from Nipah virus, as no drug therapies are effective. There is no code specific to Nipah virus, nor is it indexed in ICD-9-CM. Report Nipah virus with ICD-9-CM other specified virus code 079.89, and also report any accompanying encephalitis.

NIPD Nocturnal intermittent peritoneal dialysis. A mechanized cycler is used to perform six or more exchanges of dialyzing fluid overnight. No exchange is performed during the day. This type of dialysis is normally used by patients who still have considerable renal function, or those whose peritoneum has the ability to quickly transport waste products.

Nipent Injectable chemotherapeutic drug of the antimetabolite group used to treat hairy cell leukemia by interfering with the growth of cancer cells. Supply is reported with HCPCS Level II code J9268. Nipent contains pentostatin.

nipple inversion Nipples that draw inward and do not protrude when compressed or cold, reported with ICD-9-CM code 611.79. If specified as congenital, report 757.6 and if occurring in pregnancy, report a code from subcategory 676.3.

NIPS *1)* Neonatal infant pain scale. Scale based on facial expression (relaxed, grimacing), cry (none, whimper, vigorous), breathing patterns, arm and leg tension, and state of arousal. *2)* Noninvasive programmed electrical stimulation, reported with ICD-9-CM procedure code 37.20. NIPS allows noninvasive evaluation of the defibrillation threshold of implantable cardioverter-defibrillators.

NIR Near infrared spectroscopy. Infrared light is passed through tissue and a computerized image of a cross section of that tissue is created.

NIRflex Brand name coronary stent system.

Nissen fundoplasty Surgical repair technique that involves the fundus of the stomach being wrapped around the lower end of the esophagus to treat reflux esophagitis.

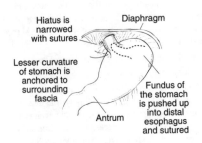

Nissen Fundoplication

Hiatus is narrowed with sutures

Diaphragm

Lesser curvature of stomach is anchored to surrounding fascia

Fundus of the stomach is pushed up into distal esophagus and sutured

Antrum

The Nissen procedure involves various techniques to plicate the fundus of the stomach to the distal esophagus. The CPT code is the same regardless of the technique employed

Nissen fundoplication Procedure to treat gastric reflux disease. The stomach is sutured in pleats around the distal esophagus. Nissen fundoplication is reported with CPT code 43327 or 43328 for an open procedure or 43280 for a laparoscopic procedure. The inpatient code for Nissen fundoplication is ICD-9-CM procedure code 44.66 for an open procedure or 44.67 for a laparoscopic procedure.

nitrogen mustard See Mechlorethamine HCl.

NJ Nasojejunal.

NKA No known allergies.

NKDA *1)* No known drug allergies. *2)* Non-ketotic diabetic acidosis.

NKHC Non-ketotic hyperglycemic coma.

NKHHC Nonketotic hyperglycemic-hyperosmolar coma.

NKMA No known medical allergies.

NM Nodular melanoma.

NMES Neuromuscular electrical stimulation. Technology that uses percutaneous stimulation to deliver electrical impulses for muscle flexion to trigger action. NMES can, in some cases, create an ability to ambulate among paraplegic patients. *NCD References: 160.12, 160.13.*

NMM Nodular malignant melanoma.

NMO Neuromyelitis optica. Syndrome that includes inflammation of the optic nerve and spinal cord. Its relationship with multiple sclerosis is not proven. NMO can occur as a single episode, or continue for years with relapses and remissions. Its symptoms can be mild or acute. NMO is reported with ICD-9-CM code 341.0. *Synonym(s): Devic's disease.*

NMSC Nonmelanoma skin cancer.

NNR New and nonofficial remedies.

noble intestinal plication Suturing the intestine.

NOC *1)* Not otherwise classified. *2)* Nursing outcomes classification.

noc. Night.

nocardiosis Rare bacterial infection occurring most often in those with weakened immune systems. It typically begins in the lungs and has a tendency to spread to other body systems, particularly the brain and skin. Involvement of the kidneys, joints, heart, eyes, and bones may also occur. Report this condition with a code from ICD-9-CM rubric 039.

noci- Relating to injury or pain.

nocturia Frequent urination during the night, affecting sleep patterns; reported with ICD-9-CM code 788.43. *Synonym(s): nycturia.*

nocturnal enuresis Bed-wetting.

nocturnal hyperhidrosis Profuse sweating occurring during sleep. Underlying causes may include menopause, andropause, HIV, tuberculosis, diabetes, sleep apnea, certain foods or drugs, or alcohol. Report this condition with ICD-9-CM code 780.8 if underlying cause is unknown. *Synonym(s): night sweats.*

nodular prostate Small mass of tissue that swells, knots, or is a protuberance in the prostate. Report ICD-9-CM code 600.10 if urinary obstruction is not documented and 600.11 if the condition is described as impeding the flow of urine.

no-fault insurance Insurance that pays for medical expenses for injuries sustained in or on the property or premises of the insured, or in the use, occupancy, or operation of an automobile, regardless of who may have been responsible for causing the accident.

NOI Notice of intent. Document that describes a subject area for which the federal government is considering developing regulations. It may describe the presumably relevant considerations and invite comments from interested parties. These comments can then be used in developing a notice of proposed rule making (NPRM) or a final regulation.

noma Severe, invasive, often gangrenous inflammation and ulceration most frequently occurring in the mouth or genital area of malnourished children. Serious disfigurement or death may result. If the ulceration is occurring in the mouth, report ICD-9-CM code 528.1; vulvae, report 616.10.

nomenclature Assignment of a name or the description of a term or procedure such as a HCPCS code description.

nonabsorbable sutures Strands of natural or synthetic material that resist absorption into living tissue and are removed once healing is under way. Nonabsorbable sutures are commonly used to close skin wounds and repair tendons or collagenous tissue. Examples include surgical silk, surgical cotton, linen, stainless steel, surgical nylon, polyester fiber, polybutester (Novofil), polyethylene (Dermalene), and polypropylene (Prolene, Surilene).

nonautogenous Derived from a source other than the same individual or recipient (e.g., cells, tissue, blood vessels, and other organs donated from another human). *Synonym(s): nonautologous.*

non-autogenous graft Cells or tissue taken from a cadaver or human source other than the recipient and transplanted into another individual. *Synonym(s): nonautologous.*

nonclinical or nonmedical code sets Code sets that characterize a general business situation, rather than a medical condition or service. Under HIPAA, these are sometimes referred to as nonclinical or nonmedical code sets. *Synonym(s): administrative code sets.*

noncovered inpatient days Inpatient days of care not covered by the primary payer. Under Medicare, noncovered days are not claimable as Medicare patient days for cost reporting purposes, and the beneficiary will not be charged for utilizing Part A services.

noncovered procedure Health care treatment not reimbursable according to provisions of a given insurance policy, or in the case of Medicare, in accordance with Medicare laws and regulations.

noncovered services Health care services not reimbursable according to provisions of a given insurance policy.

nonessential modifiers Subterms listed to the right of the ICD-9-CM main term and enclosed in parentheses.

nonexudative macular degeneration Age-related, atrophic (dry, nonexudative) macular degeneration characterized by variable degrees of atrophy and progressive degeneration of the outer retina, retinal pigment epithelium, Bruch's membrane, and choriocapillaris. Report this degeneration with ICD-9-CM code 362.51. *Synonym(s): Drusinoid macular degeneration.*

nonfacility practice expense Physician's direct and indirect practice costs related to each service when that service is provided in the physician's office, patient's home, or other nonhospital setting, such as a residential care facility.

noninstitutional setting All settings other than a hospital or skilled nursing facility.

noninvasive diagnostic test Procedure that does not require insertion of an instrument or device through the skin or body orifice for diagnosis.

Nonne-Milroy-Meige syndrome Lymphatic edema of the legs (and face and arms in severe cases) caused by obstruction of lymphatic ducts. Report this disorder with ICD-9-CM code 757.0. *Synonym(s): Milroy syndrome.*

nonoperating room procedure Procedure that does not normally require the use of the operating room and that can affect DRG assignment.

non-par Non-participating provider.

nonpatient services Services that are not rendered to a patient seen at the hospital. This typically refers to laboratory tests performed on samples sent to the hospital laboratory from an outside source to process. The account is established, but the services are rendered on the specimen rather than to a patient seen at the hospital.

nonpayment claim Claim submitted to the payer for which the provider does not expect payment. These claims are submitted to the third-party payer to inform it of reimbursable periods of confinement or termination dates of care. For Medicare purposes, examples of no-payment situations include the following: benefits are exhausted; lifetime reserve days are exhausted or the beneficiary elected not to use them; services are not otherwise covered under Part A; the hospital fails to submit needed information to assist in making a final determination on the bill for the period covered fully by workers compensation, including black lung, automobile medical, no-fault, or other liability insurance. *Synonym(s): no-payment claim.*

nonpsychotic syndrome   Persistent personality disturbance of nonpsychotic origin following blow to the head with affective instability, bursts of aggression, apathy and indifference, impaired social judgment, and suspiciousness or paranoid ideation. Report this disorder with ICD-9-CM code 310.2.

nonpurulent mastitis   Inflammation of the breast without the formation of infected discharge.

nonreportable procedure   Diagnostic service, as described by HCPCS codes, that should not be billed because they consist of supervision, interpretation, technical, or professional services only. Hospitals should always use the codes for the complete procedure, which are reportable. Exceptions to this rule are noted as coding tips under the applicable revenue codes.

nonselective placement   Insertion of a large needle with passage of a guidewire via the needle into the punctured vein or artery. The needle is removed leaving the guidewire and catheter in place. In direct punctures to peripheral veins or arteries, the catheter is not manipulated further after the initial stick is secured. Regardless of the site of the puncture, catheterization of the aorta or of the vena cava is considered nonselective placement.

nonspecific code   Catch-all code that identifies the diagnosis as ill-defined, other, or unspecified. A nonspecific code may be a valid choice if no other code closely describes the diagnosis.

nonunion   Failure of two ends of a fracture to mend or completely heal.

nonviable   Unable to live.

Noonan syndrome   Genetic disorder characterized by atypical facial features, short stature, congenital heart defects, musculoskeletal and lymphatic anomalies, and abnormalities of the eyes and eyelids. Since there is no specific treatment, the focus of care is directed toward treating the individual associated symptoms and complications of the disease. Report Noonan syndrome with ICD-9-CM code 759.89. *Synonym(s): NS.*

no-payment bill   Claim submitted to the payer for which the provider does not expect payment. These claims are submitted to the third-party payer to inform it of reimbursable periods of confinement or termination dates of care.

no-payment claim   Claim submitted to the payer for which the provider does not expect payment. These claims are submitted to the third-party payer to inform it of reimbursable periods of confinement or termination dates of care.

Nordryl   See diphenhydramine HCl.

normal delivery   Baby delivered without complication.

North Carolina Healthcare Information and Communications Alliance   Organization that promotes the advancement and integration of information technology into the health care industry. *Synonym(s): NCHICA.*

Norwalk virus   Virus causing gastroenteritis in epidemic proportions, passed through fecal-oral route in contaminated food and water. Nausea, vomiting, and diarrhea begin 24 to 48 hours after exposure and lasts approximately two days from onset. The virus attacks the mucosa of the proximal portion of the small intestine causing abnormal intestinal motility and malabsorption of D-xylose, lactose, and fat. Report with ICD-9-CM code 008.63, which also includes a new genus of Norwalk like viruses (NLVs).

Norwood procedure   Surgical correction to widen the diameter of the aorta and repair single ventricle with aortic outflow obstruction. The pulmonary valve is transformed into the systemic arterial heart valve by means of encircling it with the application of a large pericardial patch, used to enlarge the aorta and sewn as a tube along the sides of the hypoplastic ascending aorta and aortic arch. This procedure is reported with CPT code 33619.

NOS   Not otherwise specified. Condition or diagnosis remains ill defined and is unspecified without the necessary information for selecting a more specific code.

nosology   Science of disease classification; nosologist is the professional who performs this function.

not elsewhere classified   Condition or diagnosis is not provided with its own specified code in ICD-9-CM, but included in a more broadly defined code for other specified conditions. *Synonym(s): NEC.*

not otherwise specified   Condition or diagnosis remains ill defined and is unspecified without the necessary information for selecting a more specific code. *Synonym(s): NOS.*

notalgia paresthetica   Condition in which the skin of the upper back becomes pruritic (itches), and is often accompanied by hyperpigmentation due to persistent rubbing and scratching of the affected area. This chronic sensory neuropathy may be manifested by pain, increased sensitivity, and/or a feeling of pins and needles (paresthesia). Treatments vary, and may include topical corticosteroids or capsaicin, local anesthetics, or intradermal injections of botulinum toxin type A (Botox).

notice of intent   Document that describes a subject area for which the federal government is considering developing regulations. It may describe the presumably relevant considerations and invite comments from interested parties. These comments can then be used in

J-N

developing a notice of proposed rule making (NPRM) or a final regulation. *Synonym(s): NOI.*

notice of proposed rule making Document that describes and explains regulations the federal government proposes to adopt at some future date, and invites interested parties to submit comments related to them. These comments can then be used in developing a final regulation. *Synonym(s): NPRM.*

NovaSilk Brand name synthetic mesh for treatment of pelvic organ prolapse. Insertion of mesh during pelvic floor repair is reported with CPT add-on code 57267.

NovaSure Brand name endometrial ablation system using radiofrequency energy to treat excessive menstrual bleeding. The use of this device is reported with CPT code 58563.

novem. Nine.

NP 1) Nurse practitioner. 2) Neuropsychiatry.

NPA Nasopharyngeal airway.

NPC Nasopharyngeal carcinoma.

NP-CPAP Nasopharyngeal continuous positive airway pressure.

NPD Nightly peritoneal dialysis.

NPEP Non-occupational post exposure prophylaxis. Treatment, often with pharmaceuticals, is intended for a patient who has been exposed outside of the workplace to a disease but has not yet contracted it. NPEP is reported with codes from ICD-9-CM category V01.

NPF National provider file.

NPI National provider identifier. Standard eight-digit alphanumeric provider identifier implemented under the Health Insurance Portability and Accountability Act of 1996 (HIPAA) requirements. The first seven digits identify the provider and the eighth position is a check digit. Providers are required to report their NPI number for electronic and paper billing.

Nplate Brand name for romiplostim, an injectable thrombopoietin receptor agonist used to treat low platelet counts (thrombocytopenia) in patients with idiopathic thrombocytopenic purpura (ITP) who have not responded well to immunoglobulins, steroids, or removal of the spleen. Supply is reported with HCPCS Level II code J2796.

NPN 1) Non-par not approved. 2) Nonprotein nitrogen.

NPO Nothing by mouth.

NPPES National Plan and Provider Enumeration System. System that uniquely identifies a health care provider and assigns it an NPI.

NPQ Not physically qualified.

NPRM Notice of proposed rule making. Document that describes and explains regulations the federal government proposes to adopt at some future date, and invites interested parties to submit comments related to them. These comments can then be used in developing a final regulation.

NPS National provider system.

npt Normal pressure and temperature.

NPWT Negative pressure wound therapy, reported with CPT codes 97605 and 97606. NPWT is used to promote healing of acute or chronic wounds. The electrical pump required for NPWT is reported with HCPCS Level II code E2402, and the wound care set, with A6550.

NS 1) Normal saline. 2) Not significant.

NSAID Non-steroidal antiinflammatory drug. Analgesic and antiinflammatory drug commonly used to mitigate inflammatory conditions. NSAIDs include aspirin, ibuprofen, naproxen, and nabumetone.

NSC Non-service connected, as noted on a veteran's chart regarding his ailment.

NSD Nominal standard dose.

NSF National standard format.

NSR Normal sinus rhythm.

NST Nonstress test.

NSU Nonspecific urethritis. Infection and inflammation of the urethra, most commonly seen in males. Though commonly considered a sexually transmitted disease, NSU can occur as a result of a urethral stricture or trauma or spreading of another urinary tract infection. If sexually transmitted, NSU is reported with a code from ICD-9-CM subcategory 099.4. If not sexually transmitted, report with 597.80. If occurring as a complication of pregnancy, childbirth, or the puerperium, report in addition to the appropriate code from subcategory 646.6 or 647.2. A discussion with clinicians regarding NSU is advised to ensure coding reflects intent of documentation.

NSV Nonspecific vaginitis, reported with ICD-9-CM code 616.10. If complicating pregnancy, childbirth, or the puerperium, report in addition to the appropriate code from subcategory 646.6.

NSVB Normal spontaneous vaginal bleeding.

NSVD Normal spontaneous vaginal delivery.

NT 1) Nasotracheal. 2) Nontender.

NTD Nitroblue tetrazolium dye test, reported with CPT code 86384.

NTE Neutral thermal environment.

NTL Near total laryngectomy. This procedure is reported with CPT code 31367 or 31368.

NTP Normal temperature and pressure.

NTT Near total thyroidectomy. This procedure is reported with CPT code 60252 or 60271.

N-J

Nubain Synthetic injectable opiate analgesic used to relieve moderate to severe pain caused by acute or chronic medical conditions including cancer, colic, certain forms of headaches, and postoperative pain. It may also be used for labor and delivery analgesia. Supply is reported with HCPCS Level II code J2300. Nubain contains nalbuphine HCl.

NUBC National Uniform Billing Committee. Organization, chaired and hosted by the American Hospital Association, that maintains the UB-92 hardcopy institutional billing form and the data element specifications for both the hardcopy form and the 192-byte UB-92 flat file EMC format. The NUBC has a formal consultative role under HIPAA for all transactions affecting institutional health care services.

NUBC EDI TAG The National Uniform Billing Committee's Electronic Data Interchange Technical Advisory Group. NUBC EDI TAG coordinates issues affecting both the NUBC and the X12 standards.

NUCC National Uniform Claim Committee. Organization, chaired and hosted by the American Medical Association, that maintains the CMS-1500 claim form and a set of data element specifications for professional claims submission via the CMS-1500 claim form, the Professional EMC NSF, and the X12 837. The NUCC also maintains the provider taxonomy codes and has a formal consultative role under HIPAA for all transactions affecting nondental, noninstitutional professional health care services.

nuclear medicine Radioactive elements used for diagnostic imaging or radiopharmaceutical imaging. A radioactive element, such as uranium, spontaneously emits energetic particles by the disintegration of the nuclei.

nucleus ambiguous-hypoglossal syndrome Unilateral lesions of the ninth, tenth, eleventh, and twelfth cranial nerves producing paralysis of vagal, glossal, other nerves, and tongue on the same side. Usually a result of injury. Report this disorder with ICD-9-CM code 352.6. *Synonym(s): Collet-Sicard syndrome.*

nucleus pulposus Semi-gelatinous mass of fine white and elastic fibers forming the central portion of the intervertebral disk, contained within the annulus fibrosus, preventing it from protruding out of the disk space. Percutaneous aspiration of the nucleus pulposus is reported with CPT code 62287.

nulligravida Obstetric status of a female who has never been pregnant. This includes abortions, ectopic pregnancies, and molar pregnancies.

nulliparous Obstetric status of a female who has never given birth to a child.

number of units Quantitative measure of the procedures, services, items, tests, accommodation days, treatments, etc., identified by a particular revenue code. Not all revenue codes require reporting the number of units.

nurse practitioner Specially trained, degreed nurse who assesses, treats, and prescribes medication.

nursemaid elbow Form of radial head subluxation common in children between the ages of 1 and 3. Nursemaid elbow is usually the result of a sudden pull on the extended arm.

nutrition Enteral and parenteral nutrition describe the administration of nutrients. Enteral nutrition: Nutrients are provided by a nasogastric or gastric tube for patients who cannot ingest, chew, or swallow food, though their bodies are able to absorb the nutrients. Parenteral nutrition: Nutrients are provided subcutaneously, intravenously, intramuscularly, or intradermally for patients during the postoperative period and in other conditions, such as shock, coma, and renal failure.

nutritional marasmus Protein-calorie malabsorption or malnutrition of children, characterized by tissue wasting, dehydration, and subcutaneous fat depletion that may occur with infectious disease. *Synonym(s): infantile atrophy.*

NV Nausea and vomiting.

NVHRI National Voluntary Hospital Reporting Initiative, a CMS designation

NVP Nausea and vomiting of pregnancy.

nyctalopia Impairment in the ability to see at night or in dim light. Nyctalopia is often a symptom of a variety of other medical conditions, such as vitamin A deficiency, retinitis pigmentosa, cystic fibrosis, diabetes, cataracts, or congenital disorders. Unless other medical conditions are indicated, report ICD-9-CM code 368.60 if stated as acquired or 368.61 if congenital. *Synonym(s): night blindness.*

nycto- Relating to darkness or night.

NYD Not yet diagnosed.

Nylen-Barany test Clinical observation of eye movements (nystagmus) occurring during calculated movements of the patient's head and body. The Nylen-Barany test is considered a component of evaluation and management and is not reported separately. *Synonym(s): Dix-Hallpike test.*

nymphomania Female individual with abnormal and excessive need or desire for sexual intercourse.

nystagmus Rapid, rhythmic, involuntary movements of the eyeball in vertical, horizontal, rotational, or mixed directions that can be either congenital, acquired, physiological, neurological, or due to ocular disease. Nystagmus is reported within ICD-9-CM subcategory 379.5.

o No information.

O *1)* Blood type. *2)* Oxygen.

O&P Ova and parasites.

O.D. Oculus dexter. Right eye.

o.m. *1)* Every morning. *2)* Otitis media.

o.n. Every night.

O.S. Oculus sinister. Left eye.

O.U. Oculus uterque. Each eye.

O2 Oxygen.

OA *1)* Open access. *2)* Osteoarthritis.

OAB Overactive bladder. Chronic frequency and urgency in urination due to abnormal muscle contractions within the bladder's elastic and muscular walls. OAB is reported with ICD-9-CM code 596.51.

OAE test Otoacoustic emission test. Performed to determine the status of cochlear hair cell function by four types of OAE testing. Spontaneous otoacoustic emissions (SOAEs): Sounds emitted spontaneously without an acoustic stimulus. Transient otoacoustic emissions (TOAEs) or transient evoked otoacoustic emissions (TEOAEs): Sounds emitted in response to an acoustic stimuli of very short duration, usually clicks or tone-bursts. Distortion product otoacoustic emissions (DPOAEs): Sounds emitted in response to two simultaneous tones of different frequencies. Sustained frequency otoacoustic emissions (SFOAEs): Sounds emitted in response to a continuous tone. Report CPT code 92587 if the test is limited to a single stimulus level and 92588 if the test is comprehensive or uses multiple stimulations. *Synonym(s): DPOAE, otoacoustic emission test, SFOAE, SOAE, TEOAE, TOAE.*

OAG Open angle glaucoma.

Oasis Brand name, acellular wound management material made from porcine-derived acellular small intestine mucosa. Its application is reported with CPT codes 15430 and 15431. Supply is reported with HCPCS Level II codes Q4102 and Q4103.

OAV syndrome Oculoauriculovertebral dysplasia. Number of anomalies, including epibulbar dermoids, preauricular appendages, micrognathia, and vertebral. Report this disorder with ICD-9-CM code 756.0. *Synonym(s): Goldenhar's syndrome.*

Ob Obstetrician. *Synonym(s): OB.*

OB-GYN Obstetrics and gynecology.

objectives Measurable behavioral statements of expected behavior or outcome.

obligate anaerobe Bacterium that can grow only in a non-oxygenated environment. Identification of this microorganism does not directly drive code selection, although it does drive treatment decisions.

oblique facial cleft Rare congenital abnormality in which a facial cleft extends from the lip to the eye's inner canthus, usually separating the underlying bone. It may occur in conjunction with a cleft lip or palate, or with a lateral facial cleft. Report this abnormality with ICD-9-CM code 744.83. *Synonym(s): meloschisis, prosopoanoschisis.*

oblique x-ray view Slanted view of the object being x-rayed.

obliterate Get rid or do away with completely.

OBRA Omnibus Budget Reconciliation Act.

observation Perception of events.

observation patient Patient who needs to be monitored and assessed for inpatient admission or referral to another site for care

observation services Services furnished on a hospital's premises, including use of a bed and periodic monitoring by a hospital's nursing or other staff, that are reasonable and necessary to evaluate an outpatient's condition or determine the need for a possible admission to the hospital as an inpatient. Such services are covered only when provided by the order of a physician or another individual authorized by state license laws and hospital staff bylaws to admit patients to the hospital or to order outpatient tests. Observation services normally do not extend beyond 23 hours.

obsessional personality Feelings of personal insecurity, excessive doubt, and incompleteness leading to excessive conscientiousness, stubbornness, perfectionism, meticulous accuracy, and caution with persistent checking in an individual who may also have intrusive thoughts or impulses.

obsessive-compulsive Feeling of great anxiety or inner struggle as a result of subjective compulsions to carry out some action, dwell on an idea, recall an experience, or ruminate on an abstract topic that is manifested by performance of quasi-ritual acts.

obstetric cerclage Surgical procedure that encircles an incompetent cervix with suture material for support in an attempt to retain a pregnancy, usually performed between 12 and 14 weeks' gestation and often employed in patients with a history of spontaneous abortion in otherwise normal pregnancies.

obstetric tamponade Insertion and inflation of a balloon inside the uterus in order to control postpartum hemorrhage.

obstruction Act or state of being clogged or blocked from allowing through passage.

obstructive hydrocephalus Excess cerebrospinal fluid filling dilated cavities of the brain, caused by an acquired obstruction of the cerebrospinal fluid pathways.

obturate To occlude or close off an opening.

O-R

obturator Prosthesis used to close an acquired or congenital opening in the palate that aids in speech and chewing.

obturator nerve Lumbar plexus nerve with anterior and posterior divisions that innervate the adductor muscles (e.g., adductor longus, adductor brevis) of the leg and the skin over the medial area of the thigh or a sacral plexus nerve with anterior and posterior divisions that innervate the superior gemellus muscles.

OC 1) Office call. 2) Open crib. 3) Oral contraceptive.

occiput Bone at the base of the skull that contains the foramen magnum, the opening in the bone that allows the spinal cord to join the brain.

occlusal Biting surfaces of premolar and molar teeth or the areas of contact between opposing teeth in the maxilla and mandible.

occlusal x-ray In dentistry, radiograph taken from inside the mouth with films that are held in place by the contacting teeth in a closed jaw.

occlusion Constriction, closure, or blockage of a passage.

occlusive disease Vascular disease causing constriction, closure, or blockage of an artery or vein due to stenosis, deposits of fatty or hardened plaque, or blood clots. This would be coded according to the specific type of occlusion and the vessel involved. *Synonym(s): ASCVD, ASHD.*

occult blood test Chemical or microscopic test to determine the presence of blood in a specimen.

occupational neurosis Functional disorder of a group of muscles used chiefly in one's occupation, marked by the occurrence of spasm, paresis, or lack of coordination on attempt to repeat certain habitual movements (e.g., writer's cramp).

occupational therapy Training, education, and assistance intended to assist a person who is recovering from a serious illness or injury perform the activities of daily life.

occurrence code Two-digit number and date used to report that services are related to a specific type of accident, that the beneficiary or spouse is retired, the date on which the beneficiary was notified of the intent to bill for accommodations or procedures, or the date physical, occupational, or speech-language pathology therapy treatments started.

occurrence span code Two-digit number and the beginning and ending date used to report specific circumstances that are relevant to the claim being submitted.

OCD Obsessive-compulsive disorder.

OCE Outpatient code editor. Centers for Medicare and Medicaid Services' outpatient software program that analyzes hospital outpatient claims to detect incorrect billing and coding data, assign an ambulatory payment classification for covered services, and determine the appropriate payment. Medicare fiscal intermediaries use the OCE to test the validity of ICD-9-CM and HCPCS coding and to conduct compatibility edits. The OCE performs all editing functions related to HCPCS codes, HCPCS modifiers, and ICD-9-CM diagnosis codes. It identifies individual errors and indicates the action to take with the claim (i.e., RTP, suspend, deny).

OCR 1) Office for Civic Rights. Department of Health and Human Services entity responsible for enforcing the HIPAA privacy rules. 2) Oculocephalic response. Reflexive eye movements assessed in an unresponsive patient to determine if the brainstem is intact. OCR review would be included as part of the evaluation and management service.

OCT 1) Optical coherence tomography. 2) Ornithine carbarnyl transferase. 3) Oxytocin challenge. Stress test in pregnancy in which oxytocin is administered to evaluate the effects of contractions on the fetus, reported with CPT code 59020.

Octagam Brand name intravenous immunoglobulin solution prepared from the plasma of healthy donors. Indicated for the treatment of primary immune deficiency diseases, Octagam replaces the antibodies in patients who are unable to produce their own. Report supply with HCPCS Level II code J1568.

octo. Eight.

ocular fistula Abnormal passage in the eye through which fluids may leak, resulting in low intraocular pressure.

ocular hypotonia Low intraocular pressure.

ocular implant Implant inside muscular cone.

ocular photodynamic therapy Use of the drug Verteporfin to treat exudative macular degeneration.

ocular speculum Instrument that holds the eyelids apart to give better access to the eyeball during a surgical procedure.

oculocutaneous syndrome Uveomeningitis with patchy depigmentation of hair, eyebrows, and lashes; retinal detachment, deafness, and tinnitus may also result. Report this disorder with ICD-9-CM code 364.24. *Synonym(s): Vogt-Koyanagi syndrome.*

oculoglandular syndrome Syndrome of the eyes and glands. Report this disorder with ICD-9-CM code 372.02.

oculomotor syndrome Paralysis of conjugate movement of the eyes without paralysis of convergence. Caused by lesions of the midbrain. Report this disorder with ICD-9-CM code 378.81. *Synonym(s): Parinaud's syndrome.*

O-R

ODM Ophthalmodynamometry. Measurement of the blood pressure in the retinal vessels.

odont- Relating to the teeth.

odontectomy Extraction of a tooth.

odontoplasty Adjustment of tooth shape, size, or length.

-odynia Indicates pain or discomfort.

OFC Occipitofrontal circumference.

Office for Civil Rights Department of Health and Human Services entity responsible for enforcing the HIPAA privacy rules. *Synonym(s): OCR.*

Office of Audit Services Conducts comprehensive audits to promote economy and efficiency and to prevent and detect fraud, abuse, and waste in operations and programs. The OAS may request data for use in auditing aspects of Medicare and other Health and Human Service (HHS) programs, and is often involved in assisting the Office of Inspector General (IOG) or Office of Investigations (OI) in its role in investigations and prosecutions. *Synonym(s): OAS.*

Office of Civil Fraud and Office of Administrative Adjudication Responsible for coordinating activities that result in the negotiation and imposition of civil monetary penalties (CMP), assessments, and other program exclusions. It works with the Office of Investigations, Office of Audit Services (OAS), CMS, and other organizations in the development of health care fraud and exclusion cases. *Synonym(s): OCFAA.*

Office of Civil Fraud and Office of Administrative Adjudication Responsible for coordinating activities that result in the negotiation and imposition of civil monetary penalties (CMP), assessments, and other program exclusions. Works in conjunction with the Office of Investigations, Office of Audit Services (OAS), CMS, and other organizations in the development of health care fraud and exclusion cases. *Synonym(s): OCFAA.*

Office of Inspector General Agency within the Department of Health and Human Services ultimately responsible for investigating instances of fraud and abuse in the Medicare and Medicaid and other government health care programs. *Synonym(s): OIG.*

Office of Investigations Staffed with professional criminal investigators, the Office of Investigations is responsible for all HHS criminal investigations, including Medicare fraud. OIG/OI investigates allegations of fraud or abuse whether committed by contractors, grantees, beneficiaries, or providers of service (e.g., fraud allegations involving physicians and other providers, contract fraud, and cost report fraud claimed by hospitals). OIG/OI presents cases to the United States Attorney's Office within the Department of Justice (DOJ) for civil or criminal prosecution. When a practitioner or other person is determined to have failed to comply with its obligations in a substantial number of cases or to

have grossly and flagrantly violated any obligation in one or more instances, OIG/OI may refer the case to OCFAA for consideration of one or both of the following sanctions: An exclusion from participation in the Medicare program or any state health care programs as defined under sec. 1128(h) of the Social Security Act (the Act) and/or the imposition of a monetary penalty as a condition to continued participation in the Medicare program and state health care programs. *Synonym(s): OI.*

Office of Management and Budget Federal government agency that has a major role in reviewing proposed federal regulations. *Synonym(s): OMB.*

Office of Strategic Operations and Regulatory Affairs Office that maintains the official records related to CMS manuals. *Synonym(s): OSORA.*

offset Withholding payment from a provider of an established, non-Medicare overpayment.

off-site Place other than the provider's usual place of practice.

Ogilvie's syndrome Colonic obstruction with symptoms of persistent contraction of intestinal musculature. Caused by defect in sympathetic nerve supply. Report this disorder with ICD-9-CM code 560.89.

OHSS Ovarian hyperstimulation syndrome. Response to fertility drugs in which the egg production is greater than would be expected. Symptoms can include enlarged ovaries, tenderness, and nausea. OHSS is reported with ICD-9-CM code 256.1.

OIC Osteogenesis imperfecta congenital. Inherited disorder that results in fragile and brittle bones, reported with ICD-9-CM code 756.51.

-oid Indicates likeness or resemblance.

OIG Office of Inspector General. Agency within the Department of Health and Human Services that is ultimately responsible for investigating instances of fraud and abuse in the Medicare and Medicaid and other government health care programs. OIG work plan Annual plan released by the Office of Inspector General (OIG) that details the areas of focus for fraud and abuse investigations.

OIG work plan Annual plan released by the Office of Inspector General that details the areas of focus for fraud and abuse investigations.

oint Ointment.

OIT Osteogenesis imperfecta tarda. Inherited disorder that results in fragile and brittle bones, reported with ICD-9-CM code 756.51.

OJ Orange juice.

OL Outlier threshold. Component that figures in the reimbursement calculation for a DRG.

oligo- Indicates few or small.

O-R

oligohydramnios Low amniotic fluid, occurring most frequently in the last trimester. This condition is diagnosed with ultrasound and is reported with a code from ICD-9-CM subcategory 658.0. If oligohydramnios is suspected but not found, report V89.01.

oligomenorrhea Scanty or infrequent menstruation, defined as that taking place at intervals greater than 35 days. This condition is reported with ICD-9-CM code 626.1. *Synonym(s): hypomenorrhea.*

oligospermia Insufficient production of sperm in semen, a common factor in male infertility; reported with ICD-9-CM code 606.1. *Synonym(s): hypospermatogenesis.*

oliguria Deficient secretion of urine. *Synonym(s): anuria.*

Ollier's disease Disorder in which multiple enchondromas develop throughout the skeleton, reported with ICD-9-CM code 756.4. *Synonym(s): chondrodysplasia, dyschondroplasia.*

-ology Study of.

-oma Tumor.

OMB Office of Management and Budget. Federal government agency that has a major role in reviewing proposed federal regulations.

omentum Fold of peritoneal tissue suspended between the stomach and neighboring visceral organs of the abdominal cavity.

omn. hor. Every hour.

Omnilink Brand name biliary stent system.

Omnitrope FDA-approved, recombinant human growth hormone. The drug is indicated for treatment of growth disorders in children and adults. Omnitrope contains Somatropin [rDNA origin].

omo- Relating to the shoulder.

omphalo- Relating to the navel.

omphalocele Congenital protrusion of the intestine through a defect in the abdominal wall at the umbilicus, reported with ICD-9-CM code 756.79. Repair usually requires a series of surgical procedures to complete, unless the omphalocele is small. CPT codes for repair are specific to omphalocele and are found in 49600-49611.

omphalopagus Monozygotic (identical) twins who are joined at the abdomen. Report this abnormality with ICD-9-CM code 759.4. *Synonym(s): xiphopagus.*

OMS Oromaxillofacial surgery. A specialty requiring qualification in general surgery as well as dentistry.

OMT Osteopathic manipulation therapy.

ONB Olfactory neuroblastoma.

ONC *1)* Oncology. *2)* Office of the national coordinator for health information technology.

on-call physician encounter Physician who is on-call or covering for another physician classifies the patient's encounter as it would have been by the physician who is not available.

onco- Relating to a mass, tumor, or swelling.

oncofetal antigen Antigens normally produced during embryonic development and decreasing soon after birth. Oncofetal antigens are expressed by a wide number of cancer types since cancer cells tend to revert to more immature tissue and, subsequently, produce fetal antigens. Oncofetal antigens are measured to monitor a patient's progress and response to treatment over time. There are two common oncofetal antigens: alpha-fetoprotein (AFP) and carcinoembryonic antigen (CEA).

Ondine's curse Central alveolar hypoventilation, the inability of the respiratory center of the brain to react to an increase in carbon dioxide and stimulate breathing. This disorder is fatal if untreated. Ondine's curse is reported with ICD-9-CM code 327.25 when primary or 327.27 when due to an underlying condition.

Oneirophrenia Schizophrenic disorder with ideas of reference and emotional turmoil where external things, people, and events may become charged with personal significance for the patient; characterized by a dream-like state with slight clouding of consciousness and perplexity although.

ONH Optic nerve hypoplasia. Congenitally underdeveloped optic nerve. Symptoms may include photophobia, depressed visual fields, impaired depth perception, and nystagmus. ONH is reported with ICD-9-CM code 377.43.

onlay In dentistry, restoration made outside of the mouth that is cemented over a cusp or cusps of the tooth.

on-site Regular place of practice of the provider; his or her primary clinic or department location.

onychauxis Congenital condition in which the nails are hypertrophied, reported with ICD-9-CM code 757.5.

onycho- Relating to the finger- or toenails.

onychoplasty Reconstruction or repair of a nail or nail matrix that may employ the use of a graft; reported with CPT codes 11760 and 11762.

Onyx liquid embolic Artificial blocking agent that is injected through a small catheter into selective blood vessels of the brain, where it solidifies and prevents the flow of blood. Indications include obstruction of blood flow to abnormally formed blood vessels in the brain (arteriovenous malformations or AVMs) prior to surgical removal and blockage of cerebral aneurysmal spaces in

O-R

order to prevent rupture. Report Onyx liquid embolic with ICD-9-CM procedure code 39.72.

00A Out-of-area.

00B Out of bed.

oophor- Relating to the ovaries.

oophorectomy Surgical removal of all or part of one or both ovaries, either as open procedure or laparoscopically. Menstruation and childbearing ability continues when one ovary is removed.

oophoritis Inflammation or infection of one or both ovaries. Oophoritis can cause chronic pelvic pain, ectopic pregnancy, and even sterilization, and most often occurs in women younger than age 25. It is classified as acute or chronic and reported within ICD-9-CM rubric 614, unless specified as gonococcal, in which case it is reported with 098.19 or 098.39. *Synonym(s): ovaritis.*

OOPs Out-of-pocket costs/expenses.

OOX Oophorectomy.

OPA Oropharyngeal airway.

OPD Outpatient department.

open dislocation Displacement of a bone or joint with an open wound.

open enrollment period Time period during which subscribers in a health benefit program have the opportunity to re-enroll or select an alternative health plan being offered to them, usually without evidence of insurability or waiting periods.

open flap drainage Removal of fluid, blood, exudates, or other materials from the body through a tube that is left in the wound.

open fracture Exposed break in a bone, always considered compound due to its high risk of infection from the open wound leading to the fracture. Broken bone ends may protrude through the skin and contaminants or foreign bodies are often embedded in the tissues.

open panel Arrangement in which a managed care organization that contracts with providers on an exclusive basis is still seeking providers.

open reduction Treatment of a fracture or dislocation by surgically exposing the site and manipulating the fracture fragments or bone ends into proper alignment under direct vision.

open systems interconnection Multi-layered ISO data communications standard. Level Seven of this standard is industry-specific, and HL7 is responsible for specifying the level-seven OSI standards for the health industry. *Synonym(s): OSI.*

open wound Opening or break of the skin.

open-bite deformity Abnormal condition in which some of the teeth do not touch when the jaws are biting or closing. This abnormality most often occurs in the front teeth and is generally the result of an overgrowth of the back part of the upper jaw or improper growth of the lower jaw. Open-bite deformity is reported with ICD-9-CM code 524.20. *Synonym(s): apertognathia.*

operating microscope Compound microscope with two or more lens systems or several grouped lenses in one unit that provides magnifying power to the surgeon up to 40X.

operating room procedure Defined group of procedures that normally require the use of an operating room.

operculectomy Excision of a small piece of gingiva from the back or top of a tooth using a scalpel, laser, or electrocautery, in order to establish normal gingival contours around the tooth. Operculectomy is reported with CPT code 41821.

operculum Flap of tissue over a tooth that is either unerupted or only partially erupted.

OPG Oculoplethysmography.

ophth Ophthalmology.

ophthalmic biometry Noncontact technique to measure the axial length of the eye from the cornea to the retina and to calculate the power required for an intraocular lens (IOL) implant. Ultrasonography may be employed by placing a specialized transducer on the eye to acquire images and measurements, reported with CPT codes 76516 and 76519, or partial coherence interferometry using birefringent light as opposed to sound may be employed, reported with 92136. Using this technique, the eye is imaged using light sources at specific wavelengths to find the highest quality axial length display and taking measurements. This also measures the curvature of the cornea and the depth of the anterior chamber in addition to the axial length and IOL power.

ophthalmic burr Specialized surgical drill used to remove foreign body from the conjunctiva or cornea or to remove residual corneal rust rings from a metallic foreign body.

ophthalmica syndrome Any symptoms of herpes arising in eye. Report this disorder with ICD-9-CM code 053.19.

ophthalmoplegia Paralysis of the eye muscle.

ophthalmoplegia plus Condition manifested by chronic and progressive paralysis of one or more of the extraocular eye muscles and pigmentary retinal degeneration. Usually beginning before age 20, KSS produces progressive muscle weakness, deafness, dementia, and cataracts. Cardiac conduction abnormalities and cerebellar ataxia are also present. Report this condition with ICD-9-CM code 277.87. *Synonym(s): Kearns-Sayre syndrome, KSS.*

ophthalmoplegia-cerebellar ataxia syndrome Paralysis of one or more optic muscles or failure to control

O-R

muscles. Report this disorder with ICD-9-CM code 378.52.

ophthalmoplegic migraine syndrome Migraine headache accompanied by amblyopia and other visual disturbances. Report this disorder with a code from ICD-9-CM range 346.20-346.23.

opistho- Indicates behind or backwards.

OPL Other party liability. In coordination of benefits, the decision that the other plan is the primary plan.

Oppenheim-Urbach syndrome Diabetes with skin disorder. Report this disorder with ICD-9-CM subcategory 249.8 or 250.8, with additional code 709.3 to identify the manifestation.

opponensplasty Transfer of a muscle or tendon, especially the hypothenar muscle or superficialis tendon for the purpose of restoring the opposing action of the thumb.

oppositional disorder of childhood or adolescence Pervasive opposition to all in authority as demonstrated by continuous argumentativeness and an unwillingness to respond to reasonable persuasion in an individual without conduct disorder, adjustment disorder, or a psychosis of childhood.

OPPS Outpatient prospective payment system.

oprelvekin Injectable synthetic hematopoietic stimulant used to prevent chemotherapy-induced thrombocytopenia. Supply is reported with HCPCS Level II code J2355. *Synonym(s): Neumega.*

OPS Objective pain scale. Scale used in infants based on blood pressure, status of crying, amount of movement, and level of agitation.

Optease Brand name vena cava filter. Placement of a vena cava filter is reported with CPT code 37620.

optic disk Ophthalmoscopically visible portion of the optic nerve.

optic nerve Transmits visual information from the retina to the brain. *Synonym(s): cranial nerve II.*

optic nerve decompression Releasing pressure from the optic nerve by removing tissue or bone that is pressing against it, reported with CPT code 67570.

optical coherence biometry Non-contact technique that involves the use of partially coherent light to measure the axial length of the eye, the anterior chamber depth, and provide corneal curvature readings (keratometry).

OptiFlow RM Brand name, ready-made compression sleeve to relieve lymphedema in the arm or leg. Supply of OptiFlow RM for the upper extremity is reported with HCPCS Level II code S8421.

OPV Oral poliovirus vaccine. Supply of OPV is reported with CPT code 90712; its administration is reported

separately. The need for vaccination is reported with ICD-9-CM code V04.0.

OR Operating room.

oral Pertaining to the mouth.

ORAL Oral administration.

oral reconstruction Reforming, recreating, or rebuilding tissues or structures within the mouth following an injury or disease.

oral soft tissue Subcutaneous fat layers beneath oral mucosa or gingiva; excludes bone and teeth.

oral-facial-digital syndrome Defects of the oral cavity, face, and hands including bifid tongue, cleft palate, missing teeth, pug-nose, depressed nasal bridge, mental retardation, and others. Syndrome is lethal in males. Report this disorder with ICD-9-CM code 759.89. *Synonym(s): Papillon-Leage syndrome, Psaume syndrome.*

Orbasone Brand name shock wave generator for plantar fasciitis therapy. The shock waves are created by a spark plug enclosed in a soft plastic dome filled with water. During treatment, the dome is placed against the heel so the shock waves pass through the dome to the heel. The procedure is reported with CPT code 28890. Plantar fasciitis is reported with ICD-9-CM code 728.71.

orbit Bony cavity that contains the eyeball, formed by seven bones of the skull: frontal, sphenoid, maxilla, zygomatic, palatine, lacrimal, and ethmoid.

orbital Pertaining to the orbit (bony cavity containing the eyeball). *o. cellulitis* Inflammation of the connective tissue within the eye socket. *o. exenteration* Surgical removal of the entire orbital contents, including the eyeball, extraocular muscles, fat, and connective tissue. *o. fracture* Fracture of one or more of the seven bones that form the orbit of the eye. *o. hypertelorism* Abnormally increased distance between the eyes, or orbits in the skull, often due to disorders resulting in defective craniofacial formation. *o. implant* Implant outside the muscular cone of the eye.

orbital and ocular implants Usually a spherical device placed in the socket at the time of surgery to replace orbit volume after removal of the eye or its contents. *Integrated implant.* An implant that allows the muscles of the eye to be directly attached to it and transfers the motion from the implant to the artificial eye via a peg system. *Ocular implant.* Implant inside the muscular cone. *Orbital implant.* Implant outside the muscular cone.

orbitotomy Opening made into the orbital space for biopsy, abscess drainage, or tumor mass or foreign body removal.

OrCel Brand name bilayered cellular matrix composed of bovine collagen and human allogeneic skin cells used in treating burns.

O-R

orchi(do)- Relating to the testicles.

orchiectomy Surgical removal of one or both testicles via a scrotal or groin incision, indicated in cases of cancer, traumatic injury, and sex reassignment surgery. A prosthetic testis may be inserted in the scrotum at the time of surgical removal. The open procedure is reported with CPT codes 54520-54535, and laparoscopically with code 54690. **Synonym(s):** *castration, orchidectomy.*

orchiopexy Surgical fixation of an undescended testicle within the scrotum. **Synonym(s):** *orchidopexy.*

orchitis Testicular inflammation.

ordering physician Physician who orders nonphysician services (e.g., laboratory services, pharmaceutical services, imaging services, or durable medical equipment) for a patient.

oregovamab Monoclonal antibody that targets CA-125, a protein expressed in the majority of ovarian tumors. Oregovamab is currently in Phase III clinical trials for late-stage ovarian cancer. Its administration is reported with CPT code 96413 and its supply is reported with unlisted HCPCS Level II code J9999. May be sold under brand name OvaRex.

Orencia Brand name chemotherapeutic agent used in the treatment of rheumatoid arthritis. Infusion of Orencia is reported with CPT code 96413, 96415, or 96417 or for facilities, ICD-9-CM inpatient code 99.29. Supply of Orencia is reported with HCPCS Level II code J3590. Orencia contains abatacept.

organ or disease-oriented panels Panel or set of tests grouped together as a single code that neither specifies clinical parameters nor precludes performance of other tests.

organic affective syndrome Patient may exhibit a number of changes in personality such as amotivation, depression, outbursts and poor social judgment. Report this disorder with ICD-9-CM code 293.83.

organic impotence Organic erectile dysfunction in which there is partial or complete failure to attain or maintain erection until completion of intercourse. Organic impotence most often involves a vascular problem of the penis, particularly in older males. Underlying factors may include arteriosclerosis, diabetes, trauma to the arteries, or a venous leak. Organic impotence is reported with ICD-9-CM code 607.84.

organic psychotic conditions Impairment of orientation, memory, comprehension, calculation, learning capacity, and judgment that may include shallowness or liability of affect, or a more persistent disturbance of mood, lowering of ethical standards, exaggeration or emergence of personality traits, and diminished capacity for independent decision making. **Synonym(s):** *alcohol psychoses, arteriosclerotic dementia, drug psychoses, presenile dementia, senile dementia.*

mixed paranoid and affective o. Organic psychosis in which depressive and paranoid symptoms are the main features. *transient o.* Generally reversible states characterized by clouded consciousness, confusion, disorientation, illusions, and often vivid hallucinations usually due to some intra- or extracerebral toxic, infectious, metabolic, or other systemic disturbance. *transient acute delirium o.* Short-lived states, lasting hours or days, of transient organic psychotic conditions. *transient subacute delirium o.* States of transient organic psychotic conditions in which the symptoms, usually less florid than in the acute form, last for several weeks or longer with marked fluctuations in intensity.

organic reaction Generally reversible states characterized by clouded consciousness, confusion, disorientation, illusions, and often vivid hallucinations usually due to some intra- or extracerebral toxic, infectious, metabolic, or other systemic disturbance.

ORIF Open reduction internal fixation.

Orinase Brand name oral medication exclusive to lowering blood glucose in Type II diabetics; generic name tolbutamide.

oris Mouth.

Ormond's syndrome Retroperitoneal structures involving and often obstructing ureters sometimes following certain types of chemical treatment; there is no identified cause. Report this disorder with ICD-9-CM code 593.4.

Oroya fever Acute form of bartonellosis, an infectious, bacterial disease with sudden onset that is transmitted by sandflies, and usually has a short course manifested by hemolytic anemia and fever. Report this condition with ICD-9-CM code 088.0. **Synonym(s):** *Carrion's disease.*

orphan drugs Drugs that treat diseases that affect fewer than 200,000 people in the United States, as designated by the FDA. Orphan drugs follow a varied process from other drugs regulated by the FDA.

orphenadrine citrate Injectable muscle relaxant used to relieve the pain of muscle strains and spasms and also to alleviate the symptoms of Parkinson's disease. Supply is reported with HCPCS Level II code J2360. May be sold under brand name Neocyten.

-orrhaphy Suturing.

ORT Oral rehydration therapy.

ortho. Orthopedics.

orthognathia Branch of oral medicine pertaining to the cause and treatment of abnormal positioning of the jawbones.

orthognathic Causes and treatments of malpositioned jawbones.

O-R

orthopnea Shortness of breath when lying down that is relieved upon resuming an upright position. Orthopnea is reported with ICD-9-CM code 786.02.

orthoptics Treatment of defective eye coordination, binocular vision, and functional amblyopia by non-medical/surgical methods including glasses, exercises, and prisms. The treatment is focused on improving the function of the eye muscles, especially useful in strabismus. This service is reported with CPT code 92065.

orthosis Derived from a Greek word meaning "to make straight," it is an artificial appliance that supports, aligns, or corrects an anatomical deformity or improves the use of a moveable body part. Unlike a prosthesis, an orthotic device is always functional in nature.

Orthospec ECSW/OssaTron

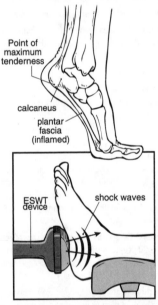

The clinician treats the patient's plantar fasciitis with extracorporeal shock waves

Orthospec ECSW Brand name extracorporeal shock wave therapy device for relief of plantar fasciitis. Its use for plantar fasciitis is reported with CPT code 28890.

orthostatic hypotension Low blood pressure that occurs when standing from a sitting or lying position, reported with ICD-9-CM code 458.0.

orthostatic hypotensive-dysautonomic dyskinetic syndrome Nerves between the striatum and pallidum are completely demyelated. Report this disorder with ICD-9-CM code 333.0. *Synonym(s): Déjérine-Thomas syndrome, Hallervorden-Spatz syndrome.*

orthotic Use of a mechanical orthopedic device that compensates for, supports, corrects, or prevents deformities.

orthotopic Natural, normal site or proper body position.

orthotopic transplant Movement or replacement of an organ or tissue in which the patient's nonfunctioning organ is removed.

Orthovisc Brand name solution of sodium hyaluronate injected into the knee joint as a lubricant to relieve osteoarthritis pain. Supply of Orthovisc is reported with HCPCS Level II code J7324. The injection is reported with CPT code 20610. Injection codes are unilateral and should be reported twice if injections are administered in both knees.

Ortolani's test Diagnostic, physical screening exam of an infant for congenital hip dislocation. It is considered part of an evaluation and management service.

os Mouth.

os trigonum syndrome Pain and inflammation as a result of the failure of a piece of the talus bone to fuse with the rest of the talus during growth, resulting in a small, round bone that can migrate to a place where it can be pinched within the ankle. Os trigonum occurs in 5 to 15 percent of the population, but only a fraction experience any complications. Symptomatic os trigonum syndrome is not indexed in ICD-9-CM but could be reported with a combination of 719.47 for the ankle pain and 755.69 for the anomaly.

OSA Obstructive sleep apnea. *NCD Reference: 240.4.*

OSAS Obstructive sleep apnea syndrome. Headaches, high blood pressure, daytime sleepiness, and mental dullness usually associated with oxygen deprivation during sleep. Snoring is also common in OSAS. Confirmation of obstructive sleep apnea requires sleep testing, reported with CPT codes 95805-95811. OSAS is reported with ICD-9-CM code 327.23.

OSCAR Online Survey Certification and Reporting, a CMS designation.

oscheo- Relating to the scrotum.

oscilloscope Instrument in which a varying electrical signal (y) vertically deflects an electron beam impinging on a fluorescent screen, while some other function (x or time) deflects the beam horizontally. The result is a visual graph of y plotted against x or time with negligible distortion by inertia.

-oscopy To examine.

OSI Open systems interconnection.

-osis Condition, process.

Osler-Weber-Rendu syndrome Post-pubescent disorder with small telangiectasia and dilated venules developing slowly on the skin and mucus membranes of the lips, nasopharynx, and tongue. Report this disorder with ICD-9-CM code 448.0.

Osmed Hydrogel tissue expanders used in oculoplastic surgery to expand the bony tissues of the deep orbit in congenitally anophthalmic patients.

Osmolite Brand name enteral nutrition. Supply of Osmolite is reported with HCPCS Level II code B4150.

OssaTron Brand name shock wave generator for plantar fasciitis therapy. The shock waves are created by a spark plug enclosed in a soft plastic dome filled with water. During treatment, the dome is placed closely against the heel so that the shock waves pass through the dome to the heel. The procedure is reported with CPT code 28890.

osseous Related to, consisting of, or resembling bone.

osseous tuberosities Nodule or tubercle that is related to, consisting of, or resembling bone.

ossicular chain Anatomic structure formed by the three small bones of the middle ear - incus, malleus, and stapes - functioning together to conduct sound vibrations through the ear.

ossification Formation of bony growth or hardening into bone-like substance.

Ost Ostomy.

OST Oxytocin stress test.

ostectomy Excision of bone.

osteitis Inflammation of the bone.

osteitis condensans Inflammation of the bones with hard, dense deposits of mineral salts.

osteitis deformans Bone disease characterized by numerous cycles of bone resorption by the body followed by accelerated repair attempts, causing bone deformities and bowing, with associated fractures and pain.

osteo- Having to do with bone.

osteoarthritis Most common form of a noninflammatory degenerative joint disease with degenerating articular cartilage, bone enlargement, and synovial membrane changes. *Synonym(s): degenerative joint disease, DJD, OA. NCD Reference: 30.3.2.*

osteoarthritis deformans endemica Endemic, chronic, and slowly progressing degenerative disease of the spine and peripheral joints believed to be caused by eating cereal grains infected with the fungus Fusarium sporotrichiella. This disease occurs mainly in children in Siberia, China, and Korea. Report this condition with a code from ICD-9-CM subcategory 716.0. *Synonym(s): Kaschin-Beck disease, Kashin-Bek.*

osteoarthrosis Most common form of a noninflammatory degenerative joint disease with degenerating articular cartilage, bone enlargement, and synovial membrane changes. *Synonym(s): degenerative joint disease.*

osteochondral defect Defect related to or composed of bone and cartilage.

osteochondritis dissecans Inflammation of the bone and cartilage that results in splinters or pieces of cartilage breaking off in the joint.

osteochondropathy Any condition in which the bone and cartilage are affected, or in which endochondral ossification occurs.

osteochondrosis Disease manifested by degeneration or necrosis of the growth plate or ossification centers of bones in children, followed by regenerating and reossification.

osteoclasis Medically guided fracture or refracture of a bone.

osteodermopathic hyperostosis syndrome Irregular linear streaks of skin atrophy, skeletal malformations, and papillomas of lips. Report this disorder with ICD-9-CM code 757.39.

osteogenesis imperfecta Hereditary collagen disorder that produces brittle, osteoporotic bones that are easily fractured, with hypermobility of points, blue sclerae and a tendency to hemorrhage. This disease varies in its manifestations and severity as well as in its molecular and genetic heterogeneity. Type 1 is the most common and mildest form, appearing with blue sclera and the affected person's stature being normal or near normal. Type II is a perinatal lethal type, causing death at or soon after birth. Type III is the progressive deforming type, and type IV is autosomal dominant as is type I, manifesting with normal sclerae. All types of osteogenesis imperfecta are reported with ICD-9-CM code 756.51.

osteogenesis stimulator Device used to stimulate the growth of bone by electrical impulses or ultrasound.

osteomalacia Bones softened by a deficiency of calcium, characterized by bone pain, muscle weakness, and weight loss. This condition is reported with ICD-9-CM code 268.2.

osteomyelitis Inflammation of bone that may remain localized or spread to the marrow, cortex, or periosteum, in response to an infecting organism, usually bacterial and pyogenic.

osteopathic manipulative treatment Form of treatment therapy that places emphasis on manually applied techniques to detect faulty structural relationships and restore normal body mechanics to allow the body to work out its own remedies.

osteopathy Diseases of the bone, but more often used for a theory of medicine based on the assumption that the human body is self-righting and capable of its own remedies against disease. Osteopathic approaches rely heavily on the "laying of hands" upon the patient for diagnostic and therapeutic purposes.

O-R

osteopetrosis Rare congenital condition in which the bones are excessively dense, resulting from a discrepancy in the formation and breakdown of bone. Osteopetrosis manifests in various types and severity and can cause optic atrophy and deafness, hepatosplenomegaly, fractures, and depleted bone marrow and nerve foramina in the skull. Osteopetrosis is often fatal. This condition is reported with ICD-9-CM code 756.52.

osteophytes Bony outgrowth.

osteoplasty Plastic surgery of a bone.

osteopoikilosis Rare genetic disorder that manifests in multiple areas of sclerotic bone density on the ends of long bones, identified by x-ray and often without symptoms. It is associated with other disorders such as dwarfism, scleroderma, syndactyly, and cleft palate. This disorder is reported with ICD-9-CM code 756.53.

osteoporosis Bone degeneration caused by the breakdown of the bony matrix without equivalent regeneration, resulting in a weak, porous, fragile bone structure.

osteoporosis-osteomalacia syndrome Osteoporosis striking middle-aged women with frequently-suffered fractures. Report this disorder with ICD-9-CM code 268.2. *Synonym(s): Debray syndrome, Looser syndrome, Milkman syndrome.*

osteoporotic Porous condition of bones from a loss of bone mass or density. *NCD Reference: 150.3.*

OSTEOSET Brand name pellets for use as a bone graft substitute, providing a biological framework into which bone can form. CPT coding of procedures including OSTEOSET beads would be selected on the base procedure performed, or reported as an unlisted code.

osteotome Tool used for cutting bone.

osteotomy Surgical cutting of a bone.

ostium primum Temporary opening between the right and left atrium between the lower margin of the septum primum and the atrioventricular canal in a fetal heart. In an adult heart, this condition results in an endocardial cushion defect of a cleft in the basal portion of the atrial septum with abnormal passage of blood through the congenital opening, usually associated with a cleft mitral valve. Ostium primum is reported with ICD-9-CM code 745.61.

-ostomy Indicates a surgically created artificial opening.

ostomy Artificial (surgical) opening in the body used for drainage or for delivery of medications or nutrients.

Ostrum-Furst syndrome Deformities of neck, platybasia and Sprengel's neck. Report this disorder with ICD-9-CM code 756.59.

OT *1)* Occupational therapy. *2)* Outlier threshold.

OTC Over-the-counter.

OTD Organ tolerance dose.

OTH Other routes of administration.

other diagnosis All conditions (secondary) that exist at the time of admission or that develop subsequently that affect the treatment received and/or the length of stay. Diagnoses that relate to an earlier episode and that have no bearing on the current hospital stay are not to be reported. *Synonym(s): comorbidity, complication.*

other Medicare-required assessment In the event that planned therapy or treatment (in a SNF) is discontinued, a new assessment is required within eight to 10 days of discontinuing the therapy or treatment in order for the care to be covered. *Synonym(s): OMRA.*

other party liability In coordination of benefits, the decision that the other plan is the primary plan. *Synonym(s): OPL.*

other specified Term in ICD-9-CM referring to codes reported when a diagnosis has been made and there is no code identifying it more specifically as with NEC, or not elsewhere classified.

oto- Relating to the ear.

otolith syndrome Ocular disturbances, deafness, nausea, thirst, anorexia, and symptoms traced to vagus centers as result of a lesion of Deiters nucleus and its connections. Report this disorder with ICD-9-CM code 386.19. *Synonym(s): Bonnier syndrome.*

-otomy Indicates a cutting.

otopalatodigital syndrome Defects of ear, oral cavity, face and hands. Report this disorder with ICD-9-CM code 759.89.

otosclerosis Pathological condition of the bony labyrinth of the ear, in which there is formation of spongy bone (otospongiosis), especially in front of and posterior to the footplate of the stapes. Ankylosis of the stapes may occur, resulting in conductive hearing loss, and cochlear otosclerosis may also develop, resulting in sensorineural hearing loss.

OTR Occupational therapist registered.

OTW Over the wire. Referring to stent deployment.

Oudard and Trillat procedure Anterior repair of the glenohumeral joint using an anterior glenoid bone buttress.

out of area Medical care received out of the geographic area that may or may not be covered depending on the plan.

out of plan In health care contracting, services of a provider who is not a member of the preferred provider network.

out of service area In health care contracting, medical care received out of the geographic area that may or may not be covered, depending on the plan.

O-R

out of service area Medical care received out of the geographic area that may or may not be covered, depending on the plan.

outcome measures Standards assessing the quality of patient care by measuring the change in a patient's performance following health services.

outcomes Condition, behavior, or attributes of a patient at the end of therapy or of a disease process, including the degree of wellness and the need for continuing care, medication, support, counseling, or education.

outlet syndrome Vascular contractions of the digits similar to Raynaud's, caused by pressure of brachial plexus and subclavian artery against first thoracic rib. Report this disorder with ICD-9-CM code 353.0. *Synonym(s): Naffziger's syndrome.*

outlier Case classified to a specific DRG but with exceptionally high costs compared with other cases classified to the same DRG. The fiscal intermediary or MAC makes a payment in addition to the original DRG amount for these situations. A cost outlier is paid an amount in excess of the cut-off threshold for a given DRG. The day outlier no longer applies.

outlier threshold Component that figures in the reimbursement calculation for a diagnostic-related group (DRG). *Synonym(s): OT.*

outpatient Patient who receives care without being admitted for inpatient or residential care.

outpatient code editor Centers for Medicare and Medicaid Services' outpatient software program that analyzes hospital outpatient claims to detect incorrect billing and coding data, assign an ambulatory payment classification for covered services, and determine the appropriate payment. Medicare fiscal intermediaries use the OCE to test the validity of ICD-9-CM and HCPCS coding and to conduct compatibility edits. The OCE performs all editing functions related to HCPCS codes, HCPCS modifiers, and ICD-9-CM diagnosis codes. It identifies individual errors and indicates the action to take with the claim (i.e., RTP, suspend, deny). *Synonym(s): OCE.*

outpatient maintenance dialysis services Outpatient services furnished by end-stage renal disease facilities that are paid under a composite payment rate and include all services, equipment, supplies, and certain laboratory tests and drugs that are necessary for dialysis treatment.

outpatient physical therapy service Physical therapy service provided to an outpatient of a hospital, clinic, CORF, rehabilitation agency, or public health agency. The attending physician must establish a plan of physical therapy or periodically review a plan developed by a qualified physical therapist. The term outpatient physical therapy services also includes physical therapy services provided by a physical therapist in office or at the patient's home and speech-language pathology services.

outpatient pricer Software used to determine the amount that will be paid for the item or service being billed, including the deductible and coinsurance amounts. This CMS-developed software determines the ambulatory payment classification line-item price. It also calculates the outlier payments on a claim-by-claim basis.

outpatient services Medical and other services provided by the hospital or other qualified supplier that are either diagnostic or help the physician treat the patient. Outpatient services are covered under Medicare Part B and include the rental or purchase of durable medical equipment prescribed by a doctor for use in the home; devices, other than dental, to replace all or part of an internal body organ; certain ambulance services; laboratory services; x-ray and other radiology services; emergency room and outpatient clinic services; medical supplies, splints, and casts; other diagnostic services; physical and occupational therapies and speech pathology services; and dialysis in the facility or home. An institutional provider supplies an outpatient service, but the beneficiary is not necessarily confined to the specific institution for periods of 24 hours or more.

outpatient surgery list List of surgical procedures that can be performed on an outpatient basis without adversely affecting the quality of care.

outpatient visit Encounter in a recognized outpatient facility.

ov. *1)* Office visit. *2)* Ovum.

OvaRex Brand name monoclonal antibody that targets CA-125, a protein expressed in the majority of ovarian tumors. OvaRex is currently in Phase III clinical trials for late-stage ovarian cancer. Its administration is reported with CPT code 96413 and its supply is reported with unlisted HCPCS Level II code J9999. OvaRex contains oregovamab.

ovarian remnant syndrome Pelvic pain typically occurring several weeks or several months following surgical removal of the ovaries, often due to the survival of an ovarian fragment after the operation. Report this disorder with ICD-9-CM code 620.8.

ovarian vein syndrome Retroperitoneal structures involving and often obstructing the ureters following certain types of chemical treatment; there is no identified cause. Report this disorder with ICD-9-CM code 593.4. *Synonym(s): Ormond's syndrome.*

OVC Ovarian cancer.

overanxious disorder Ill-defined emotional disorder of childhood involving anxiety and fearfulness.

O-R

overdenture In dentistry, prosthesis of artificial teeth that overlies and is supported by retained tooth roots or implants. It is removable.

overutilization Services rendered by providers more frequently than usual.

OVR Oculovestibular response. Reflexive eye movements assessed following the placement of cold water in one ear.

OW Open ward.

Owren's syndrome Deficiencies of clotting factors noticeable from birth. Report this disorder with ICD-9-CM code 286.3. **Synonym(s):** *Stewart-Prower syndrome.*

oxaliplatin Injectable agent used in the treatment of Stage III colon cancer and for advanced carcinoma of the colon or rectum. Supply of oxaliplatin is reported with HCPCS Level II code J9263. May be sold as brand name Eloxatin.

Oxford Meniscal System Brand name artificial knee replacing only the medial portion of the knee joint, used in patients with osteoarthritis or avascular necrosis limited to the inside of the knee.

OXY Oxytocin.

oxycephaly Type of craniosynostosis in which fusion of the coronal and sagittal sutures forms an abnormally high, cone-shaped head. Oxycephaly is reported with ICD-9-CM code 756.0.

oz Ounce.

Ozurdex Brand name dexamethasone intravitreal implant indicated for the treatment of macular edema following retinal vein occlusion (branch or central). Second only to diabetic retinopathy as the most common retinal vascular disease, retinal vein occlusion is a major cause of vision loss. Report supply with HCPCS Level II code J7312.

P *1)* After. *2)* Phosphorus. *3)* Plan. *4)* Pulse.

P&A Percussion and auscultation.

P&T Pharmacy and therapeutics.

P+PD Percussion and postural drainage.

p.c. After eating.

p.m. After noon.

p.p. Near point of visual accommodation.

p.r. *1)* Pulsefar point of visual accommodation. *2)* Through the rectum.

p.r.n. As needed for.

p/o By mouth.

P1 HCPCS Level II modifier for use with anesthesia codes to show anesthesia given to a normal healthy patient.

P2 *1)* HCPCS Level II modifier for use with anesthesia codes to show anesthesia given to a patient with mild systemic disease. *2)* Pulmonic 2nd sound.

P3 HCPCS Level II modifier for use with anesthesia codes to show anesthesia to a patient with severe system disease.

P4 *1)* HCPCS Level II modifier for use with anesthesia codes to show anesthesia given to a patient with severe systemic disease that is a constant threat to life. *2)* Progesterone. P4 levels may be monitored to track fertility in the female. Progesterone levels are measured in laboratory tests reported with CPT codes 84144 and 84234.

P5 HCPCS Level II modifier for use with anesthesia codes to show a moribund patient who is not expected to survive without the operation.

P6 HCPCS Level II modifier for use with anesthesia codes to show a patient declared brain dead whose organs are being removed for donor purposes.

PA *1)* Physician assistant. Medical professional who receives additional training and can assess, treat, and prescribe medications under a physician's review. *2)* Posteroanterior. *3)* Pulmonary artery. *4)* HCPCS Level II modifier used to denote a surgical or other invasive procedure that was performed on the wrong body part.

PAB Premature atrial beats.

PAC Premature atrial contraction. Interruption in normal heart rhythm due to a premature electrical impulse to the atrial muscle, reported with ICD-9-CM code 427.61. **Synonym(s):** *atrial ectopic beat.*

PACE Programs of all-inclusive care for the elderly.

Pacemaker

Pacemaker leads (wires)

Pacemaker generator in subcutaneous pocket is changed out

Heart

Dual chamber shown

33212: Single chamber, either
33213: Both chambers (dual)
33214: Upgrade with conversion to dual chamber

The newer pacemaker generators are quite small. The generator consists of a battery, programmable circuitry, and is attached to the wire leads to the heart. The subcutaneous pocket holding the generator is upgraded in this series of codes and the pacemaker leads tested

pacemaker Implantable cardiac device that controls the heart's rhythm and maintains regular beats by artificial electric discharges. This device consists of the pulse generator with a battery and the electrodes, or leads, which are placed in single or dual chambers of the heart, usually transvenously. Leads that are placed epicardially require a thoracotomy. A single chamber pacemaker has one lead in the atrium or ventricle. A dual chamber pacemaker has one lead in the right atrium and one in the right ventricle. An extra lead may be used for biventricular pacing of the left ventricle. The generator is placed in a subcutaneous pocket below the clavicle or in an abdominal location. Biventricular pacing is one key to differentiating between code choices, as is whether the leads are placed transvenously or epicardially. Some procedures may also be done on the leads alone or the generator alone. CPT provides codes for reporting implantation or replacement, removal, repair, and repositioning. *NCD References: 20.8, 20.8.1, 20.8.2, 20.8.3.*

pacemaker registry Registry, no longer required by the Centers for Medicare and Medicaid Services, that provides information on all pacemaker devices and leads for which Medicare payments have been made.

pacemaker syndrome Functional deficiency following heart surgery in which the triggering mechanism of the heart may be irregular. Report this disorder with ICD-9-CM code 429.4.

pachy- Indicates heavy, large, or thick.

Pachymeter Slit-lamp attachment used for measuring corneal thickness or anterior chamber depth.

Pachymetry Measuring corneal thickness with a pachymeter, a special slit-lamp camera that can photograph the endothelial cells to be used to study cell morphology and perform cell counts.

packing Material placed into a cavity or wound, such as gels, gauze, pads, and sponges.

PACU Post anesthesia care unit.

PAD Peripheral artery disease. Disorders within the arteries outside of the heart and brain, most commonly a narrowing or hardening of the arteries carrying blood and oxygen to the legs, arms, stomach, or kidneys.

PAF Platelet activating factor.

PAG Policy advisory group. Generic name for many work groups at the Workgroup for Electronic Data Interchange (EDI) and elsewhere.

Paget-Schroetter syndrome Stress thrombosis of the subclavian or axillary vein. Report this disorder with ICD-9-CM code 453.89.

Pagon syndrome Genetically linked sideroblastic anemia present from birth, reported with ICD-9-CM code 285.0. *Synonym(s): Walker-Warburg syndrome.*

pagophagia Compulsive eating of ice.

-pagus Indicates fixed or joined together.

PAH Para-aminohippurate.

pain management Initial and subsequent evaluation and management (E/M) services, trigger point injections, spine and spinal cord injections, nerve blocks, biofeedback, and psychological evaluation and treatment.

PainBuster Brand name pain management infusion kit for continuous infusion of local anesthetic directly to the postoperative site following orthopedic surgery.

PAL *1)* Progressive addition lens. Eyeglass lens that provides correction for distance, midrange, and near vision with no bi- or trifocal demarcations. This feature in eyeglass lenses is reported with HCPCS Level II code V2781. *Synonym(s): progressive power lens. 2)* Probe for aspiration/lavage.

palatal Pertaining to the palate or an area toward the palate.

palate Partition that separates the nasal from the oral cavities.

palatine bones Irregularly shaped bones that form the posterior part of the hard palate and contribute to the formation of the nasal cavity and floors of the orbits.

pali(n)- Repetition, back again, recurring.

paliperidone palmitate Generic name for Invega, an injectable drug indicated for the treatment of schizophrenia in adults. Used for both acute and

O-R

maintenance treatment, the supply is reported with HCPCS Level II code J2426.

palliative   Alleviating care or medicine that is intended to provide relief from symptoms, but not cure the disease. Palliative care is employed in cases of terminal illness or severe chronic diseases.

palliative treatment   Treatment of symptoms without treating the underlying cause or to maintain current health status.

Pallister's syndrome   Abnormal development of the ulna, mammary glands, axillary apocrine glands, and facies with an absence of breast tissue and hypergrowth of the nipples and areolas. It can occur in either sex. Pallister's syndrome is reported with ICD-9-CM code 759.89.

palmar flexion   Bending of the hand with the fingers toward the palm.

palmaris longus tendon   Tendon located in the hand that flexes the wrist joint.

PALMAZ   Brand name expandable, wire-mesh stent, mounted over a balloon on the end of a long thin flexible catheter for use in patients who have narrowing and plaque build-up in the renal artery, not successfully opened in previous balloon angioplasty. The deployment catheter is advanced to the renal artery, where the balloon is inflated, crushing the plaque and expanding the narrowed area, then deflated and removed. The stent is then deployed and left within the artery as vascular wall support.

Palomar E2000   High-speed ruby laser designed for hair removal over large areas.

palpate   Examination by feeling with the hand.

palpebral   Referring or pertaining to the eyelids.

palpebral fissure   Linear opening between the upper and lower eyelids that exposes the eyeball.

PAMI   Primary angioplasty in acute myocardial infarction.

PAN   Polyarteritis nodosa. Systemic necrotizing vasculitis seen in small to medium size arteries, for example, of the kidneys and muscles. PAN is reported with ICD-9-CM code 446.0. **Synonym(s):** *Kussmaul's disease.*

Panacryl   Brand name absorbable sutures used for soft tissue approximation and ligation, usually in orthopedic procedures for giving extended wound support that is initially as strong as nonabsorbable sutures. Panacryl lasts six months before dissolving.

Pancoast Syndrome

Pancoast syndrome describes a tumor at the apex of the lung

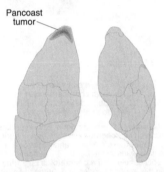

Pancoast tumor

Pancoast syndrome   Neoplasm of upper lobe of the lung. Report this disorder with ICD-9-CM code 162.3. **Synonym(s):** *Cuiffini syndrome, Hare's syndrome.*

pancreatic steatorrhea   Build up of fat in feces due to the absence of pancreatic fluids in the intestines and subsequent lack of digestion, reported with ICD-9-CM code 579.4.

pancreatitis   Inflammation of the pancreas that may be acute or chronic, symptomatic or asymptomatic. The inflammation is due to the autodigestion of pancreatic tissue by its own enzymes that have escaped into the pancreas, most often as a result of alcoholism or biliary tract disease such as calculi in the pancreatic duct. This may appear as sudden or recurring abdominal pain with nausea and vomiting, and hemorrhaging into surrounding tissue. Pancreatitis is also associated with trauma to the abdomen, hyperlipidemia, and hyperparathyroidism. Pancreatitis is reported with a code from ICD-9-CM category 577.

PANDAS   Pediatric autoimmune neuropsychiatric disorder associated with streptococcal infections. Complex of symptoms in a pediatric patient including obsessive-compulsive disorder, tic, history of strep infection, and neurological abnormalities. ICD-9-CM has no code specific to PANDAS, and guidelines instruct us in that case, to code the syndrome manifestations separately.

pandemic   Worldwide outbreak of disease within the population that exceeds normal incidence rates.

paneled   In health care contracting, provider contracted with an HMO.

panhypopituitarism Severe or complete hypopituitarism from absence or impairment of the gland, leading to manifestations including absence of gonadal function, dwarfism, regression of secondary sex characteristics, weight loss, fatigue, bradycardia, and depression with insufficient functioning of the thyroid and adrenal cortex. Panhypopituitarism is reported with ICD-9-CM code 253.2. *Synonym(s): Sheehan's syndrome.*

panhypopituitary syndrome Secretion of all anterior pituitary hormones is inadequate or absent after childbirth. Report this disorder with ICD-9-CM code 253.2.

panic disorder Episodic and often chronic, recurrent disorder manifested by discrete periods of sudden onset, intense apprehension, fearfulness, or terror often associated with feelings of impending doom.

panniculitis Inflammation of the subcutaneous fat and/or connective tissue.

panophthalmitis Infection of the eye and adnexa by bacterial or fungal agents.

panoramic x-ray X-ray that contains views of both the maxilla and mandible on a single extraoral film.

panto- Indicates the whole or all.

panuveitis Inflammation of the entire vascular layer of the eye, including the choroid, iris, and ciliary body. This condition is reported with ICD-9-CM code 360.12.

PAP *1)* Papanicolaou test or smear. *NCD References: 190.2, 210.2. 2)* Pulmonary artery pressure.

paper claim Claim that is submitted on paper, including optical character recognition (OCR) claims and claims that are converted to electronic format by Medicare. Medicare will not pay clean paper claims until the 26th day after the claim is received.

papilla of Vater Nipple-shaped opening from the pancreatic and common bile ducts into the posterior portion of the descending duodenum. Papillotomy with ERCP is reported with CPT code 43262. Report 43273 in addition to a code for the primary procedure when an endoscopic cannulation of the papilla is performed. *Synonym(s): ampulla of Vater, papilla duodenal major.*

papilloma Benign skin neoplasm with small branchings from the epithelial surface.

PapNet Brand name advanced computerized review technique to evaluate Pap or vaginal smears that were interpreted as normal in the initial screening. PapNet-generated video images are reviewed by a cytotechnologist. PapNet is performed on the original specimen and does not require additional tissue sampling. It is reported with CPT code 88152.

PAPP-A Plasma protein-A, pregnancy associated, reported with CPT code 84163.

PAPVR Partial anomalous pulmonary venous return, reported with ICD-9-CM code 747.49. *Synonym(s): Scimitar syndrome.*

papyraceous fetus Fetus that has died, but remains in utero for weeks before delivery, becoming compacted and mummified in appearance, with skin resembling parchment. This condition occurs most commonly in multigestational pregnancies in which one of the fetuses dies or intentional multigestational reduction is carried out to save another more viable fetus. Papyraceous fetus is reported with ICD-9-CM subcategory 646.0, while multiple gestation codes denoting the pregnancy with fetal loss and retention of one or more fetuses are reported under category 651. *Synonym(s): paper doll fetus.*

Par Participating provider.

PAR *1)* Parenteral. *2)* Post anesthesia recovery.

par provider Provider who is participating in a health plan or Medicare program.

para *1)* Along side of. *2)* Number of pregnancies, as para 1, 2, 3, etc.

para- Indicates near, similar, beside, or past.

parabiotic donor syndrome In a twin pregnancy, transfusion of blood from one fetus to another. Report this disorder with ICD-9-CM code 772.0.

parabiotic recipient syndrome In a twin pregnancy, polycythemia of newborn as result of blood flow from mother. Report this disorder with ICD-9-CM code 776.4.

paracentesis Surgical puncture of a body cavity with a specialized needle or hollow tubing to aspirate fluid for diagnostic or therapeutic reasons. This often refers to puncture of the abdominal cavity, although documentation should specify that it was performed on the abdomen before reporting with CPT code 49080. *ophthalmic p.* Corneal procedure to remove some anterior chamber fluid for analysis or to reduce eye pressure quickly or temporarily.

PARAFlow Brand name circulatory support system used in "beating heart" surgery.

ParaGard Brand name copper intrauterine device inserted through the cervix into the uterus by a clinician. Supply of the IUD is reported with HCPCS Level II code J7300 and insertion is reported with CPT code 58300.

Paragranuloma Another term for the lymphocyte dominant type of Hodgkin's disease.

paralysis agitans Chronic degenerative disease of the central nervous system producing resting tremor, voluntary movement disorders, and muscle weakness. Report this disorder with ICD-9-CM code 332.0. *Synonym(s): Parkinson's disease.*

paralytic ileus Intestinal obstruction due to loss of bowel motility or paralysis, usually as a result of localized

O-R

or generalized peritonitis or shock. Report this condition with ICD-9-CM code 560.1. *Synonym(s): adynamic ileus.*

paralytic lagophthalmos Palsy of the seventh cranial nerve, which prevents full closure of the eyelids.

paralytic ptosis Drooping of the upper eyelid due to nerve defect.

parametritis Inflammation and infection of the tissue in the structures around the uterus.

parametrium Connective tissue between the uterus and the broad ligament.

paranasal sinuses Air-filled spaces in the cranial bones lined with mucosa and opening into the nasal cavity and include the maxillary, frontal, ethmoid, and sphenoid sinuses.

paranoia Rare chronic psychosis in which logically constructed systematized delusions of grandeur, persecution, or somatic abnormality have developed gradually without concomitant hallucinations or the schizophrenic type of disordered thinking. *alcoholic p.* Chronic paranoid psychosis characterized by delusional jealousy and associated with alcoholism. *p. querulans* Paranoid state that may present as schizophrenic or affective state. Symptoms differ from other paranoid states and psychogenic paranoid psychosis. *senile p.* Paranoid psychosis in which there are conspicuous hallucinations, often in several modalities. May be associated with mild affective symptoms and well-preserved personality.

paranoid personality Excessive self-reference and sensitiveness to setbacks or to what are taken to be humiliations and rebuffs, a tendency to distort experience by misconstruing the neutral or friendly actions of others as hostile or contemptuous, and a combative and tenacious sense of personal rights that may be manifested as jealousy or excessive self-importance, excessive sensitivity, or aggression.

paranoid reaction Paranoid states apparently provoked by some emotional stress such as imprisonment, immigration, or strange and threatening environments. Frequently manifested as an attack or threat.

paranoid schizophrenia Pronounced affective manic or depressive features intermingled with schizophrenic features that tend toward remission without permanent defect but that are prone to recur.

paranoid state involutional Paranoid psychosis in which there are conspicuous hallucinations, often in several modalities. May be associated with mild affective symptoms and well-preserved personality.

paranoid state senile Paranoid psychosis in which there are conspicuous hallucinations, often in several modalities. May be associated with mild affective symptoms and well-preserved personality.

paranoid state simple Psychosis, acute or chronic, with fixed, elaborate, and systemized delusions, especially of being influenced, persecuted, or treated in some special way, that is not attributable to schizophrenia or affective psychosis.

paranoid traits Excessive self-reference and sensitiveness to setbacks or to what are taken to be humiliations and rebuffs, a tendency to distort experience by misconstruing the neutral or friendly actions of others as hostile or contemptuous, and a combative and tenacious sense of personal rights that may be manifested as jealousy or excessive self-importance, excessive sensitivity, or aggression.

paranoid type syndrome Organic disorder with hallucinations, beliefs about being followed, being poisoned, etc., and not meeting criteria for schizophrenia. Report this disorder with ICD-9-CM code 293.81.

paraphilia Abnormal sexual inclinations or behavior directed primarily either toward people not of the opposite sex, or toward sexual acts not associated with coitus normally, or toward coitus performed under abnormal circumstances; can take the form of exhibitionism, fetishism, homosexuality, nymphomania, pedophilia, satyriasis, sexual masochism, sexual sadism, transvestism, voyeurism, and zoophilia.

paraphrenia Paranoid psychosis in which there are conspicuous hallucinations, often in several modalities. May be associated with mild affective symptoms and well-preserved personality.

paraphrenic schizophrenia Pronounced affective manic or depressive features intermingled with schizophrenic features that tend toward remission without permanent defect but that are prone to recur.

paraplegia Paralysis (complete or incomplete) of both lower limbs, reported with ICD-9-CM code 344.1.

Parastep Brand name ambulation system using percutaneous stimulation to deliver electrical impulses for muscle flexion to trigger action. Patients also use a walker or elbow-support crutches with Parastep. Check with individual payers for coverage policy on Parastep. Supply is reported with HCPCS Level II code E0764; multiple physical therapy sessions would also be reported for the training required for use of a Parastep device.

parasympathetic nerves Nerves that function at rest decreasing heart, respiration, and metabolic rates and that stimulate digestion and urinary output.

paratenon Fatty tissue filling the gaps or space within a tendon sheath or compartment.

paratenon graft Graft composed of the fatty tissue found between a tendon and its sheath.

paratyphoid Prolonged illness with fever clinically similar to typhoid but less virulent, caused by serotypes of salmonella other than S. typhi. Paratyphoid can occur

O-R

after an outbreak of salmonella food poisoning and is reported with ICD-9-CM codes 002.1-002.9. Report carrier as V02.3 and vaccination against paratyphoid with V03.1. **Synonym(s):** *Brion-Kayser disease, Schottmüller's disease.*

Paremyd Brand name eye drop used to dilate the pupil in routine ophthalmic exams. Its use is bundled into the procedure.

parenteral Other than the alimentary canal and is usually used in a method of delivery context: total parenteral nutrition (TPN) and parenteral nutrition therapy (PNT) formulas, kits, and devices.

parenteral hyperalimentation Administration of all nutrients and vitamins required by an individual in a liquid form via a central venous catheter. **Synonym(s):** *total parenteral nutrition.* **NCD Reference:** *180.2.*

parenteral nutrition Nutrients provided subcutaneously, intravenously, intramuscularly, or intradermally for patients during the postoperative period and in other conditions, such as shock, coma, and renal failure. **NCD Reference:** *180.2.*

Parinaud's syndrome Paralysis of conjugate movement of eyes without paralysis of convergence caused by lesions of the midbrain. Report this disorder with ICD-9-CM code 378.81.

paring Cutting away an edge or a surface. For paring or cutting of benign hyperkeratotic lesions, see CPT codes 11055-11057, depending on the number of lesions treated.

PARK Photorefractive astigmatic keratectomy. Procedure that treats astigmatism with cold laser.

Parkes Weber and Dimitri syndrome Formation of multiple angiomas in skin of head and scalp. Report this disorder with ICD-9-CM code 759.6. **Synonym(s):** *Kalischer's syndrome.*

Parkinson's disease Idiopathic neurological disease resulting in degeneration and dysfunction of the basal ganglia. Toxic degeneration of a group of specialized cells in the midbrain results in signs and symptoms, including tremor, rigidity, difficulty starting movement or slowness in movement, "pill-rolling" movement of the fingers, shuffling gait, drooling, and problems with articulation. Secondary parkinsonism is a similar neurological disease that affects the central nervous system, caused by the adverse effect of certain drugs or chemicals. Report these conditions with codes from ICD-9-CM category 332.

Parlodel Brand name fertility oral medication, used to lower the level of prolactin. Parlodel may also be used to treat Parkinson's disease and to reduce or prevent the production of breast milk. Parlodel contains bromocriptine.

paronychia Infection of nail structures. For incision and drainage of paronychia, see CPT codes 10060-10061.

parotitis Inflammation of the salivary gland. Parotitis that is not infectious (i.e., allergic) is reported with ICD-9-CM code 527.2. Infectious or epidemic parotitis is the mumps and is reported with 072.9. **Synonym(s):** *sialoadenitis.*

paroxysmal nocturnal hemoglobinuria Uncommon, acquired stem cell disorder in which the red blood cells undergo premature destruction, resulting in hemoglobin in the urine and a tendency to develop recurring blood clots. Some level of bone marrow dysfunction is also present. Report this condition with ICD-9-CM code 283.2. **Synonym(s):** *Marchiafava-Micheli syndrome, PNH.*

paroxysmal supraventricular tachycardia Rapid heartbeat that starts above the ventricles and occurs sporadically.

PARR Post anesthesia recovery room

Parry fracture Common closed fracture of the ulnar shaft, resulting from blunt forearm trauma and reported with ICD-9-CM code 813.22. In a Parry fracture, there is no involvement of the radius and no dislocation, and the fracture itself is usually minimally displaced. **Synonym(s):** *Nightstick fracture.*

Parry's disease Enlargement of the thyroid gland seen mostly in women, stemming from an autoimmune process, and causing excessive secretion of thyroid hormone, goiter, and bulging eyes. The syndrome seen with hyperplasia of the thyroid and excessive hormone production consists of fatigue, nervousness, emotional lability and irritability, heat intolerance and increased sweating, weight loss, palpitations, and tremor of the hands and tongue. If there is no documentation of a thyrotoxic crisis or storm, report ICD-9-CM code 242.00; with thyrotoxic crisis or storm, report 242.01. **Synonym(s):** *Basedow syndrome, Begbie's disease, Flajani disease, Graves' disease, Marsh's disease, toxic diffuse goiter.*

Parry-Romberg syndrome Hypersomnia associated with bulimia and occurring in males between 10 to 25 years of age with ravenous appetite followed by prolonged sleep, along with behavioral disturbances, impaired thought processes, and hallucinations. Report this disorder with ICD-9-CM code 349.89.

pars planitis Chronic inflammation of the ciliary body.

Parsonage-Alden-Turner syndrome Paroxysmal pain extending length of one of many nerves. Report this disorder with ICD-9-CM code 353.5.

Part A hospital insurance coverage Hospital services covered under Medicare Part A. Part A coverage includes medically necessary and reasonable services such as bed and board (semiprivate room and all meals, including special diets, a private room when medically necessary, intensive care unit if the level of care requires it); regular nursing services, including ICU; operating room charges;

O-R

drugs furnished by the hospital; laboratory tests; x-ray and other radiology services; medical supplies such as casts and splints; appliances and equipment furnished by the hospital (e.g., wheelchairs, crutches); physical, speech and occupational therapy; respiratory therapy; inpatient stays for rehabilitation; and inpatient psychiatric hospital services. Part A also covers posthospital care provided to an inpatient in a skilled nursing facility and to a homebound patient receiving services from a home health agency or hospice.

Part A trust fund Portion of the Medicare budget allocated to pay for hospital services covered under Medicare Part A.

Part A utilization Beneficiary's use of coverage under Medicare Part A. The number of days of Part A utilization is charged based on the actual days of coverage, including grace and waiver days. The number of covered days used is posted to the beneficiary's master record. Coinsurance is applicable for the number of days charged against the master record.

Part B hospital insurance coverage Hospital services covered under Medicare Part B. Part B hospital insurance coverage applies in the following circumstances: a beneficiary receives inpatient hospital services that cannot be paid for under Part A because benefits are exhausted before or after admission and before the stay reaches outlier status; outlier days are not covered or the waiver of liability payment is not made; a noncovered level of care is received; or the patient is not entitled to Part A or elects not to use lifetime reserve days. Payment may be made under Part B for the following types of services: diagnostic x-ray, laboratory, other diagnostic tests; x-ray, radium and radioactive isotope therapy; surgical dressings, casts, splints, and other devices used for reduction of fractures and dislocations; prosthetic devices, other than dental, that replace all or part of an internal body organ or all or part of the function of a permanently inoperative or malfunctioning internal body organ, including replacement and repairs; leg, arm, back and neck braces, trusses and artificial legs, arms and eyes, including adjustments, repairs, and replacements; outpatient physical, occupational and speech pathology services; ambulance service; and dialysis services rendered to inpatients.

Part B trust fund Portion of the Medicare budget allocated to pay for hospital services covered under Medicare Part B.

part. vic. Divided doses.

partial dentures In dentistry, artificial teeth composed of a metal framework with plastic teeth and gum areas.

partial disability Congenital or acquired inability to perform part of one's job.

partial epilepsy Transient brain function disturbance resulting in episodes of seizures caused by focal, localized brain lesions. *Synonym(s): focal epilepsy.*

partial hospitalization Situation in which the patient only stays part of each day over a long period. Cardiac, rehabilitation, and chronic pain patients, for example, could use this service. *mental health p.* Intense part- or full-day controlled program for psychiatric care in the outpatient setting.

partial nephrectomy Removal of a portion of the kidney.

partial payment Payment to a provider or member with the expectation that other payments will be forthcoming before the claim is closed.

participating provider In health care contracting, provider who has contracted with the health plan to deliver medical services to covered persons. *Synonym(s): in-network provider, network provider.*

particle beam Treatment using subatomic proton and neutron particles to deliver high-energy radiation.

Parvovirus B19 Only known parvovirus to cause disease in humans. Manifestation is erythema infectiosum. This parvovirus is also associated with polyarthropathy, chronic anemia, red cell aplasia, and fetal hydrops.

PAS norms Based on a professional activity study performed regularly by the Commission on Professional and Hospital Activities and broken out by average length of stay (ALOS) by region.

PASA Proximal articular set angle. Angle between the cartilage that articulates with the big toe relative to the first metatarsal. PASA is a factor in determining what type of corrective surgery will be performed. It will not directly affect code selection. *Synonym(s): DMAA.*

PASG Pneumatic antishock garment. Inflatable trousers applied to patients in shock in an attempt to stabilize blood pressure by increasing venous blood return to the heart. *Synonym(s): MAST.*

passive mobilization Pressure, movement, or pulling of a limb or body part utilizing an apparatus or device.

passive personality Passive compliance with the wishes of elders and others and a weak inadequate response to the demands of daily life. The person may be intellectual or emotional with little capacity for enjoyment.

passive-aggressive personality Aggressive behavior manifested in passive ways, such as obstructionism, pouting, procrastination, intentional inefficiency, or stubbornness often arising from resentment at failing to find gratification in a relationship with an individual or institution upon which the individual is over dependent.

password Confidential authentication information composed of a string of characters that can include letters, numbers, and a variety of punctuation marks.

O-R

past history Record of prior illnesses or conditions occurring in childhood and adulthood, such as infectious diseases, allergies, accidents, current medications, hospitalizations, and surgical/medical procedures.

PAT *1)* Paroxysmal atrial tachycardia. *2)* Peripheral arterial tone. A physiologic signal that reflects arterial pulsatile volume changes and mirrors errors in autonomic nervous system activity. This signal may be reviewed in cardiac stress tests or in sleep-related disorder testing. Peripheral arterial tone is associated with variations in the amount of blood flowing through the peripheral arteries, such as in the finger. *Synonym(s): peripheral arterial tonometry.*

patella clunk syndrome Fibrous soft tissue accumulation, scarring, and rigidity of the knee junction caused by chronic patellar pressure following knee replacement surgery. Report this syndrome with ICD-9-CM code 719.66.

patellectomy Surgical removal of the patella, or kneecap, a sesamoid bone found in the front of the knee. Report partial patellectomy with ICD-9-CM procedure code 77.86 and total with 77.96. Report CPT code 27350.

patency State of a tube-like structure or conduit being open and unobstructed.

Patent Ductus Arteriosus

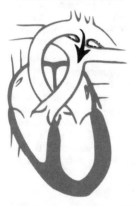

patent ductus arteriosus Condition in which the normal channel between the pulmonary artery and the aorta fails to close at birth, causing arterial blood to recirculate in the lungs and inhibiting the blood supply to the aorta. This condition is reported with ICD-9-CM code 747.0. *Synonym(s): PDA.*

patent urachus Congenital condition in which a passage, or fistula, persists between the umbilicus and the bladder, through which urine can drain out the umbilicus. This condition is reported with ICD-9-CM code 753.7.

Paterson (-Brown) (-Kelly) syndrome Condition in middle-aged women with hypochronic anemia of cracks or fissures at the corners of the mouth, painful tongue, and dysphagia due to esophageal stenosis or webs. Report this disorder with ICD-9-CM code 280.8. *Synonym(s): Kelly syndrome, Plummer-Vinson syndrome.*

Patey's mastectomy Modified radical mastectomy includes removal of the breast and axillary lymph nodes with preservation of the pectoralis major muscle.

PATH *1)* Physicians at teaching hospitals. Set up by the Office of Inspector General (OIG), initiative of the National Recovery Project targeting reimbursement practices at teaching hospitals, focusing on the use of residents and the services they perform under Medicare Part B that are paid as part of Medicare Part A. *2)* Pathology.

-pathic Indicates a feeling, diseased condition, or therapy.

patho- Indicates sensitivity, feeling, or suffering.

pathognomonic Distinct sign, symptom, or characteristic of a particular disease, from which a diagnosis can be made.

pathologic fracture Break in bone due to a disease process that weakens the bone structure, such as osteoporosis, osteomalacia, or neoplasia, and not traumatic injury. Report this type of fracture with a code from ICD-9-CM subcategory 733.1. Report a personal history of pathologic fracture with V13.51.

pathologic retraction ring Complication of labor in which the ridge that normally forms between the upper and lower portions of the uterus due to contractions (retraction ring) becomes exaggerated and visible through the abdomen above the pubic joint. This may be indicative of cephalopelvic disproportion or unstable lie, and signals pending uterine rupture if left untreated. This condition is reported on the mother's chart with a code from ICD-9-CM category 661.4. If specified as affecting the fetus or newborn, report 763.7. *Synonym(s): Bandl's ring.*

pathological alcohol intoxication Acute psychotic episodes induced by relatively small amounts of alcohol without conspicuous neurological signs of intoxication.

pathological alcohol intoxication Acute psychotic episodes induced by relatively small amounts of alcohol. These are regarded as individual idiosyncratic reactions to alcohol, not due to excessive consumption and without conspicuous neurological signs of intoxication.

pathological dislocation Displacement of a bone or joint caused by a disease process, such as infection, lesions, or muscle weakness, and not traumatic injury.

pathological drug intoxication Individual idiosyncratic reactions to comparatively small quantities of a drug,

O-R

which take the form of acute, brief psychotic states of any type.

pathological drunkenness Acute psychotic episodes induced by relatively small amounts of alcohol. These are regarded as individual idiosyncratic reactions to alcohol, not due to excessive consumption and without conspicuous neurological signs of intoxication.

pathological gambling Disorder of impulse control characterized by a chronic and progressive preoccupation with gambling and urge to gamble, with subsequent gambling behavior that compromises, disrupts, or damages personal, family, and vocational pursuits.

pathological personality Deeply ingrained maladaptive patterns of behavior generally recognizable by adolescence or earlier and continuing throughout most of adult life, although often becoming less obvious in middle or old age. The personality is abnormal either in the balance of its components, quality, and expression, or in its total aspect.

pathology Medical science, and specialty practice, regarding all aspects of disease, with special reference to the essential nature, causes, and development of abnormal conditions, as well as the structural and functional changes that result from the disease processes.

patient Individual who is receiving or who has received health care services. This could include a person who is deceased.

patient control number Patient's unique alphabetic and/or numeric identifier assigned by the provider to facilitate retrieving the patient's account and case records and posting payments.

patient education Method or process of teaching a patient about his or her health and how to manage or treat any conditions or diagnoses the patient may have.

patient problem Disease, condition, illness, injury, symptom, sign, finding, complaint, or other reason for an encounter, with or without a diagnosis being established at the time of the encounter.

patient status Patient's discharge status as of the "through" date (or discharge date) of the billing period. This information is required for both inpatient and outpatient claims for Medicare billing purposes. Patient status may be any of the following: routine discharge, discharged to another facility, still a patient, or expired.

PATOS Payment (received) at the time of service.

Patterson's test Test using blood and a reagent detects urea. Blood turns green if positive.

pauciarticular Type of juvenile rheumatoid arthritis in which four or less joints are affected, reported with ICD-9-CM code 714.32.

payer Entity that assumes the risk of paying for medical treatments. This can be an uninsured patient, a self-insured employer, a health plan, or an HMO.

PAYERID Centers for Medicare and Medicaid Services' term for its pre-HIPAA national payer ID initiative.

payers In the health care industry, entity that assumes the risk of paying for medical care. Examples of payers include public and private payers, HMOs, and self-insured employers.

payment error prevention program Program to help reduce Medicare inpatient hospital payment errors under the prospective payment system.

payment floor Minimum number of calendar days that must pass before Medicare can pay a claim, established by Omnibus Budget Reconciliation Act of 1987 for Medicare claims. Payment is made no earlier than 14 days after claim submission for electronic claims and no earlier than 27 days for paper claims submission.

payment indicator Term used in the OCE. A one-digit number that is output from the OCE indicating the type of payment that will be made. For example, 1 means "Paid standard hospital OPPS amount (status indicators K, S, T, V, X)."

payment rate Amount paid to the provider for health care services rendered to a plan member.

Payr's syndrome Bloating, gas, pain, and fullness experienced left upper abdominal quadrant with pain sometimes radiating up into left chest. Report this disorder with ICD-9-CM code 569.89.

PB *1)* HCPCS Level II modifier used to denote a surgical or other invasive procedure that was performed on the wrong patient. *2)* Pulmonary barotrauma. Complication of mechanical ventilation in which a sudden increase in intrathoracic pressure can lead to mediastinal emphysema or a tension pneumothorax. PB can also occur in scuba diving. If PB from a ventilator leads to mediastinal emphysema, report ICD-9-CM code 998.81. If PB from a ventilator leads to pneumothorax, report pneumothorax with 512.1.

PBI Protein-bound iodine.

PBM Prescription benefit managers. HMO staff who monitor amount and use of drugs prescribed.

PBO Prescription benefit manager. HMO staff that monitor amount and use of drugs prescribed.

PBSC Peripheral blood stem cell.

PBSCT Peripheral blood stem cell transplant. Procedure that restores stem cells destroyed by earlier chemotherapy or radiation therapy in treatment of a malignancy. PBSCT can be autologous, in which the patient receives his or her own stem cells; syngeneic, in which the patient receives cells from an identical twin; or allogeneic, in which the patient receives cells from another relative or non-relative. PBSCT is reported with a CPT code from range 38240-38242.

PC *1)* HCPCS Level II modifier used to denote that the wrong surgery or other invasive procedure was performed on the patient. *2)* Packed cells. *3)* Prostate cancer.

PCA *1)* Patient controlled analgesia. *2)* Posterior communicating artery.

PCD Polycystic disease.

PCG Phonocardiogram.

PCH Pouch.

PCI in AMI Percutaneous coronary intervention in acute myocardial infarction. Primary angioplasty for acute myocardial infarction.

PCL Posterior cruciate ligament.

PCN *1)* Penicillin. *2)* Primary care nurse.

PCNSL Primary central nervous system lymphoma. Lymphoma of the brain and spinal cord, definitively diagnosed with a brain biopsy.

PCOS Polycystic ovarian syndrome, reported with ICD-9-CM code 256.4.

PCP *1)* Primary care physician. Physician who makes an initial diagnosis and referral and retains control over the patient and utilization of services both in and outside of the plan. *2)* Pneumocystis pneumonia, reported with ICD-9-CM code 136.3. *3)* Phencyclidine. Illegal dissociative drug causing volatile effects in users.

PCPM Per contract per month.

PCR *1)* Physician contingency reserve. *2)* Polymerase chain reaction.

PCT *1)* Porphyria cutanea tarda. Hepatic porphyria that may be an acquired or inherited disorder caused by a deficiency in the enzyme uroporphyrinogen decarboxylase (UROD) in the liver, resulting in photosensitivity that can lead to skin blisters and crusting. PCT usually occurs in adulthood and is more common in men. PCT is reported with ICD-9-CM code 277.1. *2)* Postcoital test. Microscopic examination of cervical mucus performed following intercourse to review interaction between the sperm and mucous and the quality of the cervical mucus. PCT is reported with HCPCS Level II code Q0115.

PCTA Percutaneous transluminal angioplasty.

PCV Packed cell volume.

PCV7 Pneumococcal conjugate vaccine, a pediatric vaccine. Supply of PCV7 is reported with CPT code 90669 or HCPCS Level II code S0195. Administration is reported with HCPCS Level II code G0009. The need for vaccination is reported with ICD-9-CM code V03.82.

PCW Pulmonary capillary wedge.

PCWP Pulmonary capillary wedge pressure. Indirect indicator of left ventricular preload, useful in diagnosing such cardiac pathologies as mitral and aortic valve diseases, left ventricular failure, and abnormalities of the heart.

PD *1)* Peritoneal dialysis. *2)* Parkinson's disease. *3)* Postural drainage.

PDA *1)* Patent ductus arteriosus. *2)* Posterior descending artery.

PDD Pervasive development disorder.

PDN-SOLO Prosthetic Disc Nucleus - SOLO. Brand name artificial disc for spinal disc replacement. The natural disc is replaced with one made of a woven polyethylene jacket with a fluid-absorbent hydrogel core as a treatment for degenerative disc disease. ICD-9-CM codes appropriate to the insertion of a PDN-SOLO include 722.10, 722.52, and 722.73. The procedure is reported with ICD-9-CM hospital code 84.64 or with unlisted CPT code 22899.

PDR Physicians' Desk Reference.

PDT Percutaneous dilatational tracheostomy.

PE *1)* Practice expense. One of three components used to develop relative value units under the resource-based relative value scale. Practice expense represents the physician's direct and indirect costs associated with providing a service. *2)* Pulmonary embolism. Obstruction of the pulmonary artery resulting from a blood clot or other foreign material that broke away from its original source and traveled in the blood stream to become lodged in the pulmonary artery or one of its branches, sometimes resulting in hemorrhagic infarction and necrosis of pulmonary tissue. Pulmonary embolism is reported with ICD-9-CM subcategory 415.1. This is often seen after prolonged periods of inactivity or confinement.

PE tube Pressure equalization tube. Tympanic tube to drain fluid behind the eardrum in patients with recurrent otitis media. Placement of the tube is reported with CPT code 69433 or 69436. For an inpatient procedure, report ICD-9-CM procedure code 20.01.

Pean's amputation Arteries and veins are ligated during each step to amputate the hip joint.

PEARLA Pupils equal and react to light and accommodation.

PEC Pre-existing condition.

PECOS Provider Enrollment, Chain & Ownership System.

pectoral girdle syndrome Malignant atrophic papulosis. Report this disorder with ICD-9-CM code 447.8.

pectoralis major Chest muscle connecting at the clavicle, upper ribs, sternum, and the axilla.

pectus carinatum Congenital abnormality of the anterior chest wall with protrusion of the sternum, rounding the appearance of the chest. This abnormality is reported with ICD-9-CM code 754.82. *Synonym(s): pigeon chest.*

O-R

pectus excavatum Congenital abnormality of the anterior chest wall with depression of the sternum, sinking the appearance of the chest. This abnormality is reported with ICD-9-CM code 754.81. *Synonym(s): funnel chest.*

ped(i)- Relating to the foot.

Pederson speculum Device inserted into the vagina for viewing its walls and the cervix.

Pediarix Brand name pediatric diphtheria, tetanus, acellular pertussis, hepatitis B, and polio vaccine provided in a single-dose vial or syringe. Supply of Pediarix is reported with CPT code 90698; administration is reported separately. The need for vaccination is reported with ICD-9-CM code V06.8.

pediatric patient Patient usually younger than 14 years of age.

pedicle Stem-like, narrow base or stalk attached to a new growth.

pedicle flap Full-thickness skin and subcutaneous tissue for grafting that remains partially attached to the donor site by a pedicle or stem in which the blood vessels supplying the flap remain intact.

pedicle graft Mass of flesh and skin partially excised from the donor location, retaining its blood supply through intact blood vessels, that is grafted onto another site to repair adjacent or distant defects. *Synonym(s): flap graft.*

pedophilia Sexual deviations in which an adult engages in sexual activity with a child of the same or opposite sex.

Peds Pediatrics.

peduncle Connecting structures of the brain.

PedvaxHIB Brand name haemophilus influenzae type B vaccine provided in a single-dose vial. Supply of Code selection for PedvaxHIB is dependent upon the patient's immunization schedule. The number of doses specified does not necessarily have to be given; for children who start the Hib series late, fewer doses may be required. For children who start the schedule on time, CPT code 90647 would be reported. Administration is reported separately. Need for vaccination is reported with ICD-9-CM code V03.81.

peeling skin syndrome Congenital or acquired skin condition in which the palms and sometimes the soles develop blisters, followed by peeling of the outer layer of epidermis. Young adults are often affected during the summer months. If specified as congenital, report this condition with ICD-9-CM code 757.39, otherwise report 695.89. *Synonym(s): keratolysis exfoliativa.*

peer review Evaluation of the quality of the total health care provided by medical staff with equivalent training,

such as a physician-to-physician or nurse-to-nurse evaluation.

peer review organization Organization that contracts with CMS to conduct preadmission, preprocedure, and postdischarge medical reviews and determine medical necessity, appropriateness, and quality of certain inpatient and outpatient surgical procedures for which payment may be made in whole or in part under the Medicare program. *Synonym(s): PRO, QIO, quality improvement organization.*

PEG Percutaneous endoscopic gastrostomy.

Pegasus Brand name Nd:YAG laser used in pulpotomies and root canals.

pegfilgrastim Injectable protein used to treat chemotherapy-induced neutropenia by stimulating production of white blood cells. Supply is reported with HCPCS Level II code J2505. May be sold under brand name Neulasta.

PEGJJ Percutaneous endoscopic gastrojejunostomy.

PEJ Percutaneous endoscopic jejunostomy.

Pelger-Huët syndrome Patients present hepatosplenomegaly, lymphadenopathy, anemia, thrombocytopenia, along with changes in bones, cardiopulmonary system, skin, and psychomotor skills. Abnormalities of granulation and nuclear structure of white cells open child to infection and result in death. Report this disorder with ICD-9-CM code 288.2.

Pelizaeus-Merzbacher disease Inherited degenerative brain disease manifested by gradually advancing white matter sclerosis of the frontal lobes, mental deficits, and vasomotor disorders. Report this disease with ICD-9-CM code 330.0. *Synonym(s): aplasia axialis extracorticalis, hereditary cerebral leukodystrophy, Merzbacher-Pelizaeus disease.*

pellagra Disease caused by a deficiency of the B-complex vitamin niacin. Manifestations include diarrhea, nausea and vomiting, mouth ulcers, dermatitis, dementia, seizures, and ataxia. Death may occur. Report this disorder with ICD-9-CM code 265.2. *Synonym(s): niacin deficiency.*

pellagra-cerebellar ataxia-renal aminoaciduria syndrome Renal tubular malfunction, including cytinosis and osteomalacia, caused by inherited disorders or the result of multiple myeloma or proximal epithelial growth. Report this disorder with ICD-9-CM code 270.0. *Synonym(s): Debre syndrome, Fanconi syndrome, Hart's syndrome, Toni syndrome.*

pellagroid syndrome Resembling pellagra or a description of pellagra. Report this disorder with ICD-9-CM code 265.2.

Pellegrini-Stieda syndrome Calcification of medial collateral ligament of knee. Report this disorder with

ICD-9-CM code 726.62. *Synonym(s):*
Kohler-Pellegrini-Stieda syndrome.

Pellizzi's syndrome Precocious development of external sexual organs, precocious development of long bones, and hydrocephalus indicating lesion of pineal body. Report this disorder with ICD-9-CM code 259.8.

pelvic bones Ilium, ischium, pubis, and sacrum together forming a bony circle to protect the pelvic contents, provide stability for the vertebral column (sacrum), and provide an appropriate surface for femoral articulation for ambulation.

pelvic congestion syndrome Varicose veins of the pelvis that become distended and engorged, resulting in an excessive accumulation of blood in those vessels. Symptoms may include dull pelvic pain, abnormal menstruation, abdominal distention, and ovarian tenderness. This syndrome is reported with ICD-9-CM code 625.5. *Synonym(s): congestion-fibrosis syndrome, PCS, Taylor's syndrome.*

pelvic exenteration Radical removal of all the organs and adjacent structures of the pelvic cavity: bladder, lower ureters, lymph nodes, urethra, prostate or cervix, uterus, vagina, colon, and rectum, due to prostatic, gynecological, or vesical, or urethral malignancy. Pelvic exenteration is reported with CPT codes 51597 and 58240.

pelvis Distal anterior portion of the trunk that lies between the hipbones, sacrum, and coccyx bones; the inferior portion of the abdominal cavity.

Pemberton osteotomy Osteotomy is performed to position triradiate cartilage as a hinge for rotating the acetabular roof in cases of dysplasia of the hip in children.

pemphigoid (ophthalmic) Progressive scarring of the eyes' mucous membranes that leads to adhesions, drying-out, and opacification of the cornea, and vision loss.

pemphigus contagiosus Infection most often caused by pus-producing bacteria and manifested by a severe localized inflammatory pustular response. Report this condition with ICD-9-CM code 684. *Synonym(s): Manson's pyosis.*

pemphigus vegetans Rare form of pemphigus bulgaris, a chronic dermatologic disease manifested by serous fluid-filled vesicles, bullae in the outermost layer of the skin, and persistent erosions. The lesions are predominantly on the face and within body folds. Bare areas heal with enlarged warty granulations. This condition is reported with ICD-9-CM code 694.4. *Synonym(s): Neumann's disease.*

pemphigus vulgaris Most common, severe form of a group of chronic, relapsing skin diseases that may become fatal. Beginning around age 40, easily ruptured

bullae appear on otherwise normal skin and mucous membranes, spreading more generally and becoming large, open, weeping areas with some crusting, but no tendency to heal. The affected areas may cause sepsis, electrolyte imbalances, or cachexia and become fatal. Report this condition with ICD-9-CM code 694.4.

PEN Parenteral and enteral nutrition.

Pendred's syndrome Autosomal recessive goiter and congenital deafness as a result of a defect in pendrin, a protein involved in transport of chloride and iodide. This syndrome is reported with ICD-9-CM code 243.

penetrate Pierce.

penetrating wound Wounds resulting from a traumatic injury piercing the skin to the inside of the body such as a gunshot or stab wound.

Penfield's syndrome Epilepsy with unilateral clonic movements starting in one group of muscles and spreading to adjacent groups, following the movement of the epilepsy through the contralateral motor cortex. Report this disorder with a code from ICD-9-CM range 345.50-345.51.

-penia Indicates a deficiency, less than normal.

penile plethysmography Procedure that measures the physiological potential of the penis to attain and maintain an erection, using a plethysmograph, an instrument that measures variations in the volume of an organ or limb and the amount of blood passing through it or within it. The volume change of the penis is measured in response to external stimuli. Penile plethysmography is reported with CPT code 54240. *NCD References: 20.14, 160.26.*

penis Male reproductive and urinary excretion organ, the body of which is composed of three structures enclosed by fascia and skin: two parallel cylindrical bodies--the corpora cavernosa--and the corpus spongiosum lying underneath them, through which the urethra passes.

penis leukoplakia White, thickened patches on the glans penis considered to be precancerous lesions. Penis leukoplakia is reported with ICD-9-CM code 607.0.

PENS Percutaneous electrical nerve stimulation. *NCD Reference: 160.7.1.*

Penta X syndrome Pentasomy. Presence of three additional chromosomes of one type. Report this disorder with ICD-9-CM code 758.81.

pentamidine isethionate Inhalation solution used as a preventive treatment for pneumoocystis carinii pneumonia, a serious form of pneumonia commonly occurring in those with impaired immune systems. Supply is reported with HCPCS Level II code J2545. May be sold as brand name Nebupent.

pentobarbital sodium Injectable short-acting barbiturate used primarily as a sedative hypnotic or

O-R

anticonvulsant agent. Supply is reported with HCPCS Level II code J2515. May be sold under brand name Nembutal sodium solution.

pentostatin Injectable chemotherapeutic drug of the antimetabolite group used to treat hairy cell leukemia by interfering with the growth of cancer cells. Supply is reported with HCPCS Level II code J9268. May be sold under brand name Nipent.

PEP Post-exposure prophylaxis. Treatment, often with disease-specific immune globulin, is intended for a patient who has been exposed to a disease but has not yet contracted it. PEP is reported with codes from ICD-9-CM category V01.

PEPM Per employee per month.

PEPP Payment error prevention program. Program to help reduce Medicare PPS inpatient hospital payment errors.

per diem rate In health care contracting, payment made to the hospital from which a patient is transferred for each day of stay. Per diem rate is determined by dividing the full DRG payment by the geometric mean for the DRG. The payment rate for the first day of stay is twice the per diem rate, and subsequent days are paid at the per diem rate up to the full DRG amount.

per diem reimbursement In health care contracting, reimbursement to an institution based on a set rate per day rather than on a charge-by-charge basis.

per member per month One of two basic methods used to calculate a capitation payment. The amount paid for each covered member each month in lieu of another payment method such as fee for service. *Synonym(s): PMPM.*

per member per year In capitation, amount paid for each covered member over a one-year period.

per visit fee In health care contracting, flat-rate payment made to a provider for a single patient encounter.

perabduction syndrome Malignant atrophic papulosis. Report this disorder with ICD-9-CM code 447.8.

percent of premium In health care contracting, one of two basic methods used to compute a capitation payment. With percent of premium, a fixed amount calculated as a percentage of the average monthly premium paid by each plan enrollee is paid to the provider each month in lieu of another payment method such as fee for service.

percutaneous Through the skin.

percutaneous intradiscal electrothermal annuloplasty Procedure corrects tears in the vertebral annulus by applying heat to the collagen disc walls percutaneously through a catheter. The heat contracts

and thickens the wall, which may contract and close any annular tears.

percutaneous skeletal fixation Treatment that is neither open nor closed. In this procedure, the injury site is not directly visualized. Instead, fixation devices (pins, screws) are placed to stabilize the dislocation using x-ray guidance.

percutaneous transluminal coronary angioplasty Procedure used to treat coronary artery obstruction. A balloon catheter is placed in the affected artery and the balloon is inflated to flatten the plaque against the wall of the artery and open the obstruction. *Synonym(s): PTCA.*

Percutaneous Vertebroplasty

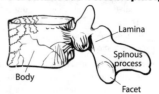

Lateral view of fractured body of thoracic vertebra

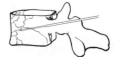

The fracture is injected percutaneously with methylmethacrylate cement

A percutaneous injection is performed on a fractured vertebral body, from one side of the lamina, or from both sides (bilateral). Report 22520 for an injection into a thoracic body. Report 22521 for a lumbar body. And report 22522 for injection into each additional thoracic or lumbar body

percutaneous vertebroplasty Minimally invasive procedure for treatment of vertebral compression fractures in which orthopedic cement is injected percutaneously into the fractured vertebrae. Report percutaneous vertebroplasty with ICD-9-CM procedure code 81.65 or a code from CPT range 22520-22522. *Synonym(s): PV, vertebroplasty.*

peregrinating patient Someone who fakes or grossly exaggerates a physical or psychiatric illness, apparently under voluntary control, to avoid work, military service, or prosecution, or to obtain financial gain or drugs. The behavior is recognizable and understandable in light of the individual's circumstances.

perforation Hole in an object, organ, or tissue, or the act of punching or boring holes through a part.

perfusion Act of pouring over or through, especially the passage of a fluid through the vessels of a specific organ.

Pergonal Injectable drug consisting of a mixture of follicle-stimulating hormone (FSH) and luteinizing hormone (LH), used to stimulate ovulation in instances when the ovaries are capable of producing a follicle but there is inadequate hormonal stimulation. This drug is also used to prompt the growth of multiple eggs for in vitro fertilization, as well as to stimulate sperm production in men who have inadequate hormonal stimulation but functioning testes. Supply is reported with HCPCS Level II code S0122.

peri- About, around, or in the vicinity.

periapical Anatomical area around the terminal end of a tooth root.

periapical x-ray X-ray of the terminal end of the root of a tooth.

pericardial window Incision made in the pericardium to create an opening large enough to allow drainage of pericardial fluid into the pleural space, reported with CPT code 33025.

Pericardiocentesis

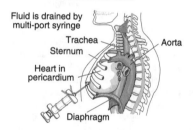

Fluid is drained by multi-port syringe
Trachea
Sternum
Aorta
Heart in pericardium
Diaphragm

pericardiocentesis Puncture of a cavity for the purpose of removing fluid from the pericardial sac.

pericarditis Inflammation affecting the pericardium.

pericardium Thin and slippery case in which the heart lies that is lined with fluid so that the heart is free to pulse and move as it beats.

perinatal death Stillborn births and neonatal deaths.

perineal Pertaining to the pelvic floor area between the thighs; the diamond-shaped area bordered by the pubic symphysis in front, the ischial tuberosities on the sides, and the coccyx in back.

periodic interim payment In health care contracting, payment method in which providers are reimbursed for services more quickly than in other arrangements. *Synonym(s): PIP.*

periodontal Relating to the tissues that support and surround the teeth.

periodontal pocket Inflammatory process of the gingiva in periodontal disease that results in deepened furrows around teeth.

periodontitis Inflammation of the tissue structures supporting the teeth leading to a loss of connective tissue attachments.

periodontosis Periodontitis occurring with the onset of puberty.

periorbital approach Surgical approach around the orbital area.

periosteum Double-layered connective membrane on the outer surface of bone.

periostitis Inflammation of the outer layers of bone.

peripheral Outside of a structure or organ.

peripheral nerve block Introduction or injection of an anesthetic agent into an individual nerve or nerve networks rather than all nerves as in an anatomical region.

peripheral neuropathy Known or unknown functional disturbance, disease process, or pathological change within the peripheral nervous system. It may be due to a noninflammatory lesion, nerve diseases, nerve injury or compression, or the result of another systemic illness such as diabetes, AIDs, uremia, or nutritional disorders.

peripherally inserted central venous catheter Catheter that originates in the basilic or cephalic vein in the arm and is threaded into the superior vena cava above the right atrium. A peripherally inserted central venous catheter is reported with CPT code 36568. *Synonym(s): PICC.*

periradicular Surrounding part of the tooth's root.

peristalsis Smooth muscle action of automatic contractions that propel substances through the body, such as urine into the bladder and food through the digestive tract.

peritoneal Space between the lining of the abdominal wall, or parietal peritoneum, and the surface layer of the abdominal organs, or visceral peritoneum. It contains a thin, watery fluid that keeps the peritoneal surfaces moist. *p. dialysis* Dialysis that filters waste from blood inside the body using the peritoneum, the natural lining of the abdomen, as the semipermeable membrane across which ultrafiltration is accomplished. A special catheter is inserted into the abdomen and a dialysis solution is drained into the abdomen. This solution extracts fluids and wastes, which are then discarded when the fluid is drained. Various forms of peritoneal dialysis include CAPD, CCPD, and NIDP. *p. effusion* Persistent escape of fluid within the peritoneal cavity.

peritoneocentesis Surgical puncture of the peritoneum with a specialized needle or hollow tubing to aspirate fluid from within the peritoneal space for diagnostic or

O-R

therapeutic reasons. This procedure is reported with CPT code 49080.

peritoneum Strong, continuous membrane that forms the lining of the abdominal and pelvic cavity. The parietal peritoneum, or outer layer, is attached to the abdominopelvic walls and the visceral peritoneum, or inner layer, surrounds the organs inside the abdominal cavity. The peritoneum is closed in the male and continuous with the uterine tubes' mucous membrane in the female. The membrane forms a double-layer sac with a space between the parietal and visceral peritoneum, the peritoneal cavity.

peritonitis Inflammation and infection within the peritoneal cavity, the space between the membrane lining the abdominopelvic walls and covering the internal organs. Peritonitis is reported with ICD-9-CM category 567. Pneumococcal, gonococcal, syphilitic, and tuberculous peritonitis each have a specific code for reporting the condition, other infectious agents identified as the cause are identified with a separate code, followed by an ICD-9-CM code from subcategory 567.0 for the peritonitis in infectious diseases classified elsewhere. Peritonitis is also a common and serious complication of a ruptured appendix.

periurethral fibrosis syndrome Retroperitoneal structures involving and often obstructing the ureters. Report this disorder with ICD-9-CM code 593.4. *Synonym(s): Ormond's syndrome.*

PermaCath Brand name catheter implanted just under the skin to gain access through a vein for kidney dialysis.

Permacol Brand name porcine dermal collagen implant used for hernia repair and other abdominal wall defects. Supply is reported with HCPCS Level II code C9364.

Perma-flow graft Brand name synthetic blood vessel used as a graft in coronary bypass procedures.

permanent tooth One of 32 adult teeth that usually erupt between 6 years and adulthood with the third molar.

Permapen Bicillin L-A Natural penicillin antibiotic that prevents bacteria cell wall formation during multiplication. It is used to treat syphilis and Group A streptococcal respiratory infections as well as for the prevention of postinfection streptococcal rheumatic fever. May be sold under brand names Bicillin L-A, Permapen.

pernicious anemia Chronic, progressive anemia due to Vitamin B12 malabsorption; caused by lack of a secretion known as intrinsic factor, which is produced by the gastric mucosa of the stomach. Report pernicious anemia with ICD-9-CM code 281.0.

pero- Indicates being maimed or deformed.

peroneal muscular atrophy Weakness and reduction in the size of the muscles of the hands and lower limbs, reported with ICD-9-CM code 356.1.

PERRLA Pupils equal, regular, reactive to light and accommodation.

persistent trophoblastic disease Local invasion of the myometrium by the villi of a hydatidiform mole, occurring in about 15 percent of hydatidiform moles. *Synonym(s): chorioadenoma, invasive mole, PTD.*

personal representative Someone who is legally authorized to make decisions related to health care on behalf of an individual. A personal representative may consent to or authorize the use or disclosure of another person's protected health information under certain circumstances, and may exercise the right of that other individual to inspect, copy, and correct protected health information in the possession of a covered entity.

personality disorders Deeply ingrained maladaptive patterns of behavior generally recognizable by adolescence or earlier and continuing throughout most of adult life, although often becoming less obvious in middle or old age. The personality is abnormal either in the balance of its components, quality, and expression, or in its total aspect. *affective p. d.* Chronic, intermittent personality disorder without clear onset that is characterized by lifelong predominance of a pronounced mood. *anancastic p. d.* Feelings of personal insecurity, excessive doubt, and incompleteness leading to excessive conscientiousness, stubbornness, perfectionism, meticulous accuracy, and caution with persistent checking in an individual who may also have intrusive thoughts or impulses. *antisocial p. d.* Disregard for social obligations, lack of feeling for others, and impetuous violence or callous unconcern and self-rationalization of behavior. *avoidant p. d.* Excessive social inhibitions and shyness, a tendency to withdraw from opportunities for developing close relationships, and a fearful expectation that the individual will be belittled and humiliated. *borderline p. d.* Instability in behavior, mood, self-image, and interpersonal relationships that are intense, unstable, and may shift dramatically. Manifested by impulsive and unpredictable behavior or expressions of boredom, emptiness, or fear of being alone. *chronic depressive p. d.* Affective personality disorder characterized by lifelong predominance of a chronic, nonpsychotic disturbance involving intermittent or sustained periods of depressed mood manifested by worry, pessimism, low output of energy, and a sense of futility. *chronic hypomanic p. d.* Affective personality disorder characterized by lifelong predominance of a chronic, nonpsychotic disturbance involving intermittent or sustained periods of abnormally elevated mood (unshakable optimism and an enhanced zest for life and activity). *compulsive p. d.* Feelings of personal insecurity, excessive doubt, and incompleteness leading to excessive conscientiousness, stubbornness, perfectionism, meticulous accuracy, and caution with persistent checking in an individual who may also have intrusive thoughts or impulses. **cyclothymic p. d.** Chronic nonpsychotic disturbance involving depressed and elevated mood, lasting at least two years, separated by periods of normal mood. **dependent p. d.** Passive compliance with the wishes of elders and others and a weak, inadequate response to the demands of daily life. The individual may be intellectual or emotional with little capacity for enjoyment. **Synonym(s):** asthenic p. d., inadequate p. d., passive p. d. **eccentric p. d.** Oddities of behavior that do not conform to the clinical syndromes of personality disorders described elsewhere. **explosive p. d.** Instability of mood with uncontrollable outbursts of anger, hate, violence, or affection demonstrated by words or actions. **histrionic p. d.** Shallow, labile affectivity, dependence on others, craving for appreciation and attention, suggestibility, and theatricality. There may be sexual immaturity and, under stress, hysterical symptoms (neurosis) may develop. **introverted p. d.** Profound defect in the ability to form social relationships and to respond to the usual forms of social reinforcements. Often referred to as loners who do not appear distressed by their social distance and are not interested in greater social involvement. **masochistic p. d.** Personality disorder in which the individual appears to arrange life situations so as to be defeated and humiliated. **narcissistic p. d.** Interpersonal difficulties caused by an inflated sense of self-worth and indifference to the welfare of others wherein achievement deficits and social lack of responsibility are justified and sustained by a boastful arrogance, expansive fantasies, facile rationalization, and frank prevarication. **paranoid p. d.** Excessive self-reference and sensitiveness to setbacks or to what are taken to be humiliations and rebuffs, a tendency to distort experience by misconstruing the neutral or friendly actions of others as hostile or contemptuous, and a combative and tenacious sense of personal rights that may be manifested as jealousy or excessive self-importance, excessive sensitivity, or aggression. **passive-aggressive p. d.** Aggressive behavior manifested in passive ways, such as obstructionism, pouting, procrastination, intentional inefficiency, or stubbornness often arising from resentment at failing to find gratification in a relationship with an individual or institution upon which the individual is overly dependent. **schizoid p. d.** Withdrawal from social and other contacts with autistic preference for detachment, fantasy, and introspective reserve that may include slightly eccentric behavior or avoidance of competitive situations. **schizotypal p. d.** Schizoid personality disorder manifested by various oddities of thinking, perception, communication, and behavior that may be manifested as magical thinking, ideas of reference, or paranoid ideation, recurrent illusions, and derealization (depersonalization), or social isolation.

PERT Pancreatic enzyme replacement therapy. Treatment to correct steatorrhea, diarrhea, and abdominal pain in patients with cystic fibrosis.

pertinent past, family, and/or social history (PFSH) Brief narrative of the past, family, or social history elements directly related to the problems identified in the chief complaint, history of present illness, or the review of systems.

pes planus Congenital condition in which the instep, or arch, of the foot does not develop, leaving the foot flat. Congenital pes planus is reported with ICD-9-CM code 754.61 and tends to be more severe than acquired pes planus, or fallen arch, reported with 734. **Synonym(s):** flat foot.

PESA Percutaneous epididymal sperm aspiration. Fertility procedure in which a needle is passed directly into the head of the epididymis and fluid is collected.

pessary Device placed in the vagina to support and reposition a prolapsing or retropositioned uterus, rectum, or vagina. Insertion is reported by ICD-9-CM procedure code 96.18 or CPT code 57160. Supply is reported with HCPCS Level II codes A4561-A4562.

pestis bubonica Highly contagious, most common form of plague, caused by infection of Yersinia pestis. It is characterized by onset of fever, chills, headache, and swollen, tender, inflamed lymph glands called buboes, which develop intravascular coagulation, turning necrotic and gangrenous. Report this condition with ICD-9-CM code 020.0. **Synonym(s):** black death, bubonic plague, glandular plague.

PET *1)* Pressure equalizing tube. Small tube placed through the eardrum to equalize pressure within the eustachian tube. Placement of PET is reported with CPT code 69433 or 69436. These codes report bilateral procedures. *2)* Positron emission tomography. **NCD References:** 220.6, 220.6.1, 220.6.2, 220.6.3, 220.6.4, 220.6.5, 220.6.6, 220.6.7, 220.6.8, 220.6.9, 220.6.10, 220.6.11, 220.6.12, 220.6.13, 220.6.14, 220.6.15.

Petges-Cléjat syndrome Polymyositis occurring with characteristic skin changes including rash on upper eyelids with edema, a rash on the forehead, neck, shoulders, trunk, and arms, and papules on knuckles. Report this disorder with ICD-9-CM code 710.3. **Synonym(s):** Unverricht-Wagner syndrome.

petit mal status Abnormal electrical activity in the brain resulting in a temporary disturbance of function during which there is a short-term absence of conscious activity.

petrositis Inflammation occurring in the petrous portion of the lateral region (temporal bone) of the skull.

petrous apicectomy Excision of the superior aspect or tip of the petrous portion of the temporal bone.

O-R

Peutz-Jeghers syndrome Formation of multiple hematomas. Report this disorder with ICD-9-CM code 759.6.

-pexy Fixation.

Peyronie's disease Development of fibrotic hardened tissue or plaque in the cavernosal sheaths in the penis. This causes pain and a severe chordee or curvature in the penis, typically during erection. Peyronie's disease is reported with ICD-9-CM code 607.85 and may need to be treated by surgical excision of the plaques with grafting, CPT codes 54110-54112.

Pfannenstiel's incision Horizontal surgical incision used in obstetric or gynecologic surgery that is made just above the pubic bones in the lower abdomen and curved to follow the natural skin folds so that the pubic hair will cover the scar.

PFC Persistent fetal circulation.

Pfeiffer syndrome Congenital abnormality caused by a genetic mutation in which the patients have craniosynostosis, a midface that is underdeveloped, prominent eyes, large toes, and wide thumbs. Visual disturbances and hearing loss may also be present. Pfeiffer syndrome is reported with ICD-9-CM code 755.55.

PFG Percutaneous fluoroscopic gastrostomy. Procedure in which fluoroscopic guidance is used to place a tube through the skin and into the stomach for patients who cannot take food by mouth, or for patients experiencing pressure in their stomach due to intestinal obstruction. Report PFG with CPT code 49440.

PFROM Pain-free range of motion.

PFT Pulmonary function test. Tests designed to evaluate a patient's lung function and capacity, such as spirometry measuring the amount of air inhaled and exhaled, bronchodilation responsiveness and bronchospasm provocation evaluations, or respiratory flow volume loop evaluating the volume of air remaining in the lung after exhalation. Pulmonary function tests are reported with CPT codes 94010-94799 and include the laboratory procedures and interpretation of test results necessary for carrying out the pulmonary service.

PFX Pseudoexfoliation. Deposits of white material on the anterior lens capsule, zonules, iris, ciliary epithelium, or trabecular meshwork of the eye, usually without significant disruption in the visual field. PFX can lead to glaucoma. Pseudoexfoliation of the lens capsule is reported with ICD-9-CM code 366.11.

PG Prostaglandin.

PGD Pre-implantation genetic diagnosis. Genetic testing of an embryo before in vitro fertilization.

Pgraph Penile plethysmograph.

PGS Persian Gulf syndrome.

PGU Postgonococcal urethritis.

PH Patient history.

phaco- Relating to the lens of the eye.

phacoemulsification Cataract extraction in which the lens is fragmented by ultrasonic vibrations and simultaneously irrigated and aspirated. *NCD Reference: 80.10.*

phago- Relating to eating and ingestion.

phalangectomy Excision of a bone of a finger or toe.

phalanx Bones of the digits (fingers or toes).

phantom limb syndrome Itching, dull ache, or sharp, shooting pains mimicking the nerves of amputated limb. Report this disorder with ICD-9-CM code 353.6.

pharmacological agent Drug used to produce a chemical effect.

PharmD Doctor of pharmacy.

pharyngeal pouch syndrome Hypoplasia or aphasia of the thymus and parathyroid gland with congenital heart defects, anomalies of the great vessels, esophageal atresia, and facial deformities result from aphasia or hypoplasia of thymus and parathyroid glands. Seizures may accompany most severe cases. Report this disorder with ICD-9-CM code 279.11. *Synonym(s): DiGeorge's syndrome.*

pharyngo- Relating to the pharynx.

pharynx Musculomembranous passage of the throat consisting of three regions: the nasopharynx is the passage at the back of the nostrils, above the level of the soft palate, and communicating with the eustachian tube; the oropharynx is the region between the soft palate and the edge of the epiglottis; the hypopharynx is the region of the epiglottis to the juncture of the larynx and esophagus.

PHB Pharmacy benefits manager.

PHCA Profound hypothermic cardiac arrest.

PhD Doctor of philosophy.

phenylephrine HCl Injectable synthetic sympathomimetic drug that works as a vasoconstrictor to shrink blood vessels. It is used to treat specific types of tachycardia and to prevent hypotension. Supply is reported with HCPCS Level II code J2370. May be sold under brand name Neo-Synephrine.

pheresis Process of extracting blood from a donor, centrifuging or separating the desired part of the blood, and transfusing the remainder back into the donor.

PHI Protected health information.

-philia Inordinate love of or craving for something.

Philtrum

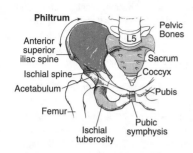

Philtrum — Pelvic Bones — L5 — Anterior superior iliac spine — Sacrum — Ischial spine — Coccyx — Acetabulum — Pubis — Femur — Ischial tuberosity — Pubic symphysis

philtrum Anatomical skin and flesh appearing as a vertical groove above the vermilion border of the median lip.

phimosis Condition in which the foreskin is contracted and cannot be drawn back behind the glans penis. Phimosis is a common medical reason for circumcision in the United States, and the most common complication of balanitis. Phimosis is reported with ICD-9-CM code 605. *Synonym(s): tight foreskin.*

phlebectasia Congenital abnormality of the peripheral vascular system manifested by dilation of the veins, reported with an ICD-9-CM code from subcategory 747.6.

phlebo- Relating to the vein.

PHN Post-herpetic neuralgia. Pain following a herpes zoster (shingles) infection. ICD-9-CM code selection for PHN is from subcategory 053.1.

PHO Physician-hospital organization.

phobia Broad-range anxiety with abnormally intense dread of certain objects or specific situations that would not normally have that effect. *acrophobia* Abnormal, intense fear of heights. *agoraphobia* Profound anxiety or fear of leaving familiar settings like home or being in unfamiliar locations or with strangers or crowds. Is almost always preceded by a phase during which there are recurrent panic attacks. *ailurophobia* Abnormal, intense fear of cats. *algophobia* Abnormal, intense fear of pain. *claustrophobia* Abnormal, intense fear of closed spaces. *isolated p.* Broad-range anxiety with abnormally intense dread of certain objects or specific situations that would not normally have that effect. *mysophobia* Abnormal, intense fear of dirt or germs. *obsessional p.* Subjective compulsion to carry out an action, dwell on an idea, recall an experience, ruminate on an abstract topic, or perform a quasi-ritual that may result in anxiety or inner struggle as the individual tries to cope with the behavior. *panphobia* Abnormal, intense fear of everything. *simple p.* Fear of a discrete object or situation, such as animals, heights, or small spaces, that is neither fear of leaving the familiar setting of the

home (agoraphobia) nor of being observed by others in certain situations (social phobia). *social p.* Fear of social situations such as public speaking, blushing, eating in public, writing in front of others, using public lavatories, or being in situations under the possible scrutiny by others with fear of acting in a fashion that will be considered shameful. *xenophobia* Abnormal, intense fear of strangers.

-phobia Abnormal fear of or aversion to.

phobic disorder Neurotic states with abnormally intense dread of certain objects or specific situations that would not normally have that effect.

Phocas' disease Multiple, benign cysts of the breast, colored brown or blue, caused by hyperplasia of the ductal epithelium. Occurs in women, usually after the age of 30. Phocas' disease is reported with ICD-9-CM code 610.1. *Synonym(s): Bloodgood's disease, Reclus syndrome, Schimmelbusch disease, Tillaux-Phocas disease.*

phocomelia Congenital abnormality usually occurring from ingestion of a teratogen, such as thalidomide, in which the upper part of an arm or leg is missing so that the hands and feet are attached to the body trunk like stubs. Phocomelia is reported with a code from ICD-9-CM category 755. *Synonym(s): seal limbs.*

phonophoresis Use of ultrasound to increase the diffusion of a drug into the skin.

PhotoAppeal Brand name YAG laser used in skin resurfacing.

photocoagulation Application of an intense laser beam of light to disrupt tissue and condense protein material to a residual mass, used especially for treating ocular conditions. CPT provides codes based on the laser's application purpose, such as for vitrectomy, to treat retinal detachment, destroy lesions of the cornea and retina, or for iridoplasty.

photodensitometry Noninvasive radiological procedure that provides a quantitative measurement of the bone mineral density of cortical bone mass by measuring the optical density of extremity radiographs with a photodensitometer, usually with reference to a standard-density wedge placed on the film at the time of exposure. It is used for monitoring gross bone change. *Synonym(s): radiographic absorptiometry.* **NCD Reference:** *150.3.*

photography Still image pictures that may be digital or film generated.

photon Particle of an atom having no mass and no charge; a quantum of electromagnetic radiation.

photopheresis Extracorporeal process for eliminating destructive elements from circulating blood stream. The blood is cycled outside the body through a specialized machine that exposes it to therapeutic wavelengths of

O-R

light and returns the treated blood to the patient. This process is reported with CPT code 36522.

photophobia Sensitivity to light.

photorefractive therapy Procedure involving the removal of the surface layer of the cornea (epithelium) by gentle scraping and use of a computer-controlled excimer laser to reshape the stroma. *Synonym(s): PKR.*

PHP *1)* Partial hospitalization program. *2)* Pre-paid health plan. *3)* Physician hospital plan.

PHPT Primary hypoparathyroidism.

phrenic nerves Two nerves that arise mainly from the fourth cervical nerve, providing motor nerve function to a side of the diaphragm, and serve in the breathing function. The right nerve plays a role in liver function. *NCD Reference: 160.19.*

phreno- *1)* Relating to the diaphragm. *2)* Head or mind.

PHS Public Health Service.

phthisis bulbi Shrinking of the eyeball following injury, infection, or disease.

physical status modifiers Alphanumeric modifier used to identify the patient's health status as it affects the work related to providing the anesthesia service.

physical therapy modality Therapeutic agent or regimen applied or used to provide appropriate treatment of the musculoskeletal system.

physically present Teaching physicians must be in the same room, or a partitioned or curtained area, as the patient and resident and/or perform a face-to-face service.

physician Legally authorized practitioners including a doctor of medicine or osteopathy, a doctor of dental surgery or of dental medicine, a doctor of podiatric medicine, a doctor of optometry, and a chiropractor only with respect to treatment by means of manual manipulation of the spine (to correct a subluxation).

physician assistant Medical professional who receives additional training and can assess, treat, and prescribe medications under a physician's review.

physician services Professional services performed by physicians, including surgery, consultations, and home, office, and institutional calls.

physician work One of three components used to develop relative value units (RVU) under the resource-based relative value scale. Physician work represents the value of the skill and time required to perform a service.

physician's assistant Medical professional who receives additional training and can assess, treat, and prescribe medications under a physician's review. *Synonym(s): PA.*

physician-directed clinic Clinic where 1) a physician (or a number of physicians) is present to perform medical (rather than administrative) services at all times; 2) each patient is under the care of a clinic physician; and 3) the nonphysician services are under medical supervision.

physicians at teaching hospitals Set up by the Office of Inspector General (OIG), initiative of the National Recovery Project targeting reimbursement practices at teaching hospitals, focusing on the use of residents and the services they perform under Medicare Part B that are paid as part of Medicare Part A. *Synonym(s): PATH.*

Physicians' Current Procedural Terminology Definitive procedural coding system developed and owned by the American Medical Association that is a listing of descriptive terms and identifying codes used for reporting medical services and procedures. *Synonym(s): CPT.*

physiologic studies Evaluation of bi-directional blood flow, blood pressure, plethysmography, or oxygen tension measurements using non-invasive, non-imaging Doppler.

physis Growth plate segment of bone.

PI *1)* Present illness. *2)* Patient information.

PICA Porch Index of Communicative Abilities. Standardized diagnostic test for aphasia.

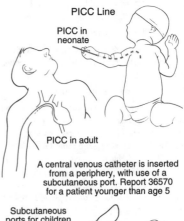

PICC Line

PICC in neonate

PICC in adult

A central venous catheter is inserted from a periphery, with use of a subcutaneous port. Report 36570 for a patient younger than age 5

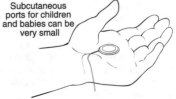

Subcutaneous ports for children and babies can be very small

PICC Peripherally inserted central catheter. The catheter is inserted into one of the large veins of the arm and threaded through the vein until the tip sits in a large vein just above the heart. The space in the middle of the tube is called the lumen. If a tube has more than one lumen, this allows different treatments to be given at the same time. At the end of the tube, which remains outside the body, each lumen is capped so a drip line or syringe can be attached. A clamp keeps the tube closed when not in use. Refer to CPT codes 36560-36571 for insertion of an implantable catheter; 36575-36585 for replacement procedures; 36589-36590 for removal; and 36595-36597 for other procedures on a central venous catheter device.

PICD Primary irritant contact dermatitis.

PICHI Pulse-inversion contrast harmonic imaging.

Pick-Herxheimer syndrome Atrophy of skin throughout body and of unknown cause. Report this disorder with ICD-9-CM code 701.8.

Pickwickian syndrome Obesity, hypoventilation, somnolence, and erythrocytosis. Report this disorder with ICD-9-CM code 278.03.

Pico-ST Brand name angiography balloon catheter for use in percutaneous transluminal angioplasty.

PICT Pancreatic islet cell transplantation.

PID Pelvic inflammatory disease.

PIE *1)* Pulmonary interstitial emphysema, reported with ICD-9-CM code 518.1. *2)* Pulmonary infiltration with eosinophilia, reported with ICD-9-CM code 518.3. *3)* Postirradiation examination.

PIE syndrome Pulmonary infiltration with eosinophilia. Transient infiltrations of lungs by eosinophilia, resulting in coughing, fever, and dyspnea. Report this disorder with ICD-9-CM code 518.3. *Synonym(s): Loffler's syndrome.*

Pierre Marie-Bamberger syndrome Symmetrical osteitis of limbs localized to phalanges, terminal epiphyses of long bones of forearm and leg, kyphosis of the spine, and affection of the joints. Report this disorder with ICD-9-CM code 731.2. *Synonym(s): Mankowsky's syndrome.*

Pierre Mauriac's syndrome Endocrine dysfunction causing diabetes and affecting growth and weight. Report this disorder with ICD-9-CM code 258.1.

PIFG Poor intrauterine fetal growth.

pigmentation Coloration.

PIH Pregnancy-induced hypertension. High blood pressure in pregnant women who do not have a preexisting diagnosis of hypertension. It most often begins in the third trimester of pregnancy and usually resolves after delivery. It is most common in first pregnancies and is reported with a code from ICD-9-CM subcategory 642.3. *Synonym(s): gestational hypertension, transient hypertension of pregnancy.*

Pillar procedure Minimally invasive procedure in which three small polyester implants are inserted into the back of the roof of the mouth (soft palate). Indicated for the treatment of upper airway obstruction in patients with mild to moderate obstructive sleep apnea (OSA), and/or the reduction of snoring caused by the fluttering of tissue in the soft palate. Combined with the body's natural fibrotic response, the implants eventually add structural support by stiffening the soft palate, thereby reducing the tissue vibration and collapse of palatal tissue that causes snoring and/or OSA. Report this procedure with CPT code 42299; hospitals report the supply of the implants with HCPCS Level II code C9727.

PillCam ESO Brand name esophageal video capsule. The swallowed device captures images that are transmitted to sensor arrays placed on the patient's chest. The PillCam ESO identifies gastric abnormalities. The use of PillCam ESO is reported with ICD-9-CM hospital procedure code 42.29 or 87.69 for inpatient use or with CPT code 91111 for physicians in outpatient or office settings.

PILO Pilocarpine.

pilomatricoma Benign follicular tumor containing features of the follicle matrix. Most often found in the head and neck area, these firm, button-like lesions are attached to the skin and underlying subcutaneous tissue. Report pilomatricoma with a code from ICD-9-CM category 216. *Synonym(s): Malherbe tumor, pilomatrixoma.*

pilonidal Containing a tuft of hair. *p. cyst* Sac or sinus cavity of trapped epithelial tissues in the sacrococcygeal region, usually associated with ingrown hair. *p. sinus* Fistula, tract, or channel that extends from an infected area of ingrown hair to another site within the skin or out to the skin surface.

pimel- Relating to fat.

PIN *1)* Prostatic intraepithelial neoplasia. Premalignant dysplasia or atypical hyperplasia of the prostate in which the cells are abnormal in shape and size. PIN I and PIN II are reported with ICD-9-CM code 602.3 as dysplasia, while PIN III is reported as carcinoma in situ of the prostate with 233.4. *2)* Physician identification number. *3)* In dentistry, a restoration retention aid consisting of a metal rod that has been cemented or driven into the dentin.

pinch graft Split-thickness skin graft very small in size.

pineal syndrome Precocious development of external sexual organs, precocious development of long bones, and hydrocephalus indicating lesion of pineal body. Report this disorder with ICD-9-CM code 259.8. *Synonym(s): Pellizi's syndrome.*

pinguecula Proliferation on the conjunctiva near the sclerocorneal junction, usually of the side of the nose and usually in older patients. Report pinguecula with ICD-9-CM code 372.51.

pingueculitis Conjunctival inflammatory condition that occurs when pinguecula form vessels and become red

O-R

and irritated. Report this condition with ICD-9-CM code 372.34.

pink eye   Acute contagious inflammation and irritation of the conjunctiva that normally occurs in the spring or fall and is caused by a variant of the H. influenzae bacteria. Report this condition with ICD-9-CM code 372.03. **Synonym(s):** *Koch-Weeks conjunctivitis.*

pink puffer syndrome   Acquired unilateral hyperlucent lung with severe airway obstruction during expiration, oligemia, and a small hilum. Report this disorder with ICD-9-CM code 492.8. **Synonym(s):** *Swyer-James syndrome.*

pinna   Outer portion of the ear attached to the side of the head that collects sound by amplifying and directing the sound waves into the external auditory canal.

pinning   Bone fastening.

PIOL   Phakic intraocular lens. Lens implanted in the anterior segment of the eye to correct nearsightedness. The eye retains its natural lens. PIOL placement is considered a cosmetic procedure.

PION   Posterior ischemic optic neuropathy. Less common type of optic neuropathy due to a serious shortage of blood supply to the posterior optic nerve causing damage to the nerve and vision loss. PION is reported with ICD-9-CM code 377.41.

PIP   *1)* Proximal interphalangeal joint. *2)* Periodic interim payment. Payment method in which providers are reimbursed for services more quickly than in other arrangements.

PIP-DCG Model   Principal inpatient diagnostic cost group. Initial risk adjustment model for capitation payments to Medicare Managed Care Organizations (MCOs), phased out in 2003 and replaced by the CMS-HCC model. The PIP-DCG model was based on data derived from inpatient diagnostic data and was limited by the fact that the data included only diagnoses that resulted in inpatient hospital admission. The PIP-diagnostic cost groups were similar to the inpatient diagnosis related groups (DRGs). Since the data did not include other diagnosis groupings not associated with inpatient admissions, payment for those cases was predicted based upon demographic adjusters only.

pipette   Small, narrow glass or plastic tube with both ends open used for measuring or transferring liquids.

Piskacek's sign   Asymmetry in a pregnant uterus before 12 weeks gestation. A normal condition seen as a sign of pregnancy.

pituitary dwarfism   Dwarfism with infantile physical characteristics due to abnormally low secretion of growth hormone and gonadotropin deficiency. Report this disorder with ICD-9-CM code 253.3. **Synonym(s):** *Burnier syndrome, GHD, growth hormone deficiency, Lorain-Levi syndrome.*

pituitary gigantism   Pituitary secretions causing gigantism beginning before puberty with eosinophilic cell hyperplasia, eosinophilic adenoma, or chromophobe adenoma. Report this disorder with ICD-9-CM code 253.0. **Synonym(s):** *Launois' syndrome*

pituitary gland   Hormone-controlling epithelial body located within the sella turcica at the base of the brain that secretes most of the body's hormones and regulates neurohormones received from the hypothalamus.

pityriasis nigra   Minor fungal infection caused by cladosporium mansoni or Exophiala werneckii, producing lesions that most commonly appear on the hands and rarely on other areas. The lesions look like the characteristic dark ink or dye stain that occurs when silver nitrate is spilled on the skin. Report this condition with ICD-9-CM code 111.1. **Synonym(s):** *cladosporiosis epidermica, keratomycosis nigricans, microsporosis nigra, tinea nigra, tinea palmaris nigra.*

PJRT   Permanent junctional reciprocating tachycardia. Nearly incessant tachycardia in a child, a condition that puts the patient at risk for developing cardiomyopathy. It is usually treated with laser ablation of the His bundle or accessory pathway.

pk.   Pack.

PKD   Polycystic kidney disease. Congenital condition in which multiple cysts form on the kidneys, impairing kidney function, often accompanied by chronic high blood pressure, kidney infections, and liver cysts. The various forms of PKD are reported with codes from ICD-9-CM category 753.1. **Synonym(s):** *PCKD.*

PKP   Penetrating keratoplasty. When performed for reasons other than refractive correction, PKP is reported with CPT code 65730 for patients with their own natural lens; 65750 for patients with no lens; or 65755 for patients with an artificial lens.

PKR   Photorefractive therapy. Procedure involving the removal of the surface layer of the cornea (epithelium) by gentle scraping and use of a computer-controlled excimer laser to reshape the stroma.

PKU   Phenylketonuria.

PL   Public Law, as in PL 104-191 (HIPAA).

placenta   Temporary organ within the uterus during pregnancy, joining the mother and fetus. It is attached to the fetus via the umbilical cord and provides oxygen and nutrients and helps to eliminate carbon dioxide and waste through the selective exchange of soluble substances carried via the blood. The placenta is expelled from the uterus after the baby is delivered, and is then termed the afterbirth.

O-R

Placenta Abruptio

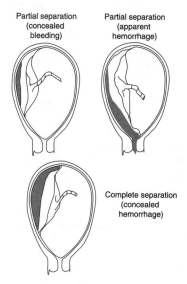

Partial separation
(concealed
bleeding)

Partial separation
(apparent
hemorrhage)

Complete separation
(concealed
hemorrhage)

placenta abruptio Partial or total detachment of the placenta from the site of uterine implantation prior to delivery of the fetus. The placental separation may be concealed with hemorrhaging confined to the uterine cavity, or it may result in blood escaping through the cervix. Symptoms include back and abdominal pain, vaginal bleeding, even shock. This condition is reported with a code from ICD-9-CM category 641.2, with fifth digits to indicate the current episode of care. *Synonym(s): ablatio placentae, abruptio placentae, accidental antepartum hemorrhage, Couvelaire uterus, placental abruption, placental apoplexy, premature detachment of placenta, premature separation of placenta.*

placenta previa Implantation of the placenta in the lower segment of the uterus, over or near the internal cervical os. In total previa, the cervical os is completely covered by the placenta; in partial previa, only a portion is covered. This condition is reported with a code from ICD-9-CM subcategory 641.0 if it occurs without hemorrhage and a code from subcategory 641.1 if hemorrhage is present. *Synonym(s): low implantation of placenta, low lying placenta, placenta centralis.*

placental dysfunction syndrome Fetal hypoxia and malnutrition resulting from lack of nutrition and oxygen transferred from mother. Due to degeneration of placenta and identified by yellow vernix. Report this disorder with ICD-9-CM code 762.2. *Synonym(s): placental insufficiency.*

placental transfusion syndrome Birth of one anemic twin and one plethoric twin due to forcing of blood of

one twin into other. Report this disorder with ICD-9-CM code 762.3.

plagiocephaly Form of craniosynostosis caused by premature fusion of one of the coronal or lambdoid sutures, resulting in asymmetry in the skull and face that is often described as lopsided. Plagiocephaly is reported with ICD-9-CM code 754.0.

plague Broad term for a group of bacterial infections caused by yersinia pestis, a genus of gram negative, facultative anaerobes, responsible for bubonic and pneumonic plague. The infective agent is carried by rats with the communicating vector between humans and rats being the infected flea of three main species: Leptopsylla, Nosopsylla, and Xenopsylla. Bubonic Plague starts with flu like symptoms such as fever, chills, headache and weakness, progressing to markedly enlarged lymph nodes, and concluding with vascular hypercoagulopathy causing gangrene and necrotic purpura. Pneumonic plague is a form of pneumonia marked by bloody productive cough, filled with the contagious bacteria. Septicemic plague references a severe infection in the blood during the acute phase of bubonic or pneumatic plague and can occur prior to the symptoms in some cases. Plague is reported with a code from ICD-9-CM category 020. Report V74.8 for plague screening. Vaccination against the plague is reported with V03.3. *Synonym(s): black death.*

Plan ID System for uniquely identifying all organizations that pay for health care services. *Synonym(s): national payer ID.*

plan manager Payer employee managing all of the contracts and contract negotiations for one or more specific plans.

plan of treatment Written documentation of the type of therapy services (e.g., physical, occupational, speech-language pathology, cardiac rehabilitation) to be provided to a patient and of the amount, frequency, and duration (in days, weeks, months) of the services to be provided. An active treatment plan must identify the diagnosis, the anticipated goals of the treatment, the date the plan was established, and the type of modality or procedure to be used.

plan sponsor Entity that sponsors a health plan. This can be an employer, a union, or some other entity.

plantar fascia syndrome Disorder of the fascia at the bottom of the foot. Report this disorder with ICD-9-CM code 728.71.

plantar fasciitis Inflammation of the tough band of tissue that connects the heel bone to the toes, with pain occurring along the inside of the foot. The pain is typically worse in the morning and with weight bearing.

plaque Accumulation of a soft sticky substance on the teeth largely composed of bacteria and its byproducts.

O-R

plasma Liquid portion of the blood, lymph, or milk.

plasma cell myeloma Rare form of cancer in which the bone marrow's plasma cells are produced at an increased rate, forming multiple bone marrow tumors and bone-destroying lesions that progress to other parts of the body in advanced stages. Symptoms involve bone pain, weakness, spontaneous fractures, anemia, fatigue, and hypercalcemia causing renal cast formation, nephropathy, and kidney failure. This condition is diagnosed by the presence of Bence-Jones protein in the urine. Report this condition with a code from ICD-9-CM subcategory 203.0. *Synonym(s): Kahler (-Bozzolo) disease, multiple myeloma.*

Plastibell Brand name male circumcision clamp device. It is intended for one-time use. Typically, its use is reserved for newborn circumcision, reported with CPT code 54150.

-plasty Indicates surgically formed or molded.

plateau iris syndrome *1)* Primary angle-closure glaucoma in the absence of classic pupillary block, identifiable by an angle-closure attack. Occurs in the presence of a patent iridectomy caused by an abnormality of the peripheral iris. Report this disorder with ICD-9-CM code 364.89. *2)* Post-iridectomy condition in which the relative pupillary block, important in causing angle closure, has been removed, but in which angle closure recurs without axial shallowing of the anterior chamber. This closure typically occurs in the early postoperative period but may also occur much later when the pupil dilates due to dilating agents or spontaneously. Report this condition with ICD-9-CM code 364.82.

platelet Disk-shaped structure found in the blood. Platelets are important for normal blood coagulation. *Synonym(s): thrombocyte.*

platy- Indicates wide or broad.

platybasia Congenital condition in which the skull base is flattened, caused by a deformity of the upper cervical spine and the occipital bone. Platybasia is reported with ICD-9-CM code 756.0. *Synonym(s): basilar impression.*

platysma Muscle originating from the neck region attached to the mandible that opens the jaw.

PLED Periodic lateralized epileptiform discharge. Repetitive paroxysmal slow or sharp waves denoting epilepsy, limited to one hemisphere of the brain, as seen on an EEG.

-plegia Indicates a stroke or paralysis.

pleio- More, additional.

pleiomorphic nuclei Term encountered in laboratory reports and immunology notes denoting a cell line found to have nuclei of various shapes and sizes (sometimes colors). This is a sign of irregular cell histology that can leave the cell or cells involved open to precancerous or cancerous changes. This has no direct bearing on coding. An abnormal histologic finding can be reported with ICD-9-CM code 795.39.

Plenaxis See abarelix.

pleoptics Treatment of defective eye coordination, vision, or function when there is no evidence of organic eye disease. It is less common than orthoptics because it is seen as having less of a scientific basis. Pleoptics and orthoptics training is reported with CPT code 92065.

plerixafor Injectable drug used in combination with G-CSF (granulocyte-colony stimulating factor) in patients with non-Hodgkin lymphoma and multiple myeloma. Designed to mobilize stems cells for transplant following high-dose chemotherapy, plerixafor may also be sold under the brand name Mozobil. Report the supply with HCPCS Level II code J2562.

plethysmography Recording of the volume changes in an organ or body part, particularly related to the amount of blood circulating through it. *NCD References: 20.14, 160.26.*

pleur- Relating to the side or ribs.

pleura Thin membrane covering the lungs and lining the inside of the chest wall.

pleural effusion Escape of water and lymph fluid into the pleural space. *Synonym(s): exudative effusion, pleural fluid.*

pleural pressure Negative pressure surrounding the lungs within the pleural space that is below atmospheric pressure during quiet breathing. During forced expiration when the abdominal muscles force the diaphragm, the pleural pressure can become positive and temporarily collapse the bronchi. *Synonym(s): Ppl.*

pleurectomy Surgical removal of a portion of the thin membrane covering the lungs.

pleurisy Inflammation of the serous membrane that lines the lungs and the thoracic cavity, reported with ICD-9-CM category 511. Pleurisy may cause effusion within the cavity or have exudate in the pleural space or on the membrane surface and is coded accordingly. Tuberculous pleurisy is not coded within the respiratory chapter, but to an ICD-9-CM code from subcategory 012.0.

pleurodesis Injection of a sclerosing agent into the pleural space for creating adhesions between the parietal and the visceral pleura to treat a collapsed lung caused by air trapped in the pleural cavity, or severe cases of pleural effusion. Pleurodesis by direct chemical injection is reported with CPT code 32560 and pleurodesis performed through a thoracoscope is reported with 32650.

PLEVA Pityriasis lichenoides et varioliformis acuta. Rare dermatosis that erupts suddenly and usually results in significant scars. PLEVA is reported with ICD-9-CM code 696.2. *Synonym(s): Mucha-Habermann disease.*

plexus Bundle of nerves that serve a particular region of the body that lies relatively deep in the body as opposed to superficial nerves, which are close to the surface of the skin.

PLGA Polymorphous low-grade adenocarcinoma. Uncommon and aggressive malignancy most commonly occurring in the salivary glands and palate. Diagnostic code selection would depend upon the site.

plica syndrome Pain and swelling of the knee joint and often a snapping sensation upon bending, due to a fold in the lining of the joint resulting from injury or overuse.

plication Surgical technique involving folding, tucking, or pleating to reduce the size of a hollow structure or organ.

PLIF Posterior lumbar interbody fusion. Arthrodesis to stabilize bones in the spine, reported with CPT code 22630.

PLMS Periodic limb movement in sleep. Measured by actigraphy.

plug (newborn) NEC syndrome Meconium obstruction of newborn's intestines, resulting from unusually thick or hard meconium. Report this disorder with ICD-9-CM code 777.1.

Plummer-Vinson syndrome Condition in middle-aged women with hypochronic anemia, marked by cracks or fissures at the corners of mouth, painful tongue, and dysphagia due to esophageal stenosis or webs. Report this disorder with ICD-9-CM code 280.8. *Synonym(s): Kelly syndrome, Paterson-Brown-Vinson syndrome.*

PM 1) Paramedic. 2) Program Memorandum.

PMD Progressive muscular dystrophy.

PMDC Pre-major diagnostic category. Eight DRGs to which cases are directly assigned based upon procedure codes before classification to an MDC, including DRGs for the heart, liver, bone marrow, simultaneous pancreas/kidney transplant, pancreas transplant, lung transplant, and two DRGs for tracheostomies. *Synonym(s): Pre-MDC.*

PMG Primary medical group.

PMHx Prior medical history.

PMI Point of maximal impulse. Point at which you feel the pulse the strongest, usually at the apex of the heart in the midclavicular fifth intercostal space.

PML Progressive multifocal leukoencephalopathy. Fatal nervous system disorder seen in immunocompromised patients caused by the JC papovavirus and affecting the cerebral cortex. PML is reported with ICD-9-CM code 046.3.

PMMA Polymethylmethacrylate. Bone cement that may be used for percutaneous vertebral augmentation, a procedure reported with ICD-9-CM procedure code 81.65 or CPT codes 22523-22525.

PMN Polymorphonuclear neutrophil leukocytes.

PMP Previous menstrual period.

PMPM Per member per month.

PMPY Per member per year.

PMR Polymyalgia rheumatica. Pain and stiffness of proximal limbs, neck, and back, most prevalent in the morning, accompanied by elevated sedimentation rate and temporal arteritis. It is usually seen in people 50 years and older. PMR is reported with ICD-9-CM code 725.

PMS Premenstrual syndrome. Hormonal disorder that manifests in symptoms of anxiety, emotional lability, edema, bloating, constipation, depression, headache, fatigue or lethargy, food cravings, and breast swelling and tenderness. PMS typically occurs from the time of ovulation until the onset of menses. PMS is reported with ICD-9-CM code 625.4. *Synonym(s): late-luteal phase dysphoria, premenstrual tension syndrome.*

PNB Pulseless, not breathing.

PNC Premature nodal contraction.

PND 1) Paroxysmal nocturnal dyspnea. 2) Post nasal drip.

PNE Peripheral neuroepithelioma. Uncommon malignant neoplasm of the peripheral nervous system presenting in older children and young adults. The ICD-9-CM code selected would be appropriate to the site of the tumor. *Synonym(s): peripheral neuroblastoma.*

PNET Primitive neuroectodermal tumor. Malignant tumor usually of the posterior fossa of the brain, but occasionally elsewhere in the brain. PNET is treated with surgery, radiation, and chemotherapy, and reported with an ICD-9-CM code from category 191, according to site. *Synonym(s): medulloblastoma.*

pneum(o)- Relating to respiration, air, the lungs.

pneumatic splint Splint filled with air or gas to provide circumferential protection and support.

pneumolysis Breakdown of tissue attaching the lungs to the wall of the chest cavity, causing lung collapse.

pneumonectomy Surgical removal of a lung or lung tissue.

pneumonotomy Surgical incision into a lung.

pneumoperitoneum Air or gas present within the peritoneal cavity and reported with ICD-9-CM code 568.89 as other specified disorder for the peritoneum, since there is no code specifically for pneumoperitoneum provided in ICD-9-CM. When this condition occurs in a newborn, it is reported with 770.2.

O-R

pneumoretinopexy Gas tamponade technique used to treat retinal defects. Follow-up care positioning is based upon the path of the gas bubble, which may be maintained over the retinal defect until healed. *Synonym(s): pneumatic retinopexy.*

pneumothorax Collapsed lung due to air or gas trapped in the pleural space formed by the membrane that encloses the lungs and lines the thoracic cavity. Pneumothorax codes are found in different chapters based on the cause. When it happens spontaneously, it is reported with ICD-9-CM code 512.8. When this occurs as a result of surgery, it is coded as iatrogenic, 512.1. Tuberculosis as a current condition causing pneumothorax is reported with an ICD-9-CM code from subcategory 011.7. Traumatic causes are found in category 860, and the congenital condition is reported with 770.2. *Synonym(s): postoperative pneumothorax.*

Pneumovax 23 Brand name pneumococcal polysaccharide vaccine provided in a single-dose or five-dose vial. Supply of Pneumovax 23 is reported with CPT code 90732. Administration is reported with HCPCS Level II code G0009. The need for vaccination is reported with ICD-9-CM code V03.82.

PNH Paroxysmal nocturnal hemoglobinuria. Acquired blood disorder with intermittent autodestruction of blood cells. PNH is reported with ICD-9-CM code 283.2.

PNS Peripheral nervous system.

PO By mouth; per oral.

POAG Primary open angle glaucoma. High intra-ocular pressure that can damage the eye, this chronic condition can usually be treated with medication. Ninety percent of glaucoma cases are POAG, which is reported with ICD-9-CM code 365.11.

POD Postoperative day.

pod(o)- Relating to the feet.

-poietic Indicates producing or making.

point of service plan Health benefit plan allowing the covered person to choose to receive a service from a participating or nonparticipating provider, with different benefit levels associated with the use of participating providers. *Synonym(s): POS.*

policy advisory group Generic name for many work groups at the Workgroup for Electronic Data Interchange (EDI) and elsewhere. *Synonym(s): PAG.*

pollen extracts Used in skin testing for pollen sensitivity and immunotherapy (desensitization) for pollen allergy.

pollicization Surgical creation of a thumb from another digit.

poly- Much or many.

polya anastomosis Anastomosis of the transected stomach to the side of the jejunum following gastrectomy. Report polya anastomosis with CPT code 43632.

polyarteritis nodosa Systemic necrotizing vasculitis of small and medium arteries that results in the infarction and scarring within the affected organs.

polyarticular Form of juvenile rheumatoid arthritis affecting five or more joints, reported with ICD-9-CM codes 714.30 or 714.31.

polycystic Multiple cysts.

polycystic ovary Fluid-filled sacs, or cysts, that accumulate on the ovaries. These are associated with increased levels of male hormones, absence of ovulation, irregular menstrual cycles, excessive hair growth, and other disturbances in the metabolism. This condition is reported with ICD-9-CM code 256.4. *Synonym(s): isosexual virilization, PCOS, sclerocystic ovarian disease, Stein-Leventhal syndrome.*

polycythemic syndrome Gaisböck's syndrome. Report this disorder with ICD-9-CM code 289.0.

polydactyly Congenital condition in which there are six or more digits on the hand or foot. This condition is reported with a code from ICD-9-CM category 755.0. *Synonym(s): hyperdactyly, polydactylia, polydactylism.*

polyhydramnios Excess amniotic fluid surrounding the fetus, typically defined as a total fluid volume of greater than 24 cc, reported with a code from ICD-9-CM subcategory 657.0. This condition may require therapeutic amniocentesis to reduce the fluid volume, which is reported with CPT code 59001. If polyhydramnios is suspected but not found, report ICD-9-CM code V89.01. *Synonym(s): hydramnios syndrome.*

polymethylmethacrylate Bone cement that may be used for percutaneous vertebral augmentation, a procedure reported with ICD-9-CM procedure code 81.65 or CPT codes 22523-22525. *Synonym(s): PMMA.*

polyneuropathy Disease process of severe inflammation of multiple nerves.

polyorchism Congenital anomaly in which there are more than two testes. Polyorchism is reported with ICD-9-CM code 752.89. *Synonym(s): polyorchidism.*

polyostotic fibrous dysplasia Fibrous tissue displaces bone and results in segmented, ragged-edge cafe-au-lait spots. Polyostotic fibrous dysplasia occurs in girls during early puberty. Report this disorder with ICD-9-CM code 756.54.

polyotia Congenital anomaly in which there are more than two ears, reported with ICD-9-CM code 744.1.

polyp Small growth on a stalk-like attachment projecting from a mucous membrane.

polyphagia Intake or ingestion of amounts of food excessive to the body's caloric requirements, reported with ICD-9-CM code 783.6. *Synonym(s): hyperalimentation, excessive eating.*

polypoid lesion Lesion with a stalk, usually removed with a snare or loop forceps.

polys Polymorphonuclear neutrophil leukocytes.

polysomnography Test involving monitoring of respiratory, cardiac, muscle, brain, and ocular function during sleep.

polysplenia syndrome Organs of left side of body are mirror image of organs on right side. Splenic agenesis and cardiac malformation are associated. Report this disorder with ICD-9-CM code 759.0.

polyuria Excessive urination.

Pompe's disease Rare genetic disorder caused by an enzyme deficiency. In Pompe's disease, the patient has a build-up of glycogen that causes progressive muscle weakness. Pompe's disease is reported with ICD-9-CM code 271.0. *Synonym(s): infantile acid maltase deficiency, Type 2 glycogen storage disease.*

pontic Artificial tooth on a bridge.

pontine syndrome Quadriplegia, anesthesia, and nystagmus due to the obstruction of twigs of the basilar artery, causing lesions in pontine region. Report this disorder with a code from ICD-9-CM range 433.80-433.81.

PONV Postoperative nausea and vomiting. Common cause of discharge delay or unanticipated hospital admission from ambulatory procedures.

pooling Health payers' practice of combining risk.

POP Progestin-only pill. Form of prescription birth control, taken orally. *Synonym(s): Mini-pill.*

POPmesh Brand name synthetic mesh for treatment of pelvic organ prolapse. Insertion of mesh during pelvic floor repair is reported with CPT add-on code 57267.

POR *1)* Postoperative recovery. *2)* Problem oriented record.

porencephaly Congenital central nervous system abnormality in which cysts or cavities are located in a cerebral hemisphere, usually evident shortly after birth. Symptoms include delayed development, poor muscle tone, spastic hemiplegia, seizures, and abnormally large or small head. Porencephaly is reported with ICD-9-CM code 742.4.

PORN Progressive outer retinal necrosis. Form of herpetic retinopathy seen in immunocompromised patients.

port film Images of radiation treatment residing in the body.

portable Movable.

Port-a-cath Brand name for an implantable system used for vascular access when the patient's treatment plan requires repeat administration of drugs (e.g., chemotherapy), fluids, and/or nutrition. This system may also be used for repeated blood sampling. Refer to CPT codes 36560-36571 for insertion of an implantable catheter; 36575-36585 for replacement procedures; 36589-36590 for removal; and 36595-36597 for other procedures on a central venous catheter device.

portal Entry point in the skin where radiation treatment beams enter the body and converge upon the field of interest.

portal hypertension Abnormally high blood pressure in the portal vein.

Porter-Silber test Test to determine corticosterone, a mineral important in sodium retention.

portoenterostomy Surgical procedure in which the jejunum is connected to the bile ducts and other portal structures of the liver and gallbladder. Report this procedure with ICD-9-CM procedure code 51.37 or CPT code 47701. *Synonym(s): kasai procedure.*

POS Point of service. Health benefit plan allowing the covered person to choose to receive a service from a participating or nonparticipating provider, with different benefit levels associated with the use of participating providers.

pos. Positive.

positron emission tomography scan Tomographic imaging of metabolic and physiological functions by imaging the path of photons that are produced when positron-emitting radionuclides react with electrons in body tissue.

post *1)* Postmortem exam or autopsy. *2)* In dentistry, elongated supportive device that is fitted and cemented into the root canal of the tooth, which functions to reinforce and retain crown restorations or other restorative material.

post. cib. After meals.

postartificial syndrome Menopausal symptoms suffered by some women following destruction of their ovaries, including chills, depression, hot flashes, headache, and irritability. Report this disorder with ICD-9-CM code 627.4.

post-audit Summary of an audit or the time following an audit.

postcholecystectomy syndrome Recurrence of gall bladder pain following removal of organ. Report this disorder with ICD-9-CM code 576.0.

postcoital bleeding Bleeding that occurs after sexual intercourse, coming from the vagina or cervix rather than the endometrium. Postcoital bleeding can be an indication of cervical or vaginal cancer, vaginal infections,

O-R

cervicitis, or polyps, and is reported with ICD-9-CM code 626.7.

postconcussion syndrome States occurring after generalized contusion of the brain that may resemble frontal lobe syndrome or neurotic disorders, and may include headache, giddiness, fatigue, insomnia, mood fluctuation, and a subjective feeling of impaired intellectual function with extreme reaction to normal stressors.

postconcussional syndrome Persistent personality disturbance of nonpsychotic origin following blow to head and featuring affective instability, bursts of aggression, apathy and indifference, impaired social judgment, and suspiciousness or paranoid ideation. Report this disorder with ICD-9-CM code 310.2. *Synonym(s): postcontusional syndrome, postcephalitic syndrome.*

postcontusion syndrome or encephalopathy States occurring after generalized contusion of the brain that may resemble frontal lobe syndrome or neurotic disorders, and may include headache, giddiness, fatigue, insomnia, mood fluctuation, and a subjective feeling of impaired intellectual function with extreme reaction to normal stressors.

postencephalitic syndrome Nonpsychotic organic mental disorder resembling the postconcussion syndrome associated with central nervous system infections.

posterior Located in the back part or caudal end of the body.

posterior cranial fossa Posterior cranial fossa supports both the occipital lobe and the cerebellum. It comprises the dorsum sellae of the sphenoid (anterior and medial), the petrous portions of the temporal bones (laterally), and the occipital bone (posteriorly). It is further subdivided into the internal occipital crest and cerebellar fossae.

posterior pigmentations of cornea Color deposits in the innermost layers of the cornea.

posterior symblepharon Adhesions between the eyelid and the eyeball extending into the fornix. May resemble a pterygium.

posterior synechiae Adhesion binding the iris to the lens.

posterior teeth Teeth that are located toward the back of the mouth, distal to the canines; includes maxillary and mandibular premolars and molars.

posteroanterior x-ray X-ray view taken from back to front.

posterolateral Located in the back and off to the side.

post-gastric surgery syndrome Emptying of contents of jejunum with nausea, sweating, weakness, palpitation, syncope, warmth, and diarrhea. Occurs after eating in patients who have had partial gastrectomy and

gastrojejunostomy. Report this disorder with ICD-9-CM code 564.2. *Synonym(s): dumping syndrome.*

posthepatitis syndrome Marked by persistent or relapsing fatigue not resolved by bed rest that significantly reduces daily activity. Causes listlessness, drowsiness, stupor and apathy following acute viral infection. Report this disorder with ICD-9-CM code 780.79. *Synonym(s): postviral (asthenic) syndrome.*

postherpetic syndrome Description of any symptoms of herpes arising in parts of body after an acute case of herpes. Report this disorder with ICD-9-CM code 053.19.

postinfarction syndrome Fever, leukocytosis, chest pain, evidence of pericarditis, pleurisy and pneumonia occurring days or weeks after a myocardial infarction. Report this disorder with ICD-9-CM code 411.0. *Synonym(s): Dressler syndrome.*

posting date Date a charge is posted to a patient account by the provider, frequently not the same as the actual date of service, but usually within five days of the actual date of service.

postleucotomy syndrome Changes in behavior following damage to the frontal areas of the brain resulting in general diminution of self-control, concentration, memory, intellect, foresight, creativity, and spontaneity, which may be manifested as increased irritability, selfishness, restlessness, slowness, dullness, loss of drive, and lack of concern for others.

postleukotomy syndrome Klüver-Bucy or postlobotomy syndrome. Report this disorder with ICD-9-CM code 310.0.

postmastectomy lymphedema syndrome Edema of arms and hands following a mastectomy requiring removal of adjacent lymph nodes. Report this disorder with ICD-9-CM code 457.0.

postmature syndrome Effect of placental dysfunction in the postmature newborn. Report this disorder with ICD-9-CM code 766.22.

postmyocardial infarction syndrome Fever, leukocytosis, chest pain, evidence of pericarditis, pleurisy, and pneumonia occurring days or weeks after myocardial infarction. Report this disorder with ICD-9-CM code 411.0. *Synonym(s): Dressler syndrome.*

postpartum Period of time following childbirth.

postpartum panhypopituitary syndrome Secretion of all anterior pituitary hormones is inadequate or absent after childbirth. Report this disorder with ICD-9-CM code 253.2.

postphlebitic syndrome Deep vein thrombosis with edema, pain, purpura, and increased cutaneous pigmentation, eczema dermatitis, pruritus, ulceration, and cellulitis. Report this disorder with a code from ICD-9-CM range 459.10-459.19.

postpolio syndrome Inflammation of spinal cord following polio. Symptoms vary. Report this disorder with ICD-9-CM code 138.

postprandial After meals. *Synonym(s): postcibal.*

postsurgical syndrome Hypoglycemia and malabsorption following surgery. Report this disorder with ICD-9-CM code 579.3.

postterm infant Neonate born after 40 weeks gestation. Postmaturity is reported in the infant's chart with a code from ICD-9-CM subcategory 766.2. Prolonged pregnancy is a post-term pregnancy that exceeds 42 weeks, and increases the likelihood of complications for the fetus and mother. A post-term or prolonged pregnancy would be reported in the mother's chart with a code from ICD-9-CM category 645.

postterm pregnancy Normal pregnancy of more than 40 weeks up to 42 completed weeks of gestation. Postterm babies may require no intervention if there are no indications of fetal risk. This diagnosis is reported with a code from ICD-9-CM subcategory 645.1.

post-transplant lymphoproliferative disorder Life-threatening complication of solid organ and allogeneic bone marrow transplantation. Featuring many of the traits of immune system malignancy, it is frequently associated with the Epstein-Barr virus and manifests as an uncontrolled production of B cells in post-transplant immunosuppression. Report this disorder with ICD-9-CM code 238.77 after first assigning a code from range 996.80-996.89 to identify the transplant complication.

posttraumatic brain syndrome, nonpsychotic States occurring after generalized contusion of the brain that may resemble frontal lobe syndrome or neurotic disorders that may include headache, giddiness, fatigue, insomnia, mood fluctuation, and a subjective feeling of impaired intellectual function with extreme reaction to normal stressors.

posttraumatic organic psychosis Generally reversible states characterized by clouded consciousness, confusion, disorientation, illusions, and often vivid hallucinations usually due to some intra- or extracerebral toxic, infectious, metabolic, or other systemic disturbance.

posttraumatic stress disorder Development of characteristic symptoms (re-experiencing the traumatic event, numbing of responsiveness to or involvement with the external world, and a variety of other autonomic, dysphoric, or cognitive symptoms) after experiencing a psychologically traumatic event or events outside the normal range of human experience (e.g., rape or assault, military combat, natural catastrophes such as flood or earthquake, or other disasters, such as an airplane crash, fires, or bombings).

posttraumatic stress disorder acute Brief, episodic, or recurrent disorders lasting less than six months after the onset of trauma.

posttraumatic stress disorder prolonged Brief, episodic, or recurrent disorders lasting six months or more following the trauma.

posttraumatic syndrome Amnestic dementia in which patient cannot remember short-term or long-term memories but is not delirious. Report this disorder with ICD-9-CM code 294.0.

postural proteinuria Excessive excretion of protein in the urine caused by the body position (standing to upright position), but with normal excretion when lying down. This diagnosis is reported with ICD-9-CM code 593.6. *Synonym(s): orthostatic proteinuria.*

postural reactions Adjustments of the body to gravity that are essential for normal functions.

postvagotomy syndrome Emptying of contents of jejunum with nausea, sweating, weakness, palpitation, syncope, warmth, and diarrhea. Occurs after eating in patients who have had partial gastrectomy and vagotomy. Report this disorder with ICD-9-CM code 564.2. *Synonym(s): dumping syndrome.*

post-void dribbling Inability to control urine flow after urination.

Potain's syndrome Dilation of stomach with indigestion. Report this disorder with ICD-9-CM code 536.1.

potassium hydroxide examination Diagnostic laboratory test used to detect a fungal or yeast infection of the skin. A scraping of the lesion is obtained, placed in a potassium hydroxide (KOH) solution, and examined under a microscope, where the fungus is visible if present. Report this test with CPT code 87220. *Synonym(s): fungal wet prep, KOH examination.*

potassium intoxication syndrome Excessive potassium, causing a number of symptoms. Report this disorder with ICD-9-CM code 276.7. *Synonym(s): potassium overload.*

POTS Postural orthostatic tachycardia syndrome. Orthostatic intolerance associated with increased heart rate, hypotension, dizziness, nausea, and fatigue, usually seen in young female patients. POTS is caused by a dysfunction in the autonomic nervous system. POTS is reported with ICD-9-CM code 427.89. Orthostatic hypotension is recorded secondarily with 458.0. Code also any neurological manifestations. *Synonym(s): chronic orthostatic intolerance.*

Potter's syndrome Renal agenesis with hypoplastic lungs and associated neonatal respiratory distress, hemodynamic instability, acidosis, cyanosis, edema, and characteristic facial features. Death usually occurs from lack of oxygen. Report this disorder with ICD-9-CM code 753.0.

O-R

Potts-Smith operation Side-to-side anastomosis of the descending aorta to the left pulmonary artery creating a shunt that enlarges as the child grows, reported with CPT code 33762.

Potts-Smith-Gibson procedure Side-to-side anastomosis of the aorta and left pulmonary artery creating a shunt that enlarges as the child grows.

pound Weight measurement. One pound is equal to 16 ounces or 452.59 grams.

Pow Powder.

POWERSAIL Brand name coronary dilatation catheter used in percutaneous intraluminal balloon angioplasty as a treatment approach for blocked coronary arteries. The procedure is reported with CPT code 92982 for one vessel and 92984 for each additional vessel. If performed with atherectomy, 92995 would be reported, with 92996 for each additional vessel. Inpatient procedures would be reported with ICD-9-CM procedural codes 00.40-00.43 and 00.66.

POX Point of exit.

PP Postprandial.

PPA Preferred provider arrangement. Similar to a PPO.

PPBS Postprandial blood sugar. Glucose measurement in blood after a meal. Commonly diabetic patients will be asked to test PPBS two hours after eating.

PPD *1)* Percussion and postural drainage. *2)* Purified protein derivative. Standard concentration of tuberculin derivative that is injected under the skin intradermally to determine tuberculosis exposure. For intradermal testing, report CPT code 86580. *Synonym(s): TB test.*

PPE Palmar-plantar erythrodysesthesia. Adverse effect of certain types of chemotherapy whereby leakage of the chemotherapeutic drug from the capillaries damages the surrounding tissues of the hands and feet, causing swelling and pain. Report PPE with ICD-9-CM code 693.0.

PPH Postpartum hemorrhage.

PPK Palmoplantar keratoderma. Callous patches of skin on the palms of the hands and soles of the feet. Acquired PPK is reported with ICD-9-CM code 701.1; congenital PPK with 757.39.

Ppl Pleural pressure. Negative pressure surrounding the lungs within the pleural space that is below atmospheric pressure during quiet breathing. During forced expiration when the abdominal muscles force the diaphragm, the pleural pressure can become positive and temporarily collapse the bronchi.

PPO Preferred provider organization. Program that establishes contracts with providers of medical care. Usually the benefit contract provides significantly better benefits and lower member cost for services received from preferred providers, encouraging covered persons

to use these providers, who may be reimbursed on a discounted basis.

PPP Protamine paracoagulation.

PPPD

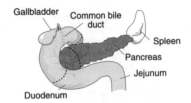

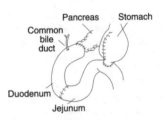

PPPD is an actonm for pylorus-preserving pancreaticduodenectomy, a procedure usually related to a pancreatic malignancy

PPPD Pylorus-preserving pancreaticoduodenectomy. Alternative to the Whipple procedure in cases of pancreatic cancer. Surgery includes duodenectomy, partial gastrectomy, choledochoenterostomy, and duodenojejunostomy.

PPS Prospective payment system. Reimbursement methodology that uses predetermined rates for each type of discharge, procedure, service, or item based on a standard type of case. For hospital inpatients, the Medicare PPS system of DRGs was implemented in 1983 to hold down the rising cost of health care. For hospital outpatients, OPPS has been based on ambulatory payment classifications effective August 1, 2000. For skilled nursing facilities, it is based on the RUG-IV system, and for home health it is based on the HHRGs.

PPV Pneumococcal polysaccharide vaccine. Supply of PPV is reported with CPT code 90732. Administration is reported with HCPCS Level II code G0009. The need for vaccination is reported with ICD-9-CM code V03.82. *Synonym(s): PPV23.*

PQRI Physician quality reporting initiative. Program includes an incentive payment for eligible professionals who satisfactorily report data on specific quality measures for covered services furnished to Medicare beneficiaries.

PQRS Physician Quality Reporting System: A voluntary CMS reporting mechanism used to measure physician

O-R

quality that will be mandatory as of January 1, 2015. Eligible providers submit quality data for set measures through approved reporting options.

PR Per rectum.

P-R interval syndrome Electrocardiographic disorder indicated by a short P-R interval with normal duration of the QRS complex. Report this disorder with ICD-9-CM code 426.81. *Synonym(s): Lown-Ganong syndrome.*

PRA *1)* Paperwork Reduction Act. *2)* Per resident amount.

practice expense One of three components used to develop relative value units under the resource-based relative value scale. Practice expense represents the physician's direct and indirect costs associated with providing a service.

practitioner Physician or nonphysician practitioner authorized to receive payment for services or incident-to services rendered.

-praxis Indicates activity, action, condition, or use.

PRBC Packed red blood cells.

preadmission and preprocedure review Review conducted by a quality improvement organization as defined by its contract with the CMS. For certain surgical procedures and scheduled inpatient services, the conditions must be reviewed and approved before they are provided.

preauthorization Requirement that approval for requested services be obtained before providing those services.

precertification Preadmission certification. Approval in advance of a procedure or hospital stay by a payer employee, who considers the diagnosis, the planned treatment, and expected length of stay.

precipitate labor Rapid labor and delivery marked by cervical dilation of 5 cm or more an hour in primigravida patients and 10 cm or more per hour in multigravida patients, reported with a code from ICD-9-CM subcategory 661.3.

precision attachment In dentistry, an interlocking device in which one component is attached to an abutment and the other is incorporated into a prosthesis (fixed or removable) to stabilize or retain it.

Precose Brand name oral medication exclusive to lowering blood glucose in Type II diabetics. Precose contains acarbose.

preeclampsia Complication of pregnancy manifesting in the development of borderline hypertension, protein in the urine, and unresponsive swelling between the 20th week of pregnancy and the end of the first week following birth in mild to moderate cases. Severe preeclampsia presents with hypertension (blood pressure greater than 150/100), associated with marked swelling,

proteinuria, abdominal pain, and/or visual changes. If untreated, it can progress to eclamptic toxemia and convulsions. Mild or unspecified preeclampsia is reported with a code from ICD-9-CM subcategory 642.4. If superimposed on preexisting hypertension, it is reported with a code from subcategory 642.7. *Synonym(s): mild toxemia.*

pre-excitation syndrome Pre-excitation associated with paroxysmal tachycardia or atrial fibrillation with a short P-R interval on EKG and an early delta wave. The normal conduction pathway is bypassed. This syndrome is reported with ICD-9-CM code 426.7. *Synonym(s): anomalous atrioventricular excitation, Wolff-Parkinson-White syndrome, WPW syndrome.*

preexisting condition Symptom that causes a person to seek diagnosis, care, or treatment for which medical advice or treatment was recommended or received by a physician within a certain time period before the effective date of medical insurance coverage. The preexisting condition waiting period is the time the beneficiary must wait after buying health insurance before coverage begins for a condition that existed before coverage was obtained.

preferred provider arrangement Program that establishes contracts with providers of medical care. Usually the benefit contract provides significantly better benefits and lower member cost for services received from preferred providers, encouraging covered persons to use these providers, who may be reimbursed on a discounted basis. *Synonym(s): PPA, PPO, preferred provider organization.*

preferred provider organization Program that establishes contracts with providers of medical care. Usually the benefit contract provides significantly better benefits and lower member cost for services received from preferred providers, encouraging covered persons to use these providers, who may be reimbursed on a discounted basis. *Synonym(s): PPO.*

preg Pregnant.

PreGen-Plus Brand name fecal DNA assay intended for use as a colorectal cancer screening test, reported with HCPCS Level II code S3890.

pregnancy Conception until the birth of a child, usually 40 weeks.

pregnancy ptyalism Excessive saliva production that is a rare side effect of pregnancy, reported with a code from ICD-9-CM subcategory 646.8 and code 527.7.

premature delivery Infant delivered with time of gestation less than 37 weeks.

premature ejaculation Form of psychosexual dysfunction in which ejaculation occurs before the individual wishes it, because of recurrent and persistent absence of reasonable voluntary control of ejaculation and orgasm during sexual activity.

O-R

premature infant Neonate born before 37 weeks gestation. A premature infant is more susceptible to complications. Prematurity is reported in the infant's chart with two codes from ICD-9-CM category 765. One code will provide information on birth weight while the second code identifies completed weeks of gestation. A diagnosis of prematurity must be documented by the physician and may not be assumed based on birth weight or gestational age. Threatened premature labor or early onset of delivery would be reported in the mother's chart with a code from ICD-9-CM subcategory 644.0 or 644.2.

premenstrual tension syndrome Monthly physiological and emotional distress during the days preceding menses with symptoms of nervousness, fluid retention, weight gain, and depression. Report this disorder with ICD-9-CM code 625.4. *Synonym(s): PMS, premenstrual syndrome.*

premium Amount paid by the insured and/or the employer or other group to cover the cost of the benefits provided by an insurance policy.

prentice orchiopexy Treatment of an undescended testicle in which an inguinal incision is made to move it to the scrotum.

preprandial Before meals. *Synonym(s): ac.*

prepuce Fold of penile skin covering the glans. *Synonym(s): foreskin.*

PRES *1)* Posterior reversible encephalopathy syndrome, reported with ICD-9-CM code 348.39. *2)* Progressive resistive exercises.

presbyophrenia Psychotic, chronic, mild states of memory disturbance and intellectual deterioration accompanied by increased irritability, querulousness, lassitude, and complaints of physical weakness associated with old age and brain damage classifiable as organic, senile, or presenile dementia, delirium, delusions, hallucinosis, and depression.

presbyopia Age-related visual impairment due to loss of elasticity in the crystalline lens and errors of accommodation that cause the near point of clear vision to be removed farther from the eye. Presbyopia is reported with ICD-9-CM code 367.4.

prescription benefit manager HMO staff that monitor amount and use of drugs prescribed. *Synonym(s): PBO.*

presenile dementia Dementia occurring usually before the age of 65 in patients with the relatively rare forms of diffuse or lobar cerebral atrophy usually caused by an associated neurological condition.

present illness Current problem, from the onset of symptoms to the time of the encounter.

present on admission indicator Single character appended to the end of certain ICD-9-CM diagnosis codes that indicates whether the condition was present at the time of an inpatient hospital admission. Valid indicators

are: Y (yes), N (no), U (no information in the record), W (clinically undetermined), and a blank or 1 (exempt from POA reporting).

presenting problem Disease, condition, illness, injury, symptom, sign, finding, complaint, or other reason for the patient encounter

pressure dressing Wound dressing used to apply pressure to the injured area, often used after skin grafting procedures.

pressure ulcers Progressively eroding skin lesion produced by inflamed necrotic tissue as it sloughs off, caused by continual pressure impeding blood circulation, especially over bony areas, when a patient lies still for too long without changing position. Report pressure ulcers with a code from ICD-9-CM subcategory 707.0. Report an additional code from subcategory 707.2 to identify the stage of pressure ulcer. *Synonym(s): bed sore, decubitus ulcer.*

presumptive identification Identification of microorganisms using media growth, colony morphology, gram stains, or up to three specific tests (e.g., catalase, indole, oxidase, urease).

pre-ulcer syndrome Excessive secretion of gastric juice either constantly or during digestion only. Report this disorder with ICD-9-CM code 536.8. *Synonym(s): Reichmann's syndrome.*

prevailing charge Charge at the 75th percentile in an array of weighted customary charges made for the same services in the same geographic area. This is the upper limit of charges deemed reasonable for Medicare reimbursement under Part B.

preventive medicine service Evaluation and management service provided as a periodic health screening and/or prophylactic service that does not typically include management of new or existing diagnoses or problems.

previa In obstetrics, placenta previa.

Prevnar Brand name pediatric pneumococcal conjugate vaccine provided in a single-dose vial. Supply of Prevnar is reported with CPT code 90669 or HCPCS Level II code S0195. Administration is reported with HCPCS Level II code G0009. The need for vaccination is reported with ICD-9-CM code V03.82.

PRG Procedure-related group.

priapism Persistent, painful erection lasting more than four hours and unrelated to sexual stimulation, causing pain and tenderness. This condition can occur in all age groups, and does not diminish following ejaculation. Causative factors include trauma to the perineum, penis, or spinal cord, and drug injection therapy. Secondary priapism is a result of obstructed venous outflow in the dorsal vein of penile vasculature. Priapism can often be treated with medication, although aspiration or shunting

O-R

may be required. Priapism is reported with ICD-9-CM code 607.3.

pricer Person, organization, or software package that reviews procedures, diagnoses, fee schedules, and other data and determines the eligible amount for a given health care service or supply. Additional criteria can then be applied to determine the actual allowance, or payment, amount.

primary Principal or first in the order of occurrence or importance.

primary care Basic or general health care, traditionally provided by family practice, pediatrics, and internal medicine practitioners.

primary care physician Physician who makes an initial diagnosis and referral and retains control over the patient and utilization of services both in and outside of the plan. *Synonym(s): PCP.*

primary cerebellar degeneration Hereditary neurologic condition characterized by uncontrolled movements of the extraocular muscles, internal paralysis of the eye muscles, and optic wasting. Report this disorder with ICD-9-CM code 334.2. *Synonym(s): Marie's cerebellar ataxia.*

primary diagnosis Current, most significant reason for the services or procedures provided.

primary localized osteoarthrosis Degenerative joint disease confined to a specific area.

primary or idiopathic syndrome Increased thickening of skin on extremities and face with clubbing of fingers and deformities in bone of limb. Report this disorder with ICD-9-CM code 757.39.

primary payer Insurance company whose coverage of the insured individual takes precedence (i.e., the company that is the first to pay) in the payment of a hospital or medical bill when two or more insurers may be responsible for paying the claim.

primary tooth Any of 20 deciduous teeth that usually erupt between the ages of 6 and 24 months.

Primaxin See cilastatin sodium, imipenem.

primigravida Female currently in her first pregnancy. *elderly p.* Female in her first pregnancy who will be 35 years or older at her expected date of delivery. Women in this category are considered to be at high risk during pregnancy. Elderly primigravida is reported with a code from ICD-9-CM subcategory 659.5. *young p.* Female who is pregnant for the first time who will be younger than age 16 at the expected date of delivery. Patients in this category are considered to be at high risk during pregnancy. Young primigravida is reported with a code from subcategory 659.8.

primip Primipara.

primipara Female who has delivered for the first time.

principal diagnosis Condition established after study to be chiefly responsible for occasioning the admission of the patient to the hospital for care.

principal diagnosis code Code that identifies the condition established after study to be chiefly responsible for occasioning the patient's visit to the facility for care. The principal diagnosis exists at the time of admission or develops subsequently and has an effect on the length of stay and the resources used to treat the patient.

principal procedure Procedure performed for definitive treatment rather than for diagnostic or exploratory purposes, or that was necessary to treat a complication. Usually related to the principal diagnosis.

principal procedure code ICD-9-CM code that describes a procedure performed for the treatment of an illness or injury and not for diagnostic, testing, or assessment purposes. The principal procedure is usually related to the principal diagnosis.

prinzmetal syndrome Chest pain secondary to large vessel spasm that may interfere with breathing. Report this disorder with ICD-9-CM code 786.52.

prion Abnormal infectious agent that can produce rare, progressive neurodegenerative disorders that can affect both humans and animals. Marked by long incubation periods and distinctive changes in the brain due to neuronal loss, prion diseases lead to brain damage and are typically rapidly progressive. Examples of prion diseases include Creutzfeldt-Jakob disease, fatal familial insomnia, Gerstmann-Straussler-Scheinker syndrome, and kuru.

prior-stay dates "From" and "through" dates provided by the patient or other facility to account for any hospital, skilled nursing facility, or nursing home stay that ended within 60 days of the current hospital or SNF admission.

PRITS Partial resection inferior turbinates, reported with CPT code 30140.

PRK Photoreactive keratectomy.

PRN Pro re nata. Latin for whenever necessary or as needed.

PRO Peer review organization. Organization that contracts with CMS to conduct preadmission, preprocedure, and postdischarge medical reviews and determine medical necessity, appropriateness, and quality of certain inpatient and outpatient surgical procedures for which payment may be made in whole or in part under the Medicare program. *Synonym(s): QIO, quality improvement organization.*

probing Exploration using a slender, often flexible rod.

problem focused physical examination Under the 1995 guidelines, an examination of one organ system or body area. Under the 1997 guidelines, examination of one to

O-R

five bullet point elements in one or more organ system or body areas.

problem pertinent system review Narrative of the organ systems reviewed related to the system identified in the chief complaint and/or history of present illness.

problem-oriented V codes ICD-9-CM codes that identify circumstances that could affect the patient in the future but are neither a current illness nor an injury. Use these codes to describe an existing circumstance or problem that may influence future medical care.

procedure Diagnostic or therapeutic service provided for the care and treatment of a patient, usually conforming to a specific set of steps or instructions.

procedure in detail Step-by-step report of an operation that includes the structures and layers of tissue involved as well as the length of all incisions and the size of all pertinent normal or abnormal structures.

process Anatomical projection or prominence on a bone.

proctectomy Surgical resection of the rectum.

procto- Relating to the rectum and/or anus.

proctosigmoidoscope Instrument used for examination of the sigmoid colon and rectum.

prodromal schizophrenia Seldom recognized term to describe a condition of eccentric or inconsequent behavior and anomalies of affect that give the impression of schizophrenia though no definite and characteristic schizophrenic anomalies, present or past, have been manifested. *Synonym(s): latent schizophrenia.*

prodrug Inactive drug that goes through a metabolic process when given resulting in a chemical conversion that changes the drug into an active pharmacological agent.

professional association plans Plan provided by a professional association that affords self-employed professionals (e.g., physicians, CPAs, lawyers) less expensive coverage.

professional component Portion of a charge for health care services that represents the physician's (or other practitioner's) work in providing the service, including interpretation and report of the procedure. This component of the service usually is charged for and billed separately from the inpatient hospital charges.

professional courtesy discount Accepting payment by a third-party payer as full payment without collecting co-pay or deductible or discounting services billed at a higher rate to a payer.

Profichet's syndrome Calcareous nodules in the subcutaneous tissues primarily around larger joints. The nodules ulcerate and exhibit nervous system symptoms. Report this disorder with ICD-9-CM code 729.90.

profunda Denotes a part of a structure that is deeper from the surface of the body than the rest of the structure.

progeria Syndrome of premature aging in a child. The child has an aged appearance along with small stature, loss of hair, thick and immobile skin, high-pitched voice, and infantile sex organs with a lifespan of 12 to 13 years. This syndrome is reported with ICD-9-CM code 259.8.

progeria syndrome Precocious senility with death from coronary artery disease occurring before 10 years of age. Report this disorder with ICD-9-CM code 259.8. *Synonym(s): Hutchinson-Gilford syndrome.*

Progestasert Brand name intrauterine device inserted through the cervix into the uterus by a clinician. Supply is reported with HCPCS Level II code S4989 and insertion is reported with CPT code 58300.

progesterone Steroid hormone, secreted by the corpus luteum of the ovary and by the placenta, that acts to prepare the uterus for implantation of the fertilized ovum, to maintain pregnancy, and to promote development of the mammary glands.

prognathism Condition in which the mandible protrudes abnormally with misalignment of the teeth; reported with ICD-9-CM code 524.10. *Synonym(s): extended chin, type 3 malocclusion, underbite.*

prognosis Forecast of the probable outcome of a condition or disease, and the prospects of recovery and disease residual, dependant on the nature of the disease and the patient's response to treatment.

Prograf Brand name immunosuppressant prescribed to organ transplant patients. Prograf contains tacrolimus.

program memorandum Communication from CMS to its contractors containing information about the Medicare coverage, claim processing, billing instructions, and operational management. The identifying scheme is X-XX-XXX. The first character is a letter that indicates the intended audience: A = fiscal intermediary, B = carrier, AB = both intermediary and carrier. The second two numbers represent the year that the PM was released, e.g., 03 = 2003. The last three numbers represent the sequence in which the PM was released, e.g., A-03-010 is the 10th PM released in 2003 for intermediaries. Most contractors simply reprint this communication on their own letterhead and release it to providers and suppliers.

program safeguard coordinator Contractor charged with maintaining the integrity of the Medicare program. Duties include data analysis, audit, review, and monitoring related to beneficiary information (such as COB data), medical review, cost reports, provider education, and fraud detection and prevention.

progress note Providers documentation of the encounter, treatment, or interaction with the patient and

O-R

caregiver and retained as part of the permanent medical record.

progressive pallidal degeneration syndrome Condition in which the nerves between the striatum and pallidum are completely demyelated. Report this disorder with ICD-9-CM code 333.0. **Synonym(s):** *Dejerine-Thomas syndrome, Hallervorden-Spatz syndrome.*

prolapse Falling, sliding, or sinking of an organ from its normal location in the body.

Prolieve Brand name transurethral thermodilation system using microwaves combined with compression to treat benign prostatic hypertrophy (BPH). The Prolieve device uses a balloon to compress prostatic tissue as microwave energy heats it, resulting in a reduction in prostatic tissue. CPT code 53850 reports microwave therapy, although there is no code specific to thermodilation. Check with payers to determine how to report appropriately.

proliferating capillary hemangioma (strawberry nevus) Most common type of hemangioma appearing as a firm, red, dome-like mark on the head or neck that grows rapidly and then regresses. It is composed of proliferating immature capillaries closely grouped within scant connective stroma.

prolonged physician services Extended pre- or post-service care provided to a patient whose condition requires services beyond the usual.

prolonged pregnancy Normal pregnancy that has advanced beyond 42 completed weeks of gestation. An increased risk of stillbirth, neonatal death, and neonatal seizures has been reported in cases of prolonged pregnancy. When no signs of postmaturity syndrome exist, the pregnancy may be allowed to continue; if there are signs, labor may be induced. Prolonged pregnancy is reported with a code from ICD-9-CM subcategory 645.2.

prolonged QT interval syndrome Potentially fatal condition precipitated by vigorous exertion, emotional upset, or startling moments due to an imbalance in the electrical timing mechanism that controls the pumping action of the heart's ventricles. This syndrome causes the patient to be susceptible to recurrent episodes of syncope, collapse, and possible ventricular fibrillation that can cause sudden death. Report this condition with ICD-9-CM code 426.82. **Synonym(s):** *long QT syndrome, Romano-Ward syndrome.*

PROM Premature rupture of membranes. When the fetal sac bursts and the amniotic fluid is lost, labor usually begins within 24 hours. In preterm cases, premature rupture is clinically significant and can cause mortality or morbidity complications for the fetus. PROM is reported with ICD-9-CM code 761.1 on the newborn chart and with a code from subcategory 658.1 on the mother's chart.

Pronation

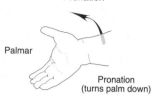

Palmar

Pronation
(turns palm down)

pronation Lying on the stomach or in a face down position; turning the palm toward the back or downward; lowering of the medial margin of the foot by an everting and abducting movement.

prone Lying face downward.

ProPAC Prospective Payment Assessment Commission.

prophylactic Agent or treatment measure intended to prevent or ward off a disease condition.

prophylaxis Intervention or protective therapy intended to prevent a disease.

ProQuad Brand name measles, mumps, rubella, and varicella vaccine provided in a single-dose vial. Supply of ProQuad is reported with CPT code 90710; administration is reported separately. The need for vaccination is reported with ICD-9-CM code V06.4.

prosencephalon Forebrain of the embryo.

proso- Indicates toward the front, anterior, forward.

prosopoanoschisis Rare congenital abnormality in which a facial cleft extends from the lip to the eye's inner canthus, usually separating the underlying bone. It may occur in conjunction with a cleft lip or palate, or with a lateral facial cleft. Report this abnormality with ICD-9-CM code 744.83. **Synonym(s):** *meloschisis, oblique facial cleft.*

prospective payment system Reimbursement methodology that uses predetermined rates for each type of discharge, procedure, service, or item based on a standard type of case. For hospital inpatients, the Medicare PPS system of DRGs was implemented in 1983 to hold down the rising cost of health care. For hospital outpatients, OPPS has been based on ambulatory payment classifications effective August 1, 2000. For skilled nursing facilities, it is based on the RUGs-III system, and for home health it is based on the HHRGs. **Synonym(s):** *PPS.*

PROST Pronuclear stage tube transfer. In vitro fertilization technique in which the fertilized egg is transferred to the fallopian tube before cell division occurs. PROST is reported with CPT code 58976. **Synonym(s):** *ZIFT.*

PROSTALAC Prosthesis with antibiotic-loaded acrylic cement. Temporary hip or knee prosthesis providing a functional spacer when a joint replacement must be

O-R

removed due to infection. The prosthesis keeps the internal wound from closing while the infection resolves. A subsequent surgery, months later, would place a permanent prosthesis.

ProstaLund CoreTherm Brand of medical device using microwave therapy to heat and shrink prostate tissue in patients with benign prostatic hypertrophy (BPH). The device accesses the prostrate with a transurethral approach. The procedure is reported using CPT code 53850.

ProstaSeed

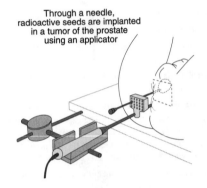

Through a needle, radioactive seeds are implanted in a tumor of the prostate using an applicator

Several seeds may be implanted at one session

ProstaSeed Brand name radioactive implants used in brachytherapy for the treatment of prostate cancer.

prostate Male gland surrounding the bladder neck and urethra that secretes a substance into the seminal fluid. *NCD Reference: 230.9.*

prostate cancer screening tests Test that consists of any (or all) of the procedures provided for the early detection of prostate cancer to a man 50 years of age or older who has not had a test during the preceding year. The procedures are as follows: A digital rectal examination; A prostate-specific antigen blood test. After 2002, the list of procedures may be expanded as appropriate for the early detection of prostate cancer, taking into account changes in technology and standards of medical practice, availability, effectiveness, costs, and other factors.

prostate hyperplasia Enlargement of the prostate gland from an abnormal proliferation of fibrostromal tissue in the paraurethral glands. The outer prostate glands are pushed against the prostate capsule, resulting in a thick pseudocapsule and as enlargement continues and the intracapsular pressure increases, impingement of the urethra results in obstructed urinary flow. This condition is reported with a code from ICD-9-CM category 600. *Synonym(s): BPH.*

prostatic hypertrophy Overgrowth of the normal prostate tissue.

prostatitis Inflammation of the prostate that may be acute or chronic. Symptoms include urinary frequency, urgency, and dysuria, often accompanied by pain in the pelvis, groin, or low back. Acute prostatitis is reported with ICD-9-CM code 601.0 and chronic with 601.1.

prostatosis Buildup of prostatic fluid causing congestion of the prostate. This is a benign condition, but can cause pain upon urination, frequent urination, or slowing of the urinary stream.

prosthesis Man-made substitute for a missing body part. *NCD Reference: 280.10.*

prosthetic Device that replaces all or part of an internal body organ or body part, or that replaces part of the function of a permanently inoperable or malfunctioning internal body organ or body part. *NCD Reference: 280.10.*

prosthodontics Branch of dentistry that specializes in the replacement of missing or damaged teeth.

Prostigmin Injectable parasympathomimetic agent used to diagnose and treat acute exacerbations of myasthenia gravis. It is also used to reverse the effects of neuromuscular blocking agents, and to treat ileus and urinary retention. Supply is reported with HCPCS Level II code J2710. Prostigmin contains neostigmine methylsulfate.

prostrate Recline on one's front.

prostration State of extreme exhaustion or collapsed in powerlessness.

protected health information Information that identifies an individual and describes his or her health status, age, sex, ethnicity, or other demographic characteristics. *Synonym(s): PHI.*

proteus Genus of gram positive, facultative anaerobes that are actively motile and often exhibit a swarming activity by spreading out across the top of a culture. The name is derived from the Greek god proteus, since these bacteria can take on many forms. They are especially prevalent in patients treated with antibiotics for urinary tract infections, with P. mirabilis being the most frequently encountered as the leading cause of UTI. They are also found in abdominal and wound infections and can cause septicemia, cystitis, meningitis, and pneumonia. Proteus are coded to the disease, with ICD-9-CM code 041.6 used to report the causative agent in infections classified elsewhere.

protozoa Subkingdom in animal taxonomy comprised of the simplest, single celled organisms, ranging in size from micro to macroscopic. They can live alone or in colonies, and do not show any differentiation in tissues. Most are motile and can live free in nature, but some

O-R

are parasitic, causing disease in the variety of hosts they inhabit.

proud flesh Large amounts of soft, edematous, granulation tissue that may develop during the healing of large surface wounds.

Provenge Brand name cellular immunotherapy vaccine currently in Phase II clinical trials for the treatment of prostate cancer. Outpatient administration of Provenge is reported with CPT code 96413 or inpatient ICD-9-CM code 99.28. Supply is reported with HCPCS Level II code J9999. Provenge contains sipuleucel-T.

provider Institution, entity, organization, or person that administers health care services. *p. identification number* Number assigned by CMS that identifies the provider (an institution, individual physician, clinic, or organization) of health care services. *p. statistical and reimbursement report* Report completed by the provider to reconcile costs and expenses, as reported on annual cost reports, incurred in treating Medicare beneficiaries. The PS&R report is required by Medicare for all fiscal years after October 1, 1987. Medicare accumulates all processed claim information in the PS&R reporting system. UB-04 revenue codes identify the bill types and types of services, and the PS&R identifies each reimbursement method used to pay for Medicare services (e.g., ambulatory surgery, radiology, laboratory, other outpatient diagnostic services, end-stage renal disease, orthotic and prosthetics, all other outpatient). Providers must ensure that UB-04 billing information is accurate because it affects the reimbursement the provider receives through the PS&R reporting system and cost-report settlement process. *p. taxonomy codes* Administrative code set for identifying the provider type and area of specialization for all health care providers. A given provider can have several provider taxonomy codes. This code set is used in the X12 278 Referral Certification and Authorization and the X12 837 Claim Transactions, and is maintained by the National Uniform Claim Committee. *p. self-disclosure protocol* Protocol, provided by the Office of Inspector General, that gives providers the opportunity to disclose any misconduct related to federal health care agencies whereby the provider may face a lesser restitution than had the information not been disclosed.

provider identification number Number assigned by the Centers for Medicare and Medicaid Services that identifies the provider (an institution, individual physician, clinic, or organization) of health care services. *Synonym(s): PIN, unique provider identification number, UPIN.*

provider number Number assigned by CMS that identifies the provider (an institution, individual or organization) of health care services.

provider of services Institution, individual, or organization that provides health care.

provider statistical and reimbursement report Report completed by the provider to reconcile costs and expenses, as reported on annual cost reports, incurred in treating Medicare beneficiaries. The PS&R report is required by Medicare for all fiscal years after October 1, 1987. Medicare accumulates all processed claim information in the PS&R reporting system. UB-92 revenue codes identify the bill types and types of services, and the PS&R identifies each reimbursement method used to pay for Medicare services (e.g., ambulatory surgery, radiology, laboratory, other outpatient diagnostic services, end-stage renal disease, orthotic and prosthetics, all other outpatient). Providers must ensure that UB-92 billing information is accurate because it affects the reimbursement the provider receives through the PS&R reporting system and cost-report settlement process. *Synonym(s): PS&R.*

provider taxonomy codes Administrative code set for identifying the provider type and area of specialization for all health care providers. A given provider can have several provider taxonomy codes. This code set is used in the X12 278 Referral Certification and Authorization and the X12 837 Claim Transactions, and is maintained by the National Uniform Claim Committee.

provider tracking system Identifies all individual providers and tracks all contacts made as a result of actions to correct identified problems such as eligibility, medical necessity issues, and repeated billing abusers who frequently change the way they code bills to their financial advantage. All fiscal intermediaries were required to have such a system in place by January 1, 2002. *Synonym(s): PTS.*

provider's self-disclosure protocol Protocol, provided by the Office of Inspector General, that gives providers the opportunity to disclose any misconduct related to federal health care agencies whereby the provider may face a lesser restitution than had the information not been disclosed.

proximal Located closest to a specified reference point, usually the midline.

PRRB Provider Reimbursement Review Board.

PRS Pierre Robin syndrome.

prune belly syndrome Congenital absence of muscles of abdomen and genitourinary anomalies. Intestinal outlines are visible on skin. Report this disorder with ICD-9-CM code 756.71. *Synonym(s): Eagle-Barrett syndrome.*

prurigo-asthma syndrome Several itchy skin eruptions of unknown cause accompanying asthma. Report this disorder with ICD-9-CM code 691.8.

O-R

pruritus Unpleasant itching sensation of the skin, caused by various conditions that evoke the desire to scratch the skin for relief. Pruritus is coded to the affected site or type in ICD-9-CM category 698.

Prussak's Pouch

Prussak's pouch is the space near the head of the malleus and a common site for cholesteatoma

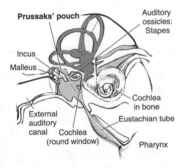

Prussaks' pouch
Auditory ossicles: Stapes
Incus
Malleus
Cochlea in bone
External auditory canal
Eustachian tube
Cochlea (round window)
Pharynx

Prussak's pouch Small space in the middle ear near the head of the malleus that is a common site for development of papillary ingrowth cholesteatoma.

PS 1) Pyloric stenosis. 2) Pulmonary stenosis.

PS&R Provider statistical and reimbursement report. Report completed by the provider to reconcile costs and expenses, as reported on annual cost reports, incurred in treating Medicare beneficiaries. The PS&R report is required by Medicare for all fiscal years after October 1, 1987. Medicare accumulates all processed claim information in the PS&R reporting system. UB-92 revenue codes identify the bill types and types of services, and the PS&R identifies each reimbursement method used to pay for Medicare services (e.g., ambulatory surgery, radiology, laboratory, other outpatient diagnostic services, end-stage renal disease, orthotic and prosthetics, all other outpatient). Providers must ensure that UB-92 billing information is accurate because it affects the reimbursement the provider receives through the PS&R reporting system and cost-report settlement process.

PSA Prostate specific antigen. Substance that is normally secreted by the prostate and is released in greater quantities found in the blood when cancer is present. Elevated PSA levels are one indication of prostate cancer, although benign prostatic hypertrophy (BPH) can also cause elevations. In a PSA test, blood is drawn from a vein in the arm and the levels are measured and reported as nanograms per milliliter. PSA testing is reported with CPT codes 84152-84154. Positive

results are reported with ICD-9-CM code 790.93. *NCD Reference: 190.31.*

PSAD PSA density. Amount of prostate specific antigen in a patient's blood. This can be useful in treating a patient with prostate cancer.

PSAV PSA velocity. The speed with which a prostate specific antigen value is increasing or decreasing; a health indicator in prostate cancer risk.

PSC Program safeguard coordinators.

pseudo- Indicates false or imagined.

pseudoaneurysm False aneurysm produced by a dilated vessel wall, or a ruptured blood vessel that has formed a clot that pulsates, mimicking a true aneurysm. For coding classification purposes, pseudoaneurysm is coded as an aneurysm to the site and/or type. The index entry directs the coder to aneurysm, for which "false" is a nonessential modifier. *Synonym(s): false aneurysm.*

pseudoarthrosis Pathologic false joint created by the deossification of a long bone, with subsequent bending and fracture and no formation of normal bone meshwork after fracturing. Report pseudoarthrosis with ICD-9-CM code 733.82.

pseudocarpal tunnel syndrome Pain and tingling, numbness, or burning in the hand as result of compression of median nerve by tendons. Report this disorder with ICD-9-CM code 354.0.

pseudocyst Enlarged, abnormal cavity resembling a cyst but without epithelial lining; a complication of acute pancreatitis, fluid and dead cell debris that collect within the walls of the pancreas.

pseudoexfoliation of lens Deposits of unknown composition and origin appearing on lens surfaces of the eye.

pseudohermaphroditism Presence of gonads of one sex and external genitalia of another sex. Report this disorder with ICD-9-CM code 752.7.

pseudohermaphroditism-virilism-hirsutism syndrome Possession of mature masculine somatic characteristics by a prepubescent male, girl, or woman. This syndrome may show at birth or develop later as result of adrenocortical dysfunction. Report this disorder with ICD-9-CM code 255.2.

pseudoinflammatory macular dystrophy Juvenile macular degeneration usually beginning between the ages of 20 and 40, resulting in vision impairment with possible color vision abnormality. This condition is inherited and progressive in nature. Report this condition with ICD-9-CM code 362.77. *Synonym(s): Sorsby's macular dystrophy.*

pseudomeningocele Pocket of cerebrospinal fluid (CSF) in the base of the neck, which sometimes extends into the upper axillary region and may denote a detachment

O-R

of a nerve root from the spinal cord. Pseudomeningocele can be the result of a CSF leak through a dural and arachnoidal rupture at the level of a lower cervical or upper thoracic neuroforamen, caused by a brachial plexus injury.

pseudomonas Large genus of anaerobic, gram negative bacteria, with more than 100 species, some producing toxins, responsible for causing diseases such as glanders or melioidosis, septicemia, pyogenic arthritis, and bacterial meningitis.

pseudoparalytica syndrome Progressive muscular weakness beginning in face and throat and caused by a defect in myoneural conduction. Report this disorder with ICD-9-CM code 358.00. *Synonym(s): Erb syndrome, Goldflam syndrome, Hoppe syndrome.*

pseudosclerosis of Westphal Rare, progressive, chronic disease caused by an inherited copper metabolism defect that results in the poisonous accumulation of copper in certain organs and tissues, such as the brain, kidneys, cornea, and liver. The disease causes cirrhosis, brain degeneration with progressive neurological dysfunction, and pigmented Kayser-Fleischer corneal ring. Report this condition with ICD-9-CM code 275.1. *Synonym(s): familial hepatitis, hepatolenticular degeneration, Kinnier Wilson's disease, Westphal-Struempell disease, Wilson's disease.*

pseudotumor cerebri Condition manifested by cerebral edema and fluid retention in the brain cavities, causing increased intracranial pressure with headache, nausea, vomiting, and papilledema, often no neurological signs present, although sixth-nerve palsy can occur. This condition is reported as benign intracranial hypertension, ICD-9-CM code 348.2. *Synonym(s): benign intracranial hypertension, meningeal hydrops intracranial hypertension.*

pseudo-Turner's syndrome Congenital disorder with short stature, mental retardation, and a webbed neck but, unlike Turner's, patients can be of either sex and have normal chromosomes and no renal abnormalities. Report this disorder with ICD-9-CM code 759.89. *Synonym(s): Bonnevie-Ullrich syndrome.*

PSM Presystolic murmur. Heart murmur at the end of ventricular diastole, during atrial systole. PSM may be due to an obstruction at an atrioventricular orifice. Typically, coding should focus on the cause of the murmur.

PSMS Physical Self Maintenance Scale. Tool to assess the functional abilities of patients age 60 or older. The functions tested include ambulation, toilet, feeding, grooming, dressing, and bathing.

psoas Muscles of the loins, the part of the side and back between the ribs and the pelvis.

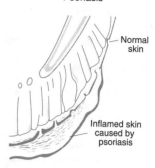

Psoriasis

Normal skin

Inflamed skin caused by psoriasis

psoriasis Chronic desquamating skin disease characterized by raised, rounded erythematous lesions covered by dry, silvery scaling patches. Psoriasis may affect any area of the body but most commonly is found on the scalp, elbows, knees, hands, feet, and genitals. There are many forms of the disease, but all of these are coded to ICD-9-CM subcategory 696.1, with the exception of psoriatic arthritis or psoriatic arthropathy, a genetically driven autoimmune disease affecting large and small joints, coded to subcategory 696.0. *Synonym(s): erythrodermic psoriasis, guttate psoriasis, nail psoriasis, plaque psoriasis, pustular psoriasis. NCD Reference: 250.1.*

psoriasis plaque Rounded, circumscribed, erythematous lesion on the skin that is slightly elevated and covered by a patch of silvery scales.

PSP Phenolsulfonphthalein.

PSVT Paroxysmal supraventricular tachycardia.

psychalgia Pains of mental origin, such as headache or backache, for which a more precise medical or psychiatric diagnosis cannot be made.

psychiatric hospital Specialized institution that provides, under the supervision of physicians, services for the diagnosis and treatment of mentally ill persons.

psychic factors associated with physical diseases Mild mental disturbances or psychic factors of any type thought to have played a major part in the etiology of physical conditions that usually involve tissue damage but that may include asthma, dermatitis, eczema, duodenal ulcer, ulcerative colitis, and urticaria. Describes conditions not classifiable elsewhere.

psychic shock Sudden disturbance of mental equilibrium produced by strong emotional response to physical or mental stress.

psychogenic amnesia Sudden onset of dissociative hysteria in the absence of an organic mental disorder where there is a temporary disturbance in the ability to recall important personal information that has already

O-R

been registered and stored in memory that is greater than ordinary forgetfulness.

psychogenic asthenia Neurotic disorder characterized by fatigue, irritability, headache, depression, insomnia, difficulty in concentrating, and lack of capacity for enjoyment (anhedonia).

psychogenic confusion Psychological factors usually provoked by emotional stress, causing symptoms such as clouded consciousness, mild to moderate disorientation, and diminished accessibility, often accompanied by excessive activity.

psychogenic excitation Psychological factors usually provoked by emotional stress, causing affective psychosis, with symptoms similar to manic-depressive psychosis, manic type.

psychogenic fugue Rapid onset form of dissociative hysteria characterized by an episode of wandering with the inability to recall one's prior identity, followed by a quick recovery and no recollection of events that took place during the fugue state.

psychogenic stupor Psychotic condition that is largely or entirely attributable to a recent life experience.

psychoneurosis Mental disorders without any demonstrable organic basis in which the individual may have considerable insight and has unimpaired reality testing, in that he or she usually does not confuse his morbid subjective experiences and fantasies with external reality and usually remains within socially acceptable limits. Manifestations include excessive anxiety, hysterical symptoms, phobias, obsessional and compulsive symptoms, and depression.

psycho-organic syndrome Generally reversible states characterized by clouded consciousness, confusion, disorientation, illusions, and often vivid hallucinations usually due to some intra- or extracerebral toxic, infectious, metabolic, or other systemic disturbance and are generally reversible.

psychopathic constitutional state Deeply ingrained maladaptive patterns of behavior generally recognizable by adolescence or earlier and continuing throughout most of adult life, although often becoming less obvious in middle or old age. The personality is abnormal either in the balance of its components, quality, and expression, or in its total aspect.

psychopathic personality Deeply ingrained maladaptive patterns of behavior generally recognizable by adolescence or earlier and continuing throughout most of adult life, although often becoming less obvious in middle or old age. The personality is abnormal either in the balance of its components, quality, and expression, or in its total aspect.

psychophysiological disorders Various physical symptoms or types of physiological malfunctions of mental origin, usually manifested in the autonomic nervous system.

psychosexual dysfunctions Recurrent and persistent dysfunction encountered during sexual activity that may be lifelong or acquired, generalized or situational, and total or partial. *functional dyspareunia* Recurrent and persistent genital pain associated with coitus. *functional vaginismus* Recurrent and persistent involuntary spasm of the musculature of the outer one-third of the vagina that interferes with sexual activity. *gender identity disorder* Preferring to be of the other sex and strongly preferring the clothes, toys, activities, and companionship of the other sex. May include cross-dressing in children or adults. *inhibited female orgasm* Recurrent and persistent inhibition of the female orgasm as manifested by a delay or absence of orgasm following a normal sexual excitement phase during sexual activity. *inhibited male orgasm* Recurrent and persistent inhibition of the male orgasm as manifested by a delay or absence of either the emission or ejaculation phases or, more usually, both, following an adequate phase of sexual excitement. *inhibited sexual desire* Persistent inhibition of desire for engaging in a particular form of sexual activity. *inhibited sexual excitement* Recurrent and persistent inhibition of sexual excitement during sexual activity, manifested either by partial or complete failure to attain or maintain erection until completion of the sexual act (impotence), or partial or complete failure to attain or maintain the lubrication-swelling response of sexual excitement until completion of the sexual act (frigidity). *premature ejaculation* Ejaculation that occurs before the individual wishes it, because of recurrent and persistent absence of reasonable voluntary control of ejaculation and orgasm during sexual activity. *psychosexual gender identity disorders* Behavior occurring in preadolescents of immature psychosexuality, or in adults, in which there is incongruity between the individual's anatomic sex and gender identity. *transsexualism* Fixed belief that the overt anatomical sex is wrong, resulting in behavior that is directed toward either changing the sexual organs by operation or completely concealing the anatomical sex by adopting both the dress and behavior of the opposite sex.

psychosexual gender identity disorder Form of psychosexual dysfunction in which there is behavior occurring in preadolescents of immature psychosexuality, or in adults, in which there is incongruity between the individual's anatomic sex and gender identity.

psychosis Impairment of mental function that has progressed to a degree that interferes grossly with insight, ability to meet some ordinary demands of life, or to maintain adequate contact with reality. *acute p.* Affective psychosis with symptoms similar to manic-depressive psychosis, manic type, but apparently

O-R

provoked by emotional stress. *affective p.* Severe disturbance of mood or emotion that adversely affects the thinking process. May be accompanied by delusions or hallucinations. *alcoholic p.* Organic psychotic states due mainly to excessive consumption of alcohol that may be exacerbated by nutritional defects. *atypical childhood p.* Atypical infantile psychosis manifested by stereotyped repetitive movements, hyperkinesis, self-injury, retarded speech development, echolalia, or impaired social relationships that is particularly common in those with mental retardation and is not as severe as infantile autism. *Synonym(s): borderline p. of childhood.* *child p.* Group of disorders in children, characterized by distortions in the timing, rate, and sequence of many psychological functions involving language development and social relations in which the severe qualitative abnormalities are not normal for any stage of development. *disintegrative p.* Congenital or acquired condition in which normal or near-normal development for the first few years is followed by the rapid loss of social skills and of speech, together with a severe disorder of emotions, behavior, overactivity, repetitive motion, and relationship problems. *epileptic p.* Organic psychotic condition associated with epilepsy. *excitative type p.* Affective psychosis with symptoms similar to manic-depressive psychosis, manic type, but apparently provoked by emotional stress. *hypomanic p.* States of elation or excitement out of keeping with the individual's circumstances and varying from enhanced liveliness (hypomania) to violent, almost uncontrollable, excitement. Aggression and anger, flight of ideas, distractibility, impaired judgment, and grandiose ideas are common. *hysterical p.* Psychotic condition that is largely or entirely attributable to a recent life experience. *induced p.* Mainly delusional psychosis, usually chronic and often without florid features, that appears to have developed as a result of a close, if not dependent, relationship with another person who already has an established similar psychosis. *infantile p.* Syndrome beginning in the first 30 months of life affecting interaction with others, characterized by abnormal response to auditory and visual stimuli accompanied by difficulty understanding spoken language and limiting the ability to communicate or develop social skills. *infective p.* Generally reversible states characterized by clouded consciousness, confusion, disorientation, illusions, and often vivid hallucinations usually due to some intra- or extracerebral toxic, infectious, metabolic, or other systemic disturbance. *Korsakoff's alcoholic p.* Syndrome of prominent and lasting reduction of memory span, including striking loss of recent memory, disordered time appreciation, and confabulation, occurring in alcoholics as the sequel to an acute alcoholic psychosis or, more rarely, in the course of chronic alcoholism. It is usually accompanied by peripheral neuritis and may be associated with Wernicke's

encephalopathy. *Korsakoff's nonalcoholic p.* Syndrome of prominent and lasting reduction of memory span, including striking loss of recent memory, disordered time appreciation, and confabulation frequently caused by substance abuse and malnutrition. An amnestic syndrome may be present in early states of presenile and senile dementia, arteriosclerotic dementia, and in encephalitis and other inflammatory and degenerative diseases and certain temporal lobe tumors. *manic-depressive p.* Severe disturbance of mood or emotion that adversely affects the thinking process and that may be accompanied by delusions or hallucinations. *paranoid chronic p.* Rare chronic psychosis in which logically constructed systematized delusions of grandeur, persecution, or somatic abnormality have developed gradually without concomitant hallucinations or the schizophrenic type of disordered thinking. *paranoid psychogenic acute p.* Paranoid states apparently provoked by some emotional stress such as imprisonment, immigration, or strange and threatening environments. Frequently manifested as an attack or threat. *postpartum p.* Any psychosis occurring within a fixed period (approximately 90 days) after childbirth. *Synonym(s): puerperal p.* *psychogenic depressive p.* Depressive psychosis with severe behavioral disturbance, apparently provoked by saddening stress such as a bereavement or a severe disappointment or frustration. The delusions are more often understandable in the context of life experiences. *reactive brief p.* Florid psychosis of at least a few hours' duration but lasting no more than two weeks, with sudden onset immediately following a severe environmental stress and eventually terminating in complete recovery to the pre-psychotic state. *reactive confusional p.* Mental disorders with clouded consciousness, mild to moderate disorientation, and diminished accessibility often accompanied by excessive activity and apparently provoked by emotional stress. *reactive depressive p.* Depressive psychosis with severe behavioral disturbance, apparently provoked by saddening stress such as a bereavement or a severe disappointment or frustration. The delusions are more often understandable in the context of life experiences. *schizoaffective p.* Pronounced affective manic or depressive features are intermingled with schizophrenic features that tend toward remission without permanent defect but that are prone to recur. *schizophrenic p.* Fundamental disturbance of personality, and characteristic distortion of thinking, often a sense of being controlled by alien forces, delusions, disturbed perception, abnormal affect out of keeping with the real situation, and auditory or visual hallucinations with fear that intimate thoughts, feelings, and acts are known by others although clear consciousness and intellectual capacity are usually maintained. *senile p.* Progressive type of senile dementia characterized by development in advanced old age, with delusions, varying from simple,

O-R

poorly formed paranoid delusions to highly formed paranoid delusional states, and hallucinations.

psychosomatic disorders Variety of physical symptoms or types of physiological malfunctions of mental origin, usually manifested in the autonomic nervous system.

psychotherapy Treatment for mental illness and behavioral disturbances in which the clinician establishes a professional contract with the patient and, through definitive therapeutic communication, attempts to alleviate the emotional disturbances, reverse or change maladaptive patterns of behavior, and encourage personality growth and development.

PsyD Doctor of psychology.

PT *1)* Physical therapy. *2)* Prothrombin time. *NCD References:* 190.11, 190.17.

PTA *1)* Percutaneous transluminal angioplasty. *NCD Reference:* 20.7. *2)* Physical therapy assistant. *3)* Prior to admission.

PTB Patellar tendon bearing.

PTC assay Blood test that measures the activity for factor IX, a plasma thromboplastin component, one of the substances involved in the intrinsic pathway of coagulation or blood clotting. This test is performed on people with bleeding problems as a deficiency in this factor causes hemophilia B. *Synonym(s): Christmas factor assay, factor IX assay.*

PTCA Percutaneous transluminal coronary angioplasty. Procedure performed by threading a balloon catheter through an access artery up to the affected artery of the heart and inflating the balloon to flatten obstructive plaque against the wall of the artery and open the passage. This procedure is reported with CPT codes 92982 and 92984.

PTE

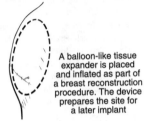

PTE is the acronym for prolonged tissue expansion

A balloon-like tissue expander is placed and inflated as part of a breast reconstruction procedure. The device prepares the site for a later implant

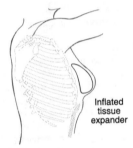

Inflated tissue expander

PTE Prolonged tissue expansion. Tissue expansion that occurs over one to six weeks, allowing resurfacing of even wider defects with adjacent skin. Typically, PTE requires two surgeries: One to place the expander, reported with CPT code 11960 for most skin, except 19357 for the breast, and one to remove it and perform the reconstruction.

pterygium Benign, wedge-shaped, conjunctival thickening that advances from the inner corner of the eye toward the cornea.

pterygolymphangiectasia syndrome Congenital disorder characterized by short stature and webbed neck. Patients of either sex suffer congenital heart disease, mental retardation, and other symptoms. Report this disorder with ICD-9-CM code 758.6. *Synonym(s): XO syndrome.*

pterygomaxillary fossa Wide depression on the external surface of the maxilla above and to the side of the canine tooth socket.

PTH Parathyroid hormone.

PTHC Percutaneous transhepatic cholangiography. Diagnostic procedure to identify obstructions in the liver or bile ducts, reported with CPT code 74320.

PTK Phototherapeutic keratectomy. Removal by laser of diseased outer layers of the cornea, reported with HCPCS Level II code S0812 or CPT code 65400.

O-R

PTLD Post-transplant lymphoproliferative disorder.

PTMPY Per thousand members per year.

Ptosis

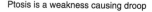

Ptosis is a weakness causing droop

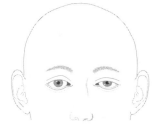

Patient has ptosis in his right eye

ptosis Drooping or displacement of the upper eyelid, caused by paralysis, muscle problems, or outside mechanical forces. For acquired ptosis, report ICD-9-CM codes 374-30-374.33. For congenital ptosis, report 743.61. **Synonym(s):** *blepharoptosis.*

ptosis-epicanthus syndrome Eyebrow or upper or lower eyelid sags. Report this disorder with ICD-9-CM code 270.2. **Synonym(s):** *Mendes syndrome, van der Hoeve-Halbertsma-Waardenburg syndrome, Waardenburg-Klein syndrome.*

PTPN Peripheral total parenteral nutrition. When a patient cannot tolerate enteral feeding (a tube into the stomach), nutrients are provided intravenously, through a peripheral vein. PTPN has a lower concentration of dextrose, because peripheral veins are irritated by higher concentrations. PTPN is usually associated with short-term parenteral feeding.

PTSD Post traumatic stress disorder, reported with ICD-9-CM code 309.81.

PTT Partial thromboplastin time. **NCD Reference:** *190.16.*

pubiotomy Surgical division of the pubic bone laterally to the symphysis pubis, performed in order to facilitate delivery of an infant. This procedure is reported with ICD-9-CM procedure code 73.94. **Synonym(s):** *Gigli's operation, obstetrical symphysiotomy, pelviotomy.*

PUBS

PUBS is an acronym for percutaneous umbilical blood sampling

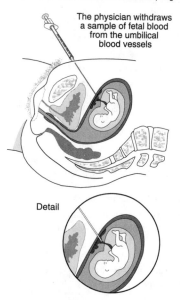

The physician withdraws a sample of fetal blood from the umbilical blood vessels

Detail

PUBS Percutaneous umbilical blood sampling. Blood is removed by aspiration from the fetal umbilical cord for testing. A needle is inserted through the mother's abdomen and uterus, and with ultrasound guidance, into the fetal umbilical cord. PUBS is reported with CPT code 59012, with radiologic guidance reported with 76941. **Synonym(s):** *cordocentesis.*

PUD *1)* Peptic ulcer disease. *2)* Periurethral diathermy.

pudendal nerve Nerve that serves most of the perineum and the external anal sphincter and provides sensation to the external genitalia.

puerperal Pertaining to the time from the end of the third stage of labor until the uterus and other reproductive organs return to their normal state, which is approximately three to six weeks following childbirth.

puerperium Postpartum period that begins immediately following delivery and continuing for six weeks.

pulmo- Relating to the lungs and respiration.

Pulmo-Aide compressor Brand name for a compressor/nebulizer for inhalation therapy treatments. Its supply is reported with HCPCS Level II code E0570.

pulmonary artery banding Surgical constriction of the pulmonary artery to prevent irreversible pulmonary vascular obstructive changes and overflow into the left ventricle.

O-R

pulmonary bifurcation Split of the left pulmonary veins that branch off from the left atrium to carry oxygenated blood away from the heart.

pulmonary collapse Condition in which all or part of a lung remains airless and cannot completely expand and fill with air. Report this condition with ICD-9-CM code 518.0. *Synonym(s): atelectasis, collapsed lung.*

pulmonary congestion Excessive retention of interstitial fluid in the lungs and pulmonary vessels.

pulmonary decortication Removal of a constricting membrane or layer of pleural tissue from a portion of the lung surface to allow for lung expansion. This procedure is reported with CPT codes 32220 and 32225. These are separate procedures and are not reported when performed in conjunction with another related service or procedure. When decortication is performed together with a parietal pleurectomy, report 32320. Decortication procedures performed via thoracoscopy are classified to 32651 and 32652. *Synonym(s): VATS.*

pulmonary eosinophilia Infiltration of eosinophils (nucleated, granular leukocytes) into the parenchyma of the lungs, resulting in cough, fever, and dyspnea. Report this condition with ICD-9-CM code 518.3.

pulmonary sulcus syndrome Neoplasm of upper lobe of lung. Report this disorder with ICD-9-CM code 162.3. *Synonym(s): Cuiffini-Pancoast syndrome, Hare's syndrome.*

pulmonary venolobar syndrome Congenital anomalous connection of the pulmonary veins in one lung to the inferior vena cava. Generally includes hypoplasia to some degree of the lung. Pulmonary venolobar syndrome may be asymptomatic with no treatment required, or it can require correction early in life. Pulmonary venolobar syndrome is reported with ICD-9-CM code 747.49, and its surgical correction is reported with CPT code 33724.

pulp Living connective tissue within the tooth's root canal space that supplies blood vessels and nerves to the tooth.

pulpectomy In dentistry, complete excision of both vital and devitalized pulp from a tooth's root canal space.

pulpotomy In dentistry, partial excision or amputation of pulp from a root canal, with some vital tissue remaining in the rest of the pulp.

Pulsar Max II Brand name cardiac pacing system.

pulse generator Component of a pacemaker or an implantable cardioverter defibrillator that contains the battery and the electronics for producing the electrical discharge sent to the heart to control cardiac rhythm. Insertion or replacement of the pulse generator may be done alone, not in conjunction with insertion or replacement of the entire pacemaker system.

pulv. Powder.

pump Forcing gas or liquid from a body part.

punch biopsy Technique to remove tissue samples by a small, round cutting tool that is screwed or punched into the tissue.

punctate keratitis Small, superficial corneal lesion of unknown cause or inflammatory cells creating the sensation of having a foreign body in the eye and sensitivity to bright light.

puncture Creating a hole.

puncture aspiration Use of a knife or needle to pierce a fluid-filled cavity and then withdraw the fluid using a syringe or suction device.

PUNL Percutaneous ultrasonic nephrolithotripsy.

PUO Pyrexia of unknown origin. Elevated body temperature or fever without known cause, reported with ICD-9-CM code 780.6. *Synonym(s): FUO.*

pupil Opening in the center of the colored iris ring through which light reaches the retina. A reaction to light is what causes the normal contraction or expansion of the pupil, changing the size of the opening so as to optimize light entry and prevent harm.

pupillary block glaucoma Progressive optic nerve disease associated with high intraocular pressure that can lead to irreversible vision loss. The aqueous humor is the clear fluid filling the chambers of the eye that is continually drained and renewed, produced by the ciliary body and passing out through the pupil and trabecular meshwork. Pupillary block glaucoma causes an increase in intraocular pressure due to an impairment of aqueous outflow caused by a narrowing or closing of the anterior chamber angle as the iris comes into contact with the trabecular meshwork. This type of glaucoma is identified in four stages: latent, intermittent, acute, and chronic. In the latent and intermittent phases, minor or transient attacks of varying severity, duration, and frequency occur in which intraocular pressure (IOP) rises with accompanying pain and edema. Acute angle closure glaucoma is a grave medical emergency as IOP rises, the cornea swells, and excruciating pain radiates through the eye. Visual acuity falls rapidly as the eye swells and blindness may result if the IOP is not lowered. The chronic stage manifests as irreversible IOP increases from progressive damage and scar tissue closing the anterior angle. Pupillary block glaucoma is reported with ICD-9-CM codes 365.20-365.24. *Synonym(s): angle closure glaucoma, closed angle glaucoma, narrow angle glaucoma.*

PUPPP syndrome Pruritic urticarial papules and plaques of pregnancy. Temporary and benign condition that resolves following delivery. PUPPP syndrome is not specifically indexed in ICD-9-CM, but is reported with a pregnancy code from subcategory 646.8 and a code for other specified urticaria, 708.8.

O-R

purpura Latin for purple. Refers to multiple pinpoint hemorrhages and accumulation of blood under the skin. Bleeding into the skin produces red-purple discoloration of the skin. Report this disorder with ICD-9-CM codes from rubrics 286, 287, and 709 or codes 446.6, 666.34, and 776.1.

purse-string suture Continuous suture placed around a tubular structure and tightened, to reduce or close the lumen.

Purtscher's retinopathy Hemorrhage, edema, or whitening of the retinal secondary to compression injury of the head.

purulent ophthalmia Infection and inflammation of the eye manifested by a discharge of pus, normally as a result of a gonorrheal infection. Report this condition with ICD-9-CM code 098.49. *Synonym(s): blepharopyorrhea.*

PUS Percutaneous ureteral stent.

Putnam-Dana syndrome Numbness and tingling, weakness, a sore tongue, dyspnea, faintness, pallor of the skin and mucous membranes, anorexia, diarrhea, loss of weight, and fever. Strikes in fifth decade. Report this disorder with ICD-9-CM code 281.0 and 336.2.

Putti-Platt procedure Realignment of the subscapularis tendon to treat recurrent anterior dislocation, thereby partially eliminating external rotation. The anterior capsule is also tightened and reinforced.

PUV Posterior urethral valves.

PV Percutaneous vertebroplasty. Minimally invasive procedure for treatment of vertebral compression fractures in which orthopedic cement is injected percutaneously into the fractured vertebrae. Report PV with ICD-9-CM procedure code 81.65 or a code from CPT range 22520-22522. *Synonym(s): vertebroplasty.*

PVA

PVA is the acronym for percutaneous vertebral augmentation

Physician injects material into spine

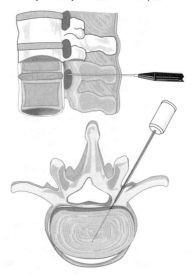

PVA Percutaneous vertebral augmentation. Surgical injection of polymethylmethacrylate into a fractured vertebral body to affix the fracture, performed under fluoroscopic guidance. Report PVA with ICD-9-CM procedure code 81.65 or CPT codes 22523-22525.

PVC *1)* Premature ventricular contraction. *2)* Polyvinyl chloride.

PVD Peripheral vascular disease. Disorders within the blood vessels outside of the heart and brain, most commonly a narrowing of the vessels carrying blood and oxygen to the legs, arms, stomach, or kidneys.

PVDA Prednisone, vincristine, daunorubicin, and asparaginase.

PVL Periventricular leukomalacia. Necrosis of white matter adjacent to lateral ventricles with the formation of cysts in infants. Cause of PVL has not been firmly established, but thought to be related to ischemia and is a common brain injury in premature infants. PVL is reported with ICD-9-CM code 779.7.

PVS *1)* Peripheral vascular system. *2)* Persistent vegetative state. Clinical condition in which a patient has no detectable awareness; it is usually associated with brain damage. PVS differs from coma in that a patient with PVS may seem to be awake, but is unconscious of surroundings and unresponsive to stimuli other than pain. PVS requires at least a month of persistent non-awareness before a diagnosis can be

O-R

made. PVS is reported with ICD-9-CM code 780.03. **Synonym(s):** *cortical death.*

PWA Person with AIDS (autoimmune deficiency syndrome).

PWI Posterior wall infarct.

Px Pneumothorax.

PXA Pleomorphic xantroastrocytoma. Low-grade astrocytoma or brain tumor. PXAs are usually localized and slow growing.

pyelo- Relating to the pelvis.

pyelolithotomy Removal of a renal calculus through an incision into the pelvis of the kidney.

pyelonephritis Infection of the renal pelvis and ureters that may be acute or chronic, often occurring as a result of a urinary tract infection, particularly in instances of vesicoureteric reflux, the backflow of urine from the bladder into the kidney pelvis or ureters. Pyelonephritis is reported with a code from ICD-9-CM category 590. **Synonym(s):** *pyelonephrosis.*

pyelonephrosis Infection of the renal pelvis and ureters that may be acute or chronic, often occurring as a result of a urinary tract infection, particularly in instances of vesicoureteric reflux, the backflow of urine from the bladder into the kidney pelvis or ureters. Pyelonephrosis is reported with a code from ICD-9-CM category 590. **Synonym(s):** *pyelonephritis.*

pyeloplasty Surgical correction of an obstruction or defect in the renal pelvis of the kidney or its junction with the ureter. This procedure is performed openly, reported with CPT code 50400 and 50405, or laparoscopically, reported with 50544.

pyelostolithotomy Removal of a renal calculus via a tube placed through an opening in the abdominal wall into the pelvis of the kidney.

pyelostomy Surgical creation of an opening through the abdominal wall into the renal pelvis.

pyelotomy Incision or opening made into the renal pelvis. Pyelotomies are performed to accomplish other procedures such as exploration, drainage, removal of a kidney stone, instill medications, or perform ureteropyelography or renal endoscopy. The pyelotomy is included as part of the procedure or method of access.

pyeloureteritis cystica Inflammation and formation of many small fluid-filled submucosal cysts in the ureter and renal pelvis. Most commonly affected individuals are between the ages of 50-60, with a small predominance of females.

pygo- Relating to the buttocks or rump.

pygopagus Monozygotic (identical) twins who are joined at the buttocks. Report this abnormality with ICD-9-CM code 759.4.

pyle- Relating to an opening/orifice of the portal vein.

pyloro- Relating to the pylorus (the stomach opening into the duodenum).

pyloroduodenal syndrome Distended efferent loop causing illness and pain with acute or chronic obstruction of the duodenum and jejunum proximal to a gastrojejunostomy. Report this disorder with ICD-9-CM code 537.89. **Synonym(s):** *gastrojejunal loop obstruction.*

pyloroplasty Enlargement and reconstruction of the lower portion of the stomach opening into the duodenum performed after vagotomy to speed gastric emptying and treat duodenal ulcers.

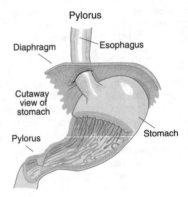

pylorus Lower portion of the stomach, which opens into the duodenum.

pyo- Relating to pus.

pyoderma Any skin disease commonly characterized by the discharging of pus.

pyogenic granuloma Small, erythematous papule on the skin and oral or gingival mucosa that increases in size and may become pendulum-like, infected, and/or ulcerated.

pyonephrosis Destruction of the kidney parenchyma wherein pus is produced and there is partial or total loss of kidney function. Report pyonephrosis with ICD-9-CM code 590.2. **Synonym(s):** *nephropyosis.*

pyreto- Indicates a fever, heat.

pyriformis syndrome Lesion on the sciatica nerve causing a pear shaped area of pain and paresthesia. Report this disorder with ICD-9-CM code 355.0.

pyromania Recurrent failure to resist impulses to set fires without regard for the consequences, or with deliberate destructive intent and an intense fascination with the setting of fires, seeing fires burn, and a satisfaction with the resultant destruction.

PZI Protamine zinc insulin.

O-R

Q fever Infection of *Coxiella burnetii* commonly found in livestock and usually acquired through airborne organisms. Most patients experience the sudden onset of one or more of the following: high fevers (up to 104-105⬚ F), severe headache, general malaise, myalgia, confusion, sore throat, chills, sweats, non-productive cough, nausea, vomiting, diarrhea, abdominal pain, and chest pain. A majority of patients infected with *Coxiella burnetii* have abnormal results on liver function tests and may develop hepatitis. Report this condition with ICD-9-CM code 083.0.

Q. Every.

q.2h Every two hours.

q.a.m. Every morning.

q.d. Every day.

q.h. Every hour.

q.h.s. Every night.

q.i.d. Four times daily.

q.n. Every night.

q.o.d. Every other day.

q.q.h. Every four hours.

Q3 HCPCS Level II modifier for use with CPT or HCPCS Level II codes, that identifies a live kidney donor surgery and related services. Postoperative live kidney donor services are reimbursed at 100 percent of the Medicare fee schedule amount.

Q4 HCPCS Level II modifier for use with CPT or HCPCS Level II codes, that identifies a service for the ordering/referring physician that qualifies as a service exemption. The ordering or referring provider has a financial relationship with the entity performing the service, for which the service qualifies as one of the service-related exemptions.

Q5 HCPCS Level II modifier for use with CPT or HCPCS Level II codes, that identifies a service furnished by a substitute physician under a reciprocal billing arrangement. This modifier has no effect on reimbursement.

Q6 HCPCS Level II modifier for use with CPT or HCPCS Level II codes, that identifies a service furnished by a locum tenens physician, or one that usually has no practice of his/her own and travels where needed. The patient's regular physician may submit a claim and receive Medicare Part B payment for a covered and medically necessary visit of a locum tenens physician who is not an employee of the regular physician and whose services for patients of the regular physician are not restricted to the regular physician's office.

Q7 HCPCS Level II modifier for use with CPT or HCPCS Level II codes, that identifies one class A finding on foot care procedures to indicate the severity of the patient's systemic condition without having to write a narrative description. This is a nontraumatic amputation of foot or integral skeletal portions.

Q8 HCPCS Level II modifier for use with CPT or HCPCS Level II codes, that identifies two class B findings on foot care procedures to indicate the severity of the patient's systemic condition without having to write a narrative description. Class B findings are absent posterior tibial pulse, absent dorsalis pedis pulse, advanced trophic changes, such as hair growth (decrease, absence), nail changes (thickening), pigmentary changes (discoloration), skin texture (thin, shiny), and/or skin color (rubor, redness).

Q9 HCPCS Level II modifier for use with CPT or HCPCS Level II codes, that identifies one class B and two class C findings on foot care procedures to indicate the severity of the patient's systemic condition without having to write a narrative description. Class C findings include claudication, temperature changes, edema, paresthesia, and burning.

QA Quality assurance. Monitoring and maintenance of established standards of quality for patient care.

QCT Quantitative computed tomography.

QD HCPCS Level II modifier for use with CPT or HCPCS Level II codes, that identifies recording and storage in solid state memory by a digital recorder. Has no effect on reimbursement.

QE HCPCS Level II modifier for use with HCPCS Level II codes that indicates that a prescribed amount of oxygen is less than one liter per minute (LPM). The Medicare allowed amount will be reduced by 50 percent.

QF HCPCS Level II modifier for use with HCPCS Level II codes that indicate that a prescribed amount of oxygen exceeds four liters per minute (LPM) and portable oxygen is prescribed. The Medicare allowed amount will increase by 50 percent monthly.

Qflow Brand name monitor to evaluate blood flow in the brain following head trauma or stroke. The monitor consists of a probe that is inserted via a twist hole or burr hole into the area of interest in the brain. Implanting and securing a Qflow device is reported with CPT codes 61107 or 61210.

QG HCPCS Level II modifier for use with HCPCS Level II codes that indicates that a prescribed amount of oxygen is greater than four liters per minute (LPM).

QH HCPCS Level II modifier for use with HCPCS Level II codes that indicates that an oxygen conserving device is being used with an oxygen delivery system.

QID Quarter in die. Latin for four times a day.

QIO Quality improvement organization. Entity established by TEFRA to review, monitor, educate, and improve the care given to patients. A QIO primarily performs this function for Medicare, but may also review

Q-R

Medicaid and private insurers under separate contracts. **Synonym(s):** *peer review organization, PRO.*

QK HCPCS Level II modifier for use with CPT anesthesia codes, that identifies medical direction of two, three, or four concurrent anesthesia procedures involving qualified individuals.

QM *1)* Quality management. Monitoring and maintenance of established standards of quality. *2)* HCPCS Level II modifier for use with HCPCS Level II codes that identifies an ambulance service provided under arrangement by a provider of services. Is payable under Medicare Part A, not Medicare Part B.

QN HCPCS Level II modifier for use with HCPCS Level II codes that identifies an ambulance service furnished directly by a provider of services. Is payable under Medicare Part A, not Medicare Part B.

qns Quantity not sufficient.

QOD Every other day.

qoh Every other hour.

QOL Quality of life.

QP HCPCS Level II modifier for use with CPT codes, that indicates that documentation is on file showing that the laboratory test was ordered individually or ordered as a CPT-recognized panel other than automated profiles. CMS does not require laboratories to use this modifier.

QPIT Quantitative pilocarpine iontophoresis test. Method of localized transdermal delivery of pilocarpine to a patient to stimulate sweat production. The sweat is evaluated to determine if the patient has cystic fibrosis.

qs Quantity sufficient.

QST Quantitative sensory testing. Helps in diagnosing and monitoring the function of nerve fibers in the somatosensory system, reported with CPT codes 0106T-0110T.

QT HCPCS Level II modifier for use with CPT or HCPCS Level II codes, that indicates recording and storage on tape by an analog tape recorder. Has no effect on Medicare reimbursement.

Q-T interval prolongation syndrome Prolonged Q-T interval and syncope, sometimes leading to ventricular fibrillation and sudden death. Report this disorder with ICD-9-CM code 794.31. **Synonym(s):** *Romano-Ward syndrome.*

quadriplegia Loss or impairment of the nerves and muscles of the arms and legs that impedes normal activity or movement or results in paralysis.

qualifying circumstance modifiers CPT add-on codes 99100, 99116, 99135, and 99140 for use with primary anesthesia procedure codes to show extreme age, complication of total body hypothermia, controlled hypotension, or emergency conditions.

qualitative To determine the nature of the component of substance.

quality assurance Monitoring and maintenance of established standards of quality for patient care. **Synonym(s):** *QA.*

quality health care Keeping members healthy or treating them when they are sick by doing the right thing at the right time, in the right way, for the right person, and getting the best possible results.

Quality Improvement Organization Entity established by TEFRA to review, monitor, educate, and improve the care given to patients. A QIO primarily performs this function for Medicare, but may also review Medicaid and private insurers under separate contracts. **Synonym(s):** *peer review organization, PRO, QIO.*

quality management Monitoring and maintenance of established standards of patient care to ensure that the most effective services are provided in the most effective and safest manner. **Synonym(s):** *QM.*

quantitative To determine the amount and nature of the components of a substance.

quattour Four.

query fever Disease caused by infection with Coxiella burnetii, a rickettsial bacteria spread by inhaling contaminated dust or aerosols or contact with infected livestock or articles such as wool, hair, and hides. It most often affects workers in stockyards, textile plants, or meat packing plants. Symptoms are usually mild and flu-like, but may manifest with high fever, muscle pain, and severe headache and may require antibiotic treatment. Report this condition with ICD-9-CM code 083.0. **Synonym(s):** *abattoir fever, Balkan grippe, Q fever.*

questionable covered procedures For Medicare purposes, procedures that may be covered depending on the medical circumstances involved. When one of these codes is billed, the fiscal intermediary is required to conduct a medical review of the claim to make a coverage decision. These procedures were formerly called "development-needed procedures."

qui tam actions Legal action against an individual or entity believed to be involved in fraud against the government. Under the False Claims Act, any individual who has such knowledge can file a lawsuit in his or her own name and in the name of the United States government. An employee usually brings these types of lawsuits for actions he or she believes constitute fraud or abuse on the part of the employer.

quicdecem Fifteen.

Quinquaud's syndrome Miliary abscesses in the scalp's hair follicles, resulting in scars and bald patches. Quinquaud's syndrome is reported with ICD-9-CM code 704.09. **Synonym(s):** *acne decalvans, Arnozan's syndrome, Brocq's lupoid sycosis.*

Q-R

quinque Five.

quotid Daily.

QW HCPCS Level II modifier for use with CPT or HCPCS Level II codes, that identifies a clinical laboratory improvement amendment (CLIA) waived test. The Centers for Medicare and Medicaid Services established standards to ensure accuracy, reliability, and timeliness of laboratory services. These apply to all lab tests, regardless of whether the payment is provided by Medicare, Medicaid, another third-party payer, or the patient.

QX HCPCS Level II modifier for use with CPT codes, that identifies a certified registered nurse anesthetist (CRNA) service with medical direction by a physician. Reimbursement is up to 55 percent of the amount that would have been allowed if personally performed by a physician.

QY HCPCS Level II modifier for use with CPT codes, that identifies medical direction of one certified registered nurse anesthetist (CRNA) by an anesthesiologist. Has no effect on Medicare reimbursement.

QZ HCPCS Level II modifier for use with CPT codes, that identifies a certified registered nurse anesthetist (CRNA) service without medical direction by a physician. Has no effect on Medicare reimbursement.

r Roentgen units (x-rays).

R *1)* Respiration. *2)* Right atrium. *3)* Right.

R&C Reasonable and customary.

R,R,& E Round, regular, and equal.

R/O Rule out.

RA *1)* Remittance advice. *2)* Risk assessment. *3)* Rheumatoid arthritis.

RabAvert Brand name rabies vaccine provided in a single-dose vial. RabAvert is administered to people who are at risk to be exposed to rabies, but have not been exposed. Supply of RabAvert is reported with CPT code 90675 and administration is reported with 90471. The need for immunization is reported with ICD-9-CM code V04.5.

rabbit fever Infection caused by the *Francisella tularensis* organism. It usually enters the body through the fingers and hands. The signs and symptoms of rabbit fever vary depending on how the bacteria enters the body but can include skin ulcers, swelling of lymph glands, inflammation of the eye, sore throat, mouth ulcers, tonsillitis, and pneumonia. All forms are accompanied by fever, which can be as high as 104□F. Report this condition with ICD-9-CM code 021.0. *Synonym(s): tularemia.*

rachi(o)- Relating to the spine.

RAD Reactive airway disease.

Radial Keratotomy

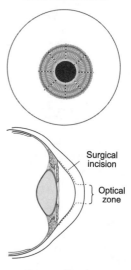

Radial incisions extend from optical zone to limbus

Surgical incision

Optical zone

Cross-section view

radial keratotomy Procedure consisting of multiple, nonpenetrating cuts made into the cornea in a spoke-like fashion to treat myopia, or in a variety of peripheral tangential cuts to treat astigmatism. The multiple cuts allow the cornea to stretch and flatten, changing the curvature and the refractive property of the eye.

radical Extensive surgery.

radical resection Removal of an entire tumor (e.g., malignant neoplasm) along with a large area of surrounding tissue, including adjacent lymph nodes that may have been infiltrated.

radicular cyst Cyst lined in stratified squamous epithelium that is attached to the apex of the root of a tooth.

radicular syndrome Disorder presenting symptoms similar to Raynaud's, caused by pressure of brachial plexus and subclavian artery against first thoracic rib. Report this disorder with ICD-9-CM code 353.0. *Synonym(s): Naffziger's syndrome.*

radiculitis Pain along an inflamed nerve, with inflammation of the root of the associated spinal nerve.

radioactive substances Materials used in the diagnosis and treatment of disease that emit high-speed particles and energy-containing rays.

radioelement Any element that emits particle or electromagnetic radiations from nuclear disintegration,

O-R

occurring naturally in any element with an atomic number above 83.

radiograph Image made by an x-ray.

radiological examination Plain films of specific sites. *Synonym(s): conventional film, standard film.*

radiology services Services that include diagnostic and therapeutic radiology, nuclear medicine, CT scan procedures, magnetic resonance imaging services, ultrasound, and other imaging procedures. HCPCS codes are required for billing outpatient radiology procedures.

radiopaque dye Medium injected into the body that is impenetrable by x-rays.

radiotherapy External source of high-energy rays (x-rays or gamma rays) or internally implanted radioactive substances used in destroying tissue and stopping the growth of malignant cells.

radiotherapy afterloading Part of the radiation therapy process in which the chemotherapy agent is actually instilled into the tumor area subsequent to surgery and placement of an expandable catheter into the void remaining after tumor excision. The specialized catheter remains in place and the patient may come in for multiple treatments with radioisotope placed to treat the margin of tissue surrounding the excision. After the radiotherapy is completed, the patient returns to have the catheter emptied and removed. This is a new therapy in breast cancer treatment. Placement of the radiotherapy afterloading catheter is reported with CPT codes 19296-19298. The isotope planning (77326-77328) and afterloading process itself (77785-77787) are each reported separately in addition to the catheter implant.

RAE Right atrial enlargement. *Synonym(s): RVH.*

RAEB Refractory anemia with excessive blasts. Insufficient red blood cells, with changes in the white blood cells and platelets. Between 5 and 19 percent of the cells in the bone marrow are blasts. RAEB is reported with ICD-9-CM code 238.73.

RAEBT Refractory anemia with excessive blasts in transformation. Insufficient red blood cells, white blood cells, and platelets in the blood. Between 20 and 30 percent of the cells in the bone marrow are blasts. Active RAEBT is reported with ICD-9-CM code 205.00. *Synonym(s): acute myeloid leukemia.*

Raeder-Harbitz syndrome Progressive obliteration of brachiocephalic trunk and left subclavian and left common carotid arteries above their source in the aortic arch. Symptoms include ischemia, transient blindness, facial atrophy, and many others. Report this disorder with ICD-9-CM code 446.7. *Synonym(s): Marorell-Fabre syndrome, Takayasu-Onishi syndrome.*

RAI *1)* Radioactive iodine. *2)* Resident assessment instrument, an evaluation form for residents of skilled nursing facilities.

Railroad Retirement Board Manages health insurance entitlement and investigates entitlement problems and issues affecting Railroad Retirement beneficiaries (i.e., those entitled to Part A and/or Part B coverage based on the Railroad Retirement Act). *Synonym(s): RRB.*

RAIU Radioactive iodine uptake.

range of motion Action of a body part throughout its extent of natural movement, measured in degrees of a circle.

ranibizumab Injectable drug to treat subfoveal neovascularization due to age-related macular degeneration. The injection procedure is reported with CPT code 67028, with modifier RT or LT appended to indicate which eye. Supply of ranibizumab is reported with HCPCS Level II code J2778. May be sold under the brand name Lucentis.

RAO Retinal artery occlusion. Ocular stroke or stenosis that presents with painless loss of visual acuity. RAO is reported with ICD-9-CM codes 362.30-362.35.

RAP Resident assessment protocol, an evaluation criteria for residents of skilled nursing facilities.

rapid time-zone change syndrome Imbalance of normal sleep patterns resulting from airplane travel through a number of time zones. Leads to fatigue, irritability, and other constitutional disturbances. Report this disorder with ICD-9-CM code 307.45. *Synonym(s): jet lag.*

RARS Refractory anemia with ringed sideroblasts. Too few red blood cells and the cells have too much iron in them. RARS is reported with ICD-9-CM code 238.72.

Rashkind Procedure

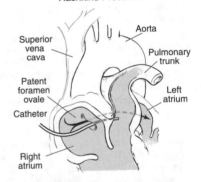

Depiction of patent foramen ovale. The procedure involves placing a catheter through the foramen ovale and enlarging the opening to allow mixing of blood between the atria. A balloon catheter may be used, or a cutting device may be required to create an opening (septostomy)

Rashkind procedure Transvenous balloon atrial septectomy or septostomy performed by cardiac

O-R

catheterization. A balloon catheter is inserted into the heart either to create or enlarge an opening in the interatrial septal wall. In cases where the foramen ovale has not closed, the deflated balloon is passed through it, then inflated and withdrawn, pulled through the atrial septum to enlarge the opening. When the septum remains intact, the deflated balloon is passed from the right to the left atrium, inflated, and pulled across the septum to create an interatrial septal defect. This improves blood flow and oxygenation and is reported with CPT code 92992.

RAST Radioallergosorbent test. Quantitative laboratory test for specific IgE to avoid exposing a patient to potentially harmful skin testing. RAST is reported with CPT codes 86003 and 86005.

Rastelli Operation

Two types of truncus arteriosus

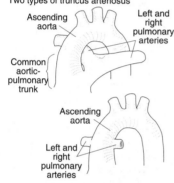

The complex surgery involves closing the VSD while ligating off the pulmonary artery at its source on the aorta. A conduit is then constructed from the right ventricle to the pulmonary system beyond the anomalous area

Rastelli operation Correction of persistent truncus arteriosus in which the pulmonary artery is separated from the primitive truncus to create a right ventricle-to-pulmonary artery conduit. Rastelli operation is reported with ICD-9-CM procedure code 35.83 and CPT code 33786.

rat bite fever Febrile illness, spirillary and streptobacillary, caused by two different types of bacteria found in the nasopharynx of rats. The infection is spread via rat bite, contact with secretions, or ingestion of food or water contaminated by secretions. In Japan and other parts of Asia, the infection is caused by spirillum minus, and the disease is called sodoku. The other organism responsible for rat bite fever is a gram-negative facultative anaerobe, Streptobacillus moniliformis Rat bite fever is reported with a code from ICD-9-CM category 026. *Synonym(s): epidemic arthritic erythema, Haverhill fever, Streptobacillosis.*

RATx Radiation therapy.

Raymond (-Céstan) syndrome Identified through symptoms of quadriplegia, anesthesia, and nystagmus due to the obstruction of twigs of the basilar artery, causing lesions in the pontine region. Report this disorder with a code from ICD-9-CM range 433.80-433.81.

Raynaud's phenomenon Vascular disorder resulting in bilateral decreased circulation of the fingers and toes causing a pale or bluish appearance, numbness, tingling, and pain brought on by cold or emotions and relieved with heat.

Raynaud's syndrome Constriction of the arteries of the digits caused by cold or emotion. Temperature drops in extremities as much as 30 degrees Fahrenheit, and skin turns white with red and blue mottling. Caused by nerve or arterial damage and can be prompted by stress. Report this disorder with ICD-9-CM code 443.0. *Synonym(s): Patriots disease.*

Raz procedure Abdominovaginal vesicle neck suspension procedure to control female urinary stress incontinence. The bladder neck is suspended by suturing surrounding tissue through an incision in the vagina near the base of the bladder to the fibrous membranes (fascia) of the abdomen. This procedure is reported with CPT code 51845.

RBB Right branch bundle or right bundle branch. Part of the heart's electrical system carrying nerve impulses that cause the right ventricle to contract. If the impulses are blocked, the heart rate slows or fails.

RBBB

RBBB is the acronym for right branch bundle block

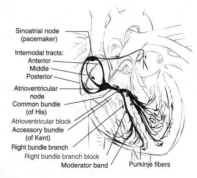

RBBB Right bundle branch block.

RBC Red blood cell.

O-R

RBL

RBL is an acronym for rubber band ligation

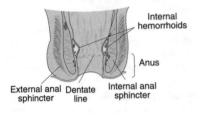

Internal hemorrhoids
Anus
External anal sphincter Dentate line Internal anal sphincter

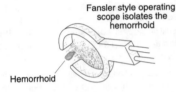

Fansler style operating scope isolates the hemorrhoid

Hemorrhoid

The hemorrhoid is identified and isolated. The physician ties suture material around the base of the hemorrhoid. The hemorrhoid is left to slough off as the suture strangulates blood flow

RBL Rubber band ligation. Treatment of a defect in skin or mucosal tissue by trapping the defective tissue with a rubber band that cuts off its blood supply. The trapped tissue dies and falls off and the surrounding tissue in the banded area heals. RBL is a common treatment for internal hemorrhoids or large skin tags. RBL of internal hemorrhoids is reported with CPT codes 46945 and 46946. RBL of skin tags is reported with 11200 and 11201.

RBN Retrobulbar neuritis. Inflammation of the optic nerve between the eye and the brain. RBN is usually the result of infection, multiple sclerosis, tumors, allergies, or toxins and is reported with ICD-9-CM code 377.32 unless syphilitic in origin, in which case it is reported with 094.85.

RBOW Ruptured bag of water.

RBRVS Resource-based relative value scale. Fee schedule introduced by CMS to reimburse physician Medicare fees based on the amount of time and resources expended in treating patients with adjustments for overhead costs and geographical differences.

RC HCPCS Level II modifier, for use with CPT codes, that identifies the right coronary artery. Used to indicate specific vessel involvement in a stent placement, balloon angioplasty, and/or atherectomy.

RCA Right coronary artery.

RCC Renal cell carcinoma.

RCCA Right common carotid artery.

RCD Relative cardiac dullness.

RCE Reasonable compensation equivalent.

RCL Renal clearance. Rate at which a chemical is removed from plasma and an indicator of kidney efficiency.

RCM Radiocontrast media. Radiopharmaceutical injected into a patient to enhance diagnostic imaging.

RCT Randomized controlled trials.

RDI Respiratory disturbance index. Frequency of respiratory abnormalities during an hour of sleep, used as an evaluation in sleep apnea. An RDI of 30 would indicate that during one hour of sleep the patient experienced 30 incidences of sleep flow disruption.

RDS Respiratory distress syndrome. Reduced amounts of lung surfactant in premature neonates with respiratory distress. Frequently fatal. Report this disorder with ICD-9-CM code 769. **Synonym(s):** *hyaline membrane.*

rDSPA 1-a Genetically engineered form of the clot-dissolving protein found in the saliva of the vampire bat in Phase III clinical trials as a therapeutic treatment for ischemic stroke. Infusion of rDSPA 1-a would be reported with CPT code 37195 or inpatient ICD-9-CM code 99.10.

RDW Red cell distribution width.

reactive confusion Psychological response apparently provoked by emotional stress that leads to clouded consciousness, mild to moderate disorientation, and diminished accessibility, often accompanied by excessive activity.

reactive excitation Affective psychosis, usually a response to emotional stress with symptoms similar to manic-depressive psychosis, manic type.

reagent Substance used to produce a chemical reaction in order to detect, measure, or create another substance.

real-time Immediate imaging, with movement as it happens.

real-time scan Two-dimensional procedure with display of both structure and motion with time.

ream Shape or enlarge a hole.

reasonable and customary Fees charged for medical services that are considered normal, common, and in line with the prevailing fees in the provider's geographical area.

reasonable charge Under Medicare, lowest of either the actual charge, the charge customarily billed to patients, or the prevailing charge for the service. The reasonable charge represents the charge determination made by a carrier on a covered Part B medical service or supply.

O-R

reasonable cost methodology Methodology used by fiscal intermediaries, under guidelines from CMS, to determine the reasonable cost incurred by the provider when furnishing covered services to a beneficiary. Reasonable costs are based on the actual cost of providing services, including direct and indirect costs incurred in furnishing covered hospital services to Medicare beneficiaries, and are intended to exclude unnecessary costs.

reattachment Joining together parts that have been separated.

rebase In dentistry, refitting of a denture by replacement of the base materials.

recess Small empty cavity in a body part.

recession Drawing away or back from the normal position; displacing tissue surgically to a point posterior to the normal location or insertion.

recipient twin syndrome Polycythemia of newborn as result of blood flow from mother. Report this disorder with ICD-9-CM code 776.4.

Reclus syndrome Multiple, benign cysts of the breast, colored brown or blue, caused by hyperplasia of the ductal epithelium. Occurs in women, usually after the age of 30. Reclus syndrome is reported with ICD-9-CM code 610.1. *Synonym(s): Bloodgood's disease, Phocas' disease, Schimmelbusch disease, Tillaux-Phocas disease.*

Recombivax HB Brand name hepatitis B vaccine provided in a single-dose vial. Supply of Recombivax HB is reported with CPT codes 90743 and 90746. Administration is reported with HCPCS Level II code G0010. Need for vaccination is reported with ICD-9-CM code V02.61.

reconstruct Tissue rebuilding.

reconstruction Recreating, restoring, or rebuilding a body part or organ.

reconstructive surgery Blepharoplasty involving more than skin (i.e., involving lid margin, tarsus, and/or palpebral conjunctiva).

recoupment Recovery by a payer of any debt by reducing present or future payments and applying the amount withheld to the indebtedness.

rectal Pertaining to the rectum, the end portion of the large intestine.

recto- Meaning straight or relating to the rectum.

rectocele Rectal tissue herniation into the vaginal wall. *Synonym(s): proctocele.*

rectovaginal fistula Abnormal communication between the rectum and the vagina that may follow obstetrical laceration repair, vaginal or rectal surgery, radiation therapy, trauma, or infection with fecal incontinence or leakage into the vaginal canal.

rectum End portion of the large intestine from the rectosigmoid junction to the anus.

recurrent corneal erosion Painful periodic loss of the outer layer of corneal epithelium due to its failure to properly adhere to the Bowman's membrane.

recurring outpatient (repetitive outpatient services, or series outpatient) Part B services that recur for an individual outpatient. These services are billed monthly or at the conclusion of the individual's treatment. They include durable medical equipment rental; therapeutic radiology; therapeutic nuclear medicine; respiratory, physical, and occupational therapy; speech pathology; home health visits; kidney dialysis treatments; cardiac rehabilitation services; and psychological services. *Synonym(s): repetitive outpatient services, series outpatient.*

reduce Restoration to normal position or alignment.

reducible hernia Protrusion of tissue through the wall of another structure that can be manually returned to the correct anatomical position.

reduction Correction of a fracture, dislocation, or hernia to the correct place and alignment, manually or by surgery.

REEDA Redness, edema, ecchymosis, drainage, approximation.

refer Recommendation to another source.

referenced diagnostic laboratory services Tests performed on samples that are referred to the hospital laboratory for diagnostic work.

referral Approval from the primary care physician to see a specialist or receive certain services. May be required for coverage purposes before a patient receives care from anyone except the primary physician.

referred outpatient Person sent to a special diagnostic facility or to a hospital service department for the diagnostic tests or procedures.

referring physician Physician who requests an item or service for a patient.

reflex Involuntary action, movement, or activity brought about by triggering the corresponding stimulus.

reflex sympathetic dystrophy Condition marked by an abnormal response of the nerves of the face or extremities that causes pain, autonomic dysfunction, vasomotor instability, and tissue swelling.

reflux Return or backward flow.

reflux esophagitis Inflammation of the lower esophagus as a result of regurgitated gastric acid, reported with ICD-9-CM code 530.11. Reflux esophagitis is not the same as gastroesophageal reflux disease (GERD). They are not coded together since inflammation of the esophagus from regurgitated stomach acid appears as a symptomatic part of the disorder.

O-R

Refsum's syndrome Deafness, retinitis pigmentosa, polyneuritis, nystagmus, and cerebellar signs. Report this disorder with ICD-9-CM code 356.3.

regeneration Process of reproducing or regrowing tissue.

Regenstrief Institute Research foundation for improving health care by optimizing the capture, analysis, content, and delivery of health care information. Regenstrief maintains the logical observation identifiers, names, and codes (LOINC) coding system that is being considered for use as part of the HIPAA claim attachments standard.

regional anesthesia Anesthesia administered to a nerve or nerve plexus to provide a loss of sensation in a particular region, without inducing unconsciousness. Sometimes sedative agents are administered, such as Valium, prior to administration of the regional anesthesia. *Synonym(s): Bier block, caudal, epidural, nerve root injection, peripheral nerve block, spinal, trigger point injection.*

regional enteritis Chronic inflammation of unknown origin affecting the ileum and/or colon. *Synonym(s): Crohn's disease.*

regional home health intermediary Five fiscal intermediaries nationally designated to process all Medicare home health and hospice claims. *Synonym(s): RHHI.*

regional medical center Hospital that provides comprehensive services to a large regional area but that may not be a tertiary care facility. Largely used in the west where facilities may serve hundreds of square miles.

registered health information administrator Accreditation for medical record administrators, previously known as a registered records administrator (RRA), through AHIMA. *Synonym(s): RHIA.*

registered health information technician Accreditation for medical records practitioners, previously known as accredited records technician (ART), through AHIMA. *Synonym(s): RHIT.*

Regnolli's excision Partial or total surgical excision of the tongue.

regulation Directive, order, ruling, or law put forth by an executive authority granted such powers by law.

regurgitation Abnormal backward flow.

rehabilitation Restoration of physical and mental functions to allow the usual daily activities of life.

rehabilitation hospital Institution that serves inpatients of whom the vast majority require intensive rehabilitative services for the treatment of certain conditions (e.g., stroke, amputation, brain or spinal cord injuries, and neurological disorders).

rehabilitation services Therapy services provided primarily for assisting in a rehabilitation program of evaluation and service including cardiac rehabilitation, medical social services, occupational therapy, physical therapy, respiratory therapy, skilled nursing, speech therapy, psychiatric rehabilitation, and alcohol and substance abuse rehabilitation.

Rehfuss' test Gastric secretion determined by drawing specimens of digestion every 15 minutes after eating. *NCD Reference: 300.1.*

Reichmann's syndrome Excessive secretion of gastric juice either constantly or during digestion only. Report this disorder with ICD-9-CM code 536.8.

ReidSleeve Brand name custom compression sleeve for the arm or leg to relieve lymphedema. Supply of ReidSleeve for the upper extremity is reported with HCPCS Level II code S8420.

Reifenstein's syndrome Hypogonadism with gynecomastia, hypospadias, and postpubertal testicular atrophy caused by an inherited defect of androgen receptors and insensitivity to testosterone. Report this disorder with ICD-9-CM code 259.52.

Reilly's syndrome Pain and stiffness in the shoulder, with puffy swelling and pain in the hand following a heart attack. Report this disorder with ICD-9-CM code 337.9. *Synonym(s): Claude Bernard-Horner syndrome, Steinbrocker's syndrome.*

reimbursement Payment of actual charges or allowable incurred as a result of accident or illness.

reimplant Reinsert or reattach tissue.

reinforce Enhancement of strength.

reinnervation Restoration of nerve function.

Reinsch test Test determines level of heavy metals in body tissue.

reinsurance Insurance purchased by an HMO, insurance company, or self-funded employer from another insurance company to protect itself against all or part of the losses that may be incurred in the process of honoring the claims of its participating providers, policy holders, or employees and covered dependents. *Synonym(s): risk-control insurance, stop-loss insurance.*

Reiter's syndrome Arthritis, iridocyclitis, and urethritis, sometimes with diarrhea. While symptoms may recur, arthritis is constant. Report this disorder with ICD-9-CM code 099.3. *Synonym(s): Fiessinger-Leroy-Reiter syndrome.*

relapsing fever Infection of *Borrelia*. Symptoms are episodic and include fever and arthralgia. This condition is reported with ICD-9-CM codes 087.0-087.9.

related cases Procedures with the same diagnosis, same operative area, and same indication.

relationship problems of childhood Emotional disorders characteristic of childhood that involve a state

O-R

of affairs existing between two parties' problems and issues.

relative value scale Numeric ranking of physician and ancillary services based on the intensity of the procedure or service being performed. *Synonym(s): RVS.*

relative value study Guide that shows the relationship between the time, resources, competency, experience, severity, and other factors necessary to perform procedures that is multiplied by a dollar conversion factor to determine a monetary value for the procedure. *Synonym(s): RVS.*

relative value unit Value assigned a procedure based on difficulty and time consumed. Used for computing reimbursement under a relative value study. *Synonym(s): RVU.*

relative weight Assigned weight that is intended to reflect the relative resource consumption associated with each DRG. The higher the relative weight, the greater the payment to the hospital. The relative weights are calculated by CMS and published in the final prospective payment system rule. *Synonym(s): RW.*

relaxin Female hormone secreted by the corpus luteum that helps soften the cervix and relax the pelvic ligaments in childbirth.

release Disconnection of a tendon or ligament.

release of information Authorization from the patient that allows the hospital to release to the insurer or other payer the medical and billing information for determining coverage eligibility, medical necessity, the final diagnosis, and any procedures performed or as needed to process a claim for reimbursement.

reliable information All credible allegations, oral or written, and/or other material facts that would likely cause a non-interested third party to think that there is a reasonable basis for believing that a certain set of facts exists; for example, that claims are or were false or were submitted for non-covered or miscoded services.

reline Adjust the fit of a denture by filling in or resurfacing the part that makes contact with mucosal tissue.

REM Rapid eye movement.

remittance advice Statement, voucher, or notice that a provider of services receives from a payer that reflects adjudicated claims, either paid or denied. *Synonym(s): EOB, ERA, RA.*

Remodulin Brand name continuous subcutaneous or intravenous infusion agent for treating pulmonary arterial hypertension, reported with ICD-9-CM code 416.8. Supply of Remodulin is reported with HCPCS Level II code J3285. Remodulin contains treprostinil sodium.

remote afterloading Form of brachytherapy in which the radioactive sources are loaded into the patient from a remote location.

removal Process of moving out of or away from, or the fact of being removed.

remuneration Pay an equal amount for a service, loss, or expense.

renal Referring to the kidney.

renal ablation Destruction or removal of renal tissue or a mass or lesion of the kidney using cryosurgery, radiofrequency, or high-energy electrical current. Renal ablation may be laparoscopic or open. Renal cyst ablation is reported with CPT code 50541.

renal calyces Cuplike structures formed by the papilla, where urine is collected for transfer via the renal pelvis out of the kidney and into the ureter.

renal failure Inability of a kidney to eliminate metabolites and retain electrolytes at a normal level.

renal glomerulohyalinosis-diabetic syndrome High blood pressure and kidney failure resulting from a form of diabetes in which carbohydrate utilization is reduced and that of lipid and protein enhanced. Report this disorder with a code from ICD-9-CM subcategory 249.4 or 250.4, and 581.81.

renal hemorrhage Kidney hemorrhage, reported with ICD-9-CM code 593.81. *Synonym(s): nephrorrhagia.*

renal osteodystrophy Bone disorder manifested by various bone diseases occurring when kidney function is impaired or fails. Osteomalacia, osteoporosis, or osteosclerosis can be present. Abnormal levels of phosphorous and calcium are seen in the blood with impaired stimulation of the parathyroid gland. This disorder is reported with ICD-9-CM code 588.0.

renal sclerosis Atrophy, fibrosis, or other hardening of tissue in the kidney caused by inflammation, mineral deposits, or other causes. Renal sclerosis is reported with ICD-9-CM code 587, excluding arteriosclerotic induced nephrosclerosis or that associated with hypertension (403.00-403.91). *Synonym(s): atrophy of kidney, contracted kidney, renal cirrhosis, renal fibrosis.*

renal syndrome Renal condition in which nephritis progresses rapidly to death, with lungs showing extensive hemosiderosis or bleeding. Report this disorder with ICD-9-CM code 446.21. *Synonym(s): Goodpasture's syndrome.*

Rendu-Osler-Weber disease Post-pubescent appearing genetic disorder with small telangiectasia and dilated venules developing slowly on the skin and mucus membranes of the lips, nasopharynx, and tongue with recurrent bleeding. Report this disorder with ICD-9-CM code 448.0. *Synonym(s): Babington's disease, hereditary hemorrhagic telangiectasia.*

O-R

Renessa Brand name treatment system or female urinary stress incontinence in which controlled heat is administered with a transurethral probe. There is no code specific to this procedure, which should be reported with an unlisted procedure code.

renofacial syndrome Renal agenesis with hypoplastic lungs and associated neonatal respiratory distress, hemodynamic instability, acidosis, cyanosis, edema, and characteristic facial features. Death usually occurs from lack of oxygen. Report this disorder with ICD-9-CM code 753.0.

Rénon-Delille syndrome Obesity and hypogonadism in adolescent boys. Rare accompanying dwarfism is thought to indicate hypothyroidism. Report this disorder with ICD-9-CM code 253.8. *Synonym(s):* Babinski-Frolich syndrome, Launois-Cleret syndrome.

reopening Action taken, after all appeal rights are exhausted, to re-examine or question the correctness of a final determination, decision, or cost report.

reoperation Repeat performance of operation.

repair Surgical closure of a wound. The wound may be a result of injury/trauma or it may be a surgically created defect. Repairs are divided into three categories: simple, intermediate, and complex. Simple repair is performed when the wound is superficial and only requires simple, one layer, primary suturing. Intermediate repair is performed for wounds and lacerations in which one or more of the deeper layers of subcutaneous tissue and non-muscle fascia are repaired in addition to the skin and subcutaneous tissue. Complex repair includes repair of wounds requiring more than layered closure.

repeated infarct dementia Dementia attributable, because of physical signs (confirmed by examination of the central nervous system), to degenerative arterial disease of the brain.

repetitive outpatient services Part B services that recur for an individual outpatient. These services are billed monthly or at the conclusion of the individual's treatment. They include durable medical equipment rental; therapeutic radiology; therapeutic nuclear medicine; respiratory, physical, and occupational therapy; speech pathology; home health visits; kidney dialysis treatments; cardiac rehabilitation services; and psychological services.

Repl Replace.

replacement Insertion of new tissue or material in place of old one.

replantation Surgical reattachment or replacement of a body part or structure to its previous site, such as a digit or tooth.

Repliderm Brand name, collagen-based powder for treatment of pressure, stasis, diabetic and foot ulcers,

first and second-degree burns, surgical incisions, cuts, abrasions, partial-thickness wounds, and for absorbing exudates.

report of benefit savings Required medical review report detailing savings realized each quarter as a direct result of medical review activities by contractors. *Synonym(s):* RBS.

reposition Placement of an organ or structure into another position or return of an organ or structure to its original position.

Repronex Brand name fertility drug that prepares the body for ovulation. Its active ingredient is a menotropin and it is administered by injection. Supply is reported with HCPCS Level II code S0122.

request for anticipated payment Request submitted by a home health agency to its regional home health intermediary to request the initial split percentage payment for a home health prospective payment system episode. A RAP may be submitted after receiving verbal orders and delivering at least one service to the beneficiary. Though submitted on Form CMS-1450 (UB-92) and resulting in Medicare payment for home services, the RAP is normally not considered a Medicare home health claim and is not subject to many of the stipulations applied to such claims in regulations. *Synonym(s):* RAP.

RESA Radial cryosurgical ablation.

resect Cutting out or removing a portion or all of a bone, organ, or other structure.

resection Surgical removal of a part or all of an organ or body part.

reservoir Space or body cavity for storage of liquid.

resident Individual participating in an approved graduate medical education (GME) program or a physician who is not in an approved GME program but who is authorized to practice only in a hospital setting including interns and fellows but not medical students.

residual root Remaining root portion after loss of 75 percent or more of the tooth crown.

residual schizophrenia Continued disturbance of personality with flat affect, odd beliefs or perceptions, and speech poverty without delusions, without hallucinations, and without disorganized speech or behavior and a history of schizophrenia. Emotional response is blunted, but this thought disorder does not prevent the accomplishment of routine work.

resistance exercise Any form of active exercise in which a dynamic or static muscular contraction is resisted by an outside manual or mechanical force.

resource utilization group In health care contracting, patient classification system that uses patients' characteristics and health status information from the

O-R

minimum data set (MDS), such as diagnoses, ability to perform activities of daily living (ADL), and treatments received, to assign the patient to a resource group for payment under the Medicare prospective payment system for skilled nursing facilities. The RUG-III system is a hierarchy of major patient types consisting of seven major categories that represent the first level of patient classification. The major categories are rehabilitation, extensive services, special care, clinically complex, impaired cognition, behavior problems, and reduced physical function. These major categories are further differentiated into 44 more specific patient groupings. **Synonym(s):** *RUG-III.*

resource-based relative value scale Fee schedule introduced by the Centers for Medicare and Medicaid Services to reimburse physician Medicare fees based on the amount of time and resources expended in treating patients with adjustments for overhead costs and geographical differences. **Synonym(s):** *RBRVS.*

resource-based relative value study Relative value scale originally developed by Harvard for use in Medicare. The scale assigns value to procedures based on the related resources rather than on historical data. **Synonym(s):** *RBRVS.*

resp Respiration, respiratory.

respiratory distress syndrome Premature neonates with respiratory distress and associated with reduced amounts of lung surfactant. Frequently fatal. Report this disorder with ICD-9-CM code 769. **Synonym(s):** *hyaline membrane syndrome.*

response Reaction to stimulus.

restless leg syndrome Indescribable uneasiness, restlessness, or twitching in the legs after going to bed. Often caused by poor circulation or antipsychotic medications, it can lead to insomnia. Report this disorder with ICD-9-CM code 333.99. **Synonym(s):** *Ekborn's syndrome.*

Restylane Brand name, transparent gel injected into facial tissue to smooth wrinkles and folds, especially around the nose and mouth, composed of hyaluronic acid.

Restzustand (schizophrenia) Continued disturbance of personality with flat affect, odd beliefs or perceptions, and speech poverty without delusions, without hallucinations, and without disorganized speech or behavior and a history of schizophrenia. Emotional response is blunted, but this thought disorder does not prevent the accomplishment of routine work.

resubmitted claim Claim that has been sent more than once to the payer for a response.

resuscitation Restoration to life or consciousness of one apparently dead, it includes such measures as artificial respiration and cardiac massage or electrical shock.

Retaane Brand name injectable drug to treat subfoveal neovascularization due to macular degeneration. The injection of Retaane is reported with CPT code 0124T, with modifier RT or LT. Supply of Retaane is reported with HCPCS Level II code J3490. Retaane contains anecortave acetate.

retainer In dentistry, portion of a fixed partial denture that attaches an artificial tooth to the abutment tooth or implant.

retention suture Secondary stitching that bridges the primary suture, providing support for the primary repair. A plastic or rubber bolster may be placed over the primary repair and under the retention sutures.

retina Layer of tissue located at the back of the eye that is sensitive to light similar to that of film in a camera.

retinal edema Retinal swelling due to fluid accumulation.

retinal neovascularization New and abnormal vascular growth in the retina.

retinal tear Vitreous detachment that disengages in such a way as to cause a tear in the retina.

retinochoroiditis juxtapapillaris Eye condition characterized by small areas of inflammation on the interior back portion of the eyeball (fundus) near the optic disc or papilla, found in young, healthy individuals. Report this condition with ICD-9-CM code 363.05. **Synonym(s):** *Jensen's disease, Jensen's retinitis.*

retinopathy of prematurity Disease of the eye found in premature infants and occurring when aberrant blood vessels grow and spread through the tissue lining the back of the eye (retina). When these fragile blood vessels leak, the retina is scarred and displaced, causing retinal detachment. Retinopathy of prematurity is the leading cause of blindness in children, and is reported with a code from ICD-9-CM subcategory 362.2.

retirement date Date the patient and/or the patient's spouse retired from active employment. The retirement date is important for Medicare billing purposes to determine primary and secondary insurance coverage.

retractile Capable of being drawn back. r. testis Congenital condition in which the testicle is located near the groin or high in the scrotum, although it can move down into the scrotum at times. Surgery is rarely required, although the condition may be treated with chorionic gonadotropin to encourage complete descent of the testicles. This condition is reported with ICD-9-CM code 752.52. **Synonym(s):** *hypermobile testis.*

retraction Act of holding tissue or a structure back away from its normal position or the field of interest.

O-R

retraction syndrome Simultaneous retraction of eye muscles causing an inability to abduct the affected eye with retraction of the globe. Report this disorder with ICD-9-CM code 378.71. **Synonym(s):** *Still-Turk-Duane syndrome.*

Retro Retrospective rate derivation.

retro- Indicates behind, backward, in a reverse direction.

retrognathism Condition in which the maxilla and upper teeth overlap the mandible and bottom teeth due to the lower jaw being set back further than a normal jaw. This condition is reported using ICD-9-CM code 524.10. **Synonym(s):** *overbite, type 2 malocclusion.*

retrograde Moving against the usual direction of flow.

retrograde ejaculation Condition in which the semen enters the bladder rather than exiting the urethra during ejaculation due to damaged nerves that cause the bladder neck to remain open. Underlying causes include diabetes, prior genitourinary tract surgery, and certain medications. Retrograde ejaculation is reported with ICD-9-CM code 608.87.

retrograde filling Filling of a root canal by sealing it from the root apex.

retrograde pyelogram X-ray study of the renal pelvis after injection of a radiopaque contrast material through the ureter in order to determine a blockage or other abnormality. Through a catheter inserted into the ureter via a cystoscope, dye is injected, and x-rays are taken as the dye moves into the renal pelvis through the ureter. This procedure is reported with both an injection code (52005) and a radiological and supervision code (74420). Report 87.74 for the ICD-9-CM procedure.

retroperitoneal Located behind the peritoneum, the membrane that lines the abdominopelvic walls and forms a covering for the internal organs.

retroperitoneal fibrosis syndrome Retroperitoneal structures obstructing ureters following certain types of chemical treatment; there is no identified cause. Report this disorder with ICD-9-CM code 593.4. **Synonym(s):** *Ormond's syndrome.*

Retrovir Brand name oral or intravenous antiviral for the treatment of human immunodeficiency virus (HIV) that causes AIDS. Retrovir is used with other antiretrovirals to prevent HIV transmission by pregnant women to the baby, for health care workers with needle stick exposure, and in some rape cases. Its supply is reported with HCPCS Level II code J3485 or S0104. Generic Retrovir may be known as azidothymine, AZT, zidovudine.

RetroX Brand name transcutaneous air conduction hearing aid system. Behind-the-ear hearing aid that works without an ear mold, leaving the ear canal totally open. A titanium tube is implanted in the soft tissue between the back of the outer ear and the outer ear canal. It improves hearing in people with mild to moderate high-frequency hearing loss by amplifying sounds while leaving the ear canal open. This is a hearing aid device and is not considered a cochlear implant.

Rett's syndrome Progressive disease affecting grey matter of the brain, where infant females present ataxia, autism, dementia, seizures, loss of purposeful use of the hands, and cerebral atrophy. Report this disorder with ICD-9-CM code 330.8.

return to provider Entire claim is returned to the provider for correction and resubmission. **Synonym(s):** *RTP.*

rev. Revise, revision.

revascularization Restoration of blood flow and oxygen supply to a body part. This may apply to an extremity, the heart, or penis.

revascularize Restoring blood flow or blood supply to a body part.

revenue code Identifies a specific accommodation or ancillary charge on the bill. The revenue code field was expanded to allow four-digit codes for use in the future.

Reverdin Bunion correction. In a Reverdin osteotomy, a wedge of metatarsal bone is removed and the bones repositioned to correct angulation. A simple Reverdin operation is reported with CPT code 28296. The bunion is reported with ICD-9-CM code 727.1.

review committee Multidisciplinary committee that considers denied cases being appealed, catastrophic cases, or fee-for-service cases.

revision Reordering or rearrangement of tissue to suit a particular need or function.

Reye's syndrome Condition of childhood spawned by a spirochetic or viral disease of the upper respiratory system. Symptoms include recurrent vomiting, brain swelling, disturbances of consciousness, and seizures. Often fatal. Reye's syndrome can be prompted by use of aspirin. Report this disorder with ICD-9-CM code 331.81.

Reye-Sheehan's syndrome Secretion of all anterior pituitary hormones is inadequate or absent presenting after childbirth. Report this disorder with ICD-9-CM code 253.2. **Synonym(s):** *Sheehan's syndrome.*

RFA *1)* Radiofrequency ablation. *2)* Regulatory Flexibility Act.

RGO Reciprocating gait orthosis. Orthosis designed to allow ambulation in paraplegic patients, using hip flexion and pivot points. RGO components are reported using HCPCS Level II L codes.

Rh Rhesus.

Rh neg Rhesus factor negative.

O-R

-rhage Indicates bleeding or other fluid discharge. *Synonym(s): -rhagia.*

-rhaphy Indicates a suture or seam joining two structures.

RHB Right heart bypass.

RHC *1)* Right heart catheterization. *2)* Rural health center.

RHD *1)* Relative hepatic dullness. *2)* Rheumatic heart disease.

rheo- Indicates a flow or stream of fluid.

rheumatic heart disease Manifestation of and sequel to rheumatic fever; any cardiac involvement in rheumatic fever.

rheumatoid pneumoconiosis Pulmonary condition in rheumatoid arthritis patients in which the lungs have multiple, spherical nodules, or lesions throughout both lungs. Report this condition with ICD-9-CM code 714.81. *Synonym(s): Caplan's syndrome.*

RHF Right heart failure.

RHHI Regional home health intermediary. Five fiscal intermediaries nationally designated to process all Medicare home health and hospice claims.

RHIA Registered health information administrator. Accreditation for medical record administrators, previously known as a registered records administrator (RRA), through AHIMA.

rhino- Relating to the nose.

rhinodynia Pain in the nose. *Synonym(s): Rhinalgia.*

Rhinolight Brand name device for performing rhinophototherapy, a procedure in which visible and ultraviolet light is applied to the mucosal lining of the nose and sinus to mitigate allergic rhinitis. Treatment with Rhinolight is reported with CPT code 0168T.

rhinomanometry Technique using sound wave analysis as the waves are reflected from the nasal cavities in order to evaluate nasal obstruction and assess the geometry of the nasal cavity. Acoustic rhinometry is used prior to nasal surgery and to compare the decongestive action of corticosteroids and antihistamines. Report rhinomanometry with ICD-9-CM procedure code 89.12 and CPT code 92512. *Synonym(s): acoustic rhinometry.*

rhinophototherapy Application of visible and ultraviolet light to the mucosal lining of the nose and sinus to mitigate allergic rhinitis. Rhinophototherapy is reported with CPT code 0168T.

rhinophyma Severe rosacea appearing as red, thickened, overgrown, and edematous lobules of the skin and sebaceous glands of the nose and cheeks, most often seen in men. Rhinophyma is reported with a code from ICD-9-CM subcategory 695.3. *Synonym(s): rosacea.*

rhinoplasty Reconstructive, restorative, or cosmetic plastic surgery of the nose. Code selection is dependent upon the intensity of and reason for the procedure. Rhinoplasty to repair a deformity due to congenital cleft lip and/or palate is assigned the appropriate CPT code from 30460-30462. Secondary rhinoplasty procedures are classified to 30430-30450 and primary rhinoplasty procedures to 30400-30410.

rhinotomy Incision into the nose.

RHIO Regional health information organization.

RHIT Registered health information technician. Accreditation for medical records practitioners, previously known as accredited records technician (ART), through AHIMA.

rhizotomy Procedure to interrupt the roots of cranial or spinal nerves. Posterior rhizotomy separates the sensory spinal nerve roots to relieve intractable pain. Anterior rhizotomy separates the motor spinal nerve roots to stop involuntary spasmodic movements associated with conditions like cerebral palsy, torticollis, or paraplegia. Trigeminal rhizotomy destroys part of the fifth cranial nerve sensory root or ganglion to relieve trigeminal neuralgia.

rhonchus(i) Abnormal continual wheeze heard when listening to the chest as a person breathes. Wheeze is usually caused by airway obstruction from swelling or secretions. Wheeze can be high or low pitched. Report this condition with ICD-9-CM code 786.07. *Synonym(s): wheeze.*

rhytidectomy Facelift. Surgical removal of wrinkles from the face. Code selection is dependent upon the areas involved, such as the forehead alone, the glabellar frown lines, or the neck. Rhytidectomy is reported with CPT codes 15824-15829.

rhytids Wrinkles. Wrinkling of the skin is classified to ICD-9-CM code 701.8.

RIA Radioimmunoassay.

rib belt Device that encircles the abdomen and provides support for injured ribs while they heal.

ribbons In oncology, small plastic tubes containing radioactive sources for interstitial placement that may be cut into specific lengths tailored to the size of the area receiving ionizing radiation treatment.

RICA Right internal carotid artery.

rice disease Disease caused by a lack of vitamin B1 (thiamine) causing cardiac damage, polyneuritis, and edema. The disease is found mostly in areas where white, polished rice is the main staple of the diet. Report this disorder with ICD-9-CM code 265.0. *Synonym(s): beriberi, dietetic neuritis, endemic polyneuritis.*

Rickets Softening or weakening of the bones due to a lack of vitamin D, calcium, and phosphate.

0-R

Riddoch's syndrome   Cortical paralysis of visual fixation, optic ataxia, and disturbance of visual attention. Eye movements are normal. Report this disorder with ICD-9-CM code 368.16. *Synonym(s): Balint's syndrome, Holmes' syndrome, Riddoch's syndrome.*

Ridell sinusotomy   Frontal sinus tissue is destroyed to eliminate tumors.

Ridley's syndrome   Left heart failure marked by acute edema of lung. Report this disorder with ICD-9-CM code 428.1.

Riedel's lobe   Variation in liver anatomy presenting as a tongue-like accessory projecting from the right lobe, most likely seen documented in gastrointestinal imaging studies. Riedel's lobe is of itself of no clinical significance, but may cause problems if it undergoes torsion.

Rieger's syndrome   Dysgenesis of eye marked through widened trabecular meshwork, large iridial bands, and glaucoma. Report this disorder with ICD-9-CM code 743.44.

Rietti-Greppi-Micheli syndrome   One of a group of hemolytic anemias sharing a common decreased rate of synthesis of one or more hemoglobin polypeptide chains and are classified according to chain involved. Report this disorder with ICD-9-CM code 282.49.

RIG   Rabies immune globulin, usually in reference to a vaccine. RIG is administered to patients exposed to rabies. Supply of RIG is reported with CPT codes 90375 and 90376; administration is reported separately. The need for treatment is reported with ICD-9-CM code V01.5.

Right Heart

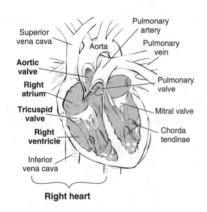

Right heart

The right heart receives deoxygenated blood and sends it to the lungs

right heart   Areas of the right heart, including the right atrium and right ventricle.

Rigler's sign   Indication of pneumoperitoneum; the bowel is well defined because it is outlined by air on x-ray. Pneumoperitoneum is reported with ICD-9-CM code 568.89. *Synonym(s): double wall sign.*

RIH

RIH is the acronym for right inguinal hernia

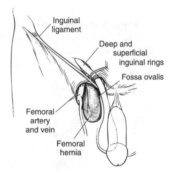

RIH   Right inguinal hernia. *Synonym(s): bubonocele, scrotal hernia.*

RIJ   Right internal jugular.

Riley-Day syndrome   Congenital anomaly primarily found in families of European-Jewish extraction, characterized by poor sucking ability, sweating while eating, hypotonia, and insensitivity to pain. This syndrome is reported with ICD-9-CM code 742.8. *Synonym(s): familial dysautonomia.*

rilonacept   Injectable interleukin-1 (IL-1) blocker indicated for the treatment of cryopyrin-associated periodic syndromes (CAPS), a group of rare hereditary autoinflammatory disorders. Rilonacept may also be sold under the brand name Arcalyst. Report supply with HCPCS Level II code J2793.

RIND   Reversible ischemic neurologic event.

risk adjustment   Method of predicting and adjusting payment for expenditures relating to health care services based upon patient diagnoses and certain demographic adjusters.

risk contract   Contract between Medicare and a payer or a payer and a provider in which the payer (in the case of Medicare) and the provider (in the case of the payer contracts) receive a set amount for care of a patient base. If costs exceed the amount the payer or provider was paid, the patients still receive care during the term of the contract.

risk factor reduction Reduction of risk in the pool of health plan members.

risk manager Person charged with keeping financial risk low, including malpractice cases.

risk pool Pool of people who will be in the insured group, their medical and mental histories, other factors such as age, and their predicted health.

Risser jacket Extended body cast with hinges and buckles that covers the neck, extends down to one knee, and sometimes includes an arm to the elbow. This is applied in cases of scoliosis, reported with CPT codes 29010-29015. *Synonym(s): Reiser jacket, Turnbuckle jacket.*

RIST Radioimmunosorbent test. Laboratory test measuring total IgE, reported with CPT code 82785.

RITE Rapid intraoperative tissue expansion. Minor (up to 3 cm) tissue expansion occurring in the operating room, usually because sufficient skin is not available to close a wound. The tissue is typically stretched using a silicone balloon, or in some cases, a Foley catheter.

Rithron-XR Brand name coronary stent system.

Ritter's disease Skin infection most commonly found in infants and children under the age of five. It is caused by certain strains of *Staphylococcus* bacteria, which damages the skin and results in shedding. Symptoms include fever, exfoliation of large areas of skin, pain, and redness over most of the body. Gentle pressure may cause the skin to slip off, leaving red, wet areas known as Nikolsky's sign. Report this disorder with ICD-9-CM code 695.81, and use an additional code from range 695.50-695.59 to identify the percentage of skin exfoliation. *Synonym(s): Staphylococcal scalded skin syndrome, SSS.*

RL Ringer's lactate.

RLE Right lower extremity.

RLF Retrolental fibroplasia.

RLL Right lower lobe.

rlq Right lower quadrant.

RLS Restless legs syndrome.

RM Respiratory movement.

RMA Right mentum anterior position.

RMC Rating method code.

RML Right middle lobe.

RMP Right mentum posterior position.

RMS Rhabdomyosarcoma.

RMT Right mentum transverse position.

RN Registered nurse.

RNA Ribonucleic acid.

RNFL Retinal nerve fiber layer. Layer of the retina that is examined using a slit lamp, photography, or scanning laser polarimetry. RNFL thickness can be a predictor of future field loss or disc changes caused by the presence of glaucoma. *Synonym(s): NFL.*

RNV Radionuclide ventriculography. Noninvasive test that produces a moving image of the heart to assess the pumping function of the left ventricle. Technetium 99 is mixed with the patient's red blood cells, the cells are injected into the patient's bloodstream, and the patient is placed under a gamma camera so the ejection fraction of the left ventricle of the heart, an overall indicator of cardiac function, can be measured. MUGA scans identify the area of damage following a myocardial infarct or monitor the effects of chemotherapy upon the heart, as some drugs are toxic to heart muscle. *Synonym(s): MUGA.*

ROA Right occiput anterior position.

Robin's syndrome Brachygnathia and cleft palate, upward displacement of the larynx, and angulation of the manubrium sterni. May be paired with others or the sole hyperplasia. Report this disorder with ICD-9-CM code 756.0. *Synonym(s): Pierre Robin's syndrome.*

robotic assisted surgery New technology that is used to assist the surgeon which involves instrumentation combined with the use of robotic arms, devices, or systems. Through the use of a robotic system the surgeon guides the instrumentation from a console maintaining direct visualization. Robotic assisted surgery can be performed with many minimally invasive procedures, such as laparoscopic or thorascoscopic procedures. Two systems that have received FDA approval are daVinci and Zeus.

Rocephin See ceftriaxone sodium.

rod Straight, slim, cylindrical metal instrument for therapeutics.

roentgenogram Film produced by x-ray. *Synonym(s): radiograph.*

Rokitansky-Kuster-Hauser syndrome Absence of vagina and uterus with normal karyotype and ovaries. Amenorrhea. Report this disorder with ICD-9-CM code 752.49.

Rolando's fracture Comminuted intra-articular fracture at the base of the thumb metacarpal, reported with ICD-9-CM code 815.01 or 815.11.

role-based access control Method of limiting access to information that assigns each user to one or more predefined roles. *Synonym(s): RBAC.*

ROM Range of motion.

Romano-Ward syndrome Potentially fatal condition precipitated by vigorous exertion, emotional upset, or startling moments due to an imbalance in the electrical

O-R

timing mechanism that controls the pumping action of the heart's ventricles. This syndrome causes the patient to be susceptible to recurrent episodes of syncope, collapse, and possible ventricular fibrillation that can cause sudden death. Report this condition with ICD-9-CM code 426.82. **Synonym(s):** *long QT syndrome, prolonged QT interval syndrome.*

Romberg's syndrome Hypersomnia associated with bulimia and occurring in males between 10 to 25 years of age. Ravenous appetite following prolonged sleep, along with behavioral disturbances, impaired thought processes, and hallucinations. Report this disorder with ICD-9-CM code 349.89. **Synonym(s):** *Kleine-Levin syndrome, Parry-Romberg syndrome.*

romiplostim Generic name for Nplate, an injectable thrombopoietin receptor agonist used to treat low platelet counts (thrombocytopenia) in patients with idiopathic thrombocytopenic purpura (ITP) who have not responded well to immunoglobulins, steroids, or removal of the spleen. Supply is reported with HCPCS Level II code J2796.

rongeur Sharp-edged instrument with a scoop-tip used to cut through tissue and bone.

root Part of the tooth located in the socket, covered by cementum, and attached by the periodontal structures.

root canal Inner soft tissue, or pulp, of the tooth containing the lymph vessels, veins, arteries, and nerves of the tooth within small channels (up to five) running from the top of the tooth down to the tip of the root. When the tooth is cracked or decayed, bacteria enter the pulp and infect it, causing damage or death to the pulpal tissue and possibly an abscess that can infect bone. Root canal therapy repairs the root canal by removing the damaged pulp and cleaning out bacteria to prevent further damage and save the tooth. Root canals are reported with a code from HCPCS Level II series D3310-D3353.

root planing Smoothing a root surface by abrasion or filing of the exposed root surface.

ROP *1)* Retinopathy of prematurity. *2)* Right occiput posterior position.

ROS Review of systems. Inventory of body systems obtained through a series of questions seeking to identify signs and/or symptoms that the patient may be experiencing or has experienced. For purposes of ROS, the following systems are recognized: constitutional symptoms (e.g., fever, weight loss); eyes; ears, nose, mouth, throat; cardiovascular; respiratory; gastrointestinal; genitourinary; musculoskeletal; integumentary; neurological; psychiatric; endocrine; hematologic/lymphatic; and allergic/immunologic.

rosacea Skin disease involving the face, characterized by redness and permanent dilation of small blood vessels,

with outbreaks of edema and pustule formation. Rosacea is classified to ICD-9-CM code 695.3.

ROSE Rapid onsite cytology.

Rosen-Castleman-Liebow syndrome Chronic disease of lungs marked by chest pain, weakness, hemoptysis, dyspnea, and productive cough. Ventilation of affected areas is prevented by a proteinaceous material. Report this disorder with ICD-9-CM code 516.0.

roseola infantum Sixth of the customary exanthems of childhood, roseola infantum is typically an acute, benign disease manifested by a short-lived high fever followed by the appearance of a light pink maculopapular or erythematous rash. Since the identification of the etiologic agent human herpesvirus 6 (HHV-6), cases of roseola infantum have also been documented that lack the characteristic rash, instead presenting as an acute febrile illness with associated gastrointestinal or respiratory manifestations. Although the full range of clinical manifestations of HHV-6 is unclear, other recently recognized clinical signs include hepatitis, encephalitis, hemophagocytic syndrome, and adult mononucleosis-like illness. HHV-7, closely related to both HHV-6 and cytomegalovirus (CMV), has also been found to be the causative agent in a small number of roseola cases. Believed to affect more than 95 percent of the population, HHV-7 is the least pathogenic of the three viruses and is most often acquired prior to age 5. As with other herpesviruses, it becomes latent in the host following the primary infection, predisposing individuals to later reactivation. Report roseola infantum with an ICD-9-CM diagnosis code from range 058.10-058.12. **Synonym(s):** *exanthema subitum, sixth disease.*

rosiglitazone Oral medication exclusive to lowering blood glucose in Type II diabetics. May be sold as brand name Avandia.

RotaTeq Brand name oral vaccine against rotavirus, administered as part of the childhood immunization schedule at ages 2, 4, and 6 months. RotaTeq is a new vaccine approved by the FDA in 2006. Check with individual payers for coverage policies. Supply of the vaccine is reported with CPT code 90680.

rotator cuff Four muscles that originate on the scapula and form a single tendon that inserts on the head of the humerus. The supraspinatus, infraspinatus, subscapulari, and teres minor are the four muscles that come together to help lift and rotate the arm.

rotavirus Genus of viruses having a wheel-like shape belonging to the family Reoviridae. This is an RNA virus with six separate serotypes, only three of which-A, B, and C-cause disease in humans, namely acute, severe gastroenteritis and diarrhea in infants and young children. Transmission is fecal-oral route. Rotavirus infection is reported with ICD-9-CM code 008.61.

O-R

Roth's spot White, round spot near the optic disc, indicative of a hemorrhage that may be caused by bacterial endocarditis, pernicious anemia, diabetes, or leukemia. Coding for Roth's spot will depend on the cause of the hemorrhage. *Synonym(s): retinitis septica.*

Roth's syndrome Feeling of tingling, formication, itching, and other symptoms on the outer side of the lower part of the thigh caused by lateral femoral cutaneous nerve. Report this disorder with ICD-9-CM code 355.1.

Rothmund's syndrome Pigmentation and atrophy of the skin, along with cataracts, saddle nose, bone defects, disturbance of hair growth, and hypogonadism. Report this disorder with ICD-9-CM code 757.33.

rotoblator Instrument used to remove arterial plaque; a special catheter equipped with a high-speed burr at the tip that bores through sclerotic deposits within a vessel.

Rotor's syndrome Nonhemolytic jaundice differing from Dubin-Johnson syndrome in that it does not produce liver pigmentation. Report this disorder with ICD-9-CM code 277.4.

round ligament Ligament between the uterus and the pelvic wall.

routine Normal activity.

roux-en-Y anastomosis Y-shaped attachment of the distal end of a divided small intestine segment to the stomach, esophagus, biliary tract, or other structure with anastomosis of the proximal end to the side of the small intestine further down for reflux-free drainage. Report CPT code 43621 or 43633 for this procedure. *Synonym(s): roux-en-Y reconstruction.*

RP Radical prostatectomy. Complete removal of the prostate, including removal of attached seminal vesicles. CPT code selection for RP is determined by approach, nerve sparing, and node biopsy. Report inpatient services with ICD-9-CM procedure code 60.5 regardless of approach; lymph node excision and orchiectomy are assigned separate codes if performed.

RPG Retrograde pyelogram.

RPh Registered pharmacist.

RPP Radical perineal prostatectomy. Complete removal of the prostate through an incision in the area between the scrotum and anus, including removal of attached seminal vesicles. RPP is reported with CPT code 55810, 55812 if lymph node biopsy is included, or 55815 if a bilateral pelvic lymphadenectomy is included.

RPR Venereal disease report.

RPT Registered physical therapist.

RR *1)* HCPCS Level II modifier for use with HCPCS Level II codes that identifies rental of durable medical equipment (DME). Should be used with other rental

modifiers, KH, KI, and KJ. This modifier should be listed first, with other modifiers second. *2)* Recovery room.

RRA Registered records administrator.

RRB Railroad Retirement Board. Manages health insurance entitlement and investigates entitlement problems and issues affecting Railroad Retirement beneficiaries (i.e., those entitled to Part A and/or Part B coverage based on the Railroad Retirement Act).

RRC Rural referral center.

-rrhagia Indicates an abnormal or excessive fluid discharge.

-rrhexis Splitting or breaking.

RRP Radical retropubic prostatectomy. Procedure in which the prostate is removed through an incision in the lower abdomen. Laparoscopic RRP is reported with CPT code 55866. Open RRP is reported with 55840; 55842 if lymph node biopsy is included, and 55845 if a bilateral pelvic lymphadenectomy is included.

RRR Regular rate and rhythm.

RRT Registered respiratory therapist.

RS Reducing substances.

RSB Recurrent sinus barotrauma. Recurrent and severe sinus pain caused by poor sinus ventilation and a change in altitude, reported with ICD-9-CM code 993.1. *Synonym(s): aerosinusitis.*

RSC Right subclavian.

RSR Regular sinus rhythm.

RSS Russell Silver syndrome. Rare genetic disorder characterized by intrauterine growth retardation, unusual facial features, and other physical abnormalities. In many cases, there is asymmetry or overgrowth on one side of the body. RSS is reported with ICD-9-CM code 759.89.

RSV Respiratory syncytial virus.

RSV-IGIV Respiratory syncytial virus immune globulin intravenous. Intravenous injection given as a preventive measure for children who are at high risk of developing complications from RSV. May be sold under the brand name RespiGam.

RT *1)* HCPCS Level II modifier, for use with CPT or HCPCS Level II codes, identifying a procedure performed on the right side of the body. It does not indicate a bilateral procedure. The use of the RT modifier does not affect reimbursement, but its absence may cause payment delays. *2)* Recreational therapist. *3)* Respiratory therapist. *4)* Resting tracing. *5)* Right.

RTA Renal tubular acidosis. Condition in which the kidney tubules cannot effectively remove acid from the blood so it can be eliminated in the urine. Ingestion of a daily baking soda preparation can mitigate the

O-R

symptoms. RTA can be a primary or secondary condition, and either is reported with ICD-9-CM code 588.89.

RTC   Return to clinic.

RTI   Reproductive tract infection.

rTMS   Repetitive transcranial magnetic stimulation. Noninvasive therapeutic technique utilizing a rapidly changing magnetic field that passes through the scalp and skull, generating small electrical pulses to the pre-frontal cortex of the brain in order to alter its activity. rTMS is indicated as a potential treatment for depression and other psychiatric and neurological disorders and symptoms. Report treatment planning with CPT code 90867 and treatment delivery with 90868.

RTP   Return to provider.

RTPCR   Reverse transcriptase polymerase chain reaction. Investigational test for reviewing the levels of PSA in a patient's blood.

rubella syndrome   Developmental abnormalities of newborn baby as resulting from transplacental transference of rubella during the first trimester of pregnancy. Symptoms include ocular and cardiac lesions, deafness, microcephaly, mental retardation, hepatitis, encephalitis, and others. Report this disorder with ICD-9-CM code 771.0.

rubeosis iridis   Formation of new blood vessels on the surface of the iris.

RUCA   Rural-urban commuting area, a CMS designation.

Rud's syndrome   Dwarfism, hypogonadism, and epilepsy with scaly skin as result of inherited disorder. Report this disorder with ICD-9-CM code 759.89.

RUG   Resource utilization group.

RUG-III   Resource utilization group version III. Patient classification system that uses patients' characteristics and health status information from the minimum data set (MDS), such as diagnoses, ability to perform activities of daily living (ADL), and treatments received, to assign the patient to a resource group for payment under the Medicare prospective payment system for skilled nursing facilities. The RUG-III system is a hierarchy of major patient types consisting of seven major categories that represent the first level of patient classification. The major categories are rehabilitation, extensive services, special care, clinically complex, impaired cognition, behavior problems, and reduced physical function. These major categories are further differentiated into 44 more specific patient groupings.

Ruiter-Pompen (-Wyers) syndrome   Corneal opacities; burning pain in palms, soles, and abdomen; chronic paresthesia on hands and feet; cardiopulmonary involvement; edema of the legs; osteoporosis; retarded growth; and delayed puberty. Patients die of renal, cardiac, or cerebrovascular failure. Report this disorder

with ICD-9-CM code 272.7. **Synonym(s):** *Fabry's syndrome.*

RUL   Right upper lobe.

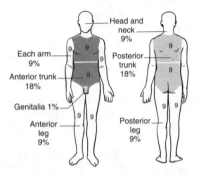

Rule of Nines
Estimation of Total Body
Surface Burned

rule of nines   Rapid measurement system used to calculate the total body surface area (TBSA) involved in burns, based upon dividing the total area into segments as multiples of 9 percent. The perineum or external genitals are 1 percent; each arm is 9 percent; the front and back of the trunk, and each leg are separately counted as 18 percent; and the head is another 9 percent in adults. For infants and children, the head is 18 percent involvement and the legs are 14 percent each, due to the larger surface area of a child's head in proportion to the body.

rumination obsessional   Constant preoccupation with certain thoughts, with the inability to dismiss them from the mind; also known as neurotic disorder, obsessive-compulsive.

rumination psychogenic   Regurgitation of food, without nausea, retching, or disgust followed by ejection or chewing with reswallowing. Frequently seen with failure to thrive or weight loss developing after a period of normal functioning. This condition may afflict any age group, but it is particularly found in the mentally retarded population,

Runge's syndrome   Placental dysfunction occurring in postmature fetuses. Report this disorder with ICD-9-CM code 766.22. **Synonym(s):** *Ballantyne syndrome.*

rupture   Tearing or breaking open of tissue.

ruq   Right upper quadrant.

rural health clinic   Clinic in an area where there is a shortage of health services staffed by a nurse practitioner, physician assistant, or certified nurse midwife under physician direction that provides routine diagnostic services, including clinical laboratory services, drugs, and biologicals and that has prompt access to

O-R

additional diagnostic services from facilities meeting federal requirements.

rush charge   Charge for expeditious test results. *Synonym(s): stat charge.*

Russell (-Silver) syndrome   Suprasellar lesions in anterior third ventricle, hampering a child's ability to thrive. Despite elevated growth hormones, child is emaciated and looses body fat. Report this disorder with ICD-9-CM code 759.89.

Russell's sign   Cuts, rashes, or calluses on the hands, especially on the knuckles or backs of the fingers. It is associated with injuries resulting from chronic binging and purging of bulimia.

Russian autumnal encephalitis   Acute mosquito-borne, epidemic viral infection seen in southern and eastern Asia, affecting the central nervous system. Although frequently asymptomatic, patients may develop fever, chills, gastrointestinal symptoms, confusion, and agitation. In the most severe cases, meningoencephalomyelitis develops with cortical damage and spinal cord lesions forming like those occurring in polio, possibly becoming fatal. Report this condition with ICD-9-CM code 062.0. *Synonym(s): Japanese B type encephalitis.*

RV   Right ventricle.

RVS   Relative value study. Guide that shows the relationship between the time, resources, competency, experience, severity, and other factors necessary to perform procedures that is multiplied by a dollar conversion factor to determine a monetary value for the procedure.

RVT   Renal vein thrombosis.

RVU   Relative value unit. Value assigned a procedure based on difficulty and time consumed. Used for computing reimbursement under a relative value study.

RW   Relative weight. Assigned weight that is intended to reflect the relative resource consumption associated with each DRG. The higher the relative weight, the greater the payment to the hospital. The relative weights are calculated by CMS and published in the final prospective payment system rule.

Rx   Take (prescription; treatment).

RX Acculink   Brand name carotid stent.

RxN   Reaction.

RYGBP-E   Roux-en-Y gastric bypass - extended. Treatment for morbid obesity in which the stomach is divided to create a gastric pouch, but the excess stomach is not removed. A long limb of small intestine is attached to the functioning stomach, thus reducing caloric absorption. The amputated stomach and proximal intestine is attached to the limb that has been secured to the new pouch. This open procedure is reported with

CPT code 43847 or ICD-9-CM procedure code 44.39. If performed laparoscopically, report CPT code 43645 or ICD-9-CM procedure code 44.38. *NCD Reference: 100.1.*

Rytand-Lipsitch syndrome   Bundle branch block in a patient with normal coronary arteries and myocardium resulting from calcification of conducting system. Report this disorder with ICD-9-CM code 426.0. *Synonym(s): Lev's syndrome.*

O-R

s Without.

S tach Sinus tachycardia, reported with ICD-9-CM code 427.89.

S&A Sugar and acetone.

s.c. Subcutaneous.

s.l. Under the tongue, sublingual.

S.O.S. If necessary (si opus sit).

S/P Status post.

S/S Signs and symptoms.

SA HCPCS Level II modifier, for use with CPT or HCPCS Level II codes, that identifies a nurse practitioner's rendering service in collaboration with a physician. It is required by some state Medicaid programs for nurse practitioner services.

SA node Sinoatrial node. Mass of specialized cardiac muscle fibers that normally acts as the "pacemaker" of the electrical conduction system, regulating contraction of the heart muscle.

SAANDS Selective apoptotic antineoplastic drugs.

SAARD Slow-acting anti-rheumatic drug. Pharmaceutical with the potential to slow the profession of rheumatic disease. An example of a SAARD is methotrexate.

SAB Spontaneous abortion.

SABA Supplied air-breathing apparatus.

SAC Short arm cast. Cast extending from the elbow to the palm or digits used for distal forearm and wrist fractures.

saccule Small pouch or sac, such as the alveolar air saccules of the lungs.

SACH Solid ankle, cushion heel.

sacral nerves Five nerves (S1-S5) on each side of the sacrum that pass from the sacral canal through the sacral foramina and form the sacral and coccygeal plexus. *NCD Reference: 230.18.*

sacralization-scoliosis-sciatica syndrome Fusion of bottom lumbar vertebra to top sacral vertebra, making a sixth sacral vertebra. Other symptoms include sciatica and scoliosis. Report this disorder with ICD-9-CM code 756.15. *Synonym(s): Bertolotti's syndrome.*

sacro- Relating to the sacrum (base of the vertebral column).

sacrum Lower portion of the spine composed of five fused vertebrae designated as S1-S5.

SACS Sleep and circadian study.

SADMERC Statistical Analysis Durable Medical Equipment Regional Carrier.

SAED Semiautomatic external defibrillator.

Saenger's syndrome Paralysis of conjugate movement of eyes without paralysis of convergence. Caused by lesions of midbrain. Report this disorder with ICD-9-CM code 379.46.

safe harbor Protected business arrangement that might otherwise constitute a violation of the antikickback statute, such as those deemed to promote competition, improve quality of care, or confer a cost savings.

Safety Glide syringe Brand name insulin syringe. Supply of a box of 100 is reported with HCPCS Level II code S8490 or A4206 x 100 for Medicare claims.

SAFHS Sonic accelerated fracture healing system.

Safire Brand name bi-directional ablation catheter used in cardiac electrophysiology mapping or in cardiac ablation procedures to treat arrhythmias.

Sager traction splint Emergency traction splint used for femoral fractures having a unit that measures the force of traction at the ankle and maintains position and alignment without excessive pressure around the ankle or sciatic nerve injury.

SAGES Society of American Gastrointestinal Endoscopic Surgeons.

sagittal Up and down along the length of the body, as opposed to across it (transverse).

sagittal plane Imaginary plane in the human body that travels from the top to the bottom of the body, dividing it into left and right portions.

SAH Subarachnoid hemorrhage.

Sahara sonometer Brand name of a portable bone density meter for testing patients for risk of osteoporosis.

SAL Suction assisted lipectomy.

salabrasion Tattoo removal in which the skin is first soaked with a highly concentrated saline solution and then abraded.

salmonella Group of more than 1,500 serotypes of a genus of gram negative, facultative anaerobic bacteria of the family Enterobacteriacae. The major clinical symptom is food poisoning. Salmonella causes enteric fevers like typhoid and paratyphoid, acute gastroenteritis, and septicemias. Spread through contaminated food, infected turtles or lizards, infected dyes, or contaminated marijuana. Salmonella is reported within ICD-9-CM category 003, based on the disease process caused by any serotype, e.g., gastroenteritis, septicemia, meningitis, pneumonia, arthritis, osteomyelitis. A suspected carrier is reported with ICD-9-CM code V02.3.

salmonellosis Infection with the Salmonella bacteria. Common symptoms include diarrhea, fever, and abdominal cramps within 12 to 72 hours after infection with duration of four to seven days. Most persons infected with Salmonella recover without treatment, however patients with severe symptoms may need medical management in the hospital setting, particularly for hydration. In some instances, Salmonella infection may spread to the blood stream and infect other body sites resulting in death unless antibiotic treatment is started without delay. Patients with impaired immune systems, the elderly, and infants are more likely to develop severe infection. Salmonella infections are classified to ICD-9-CM category 003.

salpingectomy   Removal of all or part of one or both of the fallopian tubes. Indications include infection, ectopic pregnancy, sterilization, or cancer. This procedure is often performed in combination with other open or laparoscopic procedures.

salpingitis   Inflammation of the fallopian tubes, usually caused by a bacterial infection and occurring in conjunction with inflammation of the ovaries (oophoritis). These conditions are reported together in ICD-9-CM, depending on the status as acute or chronic. In acute salpingitis, the inflamed fallopian tubes may produce secretions that cause the inner walls to adhere to each other or to neighboring structures. Chronic salpingitis continues over time, producing milder symptoms. Salpingitis is one of the most common causes of infertility. Salpingitis is reported within category 614 unless it is specifically stated as gonococcal, in which case it is reported with 098.17 or 098.37.

salpingo-   Relating to the fallopian or eustachian tubes.

salpingo-oophorectomy   Surgical removal of both the fallopian tube and ovary.

SALT   *1)* Sequential aggressive local therapy, as it applies to chemotherapy. *2)* Skin associated lymphoid tissue.

Salter osteotomy   Innominate bone of the hip is cut, removed, and repositioned to repair a congenital dislocation, subluxation, or deformity.

same-day transfer   Patient admitted to a hospital as an inpatient and transferred the same day to another acute care or skilled nursing facility as an inpatient.

sanction   Imposition of penalties or exclusion of a provider for fraud or infractions such as an inappropriate use of services, providing procedures that may harm the patient, or applying inferior techniques.

sand flea disease   Disease spread by the parasitic flea, Tunga penetrans, the pregnant female of which burrows into the host's skin, often the lower limbs and under nails, causing inflammation, swelling, and cyst formation that turns ulcerative. Gas gangrene, bacteremia, or tetanus may occur in cases of severe infestation, as well as spontaneous loss of a digit. Report this condition with ICD-9-CM code 134.1. **Synonym(s):** *burrowing flea disease, chigoe disease, jigger disease.*

sand process   Thermal modification of the collagen of the cornea.

Sander's disease   Rare, chronic psychosis in which logically constructed systematized delusions of grandeur or persecution, or somatic abnormality have developed gradually without concomitant hallucinations or the schizophrenic type of disordered thinking.

Sanfilippo's syndrome   Results from accumulation of mucopolysaccharide sulfates affecting the eye, ear, skin, teeth, skeleton, joints, liver, spleen, cardiovascular system, respiratory system, and central nervous system. Report this disorder with ICD-9-CM code 277.5.

SANS   Stoller afferent nerve stimulation. Brand name device used for treatment of incontinence using electricity.

SAPHO syndrome   Synovitis, acne, pustulosis, hyperostosis, osteitis. Chronic disorder involving the skin, joints, and bones, possibly related to spondyloarthropathies and treated with anti-inflammatories. No specific code is indexed to SAPHO syndrome in ICD-9-CM. Report each manifestation separately.

sarco-   Relating to flesh.

-sarcoma   Malignant tumor of flesh or connective tissue.

SAS   Signs and symptoms.

SAST   Serum aspartate aminotransferase.

Satyriasis   Pathologic or exaggerated sexual desire or excitement in males.

saucerization   Creation of a shallow, saucer-like depression in the bone to facilitate drainage of infected areas.

S-U

SAVER

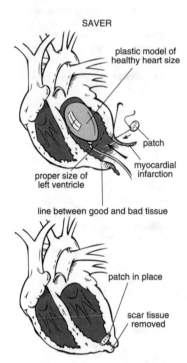

plastic model of
healthy heart size

patch

myocardial
infarction

proper size of
left ventricle

line between good and bad tissue

patch in place

scar tissue
removed

SAVER Surgical anterior ventricular endocardial restoration. Treatment of congestive heart failure by restoring the heart to a more normal size and shape. The ventricular muscle and chamber are resized with the aid of a plastic model, in hopes of improving heart function. This procedure is often performed with bypass or valve repair, which is reported separately. SAVER is reported with CPT code 33548. *Synonym(s): Dor procedure, LV reconstruction, SVR, TR3SVR.*

SB *1)* HCPCS Level II modifier, for use with CPT or HCPCS Level II codes, that identifies a service or supply provided by a nurse midwife. It is required by some state Medicaid programs for nurse midwife services. *2)* Spina bifida. *3)* Sinus bradycardia.

SBA Standby assist.

SBE Subacute bacterial endocarditis.

SBFT Small bowel follow-through.

SBGM Self blood glucose monitoring.

SBO *1)* Small bowel obstruction. *2)* Side branch occlusion.

SBP Systolic blood pressure.

SBRT Stereotactic body radiation therapy, reported with CPT code 77373.

SC *1)* Subcommittee. *2)* Subcutaneous.

S-C disease Sickle cell hemoglobin-c disease.

Scaglietti-Dagnini syndrome Arthritis of spine accompanying acromegaly, resembling rheumatoid arthritis, and progressing to bony ankylosis with lipping of vertebral margins. Report this disorder with ICD-9-CM code 253.0.

scalded skin syndrome Skin infection most commonly found in infants and children under the age of five. It is caused by certain strains of *Staphylococcus* bacteria, which damages the skin and results in shedding. Symptoms include fever, exfoliation of large areas of skin, pain, and redness over most of the body. Gentle pressure may cause the skin to slip off, leaving red, wet areas known as Nikolsky's sign. Report this disorder with ICD-9-CM code 695.81, and use an additional code from range 695.50-695.59 to identify the percentage of skin exfoliation. *Synonym(s): Staphylococcal scalded skin syndrome, SSS, Ritter's disease.*

scalenus anticus syndrome Disorder presenting symptoms similar to Raynaud's, caused by pressure of brachial plexus and subclavian artery against first thoracic rib. Report this disorder with ICD-9-CM code 353.0. *Synonym(s): Naffziger's syndrome.*

scaling Removal of plaque, calculus, and stains from teeth.

scapho- Indicates deformed condition, shaped like a boat.

scaphocephaly Most common form of craniosynostosis, manifested by a boat-shaped head. It is caused by early closure of the fontanel and the sagittal suture. This condition is reported with ICD-9-CM code 756.0.

Scapula

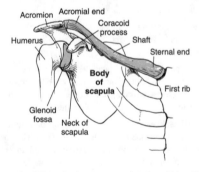

Acromion   Acromial end
                        Coracoid
                        process
Humerus   Shaft
                                  Sternal end

                        Body
                        of
                        scapula   First rib

Glenoid
fossa   Neck of
         scapula

scapula Triangular bone commonly referred to as the shoulder blade.

scapular region Pertaining to the shoulder blade area.

scapulo- Relating to the shoulder.

scapulocostal syndrome Pain in upper and posterior part of the shoulder radiating into neck and occiput, down the arm, and around the chest. Caused by abnormal positioning between scapula and thorax, pain can include tingling in the fingers. Report this disorder with ICD-9-CM code 354.8.

scapuloperoneal syndrome Position of fetus in which the scapula rests closest to the perineal area. Report this disorder with ICD-9-CM code 359.1.

scapulopexy Surgical fixation of the scapula.

scar tissue Fibrous connective tissue that forms around a wounded area or injury, composed mainly of fibroblasts or collagenous fibers. *Synonym(s): cicatrix.*

scarification Process of making scratches or small cuts in the skin or tissue.

SCBE Single contrast barium enema. Radiology exam for viewing the intestine that utilizes a suspension of barium sulfate, a chalk-like substance that appears white in an x-ray, to delineate the lining of the colon and rectum. The barium is administered via the rectum and held inside the colon while x-rays are taken. Report SCBE with ICD-9-CM procedure code 87.64 or CPT code 74270.

SCC Squamous cell carcinoma.

SCCHN Squamous cell carcinoma of the head and neck

SCD Sudden cardiac death, sickle cell disease, or systemic carnitine deficiency. Sudden cardiac death describes unexpected loss of heart function most often due to coronary artery disease or irregularities in the heart's electrical system and is reported with ICD-9-CM code 427.5. Sickle cell disease is reported with codes in ICD-9-CM category 282. Systemic carnitine deficiency is reported with ICD-9-CM code 277.81.

SCFE Slipped capital femoral epiphysis. Condition occurring in childhood, usually among boys, in which the growth end of the upper femur slips off the rest of the bone, causing pain or stiffness and putting the bone at risk for necrosis. SCFE is reported with ICD-9-CM code 732.3.

SCH Sole community hospital, as designated by CMS. Sole source of care in a locality.

Schatzki's ring Abnormal anatomic narrowing ring in the lower esophagus. Schatzki's ring is reported with ICD-9-CM code 750.3 if congenital or 530.3 if acquired.

Schaumann's syndrome Involves the lungs with resulting fibrosis, lymph nodes, skin, liver, eyes, spleen, phalangeal bones, and parotid glands. Identified by systemic granulomas composed of epithelioid and multinucleated giant cells. Report this disorder with ICD-9-CM code 135. *Synonym(s): Besnier-Boeck-Schaumann syndrome, Hutchinson-Boeck syndrome, Lofgren's syndrome.*

schedule Listing of amounts payable for specific procedures.

Scheie's syndrome Accumulation of mucopolysaccharide sulfates affecting the eye, ear, skin, teeth, skeleton, joints, liver, spleen, cardiovascular system, respiratory system, and central nervous system. Report this disorder with ICD-9-CM code 277.5.

Scheuer staging Scoring system for chronic hepatitis, with scores of 0 to 4. No fibrosis is present in stage 0; portal fibrosis is present in stage 1; expanded portal fibrosis is present in stage 2; bridging fibrosis is present in stage 3; and cirrhosis is present in stage 4.

Scheuermann's disease Increased curvature of the thoracic spine (kyphosis) usually occurring during growth spurts through adolescence and puberty. Most patients with Scheuermann's disease will have an increased roundback (e.g., hunch back or hump back), poor posture or slouching, and mild to moderate pain. Report this disease with ICD-9-CM code 732.0. *Synonym(s): juvenile kyphosis.*

Scheuthauer-Marie-Sainton syndrome Defective bone formation in skull, often associated with other symptoms. Report this disorder with ICD-9-CM code 755.59.

Schilder's disease Rare disorder affecting the white matter of the brain, occurring in childhood in both sexes and manifested by increased mental deterioration, spastic paralysis, blindness, and deafness. The portion of the brain that is affected determines the signs and symptoms of the neurological disorder. This condition is reported with ICD-9-CM code 341.1. *Synonym(s): Baló's concentric sclerosis, Baló's disease, chronic leukoencephalopathy.*

Schimmelbusch disease Multiple, benign cysts of the breast, colored brown or blue, caused by hyperplasia of the ductal epithelium. Occurs in women, usually after the age of 30. Schimmelbusch disease is reported with ICD-9-CM code 610.1. *Synonym(s): Bloodgood's disease, Phocas' disease, Reclus syndrome, Tillaux-Phocas disease.*

Schiotz tonometer Instrument that measures intraocular pressure by recording the depth of an indentation on the cornea by a plunger of known weight.

SCHIP State Children's Health Insurance Program.

Schirmer test Test for moisture in the eye, using sterile paper strip between the lower lid and globe and measuring how much moisture is wicked into the strip within five minutes. If local anesthesia is applied, it is called a basic Schirmer test.

Schirmer's syndrome Formation of multiple angiomas in skin of the head and scalp. Report this disorder with ICD-9-CM code 759.6. *Synonym(s): Kalischer's syndrome.*

schisto- 1) Indicates cleft or split. 2) Fissure.

schistosomiasis Parasitic infection caused by blood flukes of the genus Schistosoma, a worm that is typically found in infested waters. The larva enters through the

S-U

skin and eggs from the parasite lodge in various places such as portal venules, liver, mesenteric vein, intestines, and urinary tract. It causes inflammatory response in the organ, fibrosis, abdominal pain, diarrhea, bloody stools, and hematuria. Report this condition with a code from ICD-9-CM rubric 120. **Synonym(s): bilharziasis.**

schizencephaly Abnormal clefts in one or both of the cerebral hemispheres. Most schizencephalic patients experience seizures and some have hydrocephalus. Abnormally small head, complete or partial paralysis, and mental retardation may also be present. Schizencephaly is reported with ICD-9-CM code 742.4.

schizoid personality disorder Withdrawal from social and other contacts with autistic preference for detachment, fantasy, and introspective reserve that may include slightly eccentric behavior or avoidance of competitive situations.

schizophrenia acute episode Schizophrenic disorder with ideas of reference and emotional turmoil where external things, people, and events may become charged with personal significance for the patient. Characterized by a dreamlike state with slight clouding of consciousness and perplexity. External things, people, and events may become charged with personal significance for the patient.

schizophrenia atypical Schizophrenia of florid nature that cannot be classified as simple, catatonic, hebephrenic, paranoid, or any other type.

schizophrenia borderline Eccentric or inconsequent behavior and anomalies of affect that give the impression of schizophrenia though no definite and characteristic schizophrenic anomalies, present or past, have been manifested.

schizophrenia catatonic type Psychomotor disturbances often alternating between extremes such as hyperkinesis or excitement and stupor or automatic obedience and negativism. May be accompanied by depression, hypomania, or submission to physical constraints.

schizophrenia cenesthopathic Schizophrenia of florid nature that cannot be classified as simple, catatonic, hebephrenic, paranoid, or any other type.

schizophrenia childhood type Group of disorders in children, characterized by distortions in the timing, rate, and sequence of many psychological functions involving language development and social relations in which the severe qualitative abnormalities are not normal for any stage of development.

schizophrenia chronic undifferentiated Continued disturbance of personality with flat affect, odd beliefs or perceptions, and speech poverty without delusions, without hallucinations, and without disorganized speech or behavior and a history of schizophrenia. Emotional

response is blunted, but this thought disorder does not prevent the accomplishment of routine work.

schizophrenia cyclic Pronounced affective manic or depressive features intermingled with schizophrenic features that tend toward remission without permanent defect but that are prone to recur.

schizophrenia disorganized type Solitary, disorganized schizophrenic state with prominent affective changes, delusions, hallucinations, and fleeting, fragmented, irresponsible or unpredictable behavior that is manifested by purposeless giggling or self-satisfied, self-absorbed smiling, or by a lofty manner, grimaces, mannerisms, pranks, hypochondriacal complaints, and reiterated phrases. Also known as hebephrenic schizophrenia.

schizophrenia hebephrenic type Solitary, disorganized schizophrenic state with prominent affective changes, delusions, hallucinations, and fleeting, fragmented, irresponsible or unpredictable behavior that is manifested by purposeless giggling or self-satisfied, self-absorbed smiling, or by a lofty manner, grimaces, mannerisms, pranks, hypochondriacal complaints, and reiterated phrases. Also known as disorganized schizophrenia.

schizophrenia latent Eccentric or inconsequent behavior and anomalies of affect that give the impression of schizophrenia though no definite and characteristic schizophrenic anomalies, present or past, have been manifested.

schizophrenia paranoid type Schizophrenia with relatively stable delusions, which may be accompanied by hallucinations and erratic behavior, disturbed conduct, gross thought disorder, flat affect, and fragmentary delusions of persecution, jealousy, anatomic change, exalted birth, or messianic mission.

schizophrenia paranoid type prepsychotic Eccentric or inconsequent behavior and anomalies of affect that give the impression of schizophrenia though no definite and characteristic schizophrenic anomalies, present or past, have been manifested.

schizophrenia paranoid type prodromal Eccentric or inconsequent behavior and anomalies of affect that give the impression of schizophrenia though no definite and characteristic schizophrenic anomalies, present or past, have been manifested.

schizophrenia paranoid type pseudoneurotic Eccentric or inconsequent behavior and anomalies of affect that give the impression of schizophrenia though no definite and characteristic schizophrenic anomalies, present or past, have been manifested.

schizophrenia paranoid type pseudopsychopathic Eccentric or inconsequent behavior and anomalies of affect that give the impression of schizophrenia though no definite and characteristic schizophrenic anomalies, present or past, have been manifested.

schizophrenia paranoid type residual Continued disturbance of personality with flat affect, odd beliefs or perceptions, and speech poverty without delusions, without hallucinations, and without disorganized speech or behavior and a history of schizophrenia. Emotional response is blunted, but this thought disorder does not prevent the accomplishment of routine work.

schizophrenia paranoid type schizoaffective type Pronounced affective manic or depressive features that are intermingled with schizophrenic features and that tend toward remission without permanent defect but that are prone to recur.

schizophrenia paranoid type simple type Insidious development of oddities of conduct, inability to meet the demands of society, and decline in total performance with increasing social impoverishment, self-absorption, idleness, and aimless.

schizophrenia paranoid type simplex Insidious development of oddities of conduct, inability to meet the demands of society, and decline in total performance with increasing social impoverishment, self-absorption, idleness, and aimless. Also known as simple paranoid schizophrenia type.

schizophrenia residual type Continued disturbance of personality with flat affect, odd beliefs or perceptions, and speech poverty without delusions, without hallucinations, and without disorganized speech or behavior and a history of schizophrenia. Emotional response is blunted, but this thought disorder does not prevent the accomplishment of routine work.

schizophrenia undifferentiated acute Schizophrenia of florid nature that cannot be classified as simple, catatonic, hebephrenic, paranoid, or any other types.

schizophrenic syndrome of childhood Group of disorders in children, characterized by distortions in the timing, rate, and sequence of many psychological functions involving language development and social relations in which the severe qualitative abnormalities are not normal for any stage of development.

schizophreniform attack Schizophrenic disorder with ideas of reference and emotional turmoil in which external things, people, and events may become charged with personal significance for the patient. Characterized by a dreamlike state with slight clouding of consciousness and perplexity. External things, people, and events may become charged with personal significance for the patient.

schizophreniform disorder Schizophrenic disorder with ideas of reference and emotional turmoil in which external things, people, and events may become charged

with personal significance for the patient. Characterized by a dreamlike state with slight clouding of consciousness and perplexity. External things, people, and events may become charged with personal significance for the patient.

schizophreniform psychosis Fundamental disturbance of personality and characteristic distortion of thinking, often a sense of being controlled by alien forces, delusions, disturbed perception, abnormal affect out of keeping with the real situation, and auditory or visual hallucinations with fear that intimate thoughts, feelings, and acts are known by others although clear consciousness and intellectual capacity are usually maintained. *s. p. affective type* Pronounced affective manic or depressive features intermingled with schizophrenic features that tend toward remission without permanent defect but that are prone to recur. *s. p. confusional type* Schizophrenic disorder with ideas of reference and emotional turmoil where external things, people, and events may become charged with personal significance for the patient. Characterized by a dream-like state with slight clouding of consciousness and perplexity. External things, people, and events may become charged with personal significance for the patient.

schizophreniform psychosis affective type Pronounced affective manic or depressive features that are intermingled with schizophrenic features and that tend toward remission without permanent defect but that are prone to recur.

schizophreniform psychosis confusional type Schizophrenic disorder with ideas of reference and emotional turmoil in which external things, people, and events may become charged with personal significance for the patient. Characterized by a dreamlike state with slight clouding of consciousness and perplexity. External things, people, and events may become charged with personal significance for the patient.

schizotypal personality Schizoid personality disorder manifested by various oddities of thinking, perception, communication, and behavior that may be manifested as magical thinking, ideas of reference, or paranoid ideation, recurrent illusions and derealization (depersonalization), or social isolation.

S-U

Schlemm's Canal

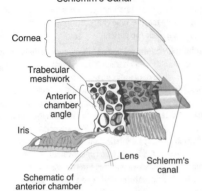

Schematic of
anterior chamber

Schlemm's canal Canal imbedded in the corneoscleral junction (limbus) and carrying aqueous humor from the anterior segment of the eye to the bloodstream. Obstructions in Schlemm's canal lead to glaucoma. Trabeculectomy or trabeculoplasty is often the treatment of choice for these obstructions.

Schmidt's syndrome Hypofunction of endocrine glands involving Hashimoto's thyroiditis, hypoparathyroidism, adrenal insufficiency, and underfunctioning gonads Report this disorder with ICD-9-CM code 258.1.

Schneider's syndrome Form of viral meningitis. Report this disorder with ICD-9-CM code 047.9.

Schocket shunt Eponym for a silastic tube implanted as a treatment for glaucoma. Insertion of the shunt is reported with CPT code 66180; revision with 66185; and removal with 67120.

Scholte's syndrome Carcinoid tumors causing cyanotic flushing of skin, diarrheal watery stools, bronchoconstrictive attacks, hypotension, edema, and ascites. Report this disorder with ICD-9-CM code 259.2. *Synonym(s): Bjorck-Thorson syndrome, Cassidy-Scholte syndrome, Hedinger's syndrome.*

Scholz (-Bielschowsky-henneberg) syndrome Metachromatic leukodystrophy, a disturbance of white substance of brain. Report this disorder with ICD-9-CM code 330.0.

Schroeder's syndrome Disorder of adrenal medullary tissue resulting in hypertension accompanied with attacks of palpitation, headache, nausea, dyspnea, anxiety, pallor, and profuse sweating. Report this disorder with ICD-9-CM code 255.3. *Synonym(s): Slocumb's syndrome.*

Schüller-Christian syndrome Histiocytosis with occasional accumulation of cholesterol. Symptoms include defects of the membranous bones, exophthalmos and diabetes insipidus. There is often also a multiple-system, soft tissue, and skeletal involvement.

Report this disorder with ICD-9-CM code 277.8. *Synonym(s): Hand-Schuller-Christian syndrome.*

Schultz's syndrome Bronchiectasis and pancreatic insufficiency, resulting in malnutrition, sinusitis, short stature, and bone abnormalities. Report this disorder with ICD-9-CM code 288.09.

Schwartz (-Jampel) syndrome Dysplasia of fingernails and toenails, hypoplasia of patella, iliac horns, thickening of glomerular lamina densa, and flask-shaped femur. Report this disorder with ICD-9-CM code 756.89.

Schwartz-Bartter syndrome Found in children with hypokalemic alkalosis and elevated renin or angiotensin levels with low or normal blood pressure, no edema, and retarded growth. Report this disorder with ICD-9-CM code 253.6.

SCI Spinal cord injury.

sciatic nerve Largest nerve in the body that arises from the sacral plexus and innervates all of the muscles of the leg and foot.

sciatica Low back, buttock, and hip pain that radiates down the leg, sometimes accompanied by paresthesia and weakness, usually caused by a herniated disk in the lumbar spine or neuropathy affecting the sciatic nerve. Report sciatica with ICD-9-CM code 724.3. *Synonym(s): Cotugno's disease.*

SCID Severe, combined immunodeficiency disease. Combined deficiency of T cells and antibodies, congenital or acquired, reported with ICD-9-CM code 279.2. *Synonym(s): boy-in-the-bubble disease, bubble boy disease.*

S-U

Scimitar Syndrome

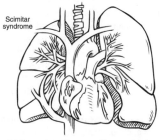

Scimitar syndrome is so named because the aberrant vein casts a shadow shaped like a curved Turkish sword, a scimitar, upon x-ray

The defect can be repaired in various ways through patching, division, or securing a baffle

Scimitar syndrome Congenital anomalous connection of the pulmonary veins in one lung to the inferior vena cava, creating an x-ray image appearing like a curved Turkish sword, a scimitar. Generally includes hypoplasia to some degree of the lung. Scimitar syndrome may be asymptomatic with no treatment required, or it can require correction early in life. Scimitar syndrome is reported with ICD-9-CM code 747.49, and its surgical correction is reported with CPT code 33724.

scintigraphy Exam using a low level injection of radionuclides to view various parts of the body by radioactive emission.

scintillating scotoma Transient blind spot within the visual field or an area of lost or diminished vision surrounded by more sensitive or normal vision. This condition is reported with ICD-9-CM code 368.12. *Synonym(s): concentric fading, scotoma.*

SCIWORA Spinal cord injury without radiologic abnormality.

sclera White, fibrous, outer coating of the eye continuous with the cornea anteriorly and the optic nerve sheath posteriorly that is covered with conjunctival tissue.

sclera syndrome Blue sclera, little growth, brittle bones, and deafness. Report this disorder with ICD-9-CM code 756.51. *Synonym(s): van der Hoeve's syndrome.*

Scleral Buckle

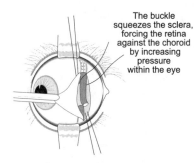

The buckle squeezes the sclera, forcing the retina against the choroid by increasing pressure within the eye

scleral buckle Surgery to treat retinal detachment in which a piece of silicone rubber or sponge-like material is placed on the outer layer of the eye (sclera). Placement is usually against the surface, but may be placed within scleral tissue. The buckling element usually remains permanently. The buckle pushes in or "buckles" the sclera in toward the middle, forcing the two layers of the retina together and allowing retinal tears or breaks to settle against the wall. The buckling may exert its effect only on the area of detachment, or the buckle may encircle the eyeball like a ring. Scleral buckling is reported with ICD-9-CM procedure code 14.41 or 14.49 or CPT code 67107 or 67112.

scleral ectasia Bulging of the eyeball contents at a site of scleral thinning, reported with ICD-9-CM code 379.11. *Synonym(s): scleral staphyloma.*

scleral staphyloma Bulging of the eyeball contents at a site of scleral thinning, reported with ICD-9-CM code 379.11. *Synonym(s): scleral ectasia.*

sclerocystic ovary syndrome Oligomenorrhea or amenorrhea, anovulation and infertility, and hirsutism. Most often caused by bilateral polycystic ovaries. Report this disorder with ICD-9-CM code 256.4. *Synonym(s): Stein syndrome, Stein-Leventhal syndrome.*

scleroderma Systemic disease characterized by excess fibrotic collagen build-up, turning the skin thickened and hard. Fibrotic changes also occur in various organs and cause vascular abnormalities and affect more women than men. Report this condition with ICD-9-CM code 710.1.

sclerose To become hard or firm and indurated from increased formation of connective tissue or disease.

sclerotherapy *1)* Injection of a chemical agent that will irritate, inflame, and cause fibrosis in a vein, eventually obliterating hemorrhoids or varicose veins. *NCD References: 100.10, 150.7. 2)* Instillation of a chemical agent into the chest cavity to artificially create the adhesion between the parietal and the visceral pleura for treating a collapsed lung.

S-U

Scoliosis

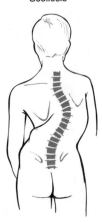

scoliosis Congenital condition of lateral curvature of the spine, often associated with other spinal column defects, congenital heart disease, or genitourinary abnormalities. It may also be associated with spinal muscular atrophy, cerebral palsy, or muscular dystrophy. Congenital scoliosis is reported with ICD-9-CM code 754.2. Most cases will require treatment with bracing or surgical correction.

scope of service Services included in and covered under the contract. *Synonym(s): SOS.*

scope of work Document describing the specific tasks and methodologies that will be followed to satisfy the requirements of an associated contract or memorandum of understanding. *Synonym(s): SOW.*

SCORE Simple calculated osteoporosis risk estimation. Review of age and weight, history of fractures, rheumatoid arthritis hormone replacement therapy, and race. The resulting calculation estimates current bone marrow density.

scoto- *1)* Relating to darkness. *2)* Visual field gap.

scotoma Blind spot within the visual field or an area of lost or diminished vision surrounded by more sensitive or normal vision. Transient or scintillating scotoma is reported with ICD-9-CM code 368.12 or with a code from subcategory 368.4 if permanent. *Synonym(s): concentric fading, scintillating scotoma.*

SCR Standard class rate.

screen Examination involving scanning data from body systems to identify any areas of deficit requiring more detailed assessment.

screening mammography Radiologic images taken of the female breast for the early detection of breast cancer. *NCD Reference: 220.4.*

screening mammography services Radiological procedures provided to women for early detection of breast cancer. A physician must interpret the results of the procedure. No symptoms need to be present for a screening mammography to be covered. Coverage for this service was added to the Medicare program effective January 1, 1991. *NCD Reference: 220.4.*

screening pap smear Diagnostic laboratory test consisting of a routine exfoliative cytology test (Papanicolaou test) provided to a woman for the early detection of cervical or vaginal cancer. The exam includes a clinical breast examination and a physician's interpretation of the results. *NCD Reference: 210.2.*

Scribner cannula Short-term hemodialysis access portal created in an artery and a vein, usually in the nondominant forearm, with the insertion of a needle through the skin and into each vessel. An end of a single cannula is inserted into each puncture. A Scribner cannula remains external and may be left in place for several days. Report Scribner cannula with ICD-9-CM procedure code 39.93 or CPT code 36810.

Scribner type arteriovenous access External cannula or shunt with the ends inserted into both an artery and a vein, at a puncture site made into the vessels through the skin, usually in the forearm. The Scribner cannula remains external and may be left in place for several days and is generally placed to route blood outside the body for hemodialysis purposes. This procedure is reported with CPT code 36810.

scrotal transposition Congenital abnormality in which the scrotum is located above the penis, reported with ICD-9-CM code 752.81.

Scrotoplasty

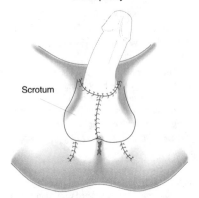

Scrotum

scrotoplasty Repair of defects and developmental abnormalities of the scrotum by plastic surgery techniques such as wound revision and the creation of simple scrotal skin flaps (CPT code 55175), free skin grafts, mesh grafts, and/or rotational pedicle grafts from adjacent skin (55180).

scrotum Skin pouch that holds the testes and supporting reproductive structures.

scrub typhus Acute infectious disease resembling typhus, caused by rickettsia bacteria and transmitted by the bite of infected larval mites, called chiggers. This disease occurs chiefly in Asia and the Pacific and is manifested by a specific telltale lesion or eschar at the site of the bite, fever, regional lymphadenopathy, and skin lesions and rashes. Report this disease with ICD-9-CM code 081.2. *Synonym(s): akamushi disease, inundation fever, island fever, Japanese flood fever, Japanese river fever, kedani fever, mite-borne typhus, Mossman fever, shimamushi disease, tropical typhus, tsutsugamushi disease.*

SCT Specialty care transport.

Sculptra Brand name injectable subcutaneous implant to temporarily reverse the effects of wasting on the face. The effect lasts for about one year, and can be repeated, used as a treatment for patients with human immunodeficiency virus (HIV) who have facial lipoatrophy. Sculptra injections were only recently approved for use in the United States. Check with individual payer policies as injections may be considered cosmetic.

SD Still's disease. Systemic juvenile rheumatoid arthritis characterized by a transient rash and spiking fevers that may affect internal organs, as well as joints. SD is reported with ICD-9-CM code 714.30.

SDO Standards development organization.

sea-blue histiocyte syndrome Corneal opacities; burning pain in palms, soles, and abdomen; chronic paresthesia of hands and feet; cardiopulmonary involvement; edema of the legs; osteoporosis; retarded growth; and delayed puberty. Patients die of renal, cardiac or cerebrovascular failure. Report this disorder with ICD-9-CM code 272.7. *Synonym(s): Fabry's syndrome, Ruiter-Pompen-Wyers syndrome.*

Seabright-Bantam syndrome Similar to hypoparathyroidism, caused by failure to respond to parathyroid hormone with short stature, obesity, short metacarpals, and ectopic calcification. Report this disorder with ICD-9-CM code 275.49. *Synonym(s): Albright-Martin syndrome, Martin-Albright syndrome.*

SEB Scleral expansion band.

sebaceous cyst Benign cyst of the skin or hair follicle filled with keratin and debris rich in lipids. Cysts of the integumentary system may be treated by incision and drainage (CPT codes 10060-10081) or puncture aspiration (10160).

seborrheic dermatitis Chronic, inflammatory skin disease primarily on the face and scalp that produces crusted, yellow eruptions, that may be moist or oily and leads to dry, scaly patches (dandruff) covering the scalp. Seborrheic dermatitis is reported with a code from ICD-9-CM subcategory 690.1. *Synonym(s): cradle cap, eczema.*

seborrheic keratosis Common, benign, noninvasive, lightly pigmented, warty growth composed of basaloid cells that usually appear at middle age as soft, easily crumbling plaques on the face, trunk, and extremities. Correct code assignment is dependent upon the presence of inflammation. If inflammation is present, assign ICD-9-CM code 702.11, if not 702.19.

Seckel's syndrome Dwarfism with low birth weight, microcephaly, large eyes, beaked nose, receding mandible, and moderate mental retardation. Report this disorder with ICD-9-CM code 759.89.

second look Computer-aided detection (CAD) system used by radiologists to read mammograms by highlighting suspicious tissue in the film and changing the mammogram into a digital read-out. The use of a MammoReader does not affect reimbursement.

second opinion Medical opinion obtained from another health care professional, relevant to clinical evaluation, before the performance of a medical service or surgical procedure. Includes patient education regarding treatment alternatives and/or to determine medical necessity.

second order catheter placement Catheter manipulation into a vessel that branches off the aorta. May be noted in the record as a second branch or second family placement. Code assignment depends upon site.

second skin Brand of hydrogel dressing to promote healing and protect against infection.

secondary Second in order of occurrence or importance, or appearing during the course of another disease or condition. *s. payer* Insurer who pays, according to its coverage guidelines, any residual balance remaining after another insurer pays the claim. When Medicare is the secondary payer, it will not pay for medical expenses that are reimbursable by another primary health insurance plan, including employer group health plans, workers' compensation, black lung, automobile liability, etc. *s. repair* Delayed repair of a wound performed 10 or more days out from the initial injury or a subsequent repair done after the first procedure failed to restore function or achieve the desired results. Secondary closure of a surgical wound dehiscence is assigned CPT code 13160. *s. syndrome* Symmetrical osteitis of limbs localized to phalanges and terminal epiphyses of long bones of forearm and leg. Symptoms include kyphosis of the spine and affection of joints. Report this disorder with ICD-9-CM code 731.2.

secondary care Services provided by medical specialists, such as cardiologists, urologists, and

S-U

dermatologists who generally do not have first contact with patients.

secondary insurer In a COB arrangement, the insurer that reimburses for benefits pending after payment by the primary insurer.

secondary payer Organization that pays, according to its coverage guidelines, any residual balance remaining after another insurer pays the claim.

secondary repair Repeat or delayed repair of a wound.

second-degree burn Deep partial-thickness burn with destruction of the epidermis, the upper portion of the dermis, possibly some deeper dermal tissues, and blistering of the skin with fluid exudate. Dressing and debridement of burns are reported with CPT codes 16020-16030. Burns that are the result of hot objects, flames, chemicals, or radiation are classified to ICD-9-CM categories 940-949. Appropriate code selection is dependent upon the degree and site of the burn. Second-degree burns resulting from exposure to solar radiation (sunburn) are classified to 692.76.

Secretan's syndrome Traumatic, recurrent edema or hemorrhage of the back of the hand. Report this disorder with ICD-9-CM code 782.3.

secretary Under HIPAA, secretary of the Department of Health and Human Services or his or her designated representatives.

secretoinhibitor syndrome Complex of symptoms of unknown source in middle aged women in which the following triad exists: keratoconjunctivitis sicca, zerostomia, and connective tissue disease (usually rheumatoid arthritis but sometimes systemic lupus erythematosus. Cause may be an abnormal immune response. Report this disorder with ICD-9-CM code 710.2. *Synonym(s): Gougerot-Houwer syndrome, Sjögren syndrome.*

section Process of cutting a division or segment out of a part.

secundines Placenta and membranes; the afterbirth.

SECURE-C Brand name artificial cervical disc, an alternative to spinal fusion for discs C3-C7 in patients with herniated nucleus pulposus, radiculopathy, myelopathy, or spondylosis. Insertion of a SECURE-C disc is reported with CPT codes 22856 and 0092T.

sed rate Sedimentation rate of erythrocytes.

sedation Induced state of calmness or tranquilized consciousness.

seeds Small (1 mm or less) sources of radioactive material that are permanently placed directly into tumors.

SEER Surveillance, epidemiology, and end results.

segment Group of related data elements in a transaction.

Segond fracture Avulsion fracture of the lateral tibial plateau at the site of the attachment of the lateral capsular ligament, usually indicative of an anterior cruciate ligament (ACL) or meniscal tear.

Seidel's test Use of sodium fluorescein to check for leaks following corneal trauma or post trabeculectomy.

seizure Sudden, abnormal electrical activity in the brain due to any number of causes including medication, high fever, head injuries, epilepsy, and other diseases. Seizures fall into two main groups. Focal seizures, also called partial seizures, happen in just one section of the brain. Generalized seizures are the result of abnormal activity on both sides of the brain.

selective Separation.

selective abortion Selective reduction, most often using potassium chloride injections, performed to eliminate one or more fetuses of a multiple pregnancy in an attempt to increase the viability of the remaining fetuses. Fetuses are usually eliminated in this procedure until only a twin or triplet pregnancy remains. Report this procedure with ICD-9-CM procedure code 75.0 or CPT code 59866. *Synonym(s): MPR, multifetal pregnancy reduction.*

selective placement Introduction and manipulation of a catheter or guidewire within a vascular tree or family into a specified target area that is identified and monitored by radiographic imaging in order to carry out a diagnostic or therapeutic procedure.

self-disclosure Admitting or providing information that an individual or entity has performed an act that is improper or illegal.

self-funded plan Plan where the risk is assumed by the employer rather than the insurer. The employer generally pays claims directly from a general fund account that may be managed by a third party. *Synonym(s): self-insured plan.*

self-funding Health care program in which employers fund benefit plans from their own resources without purchasing insurance. May be self-administered, or the employer may contract with an outside administrator.

self-insured Individual or organization that assumes the financial risk of paying for health care.

self-pay patients Patients who pay for medical care out-of-pocket.

self-referral Patient who was not referred by a physician or other health care practitioner, but who chose that facility or provider on his or her own.

SEM Systolic ejection murmur.

semi-circular canals Passages in the inner ear associated with maintaining equilibrium.

seminal vesicles Paired glands located at the base of the bladder in males that release the majority of fluid

S-U

into semen through ducts that join with the vas deferens forming the ejaculatory duct.

seminal vesiculitis Inflammation or infection of the seminal vesicles that may occur alone but is often a result of prostatitis. Seminal vesiculitis is reported with ICD-9-CM code 608.0 unless specified as gonococcal, in which case it is reported with 098.14 or 098.34.

seminiferous tubules Small tubes found in the testes where the spermatozoa develop.

seminoma Malignant tumor of the testis. Seminomas are slow-growing, immature germ cells that spread relatively slowly. It is not uncommon for a patient to be diagnosed with both seminoma and nonseminoma tumors. Report this condition with the site-specific code from ICD-9-CM category 186.

Semont maneuver Therapy for benign positional paroxysmal vertigo. In the Semont maneuver, the clinician has the patient lie down and rotate his head to displace canaliths in the inner ear. The canaliths may be the source of dizziness in the patient. The Semont maneuver is reported with CPT code 95992.

Senear-Usher syndrome Eruption of the skin on the face, scalp, and trunk with lesions scaling erythematosus. Report this disorder with ICD-9-CM code 694.4.

senile dementia Dementia occurring usually after the age of 65 in which any cerebral pathology other than that of senile atrophic change can be reasonably excluded. *s. d. delirium* Senile dementia with a superimposed reversible episode of acute confusional state. *s. d. delusional type* Progressive type of senile dementia characterized by development in advanced old age, with delusions, varying from simple, poorly formed paranoid delusions to highly formed paranoid delusional states, and hallucinations. *s. d. depressed type* Progressive type of senile dementia characterized by development in advanced old age, with depressive features, ranging from mild to severe forms of manic-depressive affective psychosis. May include disturbance of the sleep-waking cycle and preoccupation with dead people. *s. d. paranoid type* Progressive type of senile dementia characterized by development in advanced old age, with delusions, varying from simple, poorly formed paranoid delusions to highly formed paranoid delusional states, and hallucinations. *s. d. simple type* Dementia occurring usually after the age of 65 in which any cerebral pathology other than that of senile atrophic change can be reasonably excluded.

senile entropion Eyelid that sags away from normal contact with the eyeball because some portions have become stretched or weakened. Usually occurs in the elderly. **Synonym(s):** *involutional entropion.*

senilism syndrome Progeria syndrome which includes marked senility by 10 years of age. Report this disorder with ICD-9-CM code 259.8.

senning procedure Flaps of intra-atrial septum and right atrial wall are used to create two interatrial channels to divert the systemic and pulmonary venous circulation.

Seno supp Senokot suppository.

sensitiver Beziehungswahn Paranoid state that may present as schizophrenic or affective state symptoms. Different from other paranoid states and psychogenic paranoid psychosis.

sensitivity reaction of childhood or adolescence Persistent and excessive shrinking from familiarity or contact with all strangers of sufficient severity as to interfere with peer functioning, yet there are warm and satisfying relationships with family members.

sensitivity tests Number of methods of applying selective suspected allergens to the skin or mucous.

sensorineural conduction Transportation of sound from the cochlea to the acoustic nerve and central auditory pathway to the brain.

sentinel lymph node First node to which lymph drainage and metastasis from a cancer can occur. Surgery for excisional biopsy of a sentinel node is reported according to site, with CPT codes 38500-38542. Identification of sentinel node is reported with CPT code 38792.

sentinel node biopsy Tissue or fluid removed from the first lymph node from the breast for analysis of the cells and diagnosis.

SEO Shoulder-elbow orthosis.

SEP Somatosensory evoked potentials. Test evaluating the pathways of nerves in the extremities through the spinal cord and to the brainstem or cerebral cortex, especially useful in spinal cord trauma, nontraumatic spinal cord lesions, cervical spondylosis, multiple sclerosis, coma, and intraoperative monitoring of spinal cord. SEP is reported with CPT codes 95925, 95926, and 95927.

separate procedures Services commonly carried out as a fundamental part of a total service, and as such usually do not warrant a separate identification. They are noted in the CPT book with the parenthetical phrase (separate procedure) at the end of the description, and are payable only when they are performed alone.

SEPS Subfascial endoscopic perforator surgery. Minimally invasive ligation of incompetent calf perforator veins through an endoscope. SEPS is usually performed with two points of entry, one for the endoscope and one for dissecting or dividing instrumentation. The

S-U

perforating veins are divided using endoscopic scissors. Another option is to interrupt the diseased vein using a harmonic scalpel. Report this surgery with ICD-9-CM procedure code 38.89 or CPT code 37500. **Synonym(s):** *vascular endoscopy.*

sepsis Phase following septicemia in the infectious illness continuum, not to be used interchangeably with septicemia. Sepsis is defined for clinical coding purposes as septicemia that has advanced to involve the presence of two or more manifestations of systemic inflammatory response syndrome (SIRS), without organ dysfunction. This is a different clinical picture than septicemia, which has a different outcome. Sepsis (generalized) is coded as the appropriate septicemia code (ICD-9-CM category 038), as well as the SIRS code (995.91-995.92).

septate hymen Congenital condition in which the hymenal membrane has a thin band of extra tissue in the middle, which creates two small vaginal openings rather than one. Minor surgery is done to remove the extra band of tissue and create a normal vaginal opening. Septate hymen is reported with ICD-9-CM code 752.49 and hymenotomy with CPT code 56442.

septate uterus Congenital abnormality of the uterus in which the body is divided by a wall or septum. Complications of this condition include infertility and miscarriage. Surgery may be necessary to reshape the uterus and remove the septum. Congenital septate uterus is reported with ICD-9-CM code 752.35. In pregnancy, it is reported with a code from subcategory 654.0.

septectomy *1)* Surgical removal of all or part of the nasal septum. *2)* Submucosal resection of the nasal septum.

septem Seven.

septic shock Progression from septicemic infection to severe sepsis with shock, which carries a greater than 50 percent mortality rate. Septic shock presents with severe sepsis with low blood pressure, decreased urine output, increased oxygen demands, followed by major organ failure, manifesting systemic inflammatory disease from bacterial toxins. Coding septic shock correctly requires at least three codes to be assigned: Since septic shock is a systemic inflammatory response syndrome (SIRS) with organ dysfunction that has progressed from septicemic infection and not from trauma, the septicemia is coded first with ICD-9-CM code 038.x, to identify the type of bacteria, if known. The SIRS is coded secondarily with 995.92, followed by the additional code for septic shock, 785.52. When the specific organ failure is known, a fourth code is assigned to identify the type. **Synonym(s):** *endotoxic shock.*

septicemia Systemic disease associated with the presence and persistence of pathogenic microorganisms and their toxins in the blood. Septicemia is not interchangeable with sepsis, nor with bacteremia. Septicemia is a more acute illness than bacteremia and is also a clinically distinct condition presenting with a different clinical picture and outcome than sepsis. Septicemia is coded to ICD-9-CM category 038 with fourth and fifth digit assignment to identify the casual organism. Septicemia becomes sepsis when it is present with two or more manifestations of systemic inflammatory response syndrome.

septostomy Surgical creation of a septal defect or opening.

Septra IV Injectable combination antibacterial drug used in the treatment and prevention of Pneumocystis carinii. It is also used to treat certain other bacterial infections including UTI, bronchitis, gastrointestinal infection, and otitis media infections. Supply is reported with HCPCS Level II code S0039. May be sold under brand name Bactrim IV, SMZ-TMP, sulfamethoxazole-trimethoprim, Sulfutrim.

septum Anatomical partition or dividing wall.

sequela Abnormality, dysfunction, or other residual condition produced after the acute phase of an illness, injury, or disease is over. There is no time limit on when sequelae can appear. It may be apparent early, as with a stroke, or it can occur years later, as in arthritis following an injury. The code for the condition is sequenced first, and then the sequelae or late effect code, unless the late effect code is combined with the manifestation in one code or the late effect is followed by the manifestation. **Synonym(s):** *late effect.*

sequencing codes Codes reported according to ranking guidelines defining severity, time, and skill required to treat the diagnosed condition and cost of the service for procedures.

sequestrectomy Surgical excision of a nonviable piece of bone that has become walled off, or sequestered, away from living bone during necrosis.

SERM Selective estrogen receptor modulator. Pharmaceutical class that acts on the estrogen receptor. SERMs include clomiphene, raloxifene, tamoxifen, toremifene, bazedoxifene, and lasofoxifene. SERMs are used in treatments for anovulation, menopause, breast cancer, and osteoporosis. Report prophylactic use with ICD-9-CM code V07.51.

seroma Tumor-like swelling caused by the collection of serum, or clear fluid, in the tissues. Report post-traumatic seroma with ICD-9-CM code 729.91 and seroma complicating a procedure with code 998.13. For incision and drainage of a seroma, see CPT code 10140.

serous detachment of retinal pigment epithelium Blister of fatty fluid causing localized detachment of retina from pigment epithelium.

serous meningitis syndrome Meningitis with serious inflammation in subarachnoid and ventricle spaces and little change in cerebrospinal fluid. Report this disorder with ICD-9-CM code 348.2.

SERPACWA Skin exposure reduction paste against chemical warfare agents, seen in military use.

sertoli cell syndrome Congenital germinal epithelium absence of the testes. Report this disorder with ICD-9-CM code 606.0.

service date Date a charge is incurred for a service.

service indicator Term used in the OCE that means the same as status indicator.

service line Charge information that would be submitted on a single charge line. This corresponds to one line on a UB-92 claim form.

service plan *1)* Plan that has contracts with providers but is not a managed care plan. *2)* Another name for Blue Cross/Blue Shield plans.

service-oriented V codes ICD-9-CM codes that identify or define examinations, aftercare, ancillary services, or therapy. Use these V codes to describe the patient who is not currently ill but seeks medical services for some specific purpose such as follow-up visits. You can also use this type of V code as a primary diagnosis for outpatient services when the patient has no symptoms that can be coded and screening services are provided.

services Medical care, items, such as medical diagnosis and treatment, drugs and biologicals, supplies, appliances, and equipment, medical social services, and use of hospital RPCH or SNF facilities. In other sections of Medicare manuals and remittance advice records, the term item/service is used. However, throughout PIM the term service is inclusive of item/service.

sesamoidectomy Excision of a small, nodular (sesamoid) bone in tendons or joint capsules.

seton Finely spun thread or other fine material for leading the passage of wider instruments through a fistula, canal, or sinus tract.

SETTLE Spindle epithelial tumor with thymus-like element. Rare, malignant thyroid gland tumor found most often in children, adolescents, and young adults. Report this disease with ICD-9-CM code 193.

sever Separate completely.

Sever's disease Inflammation of the calcaneus at the point of Achilles tendon insertion usually occurring in boys ages 8 to 14. Pain, tenderness, and localized swelling are present. Report this condition with ICD-9-CM code 732.5. **Synonym(s):** *calcaneal apophysitis, epiphysitis of the calcaneus.*

severity of illness Relative levels of loss of function and mortality that may be experienced by patients with a particular disease.

SEWHO Shoulder-elbow-wrist-hand orthosis.

sex Six.

SEXA Single energy x-ray absorptiometry.

sextant In dentistry, one sixth of the dental arch.

sexual deviations Abnormal sexual inclinations or behavior directed primarily toward people not of the opposite sex, sexual acts not associated with coitus normally, or coitus performed under abnormal circumstances; can take the form of exhibitionism, fetishism, homosexuality, nymphomania, pedophilia, satyriasis, sexual masochism, sexual sadism, transvestism, voyeurism, and zoophilia.

sexual masochism Sexual deviation in which sexual arousal and pleasure are produced in an individual by his own physical or psychological suffering and insistent and persistent fantasies where sexual excitement is produced as a result of suffering.

sexual sadism Sexual deviation in which actual or fantasized infliction of pain on someone else causes sexual excitement.

Seymour Fracture

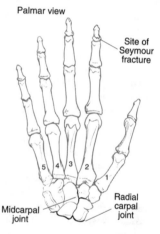

Palmar view

Site of Seymour fracture

Radial carpal joint

Midcarpal joint

5 4 3 2

1

Seymour fracture Fracture of the distal phalanx of the finger, reported with ICD-9-CM code 816.02 or 816.12.

Sezary's disease Type of cancer affecting the skin. It is a variant of cutaneous T-cell lymphoma.

SF HCPCS Level II modifier, for use with CPT or HCPCS Level II codes, that identifies a second opinion ordered by a QIO, eligible for reimbursement at 100 percent. The usual deductible and/or coinsurance amounts are not applied.

SFMS Smith-Fineman-Myers syndrome. Rare, X-linked dystrophy featuring short stature, psychomotor retardation, narrow face, and strabismus, reported with ICD-9-CM code 759.89.

S-U

SG *1)* HCPCS Level II modifier, for use with CPT or HCPCS Level II codes, that identifies an ambulatory surgery center (ASC) facility service. Physicians who provide services at ASC facilities do not need to append this modifier to their claims. Reimbursement is based on the appropriate APC. *2)* Swan-Ganz.

SGA *1)* Small for gestational age. *2)* Substantial gainful activity.

SGAP Superior gluteal artery perforator. Reconstructive surgery in which skin and fat from the upper buttock is transferred and anastomosed to feeding blood vessels in the chest following mastectomy. *NCD Reference: 140.2.*

SGC Swan-Ganz catheter. Flexible, flow-directed catheter inserted through the inferior or superior vena cava through the right side of the heart to the pulmonary artery, where it measures blood pressure in pulmonary circulation and estimate cardiac output. Report its insertion with ICD-9-CM procedure code 89.64 or CPT code 93503.

SGD Speech generating device.

SGOT Serum glutamic oxaloacetic acid.

SH *1)* HCPCS Level II modifier, for use with CPT or HCPCS Level II codes, that identifies a second concurrently administered infusion therapy. *2)* Social history.

Shaatz pessary Vaginal device inserted to treat uterine prolapse and cystocele. Shaatz pessary is made of silicone or rubber. Supply is reported with HCPCS Level II code A4561 or A4562 depending upon composition.

shadow pricing Setting rates just below a competitor's rates. Maximizes profits but raises medical costs.

shared paranoid disorder Mainly delusional psychosis, usually chronic and often without florid features, that appears to have developed as a result of a close, if not dependent, relationship with another person who already has an established similar psychosis.

shared risk Cost-control incentive whereby both the provider and the payer share risk for excessive utilization and/or excessive costs associated with the care of plan members.

Shaver's syndrome Condition resulting from the ingestion of bauxite fumes and fine particles of alumina and silica in the aluminum mining and manufacturing process. Symptoms include pulmonary emphysema and pneumothorax. Report this disorder with ICD-9-CM code 503.

shaving Sharp removal by transverse incision or horizontal slicing.

SHBG Sex hormone binding globulin.

sheath Covering enclosing an organ or part.

Sheehan's syndrome Secretion of all anterior pituitary hormones is inadequate or absent; presenting after childbirth. Report this disorder with ICD-9-CM code 253.2. *Synonym(s): Reye-Sheehan syndrome.*

shields Devices that protect specific areas of healthy tissue from radiation.

shifting sleep-work schedule Sleep disorder in which the phase-shift disruption of the 24-hour sleep-wake cycle occurs due to rapid changes in the individual's work schedule.

shigellosis Infection by the rod-shaped, nonmotile, gram-negative bacteria of the genus Shigella, from the family Enterobacteriaceae. Known to cause an acute dysenteric infection of the bowel with fever, drowsiness, anorexia, nausea, vomiting, diarrhea, abdominal pain, and distension. Blood, pus, and mucus are found in the stool. Ingestion of food contaminated by feces of infected individuals is the most common source of infection. Incubation period is one to four days. There are four species in the Shigella genus, and they differ according to their biochemical reactions. All cause dysentery in humans and some primates. Shigellosis is reported with ICD-9-CM code 004.0. A suspected Shigella carrier is reported with ICD-9-CM code V02.3.

shimamushi disease Acute infectious disease resembling typhus, caused by rickettsia bacteria and transmitted by the bite of infected larval mites, called chiggers. This disease occurs chiefly in Asia and the Pacific and is manifested by a specific telltale lesion or eschar at the site of the bite, fever, regional lymphadenopathy, and skin lesions and rashes. Report this disease with ICD-9-CM code 081.2. *Synonym(s): akamushi disease, inundation fever, island fever, Japanese flood fever, Japanese river fever, kedani fever, mite-borne typhus, Mossman fever, scrub typhus, tropical typhus, tsutsugamushi disease.*

shin bone fever Moderately severe disease borne by body lice and relatively common among the homeless. The onset of symptoms is sudden, with high fever, severe headache, back and leg pain, and a fleeting rash. Recovery takes a month or more. Relapses are common. Report this condition with ICD-9-CM code 083.1. *Synonym(s): trench fever, wolhynia fever.*

Shirodkar procedure Treatment of an incompetent cervical os by placing nonabsorbent suture material in purse-string sutures as a cerclage to support the cervix.

Shonlein-Henoch purpura Arterial capillary inflammation in the skin, kidneys, and intestinal tract, sometimes seen as an abnormal autoimmune reaction to a respiratory infection. The patient typically complains of a skin rash and joint inflammation. Shonlein-Henoch purpura is reported with ICD-9-CM code 287.0. *Synonym(s): SHP.*

short bones Bones that have a small longitudinal axis and all measure about the same in length, such as carpal and tarsal bones of the wrist and ankle.

short sleeper Individuals who typically need only four to six hours of sleep within the 24-hour cycle.

short wave diathermy Heating tissues therapeutically to a depth of about 3 cm by using high frequency oscillating electromagnetic fields.

short-stay patients Inpatients admitted for 48 hours or less, or outpatients who stay 24 hours or less.

shoulder girdle dystocia Condition causing obstructed labor that occurs when the anterior shoulder of the fetus becomes impacted against the maternal symphysis after delivery of the fetal head, requiring additional maneuvers in order to deliver the baby. Shoulder dystocia can also result from the impaction of the posterior shoulder on the sacral promontory. Fourth-degree lacerations and postpartum hemorrhage are the most common maternal complications of shoulder dystocia. Erb's palsy is the most common complication for the infant. This condition in the mother is reported with a code from ICD-9-CM category 660.4. Erb's palsy in the neonate is reported with 767.6. *Synonym(s): impacted shoulders, stuck shoulders.*

shoulder-arm syndrome Clinical disorder following a heart attack, marked by pain and stiffness in the shoulder, with puffy swelling and pain in the hand. Report this disorder with ICD-9-CM code 337.9. *Synonym(s): Claude Bernard-Homer syndrome, Reilly's syndrome, shoulder-hand syndrome, Steinbrocker's syndrome.*

SHP Shonlein-Henoch purpura. Arterial capillary inflammation in the skin, kidneys, and intestinal tract, sometimes seen as an abnormal autoimmune reaction to a respiratory infection. The patient typically complains of a skin rash and joint inflammation. SHP is reported with ICD-9-CM code 287.0.

shunt Surgically created passage between blood vessels or other natural passages, such as an arteriovenous anastomosis, to divert or bypass blood flow from the normal channel. Abnormal shunting may occur in the body when fistulas form or congenital anomalies are present that cause blood flow to be rerouted from the normal circulatory path.

Shwachman's syndrome Bronchiectasis and pancreatic insufficiency, resulting in malnutrition and sinusitis. Other symptoms include short stature and bone abnormalities. Report this disorder with ICD-9-CM code 288.02.

Shy-Drager syndrome Condition in which the nerves between the striatum and pallidum are completely demyelated. Report this disorder with ICD-9-CM code 333.0. *Synonym(s): Déjérine-Thomas syndrome, Hallervorden-Spatz syndrome.*

shyness disorder of childhood Persistent and excessive shrinking from familiarity or contact with all strangers

of sufficient severity as to interfere with peer functioning, yet there are warm and satisfying relationships with family members.

SIADH Syndrome of inappropriate antidiuretic hormone. Inappropriate antidiuretic hormone causing ongoing hypovolemia, hyponatremia, and increased urine osmolality. Often occurring as a result of head trauma, certain lung or pancreatic cancers, or pulmonary disorders, vasopressin is released in excessive amounts for the state of hydration. Report this syndrome with ICD-9-CM 253.6.

sial(o)- Relating to saliva.

sialoadenectomy Surgical removal of a salivary gland.

sialoadenitis Inflammation of the salivary gland, reported with ICD-9-CM code 527.2.

sialodochoplasty Surgical repair of a salivary gland duct.

sialography Radiographic examination of the ductal system of a salivary gland by instilling radiographic dye into a major duct and taking x-ray pictures. The injection portion of the procedure is reported with CPT code 42550 and the radiological supervision portion is reported with 70390. The same physician may perform the entire procedure, however, complete coding of what is required to carry out this procedure is not achieved by reporting a single code.

sialolith Calculus, stone, or concretion within the salivary ducts or glands.

sialolithiasis Stone or concretion in the salivary duct; reported with ICD-9-CM code 527.5.

sialolithotomy Incision in the submandibular, sublingual, or parotid ducts to remove a calculus or stone from within a salivary duct. If the stone is large, a portion of the surrounding tissue may also be removed. Sialolithotomy is reported with a code from CPT range 42330-42340 or HCPCS Level II code D7980.

SIB Severe Impairment Battery. Tool for evaluating cognitive abilities of patients who are in later stages of Alzheimer's and other dementia. The test is usually administered by a psychologist, speech language pathologist, or an occupational therapist.

sibling jealousy or rivalry Emotional disorder related to competition between siblings for the love of a parent or for other recognition or gain.

SIC Standard industry code.

Sicard's syndrome Unilateral lesions of ninth, tenth, eleventh, and twelfth cranial nerves producing paralysis of the vagal, glossal, and other nerves and tongue on same side. Usually result of injury. Report this disorder with ICD-9-CM code 352.6. *Synonym(s): Collet-Sicard syndrome.*

S-U

sicca syndrome Complex of symptoms of unknown source in middle-aged women in which the following triad exists: keratoconjunctivitis sicca, zerostomia, and connective tissue disease (usually rheumatoid arthritis but sometimes systemic lupus erythematosus). Cause may be an abnormal immune response. Report this disorder with ICD-9-CM code 710.2. *Synonym(s): Gougerot-Houwer syndrome, Sjögren syndrome.*

sick baby Infant with medical complications not resulting from premature birth.

sick sinus syndrome Range of electrophysiological abnormalities of the heart including sinus bradycardia, sinus arrest, sinus node exit block, chronic atrial fibrillation, and bradycardia-tachycardia syndrome. Most often found in older patients with a history of heart disease, it is distinguished by delayed or failed conduction between the sinus node and atria, due to inadequate sinus node pacemaking or conduction disturbances. Sick sinus syndrome is reported with ICD-9-CM code 427.81. *Synonym(s): sinus node dysfunction, SND.*

SICRET syndrome Small infarction of cochlear, retinal, and encephalic tissue. Neurological disorder characterized by disturbances of motion involving the brain and vision and hearing loss, caused by damage to small blood vessels in the affected organs. It is thought to be autoimmune in nature. There is no code specifically indexed to SICRET syndrome in ICD-9-CM. Code each manifestation individually. *Synonym(s): Susac syndrome.*

SID Sensory integration dysfunction. Inability of the brain to process sensory information correctly. A child with SID will be hyposensitive or hypersensitive to stimuli. Report SID with ICD-9-CM code 299.8. *Synonym(s): DSI.*

sideropenic syndrome Eczema, thrombocytopenia, and recurrent pyogenic infection. Patients suffer an increased susceptibility to infection with encapsulated bacteria. Report this disorder with ICD-9-CM code 280.8.

siderosis Iron pigment deposits within the tissue of the eyeball caused by high iron content in the blood. This condition is reported with ICD-9-CM code 360.23.

SIDS Sudden infant death syndrome.

SIEA Superficial inferior epigastric artery.

Siegert's sign Foreshortened and curving little finger, associated with Down syndrome.

Siemens' ectodermal dysplasia syndrome Congenitally absent sweat glands, smooth finely wrinkled skin, sunken nose, malformed teeth, sparse hair, and deformed nails. In some cases, symptoms are absent breast tissue, mental retardation, and/or syndactyly. Report this disorder with ICD-9-CM code 757.31.

Siemens' keratosis follicularis spinulosa syndrome Inherited condition in which the hair follicles are replaced by keratosis. Report this disorder with ICD-9-CM code 757.39.

Sig. Write on label (Rx) or let it be labeled.

Sig. S. (Signa) Mark or write.

Sigmoidoscopy

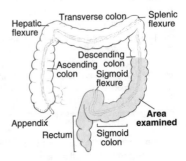

A sigmoidoscopy is an examination of the sigmoid colon and part of the descending colon. An endoscope is inserted into the anus and past the sigmoid flexure for this examination

sigmoidoscopy Endoscopic examination of the entire rectum and sigmoid colon, often including a portion of the descending colon and usually performed with a flexible fiberoptic scope in conjunction with a surgical procedure. Sigmoidoscopy is reported with CPT codes 45330-45345.

signature Physician's signature acknowledges that he/she has performed or supervised the service or procedure and that the transcription has been read and corrections made before signing. Signed or initialed laboratory and x-ray results show auditors that the physician has reviewed the information.

Silfverskiöld's syndrome Dominant inherited disease with skeletal changes in extremities. Report this disorder with ICD-9-CM code 756.50.

silver nitrate Topical antiinfective or germicide used as antiseptic and astringent.

silver's syndrome Dwarfism marked by late closure of anterior fontanel, bilateral body asymmetry, low birth weight, clinodactyly of the fifth fingers, triangular facial shape, and carp mouth. Report this disorder with ICD-9-CM code 759.89.

Silvestroni-Bianco syndrome One of a group of hemolytic anemias that shares common decreased rate of synthesis of one or more hemoglobin polypeptide chains and are classified according to chain involved. Report this disorder with ICD-9-CM code 282.49.

Simon Nitinol filter Permanent, umbrella-shaped filter implanted in the vena cava and designed to trap small clots of blood or plaque before they reach the lungs and cause pulmonary embolism. The filter is inserted intraluminally, usually through the femoral or jugular veins. Placement of a Simon Nitinol filter is reported with CPT code 37620. Radiological supervision and interpretation of filter placement is reported with CPT code 75940.

Simons' syndrome Characterized by loss of subcutaneous fat of upper torso, the arms, the neck, and the face but with an increase in fat on and below the pelvis. Report this disorder with ICD-9-CM code 272.6. *Synonym(s): Hollander-Simons syndrome.*

simple phobia Fear of a discrete object or situation, such as animals, heights, or small spaces, that is neither fear of leaving the familiar setting of the home (agoraphobia) or of being observed by others in certain situations (social phobia).

simple polyp Mucosal outgrowth of tissue that is hanging from a stalk and can easily be removed.

simple repair Surgical closure of a superficial wound, requiring single layer suturing of the skin (epidermis, dermis, or subcutaneous tissue).

Sims speculum Device inserted into the vagina for viewing its walls and the cervix.

sine Without.

single-lead device Implantable cardiac device (pacemaker or implantable cardioverter-defibrillator [ICD]) in which pacing and sensing components are placed in only one chamber of the heart.

sinistro- On or to the left.

sinoatrial node Group of cells located on the wall of the right atrium, close to the superior vena cava, that naturally discharge electrical impulses initiating heart contracture. For this reason, it is often referred to as the "physiologic pacemaker." *Synonym(s): sinus node.*

sinoatrial node dysfunction Delayed or failed conduction between the sinus node and the atria, either due to inadequate sinus node pacemaking or because of intrinsic or extrinsic conduction disturbance.

sinus *1)* Open space, cavity, or channel within the body. *2)* Abnormal cavity, fistula, or channel created by a localized infection to allow the escape of pus.

sinus node Group of cells located on the wall of the right atrium, close to the superior vena cava, that naturally discharge electrical impulses initiating heart contracture. For this reason, it is often referred to as the "physiologic pacemaker." *Synonym(s): sinoatrial node.*

sinus of Valsalva Any of three sinuses corresponding to the individual cusps of the aortic valve, located in the most proximal part of the aorta just above the cusps. These structures are contained within the pericardium and appear as distinct but subtle outpouchings or dilations of the aortic wall between each of the semilunar cusps of the valve. The coronary arteries arise from two of the sinuses. *Synonym(s): sinus aortae.*

sinus of Valsalva aneurysm Rare dilation of the proximal portion of the aorta, appearing as outpouchings just above the cusps of the aortic valve. In congenital cases, the aneurysm most often originates in the right sinus of Valsalva from separation of the aortic media and annulus fibrosis due to deficient elastic tissue or abnormal bulbus cordis development. In acquired cases, the dilatation may be the result of aging, Marfan syndrome, or syphilitic infection of the aorta. The dilated sinus can cause compression of adjacent structures, intracardiac shunting if rupture occurs into the right side of the heart, or cardiac tamponade if rupture involves the pericardial space. Congenital sinus of Valsalva aneurysm is reported with ICD-9-CM code 747.29; acquired is reported with 414.19. Surgical correction is reported with CPT code 33720.

sinus tarsi implant Titanium internal orthotic device intended to correct flat feet. The device is inserted into the sinus tarsi, the anatomical space between the inferior neck of the talus and the superior aspect of the distal calcaneus.

sinus tarsi syndrome Caused by posterior tibial nerve at ankle, syndrome can produce significant neuropathy. Report this disorder with ICD-9-CM code 726.79.

sinusitis-bronchiectasis-situs inversus syndrome Transposition or misplacement of organs or viscera. Report this disorder with ICD-9-CM code 759.3. *Synonym(s): Kartagener's syndrome.*

Sipple's syndrome Form of thyroid cancer. May cause a functional activity disorder. Report this disorder with ICD-9-CM code 193. *Synonym(s): medullary thyroid carcinoma-pheochromocytoma.*

sipuleucel-T Cellular immunotherapy vaccine currently in Phase II clinical trials for the treatment of prostate cancer. Outpatient administration of sipuleucel-T is reported with CPT code 96413 or inpatient ICD-9-CM code 99.28. Supply is reported with HCPCS Level II code J9999. May be sold under brand name Provenge.

SIR Society of Interventional Radiology. Formerly known as the Society of Cardiovascular and Interventional Radiology (SCVIR).

SIRF Severely impaired renal function.

SIRS Systemic inflammatory response syndrome.

SIR-Spheres Brand name tiny pellets or microspheres of yttrium-90 inserted into the liver through an arterial

S-U

catheter to treat secondary cancer. The radioactive pellets slow the growth of liver tumors with a new technology called selective internal radiation therapy (SIRT). This liver procedure is reported with HCPCS Level II code S2095.

SIRT   Selective internal radiation therapy.

SISI   Short increment sensitivity index. Hearing threshold measurement used in diagnosing cochlear damage. Testing for SISI is reported with CPT code 92564.

Sister Mary Joseph's nodule   Metastatic malignancy of the periumbilical region. Sister Mary Joseph's nodule is reported with ICD-9-CM code 198.2.

situational disturbance acute   Acute transient disorders of any severity and nature of emotions, consciousness, and psychomotor states (singly or in combination) that occur in individuals, without any apparent pre-existing mental disorder, in response to exceptional physical or mental stress, such as natural catastrophe or battle. Usually subside within hours or days.

situs inversus   Congenital anomaly in which the internal thoracic and abdominal organs are transposed laterally and found on the opposite side from the normal position, reported with ICD-9-CM code 759.3.

s-JIA   Systemic onset juvenile idiopathic arthritis.

Sjögren (-Gougerot) syndrome   Complex of symptoms of unknown source in middle aged women in which the following triad exists: keratoconjunctivitis sicca, zerostomia, and connective tissue disease (usually rheumatoid arthritis but sometimes systemic lupus erythematosus). Cause may be an abnormal immune response. Report this disorder with ICD-9-CM code 710.2. **Synonym(s):** *Gougerot-Houwer syndrome.*

Sjögren's syndrome/disease   Symptom complex usually occurring in middle-aged or older women of unknown etiology. Marked by the presence of connective tissue disease, usually rheumatoid arthritis, but sometimes systemic lupus erythematosus, scleroderma, or polymyositis and manifested by keratoconjunctivitis sicca and xerostomia.

Sjögren-Larsson syndrome   Congenital malformation of the skin with scaling and spastic paraplegia. Report this disorder with ICD-9-CM code 757.1.

SJS   Schwartz-Jampel syndrome. Rare recessive genetic disorder characterized by short stature, bowing of arms and legs, and permanently flexed fingers and toes. Infants may develop acute conditions. SJS is reported with ICD-9-CM code 756.89.

skeletal traction   Applying a pulling force directly on the long axis of bones by inserted wires or pins and using weights and pulleys to keep the bone in proper alignment.

Skene's gland   Paraurethral ducts that drain a group of the female urethral glands into the vestibule. Incision and drainage of a Skene's gland abscess or cyst is reported with CPT code 53060. Abscess of Skene's gland is reported with ICD-9-CM code 597.0; cyst is reported with 599.89. **Synonym(s):** *Guérin's glands, lesser vestibular gland, paraurethral glands, Schüller's ducts.*

skier's thumb   Acute injury to the ulnar collateral ligament of the thumb named for its common occurrence when a skier falls with his or her hand caught in a ski pole.

skilled nursing care   Daily care and other, related services for inpatients who require medical or nursing care or rehabilitation services for injuries, disabilities, or sickness, based on a written physician order certifying the need for such care.

skilled nursing facility   Institution or a distinct part of an institution that is primarily engaged in providing skilled nursing care and related services for residents who require medical or nursing care; or rehabilitation services for the rehabilitation of injured, disabled, or sick persons. A SNF may be a part of a hospital or a separate entity, such as a nursing home. In order for a patient to be transferred between a hospital and a SNF, the transferring facility must complete a written transfer statement. A swing-bed hospital provides skilled nursing care and related services similar to those of a SNF. **Synonym(s):** *SNF.*

skin   Outer protective covering of the body composed of the epidermis and dermis, situated above the subcutaneous tissues.

skin shaving   Slicing off or removing a thin layer of skin.

skin tag   Small skin-colored or brown appendage appearing on the neck and upper chest resembling a little epithelial polyp and reported with ICD-9-CM code 701.9. Removal of skin tags is classified to CPT codes 11200 and 11201.

skin traction   Application of a pulling force to a limb accomplished by a device fixed to felt dressings or strappings on the body surface.

skull   Cranial and facial bones that make up the skeleton of the head. The cranial bones (8) include frontal, parietal (2), temporal (2), occipital, sphenoid, and ethmoid; facial bones (14) include nasal (2), maxillae (2), zygomatic (2), mandible, lacrimal (2), palatine (2), inferior nasal conchae (2), and vomer. Skull base includes the anterior, middle, and posterior fossa; occiput bone; orbital roof; ethmoid and frontal sinus; sphenoid and temporal bones. Skull vault includes the upper, dome-like part of the cranium that includes the frontal and parietal bones.

S-U

skull base Anterior, middle, and posterior fossa; occiput bone; orbital roof; ethmoid and frontal sinus; sphenoid and temporal bones.

skull cap Dome-shaped top portion of the skull composed of the frontal and parietal bones and portions of the occipital and temporal bones. **Synonym(s):** *calvaria, cranial concha.*

skull vault Upper, dome-like part of the cranium that includes the frontal and parietal bones.

SLAP Superior labral anteroposterior (lesion).

SLB Short leg brace. Orthotic for the ankle and foot. **Synonym(s):** *AFO.*

SLC Short leg cast. Nonweight-bearing cast extending from just below the knee to the toes.

SLE Systemic lupus erythematosus.

sleep apnea Intermittent cessation of breathing during sleep that may cause hypoxemia and pulmonary arterial hypertension. Sleep apnea may be caused by respiratory centers in the brain not being stimulated or by some kind of physical airway obstruction, such as hypertrophy of the adenoids. This condition is reported based on cause. Sleep apnea of a neonate is reported with codes specific to the newborn.

sleep latency Time period between lying down in bed and the onset of sleep.

SLI Speech language impairment.

sling operation Procedure to correct urinary incontinence. A sling of fascia or synthetic material is placed under the junction of the urethra and bladder in females, or across the muscles surrounding the urethra in males. Procedure code assignment is dependent upon approach and patient sex.

Slocumb's syndrome Disorder of adrenal medullary tissue resulting in hypertension accompanied with attacks of palpitation, headache, nausea, dyspnea, anxiety, pallor, and profuse sweating. Report this disorder with ICD-9-CM code 255.3. **Synonym(s):** *Schroeder's syndrome.*

SLP Speech-language pathology.

SLR Straight-leg raising. Test for determining irritation of the nerve root. The physician elevates the supine patient's straight leg until there is ipsilateral extremity or back pain, or until the pain increases when the foot is bent backward. **Synonym(s):** *Lasègue test.*

SLUD Salivation, lacrimation, urination, defecation.

Sluder's syndrome Disorder involving facial pain manifested by a unilateral headache behind the eyes with maxillary or soft palate pain. Occasionally there is associated aching in the back of the head, neck, nose, teeth, or temple. Nasal/sinus congestion may be present, along with redness of the face and inflamed nasal mucosa, swelling, and tearing. More common in women,

this disorder appears to be caused by irritation to the sphenopalatine ganglion from intranasal infection, scarring, or deformity. **Synonym(s):** *sphenopalatine ganglion neuralgia.* Report this disorder with ICD-9-CM code 337.09.

SLWC Short leg walking cast.

SM Samarium.

small health plan Under HIPAA, health plan with annual receipts of $5 million or less.

small intestine First portion of intestine connecting to the pylorus at the proximal end and consisting of the duodenum, jejunum, and ileum.

small subscriber group aggregate Aggregate of professional associations, small business, or other entities formed to be considered a single, large subscriber group.

SMAS Superficial musculoaponeurotic system. Rhytidectomy commonly used in cosmetic surgery. Incisions are made along the margin of the face and usually within the area behind the ears. The skin is taken off and tightened. Surplus skin is removed. Underlying muscle tissue is likewise tightened and repositioned.

SMAS Flap

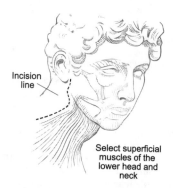

Incision line

Select superficial muscles of the lower head and neck

The interlinking musculature and fascial tissues of the face are the superficial musculoaponeurotic system, or SMAS

SMAS flap Superficial musculoaponeurotic system flap. Rhytidectomy commonly used in cosmetic surgery. Incisions are made along the margin of the face and usually within the area behind the ears. The skin is taken off and tightened. Surplus skin is removed. Underlying muscle tissue is likewise tightened and repositioned. Report this procedure with CPT code 15829.

S-U

SMBG Self-monitored blood glucose. Test of the sugar levels in the blood, typically performed by a patient with diabetes.

smear Specimen for study that is spread out across a glass slide.

Smith-Lemli-Opitz syndrome Mental retardation, small stature, ptosis, male genital anomalies, anteverted nostrils, and syndactyly of the second and third toes. Report this disorder with ICD-9-CM code 759.89.

Smith-Robinson arthrodesis Fusion procedure requiring an anterior approach to remove cervical disks and use of a bone graft fashioned to replace the disks.

SMM Smoldering multiple myeloma.

SMO *1)* Supramalleolar orthotic. Lightweight orthotic that fits inside a shoe and helps maintain foot alignment while standing or walking. *2)* Slip made out.

SMRR Submucosal resection and rhinoplasty.

SMZ-TMP Injectable combination antibacterial drug used in the treatment and prevention of Pneumocystis carinii. It is also used to treat certain other bacterial infections including UTI, bronchitis, gastrointestinal infection, and otitis media infections. Supply is reported with HCPCS Level II code S0039. SMZ-TMP contains sulfamethoxazole-trimethoprim.

snare Wire used as a loop to excise a polyp or lesion.

SNCT Sensory nerve conduction test. *NCD Reference: 160.23.*

Sneddon-Wilkinson syndrome Non-inflammatory intimal hyperplasia of medium-sized vessels. Report this disorder with ICD-9-CM code 694.1.

SNF Skilled nursing facility. Institution or a distinct part of an institution that is primarily engaged in providing skilled nursing care and related services for residents who require medical or nursing care; or rehabilitation services for the rehabilitation of injured, disabled, or sick persons. A SNF may be a part of a hospital or a separate entity, such as a nursing home. In order for a patient to be transferred between a hospital and a SNF, the transferring facility must complete a written transfer statement. A swing-bed hospital provides skilled nursing care and related services similar to those of a SNF.

SNIP Strategic national implementation process.

SNOMED Systemized nomenclature of medicine. Uniform lexicon of treatments and diseases added in 2004 into the National Library of Medicine's Unified Medical Language System. It contains more than 350,000 concepts in a hierarchal organization that reviews disease, clinical findings, therapies, and outcomes and is expected to play a role in the development of electronic health records.

SNOMED-CT Systemized nomenclature of medicine, clinical terms. Uniform lexicon of treatments and diseases added in 2004 into the National Library of Medicine's Unified Medical Language System. It contains more than 350,000 concepts in a hierarchal organization that reviews disease, clinical findings, therapies, and outcomes and is expected to play a role in the development of electronic health records.

SNS *1)* Sacral nerve stimulation. Method of managing urinary incontinence, urgency, overactive bladder, or urinary retention by electronically signaling the sacral nerve with an implanted neurostimulator. The neurostimulator is implanted subcutaneously in the upper buttock or abdomen, and a lead is placed adjacent to the sacral nerve and attached to the neurostimulator. The patient controls urination with a hand-held programmer. *2)* Sympathetic nervous system. *3)* Somatic nervous system.

SO *1)* Shoulder orthosis. *2)* Sacroiliac orthosis.

SOAP Subjective, objective, assessment, plan. When documenting patients' visits, the SOAP approach has been used historically as it standardizes physician documentation and easily adapts to history, exam, and medical decision-making. The steps are defined as follows: 1) Subjective: The information the patient tells the physician. 2) Objective: The physician's observed, objective overview, including the patient's vital signs and the findings of the physical exam and any diagnostic tests. 3) Assessment: A list the physician prepares in response to the patient's condition, including the problem, diagnoses, and reasons leading the physician to the diagnoses. 4) Plan: The physician's workup or treatment planned for each problem in the assessment.

SOB Shortness of breath.

social history Review of pertinent past and current activities of the patient including marital status, employment or occupation, use of drugs, alcohol and tobacco, educational background, sexual history, and other related social factors such as travel, avocations, and hobbies.

social phobia Fear of social situations such as public speaking, blushing, eating in public, writing in front of others, or using public lavatories or being in situations of possible scrutiny by others, with fear of acting in a fashion that will be considered shameful.

social withdrawal of childhood Emotional disturbance in children chiefly manifested by a lack of interest in social relationships and indifference to social praise or criticism.

socialized conduct disorder Acquired values or behavior of a peer group that the individual is loyal to and with whom the individual characteristically steals, is truant, stays out late at night, and is sexually promiscuous or engages in other socially delinquent practices.

sodium 2-mercaptoethane sulfonate Detoxifying agent used to prevent hemorrhagic cystitis caused by the chemotherapeutic drug ifosfamide. Supply is reported with HCPCS Level II code J9209. May be sold as brand name Mesna, Mesnex, Uromitexan.

sodium hyaluronate Substance that is similar to the naturally occurring synovial fluid found in the joints that functions as a shock absorber and lubricant. Sodium hyaluronate is indicated for the treatment of osteoarthritic knee pain and is administered as an intra-articular injection. Brand names for this indication include Euflexxa, Hyalgan, Orthovisc, Supartz, and Synvisc. Report supply with a HCPCS Level II code from range J7321-J7324.

Soemmering's ring Doughnut-shaped remnant of lens located behind the pupil caused by contact between the anterior and posterior capsules, resulting in peripherally trapped lens substance. This condition is a common occurrence following cataract surgery or trauma. Report Soemmering's ring with ICD-9-CM code 366.51.

SOF Signature on file.

soft palate Fleshy portion of the roof of the mouth extending from the back of the hard palate and from which the uvula is suspended at the posterior edge. For procedures performed on the palate, see CPT range 42000-42281.

soft tissue Nonepithelial tissues outside of the skeleton that includes subcutaneous adipose tissue, fibrous tissue, fascia, muscles, blood and lymph vessels, and peripheral nervous system tissue.

softgoods or soft goods DMEPOS industry term for medical devices such as braces, splints, joint supports and protectors, cervical pillows, and other similar orthopaedic-oriented items.

SOI Severity of illness.

Sol Solution.

solar retinopathy Macular damage from staring at the sun.

Soliris Monoclonal antibody indicated for the treatment of paroxysmal nocturnal hemoglobinuria (PNH), a disease characterized by abnormal development of the red blood cells. Report the injectable supply with HCPCS Level II code J1300. *Synonym(s): eculizumab.*

somatization disorder Chronic, but fluctuating, neurotic disorder that begins early in life and is characterized by recurrent and multiple somatic complaints for which medical attention is sought but that are not apparently due to any physical illness.

somato- Relating to the body.

somatoform disorder atypical Excessive concern with one's health in general or the integrity and functioning of some part of one's body or, less frequently, one's mind. Usually associated with anxiety and depression.

Somogyi phenomenon Almost exclusively seen in Type I diabetes, a rebound effect occurring overnight as a reaction to earlier administration of insulin. The insulin causes a low blood sugar during sleep. The low sugar causes release of countering hormones, which in turn raises the blood sugar. The patient has hyperglycemia upon awakening, unaware of nocturnal hypoglycemia. Rarely, Somogyi phenomenon may occur in an insulin-dependent Type II diabetic.

SONOCUR Brand name for a new technology for outpatient treatment of tennis elbow using shock wave therapy.

SOP Standard operation procedure.

Sorbsan Brand name calcium alginate "wet wound" dressing used on infected or non-infected wet wounds. Removal does not disrupt the healing process. When the dressing is applied in the physician office, the supply of the wound dressing is reported separately with HCPCS Level II codes A6196-A6198.

Sorsby's macular dystrophy Juvenile macular degeneration usually beginning between the ages of 20 and 40, resulting in vision impairment with possible color vision abnormality. This condition is inherited and progressive in nature. Report this condition with ICD-9-CM code 362.77. *Synonym(s): pseudoinflammatory macular dystrophy.*

Sotos' syndrome Increased birth weight and length, accelerated growth rate for the first four or five years with no elevation of serum growth hormone levels, followed by revision to normal growth rate, antimongoloid slant, prognathism, hypertelorism, dolichocephalic skull, impaired coordination, and moderate mental retardation may be present. Report this disorder with ICD-9-CM code 253.0.

sound Long, slender tool with a type of curved, flat probe at the end for dilating strictures or detecting foreign bodies.

source of admission One-digit code that identifies the referral or origination point of a patient, such as emergency room or transfer from a skilled nursing facility.

SOW Scope of work.

SPA Subperiosteal abscess of the orbit. SPA is usually a complication of sinusitis, trauma, skin infection, or foreign body. SPA is reported with ICD-9-CM code 376.02.

space maintainer In dentistry, plastic or metal appliance that is custom fit to the patient's mouth to maintain the space intended for a permanent tooth.

S-U

Spalding's sign Collapse and overlap of fetal cranial bones in the absence of labor, a sign of fetal death. Spalding's sign can be observed radiographically. The fetal death is reported with an ICD-9-CM code from subcategory 656.4 in the mother's chart.

Spanner stent Brand name temporary prostatic urethral stent to replace a urinary catheter in patients who have undergone surgical treatment of the prostate. The stent allows volitional urination and remains until swelling is reduced. Placement of the Spanner stent is reported with CPT code 53855.

SPAP Systolic pulmonary artery pressure. Right heart catheterization is required to obtain SPAP measurement, which is used in the evaluation of pulmonary hypertension.

SPARC Sling

The physician places a support sling to eliminate stress incontinence

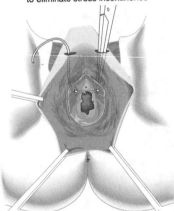

A SPARC sling is a brand name sling used in treating urinary incontinence

SPARC Sling Brand name pubourethral sling for treatment of female stress incontinence resulting from urethral hypermobility or sphincter deficiency. The sling is inserted using a suprapubic approach. Placement is reported with CPT code 57288.

spasm Involuntary muscle contraction.

-spasm Contraction.

spasmodic torticollis Neck muscle spasms and cervical dystonia, resulting in the head becoming inclined toward the affected side and the face toward the opposite side.

spastic entropion Intermittent and involuntary turning inward of the eyelid margin, reported with ICD-9-CM code 374.03. Repair of an entropion is reported with a CPT code from range 67921-67924.

spastic hemiplegia Paralytic condition affecting one side of the body marked by spasticity of the impaired muscles and an increase in tendon reflexes.

spasticity Muscular rigidity, spasms, or passive stretch resistance, synonymous with being spastic.

spatulate Cut the open end of a tubular structure with a lengthwise incision and open the end out further for greater opening size in an anastomosis.

SPD Summary plan description.

specialist in medicine Physician who has had advanced training (residency years, fellowships, etc.) in one or more clinical areas of a practice.

specific academic or work inhibition Adjustment reaction with a specific academic or work inhibition in an individual whose intellectual capacity, skills, and previous academic or work performance have been at least adequate, and in which the inhibition occurs despite apparent effort and is not due to any other mental disorder.

specified focal (partial) syndrome Persistent personality disturbance of nonpsychotic origin with one of the following symptoms: affective instability, bursts of aggression, apathy and indifference, impaired social judgment, and suspiciousness or paranoid ideation. Report this disorder with ICD-9-CM code 310.8.

specimen Tissue cells or sample of fluid taken for analysis, pathologic examination, and diagnosis.

SPECT Single photon emission computerized tomography. SPECT images are taken after the injection of a radionuclide using a special camera containing a detector crystal, usually sodium iodide. Images are captured as the gamma radiation from the radionuclide scintillates or gives off its energy in a flash of light when coming in contact with the crystal. This type of imaging is reported for the anatomical area and purpose such as detecting liver function or myocardial perfusion after an ischemic event. *NCD Reference: 220.12.*

spectral display Visual display mode in Doppler ultrasonography that shows the blood-flow velocity range present. The most common form of spectral display indicates blood flow velocity shifts.

SpectraSTIM Brand name neurostimulator providing computer-controlled sequential impulses to muscles to cause them to contract. The device is intended to prevent or retard disuse atrophy in paraplegic patients. Supply of SpectraSTIM is reported with HCPCS Level II code E0745.

SPECTRUM State Performance Evaluation and Comprehensive Test of Reimbursement Under Medicaid.

speculoscopy Viewing the cervix utilizing a magnifier and a special wavelength of light, allowing detection of abnormalities that may not be discovered on a routine

S-U

Pap smear. After washing the cervix with an acetic acid solution, a speculum is inserted that has a disposable blue-white chemiluminescent light attached. The cervix is visually examined using 5X-magnifying loupes. Abnormal epithelial cells appear white, in clear distinction to the dark blue of normal cells. Abnormal areas may be sampled for cytologic evaluation. Speculoscopy differs from colposcopy in that the latter employs visual inspection of the cervix using a lighted microscope. This new technology is reported with CPT code 58999.

speculum Tool used to enlarge the opening of any canal or cavity.

speech prosthetic Electronic speech aid device for patient who has had a laryngectomy. One operates by placing a vibrating head against the throat; the other amplifies sound waves through a tube which is inserted into the user's mouth.

speech-language pathology services Speech, language, and related function assessment and rehabilitation service furnished by a qualified speech-language pathologist. Audiology services include hearing and balance assessment services furnished by a qualified audiologist. A qualified speech pathologist and audiologist must have a master's or doctoral degree in their respective fields and be licensed to serve in the state. Speech pathologists and audiologists practicing in states without licensure must complete 350 hours of supervised clinical work and perform at least nine months of supervised full-time service after earning their degrees. *Synonym(s): audiology service.*

spell of illness Period of time used to measure the use of hospital insurance benefits. A spell of illness begins when a patient who has not been hospitalized in the past 60 days, is admitted to a Medicare-qualified facility. The patient begins the first spell of illness with 60 full days of coverage, 30 days of coinsurance coverage, and 60 days of lifetime reserve days and the inpatient deductible is due. These benefits are usually abbreviated as 60-30-60. *Synonym(s): benefit period.*

Spens' syndrome Heart block often causing slow or absent pulse, vertigo, syncope, convulsions, and Cheyne-Stokes respiration. Report this disorder with ICD-9-CM code 426.9. *Synonym(s): Morgagni's disease syndrome, Stokes-Adams syndrome.*

spermatic cord Structure of the male reproductive organs that consists of the ductus deferens, testicular artery, nerves, and veins that drain the testes.

spermatocele Noncancerous accumulation of fluid and dead sperm cells normally located at the head of the epididymis that exhibits itself as a hard, smooth scrotal mass and do not normally require treatment unless they become enlarged or cause pain. Spermatoceles may be

an acquired condition, ICD-9-CM code 608.1, or congenital, 752.89.

SpGr Specific gravity.

sphallo-pharyngo-laryngeal hemiplegia syndrome Unilateral lesions of the ninth, tenth, eleventh, and twelfth cranial nerves producing paralysis of the vagal, glossal, and other nerves and the tongue on the same side. Usually the result of injury. Report this disorder with ICD-9-CM code 352.6. *Synonym(s): Collet-Sicard syndrome.*

spheno- Relating to the sphenoid bone at the base of the skull.

sphenoid Irregular, wedge-shaped bone in the skull base.

sphenopalatine ganglion Parasympathetic group of nerve cell bodies through which sensory and sympathetic nerves pass, originating from the facial nerve and supplying the nasal, lacrimal, and palatine glands. *Synonym(s): Meckel's ganglion, pterygopalatine ganglion, sphenomaxillary ganglion.*

spherophakia-brachymorphia syndrome Abnormally round and small lens of the eyes, short stature, and brachydactyly. Report this disorder with ICD-9-CM code 759.89. *Synonym(s): Weill-Marchesani syndrome.*

sphincter Ring-like band of muscle that surrounds a bodily opening, constricting and relaxing as required for normal physiological functioning.

sphincteroplasty Surgical repair done to correct, augment, or improve the muscular function of a sphincter, such as the anus or intestines.

sphygmo- Relating to the pulse.

spica Figure-eight wrapped bandage, usually at the shoulder or hip.

spiculum Small, needle-like body or spike.

SPIDER System to Provide Immediate Data on Eligibility for Reimbursement. Outdated system that has been replaced with the Common Working File.

Spielmeyer-Vogt disease Juvenile type of neuronal ceroid lipofuscinosis or amaurotic familial idiocy. This disease is an inherited disorder in which the body stores excessive amounts of lipofuscin, the pigment that remains after damaged cells are broken down and digested, resulting in progressive nervous tissue damage, vision loss, and fatality. Vogt-Spielmeyer disease manifests between ages 5 and 10 with excessive neural tissue lipofuscin storage causing massive loss of brain tissue with accompanying cerebral and retinal decay. Death usually occurs within another 10 or 15 years. Report this disease with ICD-9-CM code 330.1.

spigelian line Curved line on the abdomen that marks the edge of each rectus abdominis muscle and the joining

S-U

of aponeuroses from the transverse abdominal and internal oblique muscles.

spike-and-wave complex Electroencephalography reading of a sharp spike followed by a slow wave, often evidence of epilepsy.

Spina Bifida

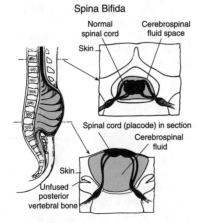

Normal spinal cord

Cerebrospinal fluid space

Skin

Spinal cord (placode) in section

Cerebrospinal fluid

Skin

Unfused posterior vertebral bone

Spinal Column

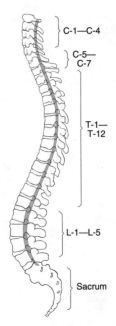

C-1—C-4

C-5—C-7

T-1—T-12

L-1—L-5

Sacrum

spina bifida Lack of closure in the vertebral column with protrusion of the spinal cord through the defect, often in the lumbosacral area. This condition can be recognized by the presence of alpha-fetoproteins in the amniotic fluid and may present alone or in conjunction with other anomalies, and with or without hydrocephalus. Spina bifida is reported with a code from ICD-9-CM category 741, with a mandatory fifth digit specifying the location of the lesion.

spina bifida cystica Defective closure of the spinal column during early fetal development with a protrusion or herniation of the cord and meninges through the defect.

spina bifida occulta Defective closure of the spinal column during early fetal development without the cord or meninges protruding through the defect.

spinal anesthesia Injection or infusion of an anesthetic agent into the vertebral column. May be epidural, subarachnoid, or pudendal.

spinal artery syndrome Occlusion of spinal artery as result of injury, disk damage, or cardiovascular disease. Report this disorder with a code from ICD-9-CM range 433.80-433.81. *Synonym(s): Beck's syndrome.*

spinal cord segment Cervical, thoracic, lumbar, sacral, and coccygeal regions of the spinal cord with their root attachments of the spinal nerves.

spinal cord syrinx Pathological tube-shaped cavity in the brain or spinal cord.

spinal stenosis Narrowing of the canal (vertebral or nerve root) or intervertebral foramina of the lumbar spine.

spindle epithelial tumor with thymus-like element Rare, malignant thyroid gland tumor found most often in children, adolescents, and young adults. Report this disease with ICD-9-CM code 193. *Synonym(s): SETTLE.*

SpineAssist Brand name, computer-controlled positioning system designed to aid surgeons in precise positioning of surgical instruments used in lumbar stabilization surgery. SpineAssist would be utilized in procedures reported with CPT code 22533, 22558, 22612, or 22630 along with 61783 or S2900.

spinnbarkeit Stretchiness of cervical mucous, associated with fertility in the ovulation cycle

spirometer Device used to determine the amount of air inhaled and exhaled from the lungs. Supply is reported with HCPCS Level II code A9284 or E0487.

spirometry Measurement of the lungs' breathing capacity.

S-U

SPJ Saphenopopliteal junction.

splanch- *1)* Relating to the intestines. *2)* Viscera.

spleen Largest organ of the lymph system located in the upper left side of the abdomen that disintegrates red blood cells and releases hemoglobin; rids the body of worn-out, damaged red blood cells and platelets; produces plasma cells and lymphocytes; and has other functions not fully understood.

splenic agenesis syndrome Congenital disorder in which organs of left side of body are a mirror image of the organs on the right side. Splenic agenesis and cardiac malformation are associated. Report this disorder with ICD-9-CM code 759.0.

splenic flexure syndrome Bloating, gas, pain, and fullness experienced in left upper abdominal quadrant with pain sometimes radiating up into left chest. Report this disorder with ICD-9-CM code 569.89.

splenic neutropenia syndrome Inherited disorder with bronchiectasis and pancreatic insufficiency, resulting in malnutrition, sinusitis, short stature, and bone abnormalities. Report this disorder with ICD-9-CM code 289.53

splint Brace or support. *Dynamic s.* Brace that permits movement of an anatomical structure such as a hand, wrist, foot, or other part of the body after surgery or injury. *Static s.* Brace that prevents movement and maintains support and position for an anatomical structure after surgery or injury.

split inventory technique Keeping highly-utilized DMEPOS easily accessible to staff, while keeping surplus in a central storage area.

split thickness skin graft Graft using the epidermis and part of the dermis.

spondylolisthesis Forward displacement of one vertebra slipping over another, usually in the fourth or fifth lumbar area, reported with ICD-9-CM code 756.12.

spondylolysis Abnormal fixation of the vertebra resulting in decreased mobility that may be acquired or congenital. Code assignment depends upon location and etiology.

spontaneous abortion Early expulsion of the products of conception from the uterus that occurs naturally, without chemical intervention or instrumentation, before completion of 22 weeks of gestation. Spontaneous abortion may be complete, in which all of the products of conception are expelled, or incomplete, in which parts of the placental material or fetus are retained. Symptoms may include lower abdominal cramping and vaginal bleeding. In cases of incomplete spontaneous abortion, surgical intervention in the form of curettage is required in order to remove the remaining tissue. Medical intervention is generally not required with complete spontaneous abortion. Spontaneous abortions are reported with a code from ICD-9-CM category 634, with fourth digits to indicate the presence or absence of complications and fifth digits to identify the stage (unspecified, incomplete, or complete). *Synonym(s): miscarriage.*

spontaneous tension pneumothorax Air leaking from the lung and trapped in the lung lining.

spousal abuse syndrome Maltreatment (abuse) of spouses and elders with emotional or physical violence. Report this disorder with a code from ICD-9-CM range 995.80-995.85.

SPR Selective posterior rhizotomy. Nerve surgery for symptoms related to cerebral palsy. In SPR, the physician identifies and selectively cuts the portions of the nerve roots (rootlets) in the cord that are causing muscle tightness and spasticity in the legs. SPR is reported with CPT codes 63185 and 63190. Cerebral palsy is reported with ICD-9-CM codes from category 343. *Synonym(s): selective dorsal root rhizotomy.*

sprain and strain Injuries to a joint, in which the fibers of supporting ligaments or muscles are overstretched or slightly ruptured, with the ligaments and muscles maintaining continuity.

Sprengel's deformity Congenital condition in which one or both shoulder blades are abnormally elevated and underdeveloped, reported with ICD-9-CM code 755.52.

Spurling's sign Pain upon rotation of the neck while axial pressure is applied. This is indicative of foraminal stenosis and nerve root irritation of the cervical spine.

Spurway's syndrome Blue sclera, little growth, brittle and malformed bones, and malformed teeth. Report this disorder with ICD-9-CM code 756.51. *Synonym(s): Eddowes' syndrome, Ekman's syndrome.*

SQ *1)* Status quo. *2)* Subcutaneous.

SR *1)* Seclusion room. *2)* Superior rectus muscle. *3)* Sedimentation rate.

SROM Spontaneous rupture of membrane.

SRP Surgical reversal of presbyopia.

SRS Stereotactic radiosurgery. Noninvasive radiation therapy technique in which focused beams of radiation are delivered precisely to a target area using three-dimensional coordinates. Stereotactic radiosurgery is often the primary source of treatment utilized when a tumor is inaccessible by surgical means or adjunctively to other treatments for a recurring or malignant tumor. Report SRS with CPT codes 61796-61800, 63620, 63621, and 77371-77373.

SRT Speech reception threshold. SRT test is reported with CPT code 92555.

SRUS Solitary rectal ulcer syndrome. Wound in the rectum causing anal pain, bleeding, and sometimes constipation that can be due to excessive straining

S-U

during a bowel movement and is reported with ICD-9-CM code 569.41.

SRVs Small round viruses. Thought to be genetically similar to astroviruses, they cause enteritis in humans. Infection is reported with ICD-9-CM code 008.64.

SS *1)* Social services. *2)* Social Security. *3)* Half. *4)* Somatostatin.

SSA Social Security Act.

SSE Soap suds enema.

SSEP Sensory evoked potential.

SSM Superficial spreading melanoma.

SSN Social security number.

SSO Standard-setting organization.

SSOP Second Surgical Opinion Program.

SSPE Subacute sclerosing panencephalitis. Progressive inflammation of the brain occurring in children and young adults secondary to a measles infection. SSPE is reported with ICD-9-CM code 046.2.

SSSGS Similarly sized subscriber groups.

ST *1)* Sinus tachycardia. *2)* Schiotz tonometry.

stabilization Fixed, firm state that is resistant to change.

staff model HMO that employs its own providers.

stage 0 breast cancer Non-invasive breast cancers, such as ductal carcinoma in situ (DCIS) and lobular carcinoma in situ (LCIS). There is no evidence of invasion into other areas of the breast except that which was initially affected.

stage I breast cancer Neoplasm less than 2 cm confined to the breast.

stage II breast cancer Neoplasm 2.1 to 5 cm, with or without axillary lymph nodes, possible extension into the pectoral fascia or muscle, no distant metastasis.

stage III breast cancer Neoplasm greater than 5 cm, palpable, fixed axillary and/or subclavicular lymph nodes, possible adherence to surrounding tissue, no distant metastasis.

stage IV breast cancer Neoplasm greater than 5 cm and fully integrated with distant metastasis, and lymphedema above and below the clavicle.

staghorn calculus Renal stone that develops in the pelvicaliceal system, and in advanced cases has a branching appearance that resembles the antlers of a stag. Report this condition with ICD-9-CM code 592.0.

staging Determination of the course of a disease, as in the case of a malignancy, to determine whether the malignancy is confined to the primary tumor, has spread to one or more lymph nodes, or has metastasized.

staging in carcinoma of the uterus

Carcinoma of the corpus uteri is classified by stage:

Stage 1A: Endometrial tumor.

Stage 1B: Invasion to less than half of the myometrium.

Stage 2A: Endocervical involvement.

Stage 2B: Cervical stromal invasion.

Stage 3A: Positive peritoneal cytology and/or serosal and/or adnexal invasion.

Stage 3B: Vaginal metastasis.

Stage 3C: Pelvic and/or paraaortic lymph node metastases.

Stage 4A: Invasion of bladder and/or rectal mucosa.

Stage 4B: Invasion of distant organs.

Note: This staging does not apply to melanoma or secondary malignancies.

staging of carcinoma of the ovary

Carcinoma of the ovary is classified by stage:

Stage 1A: Growth limited to one ovary with capsule intact and no ascites.

Stage 1B: Growth limited to both ovaries with capsule intact and no ascites.

Stage 1C: Stage 1A or 1B but with tumors on surface of ovary; positive peritoneal washings or ascites containing malignant cells.

Stage 2A: Growth on one or both ovaries with pelvic extension; tumors on surface of ovary; positive peritoneal washings or ascites containing malignant cells.

Stage 2B: Extension with metastases to uterus or tubes; tumors on surface of ovary; positive peritoneal washings or ascites containing malignant cells.

Stage 2C: Extension to other pelvic tissues; tumors on surface of ovary; positive peritoneal washings or ascites containing malignant cells.

Stage 3A: Tumor involving one or both ovaries with microscopic seeding of abdominal peritoneum; superficial liver metastasis; tumor limited to true pelvis.

Stage 3B: Tumor involving one or both ovaries with implants of abdominal peritoneum up to 2 cm in diameter; superficial liver metastasis; nodes negative.

Stage 3C: Tumor involving one or both ovaries with implants of abdominal peritoneum greater than 2 cm in diameter; superficial liver metastasis; inguinal or retroperitoneal nodes positive.

Stage 4: Distant metastases; pleural effusion; parenchymal liver metastases. *Note:* This staging does not apply to melanoma or secondary malignancies.

staging of carcinoma of the vagina

Carcinoma of the vagina is classified by stage:

Stage 0: Carcinoma in situ (intraepithelial).

S–U

Stage 1: Carcinoma limited to subvaginal wall.

Stage 2: Carcinoma involving subvaginal wall but not pelvic wall.

Stage 3: Carcinoma involving subvaginal and pelvic wall.

Stage 4: Carcinoma extending into anal or rectal mucosa, or beyond pelvis.

Stage 4A: Carcinoma spread to adjacent organs.

Stage 4B: Carcinoma spread to distant organs.

Note: This staging does not apply to melanoma or secondary malignancies.

staging of carcinoma of the vulva

Carcinoma of the vulva is classified by stage:

Stage 0: Carcinoma in situ.

Stage 1: Tumor 2.0 cm or smaller confined to vulva; nodes not palpable.

Stage 2: Tumor larger than 2.0 cm confined to vulva; nodes not palpable.

Stage 3: Tumor of any size infiltrating urethra, vagina, anus, or perineum; two nodes palpable but not fixed.

Stage 4: Tumor of any size infiltrating anal or bladder mucosa; fixed to bone or metastases; fixed nodes.

Note: This staging does not apply to melanoma or secondary malignancies.

stagnation mastitis   Local swelling of the breasts normally associated with the early weeks of nursing that forms painful lumps when the milk duct is not draining efficiently, causing the breast to become inflamed, hard, and tender. Stagnation mastitis is reported with a code from ICD-9-CM subcategory 676.2. *Synonym(s): caked breasts.*

Stamey procedure   Abdomino-vaginal vesicle neck suspension procedure to control female urinary stress incontinence. The bladder neck is suspended by suturing surrounding tissue through an incision in the vagina near the base of the bladder to the fibrous membranes (fascia) of the abdomen. This procedure is reported with CPT code 51845.

stammering   Disorders in the rhythm of speech in which the individual knows precisely what he or she wishes to say but at the time is unable to say it because of an involuntary, repetitive prolongation or cessation of a sound.

standard anesthesia formula   Reimbursement formula that consists of base units plus time units plus modifying units (e.g., physical status and qualifying circumstances) plus other allowed unit/charges that is multiplied by a conversion factor.

standard transaction   Under HIPAA, transaction that complies with the applicable HIPAA standard.

standard transaction format compliance system   HIPAA compliance certification service sponsored by the Electronic Healthcare Network Accreditation Commission and hosted by Washington Publishing Company. *Synonym(s): STFCS.*

standards   Rules that must be followed by a health plan, health care provider, or health care clearinghouse when handling protected health information.

standards of conduct   Written policies and procedures that clearly define employee conduct and the need to adhere to all statutes, regulations, and program requirements governing federal, state, and private health benefit plans.

standby anesthesia service   Requested by another physician and involves prolonged attendance without direct patient contact. This is not billable if the physician eventually does the procedure.

Stanford-Binet test   Psychological measurement of the ability to think and reason; a precursor to the development of today's IQ tests. The subject performs tasks such as following commands, copying patterns, naming things, and putting things in order. *Synonym(s): Binet test.*

Stapedectomy

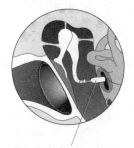

Exposed oval window may be covered by graft

An incision is made in the eardrum and the stapes, or a portion of the stapes, is removed

Prosthesic device replaces stapes (PORP)

stapedectomy   Treatment of hearing loss in which the innermost bone of the middle ear (stapes) is removed.

S-U

Report stapedectomy with ICD-9-CM procedure code 19.19 or a code from CPT range 69660-69662.

stapes Stirrup shaped, third and innermost ossicle of the middle ear, that articulates with the incus.

staph Staphylococcus.

staphylococcal scalded skin syndrome Skin infection most commonly found in infants and children under the age of five. It is caused by certain strains of *Staphylococcus* bacteria, which damages the skin and results in shedding. Symptoms include fever, exfoliation of large areas of skin, pain, and redness over most of the body. Gentle pressure may cause the skin to slip off, leaving red, wet areas known as Nikolsky's sign. Report this disorder with ICD-9-CM code 695.81, and use an additional code from range 695.50-695.59 to identify the percentage of skin exfoliation. *Synonym(s): SSS, Ritter's disease.*

staphylococcus Bacteria whose name originates from the Greek, meaning a bunch of grapes. These round clusters of gram-positive, motile, facultative anaerobes are of the family Micrococcaceae and can cause serious opportunistic infections. Staphylococcus is a major cause of extended hospital stays from nosocomial staph infections. Report staphylococcus with ICD-9-CM code 005.0 for staph-related food poisoning, 008.41 for staphylococcal enterocolitis, 038.1x for staphylococcal septicemia, and 482.4x for pneumonia secondary to staph infection. When staph is the causative organism in other conditions, use ICD-9-CM category 041 codes as appropriate. Staph colonization is reported with a code from subcategory V02.5.

Stargardt's disease Common form of inherited juvenile macular degeneration with onset in late childhood or early adulthood. Bilateral decreased central vision, central blind spot, night blindness, abnormal color visualization, and intolerance of light progressively occur. Stargardt's disease is classified to ICD-9-CM code 362.75.

Stark I & Stark II Laws named after Congressman Peter Stark (D-CA), who introduced the measures, originally enacted in 1995 and 2001, respectively. See Antikickback Act.

Starlix Brand name oral medication exclusive to lowering blood glucose in Type II diabetics. Starlix contains nateglinide.

startle disease Genetic disorder in which babies have an exaggerated startle reflex reaction. Report this disease with ICD-9-CM code 759.89. *Synonym(s): hyperexplexia.*

stat Abbreviation for Latin statim, meaning immediately.

stat charge Charge for expeditious test results. *Synonym(s): rush charge.*

state insurance commission State group that approves insurance certificates for each state and regulates the industry based on statutes.

state law Constitution, statute, regulation, rule, common law, or any other state action having the force and effect of law.

State Uniform Billing Committee State-specific affiliate of the National Uniform Billing Committee. *Synonym(s): SUBC.*

statement covers period "From" and "through" dates in FL 6 on the UB-92 claim form that represent the dates of service and charges being billed.

statement dates "From" and "through" dates on a claim or in the electronic transmission that represent the time period of the dates of service and charges being submitted.

statement of work Document describing the specific tasks and methodologies that will be followed to satisfy the requirements of an associated contract or memorandum of understanding. *Synonym(s): SOW.*

status epilepticus More than 30 minutes of continuous seizure or multiple sequential seizures without a return to consciousness in between. Treatment usually begins after five minutes of seizure, so the definition of status epilepticus is evolving. Status epilepticus does not have bearing on the type of epilepsy coded; it simply is indicative of ongoing, active seizure.

status indicator One-letter code used in OPPS to signify if a code will be paid and how it will be paid.

status migrainosus More than 72 hours of continuous migraine headache, often requiring hospitalization due to dehydration. Migraine is reported with a code from ICD-9-CM category 346. Status migrainous does not have bearing on the type of migraine coded; it is simply indicative of an ongoing, active migraine.

status modifier Required modifier to show the status of the patient's health at the time of anesthesia delivery, appended to the anesthesia code.

status postcommotio cerebri States occurring after generalized contusion of the brain that may resemble frontal lobe syndrome or neurotic disorders. May include headache, giddiness, fatigue, insomnia, mood fluctuation, and a subjective feeling of impaired intellectual function with extreme reaction to normal stressors.

statute Law enacted by a legislative branch of the government.

STB Stillborn. Late demise (22 weeks or more gestational age) of fetus in utero with subsequent delivery. As a maternal condition, stillbirth is classified to ICD-9-CM subcategory 656.4.

STD Sexually transmitted disease.

S-U

STE Subperiosteal tissue expander. Tissue expansion device placed under the layer of tissue and against the bone. Coding would depend on the site and the objective of the implant.

steal Diversion of blood to another channel.

steato- Relating to fat.

steering Providing financial incentives to plan members to use the managed care provider panel.

Stein's syndrome Oligomenorrhea or amenorrhea, anovulation and infertility, and hirsutism. Most often caused by bilateral polycystic ovaries. Report this disorder with ICD-9-CM code 256.4. *Synonym(s): Stein-Leventhal syndrome.*

Steinbrocker's syndrome Pain and stiffness in the shoulder with puffy swelling and pain in the hand following a heart attack. Report this disorder with ICD-9-CM code 337.9. *Synonym(s): Claude-Bernard-Homer syndrome, Reilly's syndrome.*

Steindler stripping Surgical release of soft tissue attached to the plantar of the calcaneus for the correction of pes cavus with claw toes.

Steinert's disease Inherited multisystem disorder characterized by progressive degeneration and weakness of muscle and abnormal muscle contracture (myotonia). Myotonia is prominent in the hand muscles and ptosis is common even in mild cases. In severe cases, marked peripheral muscular weakness occurs, often with cataracts, premature balding, hatchet facies, cardiac arrhythmias, testicular atrophy, and endocrine disorders including diabetes mellitus. Mental retardation is common. This condition is reported with ICD-9-CM code 359.21. *Synonym(s): myotonic dystrophy.*

Steinmann pin Metallic pin used for transfixing bones or bone fragments that is larger in diameter than a Kirschner wire.

stellate ganglion Sympathetic group of nerve cells at the level of the cervical and 1st thoracic vertebrae with postganglionic fibers distributing to the head, neck, upper limbs, and heart. *Synonym(s): cervicothoracid ganglion, ganglion cervicothoracicum.*

Stemmer's sign Positive test for lymphedema in which the thickened skin fold at the base of the second toe or finger cannot be lifted but only grasped as a lump. Positive or negative Stemmer's sign would be considered part of the physical exam in an evaluation and management service. Lymphedema is reported with ICD-9-CM code 457.1 when an acquired chronic condition; postmastectomy lymphedema is reported with 457.0; and hereditary edema of the legs is reported with 757.0.

Stenger test Test for hearing loss suspected as a unilateral feigned illness. The clinician presents a sound to both ears, but much louder in the ear reported to be deaf. The patient, upon hearing the dominant sound in the deaf hear, will report hearing nothing at all.

stenosis Narrowing or constriction of a passage.

Stensen's duct Duct extending from the parotid gland to an opening in the cheek, adjacent to the maxillary second molar. Stensen's duct drains saliva from the parotid gland into the oral cavity. *Synonym(s): Blasius duct, parotid papilla, steno's duct.*

stent Tube to provide support in a body cavity or lumen.

stercolith Hard intestinal concretion of fecal matter that may lead to impaction or appendicitis. Report this condition with ICD-9-CM code 560.32. *Synonym(s): coprolith, fecalith.*

stereoagnosis Type of tactile agnosia in which the ability to understand or distinguish the shape, form, or nature of objects being touched is lost or diminished. This condition is reported with ICD-9-CM code 780.99. *Synonym(s): astereocognosy, astereognosis, tactile amnesia.*

stereopsis Three-dimensional or depth perception capabilities in vision coming from both eyes.

stereoradiography Preparation of radiographs with appropriate shift of the x-ray tube or film so that the images can be viewed stereoscopically to give a three-dimensional appearance.

stereotactic radiosurgery Delivery of externally-generated ionizing radiation to specific targets for destruction or inactivation. Most often utilized in the treatment of brain or spinal tumors, high-resolution stereotactic imaging is used to identify the target and then deliver the treatment. Computer-assisted planning may also be employed. Simple and complex cranial lesions (61796-61799) and spinal lesions (63620-63621) are typically treated in a single planning and treatment session, although a maximum of five sessions may be required. No incision is made for stereotactic radiosurgery procedures.

stereotaxis Three-dimensional method for precisely locating structures.

stereotypies Voluntary repetitive stereotypical movements, which are not due to any psychiatric or neurological condition, manifested by head banging, head nodding and nystagmus, rocking, twirling, finger-flicking mannerisms, and eye poking. Common in cases of mental retardation with sensory impairment or with environmental monotony.

sterile *1)* Unable to reproduce. *2)* Aseptic condition free of microorganisms.

Sterling Monorail Brand name balloon dilatation catheter for carotid, renal, and lower extremity vessels.

S-U

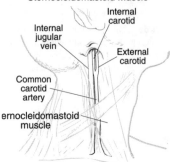

Sternocleidomastoid Muscle

Internal carotid

Internal jugular vein

External carotid

Common carotid artery

ernocleidomastoid muscle

sternocleidomastoid Large superficial muscle that passes obliquely across the anterolateral neck, originating at the sternum and clavicle and inserting at the mastoid process of the temporal bone.

sternotomy Incision into the sternum, the bone that forms the front of the chest cavity and connects with the ribs.

steroids Hormonal substances with a similar basic chemical structure, produced mainly in the adrenal cortex and gonads.

stetho- Relating to the chest.

Stevens-Johnson syndrome Necrolysis of skin caused by toxins. Report this disorder with ICD-9-CM code 695.13.

Stewart-Morel syndrome Thickening of inner table of the frontal bone associated with obesity in women nearing menopause. Report this disorder with ICD-9-CM code 733.3.

STFCS Standard transaction format compliance system. HIPAA compliance certification service sponsored by the Electronic Healthcare Network Accreditation Commission and hosted by Washington Publishing Company.

STH Somatotrophic hormone.

STICH trial Surgical treatment for ischemic heart failure trial. Clinical trial comparing three treatments for heart failure: medical therapy; medical therapy with bypass surgery; medical therapy, bypass surgery with surgical ventricular restoration (ventricular reduction).

Stickler syndrome Genetic condition causing defects in collagen development that presents with flattened facial appearance, eye abnormalities, and joint pain. Patients tend to be highly myopic. The disorder affects one in 10,000 people and is closely related to Marfan syndrome. Stickler syndrome is reported with ICD-9-CM code 759.89.

stiff-man syndrome Increasing but fluctuating rigidity of upper limb and axial muscles and increasing cerebral

and spinal disease but with increased electrical activity. Report this disorder with ICD-9-CM code 333.91.

stillborn Late demise (22 weeks or more gestational age) of fetus in utero with subsequent delivery. As a maternal condition, stillbirth is classified to ICD-9-CM subcategory 656.4. **Synonym(s):** *STB.*

Still-Felty syndrome Splenomegaly, leukopenia, arthritis, hypersplenism, anemia and other symptoms. Report this disorder with ICD-9-CM code 714.1.

Stilling-Türk-Duane syndrome Simultaneous retraction of eye muscles causing an inability to abduct affected eye with retraction of globe. Report this disorder with ICD-9-CM code 378.71. **Synonym(s):** *Duane syndrome.*

Stimson's method Use of a counterweight as traction to perform a closed reduction of an anterior shoulder dislocation with the patient placed prone on a table, reported with CPT code 23650 or 23655 depending on anesthesia use.

STJ Subtalar joint. Joint connecting the talus with the calcaneus that helps with inversion and eversion of the foot.

STM Short-term memory.

stockinet Material used to wrap an injured body part before applying a cast; usually of breathable material to wick moisture away from skin.

Stoffel rhizotomy Nerve roots are sectioned to relieve pain or spastic paralysis.

Stokes (-Adams) syndrome Heart block often causing slow or absent pulse, vertigo, syncope, convulsions, and Cheyne-Stokes respiration. Report this disorder with ICD-9-CM code 426.9. **Synonym(s):** *Morgagni's disease, Spens syndrome.*

stoma Opening created in the abdominal wall from an internal organ or structure for diversion of waste elimination, drainage, and access.

stomato- Relating to the mouth.

stop loss In health care contracting, a form of reinsurance that protects health insurance above a certain limit and minimizes risks for providers.

strabismic amblyopia Decreased or impaired vision in one or both eyes without detectable anatomic damage to the retina or visual pathways caused by purposeful suppression of vision through one eye in order to avoid diplopia (seeing double). Strabismic amblyopia is usually not correctable by eyeglasses or contact lenses. Report this condition with ICD-9-CM code 368.01. **Synonym(s):** *suppression amblyopia.*

S-U

Strabismus

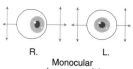

R.   L.
Monocular
(one eye only)
esotropia (inward)

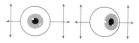

Monocular exotropia
(outward)

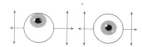

Monocular hypertropia
(upward)

Types of Strabismus

strabismus Misalignment of the eyes due to an imbalance in extraocular muscles.

straight-back syndrome Loss of the anterior concavity in the upper thoracic vertebrae causing spine to move forward and compress the heart between sternum and vertebral body. Report this disorder with ICD-9-CM code 756.19.

Straight-In Brand name sacral colpopexy system for securing the vaginal apex to the sacrum in cases of vaginal vault prolapse. Its placement is reported with CPT code 57280.

strangulated Constricted and congested area, typically in an intestine, caused by herniation that results in compromised blood supply to that area.

strap muscles Name given to several muscles located below the hyoid bone including the sternohyoid, omohyoid, sternothyroid, thyrohyoid, and the levator muscle of the thyroid gland.

strapping Application of overlapping strips of tape or bandaging to put pressure on the affected area.

strategic national implementation process Workgroup for Electronic Data Interchange program for helping the health care industry identify and resolve HIPAA implementation issues. *Synonym(s):* SNIP.

strawberry gallbladder Accumulation of cholesterol deposits in the tissues of the gallbladder, reported with

ICD-9-CM code 575.6. *Synonym(s):* cholesterolosis of gallbladder.

streak ovary Congenital anomaly in which the ovary is undeveloped, located in the broad ligament beneath the fallopian tubes and composed of fibrous connective tissue resembling ovarian stroma with no germinal or only primordial follicular cells present. Often seen in Turner's syndrome, this anomaly is reported with ICD-9-CM code 752.0. *Synonym(s):* streak gonad.

strep Streptococcus.

Streptase Brand name of streptokinase, an injectable enzyme used to break down and dissolve blood clots by stimulating extra plasmin production. This drug is primarily used to treat myocardial infarction, deep vein thrombosis, and pulmonary embolism. Supply is reported with HCPCS Level II code J2995.

streptococcus group B colonization Bacteria normally found in the vagina or lower intestine of many healthy adult women that may infect the fetus during childbirth, causing mental or physical handicaps or death. Women who test positive for streptococcus Group B during pregnancy are considered a "colonized" status and are treated with IV antibiotics at the time of delivery and may also be treated with oral antibiotics during the pregnancy. *Synonym(s):* beta Strep, GBS, Group B Strep.

stress fracture Fracture of the bone caused by repetitive overuse. Frequently occurring in the setting of heavy physical labor, sports, or strenuous exercise, these fractures are particularly common in the metatarsal bones of the foot. Treatment consists of disuse, rest, and occasionally casting or splinting to avoid reinjury during the healing process. Report stress fractures with a code from ICD-9-CM subcategory 733.9, and personal history with V13.52.

stress incontinence Involuntary escape of urine at times of minor stress against the bladder, such as coughing, sneezing, or laughing. *NCD Reference:* 30.1.1.

stress reaction Emotionally disruptive or upsetting condition occurring in response to adverse external influences and capable of affecting physical health. Often characterized by increased heart rate, a rise in blood pressure, muscular tension, irritability, and depression. This condition is reported with a code from ICD-9-CM category 308. *acute s. r.* Acute transient disorders of any severity and nature of emotions, consciousness, and psychomotor states (singly or in combination) that occur in individuals, without any apparent preexisting mental disorder, in response to exceptional physical or mental stress, such as natural catastrophe or battle, and that usually subside within hours or days. *chronic s. r.* Abnormal or maladaptive reaction with emotional or behavioral characteristics as a result of a life event or stressor that is usually temporary.

S-U

Stretta Brand name device for delivery of radiofrequency ablation to the muscle of the lower esophageal sphincter and gastric cardia as a treatment for gastroesophageal reflux disease.

stricture Narrowing of an anatomical structure. *Synonym(s): STX.*

stridor Harsh, high-pitched sound produced when breathing with an obstructed airway, like the inspiratory sound heard when laryngeal obstruction is present or heard in patients with lung or esophageal cancers that have grown to sizes that compress the airway. Stridor is reported with ICD-9-CM code 786.1.

string sign Threadlike pattern of contrast material through a filling defect seen in x-ray of the colon. *Synonym(s): Kantor's sign.*

stroboscope Device that produces an interrupted light that, when projected on moving or vibrating objects, makes them appear to be stationary.

stroke Blocked artery or a ruptured blood vessel causes a lack of blood supply and thus damage to the brain, leading to complete or partial loss of function in the area of the body that is controlled by the part of the brain that is damaged. Report this condition with a code from ICD-9-CM category 434. *Synonym(s): cerebral vascular accident, CVA.*

stromal pigmentations of cornea Color deposits in the middle layer of the cornea, reported with ICD-9-CM code 371.12. *Synonym(s): hematocornea.*

STS Serology test for syphilis.

STSG Split thickness skin graft.

STU Skin test unit.

Sturge-Kalischer-Weber syndrome Encephalocutaneous angiomatosis. Congenital condition, characterized by unilateral port-wine stain over trigeminal nerve, underlying meninges and cerebral cortex. Usually unilateral.

STWS Stuve Wiedemann syndrome. Rare recessive genetic disorder characterized by short stature, bowing of arms and legs, and permanently flexed fingers and toes. Infants may develop acute conditions including hyperthermia or respiratory distress. STWS is reported with ICD-9-CM code 756.89.

STX Stricture. Narrowing of an anatomical structure.

sub Below.

subacute Developing over days or weeks; undetermined whether acute or chronic.

subacute necrotizing lymphadenitis Benign lymphadenopathy syndrome manifested by swollen glands in the neck, fever, necrotizing lesions in the area around the thymus cortex, flu-like symptoms, and an increase in distinct types of histiocytes, monocytes, and immunoblasts. Predominantly occurring in females, this disease is sometimes considered a self-limiting form of systemic lupus erythematosus. Report this condition with ICD-9-CM code 289.3. *Synonym(s): histiocytic necrotizing lymphadenitis, Kikuchi disease, Kikuchi-Fujimoto disease, Kikuchi lymphadenitis.*

subarachnoid Located below the arachnoid meningeal layer.

SUBC State Uniform Billing Committee.

subcategory code Three-digit revenue coding structure that provides a detailed description of an accommodation or ancillary service revenue code category.

subclavian steal syndrome Obstruction of the subclavian artery proximal to the origin of the vertebral artery resulting in the subclavian artery ôstealingö cerebral blood. This condition presents with symptoms of cerebrovascular insufficiency, pain in areas at the back of the head or mastoid region, flaccid paralysis of the arm, and diminished or absent radial pulse on the affected side. This syndrome is reported with ICD-9-CM code 435.2.

subclavian-carotid obstruction syndrome Occurs in the brachiocephalic trunk and the left subclavian and left common carotid arteries above their source in the aortic arch. Symptoms include ischemia, transient blindness, facial atrophy, and many others. Report this disorder with ICD-9-CM code 446.7.

subcoracoid-pectoralis minor syndrome Malignant atrophic papulosis. Report this disorder with ICD-9-CM code 447.8.

subcortical arteriosclerotic encephalopathy Rare type of dementia manifested by deep white-matter brain lesions, memory loss, loss of cognitive ability, and alteration in mood. This is a slowly progressive condition often manifested by strokes and partial recovery. Treatment is symptomatic and consists of medication to control hyper- and hypotension, depression, and arrhythmia. Report this condition with ICD-9-CM code 290.12. *Synonym(s): Binswanger's disease, subcortical dementia.*

subcortical dementia Rare type of dementia manifested by deep white-matter brain lesions, memory loss, loss of cognitive ability, and alteration in mood. This is a slowly progressive condition often manifested by strokes and partial recovery. Treatment is symptomatic and consists of medication to control hyper- and hypotension, depression, and arrhythmia. Report this condition with ICD-9-CM code 290.12. *Synonym(s): Binswanger's disease, subcortical arteriosclerotic encephalopathy.*

subcu Subcutaneous.

subcutaneous Below the skin.

subcutaneous pocket Small space created under the skin in a suitable location for holding the battery source or pulse generator of a pacemaker or cardioverter defibrillator. This pocket is usually created under the clavicle or beneath the abdominal muscles under the ribs. Placement of an implantable cardiac device includes initial creation of this subcutaneous pocket. Sometimes the pocket itself needs to be revised or relocated, reported with CPT codes 33222-33223. Removal of such a cardiac device requires opening the pocket and subsequent closure.

subcutaneous reservoir   Space below the skin in which fluid is stored.

subcutaneous tissue   Sheet or wide band of adipose (fat) and areolar connective tissue in two layers attached to the dermis. *Synonym(s): hypodermis, superficial fascia.*

subdiaphragmatic   Below the diaphragm. *Synonym(s): subphrenic.*

subdural   Space between the dura matter and arachnoid in the brain.

subfascial   Beneath the band of fibrous tissue that lies deep to the skin, encloses muscles, and separates their layers.

subfascial endoscopic perforator surgery   Minimally invasive ligation of incompetent calf perforator veins through an endoscope. SEPS is usually performed with two points of entry, one for the endoscope and one for dissecting or dividing instrumentation. The perforating veins are divided using endoscopic scissors. Another option is to interrupt the diseased vein using a harmonic scalpel. Report this surgery with ICD-9-CM procedure code 38.89 or CPT code 37500. *Synonym(s): SEPS, vascular endoscopy.*

subind.   Immediately after.

subjective insomnia complaint   Complaint of insomnia made by the individual, which has not been investigated or proven.

subluxation   Partial or complete dislocation.

submentovertex view   Specific angle for x-ray exams used in trauma cases, in which the neck is extended and the x-ray beam enters the head under the chin (near the mental tubercle of the mandible) and exits at the vertex. The direction of the beam is perpendicular to the cantho-meatal line. This view, used with other projections, permits direct visualization of the skull base and zygomatic arches, as well as the impingement of any of these bones on the coronoid process of the mandible.

submucous resection   In otorhinolaryngology, cutting out or removing a portion of a deviated nasal septum after first laying back a flap of mucous membrane, which is replaced or repositioned after the operation.

submucous uterine leiomyoma   Benign, smooth muscle tumor beneath the inner lining of the uterus.

suboccipital   Area beneath the occipital bone in the back of the head.

subperiosteal hematoma syndrome   Anemia, spongy gums, weakness, induration of leg muscles, and mucocutaneous hemorrhages. Report this disorder with ICD-9-CM code 267. *Synonym(s): Barlow syndrome, Cheadle syndrome, Moller syndrome.*

subphrenic interposition syndrome   Interposition of colon between liver and diaphragm. Report this disorder with ICD-9-CM code 751.4.

subrogation   Recovery of monies or benefits from a third party who is liable for the payment.

subrogation clause   Contract clause that allows the substitution of one creditor for another, typically used in reference to insurance coverage where a payer may seek to recover conditional payments directly from the liability insurer."

subsequent care   All evaluation and instructions for care rendered subsequent to the inpatient admission by the admitting provider and all other providers.

subserous uterine leiomyoma   Benign, smooth muscle tumor beneath the serous membrane lining of the uterus.

subsidiary codes   Services that are not included as part of the primary procedure but that are not performed alone and may be identified as each additional, or list-in-addition-to services. Phrases that help identify subsidiary codes include, but are not limited to: each additional, list in addition to, and done at time of other major procedure

substantia propria corneae   Tough, fibrous, and transparent layer of the cornea, making up the main substance proper of the cornea. It is located between the Bowman's membrane (anterior limiting lamina) and Descemet's membrane (posterior limiting lamina).

substantial comorbidity   Preexisting condition that will, because of its presence with a specific principal diagnosis, cause an increase in the length of stay by at least one day in approximately 75 percent of the cases.

substantial complication   Condition that arises during the hospital stay that prolongs the length of stay by at least one day in approximately 75 percent of the cases.

subtalar joint   Joint connecting the talus with the calcaneus that helps with inversion and eversion of the foot. *Synonym(s): STJ.*

subtemporal   Located below the temporal bone of the skull.

subtraction   Removal of an overlying structure to better visualize the structure in question by imposing one x-ray on top of another.

subungual   Under the nail.

succulent hand   Hand that is soft, edematous, cold, and bluish in color, caused by swelling and thickening

S-U

of the subcutaneous tissues. Indication of fluid filed cyst within the spinal cord (syringomyelia). **Synonym(s):** *Marinesco's sign, Marinesco's succulent hand.*

suction   Vacuum evacuation of fluid or tissue.

SUD   Single use device. Designation for a medical device that is intended to be used once and discarded. Federal legislation allows for the reuse of some SUDs that have undergone sterilization and cleansing processes.

sudden death syndrome   Unexpected death of healthy infant typically under 12 months old. Report this disorder with ICD-9-CM code 798.0. **Synonym(s):** *SIDS.*

sudden infant death syndrome   Unexpected death of healthy infant typically under 12 months old. Report this disorder with ICD-9-CM code 798.0. **Synonym(s):** *crib death, SIDS.*

Sudeck's syndrome   Post-traumatic osteoporosis associated with vasospasm. Report this disorder with ICD-9-CM code 733.7. **Synonym(s):** *Sudeck-Leriche syndrome.*

SUI   Stress urinary incontinence. Involuntary escape of urine during times of stress against the bladder, such as coughing, laughing, sneezing, or other forms of physical exertion. The onset of symptoms is generally gradual, and there is usually a history of vaginal childbirth in women. Stress incontinence is reported with ICD-9-CM code 625.6 for females and 788.32 for males. **Synonym(s):** *genuine stress incontinence, urethral hypermobility.* **NCD Reference:** *30.1.1.*

sulfamethoxazole-trimethoprim   Injectable combination antibacterial drug used in the treatment and prevention of Pneumocystis carinii. It is also used to treat certain other bacterial infections including UTI, bronchitis, gastrointestinal infection, and otitis media infections. Supply is reported with HCPCS Level II code S0039. May be sold under brand names Bactrim IV, Septra IV, SMZ-TMP, sulfamethoxazole-trimethoprim, Sulfutrim.

Sulfatrim   Injectable combination antibacterial drug used in the treatment and prevention of Pneumocystis carinii. It is also used to treat certain other bacterial infections including UTI, bronchitis, gastrointestinal infection, and otitis media infections. Supply is reported with HCPCS Level II code S0039. May be sold under brand names Bactrim IV, Septra IV, SMZ-TMP, sulfamethoxazole-trimethoprim.

sumatriptan succinate   Neurological agent used to treat acute migraine attacks or cluster headaches. Supply is reported with HCPCS Level II code J3030. May be sold under brand name Imitrex.

SUNCT   Short-lasting, unilateral, neuralgiform headaches with conjunctival injection and tearing. Rare complex of symptoms including sharp, intermittent pain around the eye, with reddened conjunctiva, tears, and runny nose. Code according to presenting conditions.

sunrise view   Infrapatellar radiographic view of the knee in which the patella appears like a sun, rising over a horizon. This view may be ordered if the physician suspects a fracture of the patella. The radiograph is taken when the knee is flexed. A sunrise view is reported with CPT codes 73560-73564.

Supartz   Brand name solution of sodium hyaluronate injected into the knee joint as a lubricant to relieve osteoarthritis pain. Supply of Supartz is reported with HCPCS Level II code J7321. The injection is reported with CPT code 20610. These codes are unilateral and should be reported twice if injections are administered in both knees.

Super Saturated Oxygen Therapy   Used as an adjunct to other procedures that restore coronary artery blood flow, super saturated oxygen therapy involves the creation of super-oxygenated arterial blood which is infused directly to oxygen-deprived myocardial tissue in acute myocardial infarction patients.

superbill   Multipurpose sheet used for all patient encounters that typically contains a check-off list of ICD-9-CM diagnosis codes, evaluation and management codes, and procedure and HCPCS Level II codes in the outpatient setting.

superfecundation   Fertilization of two or more ova from the same cycle by sperm from separate procreative acts. Superfecundation can result in fraternal twins having different fathers. Superfecundation is reported with a code from ICD-9-CM subcategory 651.9.

superfetation   Extremely rare obstetric event in which a second ova is fertilized and established in the uterus in a cycle different from the cycle in which a first ova was fertilized and established in the uterus. This result in fetuses of differing gestational maturity, and can occur only in cases in which there are two uteri or where the menstrual cycle continues through pregnancy. Superfetation is reported with a code from ICD-9-CM subcategory 651.9.

superficial   On the skin surface or near the surface of any involved structure or field of interest. **s. dissection** Cut through the skin into the subcutaneous fat, but not through the fascia.

superficial dissection   Cutting through the skin into the subcutaneous fat, but not approaching the fascia.

superficial folliculitis   Superficial inflammation of the hair follicles most commonly caused by Staph aureus that manifests as rounded, sphere-shaped pustular eruptions in the areas of the scalp, beard, underarms, extremities, and buttocks. This condition is reported with ICD-9-CM code 704.8. **Synonym(s):** *Bockhart's impetigo.*

superficial musculoaponeurotic system flap   Rhytidectomy commonly used in cosmetic surgery.

Incisions are made along the margin of the face and usually within the area behind the ears. The skin is taken off and tightened. Surplus skin is removed. Underlying muscle tissue is likewise tightened and repositioned. Report this procedure with CPT code 15829. **Synonym(s):** SMAS flap.

superficial suppurative cheilitis glandularis One of the three types of cheilitis glandularis, an uncommon disease of the lower lip in which it becomes larger and then turns inside out. Characteristics of this disease include painless swelling, hardening, crusting, and lip ulcers. Report this condition with ICD-9-CM code 528.5. **Synonym(s):** Baelz's disease.

superior artery syndrome Complete or partial block of the superior mesenteric artery with vomiting, pain, blood in the stool, distended abdomen, and resulting in bowel infarction. Report this disorder with ICD-9-CM code 557.1. **Synonym(s):** Wilkie's syndrome.

superior hypogastric plexus Part of the autonomic nervous system, the superior hypogastric plexus is formed of parasympathetic fibers that are a continuation of the intermesenteric plexus. It divides into the left and right hypogastric nerves.

SuperSaturated oxygen therapy Treatment of acute myocardial infarction (AMI) in which superoxygenated saline solution is combined with the patient's blood to create hyperoxemic blood, which is then delivered via infusion catheter to the patient's coronary arteries, where it reestablishes vascular blood flow and tissue perfusion. This intervention is typically performed as adjunctive therapy immediately following percutaneous coronary intervention (PCI) in AMI patients. Report with ICD-9-CM procedure code 00.49. **Synonyms:** aqueous oxygen, AO therapy, myocardial salvage intervention, MSI, SuperOxygenation infusion therapy.

supervision and interpretation Radiology services that usually contain an invasive component and are reported by the radiologist for supervision of the procedure and the personnel involved with performing the examination, reading the film, and preparing the written report.

Supination

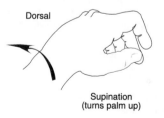

Dorsal

Supination
(turns palm up)

supination Lying on the back; turning the palm toward the front or upward; raising the medial margin of the foot by an inverting and adducting movement.

supine Lying on the back. **Synonym(s):** decubitus position, dorsal.

supp Suppository.

supplemental health services Optional services that a health plan may cover or provide.

supplementary medical insurance Also referred to as Medicare Part B insurance, it provides payment to participating providers for furnishing covered services after a yearly cash deductible is met. It is a voluntary medical insurance plan designed to supplement the basic hospital insurance coverage. It provides coverage for home health visits not available under hospital insurance (e.g., no Part A entitlement or visits after the first 100 visits) and for medical and other health services. Payment may not be made under Part B for any service that may be paid under Part A. However, where payment is not possible under Part A (e.g., no Part A entitlement or benefits are exhausted) payment may be made under Part B if the service is covered. Eligible individuals may purchase this supplement by enrolling during an open enrollment period and paying a monthly premium. Eligibility requirements include entitlement to hospital insurance (Part A) or age 65 or older and a U.S. citizen or resident alien meeting certain resident requirements. **Synonym(s):** SMI.

supplier Person or entity that furnishes or provides health care supplies, such as durable medical equipment or medical-surgical supplies.

supplies Items or accessories needed for the performance of procedures, or for the effective use of durable medical equipment, prosthetics, orthotic devices, and appliances.

support Article that provides stabilization, but not immobilization, to an injured or disabled body part.

suppository Medication in the form of a solid mass at room temperature that dissolves at body temperature, for insertion into a body orifice such as the rectal, vaginal, or urethral opening.

suppression Holding back, putting in check, or inhibiting an act, function, thought, or desire.

suppression amblyopia Decreased or impaired vision in one or both eyes without detectable anatomic damage to the retina or visual pathways caused by purposeful suppression of vision through one eye in order to avoid diplopia (seeing double). It is usually not correctable by eyeglasses or contact lenses. Report strabismic amblyopia with ICD-9-CM code 368.01. **Synonym(s):** strabismic amblyopia.

suppurative Forming pus.

S-U

supra Above.

supraglottic Located above the glottis, the sound-producing apparatus of the larynx consisting of two vocal folds and the intervening space.

supraglottis Area of the larynx superior to the vocal cords, which includes the epiglottis.

supraglottitis Infection of the lingual tonsillar area, epiglottic folds, false vocal cords, and the epiglottis, most commonly affecting children, but can appear at any age. Supraglottitis is reported with ICD-9-CM codes 464.50 and 464.51.

supraorbital nerve Ophthalmic branch of the trigeminal nerve that is sensory in nature and enervates the lateral part of the forehead and the front part of the scalp.

suprarenal cortical syndrome Disorder of adrenal medullary tissue resulting in hypertension with attacks of palpitation, headache, nausea, dyspnea, anxiety, pallor, and profuse sweating. Report this disorder with ICD-9-CM code 255.3. *Synonym(s): Schroeder's syndrome, Slocumb's syndrome.*

supraspinatus syndrome Pain on abduction of shoulder and tenderness upon deep pressure of supraspinatus tendon. Report this disorder with ICD-9-CM code 726.10.

supratentorial Located above the tentorium. The tentorium is the covering of dura mater in the brain supporting the occipital lobes and covering the cerebellum.

supraventricular tachycardia Rapid beating of the heart, usually pertains to 100 beats per minute or more. The origin of this fast beat is the atrium or the AV node. Report SVT with ICD-9-CM code 427.89. *Synonym(s): SVT.*

surgical hierarchy Ordering of surgical cases from most to least resource intensive. Application of this decision rule is necessary when patient stays involve multiple surgical procedures, each of which, occurring by itself, could result in the assignment to a different DRG. All patients must be assigned to only one DRG per admission.

surgical package Normal, uncomplicated performance of specific surgical services, with the assumption that, on average, all surgical procedures of a given type are similar with respect to skill level, duration, and length of normal follow-up care.

surgical planing Plastic surgery procedure of abrading and smoothing disfigured skin to promote re-epithelialization with minimal scarring.

surgical wound Surgical wounds fall into four categories that determine treatment methods and outcomes: *clean wound* No inflammation or contamination; treatment performed with no break in sterile technique; no alimentary, respiratory, or genitourinary tracts involved in the surgery. Infection rate: up to 5 percent. *clean-contaminated wound* No inflammation; treatment performed with minor break in surgical technique; no unusual contamination resulting when alimentary, respiratory, genitourinary, or oropharyngeal cavity is entered. Infection rate: up to 11 percent. *contaminated wound* Less than four hours old with acute, nonpurulent inflammation; treatment performed with major break in surgical technique; gross contamination resulting from the gastrointestinal tract. Infection rate: up to 20 percent. *dirty and infected wound* More than four hours old with existing infection, inflammation, abscess, and nonsterile conditions due to perforated viscus, fecal contamination, necrotic tissue, or foreign body. Infection rate: up to 40 percent. To locate the appropriate diagnosis code for a wound, see wound, open, in the ICD-9-CM index. A complicated open wound is defined as a wound that has delayed healing, delayed treatment, foreign body (including debris), or infection. For debridement of an open wound, see CPT codes 97602 and 97597-97598. For repair of wound dehiscence, see 12020-12021 and 13160. For exploration of a penetrating wound, see 20102 (abdomen), 20101 (chest), 20103 (extremity), and 20100 (neck). Repair of wounds of the integumentary system are coded based upon type of repair (simple, intermediate, or complex) and anatomical location.

SurgiMend Collagen Matrix Dermal substitute used to reinforce weak soft tissue or surgically repair damaged soft tissue membranes. SurgiMend Collagen Matrix is indicated for various forms of plastic and reconstructive surgery, as well as muscle flap reinforcement and hernia repair. Supply is reported with HCPCS Level II code C9358 or C9360.

Surgisis Brand name, acellular wound management material made from porcine-derived acellular material. Its application is reported with CPT codes 15430 and 15431.

survival Continued life.

Susac syndrome Neurological disorder characterized by disturbances of motion involving the brain and vision and hearing loss, caused by damage to small blood vessels in the affected organs. It is thought to be autoimmune in nature. There is no code specifically indexed to Susac syndrome in ICD-9-CM. Code each manifestation individually. *Synonym(s): SICRET syndrome.*

suspension *1)* Fixation of an organ for support. *2)* Temporary state of cessation of an activity, process, or experience.

suspension of payment Suspension of payment is defined in the *Code of Federal Regulations* as "the withholding of payment by the carrier or intermediary from a provider or supplier of an approved Medicare payment amount before a determination of the amount of overpayment exists.❑ In other words, contractors have received, processed, and approved claims for a provider❑s items or services; however, the provider has not been paid and the amount of the overpayment has not been established.

suture Numerous stitching techniques employed in wound closure. ***buried s.*** Continuous or interrupted suture placed under the skin for a layered closure. ***continuous s.*** Running stitch with tension evenly distributed across a single strand to provide a leakproof closure line. ***interrupted s.*** Series of single stitches with tension isolated at each stitch, in which all stitches are not affected if one becomes loose, and the isolated sutures cannot act as a wick to transport an infection. ***purse-string s.*** Continuous suture placed around a tubular structure and tightened, to reduce or close the lumen. ***retention s.*** Secondary stitching that bridges the primary suture, providing support for the primary repair; a plastic or rubber bolster may be placed over the primary repair and under the retention sutures.

SutureGroove Brand name gold eyelid weights for use in lagophthalmos treatment. Correction of lagophthalmos using a gold weight is reported with CPT code 67912. Lagophthalmos is reported with a code from ICD-9-CM subcategory 374.2.

SUZI Sub-zonal insemination. In vitro fertilization technique in which a single sperm is placed just beneath the protein shell that surrounds the ova. Most commonly a technique selected in cases in which the sperm count is low or the sperm has motility dysfunctions. SUZI is reported with CPT code 89280. Preparation of the sperm and egg and placement of the egg into the patient are all reported additionally.

Sv Scalp vein.

SVC Service.

SVCS Superior vena cava syndrome.

SVD Spontaneous vaginal delivery.

SVG Saphenous vein graft.

SVR Surgical ventricular restoration. Treatment of congestive heart failure by restoring the heart to a more normal size and shape. The ventricular muscle and chamber are resized with the aid of a plastic model, in hopes of improving heart function. This procedure is often performed with bypass or valve repair, which is reported separately. SVR is reported with CPT code 33548. ***Synonym(s):*** *Dor procedure, LV reconstruction, SAVER, TR3SVR.*

SVRS Statistically valid random sample.

SVT Supraventricular tachycardia. Rapid beating of the heart, usually pertains to 100 beats per minute or more. The origin of this fast beat is the atrium or the AV node. Report SVT with ICD-9-CM code 427.0 or 427.89.

swallowed blood syndrome Swallowed blood syndrome in the newborn, causing hematemesis and melena. Report this disorder with ICD-9-CM code 777.3.

Swan-Ganz Flexible, flow-directed catheter inserted through the inferior or superior vena cava through the right side of the heart to the pulmonary artery, where it measures blood pressure in pulmonary circulation and estimate cardiac output. Report its insertion with ICD-9-CM procedure code 89.64 or CPT code 93503. ***Synonym(s):*** *SGC.*

sweet syndrome Disease of women marked by plaque-like lesions on face, neck, and upper extremities and conjunctivitis, mucosal lesion, malaise, fever, and arthralgia. Report this disorder with ICD-9-CM code 695.89.

SWG Sub-workgroup.

swing bed Bed used for acute or long-term care, depending on the patient's need and the hospital's level of occupancy. Swing beds typically are available in small and rural hospitals. A swing-bed patient may be admitted and discharged from acute care and readmitted to a swing bed to receive skilled or intermediate levels of care. At times, the patient may remain in the same bed while changes occur in his or her care, charges, and payment.

SWISS Siblings with Ischemic Stroke Study. Study sponsored by the National Institute of Neurological Disorders and Stroke to find the genes that increase the risk of developing an ischemic stroke using DNA samples collected from siblings.

Swyer-James syndrome Acquired unilateral hyperlucent lung with severe airway obstruction during expiration, oligemia, and a small hilum. Report this disorder with ICD-9-CM code 492.8. ***Synonym(s):*** *MacLeod's syndrome.*

Sx 1) Sign. 2) Symptom.

sycosis Pus-containing rash appearing on the scalp or the bearded portion of the face, often caused by ringworm, acne, or impetigo. ***Synonym(s):*** *mentagra.*

sylvan yellow fever Acute, rare, infectious, vector-borne viral disease contracted by humans bitten by mosquitoes infected with the flavivirus through animals, usually monkeys, in the setting of tropical rain forests in Africa and South America. Manifestations include fever, jaundice, possible kidney damage, and liver necrosis. Report this disease with ICD-9-CM code 060.0. ***Synonym(s):*** *jungle yellow fever.*

sym- Indicates together with, along with, beside.

symblepharon Adhesion between the bulbar conjunctiva and the palpebral conjunctiva, resulting in the eyelids adhering to the eyeball. The adhesion can be the result of trauma, infection, or surgery. Symblepharon is reported with ICD-9-CM code 372.63.

S-U

symblepharopterygium Adhesion in which the eyelid is adhered to the eyeball by a band that resembles a pterygium, reported with ICD-9-CM code 372.63. If specified as congenital, report 743.62.

Symonds' syndrome Meningitis with serious inflammation in subarachnoid and ventricle spaces and little change in the cerebrospinal fluid. Report this disorder with ICD-9-CM code 348.2. *Synonym(s): Symonds' syndrome.*

sympathectomy Surgical interruption or transection of a sympathetic nervous system pathway.

sympathetic nerves Self-regulating nerves that are part of the autonomic nervous system and that innervate the involuntary motor systems that prepare the body for intense activity, such as the "fight-or-flight" response increasing heart, respiration, and metabolic rates and alertness, while inhibiting bodily secretions and digestion.

sympathetic nervous system One of the two peripheral visceral efferent divisions of the autonomic nervous system receiving its nerve fibers from the thoracic and upper lumbar levels of the spinal cord that regulates activity of the blood vessels, smooth muscle and glands, and the viscera of the thorax, abdomen, and pelvis. The system is responsible for the "fight or flight" reaction with restriction of the pupils; relaxation of the bronchial muscles; reduced production of saliva, urine, and mucus; the secretion of norepinephrine and epinephrine; and an increase in the rate and force of the heartbeat. Sympathectomy codes are found in CPT range 64802-64823. *Synonym(s): autonomic nervous system.*

symphysis Joint that unifies two opposed bones by a junction of bony surfaces to a plate of fibrocartilage.

syn- Indicates being joined together.

synapse Space between two nerve endings where information from one neuron flows to the other.

Syncardia TAH Brand name artificial heart used in patients awaiting transplant. *NCD Reference: 20.9.*

synchondrosis Two bones joined by hyaline cartilage or fibrocartilage. Typically, the bones fuse as they mature.

syncope Light-headedness or fainting caused by insufficient blood supply to the brain. Report syncope with ICD-9-CM code 780.2.

syndactylic oxycephaly syndrome Chromosomal condition with primary symptoms including webbing of digits and a pointed head with variations of defects. Often associated with other chromosomal abnormalities. Report this disorder with ICD-9-CM code 755.55. *Synonym(s): Apert's syndrome.*

syndactyly Congenital condition in which two or more digits fail to separate and remain fused by webbing

between the fingers or toes. The severity of the condition can vary from incomplete fusion of the skin to fusion of bone and nails. Syndactyly is reported with a code from subcategory 755.1 and often requires surgical correction. Syndactyly is reported with CPT codes 26560-26562.

syndrome of inappropriate antidiuretic hormone Inappropriate antidiuretic hormone causing ongoing hypovolemia, hyponatremia, and increased urine osmolality. Often occurring as a result of head trauma, certain lung or pancreatic cancers, or pulmonary disorders, vasopressin is released in excessive amounts for the state of hydration. Report this syndrome with ICD-9-CM code 253.6. *Synonym(s): SIADH.*

syndrome X Group of health risks that increase the likelihood of developing heart disease, stroke, and diabetes. Diagnosis of syndrome X is made if one has three or more of the following: waist measurement of 40 or more inches for men and 35 or more inches for women; blood pressure of 130/85 mm or higher; triglyceride level greater than 150 mg/dl; fasting blood sugar of more than 100 mg/dl; HDL level less than 40 mg/dl in men or less than 50 mg/dl in women. Report this condition with ICD-9-CM code 277.7, with additional codes to identify associated manifestations. *Synonym(s): dysmetabolic syndrome, insulin resistance syndrome, metabolic syndrome.*

synechia Adhesion of parts, most often used to denote adhesion of the iris to the lens or cornea, reported with ICD-9-CM codes 364.70-364.73. *intrauterine s.* Scarring and adhesions of the uterus, usually as a complication of D&C, reported with 621.5. *s. vulvae* Congenital condition in which the labia minora are sealed in the middle, reported with 752.49.

synechia vulvae Congenital condition in which the labia minora are fused, leaving a tiny opening that permits the flow of urine from the urethra. It is reported with ICD-9-CM code 752.49. *Synonym(s): fused labia.*

synonym Word having the same or nearly the same meaning as another word or other words.

synostosis Unnatural fusion of bones that are normally separate or articulate with each other, due to growth of bony tissue between them.

synovectomy Removal of the synovial membrane lining of a joint.

synovia Clear fluid lubricant of joints, bursae, and tendon sheaths, secreted by the synovial membrane.

synovitis Inflammation of the synovial membrane that lines a synovial joint, resulting in pain and swelling. Report synovitis with ICD-9-CM code 727.00 or 727.01.

syntactical aphasia Type of speech deficit in which some necessary grammatical elements for coherent sentences are lacking. *Synonym(s): ataxiaphasia.*

syntax Rules and conventions that one needs to know or follow to validly record information, or interpret previously recorded information, for a specific purpose. Thus, a syntax is a grammar. Such rules and conventions may be either explicit or implicit. In X12 transactions, the data-element separators, the subelement separators, the segment terminators, the segment identifiers, the loops, the loop identifiers (when present), the repetition factors, etc., are all aspects of the X12 syntax. When explicit, such syntactical elements tend to be the structural, or format-related, data elements that are not required when a direct data entry architecture is used. Ultimately, though, there is not a perfectly clear division between the syntactical elements and the business data content.

Synvisc Brand name solution of sodium hyaluronate injected into the knee joint as a lubricant to relieve osteoarthritis pain. Supply of Synvisc is reported with HCPCS Level II code J7325. The injection is reported with CPT code 20610. Injection codes are unilateral and should be reported twice if injections are administered in both knees.

syphilis Sexually transmitted disease caused by the treponema pallidum spirochete. Syphilis usually exhibits cutaneous manifestations and may exist for years without symptoms. Newborns may contract it via the placenta.

Syr Syrup.

syringomyelia Progressive condition that may be either from developmental origin or caused by trauma, tumor, hemorrhage, or infarction. An abnormal cavity (syrinx) forms in the spinal cord and enlarges over time, resulting in symptoms of muscle, weakness and stiffness in the back, shoulders, arms, or legs, atrophy, headaches, dissociated memory loss and a loss of sensory ability to feel pain and extremes of hot or cold temperatures. Percutaneous aspiration of a spinal cord cyst or syrinx is reported with CPT code 62268.

syrinx Cavity or fistula that develops in the spinal cord and is filled with cerebrospinal fluid, seen most often in the cervical area, but also extending into the thoracic spine, causing syringomyelia. When the cavitation extends into the brain stem, it is called syringobulbia.

systematized delusions Rare, chronic psychosis in which logically constructed systematized delusions of grandeur, persecution, or somatic abnormality have developed gradually without concomitant hallucinations or the schizophrenic type of disordered thinking. Reported with code 297.1.

systemic fibrosclerosing syndrome Widespread formation of fibrous tissue. Report this disorder with ICD-9-CM code 710.8.

systemic sclerosis Systemic disease characterized by excess fibrotic collagen build-up, turning the skin thickened and hard. Fibrotic changes also occur in various organs and cause vascular abnormalities and affect more women than men. Report this condition with ICD-9-CM code 710.1.

systole Contraction phase of the heart, especially of the ventricles, in which blood is driven through the aorta and pulmonary artery to circulate through the lungs and out to the rest of the body. Indicated physically by the first sound of the heart and by the arterial pulse.

Sz Seizure.

SZZ Sézary syndrome.

T *1)* Temperature. *2)* Tender. *3)* Thoracic vertebrae.

T&A Tonsillectomy and adenoidectomy, reported with CPT code 42820 or 42821 for the physician and ICD-9-CM procedure code 28.3 for facilities.

T&C Type and crossmatch.

T&CM Type and cross match.

T(O) Oral temperature.

t.d.s. Three times a day.

t.i.d. Ter in die. Latin for three times a day.

T/O Time out.

T1 HCPCS Level II modifier for use with CPT codes, identifying the second digit on the left foot. Do not append this modifier to procedures/services performed on the tarsals.

T2 HCPCS Level II modifier for use with CPT codes, identifying the third digit on the left foot. Do not append this modifier to procedures/services performed on the tarsals.

T3 *1)* HCPCS Level II modifier for use with CPT codes, identifying the fourth digit on the left foot. Do not append this modifier to procedures/services performed on the tarsals. *2)* Free triiodothyronine. T3 is produced by the thyroid and levels may be measured to detect thyroid dysfunction. T3 levels are measured in a laboratory test reported with CPT code 84481. *3)* Triiodothyronine.

T4 *1)* HCPCS Level II modifier for use with CPT codes, identifying the fifth digit on the left foot. Do not append this modifier to procedures/services performed on the tarsals. *2)* Thyroxine. *3)* Free thyroxine. T4 is produced by the thyroid and levels may be measured to detect thyroid or pituitary dysfunction. T4 levels are measured in a laboratory test reported with CPT code 84439.

T5 HCPCS Level II modifier for use with CPT codes, identifying the great toe on the right foot. Do not append this modifier to procedures/services performed on the tarsals.

T6 HCPCS Level II modifier for use with CPT codes, identifying the second digit on the right foot. Do not append this modifier to procedures/services performed on the tarsals.

T7 HCPCS Level II modifier for use with CPT codes, identifying the third digit on the right foot. Do not append this modifier to procedures/services performed on the tarsals.

T8 HCPCS Level II modifier for use with CPT codes, identifying the fourth digit on the right foot. Do not append this modifier to procedures/services performed on the tarsals.

T9 HCPCS Level II modifier for use with CPT codes, identifying the fifth digit on the right foot. Do not append this modifier to procedures/services performed on the tarsals.

TA *1)* HCPCS Level II modifier for use with CPT codes, identifying the great toe on the left foot. Do not append this modifier to procedures/services performed on the tarsals. *2)* Tension by applanation. *3)* Transactional analysis.

Taarnhoj procedure Gasserian ganglion nerve root is sectioned, decompressed, or compressed after being accessed through the temporal region.

tab. Tablet (tabella).

TABS Tablets.

tachy- Indicates swift or fast.

tachycardia Excessively rapid beating action of the heart, defined as more than 100 beats per minute for an adult, that is usually defined by its origin (atrial or ventricular) and whether the onset and cessation occurs in sudden attacks (paroxysmal) or in a slow pattern (nonparoxysmal).

tachycardia-bradycardia syndrome Rapid action of heart followed by protracted or transient stopping of heart. Report this disorder with ICD-9-CM code 427.81.

tachypnea Abnormal rapid respiratory rate.

TACT Trial to Assess Chelation Therapy. Clinical study looking at the use of chelating EDTA (ethylene diamine tetra-acetic acid) for coronary artery disease sponsored by the National Center for Complementary and Alternative Medicine and the National Heart, Lung and Blood Institute.

tactile Having or related to touch.

tactile amnesia Type of tactile agnosia in which the ability to understand or distinguish the shape, form, or nature of objects being touched is lost or diminished. This condition is reported with ICD-9-CM code 780.99. *Synonym(s): astereocognosy, astereognosis, stereoagnosis.*

TAG Technical advisory group.

Tagamet See cimetidine HCl.

TAH Total abdominal hysterectomy.

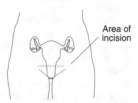

TAHBSO

Area of incision

Surgeon removes uterus, tubes, and ovaries

TAHBSO Total abdominal hysterectomy, bilateral salpingo-oophorectomy. TAHBSO is reported with CPT code 58150 when performed without node sampling or vaginectomy.

Takayasu (-Onishi) syndrome Progressive obliteration of brachiocephalic trunk and the left subclavian and left common carotid arteries above their source in the aortic arch, resulting in loss of pulse in arms and carotids. Symptoms may include ischemia, transient blindness and facial atrophy. Report this disorder with ICD-9-CM code 446.7. *Synonym(s): Marorell-Fabre syndrome, Raed-Harbitz syndrome, pulseless disease.*

Takayasu arteritis Chronic inflammatory disease of the large arteries, usually affecting the aorta, its large branches, and the pulmonary artery. Report this condition with ICD-9-CM code 446.7.

Takayasu's disease Rare inflammatory disease of the large arteries, especially affecting the aorta, that is usually fatal.

Takotsubo syndrome Complex of symptoms mimicking myocardial infarct in absence of heart disease, usually seen in postmenopausal women. Symptoms include lack of contraction in the left ventricular apex, a hypercontractile response at the base of the heart, combined with acute chest symptoms and EKG changes. Takotsubo syndrome is reported with ICD-9-CM code 429.83. *Synonym(s): broken heart syndrome.*

S-U

Talectomy

Lateral views of right ankle

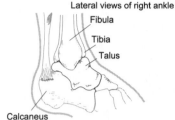

Fibula
Tibia
Talus
Calcaneus

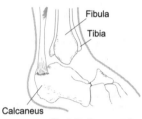

Fibula
Tibia
Calcaneus

The talus is removed

The talus (or astragalus) is surgically removed (talectomy)

talectomy Surgical removal of the astragalus (talus), the bone that forms the ankle joint by articulating with the tibia and fibula. Indications include trauma, congenital abnormalities, severe fractures, chronic infection, or tumors. Talectomy is reported with ICD-9-CM procedure code 77.98 and CPT code 28130. *Synonym(s): astragalectomy.*

talipes cavovarus Deformity in which the lateral part of the foot endures most weight bearing pressure due to an abnormally high longitudinal arch with the heel deviating inward from the midline of the leg.

talipes equinovarus Deformity in which the heel is turned inward, the foot is plantar flexed with the arch raised, causing the ball of the foot to bear the weight of the body; usual clubfoot formation.

Talipes Valgus and Varus

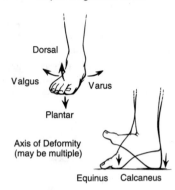

Dorsal
Valgus
Varus
Plantar

Axis of Deformity
(may be multiple)

Equinus   Calcaneus

talipes valgus Congenital condition in which the foot is bent outward with the heel inward, reported with ICD-9-CM code 754.60.

talipes varus Congenital abnormality in which the foot turns inward and the heel outward, with the outer sole making contact with the ground, reported with ICD-9-CM code 754.50. *Synonym(s): pes varus.*

tamponade heart Interference with the venous return of blood to the heart due to an extensive accumulation of blood in the pericardium (pericardial effusion). Tamponade may occur as a complication of dissecting thoracic aneurysm, pericarditis, renal failure, acute myocardial infarction, chest trauma, or a malignancy. Treatment involves the emergent removal of the fluid. Report this condition with ICD-9-CM code 423.9. *Synonym(s): cardiac tamponade.*

tangential port Radiation beam that glides across the body surface.

tank ear Inflammation of the external auditory canal as a result of irritation caused by ocean water or other seaside environmental factors. Report this condition with ICD-9-CM code 380.12. *Synonym(s): acute swimmer's ear, beach ear, otitis externa.*

tap Withdraw fluid through a needle or trocar.

Tap/H2O/E Tap water enema.

Tapia's syndrome Unilateral lesions of ninth, tenth, eleventh, and twelfth cranial nerves producing paralysis of vagal, glossal, and other nerves and tongue on the same side. Usually a result of injury. Report this disorder with ICD-9-CM code 352.6. *Synonym(s): Collet-Sicard syndrome.*

TAPVR Total anomalous pulmonary venous return.

Tara KLamp Brand name male circumcision clamp device. Tara KLamp is intended for one-time use. It can be used in infant or adult circumcision, reported with CPT code 54150.

S-U

Tarceva Brand name oral medication for the treatment of non-small cell lung cancer and pancreatic cancer. Tarceva contains erlotinib.

target tissue Specific collection of cells that responds to a given hormone treatment or tissue against which any type of immunity is directed.

tarsal bones Seven bones that make up the ankle and heel consisting of the posterior talus and calcaneus, the anterior cuboid, navicular, and three cuneiform (medial, intermediate, and lateral) bones.

Tarsal Tunnel Release

Lateral view of right ankle

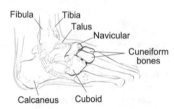

Fibula Tibia Talus Navicular Cuneiform bones Calcaneus Cuboid

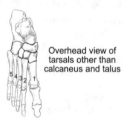

Overhead view of tarsals other than calcaneus and talus

A tarsal bone (or bone portion) other than the calcaneus or talus is surgically removed (osteotomy). Report 28305 when a bone graft harvested from elsewhere on the patient (autograft) is placed into the space

tarsal tunnel release Procedure performed to decrease pressure on the posterior tibial nerve by making an incision into the tarsal tunnel. Report this procedure with CPT code 28305.

tarsal tunnel syndrome Entrapment or compression of the posterior tibial nerve, causing tingling, pain, and numbness in the sole of the foot. Report this disorder with ICD-9-CM code 355.5.

tarsitis Inflammation of the margin of the eyelid.

tarso- 1) Relating to the foot. 2) Relating to the margin of the eyelid.

tarsocheiloplasty Plastic operation upon the edge of the eyelid for the treatment of trichiasis.

tarsomalacia Softening of the tissue of the eyelid.

tarsorrhaphy Suture of a portion or all of the opposing eyelids together for the purpose of shortening the palpebral fissure or closing it entirely. *Synonym(s): blepharorrhaphy.*

tarsus 1) Inner connective tissue framework of the eyelids that provides stiffness and shape. 2) Seven bones that make up the ankle.

TAT 1) Tetanus antitoxin. 2) Turnaround time.

tattooing Permanent method of implanting pigment into the skin to add color for the treatment of vitiligo, skin grafts, or burn scars and for cosmetic purposes. Report this procedure with CPT codes 11920-11922. *Synonym(s): micropigmentation.*

Taussig-Bing syndrome Rare cardiac congenital malformation of transposition of the great vessels in which the aorta originates in the right ventricle, and a large pulmonary artery straddles both ventricles either side of a ventricular septal defect. Cyanosis, pulmonary hypertension, and a greater oxygen concentration in the pulmonary artery than in the aorta results. Taussig-Bing syndrome is reported with ICD-9-CM code 745.11.

Tax Equity and Fiscal Responsibility Act Protects the rights of full-time employees to remain on the company's health plan to age 69. *Synonym(s): TEFRA.*

tax identification number Number an individual or organization uses to report tax information to the Internal Revenue Service, such as a Social Security Number (SSN) or employer identification number (EIN).

taxonomy code Ten-character, alphanumeric sequence code that identifies the area of specialty of a provider. CMS maintains and distributes these codes. Every type of provider can be identified with a taxonomy code. For example, an ambulatory surgery center's taxonomy code is 261QA1903X and a physician with a specialty in geriatric medicine has a taxonomy code of 207RG0300X.

TAXUS Brand name paclitaxel-eluting coronary stent system used in percutaneous intraluminal angioplasty to improve luminal diameter in coronary arteries. Insertion is reported with CPT codes 92980 and 92981 or for inpatient, ICD-9-CM procedure code 36.07.

-taxy Arrangement, grouping. *Synonym(s): -taxis.*

Taybi's syndrome Condition affecting ears, palate, mouth, and fingers. Report this disorder with ICD-9-CM code 759.89.

Tb Tubercule bacillus.

TB Tuberculosis.

TBA 1) Transluminal balloon angioplasty. Balloon-tipped catheter is placed within a narrowed artery or vein and the balloon is inflated to stretch the vessel to a larger diameter for increased blood flow. Transluminal balloon angioplasty is coded as open (CPT codes 35450-35460 and 37220-37235) or percutaneous (35471-35476 and 37220-37235), according to the specific vessel or branches, and whether it is performed on a vein or artery. Percutaneous transluminal balloon angioplasty performed on a coronary artery is done to flatten obstructive plaque against the artery wall and open the lumen and is reported with 92982 and 92984. Radiological supervision for peripheral, renal, or visceral arteries is reported with 37220-37235, 75962-75968, and 75978. *2)* To be arranged.

TBB Transbronchial biopsy. *Synonym(s): TBBX.*

TBF *1)* Total body fat. *2)* Total body failure.

TBG *1)* Thyroid binding globulin. *2)* Thyroxine.

TBI *1)* Total body irradiation. *2)* Traumatic brain injury.

TBNA Transbronchial needle aspiration. While TBNA is performed from a scope inserted into the trachea and bronchi, the sampled tissues are from parts beyond the bronchi, reaching into adjacent tissue. Report TBNA of trachea, main stem, and/or lobar bronchi with CPT code 31629 and TBNA of an additional lobe with 31633.

TBSA Total body surface area.

TBV Total blood volume.

TC *1)* HCPCS Level II modifier, for use with CPT and HCPCS Level II codes, identifying the technical component only of a procedure or service. Technical component services are only institutional and should not be billed separately by the physician. *2)* Technetium.

Tc 99m Technetium isotope.

TC&DB Turn, cough, and deep breathe.

TCC *1)* Transitional care center. Facility used in lieu of an extended care facility or before discharge to an extended care facility. *2)* Transitional cell carcinoma.

TCD Transcranial Doppler. Noninvasive ultrasound technology used to evaluate blood flow in the major intracranial arteries. TCD done with contrast is performed by intravenous microbubble injection, in which the bubbles serve to enhance ultrasound signals, thereby producing better visualization. TCD procedures are reported with a CPT code from range 93886-93893.

TCDB Turn, cough, deep breathe.

TCF Transciliary filtration. In ophthalmology, the creation of an opening in the pars plana of the ciliary body to enhance the flow of aqueous. TCF is reported with CPT code 0123T.

TCMI T cell mediated immunity. Defense against infection provided by lymphocytes developed in the thymus (T cell). Lab tests to measure a patient's T cell levels and responses include CPT codes 86359-86361.

TCR T-cell receptor.

TD *1)* HCPCS Level II modifier, for use with CPT and HCPCS Level II codes, identifying services provided by a registered nurse (RN). Required by some state Medicaid and state health departments. *2)* Tetanus.

Tdap Tetanus, diphtheria, acellular pertussis vaccine administered to patients older than 7. Supply of Tdap is reported with CPT code 90715; administration is reported separately. The need for the vaccination is reported with ICD-9-CM code V06.1.

TDD Thoracic duct drainage. *NCD Reference: 20.3*

TE HCPCS Level II modifier, for use with CPT and HCPCS Level II codes, identifying services provided by a licensed practical nurse (LPN) or licensed visiting nurse (LVN). Required by some state Medicaid and state health departments.

teaching physician Physician, other than another resident, who involves residents in the care of his or her patients.

TEB Thoracic electrical bioimpedance, reported with CPT code 93701. *NCD Reference: 20.16.*

technical component Portion of a health care service that identifies the provision of the equipment, supplies, technical personnel, and costs attendant to the performance of the procedure other than the professional services. *Synonym(s): TC.*

technique Manner of performance.

technology assessments Health care technology assessment (HTA) is a multidisciplinary field of policy analysis. It studies the medical, social, ethical, and economic implications of the development, diffusion, and use of technologies. In support of national coverage determinations (NCD), HTA often focuses on the safety and efficacy of technologies. Each NCD includes a comprehensive HTA process. For some NCDs, external HTAs are requested through the Agency for Health Research and Quality (AHRQ).

TED Thrombo-embolism deterrent.

TEDS Anti-embolism stockings.

TEE Transesophageal echocardiography.

teething syndrome Discomfort associated with eruption of teeth in small child. Report this disorder with ICD-9-CM code 520.7.

TEFRA Tax Equity and Fiscal Responsibility Act. Protects the rights of full-time employees to remain on the company's health plan to age 69.

TEG Brand name thromboelastography testing for analyzing the functional activities in cells associated with blood clotting.

tegmental syndrome Paraplegia and anesthesia over part of the body. Caused by lesions in the brain or spinal cord. Report this disorder with ICD-9-CM code 344.89. *Synonym(s): Avellis syndrome, Babinski-Nageotte syndrome, Benedikt's syndrome, Brown-Sequard syndrome, Cestan-Chenais syndrome, Cestan's syndrome, Foville's syndrome, Gubler-Millard syndrome, Jackson's syndrome, Weber-Leyden syndrome.*

S-U

Tegress Brand name urethral implant injected to remodel urethral mucosa and reduce urinary stress incontinence. Tegress injection is reported with CPT code 51715 or 52327.

telangiectasia Permanent dilation of capillaries, arterioles, or venules that appears as focal red lesions on the skin or mucous membranes.

telangiectasis-pigmentation-cataract syndrome Inherited disorder marked by pigmentation and atrophy of skin, along with cataracts, saddle nose, bone defects, disturbance of hair growth, and hypogonadism. Report this disorder with ICD-9-CM code 757.33. *Synonym(s): Rothmund's syndrome.*

TELD-3 Test of Early Language Development. Speech evaluation for patients ages 2 to 7 years.

telehealth service Care by a provider with the patient at a remote site, usually rural, utilizing electronic communication to evaluate, monitor, and treat a patient.

telemedicine Medical information exchanged from site to site via electronic communication. Examples include patient evaluation and consultation, monitoring, education, and other clinical services.

teleo- Indicates complete or perfectly formed.

teletherapy External beam radiotherapy or other treatment applied from a source maintained at a distance away from the body.

telogen effluvium Condition of alteration in the normal hair growth cycle due to a variety of causes, resulting in early hair loss and widening of the part.

Temodar See temozolomide.

temozolomide Injectable chemotherapy drug used to treat certain types of brain cancer. Temozolomide may be sold under the brand name Temodar. Report supply with HCPCS Level II code J9328.

temp Temperature.

temporal Pertaining to the temporal bone of the skull, located on both sides of the head and above the cheek prominence, or zygomatic arch.

Temporal Bone

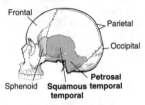

Frontal — Parietal — Occipital — Petrosal — Squamous temporal — Sphenoid

Bones of Skull Vault

Base Skull from Above

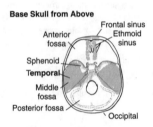

Anterior fossa — Frontal sinus — Ethmoid sinus — Sphenoid — Temporal — Middle fossa — Posterior fossa — Occipital

temporal bone One of a pair of large bones forming the lower sides and base of the cranium, and containing various cavities and recesses associated with the ear, such as the tympanic cavity and auditory tube, as well as a fossa or shallow cavity for joining with the mandible (lower jaw bone).

temporal lobe Lower lobe of the cerebral hemisphere, paired halves of the cerebrum, which is the largest part of the brain.

temporal syndrome Localized meningitis in fifth and sixth cranial nerves, causing paralysis and pain in temporal region. Report this disorder with ICD-9-CM code 383.02. *Synonym(s): Gradenigo's syndrome.*

temporalis muscle Fan-shaped muscle overlying the temporal bone that inserts into the mandible and functions together with the masseter to close the jaw.

temporary add-on payments Additional inpatient payments from CMS for designated new technologies that are 1) less than two to three years old; 2) expensive or exceeding a defined cost threshold in relation to the underlying DRG; and 3) providing clinical improvement over more standard treatments.

temporomandibular joint Joint or hinge formed by the connection of the lower jaw to the temporal bone of the cranium, located in front of the ear on both sides of the face. *Synonym(s): TMJ.*

temporomandibular joint-pain dysfunction syndrome Multiple symptoms including temporomandibular joint dysfunction, hearing difficulty,

S-U

headache, vertigo, and burning sensations in the ear, nose, tongue, and throat. Underlying causes may include overclosure of the mandible, TMJ lesions, and stress. Report this condition with ICD-9-CM code 524.60. **Synonym(s):** Costen's syndrome.

temsirolimus Injectable kinase inhibitor indicated for the treatment of advanced renal cell carcinoma (RCC). May be sold under the brand name Torisel. Supply is reported with HCPCS Level II code J9330.

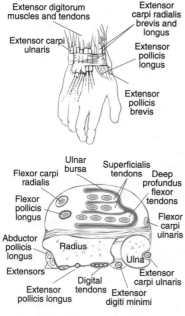

Tendons

Extensor digitorum muscles and tendons
Extensor carpi radialis brevis and longus
Extensor carpi ulnaris
Extensor pollicis longus
Extensor pollicis brevis

Ulnar bursa
Superficialis tendons
Deep profundus flexor tendons
Flexor carpi radialis
Flexor pollicis longus
Flexor carpi ulnaris
Abductor pollicis longus
Radius
Extensors
Ulna
Extensor carpi ulnaris
Digital tendons
Extensor pollicis longus
Extensor digiti minimi

tendon Fibrous tissue that connects muscle to bone, consisting primarily of collagen and containing little vasculature.

tendon allograft Allografts are tissues obtained from another individual of the same species. Tendon allografts are usually obtained from cadavers and frozen or freeze dried for later use in soft tissue repairs where the physician elects not to obtain an autogenous graft (a graft obtained from the individual on whom the surgery is being performed).

tendon suture material Tendons are composed of fibrous tissue consisting primarily of collagen and containing few cells or blood vessels. This tissue heals more slowly than tissues with more vascularization. Because of this, tendons are usually repaired with nonabsorbable suture material. Examples include surgical silk, surgical cotton, linen, stainless steel, surgical nylon, polyester fiber, polybutester (Novafil),

polyethylene (Dermalene), and polypropylene (Prolene, Surilene).

tendon transplant Replacement of a tendon with another tendon.

tennis elbow Chronic lateral epicondylitis reported with ICD-9-CM code 726.32.

teno- Relating to tendons.

tenodesis Stabilization of a joint by anchoring tendons.

tenolysis Release of a tendon from adhesions.

tenon's capsule Connective tissue that forms the capsule enclosing the posterior eyeball, extending from the conjunctival fornix and continuous with the muscular fascia of the eye. **Synonym(s):** Bonnet's ocular, bulbar fascia, bulbar sheath, capsula bulbi, sheath of eyeball, vagina bulbi.

tenonectomy Excision of a portion of a tendon to make it shorter.

tenoplasty Surgical repair of a tendon defect.

tenorrhaphy Union of a divided tendon by suture.

tenosynovectomy Excision of a tendon sheath.

tenosynovitis Inflammation of a tendon sheath due to infection or disease.

tenotomy Cutting into a tendon.

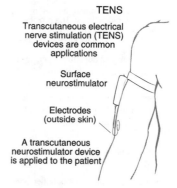

TENS

Transcutaneous electrical nerve stimulation (TENS) devices are common applications

Surface neurostimulator

Electrodes (outside skin)

A transcutaneous neurostimulator device is applied to the patient

TENS Transcutaneous electrical nerve stimulator. Applied by placing electrode pads over the area to be stimulated and connecting the electrodes to a transmitter box, which sends a current through the skin to sensory nerve fibers to help decrease pain in that nerve distribution. TENS application is reported with CPT code 64550. **NCD References:** 10.2, 160.13, 160.7.1, 280.13.

tensilon Edrophonium chloride. Agent used for evaluation and treatment of myasthenia gravis.

tension headache Headache of mental origin, such as tension or anxiety, for which a more precise medical or psychiatric diagnosis cannot be made.

S-U

tentorium cerebelli   Dual divider of dura mater that supports the occipital lobes, separating them from the underlying cerebellum.

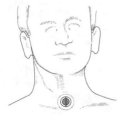

TEP

TEP is the acronym for tracheoesophageal puncture

A Blom-Singer type of voice prosthesis in place

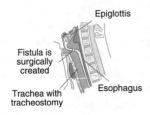

Epiglottis

Fistula is surgically created

Trachea with tracheostomy

Esophagus

A tracheal-esophageal fistula is created in order to fit a "voice button" device, usually following a laryngectomy. The prosthesis allows the patient to phonate through the esophagus by forcing air through the fistula

TEP   Tracheoesophageal puncture. Opening created between the trachea and esophagus to redirect air from the trachea to the esophagus for speech. This procedure includes insertion of a stent or one-way prosthetic valve. TEP is reported with CPT code 31611. Supply of the prosthesis is reported with HCPCS Level II code L8507 or L8509.

terato-   Indicates being seriously deformed, especially a fetus.

teratogen   Substance, including radiation and chemicals, that causes aberrant development in an embryo or fetus.

teratoma   Germ cell tumor found most often in ovaries and testicles. Teratomas may be benign or malignant. Code assignment depends upon location and type.

term   Period of time during which the contract will be in effect.

terminally ill   Individual whose medical prognosis for life expectancy is six months or less.

terminus   Ending; the final point.

Terry's syndrome   Retinopathy occurring in premature infants treated with high amounts of oxygen. Retina

converts into a fibrous mass stunting growth of eye, resulting in blindness. Report this disorder with ICD-9-CM code 362.21.

tertiary   Third in frequency or order. Tertiary care includes health care services provided by highly specialized providers such as neurosurgeons, thoracic surgeons, and intensive care units that often require highly sophisticated technologies and facilities. Tertiary payer is a third party responsible for paying a health insurance claim after the primary and secondary insurers have satisfied their payment obligations.

tertiary care   Health care services provided by highly specialized providers such as trauma units, neurosurgeons, thoracic surgeons, and intensive care units that often require highly sophisticated technologies and facilities. *Synonym(s): primary care, secondary care.*

tertiary care facility   Hospital providing specialty care to patients referred from other hospitals because of the severity of their injuries or illnesses.

tertiary payer   Third party responsible for paying a health insurance claim after the primary and secondary insurers have satisfied their payment obligations.

Terumo syringe   Brand name syringes made by Baxter-Allegiance.

TES   Threshold (or therapeutic) electrical stimulation. Form of electrical stimulation that attempts to strengthen muscles weakened by non-use.

TESA   Testicular sperm aspiration. Hollow bore needle aspiration of testicular tissue through a small incision in the scrotal skin. This technique is usually diagnostic for fertility issues; it does not usually result in collection of enough sperm to freeze for later use.

TEST   Tubal embryo stage transfer. After in vitro fertilization of an oocyte and the commencement of cell division within the egg, the transfer of the egg from the laboratory into the uterus. TEST is reported with CPT code 58974.

testes   Male gonadal paired glands located in the scrotum that secrete testosterone and contain the seminiferous tubules where sperm is produced.

testicular feminization syndrome   Male pseudohermaphroditism marked by female external genitalia. This includes an incompletely developed vagina with rudimentary uterus and fallopian tubes, scanty or absent axillary/pubic hair, and amenorrhea. Report this disorder with ICD-9-CM code 259.51. *Synonym(s): Goldberg syndrome, Goldberg-Maxwell syndrome, hairless women syndrome, Morris syndrome, nonvirilizing testis.*

testicular torsion   Twisting, turning, or rotation of the testicle upon itself, so as to compromise or cut off the blood supply and endanger the organ, normally requiring surgical intervention. This condition is more common during infancy and puberty and may be idiopathic,

S-U

caused by trauma, strenuous movement, or insufficient scrotal connective tissue. Testicular torsion is reported with ICD-9-CM code 608.2.

testosterone cypionate and estradiol cypionate Combination hormone drug used to treat vasomotor symptoms associated with menopause. Supply is reported with HCPCS Level II code J1060.

testosterone enanthate Injectable hormone used for hormonal replacement in males and as a treatment for breast cancer and postpartum mastodynia in women. Supply is reported with HCPCS Level II code J3120 or J3130.

tetanus Acute, often fatal, infectious disease caused by the anaerobic, spore-forming bacillus *Clostridium tetani*. The bacillus enters the body through a contaminated wound, burns, surgical wounds, or cutaneous ulcers. Symptoms include lockjaw, spasms, seizures, and paralysis. Report this condition with ICD-9-CM code 037.

tetanus immune globulin Injectable immunoglobulin used as a treatment for tetanus or for tetanus prophylaxis. Supply is reported with HCPCS Level II code J1670. May be sold under brand names Bay-Tet, Hyper-Tet.

tethered (spinal) cord syndrome Adhesions distorting spinal cord in the caudal area and associated with Arnold-Chiari syndrome and spina bifida. Report this disorder with ICD-9-CM code 742.59.

tetralogy of Fallot Specific combination of congenital cardiac defects: obstruction of the right ventricular outflow tract with pulmonary stenosis, interventricular septal defect, malposition of the aorta, overriding the interventricular septum and receiving blood from both the venous and arterial systems, and enlargement of the right ventricle. Tetralogy of Fallot is reported with ICD-9-CM code 745.2. **Synonym(s):** *4F repair.*

TEVAP Transurethral electro vaporization of the prostate, reported with ICD-9-CM procedure code 60.29, the same as for transurethral resection of the prostate, or TURP. Electro vaporization is done with an electric current much higher than that used in a TURP, and is applied to the prostate tissue through a roller ball mechanism as opposed to a wire loop. This procedure tends to have less occurrence of bleeding and a lower risk of blood transfusion. A TEVAP is performed to reduce the size of an enlarged prostrate that presses against the urethra, blocking or restricting the passage of urine. Diagnosis codes associated with TEVAP are those from ICD-9-CM category 600 reporting hyperplasia.

TF HCPCS Level II modifier for use with CPT and HCPCS Level II codes, identifying intermediate level of care. Required by some state Medicaid and state health departments. Definitions for the use of this modifier vary among state Medicaid providers.

TFT *1)* Tectonic fallopian tunnel. *2)* Transfer factor test.

TG *1)* HCPCS Level II modifier for use with CPT and HCPCS Level II codes, identifying a complex/high tech level of care. Required by some state Medicaid and state health departments. Definitions for the use of this modifier vary among state Medicaid providers. *2)* Task group.

TGA Transient global amnesia. Transient memory loss most often seen in patients older than 50 with no other neurological findings. Patients may be anxious, asking repeatedly about events taking place. Although symptoms usually resolve in less than 24 hours, patients may not be able to recall events occurring during the attack.

TGF Tumor growth factor.

TGV Transposition of great vessels.

TH HCPCS Level II modifier for use with CPT and HCPCS Level II codes, identifying obstetrical treatment/service, prenatal or postpartum. Required by some state Medicaid and state health departments. Definitions for the use of this modifier vary among state Medicaid providers.

THA Total hip arthroplasty.

THAD Transient hepatic attenuation differences. Phenomenon seen in contrast enhanced CT of the liver and indicative of portal vein thrombosis, reported with ICD-9-CM code 452, or any other condition in which an increased hepatic pressure results in decreased portal venous flow.

Thal Thalassemia.

thalamic syndrome Infarction of postero-inferior thalamus causing transient hemiparesis and severe loss of superficial and deep sensation with crude pain in the limbs. Limbs frequently have vasomotor or trophic disturbances. Report this disorder with ICD-9-CM code 338.0.

thalamo- Relating to the thalamus (origin of nerves in the brain).

thalassemia Group of inherited disorders of hemoglobin metabolism causing mild to severe anemia. It is usually found in people of Mediterranean, black, Chinese, or Asian descent. Report thalassemia with a code from ICD-9-CM subcategory 282.4.

thalassemia major Most severe type of beta thalassemia due to deletions in both beta chain genes and noted from birth by skeletal deformations and mongoloid facial appearance. Complete absence of hemoglobin A produces hemolytic, hypochromic, microcytic anemia and necessitates recurrent blood transfusions. If left untreated, enlargement of the liver, spleen, and heart occurs, and bones can deteriorate. Accumulation of iron in the heart and other organs may result in heart failure.

S-U

Report this condition with ICD-9-CM code 282.49. **Synonym(s):** *Cooley's anemia.*

thanato- Relating to death.

THBR Thyroid hormone binding ratio. Measurement that can be evaluated with a laboratory test, reported with CPT code 84479.

THC Tetrahydrocannabinol.

THD Total hospice days.

theleplasty Surgical repair or reconstruction of the nipple and/or areola. Report this procedure with ICD-9-CM procedure code 85.87 or CPT code 19350 or 19355. **Synonym(s):** *mammilliplasty.*

thelitis Irritation or inflammation of the nipple. Report this condition with ICD-9-CM code 611.0; when occurring in pregnancy report a code from ICD-9-CM subcategory 675.2. **Synonym(s):** *mammillitis.*

therapeutic Act meant to alleviate a medical or mental condition.

therapeutic goal Patient's expected level of performance, including the amount of independence, supervision, or assistance that will be needed and the equipment or environmental adaptation required, at the completion of the therapeutic course.

therapeutic modality Broad group of agents or any physical agent applied to produce therapeutic/physiological changes to biologic tissue, including thermal, acoustic, radiant (light), mechanical, or electric energy.

therapeutic procedure Treatment of a pathological or traumatic condition through the use of activities performed to treat or heal the cause or to effect change through the application of clinical skills or services that attempt to improve function.

therapeutic services Services performed for treatment of a specific diagnosis. These services include performance of the procedure, various incidental elements, and normal, related follow-up care.

therapeutic treatment Medical or surgical management of a patient.

TheraSphere Brand name brachytherapy seed of yttrium-90. Supply is reported with HCPCS Level II code C2616 in an outpatient facility setting, and actual administration is typically reported using CPT code 77778 or 79445.

thermocauterization Tissue destruction by means of a heated instrument point.

ThermoFlex Brand name instrumentation for water-induced thermotherapy (WIT) for treatment of benign prostatic hyperplasia by introducing heated (60ºC) water into the prostatic urethra by means of a special heat-transmitting balloon catheter. The precisely controlled heated water destroys a predictable amount

of tissue, which is reabsorbed into the body, and the obstructed urethra is reopened. WIT is an outpatient procedure requiring only topical anesthesia, reported with CPT code 55899.

thermoplastic Item that can be softened by heat, but hardens upon cooling.

thermotherapy Therapeutic elevation of body temperature between 107.6 and 113.0 degrees Fahrenheit. **NCD Reference:** *30.2.*

Thibierge-Weissenbach syndrome Systemic disorder of connective tissue marked by induration and thickening of the skin, with circulatory and organ changes. May reside in the face and hands for some time. Also includes Raynaud's phenomenon and, in some cases, esophageal problems. Report this disorder with ICD-9-CM code 710.1.

Thiersch operation Removal of thin split-thickness skin grafts using a razor, skin-graft cutting knife, or a dermatome.

ThinPrep Brand name Pap testing system that includes a fluid-based methodology for collection and preparation of cervical or vaginal Pap smear slides. The tissue sample can also be used to test for human papilloma virus and other sexually transmitted diseases. Laboratory services for ThinPrep testing are reported with CPT code 88142.

third order catheter placement Catheter placement (manipulation) into the third or greater vessel that branches off the aorta. May be noted in the record as an additional order catheterization or a third branch placement. Code assignment depends upon site.

third-degree burn Full-thickness burn with total destruction of the epidermis and dermis, while deeper underlying tissue may also be affected, including the loss of body parts (e.g., nose, ear, extremity).

third-party administrator Firm that performs administrative functions for a self-funded plan but assumes no risk. **Synonym(s):** *TPA.*

third-party liability Third-party payer liable for the cost of an illness or injury, such as an auto or homeowner's insurer.

third-party payer Public or private organization that pays for or underwrites coverage for health care expenses for another entity, usually an employer (e.g., Blue Cross Blue Shield, Medicare, Medicaid, commercial insurers).

THKAO Thoracic-hip-knee-ankle orthosis.

S-U

Thoracentesis

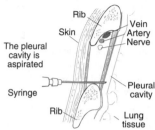

thoracentesis Surgical puncture of the chest cavity with a specialized needle or hollow tubing to aspirate fluid from within the pleural space for diagnostic or therapeutic reasons. Report this procedure with CPT code 32421 or 32422.

thoracic insufficiency syndrome Thoracic insufficiency syndrome. Congenital condition in which severe deformities of the chest, spine, and ribs prevent normal breathing and lung growth and development. TIS is reported with ICD-9-CM code 517.8 in addition to the code for the deformity or underlying disease. *Synonym(s): TIS.*

thoracic lymphadenectomy Procedure to cut out the lymph nodes near the lungs, around the heart, and behind the trachea.

thoracic outlet syndrome Constellation of symptoms resulting from compression of nerves and/or blood vessels, due to insufficient space in the thoracic outlet between the base of the neck and the axilla. Since the thoracic outlet is bordered by muscle, bone, and other tissues, any condition causing enlargement or displacement of the tissues near the thoracic outlet can result in thoracic outlet syndrome. Symptoms range in location and severity and may include pain in the neck and shoulder, arm numbness, or impaired circulation. *Synonym(s): cervical rib syndrome, costoclavicular syndrome, scalenus anticus syndrome.*

thoraco- Relating to the chest.

thoracogenous rheumatic syndrome Symmetrical osteitis of the limbs localized to the phalanges and terminal epiphyses of the long bones of the forearm and leg. Symptoms include kyphosis of the spine and affection of the joints. Report this disorder with ICD-9-CM code 731.2. *Synonym(s): Mankowsky's syndrome, Pierre Marie-Bamberger syndrome.*

thoracolumbar Thoracic and lumbar regions of the back and spine.

thoracopagus Monozygotic (identical) twins who are joined at the chest. Report this abnormality with ICD-9-CM code 759.4.

thoracostomy Creation of an opening in the chest wall for drainage.

thoracotomy Surgical procedure for opening the chest wall in order to access the lungs, esophagus, trachea, aorta, heart, and diaphragm. Depending on the disease location, thoracotomy may be done on the right or left chest. Report this procedure with a CPT code from range 32095-32160.

Thorson-Biörck syndrome Carcinoid tumors causing cyanotic flushing of skin, diarrheal watery stools, bronchoconstrictive attacks, hypotension, edema, and ascites. Report this disorder with ICD-9-CM code 259.2. *Synonym(s): Cassidy-Scholte syndrome, Hedinger's syndrome.*

THR Total hip replacement.

threatened abortion Signs and symptoms of a potential miscarriage that occur in early pregnancy, defined by ICD-9-CM as before 22 weeks of completed gestation. Primary symptoms include vaginal bleeding with or without uterine cramping, and a closed cervical os. This condition is reported with a code from subcategory 640.0. *Synonym(s): threatened miscarriage, threatened spontaneous abortion.*

three-digit diagnostic codes Codes used only when no fourth or fifth digit is available. There are only about 100 codes at the highest level of specificity in the three-digit form. Most payers, including Medicare, do not accept three-digit codes when higher levels of specificity exist.

thrombectomy Removal of a clot (thrombus) from a blood vessel utilizing various methods. Code assignment depends upon site and method.

thrombo- Relating to blood clots.

thrombocytopenia Reduced number of platelets in the blood.

thrombolysis Chemical process of dissolving or breaking down a blood clot by inducing a complex chain of events involving the action of plasminogen to solubilize fibrin clots and degrade fibrinogen. This is an infusion or injection procedure done on different vessels or targeting a clot within a catheter.

thrombolytic agent Drugs or other substances used to dissolve blood clots in blood vessels or in tubes that have been placed into the body. Code assignment depends upon location and agent utilized.

thrombopenia-hemangioma syndrome Small number of platelets in circulating blood, causing bruising. Report this disorder with ICD-9-CM code 287.39.

thrombophlebitis migrans Slowly advancing thrombophlebitis appearing in different sites, involving one vein, then appearing in another, reported with ICD-9-CM code 453.1.

thrombosed hemorrhoid Dilated, varicose vein in the anal region that has clotted blood within it.

thrombosis Condition arising from the presence or formation of blood clots within a blood vessel that may cause vascular obstruction and insufficient oxygenation.

thrombotic microangiopathy Thrombocytopenia with thrombi formation in the small arterioles and capillaries causing hemolytic anemia, purpura, azotemia, fever, and central nervous system disorders manifested by bizarre neurological effects. Report this condition with ICD-9-CM code 446.6. *Synonym(s): Baehr-Schiffrin disease, microangiopathic hemolytic anemia, Moschcowitz disease, thrombotic thrombocytopenic purpura.*

thrombotic thrombocytopenic

purpura Thrombocytopenia with thrombi formation in the small arterioles and capillaries causing hemolytic anemia, purpura, azotemia, fever, and central nervous system disorders manifested by bizarre neurological effects. Report this condition with ICD-9-CM code 446.6. *Synonym(s): Baehr-Schiffrin disease, microangiopathic hemolytic anemia, Moschcowitz disease, thrombotic microangiopathy.*

thrombus Stationary blood clot inside a blood vessel.

Thumboform Brand name, thumb supporting prefabricated orthotic for treatment of arthritis, hyperextension, or joint disorders.

thymectomy Excision of the thymus gland, situated in the anterior superior mediastinum.

thymo- Relating to the thymus.

thymus Lymphoid organ located in the front of the upper mediastinum, composed of two symmetrical pyramid-shaped lobes, that is the site where T-lymphocytes are produced.

thyroglossal duct Embryonic duct at the front of the neck, which becomes the pyramidal lobe of the thyroid gland with obliteration of the remaining duct, but may form a cyst or sinus in adulthood if it persists.

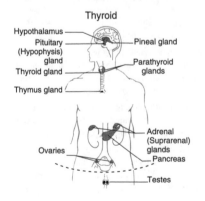

Thyroid

Hypothalamus
Pituitary (Hypophysis) gland
Thyroid gland
Thymus gland
Pineal gland
Parathyroid glands
Adrenal (Suprarenal) glands
Ovaries
Pancreas
Testes

thyroid Endocrine gland located in the front of the lower neck composed of two lobes on either side of the trachea, responsible for secreting and storing the thyroid hormones that regulate metabolism.

thyroid lobectomy Removal of an entire lobe.

thyroid-adrenocortical insufficiency

syndrome Insufficient production of hormones by the pituitary and thyroid glands. Report this disorder with ICD-9-CM code 258.1.

thyroidectomy Partial or complete removal of the thyroid gland. Code assignment is based on approach and extent of removal.

thyrotoxicosis Condition caused by excessive quantities of hormones from the thyroid gland from overproduction or loss of storage ability. *Synonym(s): hyperthyroidism.*

TI Tricuspid insufficiency.

TIA Transient ischemic attack. Intermittent or brief cerebral dysfunction from lack of oxygenation with no persistent neurological deficits; associated with occlusive vascular disease. TIA may denote an impending cerebrovascular accident and is reported with ICD-9-CM 435.9.

TIBC Total iron binding capacity.

tibia vara Leg bowed outward at the knee (or below the knee). Report this condition with ICD-9-CM code 732.4. *Synonym(s): bowleg.*

tibial syndrome Early complication of trauma. Report this disorder with ICD-9-CM code 958.8.

tic Spasmodic contraction or movement, usually of the muscles of the face or extremities. Stress is a common trigger for these repetitive, impulsive actions. Code assignment is determined by type and origin. "Tics" is also a shortened form of diverticulosis, a condition caused by the development of saclike pouches from the wall of the colon, often asymptomatic and without complications. Report this condition with ICD-9-CM code 562.10. *chronic motor t. disorder* Tic disorder (rapid, jerky movements) over which the person it affects seems to have no control. It usually starts in childhood and persists into adult life and rarely has a verbal component. *motor-verbal t. disorder (Gilles de la Tourette)* Rare disorder occurring in individuals of any level of intelligence in which facial tics and tic-like throat noises become more marked and more generalized, and as the disorder progresses, whole words or short sentences (often with obscene content) are cried out spasmodically and involuntarily. *transient t. disorder of childhood* Facial or other tics beginning in childhood but limited to one year in duration.

tidal volume Volume in a breath of air.

Tietze's syndrome Painful swelling of unknown origin of one or more costal cartilages, especially of second rib.

Patients may interpret chest pain as coronary artery disease. Report this disorder with ICD-9-CM code 733.6.

TIG Tetanus immune globulin vaccine. TIG is administered when a patient has been exposed to tetanus. Supply of TIG is reported with HCPCS code J1670 or CPT code 90389. Administration is reported separately.

TIL Tumor infiltrating lymphocytes.

Tillaux-Phocas disease Multiple, benign cysts of the breast, colored brown or blue, caused by hyperplasia of the ductal epithelium. Occurs in women, usually after the age of 30. Tillaux-Phocas disease is reported with ICD-9-CM code 610.1. *Synonym(s): Bloodgood's disease, Phocas' disease, Reclus syndrome, Schimmelbusch disease.*

tilt table test Evaluates how the body responds to the stresses of positions of the tilt table.

tilted womb Position in which the body of the uterus is tipped back instead of forward. Retroversion is considered a normal variation of female pelvic anatomy and is found in approximately 20 percent of women. Retroversion alone is usually asymptomatic and treatment is not necessary. It may also be caused by an enlarging pregnancy, tumor, or endometriosis, in which case treatment is directed at the underlying condition. Retroversion alone is reported with ICD-9-CM code 621.6; if specified as congenital, report 752.39. See appropriate ICD-9-CM sections for retroversion in pregnancy or affecting the newborn. *Synonym(s): tipped uterus, uterine retrodisplacement, uterine retroflexion, uterine retroversion.*

TIM Topical immunomodulator. Therapeutic nonsteroidal drug for use on inflamed skin to stop itching and redness. Tacrolimus ointment and pimecrolimus cream fall into this drug category. *Synonym(s): skin-selective inflammatory cytokine inhibitor.*

time limit In health care contracting, a set number of days in which a claim can be filed according to the payer or state insurance commission.

time to progression The period from which a disease is first diagnosed and treated until the period at which the disease symptoms begin to worsen.

time velocity spectral display Commonly used real-time recording of blood-flow velocity in Doppler ultrasound.

time-zone syndrome Imbalance of the normal circadian rhythm resulting from airplane travel through a number of time zones. Leads to fatigue, irritability, and other constitutional disturbances. Report this disorder with ICD-9-CM code 307.45. *Synonym(s): jet lag syndrome.*

TIMI Thrombolysis in myocardial infarction.

tin ear syndrome Triad of unilateral ear bruising, x-ray evidence of ipsilateral cerebral edema with obliteration

of the basilar cisterns, and hemorrhagic retinopathy in a child, indicative of physical abuse. Appropriate diagnostic coding would include codes specific to each of the presenting symptoms in addition to 995.54 for the child abuse.

tinct Tincture.

tinea (palmaris) nigra Minor fungal infection caused by cladosporium mansoni or Exophiala werneckii, producing lesions that most commonly appear on the hands and rarely on other areas. The lesions look like the characteristic dark ink or dye stain that occurs when silver nitrate is spilled on the skin. Report this condition with ICD-9-CM code 111.1. *Synonym(s): cladosporiosis epidermica, keratomycosis nigricans, microsporosis nigra, pityriasis nigra, tinea nigra.*

tinea cruris Fungal infection of the groin (most common in men), reported with ICD-9-CM code 110.3. *Synonym(s): jock itch.*

tinnitus Ringing in the ear, reported with a code from ICD-9-CM subcategory 388.3. *NCD Reference: 50.6.*

tipped uterus Position in which the body of the uterus is tipped back instead of forward. Retroversion is considered a normal variation of female pelvic anatomy and is found in approximately 20 percent of women. Retroversion alone is usually asymptomatic and treatment is not necessary. It may also be caused by an enlarging pregnancy, tumor, or endometriosis, in which case treatment is directed at the underlying condition. Retroversion alone is reported with ICD-9-CM code 621.6; if specified as congenital, report 752.39. See appropriate ICD-9-CM sections for retroversion in pregnancy or affecting the newborn. *Synonym(s): tilted womb, uterine retrodisplacement, uterine retroflexion, uterine retroversion.*

TIPPS Test for intermediary prospective payment system.

TIPS Transvenous intrahepatic portosystemic shunt. Life-saving procedure to improve blood flow, prevent hemorrhage, and manage the complications of portal hypertension, such as recurrent variceal bleeding and refractory ascites. The shunt may be portocaval, placed between the portal vein and the subhepatic inferior vena cava (IVC) or mesocaval, between the superior mesenteric vein (SMV) and the IVC. This procedure is reported with CPT codes 37182-37183.

TIS Thoracic insufficiency syndrome. Congenital condition in which severe deformities of the chest, spine, and ribs prevent normal breathing and lung growth and development. TIS is reported with ICD-9-CM code 517.8 in addition to the code for the deformity or underlying disease.

tissue Group of similar cells with a similar function that form definite structures and organs. Tissue types

S-U

include epithelial tissue, which lines the outside of the body and the inner surface of internal organs; muscle tissue, which can be voluntary (found in skeletal muscle) or involuntary (found in the heart and digestive system); connective tissue, such as fat, cartilage, bone, or blood; and nervous tissue.

Title I   Federal grants to states in need of assistance for aged citizens.

Title II   Federal grants to states for old age, survivors, and disability insurance benefits.

Title IV   Federal grants to states for aid and services to families and children.

Title X   Federal grants to states for aid to blind citizens.

Title XII   Federal grants for state child health programs.

Title XIV   Federal grants to states for aid to permanently and totally disabled citizens.

Title XVI   Federal grants to states for supplementary income for aged, blind, or disabled citizens.

Title XVIII   Medicare health insurance.

Title XX   Federal grants for state operated home health care.

titrant   Solution of known strength used as the additive or reagent in titration.

titration   Method for determining a certain component within a solution by adding a known reagent, such as a complexing agent, and observing the solution's final change in color. *colorimetric t.* Method of determining the concentration of hydrogen ions by adding an indicator to the sample of unknown concentration and comparing the change of color induced with prepared tubes of the indicator in known quantities of hydrogen ion concentrations.

TJ   HCPCS Level II modifier for use with CPT and HCPCS Level II codes, identifying a child and/or adolescent program group.

TK   HCPCS Level II modifier for use with CPT and HCPCS Level II codes, identifying an extra patient or passenger in a nonambulance transport. Required by some state Medicaid and state health departments. Definitions for the use of this modifier vary among state Medicaid providers.

TKA   Total knee arthroplasty.

TKE   Terminal knee extension.

TKO   To keep open.

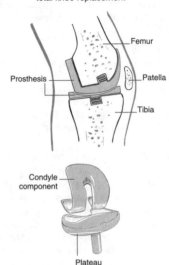

TKR

TKR is the acronym for total knee replacement

Femur

Prosthesis

Patella

Tibia

Condyle component

Plateau component

TKR   Total knee replacement.

TL   *1)* HCPCS Level II modifier for use with CPT and HCPCS Level II codes, identifying early intervention/individualized family service plan (IFSP). Required by some state Medicaid and state health departments. Definitions for the use of this modifier vary among state Medicaid providers. *2)* Triple lumen. *3)* Tubal ligation.

TLE   Temporal lobe epilepsy.

TLIF

TLIF is the acronym for
transforaminal lumbar interbody fusion

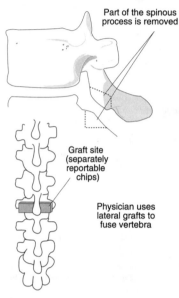

Part of the spinous
process is removed

Graft site
(separately
reportable
chips)

Physician uses
lateral grafts to
fuse vertebra

TMJ

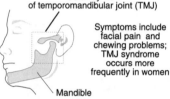

Upper joint space

Lower joint space

Articular disc
(meniscus)

TMJ syndrome is often
related to stress and
tooth-grinding; in other
cases, arthritis, injury,
poorly aligned teeth, or
ill-fitting dentures may
be the cause

Condyle

Cutaway view
of temporomandibular joint (TMJ)

Symptoms include
facial pain and
chewing problems;
TMJ syndrome
occurs more
frequently in women

Mandible

TLIF Transforaminal lumbar interbody fusion, reported with CPT code 22630 or ICD-9-CM procedure code 81.08.

TLM Torn lateral meniscus.

TLP Transitional living program.

TLS Tumor lysis syndrome, reported with ICD-9-CM code 277.88.

TLSO Thoracolumbosacral orthosis.

TLT Tonsillectomy.

TM *1)* HCPCS Level II modifier for use with CPT and HCPCS Level II codes, identifying an individualized education program (IEP). This modifier is required by some state Medicaid and state health departments. Definitions for the use of this modifier vary among state Medicaid providers. *2)* Tympanic membrane. *3)* Transcendental meditation. **NCD Reference:** *30.5.*

TME Total mesorectal excision. Nerve- and sphincter-sparing proctectomy in which part of the rectum, including fatty and lymphatic tissues, is removed as a treatment for rectal cancer. The mesorectum is the fatty tissue rich in blood and lymphatic vessels adjacent to the rectum. Coding for TME is based on approach.

TMJ Temporomandibular joint. Joint or hinge formed by the connection of the lower jaw to the temporal bone of the cranium, located in front of the ear on both sides of the face. TMJ disorder is a condition characterized by pain and dysfunction in the jaw area and limited ability to make the normal motions of speech, eating, chewing, swallowing, and facial expressions. TMJ disorders are reported with ICD-9-CM codes 524.60-524.63 and 524.69.

TML Tongue midline.

S-U

TMR

TMR is the acronym for
transmyocardial revascularization

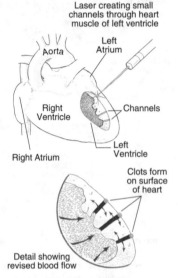

Laser creating small
channels through heart
muscle of left ventricle

Left
Atrium

Aorta

Right
Ventricle

Channels

Right Atrium

Left
Ventricle

Clots form
on surface
of heart

Detail showing
revised blood flow

TMR Transmyocardial revascularization. Laser energy directed into the heart muscle through an incision in the chest, creating small channels in the heart muscle that restore the flow of blood and oxygen. TMR relieves severe angina in patients who are not candidates for bypass surgery and is reported with ICD-9-CM procedural code 36.31 and CPT codes 33140 and 33141. *Synonym(s): MLR, myocardial laser revascularization.* *NCD Reference: 20.6.*

TMTJ Tarsometatarsal joint.

TMX Tamoxifen.

TN HCPCS Level II modifier for use with CPT and HCPCS Level II codes, identifying a service provided in a rural/outside a providers' customary service area. Required by some state Medicaid and state health departments. Definitions for the use of this modifier vary among state Medicaid providers.

TNA Total nail avulsion. While TNA usually refers to a procedure reported with CPT codes 11730 and 11732, it can also refer to an injury to the nail resulting from an open wound.

TNB Transthoracic needle biopsy.

TND Term normal delivery.

TNF Tumor necrosis factor. Protein that stimulates the death of tumor cells and causes inflammatory reactions. Blocking TNF has been beneficial in reducing

inflammation in diseases such as rheumatoid arthritis and Crohn's disease.

TNM Tumor, node, metastases.

TNR Tonic neck reflex.

TNS Transcutaneous nerve stimulator or stimulation.

TNTC Too numerous to count.

TNU Tobacco nonuser.

TO Telephone order.

TOA *1)* Time of arrival. *2)* Tubo-ovarian abscess.

tobacco use disorder Cases in which tobacco is used to the detriment of a person's health or social functioning or in which there is tobacco dependence.

Tobias' syndrome Neoplasm of the upper lobe of the lung. Report this disorder with ICD-9-CM code 162.3. *Synonym(s): Cuiffini-Pancoast syndrome, Hare's syndrome.*

toco- Relating to birth.

tocolytic Drug administered during pregnancy in order to relax the uterus and reduce or halt contractions, administered primarily to stop premature labor.

ToF Tetralogy of Fallot. Birth defect including ventricular septal defect with pulmonary stenosis or atresia, dextroposition of aorta, and hypertrophy of right ventricle, reported with ICD-9-CM code 745.2. Repairs of ToF are reported using CPT code 33692, 33694, or 33697, or for facilities, ICD-9-CM code 38.81 when a total repair is performed.

token Physical item necessary for user identification when used in the context of authentication. One example of a token is an electronic device that can be inserted in a door or a computer system to obtain access.

Token test Standardized evaluation of subtle language dysfunction like that seen in Broca's aphasia.

tolazamide Oral medication exclusive to lowering blood glucose in Type II diabetics. May be sold as brand name Tolinase.

tolbutamide Oral medication exclusive to lowering blood glucose in Type II diabetics, sold under brand name Orinase. *Synonym(s): Orinase.*

Tolinase Brand name oral medication exclusive to lowering blood glucose in Type II diabetics. Tolinase contains tolazamide.

Tolosa-Hunt syndrome Cavernous sinus syndrome produced by idiopathic granuloma. Report this disorder with ICD-9-CM code 378.55.

tomogram X-ray or radiograph of one select layer or slice of the body made by tomography.

tomograph Method of precise x-ray.

S-U

tomography Specialized type of imaging that provides slices through a body structure to obliterate overlying structures. *NCD Reference: 220.1.*

-tomy Indicates a cutting.

-tomy Incision.

Toni-Fanconi syndrome Renal tubular malfunction, including cytinosis and osteomalacia that may be caused by inherited disorders or may be the result of multiple myeloma or proximal epithelial growth. Report this disorder with ICD-9-CM code 270.0. *Synonym(s): Hart's syndrome.*

tonometry Measurement of intraocular pressure, usually by means of an instrument placed directly on the eye.

tooth bounded space Empty space in the mouth due to a missing tooth that is surrounded by a tooth on each side.

tooth erosion Wearing away of a tooth's hard substance by abrasive, not bacterial, forces.

TORCH Toxoplasma, rubella, cytomegalovirus, and herpes. These infectious agents were once bundled into a single CPT antibody test panel, but now must be reported separately: toxoplasma (86777 or 86778), rubella (86762); cytomegalovirus, (86644 or 86645); and herpes virus (86694, 86695, or 86696).

Torg classification Ranking system for stress fractures based on x-ray findings. Type I fractures are generally treated conservatively; Type II may be managed conservatively or surgically; and type III will require surgery.

Torisel Brand name for temsirolimus, an injectable kinase inhibitor indicated for the treatment of advanced renal cell carcinoma (RCC). Facilities report supply with HCPCS Level II code J9330.

torsion of ovary or fallopian tube Twisting or rotation of the ovary or fallopian tube upon itself, so as to compromise or cut off the blood supply.

torsion of testis Twisting, turning, or rotation of the testicle upon itself, so as to compromise or cut off the blood supply.

Torticollis

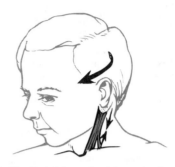

torticollis *birth injury t.* Twisted, unnatural position of the neck due to contracted cervical muscles that pulls the head to one side due to an injury at birth that turns the sternocleidomastoid muscle into a fibrous cord unable to straighten out or lengthen as the child grows, reported with ICD-9-CM 767.8. *congenital t.* Twisted, unnatural position of the neck due to contracted cervical muscles that pull the head to one side due to congenital deformity or contracture of the sternocleidomastoid muscle, reported with ICD-9-CM code 754.1. *hysterical t.* Twisted, unnatural position of the neck due to contracted cervical muscles that pull the head to one side due to a conversion mental disorder that impairs physical function without physiological basis, reported with ICD-9-CM code 300.11. *ocular t.* Twisted, unnatural position of the neck due to contracted cervical muscles that pull the head to one side due to a high degree of astigmatism or ocular muscle palsy, reported with ICD-9-CM code 781.93. *psychogenic t.* Twisted, unnatural position of the neck due to contracted cervical muscles that pull the head to one side due to a mental factor causing musculoskeletal functional disturbance with no sustained tissue damage, reported with ICD-9-CM code 306.0. *spasmodic t.* Twisted, unnatural position of the neck due to contracted cervical muscles that pull the head to one side due to sustained torsion dystonia causing neck muscle contractions, reported with ICD-9-CM code 333.6. *spastic t.* Twisted, unnatural position of the neck due to contracted cervical muscles that pull the head to one side due to intermittent dystonia from an unknown cause or accessory nerve irritation, reported with ICD-9-CM code 723.5. *traumatic t.* Twisted, unnatural position of the neck due to contracted cervical muscles that pull the head to one side due to current sprain or strain injury of the neck muscles, reported with ICD-9-CM code 847.0.

torus fracture Buckling or bowing of the bone with little or no displacement at the end and no breakage, usually occurring in children due to softer bone tissue.

S-U

torus mandibularis Bony projection or overgrowth of normal bone usually found on the floor of the mouth under the tongue.

torus palatinus Bony overgrowth or projection found on the roof of the mouth (palate).

TOS Thoracic outlet syndrome. Compression of nerves and blood vessels in the upper thorax. Symptoms can range from pain, paresthesia, and loss of dexterity or strength in the hands to more generalized symptoms of headache and pallor. TOS is reported with ICD-9-CM code 353.0 if acquired and 767.6 if congenital.

TOT collar Brand name cervical collar for treatment of torticollis.

total disc arthroplasty with artificial disc Removal of an intravertebral disc and its replacement with an implant. The implant is an artificial disc consisting of two metal plates with a weight-bearing surface of polyethylene between the plates. The plates are anchored to the vertebral immediately above and below the affected disc.

total hip replacement Joint arthroplasty in which both sides of the articulating hip joint are removed and replaced with artificial parts. The femoral head and the articulating acetabular cavity surface are replaced by insertion of a ball and socket.

total quality management Concept that quality is an organic part of a plan's service and a provider's care and can be quantified and constantly improved. *Synonym(s): TQM.*

total shoulder replacement Prosthetic replacement of the entire shoulder joint, including the humeral head and the glenoid fossa.

total symblepharon Adhesion of the entire conjunctival surface between the eyelid and the eyeball.

total therapy XV New treatment protocol for children with acute lymphoblastic anemia (ALA) that improves the cure rate and minimizes sequelae. This protocol attempts to optimize dosages of new combinations of antileukemic drugs, as well as their scheduled administration by individualizing the treatment for each patient. The plan depends on each person's response to the initial induction therapy and each patient's leukemic and host normal cell genetic characteristics.

total thyroidectomy Excision of both lobes.

total value Under the resource-based relative value scale, sum of the three components used to determine the value of each service. These include physician work, practice expense, and malpractice costs.

Touraine's syndrome Dysplasia of the fingernails and toenails, hypoplasia of the patella, iliac horns, thickening of the glomerular lamina densa, and a flask-shaped femur. Report this disorder with ICD-9-CM code 756.89.

Touraine-Solente-Golé syndrome Thickening of the skin on extremities and face with clubbing of fingers and deformities in bone of limb. Report this disorder with ICD-9-CM code 757.39.

Tourette's syndrome Familial neuropsychiatric disorder of variable expression that is characterized by multiple recurrent involuntary tics involving body movements (e.g., eye blinks, grimaces, or knee bends) and vocalizations (e.g., grunts, snorts, or utterance of inappropriate words). This syndrome often has one or more associated behavioral or psychiatric conditions (e.g., attention deficit disorder or obsessive-compulsive behavior) and is more common in males than females. It usually has an onset in childhood and often stabilizes or ameliorates in adulthood. Report this condition with ICD-9-CM code 307.23. *Synonym(s): Gilles de la Tourette's syndrome, Tourette's disease, Tourette's disorder, TS.*

tourniquet Device used to apply compressive force to a blood vessel in a limb and slow or prevent blood flow to and from the area.

Touroff ligation Neck is incised and an artery or a vein, damaged or ruptured by trauma, is isolated and tied off with sutures.

toxic amblyopia Decreased or impaired vision in one or both eyes without detectable anatomic damage to the retina or visual pathways caused by poisoning, such as from tobacco or alcohol. Toxic amblyopia is usually not correctable by eyeglasses or contact lenses. Report this condition with ICD-9-CM code 377.34.

toxic oil syndrome Pain in muscles as a result of accumulation of a large number of granular leukocytes. Report this disorder with ICD-9-CM code 710.5.

toxic shock syndrome Staphylococci producing an endotoxin, presenting a high fever, vomiting and diarrhea, decreasing blood pressure, a skin rash, and shock. Hyperemia of several mucous membranes also occurs. Report this disorder with ICD-9-CM code 040.2. *Synonym(s): TSS.*

TP *1)* HCPCS Level II modifier for use with CPT and HCPCS Level II codes, identifying Medical transport, unloaded vehicle. Required by some state Medicaid and state health departments. Definitions for the use of this modifier vary among state Medicaid providers. *2)* Tuberculin precipitation. *3)* Total protein.

TPA *1)* Third-party administrator. Firm that performs administrative functions for a self-funded plan but assumes no risk. *2)* Trading partner agreement. Agreement between the provider and the receiver of the claim transmission detailing the electronic data interchange requirements between the parties. For purposes of HIPAA, a trading partner agreement may not include any agreement to use the codes, segments, or transactions published in an implementation guide in a manner different from that prescribed in the applicable guide. The agreement does not need to be formal. It may take the form of a manual, bulletin, or memorandum. *3)* Tissue plasminogen activator.

TPAL   Term pregnancies, premature infants, abortions, living children.

TPBF   Total pulmonary blood flow.

TPC   Treatment planning conference.

TPL   Third party liability. Payer liable for the cost of an illness or injury, such as auto or homeowner insurer.

TPN   Total parenteral nutrition.

TPPV   Total pars plana vitrectomy.

TPR   Temperature, pulse, respirations.

TQ   HCPCS Level II modifier for use with CPT and HCPCS Level II codes, identifying basic life support transport by a volunteer ambulance provider. Required by some state Medicaid and state health departments. Definitions for the use of this modifier vary among state Medicaid providers.

TQM   Total quality management. Concept that quality is an organic part of a plan's service and a provider's care and can be quantified and constantly improved.

TR   *1)* HCPCS Level II modifier for use with CPT and HCPCS Level II codes, identifying school-based individualized education program (IEP) services provided outside the public school district responsible for the student. Required by some state Medicaid and state health departments. Definitions for the use of this modifier vary among state Medicaid providers. *2)* Tincture. *3)* Trace.

TR3SVR   Treatment of congestive heart failure by restoring the heart to a more normal size and shape. The ventricular muscle and chamber are resized with the aid of a plastic model, in hopes of improving heart function. This procedure is often performed with bypass or valve repair, which is reported separately. TR3SVR is reported with CPT code 33548. *Synonym(s): Dor procedure, LV reconstruction, SAVER, SVR.*

trabeculae carneae cordis   Bands of muscular tissue that line the walls of the ventricles in the heart.

trabecular meshwork   Ocular mesh structure at the juncture of the iris and sclera controlling the flow of aqueous humor from the anterior segment into the canal of Schlemm.

trabeculation   Thickening of the bladder muscle over time with enlargement of the muscle bundles in the bladder wall impressing upon the lumen and possibly leading to diverticula formation. Underlying causes include an obstruction of urinary outflow or a neurogenic bladder. Trabeculation is reported with ICD-9-CM code 596.8.

trabeculoplasty   Glaucoma treatment using lasers to coagulate the trabecular meshwork.

trabeculotomy   Surgical opening between the anterior portion of the eye and the canal of Schlemm to drain the aqueous humor.

trachea   Tube descending from the larynx and branching into the right and left main bronchi.

tracheitis   Inflammation or infection of the trachea that may result in emergency endotracheal intubation if airway obstruction persists. Acute tracheitis is reported with a code from ICD-9-CM subcategories 464.1 and 464.2.

trachelo-   Relating to the neck.

tracheloplasty   Plastic repair of the cervix uteri.

tracheoesophageal fistula   Abnormal opening between the trachea and the esophagus. There are three types of tracheoesophageal fistulas that are coded to different sections of ICD-9-CM: A congenital fistula seen in infants that causes coughing, choking, or turning blue upon feeding, is coded to 750.3. A fistula that is formed because of a previous tracheostomy is coded to 519.09. A current tracheoesophageal fistula not caused by previous surgery is coded to 530.84.

tracheoplasty   Plastic repair of the trachea, the tube descending from the larynx that branches into the right and left main bronchi.

tracheoscopy   Internal visualization of the walls of the trachea through an endoscope. Tracheoscopy is reported with CPT codes 31515-31529 when performed with a laryngoscopy, 31615 when performed through an established tracheostomy, 31630 for fracture reduction, and 31631 and 31638 for tracheal stent replacement and revision. ICD-9-CM procedure code 31.42 reports a diagnostic tracheoscopy and 31.41 reports a diagnostic tracheoscopy through an artificial stoma.

tracheostomy   Formation of a tracheal opening on the neck surface with tube insertion to allow for respiration in cases of obstruction or decreased patency. A tracheostomy may be planned or performed on an emergency basis for temporary or long-term use. Report a temporary tracheostomy that supports breathing with ICD-9-CM procedure code 31.1, a permanent tracheostomy with 31.29, mediastinal tracheostomy for long-term use with 31.21, and revision with 31.74. Tracheostomy codes in CPT are found in range 31600-31614. *Synonym(s): tracheotomy. NCD Reference: 50.4.*

tracheotomy   Formation of a tracheal opening on the neck surface with tube insertion to allow for respiration in cases of obstruction or decreased patency. A tracheotomy may be planned or performed on an emergency basis for temporary or long-term use. Report a temporary tracheotomy that supports breathing with

S-U

ICD-9-CM procedure code 31.1, a permanent tracheotomy with 31.29, mediastinal tracheotomy for long-term use with 31.21, and revision with 31.74. Tracheotomy codes in CPT are found in range 31600-31614. *Synonym(s): tracheostomy.*

trachoma Severe viral, contagious conjunctival eyelid and corneal infection that leads to corneal blood vessel formation, clouding, conjunctival scarring, and blindness.

traction Drawing out or holding tension on an area by applying a direct therapeutic pulling force.

tractor Instrument for pulling an organ.

tractotomy Ablative procedures performed to surgically sever pain-conducting fiber tracts in the spinal cord. Some procedures are of historic significance only as they have been replaced by more current procedures, such as stereotactic mesencephalic tractotomy. *Synonym(s): anterolateral cordotomy.*

trading partner agreement Agreement between the provider and the receiver of the claim transmission detailing the electronic data interchange requirements between the parties. For purposes of HIPAA, a trading partner agreement may not include any agreement to use the codes, segments, or transactions published in an implementation guide in a manner different from that prescribed in the applicable guide. The agreement does not need to be formal. It may take the form of a manual, bulletin, or memorandum. *Synonym(s): TPA.*

TRALI Transfusion related acute lung injury. Life-threatening syndrome characterized by fever, hypoxemia, hypotension, and pulmonary edema in a transfusion patient, thought to be in reaction to components in the donor blood product. TRALI is reported with ICD-9-CM code 518.7.

TRAM Transverse rectus abdominis musculocutaneous.

tranquilizer abuse Cases in which an individual has taken drugs classified as tranquilizers to the detriment of his health or social functioning, in doses above or for periods beyond those normally regarded as therapeutic.

trans Transverse.

transabdominal amnioinfusion Instillation of normal sterile saline or lactated Ringer's solution into the amniotic sac via amniocentesis needle under ultrasonic guidance. It is used to correct levels of amniotic fluid in cases of oligohydramnios; dilute thick, meconium-stained fluid; or prevent compression of the umbilical cord during labor. Transabdominal amnioinfusion is reported with ICD-9-CM procedure code 75.37 or CPT code 59070. Transabdominal amnioinfusion is excluded from the maternity care global package and should be reported separately.

transaction Exchange or transfer of information between two parties to carry out financial or administrative activities related to health care. *t. set* Complete batch of claims, including the header, trailer, and claim information. *t. standards* Defined set of rules for the transmission of electronic claims.

transaction change request system System established under HIPAA for accepting and tracking change requests for any of the HIPAA-mandated transaction standards via a single Web site. See www.hipaa-dsmo.org.

transaction standard Set of rules, conditions, or requirements describing the classification and components or a transaction. Transaction standards define the data elements and code sets that must be used in a transaction.

transantral Performed across or through a sinus, cavity, or chamber.

transcatheter Procedure or treatment performed via a catheter.

transcatheter biopsy Sampling of tissue or cells from an area of concern is removed through a catheter equipped with a suitable cutting instrument. The biopsy is reported according to the anatomic site by this method. CPT code 75970 reports the radiologic supervision and interpretation for a transcatheter biopsy.

transcatheter therapy Therapeutic procedure or treatment performed via a catheter as opposed to open access.

Transcend IGS Brand name implantable gastric stimulator designed for weight loss. Placement, replacement, or removal of IGS electrodes designed for weight loss is reported with a CPT Category III code from range 0155T-0158T. For insertion, revision, or removal of the pulse generator, report CPT code 64590 or 64595. For electronic analysis and programming, see 95980-95982.

transcranial magnetic stimulation Application of electromagnetic energy to the brain through a coil placed on the scalp. The procedure stimulates cortical neurons and is intended to activate and normalize their processes.

transcutaneous electrical nerve stimulator Device that delivers a controlled amount of electricity to an area of the body to stimulate healing and/or to mitigate postsurgical or post-traumatic pain. *Synonym(s): TENS. NCD References: 10.2, 160.13, 160.7.1, 280.13.*

TransCyte Brand name temporary wound dressing consisting of a polymer membrane of collagen and silicone used in treatment of surgically excised burns. Because it is transparent, it allows direct visual monitoring of the wound bed. When the dressing is applied in the physician office, supply of the wound dressing is reported separately. Application of TransCyte is reported with CPT codes 15360-15366.

transducer Apparatus that transfers or translates one type of energy into another, such as converting pressure to an electrical signal.

transection *1)* Transverse dissection. *2)* Cut across a long axis. *3)* Cross section.

transesophageal echocardiography Guidance of a small probe into the esophagus under sedation to closely evaluate the heart and blood vessels within the chest. *Synonym(s): heart scan with endoscopy, TEE.*

transfer Transfer between hospitals occurs when a patient is admitted to a hospital, discharged, and subsequently admitted to another for additional treatment once the patient's condition has stabilized or a diagnosis has been established. For Medicare prospective payment system hospitals, the DRG payment is made to the final discharging hospital. Payment to the transferring hospital is based on a per diem rate and the patient's length of stay.

transforaminal Across, beyond, or through a natural opening, passage, or channel within the body. Transforaminal generally refers to the large central passage within the vertebrae that forms the canal for the spinal cord. Report CPT codes 64479-64484 for transforaminal epidural injections.

transformation zone of cervix Area of the cervix at the squamocolumnar junction where squamous epithelium composing the vaginal portion of the cervix (exocervix) meets the columnar epithelium composing the endocervical (canal) portion of the cervix. The transformation zone is very thin, varying from 2 to 15 mm, and is an irregular area composed of a mixture of both epithelia, the metaplastic squamous epithelium, and the columnar or glandular epithelium. This zone is where 90 percent of cervical neoplasia develops from atypical metaplasia.

transfusion *1)* Process of transferring whole blood or blood components from one person, the donor, to another person, the recipient. Transfusions help restore lost blood and improve the ability of the blood to deliver oxygen to the body's tissues. *NCD References: 110.16, 110.5, 110.7, 110.8.* *2)* Process of taking liquid from one vessel and putting it into another.

transfusion donor syndrome Transfusion of fetus' blood across the placenta to mother's blood supply. Report this disorder with ICD-9-CM code 772.0.

transfusion recipient syndrome Polycythemia of newborn as result of blood flow from mother. Report this disorder with ICD-9-CM code 776.4.

transient global amnesia Transient memory loss most often seen in patients older than 50 with no other neurological findings. Patients may be anxious, asking repeatedly about events taking place. Although symptoms usually resolve in less than 24 hours, patients may not be able to recall events occurring during the attack. *Synonym(s): TGA.*

transient organic psychotic condition Generally reversible states characterized by clouded consciousness, confusion, disorientation, illusions, and often vivid hallucinations usually due to some intra- or extracerebral toxic, infectious, metabolic, or other systemic disturbance.

transitional care center Facility used in lieu of an extended care facility or before discharge to an extended care facility. *Synonym(s): TCC.*

transitional pass-through payment Certain drugs, biologicals, and devices that are eligible for payments in addition to the ambulatory payment classification payment under the outpatient prospective payment system.

translator Software tool for accepting an electronic data interchange (EDI) transmission and converting the data into another format, or for converting a non-EDI data file into an EDI format for transmission. *Synonym(s): EDI translator.*

transluminal balloon angioplasty Transluminal balloon angioplasty. Balloon-tipped catheter is placed within a narrowed artery or vein and the balloon is inflated to stretch the vessel to a larger diameter for increased blood flow. Transluminal balloon angioplasty is coded as open (CPT codes 35450-35460 and 37220-37235) or percutaneous (35471-35476 and 37220-37235), according to the specific vessel or branches, and whether it is performed on a vein or artery. Percutaneous transluminal balloon angioplasty performed on a coronary artery is done to flatten obstructive plaque against the artery wall and open the lumen and is reported with 92982 and 92984. Radiological supervision for peripheral, renal, or visceral arteries is reported with 37220-37235, 75962-75968, and 75978. *Synonym(s): TBA.*

transmittal Revision, addition, or deletion to a Medicare manual. The identifying number of each transmittal begins with an R. The next three to six digits represent the order in which it was released. The two last characters represent the manual to which the transmittal pertains. For example, R163-CP is revision number 163 to the Medicare Claims Processing Manual.

transmucosal Through or across the oral mucosa.

transosteal implant Dental implant composed of a plate and retentive pins or posts that are affixed to the mandible. *Synonym(s): staple bone implant, transmandibular implant.*

transpalatine Through the roof of the mouth.

transpedicular Across or through the pedicle.

transplant Insertion of an organ or tissue from one person or site into another. *NCD References: 20.3, 50.7,*

S-U

110.16, 110.8.1, 260.1, 260.2, 260.3, 260.3.1, 260.5, 260.6, 260.9.

transplantation   Grafting or movement of an organ or tissue from one person or site to another. *NCD References: 20.3, 50.7, 110.8.1, 110.16, 260.1, 260.2, 260.3, 260.3.1, 260.5, 260.6, 260.9.*

transposition   *1)* Removal or exchange from one side to another. *2)* Change of position from one place to another.

transposition of great vessels   Life-threatening congenital malformation of the two main vessels of the cardiovascular system in which the pulmonary artery branches from the left ventricle and the aorta branches from the right ventricle. This condition causes the blood being returned from the extremities to be shunted back into the systemic circulation without being oxygenated. This condition may appear in differing forms: complete or classical transposition; double outlet right ventricle in which there is incomplete transposition of the vessels or both vessels arise from the right ventricle; and corrected transposition of the great vessels in which a developmental cardiac anomaly inverts the ventricles and valves to compensate for the transposed vessels by producing mirror-image blood flow through the heart. *Synonym(s): aortopulmonary transposition, TGV.*

transsexualism   Form of psychosexual dysfunction in which there is a fixed belief that the overt anatomical sex is wrong, resulting in behavior that is directed toward changing the sexual organs by operation or completely concealing the anatomical sex by adopting both the dress and behavior of the opposite sex.

transtracheal   Through the trachea (windpipe) wall.

transvenous electrode   Electrode placed using a transvenous catheter and wedged into the endocardium of the right ventricle or atrium.

transverse   Crosswise at right angles to the long axis of a structure or part. t. lie Abnormal positioning of the fetus horizontally across the uterus rather than in the normal longitudinal or vertical position. In transverse presentation, the arm, trunk, or shoulder may exit first. When the fetus' position is not converted to a cephalic presentation prior to delivery, it is reported with a code from ICD-9-CM subcategory 652.3 and will normally be delivered via cesarean section. *Synonym(s): oblique lie.*

transvestism   Sexual deviation with recurrent and persistent dressing in clothes of the opposite sex. In the early stage, transvestism is for the purpose of sexual arousal.

trastuzumab   Antineoplastic agent used to treat metastatic breast cancer. Supply is reported with HCPCS Level II code J9355. May be sold under the brand name Herceptin.

traumatic (acute) syndrome   Acute cervical sprain caused by hyperextension of the neck (C4-C5) during an accident, usually in an automobile. Report this disorder with ICD-9-CM code 847.0.

traumatic amputation   Removal of a part or limb from accidental injury.

traumatic shock syndrome   Dangerous state of shock following a traumatic injury. Report this disorder with ICD-9-CM code 958.4.

TRCV   Total red cell volume.

Treacher Collins syndrome   Inherited condition with dysostosis of the face, characterized by bilateral malformations, deformities of the outer and middle ear, and a usually smaller lower jaw, high or cleft palate, low-set ears, unusual hair growth, and pits between mouth and ear. Report this disorder with ICD-9-CM code 756.0. Report repair and reconstruction with CPT codes 21150-21151. *Synonym(s): mandibular dysostosis, Franceschetti's syndrome.*

treatment   Management of patient.

treatment plan   Plan of care established by the provider outlining specific deficits and planned treatment that may be submitted to the case manager when seeking certification for a plan member.

treatment planning   Projected series and sequences of procedures necessary to restore the health of the patient, based on a problem or specific diagnosis and a complete evaluation of the patient.

Trelex mesh   Brand name mesh support used for reinforcement in inguinal hernia repair.

tremor   Involuntary trembling movement of a part or parts of the body due to alternate contractions of opposing muscles.

trench fever   Moderately severe disease borne by body lice and relatively common among the homeless. The onset of symptoms is sudden, with high fever, severe headache, back and leg pain, and a fleeting rash. Recovery takes a month or more. Relapses are common. Report this condition with ICD-9-CM code 083.1. *Synonym(s): shin bone fever, wolhynia fever.*

Trendelenburg position   Lying on the back with the supporting structure angled under the knees to lower the patient's head downward 30 to 40 degrees.

trephination   Cutting a circular or disc-shaped piece out of a part, such as the skull for surgical access, or the cornea for transplant purposes.

Trephine

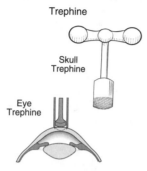

Skull
Trephine

Eye
Trephine

Trephine removes full thickness
layer of donor corneal tissue

trephine *1)* Specialized round saw for cutting circular holes in bone, especially the skull. *2)* Instrument that removes small disc-shaped buttons of corneal tissue for transplanting.

trephine Specialized round saw for cutting circular holes in bone, especially the skull.

treprostinil sodium Continuous subcutaneous or intravenous infusion agent for treating pulmonary arterial hypertension, reported with ICD-9-CM code 416.8. Supply of treprostinil sodium is reported with HCPCS Level II code J3285. May be sold under the brand name Remodulin.

tres Three.

TRF Thyrotropin releasing factor. Chemical that stimulates the release of thyroid-stimulating hormone and prolactin. TRF is used in diagnostic tests for thyroid disease and acromegaly. TRF levels are evaluated in CPT laboratory tests 80438 and 80439. *Synonym(s): TRH.*

TRH Thyrotropin releasing hormone. Chemical that stimulates the release of thyroid-stimulating hormone and prolactin. TRH is used in diagnostic tests for thyroid disease and acromegaly. TRH levels are evaluated in CPT laboratory tests 80438 and 80439. *Synonym(s): TRF.*

triage Medical screening of patients to determine priority of treatment based on severity of illness or injury and resources at hand.

Triam-A Synthetic corticosteroid used as an antiinflammatory or immunosuppressive agent to treat a wide variety of disorders, including inflammatory conditions, certain forms of arthritis, gout, and certain respiratory conditions. Supply is reported with HCPCS Level II code J3301.

triamcinolone acetonide Synthetic corticosteroid used as an anti-inflammatory or immunosuppressive agent to treat a wide variety of disorders, including inflammatory conditions, certain forms of arthritis, gout,

and certain respiratory conditions. Supply is reported with HCPCS Level II codes J3300 and J3301.

TRICARE Federal program that covers the health benefits for families of all uniformed service employees. Formerly called CHAMPUS.

trichi- *1)* Relating to hair. *2)* Hair-like shape. *Synonym(s): tricho-.*

trichiasis Condition wherein lashes are ingrown or misdirected in their growth so that they irritate the tissues of the eye.

Trichinellosis Infection by *Trichinella spiralis*, the smallest of the parasitic nematodes. *Trichinella spiralis* is transmitted by eating undercooked pork or bear meat. Report this condition with ICD-9-CM code 124. *Synonym(s): Trichinosis.*

trichoclasia Condition in which small, white nodules appear in the hair shafts where the hair shaft cortex has broken and split apart, causing the hair to break off, usually after growing only an inch or two. *Synonym(s): bamboo hair, clastothrix, trichorrhexis nodosa.*

trichomonas vaginalis Vaginal infection by a single-celled, flagellate protozoan causing discharge, inflammation, and itching.

trichomoniasis Infection with the parasitic, flagellated protozoa of the genus Trichomonas. This protozoa is found in the intestinal and genitourinary tracts of humans and in the mouth around tartar, cavities, and areas of periodontal disease. It is also found causing necrotic lesions in the upper digestive tract and liver of birds and poultry, especially pigeons. Intestinal trichomoniasis causes colitis, diarrhea, or dysentery and is reported with ICD-9-CM code 007.3. Vaginal trichomoniasis occurs in both males and females, causing severe vaginitis with burning and discharge and urethritis in the male with enlarged prostate and epididymitis. Infection with vaginal trichomoniasis is coded according to the site of infection in ICD-9-CM category 131.0 for urogenital trichomoniasis.

trichorrhexis nodosa Condition in which small, white nodules appear in the hair shafts where the hair shaft cortex has broken and split apart, causing the hair to break off, usually after growing only an inch or two. *Synonym(s): bamboo hair, clastothrix, trichoclasia.*

tricuspid atresia Congenital absence of the valve that may occur with other defects, such as atrial septal defect, pulmonary atresia, and transposition of great vessels.

trigeminal neuralgia Pain in the trigeminal nerve or branch.

trigeminal plate syndrome Progeria, which includes marked senility by 10 years of age. Report this disorder with ICD-9-CM code 259.8.

trigger finger Momentary spasmodic limitation of flexion or extension followed by a snapping into place of the

S-U

finger, due to stenosing tendovaginitis or to a nodule in the flexor tendon. Report trigger finger with ICD-9-CM code 727.03. Report CPT code 26055 for tendon sheath incision repair.

trigger point Focal, discrete spot of hypersensitivity identified within bands of muscle that causes local or referred pain. Trigger points may be formed by acute or repetitive trauma to the muscle tissue, which puts too much stress on the fibers. Injection of a therapeutic agent into trigger points is reported with CPT codes 20552-20553.

trigone Triangular, smooth area of mucous membrane at the base of the bladder, located between the ureteric openings in back and the urethral opening in front.

trigonitis Inflammation of the triangular area of mucous membrane at the base of the bladder, called the trigonum vesicae, reported with ICD-9-CM code 595.3. *Synonym(s): follicular cystitis, urethrotrigonitis.*

trigonocephaly Congenital head deformity that is caused by early fusion of the metopic suture causing a wedge-shaped appearance to the front of the head, reported with ICD-9-CM code 756.0.

TriHIBit Brand name pediatric diphtheria, tetanus, acellular pertussis, and Haemophilus influenzae type B vaccine provided in a single-dose vial. Supply of TriHIBit is reported with CPT code 90721; administration is reported separately. The need for vaccination is reported with ICD-9-CM code V06.8.

Tri-Kort Synthetic corticosteroid used as an antiinflammatory or immunosuppressive agent to treat a wide variety of disorders, including inflammatory conditions, certain forms of arthritis, gout, and certain respiratory conditions. Supply is reported with HCPCS Level II code J3301.

Trilog Synthetic corticosteroid used as an antiinflammatory or immunosuppressive agent to treat a wide variety of disorders, including inflammatory conditions, certain forms of arthritis, gout, and certain respiratory conditions. Supply is reported with HCPCS Level II code J3301.

Tripedia Brand name pediatric diphtheria, tetanus, acellular pertussis vaccine provided in a single-dose vial. Supply of Tripedia is reported with CPT code 90700; administration is reported separately. The need for vaccination is reported with ICD-9-CM code V06.1.

triple lumen Catheter with three channels; the space in the middle of the tube is called the lumen. One of the channels may be used for intravenous (IV) nutrition, the second channel for drug management, and the third channel for blood administration.

triple option Offering of an HMO, indemnity plan, and preferred provider organization by one insurance firm.

triplex X female syndrome Three X chromosomes where the only confirmed symptom is the occurrence of twin Barr bodies in a typical cell. Report this disorder with ICD-9-CM code 758.81.

Trismus Restricted ability to open the mouth stemming from muscle spasms caused by trigeminal nerve disturbance.

TRISS Trauma and injury severity score. Calculation that determines the probability of survival of a patient, based on age, site, and degree of injury for blunt or penetrating trauma, blood pressure, respiratory rate, and coma score.

tritanopia Rare type of color vision deficiency in which the sensory abilities for yellow and blue hues are lacking and only the mechanism for distinguishing the two hues of red and green are present. Tritanopia is also characterized by loss of luminance and shift of brightness of hues toward the long-wave end of the spectrum. This condition is usually associated with drugs, retinal detachment, or nervous system diseases. Tritanopia is reported with ICD-9-CM code 368.53.

tRNA Transfer ribonucleic acid.

trocar Cannula or a sharp pointed instrument used to puncture and aspirate fluid from cavities.

Troisier-Hanot-Chauffard syndrome Hypertrophic cirrhosis with pigmentation and diabetes mellitus. Report this disorder with ICD-9-CM code 275.01.

-trophy Relating to food or nutrition.

-tropic Indicates an affinity for or turning toward.

tropical typhus Acute infectious disease resembling typhus, caused by rickettsia bacteria and transmitted by the bite of infected larval mites, called chiggers. This disease occurs chiefly in Asia and the Pacific and is manifested by a specific telltale lesion or eschar at the site of the bite, fever, regional lymphadenopathy, and skin lesions and rashes. Report this disease with ICD-9-CM code 081.2. *Synonym(s): akamushi disease, inundation fever, island fever, Japanese flood fever, Japanese river fever, kedani fever, mite-borne typhus, Mossman fever, scrub typhus, shimamushi disease, tsutsugamushi disease.*

-tropism Responding to an external stimulus.

troponin Family of proteins found in skeletal and heart muscle fibers. There are three types: I, T, and C. There are cardiac-specific forms of I and T (cTnT and cTnI) that can be used as markers of myocardial damage. Report ICD-9-CM code 790.99 for elevated levels in absence of confirmed cardiac diagnosis.

Trousseau's syndrome Spontaneous development of thromboses in upper and lower limbs as a result of visceral neoplasm. Report this disorder with ICD-9-CM code 453.1.

truncus arteriosus Failure of the aorticopulmonary trunk to divide at the correct developmental stage, resulting in only one great blood vessel leaving the heart. Persistent truncus arteriosus is reported with ICD-9-CM code 745.0.

TRUSP Transrectal ultrasound of prostate. Diagnostic TRUSP is reported with CPT code 76872. For TRUSP associated with brachytherapy treatment planning, report 76873.

TS **1)** HCPCS Level II modifier for use with CPT and HCPCS Level II codes identifying follow-up service. Required by some state Medicaid and state health departments. Definitions for the use of this modifier vary among state Medicaid providers. **2)** Tourette's syndrome. **3)** Tension by Schiotz.

TSA **1)** Thermal sensory analysis. **2)** Tumor specific antigen.

TSD Tay-Sachs disease.

TSE Testicular self-exam.

TSEB Total skin electron beam. Type of radiation therapy in which the entire surface of the body is targeted.

TSH Thyroid stimulating hormone.

TSS Toxic shock syndrome.

tsutsugamushi disease Acute infectious disease resembling typhus, caused by rickettsia bacteria and transmitted by the bite of infected larval mites, called chiggers. This disease occurs chiefly in Asia and the Pacific and is manifested by a specific telltale lesion or eschar at the site of the bite, fever, regional lymphadenopathy, and skin lesions and rashes. Report this disease with ICD-9-CM code 081.2. **Synonym(s):** *akamushi disease, inundation fever, island fever, Japanese flood fever, Japanese river fever, kedani fever, mite-borne typhus, Mossman fever, scrub typhus, shimamushi disease, tropical typhus.*

TT **1)** HCPCS Level II modifier for use with CPT and HCPCS Level II codes, identifying individualized service provided to more than one patient in the same setting. Required by some state Medicaid and state health departments. Definitions for the use of this modifier vary among state Medicaid providers. **2)** Thrombin time.

TTB Third trimester bleeding.

TTD Temporary total disability.

TTE Transthoracic echocardiography.

TTN Transient tachypnea of newborn.

TTP Thrombotic thrombocytopenia purpura.

TTS Transdermal therapeutic system.

TTT Tibial tubercle transfer.

TTTS Twin-to-twin transfusion syndrome. Rare condition in which an imbalance in amniotic fluid occurs due to uneven blood flow between twins sharing a placenta. TTTS is reported with ICD-9-CM code 762.3 and 776.4.

TTWB Toe-touch weight bearing. Use of the toe only to achieve balance when standing or walking. A patient may be instructed to use TTWB when recovering from a leg, ankle, or foot injury.

TU HCPCS Level II modifier for use with CPT and HCPCS Level II codes, identifying special overtime payment rate. Required by some state Medicaid and state health departments. Definitions for the use of this modifier vary among state Medicaid providers.

tube Long, hollow cylindrical instrument or body structure.

tubed graft Mass of flesh and skin partially excised from the donor location, retaining its blood supply through intact blood vessels, that is grafted onto another site to repair adjacent or distant defects.

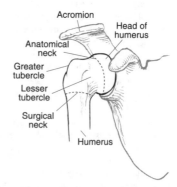

Tubercle

Acromion

Head of humerus

Anatomical neck

Greater tubercle

Lesser tubercle

Surgical neck

Humerus

tubercle Small rough prominence or rounded nodule on a bone.

Tubinstein-Taybi's syndrome Congenital defects including broad thumb and great toe, antimongoloid slant to the eyes, beaked nose, prominent forehead, low set ears, high arched palate, mental retardation, and cardiac defects. Report this disorder with ICD-9-CM code 759.89.

tularemia Infection caused by *Francisella tularensis*, a gram-negative, very small, nonmotile aerobic organism that is always pathogenic to humans and is spread through ingestion of contaminated food or water, inhalation of aerosolized *F. tularensis*, bites of flies and ticks, or through skin contact with an infected animal. It causes febrile illness with chills, weakness, headache, backache, and malaise. Tularemia is reported with a code from ICD-9-CM category 021. **Synonym(s):** *deer fly fever, Francis' disease, Ohara's disease, pahvant valley fever, rabbit fever.*

S-U

TULIP Transurethral ultrasound-guided laser-induced prostatectomy. Laser is used to coagulate or vaporize prostate tissue through an endoscope inserted in the urethra. TULIP is reported with ICD-9-CM procedure code 60.21. In CPT reporting, when a noncontact laser is utilized, report 52647; when performed with a contact laser, report 52648.

tumescence Quality or state of being swollen with blood or fluid. Tumescence often refers to engorgement with blood (vascular congestion) of the erectile tissues.

tumor Pathological swelling or enlargement; a neoplastic growth of uncontrolled, abnormal multiplication of cells.

tumor lysis syndrome Condition occurring as a result of massive doses of chemotherapy in the bloodstream, manifested by hyperkalemia, hyperuricemia, and hyperphosphatemia with secondary hypocalcemia, which can lead to renal failure. This syndrome is reported with ICD-9-CM code 277.88 and an E code to identify the specific drug. *Synonym(s): TLS.*

TUMT Transurethral microwave thermotherapy. Treatment of mild to moderate benign prostatic hypertrophy (BPH) using microwave heat applied through an antennae inserted into the prostate at the end of a balloon catheter while chilled water is circulated through the catheter to protect healthy tissue. This is a minimally invasive, nonsurgical procedure that destroys excess prostate tissue but preserves the surrounding structures. TUMT is reported with ICD-9-CM procedure code 60.96 and CPT code 53850.

TUNA Transurethral needle ablation of prostate. Destruction of prostate tissue using insulated needles inserted through the prostatic urethra. Radiofrequency energy is delivered directly to the prostate while the insulation on the needles protects the urethra. Sections of necrosis are created within the prostate while the urethral tissue is saved. A laser is not utilized in this procedure. TUNA is reported with ICD-9-CM procedure code 60.97 and CPT code 53852.

tunica vaginalis Serous membrane that partially covers the testes formed by an outpocketing of the peritoneum when the testes descend.

tunica vaginalis chylocele Accumulation or infusion of lymphatic fluid into the tunica vaginalis of the testis, reported with ICD-9-CM code 608.84.

tunica vasculosa bulbi Vascular coat of the eye located in the middle, pigmentary region composed of the iris, choroid, and ciliary body. *Synonym(s): uvea, uveal tract.*

TUOD Transurethral occlusive device.

TUR Transurethral resection.

turbinate mucosa ablation Removal or destruction of excessive or inflamed mucosal tissue of the nasal conchae by means such as application of electrical energy, chemical substances, laser beams, or excessive heat. Superficial ablation of mucosa of turbinates is assigned CPT code 30801; intramural is assigned CPT code 30802. When done at the time of another, related, more intense procedure, this service is considered incidental and is not separately reported.

turbinates Scroll or shell-shaped elevations from the wall of the nasal cavity, the inferior turbinate being a separate bone, while the superior and middle turbinates are of the ethmoid bone. *Synonym(s): conchae.*

TURBT Transurethral resection of bladder tumor.

Türk's syndrome Simultaneous retraction of eye muscles causing an inability to abduct affected eye with retraction of the globe. Report this disorder with ICD-9-CM code 378.71. *Synonym(s): Duane syndrome, Still-Turk-Duane syndrome.*

Turner syndrome Congenital disorder occurring only in females and characterized by short stature, webbed neck, congenital heart disease, nonfunctioning ovaries, and learning difficulties. Report this disorder with ICD-9-CM code 758.6. *Synonym(s): Bonnevie-Ullrich syndrome, gonadal dysgenesis, monosomy X, Ullrich-Turner syndrome, XO syndrome.*

TURP

The physician resects the prostate using a resectoscope

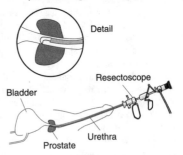

TURP Transurethral resection of the prostate. This procedure is reported with CPT code 52601. In ICD-9-CM Volume 3, the procedure is reported with 60.29. A TURP is performed to reduce the size of an enlarged prostate. Enlargement presses against the urethra, and causes difficulties in urination. Typically, diagnosis codes associated with TURP are those from the 600 rubric reporting hyperplasia, or 185, reporting a primary cancer. Similar procedures include TEVAP, done with electrovaporization; TULIP, with ultrasound guided laser ablation; TUNA, with needle ablation; or TUMT, microwave thermotherapy.

TV HCPCS Level II modifier for use with CPT and HCPCS Level II codes, identifying special holiday or weekend payment rates. Required by some state Medicaid and

S-U

state health departments. Definitions for the use of this modifier vary among state Medicaid providers.

TVCVB

TVCVB is the acronym for
transvaginal chorionic villus biopsy

The physician aspirates
placental tissue into a catheter

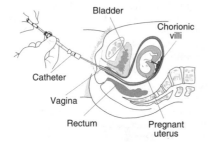

Bladder

Chorionic
villi

Catheter

Vagina

Rectum   Pregnant
                                uterus

TVCVB   Transvaginal chorionic villus biopsy. Test in early pregnancy to screen for fetal genetic disorders. Using a catheter and through a cervical approach, a sample of placental tissue (chorionic villi) is removed. TVCVB is reported with CPT code 59015. Report 76945 for any ultrasonic guidance.

TVH   Total vaginal hysterectomy. This includes removal of the uterus, ovaries, and fallopian tubes. Report a CPT code from 58262-58263, 58285, or 58291-58292.

TVS   Transvaginal sonography, reported with CPT code 76830 for the nonpregnant patient or 76817 for the obstetrical patient. Report also any concurrent transabdominal ultrasound in a nonpregnant patient. *Synonym(s): transvaginal ultrasound.*

TW   HCPCS Level II modifier for use with CPT and HCPCS Level II codes, identifying back-up equipment. Required by some state Medicaid and state health departments. Definitions for the use of this modifier vary among state Medicaid providers.

T-wave alternans   Electrocardiographic method of measuring the alternating electrical amplitude from beat to beat on an electrocardiogram that is used to evaluate ventricular arrhythmia risk. Microvolt T-wave alternans can be measured during exercise or pharmacologic stress, or during cardiac pacing, using a spectral analytic method with equipment that is able to detect as little as one microvolt of T-wave alternans.

TWB   Touch weight bar.

TWE   Tap water enema.

twilight state confusional   Short-lived organic, psychotic states, lasting hours or days, characterized by clouded consciousness, disorientation, fear, illusions, delusions, hallucinations of any kind, notably visual and tactile, restlessness, tremor, and sometimes fever.

twilight state psychogenic   Mental disorders with clouded consciousness, mild to moderate disorientation, and diminished accessibility, often accompanied by excessive activity and apparently provoked by emotional stress.

TwiLite   Brand name dental diode laser used for periodontal and soft tissue procedures as well as laser whitening of the teeth.

Twinrix   Brand name hepatitis A and B vaccine provided in a single-dose vial or syringe. Supply of Twinrix is reported with CPT code 90636; administration is reported separately. Need for vaccination is reported with ICD-9-CM code V05.3

twin-to-twin transfusion syndrome   Birth of one anemic twin and one plethoric twin due to the forcing of blood of one twin into the other. Report this disorder with ICD-9-CM code 762.3.

twist drill   Drill device with deep grooves used to create openings in bone.

Tx   Treatment.

tympanic membrane   Thin, sensitive membrane across the entrance to the middle ear that vibrates in response to sound waves, allowing the waves to be transmitted via the ossicular chain to the internal ear. *Synonym(s): eardrum.*

tympanites   Swelling from gas in the intestine or peritoneal cavity. *Synonym(s): meteorism.*

tympano-   Relating to the eardrum.

tympanolysis   Mobilization of the eardrum by division or destruction of restraining adhesions.

tympanometer   Instrument that measures the function of the middle ear and movement of the tympanic membrane by varying the pressures within the ear canal.

S-U

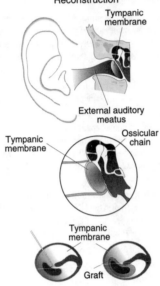

Tympanoplasty with Ossicular Chain Reconstruction

Tympanic membrane

External auditory meatus

Tympanic membrane

Ossicular chain

Tympanic membrane

Graft

The eardrum is repaired and the ossicular chain is reconstructed.

tympanoplasty Surgical repair of the structures of the middle ear, including the eardrum and the three small bones, or ossicles.

type 2 neurofibromatosis Inherited condition marked by acoustic neuromas, cutaneous lesions, benign tumors of the central and peripheral nerves, and opacities on the lenses of the eyes. This condition is reported with ICD-9-CM code 237.72. **Synonym(s):** *acoustic neurofibromatosis.*

type A emergency department Emergency department licensed and advertised to be available to provide emergent care 24 hours a day, seven days a week. Type A emergency departments must meet both the CPT book definition of an emergency department and the EMTALA definition of a dedicated emergency department.

type B emergency department Emergency department licensed and advertised to provide emergent care less than 24 hours a day, seven days a week. Type B emergency departments must meet the EMTALA definition of a dedicated emergency department.

type I syndrome Brain damage as result of compression. Report this disorder with ICD-9-CM code 348.4.

type of admission One-digit code identifying the kind of admission. It may be elective, urgent, emergent, newborn, trauma center, or unavailable.

Typhim Vi Brand name typhoid Vi polysaccharide vaccine provided in a single-dose syringe and a 20-dose vial. Report the appropriate CPT intramuscular injection code as the primary procedure and supply of the Typhim Vi secondarily, with CPT code 90691. The need for immunization is reported with ICD-9-CM code V03.1.

typhlo- 1) Relating to the cecum. **2)** Relating to blindness.

typhoid fever Infection caused by the Salmonella typhi bacteria, resulting in systemic toxic bacteremia with high fever, headache, a characteristic rose spot skin rash, abdominal pain, mesenteric lymphadenopathy, and leukopenia. Leads to an enlarged spleen, bradycardia, intestinal hemorrhage, and ultimately perforation of the intestine. It is transmitted by the ingestion of food or water contaminated from an infected person and is reported with ICD-9-CM code 002.0. Suspected carrier is reported using ICD-9-CM V02.1 and typhoid vaccination with V03.1 or V06.2.

Tysabri Brand name monoclonal antibody given in IV infusion as a treatment for relapsing forms of multiple sclerosis to reduce the frequency of clinical exacerbation. Tysabri contains natalizumab. Report supply with HCPCS Level II code J2323.

Tzank smear Test determines if there are altered epithelial cells (Tzank cells) in the fluid of the bullae of pemphigus vulgaris.

U Unit.

U&C Usual and customary.

U/A Urinalysis.

U1 HCPCS Level II modifier for use with CPT codes, identifying Medicaid level of care 1, as defined by each state. Definitions for the use of this modifier vary among state Medicaid providers.

U2 HCPCS Level II modifier for use with CPT codes, identifying Medicaid level of care 2, as defined by each state. Definitions for the use of this modifier vary among state Medicaid providers.

U3 HCPCS Level II modifier for use with CPT codes, identifying Medicaid level of care 3, as defined by each state. Definitions for the use of this modifier vary among state Medicaid providers.

U4 HCPCS Level II modifier for use with CPT codes, identifying Medicaid level of care 4, as defined by each state. Definitions for the use of this modifier vary among state Medicaid providers.

U5 HCPCS Level II modifier for use with CPT codes, identifying Medicaid level of care 5, as defined by each state. Definitions for the use of this modifier vary among state Medicaid providers.

U6 HCPCS Level II modifier for use with CPT codes, identifying Medicaid level of care 6, as defined by each state. Definitions for the use of this modifier vary among state Medicaid providers.

S–U

U7 HCPCS Level II modifier for use with CPT codes, identifying Medicaid level of care 7, as defined by each state. Definitions for the use of this modifier vary among state Medicaid providers.

U8 HCPCS Level II modifier for use with CPT codes, identifying Medicaid level of care 8, as defined by each state. Definitions for the use of this modifier vary among state Medicaid providers.

U9 HCPCS Level II modifier for use with CPT codes, identifying Medicaid level of care 9, as defined by each state. Definitions for the use of this modifier vary among state Medicaid providers.

UA HCPCS Level II modifier for use with CPT codes, identifying Medicaid level of care 10, as defined by each state. Definitions for the use of this modifier vary among state Medicaid providers.

UAC Umbilical artery catheter or catheterization.

UAE Uterine artery embolization, performed to block the blood flow to a uterine fibroid.

UAMCDS Uniform ambulatory medical care data set.

UAO Upper airway obstruction.

UAP Upper abdominal pain.

U-arm Upper arm.

UARS Upper airway resistance syndrome.

UASA Upper airway sleep apnea. Obstruction of the upper airway during sleep. It occurs more frequently in patients who are moderately or severely obese. Men are affected more often than women. Repeated nocturnal obstruction may cause repetitive sleep cycle, obstructive choking, waking with gasping, excessive daytime sleepiness, morning headache, and slowed mentation. Report this condition with ICD-9-CM code 327.23.

UAVC Univentricular atrioventricular connection.

UB *1)* HCPCS Level II modifier for use with CPT codes, identifying Medicaid level of care 11, as defined by each state. Definitions for the use of this modifier vary among state Medicaid providers. *2)* Uniform bill, as in UB-82 or UB-92.

UB-04 Uniform institutional claim form developed by the NUBC that was implemented in May 2007.

UB-82 Uniform institutional claim form developed by the National Uniform Billing Committee that was in general use from 1983-1993.

UB-92 Common paper claim form used by facilities to bill for services.

UBF Uterine blood flow.

UBO Unidentified bright object.

UBW Usual body weight.

UC *1)* HCPCS Level II modifier for use with CPT codes, identifying Medicaid level of care 12, as defined by each

state. Definitions for the use of this modifier vary among state Medicaid providers. *2)* Unit clerk. *3)* Ulcerative colitis.

UCBT Unrelated cord-blood transplant.

UCD Urine collection device.

UCDSS Uniform Clinical Data Set System.

UCF Uniform claim form, as in UCF-1500.

UCHD Usual childhood diseases.

uCi Microcurie.

UCR Usual, customary, and reasonable. Fees charged for medical services that are considered normal, common, and in line with the prevailing fees in a given geographical area.

UCTF Uniform claim task force.

UCX Urine culture, reported with CPT codes 87086-87088.

UD HCPCS Level II modifier for use with CPT codes, identifying Medicaid level of care 13, as defined by each state. Definitions for the use of this modifier vary among state Medicaid providers.

UE Upper extremity.

Uehlinger's syndrome Thickening of skin on extremities and face with clubbing of fingers and deformities in bone of limb. Report this disorder with ICD-9-CM code 757.39.

UES Upper esophageal sphincter. Cricopharyngeus muscle.

S-U

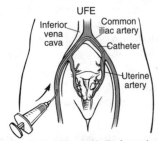

UFE

Inferior vena cava
Common iliac artery
Catheter
Uterine artery

The catheter is inserted in the femoral artery at the groin, and advanced to branches of the uterine artery

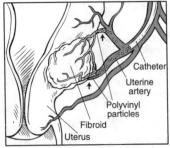

Catheter
Uterine artery
Polyvinyl particles
Fibroid
Uterus

Uterine fibroid tumors will shrink over time after granules injected into arterial branches stop the blood flow to the fibroids

UFE Uterine fibroid embolization. Treatment of a uterine fibroid tumor by occluding the blood supply to the tumor. This is done by inserting an occlusive device endoscopically through the femoral artery. UFE is reported with CPT code 37210. The fibroid is reported with ICD-9-CM codes 218.0-218.9.

UFR Uroflowmetry. Assessment of the rate that the bladder empties. In simple uroflowmetry, a stopwatch is utilized, reported with CPT code 51736. In complex uroflowmetry, calibrated electronic equipment is used, reported with 51741.

UGI Upper gastrointestinal.

UGS Urogenital sinus.

UHDDS Uniform hospital discharge data set. Minimum data set that acute-care, short-term hospitals are required to complete and report for Medicare and Medicaid discharges.

UHIN Utah Health Information Network.

Uhthoff's phenomenon Black spots in the vision of a person with multiple sclerosis, occurring when the patient is febrile or in an environment of increased temperature.

UIP Usual interstitial pneumonitis.

ulcer Open sore or excavating lesion of skin or the tissue on the surface of an organ from the sloughing of chronically inflamed and necrosing tissue.

ulcerative colitis Chronic recurrent inflammation of the large intestine (colon) causing mucosal and submucosal ulceration of unknown cause, and leading to symptoms of abdominal pain, diarrhea with passage of non-fecal discharges, and rectal bleeding. Report this condition with a code from ICD-9-CM category 556.

Ullrich (-Bonnevie) (-Turner) syndrome Congenital disorder characterized by short stature, webbed neck, congenital heart disease and mental retardation. Report this disorder with ICD-9-CM code 758.6. *Synonym(s): Turner-Varny syndrome, XO syndrome.*

Ullrich-Feichtiger syndrome Congenital abnormalities, depressed nose, small eyes, hypertelorism and protuberant ears. Report this disorder with ICD-9-CM code 759.89.

ULN Upper limits of normal.

ULO Ultra low oxygen.

ultrasound Imaging using ultra-high sound frequency bounced off body structures.

ultraviolet light Light source consisting of light rays with a higher frequency than those at the violet end of the visual spectrum.

ULV Ultra low volume.

UM *1)* Unit manager. *2)* Utilization management.

umbilicus Depression or scar left in the middle of the abdomen marking where the umbilical cord was attached in utero. *Synonym(s): navel.*

UMN Upper motor neuron.

UMO Utilization management organization.

UN/CEFACT United Nations Centre for Facilitation of Procedures and Practices for Administration, Commerce, and Transport.

UN/EDIFACT United Nations Rules for Electronic Data Interchange for Administration, Commerce, and Transport.

unbundling Separately packaging costs or services that might otherwise be billed together including billing separately for health care services that should be combined according to the industry standards or commonly accepted coding practices.

uncinate process Hook-like projection extending from the ethmoid bone.

underbilled services Uncoded or undercoded services that are often the result of medical records that lack the detail necessary to code at full reimbursement levels.

undersocialized conduct disorder Lack of concern for the rights and feelings of others resulting from a failure to establish a normal degree of affection, empathy, or

S-U

bond with others and may be manifested by self-protection with fear, timidity, whining, demanding behavior, and tantrums, or by exploitation and self-gain with lying and stealing without apparent guilt.

underwriting Evaluating and determining the financial risk a member or member group has on an insurer.

undiversion Restoration of continuity, flow, or passage through the normal channel.

undocumented services Billed service for which the supporting documentation has not been recorded or is unavailable to substantiate the service.

ung. Ointment.

uniform billing code of 1992 Common claim form used by facilities to bill for services when a paper claim is generated. *Synonym(s): UB-92.*

uniform claim task force Organization that developed the initial CMS-1500 professional claim form. The maintenance responsibilities were later assumed by the National Uniform Claim Committee. *Synonym(s): UCTF.*

uniform hospital discharge data set Minimum data set that acute-care, short-term hospitals are required to complete and report for Medicare and Medicaid discharges. *Synonym(s): UHDDS.*

unilateral Located on or affecting one side.

Unipen Injectable penicillin antibiotic used in the treatment of various infections, including those of the urinary tract, respiratory tract, skin, bones, joints, blood, and heart valves. Supply is reported with HCPCS Level II code S0032. The Unipen contains nafcillin sodium.

unique physician identification number Number unique to each physician, assigned by CMS, to identify physicians and suppliers who provide medical services or supplies to Medicare beneficiaries. It is a six-character, alphanumeric identification number designed to track payment and utilization information for individual physicians. The attending physician and operating physician identification numbers are required when billing for Medicare services. *Synonym(s): UPIN.*

unique provider identification number Number assigned by CMS that identifies the provider (an institution, individual physician, clinic, or organization) of health care services.

United Nations Centre for Facilitation of Procedures and Practices for Administration, Commerce, and Transport International organization dedicated to eliminating or simplifying procedural barriers to international commerce. *Synonym(s): UN/CEFACT.*

United Nations Rules for Electronic Data Interchange for Administration, Commerce, and Transport International electronic data interchange format. Interactive X12 transactions use the EDIFACT message syntax. *Synonym(s): UN/EDIFACT.*

universal joint, cervix syndrome Pelvic pain resulting from old laceration of broad ligament received during delivery. Report this disorder with ICD-9-CM code 620.6.

unlisted procedure Procedural descriptions used when the overall procedure and outcome of the procedure are not adequately described by an existing procedure code. Such codes are used as a last resort and only when there is not a more appropriate procedure code.

unlisted procedure code CPT codes, usually ending in 89 or 99, that typically identify surgical procedures that are rarely provided, unusual, variable, or new. When an unlisted procedure code is used, an operative report should be submitted with the claim to describe the services rendered.

unreplaced blood Blood received by a Medicare beneficiary who does not replace it. The beneficiary has the option of replacing the blood as the Part A or Part B deductible or paying the provider's charges for the unreplaced blood. Blood is replaced on a pint-for-pint or unit-for-unit basis.

unroof To remove the top, roof, or covering.

UNSM United Nations Standard Messages.

unsocialized aggressive disorder Lack of concern for the rights and feelings of others resulting from a failure to establish a normal degree of affection, empathy, or bond with others. May be manifested by self-protection with fear, timidity, whining, demanding behavior, and tantrums, or by exploitation and self-gain with lying and stealing without apparent guilt.

unspecified Term in ICD-9-CM that indicates more information is necessary to code the term to further specificity. In these cases, the fourth digit of the code is always 9.

unstable lie Frequently changing fetal position during late pregnancy, reported with a code from ICD-9-CM subcategory 652.0.

unus. One.

unusual circumstances Unusual or aberrant conditions affecting a patient encounter that should be documented.

unusual service Procedure or service that is unusual or unique, or an aberrant finding, result, response, procedure, method, or behavior that affects the patient's treatment.

Unverricht-Wagner syndrome Polymyositis occurring with characteristic skin changes that include a rash on upper eyelids with edema, a rash on the forehead, neck, shoulders, trunk, and arms, and papules on the knuckles. Report this disorder with ICD-9-CM code 710.3. *Synonym(s): Petges-Clejat syndrome.*

upcoding Practice of billing a code that represents a higher reimbursement than the code for the procedure actually performed.

S-U

UPIN Unique physician identification number. Number unique to each physician, assigned by CMS, to identify physicians and suppliers who provide medical services or supplies to Medicare beneficiaries. It is a six-character, alphanumeric identification number designed to track payment and utilization information for individual physicians. The attending physician and operating physician identification numbers are required when billing for Medicare services.

UPJ Ureteropelvic junction. Area in which the ureter connects to the renal pelvis in the kidney.

UPL Upper payment limit, in Medicaid.

UPLIFT Uterine positioning via ligament investment fixation and truncation. Laparoscopic procedure to strengthen the uterine round ligaments.

UPP Urethral pressure profile. Measures urethral pressure by pulling a transducer through the urethra and noting the pressure change. UPP is reported with ICD-9-CM procedure code 89.25 and CPT codes 51727 or 51729.

upper airway resistance syndrome Sleep disordered breathing in which repetitive increases in airflow resistance in the upper airway causes sleep arousals and daytime sleepiness. Report this disorder with ICD-9-CM code 327.8.

upper respiratory infection Common cold. Mild viral infectious disease of the nose and throat, the upper respiratory system. Its symptoms include sneezing, sniffling, and running/blocked nose; scratchy, sore, or phlegmy throat; coughing; headache; and a general feeling of illness. It is the most common of all diseases. Report this condition with ICD-9-CM code 465.9. **Synonym(s):** *URI.*

UPPP Uvulopalatopharyngoplasty. Excision of excessive or diseased tissues of the uvula, soft palate, and pharynx, reported with CPT code 42145.

upward gaze syndrome Paralysis of conjugate movement of eyes without paralysis of convergence. Caused by lesions of the midbrain. Report this disorder with ICD-9-CM code 378.81. **Synonym(s):** *Parinaud's syndrome.*

UR Utilization review. Formal assessment of the medical necessity, efficiency, and/or appropriateness of health care services and treatment plans on a prospective, concurrent, or retrospective basis.

ur. Urine.

URAC Utilization Review Accreditation Commission. Accrediting body of case management.

urachal sinus Congenital anomaly in which the urachus closes only partially during fetal development, remaining open between the bladder and umbilicus, allowing urine

to drain from the umbilicus. Urachal sinus is reported with ICD-9-CM code 753.7.

urachus Embryonic tube connecting the urinary bladder to the umbilicus during development of the fetus that normally closes before birth, generally in the fourth or fifth month of gestation.

Urbach-Oppenheim syndrome Diabetes with skin disorder. Report this disorder with ICD-9-CM code 249.8x or 250.8x, and 709.3.

Urbach-Wiethe syndrome Deposition of hyaline material in the skin and mucosa of mouth, pharynx, hypopharynx, and larynx. Skin lesions as pustules on faces and exposed surfaces of arms and legs, which heal and form scars. Report this disorder with ICD-9-CM code 272.8.

urban cutaneous leishmaniasis One of the forms of Old World cutaneous leishmaniasis. This parasitic skin disease caused by the protozoa Leishmania tropica is spread by the bite of sand flies and occurs in large urban areas in the Middle East, especially Iran and Iraq, the Mediterranean, and India. Manifestation is mainly a single, large developing boil or furuncle type lesion that persists over a year. Lymphadenopathy may be present. Report this condition with ICD-9-CM code 085.1. **Synonym(s):** *dry cutaneous leishmaniasis.*

urban yellow fever Acute, infectious, vector-borne viral disease contracted by humans bitten by mosquitoes infected with the flavivirus through other humans living in close contact with each other. Manifestations include fever, jaundice, possible kidney damage, and liver necrosis. Report this disease with ICD-9-CM code 060.1.

urecholine bethanechol chloride Cholinergic drug that stimulates receptors to increase muscle tone and contraction within the gastrointestinal tract and bladder. It is used to relieve urinary retention following surgery, childbirth, or due to atony of the bladder. Supply is reported with HCPCS Level II code J0520.

ureostomy Connection of the ureter to a stoma on the abdominal skin.

ureter Tube leading from the kidney to the urinary bladder made up of three layers of tissue: the mucous lining of the inner layer; the smooth, muscular middle layer that propels the urine from the kidney to the bladder by peristalsis; and the outer layer made of fibrous connective tissue. Each ureter leaves the kidney from the hilum, a concave notch on the middle surface, and enters the bladder through a narrow valve-like orifice that prevents the backflow of urine to the kidney.

ureterectomy Excision of all or part of a ureter. This procedure may be performed alone or as part of another procedure, such as urinary diversion or nephrectomy. Ureterectomy is reported with ICD-9-CM procedure codes 56.40-56.42 or CPT codes 50650 or 50660.

S-U

ureterocele Saccular formation of the lower part of the ureter, protruding into the bladder.

ureteroileal conduit Surgical procedure to connect the ureters to a segment of the ileal colon to divert urine flow through the bowel. *Synonym(s): Bricker operation.*

ureterolithiasis Calculus or stone that passes from the kidney into the ureter, causing common symptoms like hematuria, nausea and vomiting, and extreme pain, reported with ICD-9-CM code 592.1. *Synonym(s): calculus of ureter, ureteric stone.*

ureterolithotomy Surgical removal of a calculus or stone from the ureter. Different methods of removal are distinguished in CPT: for laparoscopic removal, see 50945; transvesical removal, see 51060; and for stone basket removal, see 51065. Ureterolithotomy is reported in ICD-9-CM with procedure code 56.2.

ureterolysis Surgical procedure to release or free the ureter from surrounding obstructive retroperitoneal fibrotic tissue (CPT code 50715), free the ureter from adhesions caused by obstructive ovarian veins (50722), or divide and reconnect to free the ureter from an obstructive aberrant position behind the vena cava (50725).

ureteroneocystostomy Surgical procedure that divides the ureter at a point of disease or obstruction and reconnects it to the bladder to form a new junction with the bladder and allow for urinary drainage and prevent vesicouteral reflux.

ureteroplasty Plastic surgery to reconstruct a ureter when a congenital malformation or acquired narrowing blocks the normal flow of urine. Ureteroplasty is reported with ICD-9-CM procedure code 56.89 or CPT code 50700.

ureteropyelogram Radiologic study of the renal pelvis and the ureter.

ureterorrhaphy Surgical repair using sutures to close an open wound or injury of the ureter.

ureterotomy Incision made into the ureter for accomplishing a variety of procedures such as exploration, drainage, instillation, ureteropyelography, catheterization, dilation, biopsy, or foreign body removal.

ureteroureterostomy Surgical procedure to divide and reconnect a damaged or diseased ureter to bypass a defect or obstruction. The ureter may be anastomosed after excision of the defect or it may be connected to the other ureter in a contralateral ureteroureterostomy. Ureteroureterostomy is reported with ICD-9-CM procedure codes 56.41 and 56.75 or CPT codes 50760 and 50770.

urethra Small tube lined with mucous membrane that leads from the bladder to the exterior of the body. In the male, it is approximately 20 cm long and passes through the prostate gland just below the bladder, where it joins the ejaculatory ducts. Urine is prevented from mixing with semen during ejaculation by the reflex closure of the sphincter muscles guarding the opening into the bladder. In the female, the urethra lies directly behind the symphysis pubis and in front of the vagina, and is only about 3 cm long.

urethral caruncle Small, polyp-like growth of a deep red color found in women on the mucous membrane of the urethral opening, reported with ICD-9-CM code 599.3.

urethral diverticulum Abnormal outpouching in the urethral wall that causes urinary urgency and frequency, persistent urinary tract infections, a weak stream with post-void dribbling, discomfort, or incontinence. This condition is reported with ICD-9-CM code 599.2.

urethral hypermobility Inferior and posterior motion of the urethra into the potential space of the vagina caused by a loss of urethral supporting structures in the pelvis and pelvic floor. It is associated with vaginal prolapse and cystoceles and is commonly seen in women with urinary stress incontinence. This condition is reported with ICD-9-CM code 599.81.

urethral pressure profile Measures urethral pressure by pulling a transducer through the urethra and noting the pressure change.

urethral stricture Narrowing of the urethra, which may be due to infection, trauma, catheterization, or a congenital anomaly. Acquired stricture is reported with a code from ICD-9-CM rubric 598, with additional codes to indicate infectious origins or urinary incontinence. Report congenital urethral stricture with 753.6.

urethrectomy Excision of the urethra, which includes a cystostomy to create an opening for drainage from the bladder out through the skin surface. Urethrectomy is reported with CPT codes 53210 and 53215 respectively for male and female operations.

urethrocele Urethral herniation into the vaginal wall.

urethrolysis Procedure performed to cut obstructive adhesions, fibrous bands, or periurethral scar tissue that affix the urethra to the pubic bone, obstructing voiding. This is often caused by previous surgical repair of stress incontinence, such as bladder neck suspension. Urethrolysis is reported with CPT code 53500.

urethromeatoplasty Procedure to open or reconstruct a narrowed or congenitally small meatus, the opening of the urethra. This procedure is reported with CPT codes 53450-53460. *Synonym(s): Richardson procedure.*

urethro-oculoarticular syndrome Association of arthritis, iridocyclitis, and urethritis, sometimes with diarrhea. While symptoms may recur, the arthritis is constant. Report this disorder with ICD-9-CM code 099.3. *Synonym(s): Fiessinger-Leroy-Reiter syndrome, urethro-oculosynovial syndrome.*

S-U

urethropexy Surgical suspension of the urethra, often with a bladder suspension or vaginal repair. Sutures may be placed within the fascial tissues along each side of the urethra to the urethrovesical junction and then elevated by pulling up on special ligatures placed above the pubis and around the supporting muscles. Sutures may also be placed in tissue surrounding the urethra into the vaginal wall and pulled tight to the symphysis pubis. Urethropexy is reported with ICD-9-CM procedure codes 58.49 and 59.79 or CPT codes 51840, 51841, and 57289.

urethroplasty Surgical repair or reconstruction of the urethra to correct a stricture or problem caused congenitally, from previous surgical repair, trauma, or prolapse. There are many different types of urethroplasty performed on both males and females. CPT codes for urethroplasty are found in the digestive system, urinary system, and male genital system chapters of the CPT book.

urethrorrhaphy Suture of urethral wound or injury. Urethrorrhaphy is reported with CPT codes 53502-53515 based on gender and type of repair.

urethrovaginal fistula Abnormal communication between the urethra and the vagina resulting in urinary leakage from the vagina.

urge incontinence Involuntary escape of urine coming from sudden, uncontrollable impulses. *NCD Reference: 30.1.1.*

urgent Admission category for patients who should be admitted as soon as a bed is available, within 24 to 48 hours. Prolonged delay of this admission type would threaten the patient's life or well-being.

urgent admission Admission in which the patient requires immediate attention for treatment of a physical or psychiatric problem.

URI Upper respiratory infection. Common cold. Mild viral infectious disease of the nose and throat, the upper respiratory system. Its symptoms include sneezing, sniffling, and running/blocked nose; scratchy, sore, or phlegmy throat; coughing; headache; and a general feeling of illness. It is the most common of all diseases. Report this condition with ICD-9-CM code 465.9.

urine sensitivity test Urine bacterial culture with isolation and presumptive identification of bacteria found (CPT code 87088) or quantified colony count (87086). *NCD Reference: 190.12.*

URN Utilization review nurse.

urodynamics Diagnostic procedures performed to evaluate voiding disorders. Urodynamics also pertains to the study of bladder function as it relates to control (continence) and urination or voiding. It is performed on men and women through the use of equipment with small catheters and electrodes. Sometimes x-rays are taken during this study (video urodynamics). Report this procedure with CPT codes 51725-51798.

uroflowmetry Recording of the rate of bladder emptying by manual or electronic methods.

urohepatic syndrome Acute renal failure in patients with disease of biliary or liver tract. Cause seems to be decreased renal blood flow, damaging both organs. Report this disorder with ICD-9-CM code 572.4. *Synonym(s): Heyd's syndrome.*

urokinase Plasminogen activator responsible for dissolving blood clots.

UroLume Brand name endoprosthesis surgically implanted for the treatment of urinary obstruction secondary to recurrent bulbar urethral strictures, detrusor external sphincter dyssynergia, or benign prostatic hypertrophy (BPH). Its use is typically associated with cystourethroscopic procedures reported with CPT codes 52282, 52310, and 52315.

Uromitexan Brand name detoxifying agent used to prevent hemorrhagic cystitis caused by the chemotherapeutic drug ifosfamide. Supply is reported with HCPCS Level II code J9209. Uromitexan contains sodium 2-mercaptoethane sulfonate.

urosepsis Pus or bacteria in the urine. This is a nonspecific term that requires further clarification. When the documentation indicates only urosepsis, the physician should be contacted to clarify whether this term is meant as generalized sepsis or septicemia or whether the urine alone is contaminated by bacteria or other toxic material without other findings. When no further clarification is made, the default code for a diagnosis of urosepsis must be used to report it as a urinary tract infection, ICD-9-CM code 599.0.

urostomy Creation of an opening from the ureter to the abdominal surface to divert urine flow.

URT Upper respiratory tract.

urticaria pigmentosa Congenital condition in which mastocytosis causes cells to accumulate in the dermis, characterized by persistent, small, reddish brown itchy macules and papules mostly on the trunk. The condition often goes away by puberty. This condition is reported with ICD-9-CM code 757.33. *Synonym(s): mastocytoma, mastocytosis.*

US *1)* Ultrasound. *2)* Unstable spine.

USC United States Code.

USDHHS United States Department of Health and Human Services.

use Sharing, employing, applying, examining, or analyzing individually identifiable health information by employees or other members of an organization's workforce.

user-based access Method of limiting access to information that gives each individual authority to access specific pieces or types of information.

USG Ultrasonography.

Usher syndrome Congenital deafness and retinitis pigmentosa caused by an autosomal disorder, sometimes also presenting with disturbances in gait and mental retardation. This syndrome is reported with ICD-9-CM code 759.89. **Synonym(s):** *USH.*

USP United States pharmacopoeia.

USPHS United States Public Health Service.

USRDS United States renal data system.

U-stitch Surgical closure that has a "U" shape.

usual, customary, and reasonable Fees charged for medical services that are considered normal, common, and in line with the prevailing fees in a given geographical area.

ut dict. As directed.

Utah Health Information Network Public-private coalition for reducing health care administrative costs through the standardization and electronic exchange of health care data. **Synonym(s):** *UHIN.*

uterine atony Failure of the uterine muscle to contract after the fetus and placenta are delivered, often resulting in postpartum hemorrhaging. Indications of uterine atony are excessive bleeding following delivery and a large, distended uterus. Treatment may consist of uterine massage and the intravenous administration of medications that promote uterine contractions, such as oxytocin, prostaglandins, or methylergonovine. This condition is reported under ICD-9-CM subcategory 666.1.

uterine fibroid tumor Benign tumor consisting of smooth muscle in the uterus. Fibroid types are classified according to the site of the growth: intramural or interstitial tumors are found in the wall of the uterus; subserous fibromas are found beneath the serous membrane lining the uterus; and submucosal fibromas are found beneath the inner lining of the uterus. Although often asymptomatic, these fibroid tumors can cause reproductive problems, pain and pressure, and abnormal menstruation. This condition is reported with a code from ICD-9-CM category 218. **Synonym(s):** *leiomyoma, uterine fibroma, uterine fibromyoma, uterine myoma.*

uterine fibroma See uterine fibroid tumor.

uterine fibromyoma See uterine fibroid tumor.

uterine inertia Weak or poorly coordinated contractions of the uterus during labor. Primary uterine inertia is the lack of efficient contractions initiated during labor, prolonging it with a failure of the cervix to dilate, reported with ICD-9-CM subcategory 661.0. Secondary uterine inertia is manifested by weakness and uterine dysfunction causing an arrested active phase of labor, reported with an ICD-9-CM code from subcategory 661.1. **Synonym(s):** *failure of cervical dilation, primary hypotonic uterine dysfunction, prolonged latent phase of labor.*

uterine isthmus Narrow portion of the uterus between the cervix and the main body of the uterus.

uterine myoma See uterine fibroid tumor.

uterine retrodisplacement Position in which the body of the uterus is tipped back instead of forward. Retroversion is considered a normal variation of female pelvic anatomy and is found in approximately 20 percent of women. Retroversion alone is usually asymptomatic and treatment is not necessary. It may also be caused by an enlarging pregnancy, tumor, or endometriosis, in which case treatment is directed at the underlying condition. Retroversion alone is reported with ICD-9-CM code 621.6; if specified as congenital, report 752.39. See appropriate ICD-9-CM sections for retroversion in pregnancy or affecting the newborn. **Synonym(s):** *tilted womb, tipped uterus, uterine retroflexion, uterine retroversion.*

uterine retroflexion See uterine retrodisplacement.

uterine retroversion See uterine retrodisplacement.

uterovaginal prolapse Uterus displaces downward and is exposed in the external genitalia.

uterus retroversion See uterine retrodisplacement.

UTI Urinary tract infection.

utilization management Process of integrating clinical review and case management of services in a cooperative effort with other parties, including patients, employers, providers, and payers.

utilization review Formal assessment of the medical necessity, efficiency, and/or appropriateness of health care services and treatment plans on a prospective, concurrent, or retrospective basis. **Synonym(s):** *UR.*

Utilization Review Accreditation Commission Accrediting body of case management. **Synonym(s):** *URAC.*

utilization review nurse Nurse who evaluates cases for appropriateness of care and length of service and can plan discharge and services needed after discharge.

UV Ultraviolet light.

UVC Umbilical vein catheter.

uvea Vascular coat of the eye located in the middle, pigmentary region composed of the iris, choroid, and ciliary body. **Synonym(s):** *tunica vasculosa bulbi, uveal tract.*

uveal tract Vascular coat of the eye located in the middle, pigmentary region composed of the iris, choroid, and ciliary body. **Synonym(s):** *tunica vasculosa bulbi, uvea.*

S-U

uveocutaneous syndrome Uveomeningitis marked by patchy depigmentation of hair, eyebrows, and lashes. Retinal detachment, deafness, and tinnitus may also result. Report this disorder with ICD-9-CM code 364.24. *Synonym(s):* *Vogt-Koyanagi syndrome.*

UVR Ultraviolet radiation.

UW Unilateral weakness. Weakness on one side of the body.

V Largest cranial nerve at the surface of the pons, responsible for muscles of mastication and somatic sensation of face.

V code Part of ICD-9-CM codes, V codes describe circumstances that influence a patient's health status and identify reasons for medical encounters resulting from circumstances other than a disease or injury already classified in the main part of ICD-9-CM. *Synonym(s): Supplementary Classification of Factors Influencing Health Status and Contact with Health Services (V01-V82).*

V fib Ventricular fibrillation, reported with ICD-9-CM code 427.41. *Synonym(s): VF.*

V tach Ventricular tachycardia. Excessively rapid ventricular rhythm of the heart, usually more than 150 beats per minute, with an origin beat generated in the ventricle, commonly from atrioventricular dissociation. Ventricular tachycardia is reported with ICD-9-CM code 427.1. *Synonym(s): VT.*

Va Visual acuity.

VA Veterans Administration.

VABRA aspirator Disposable vacuum aspirator used to collect samples of uterine tissue to test for endometrial cancer. Supply is reported with HCPCS Level II code A4480. *NCD Reference: 230.6.*

vaccine Preparation formed by microorganisms or viruses that have been altered to reduce their virulence but retain their ability to trigger the immune response.

VACTERL Vertebral, anal, cardiac, tracheal, esophageal, renal, and limb. Used as a descriptor for a complex of congenital anomalies. Report VACTERL with ICD-9-CM code 759.89. *Synonym(s): VATER.*

VAD Ventricular assist device. Temporary measure used to support the heart by substituting for left and/or right heart function. The device replaces the work of the left and/or right ventricle when a patient has a damaged or weakened heart. A left ventricular assist device (VAD) helps the heart pump blood through the rest of the body. A right VAD helps the heart pump blood to the lungs to become oxygenated again. Catheters are inserted to circulate the blood through external tubing to a pump machine located outside of the body and back to the correct artery. Report VAD-related procedures with CPT codes 33975-33983, 0048T, and 0050T. *NCD Reference: 20.9.*

VADCS Ventricular atrial distal coronary sinus.

vaginal caruncle Small, mucous membrane elevations around the vaginal orifice, left from the torn hymen, reported with ICD-9-CM code 616.89.

vaginectomy Surgical excision of all or a portion of the vagina.

vaginosis Condition in which there is a disturbance in the normal balance of bacteria in the vagina, causing an increase in the percentage of harmful bacteria. This is the most common vaginal infection in females of childbearing age. It may occur along with itching, burning, pain, swelling, odor, and discharge. Vaginosis is reported with ICD-9-CM code 616.10, with an additional code to identify the bacteria, if specified.

vagoaccessory syndrome Unilateral lesions of the ninth, tenth, eleventh, and twelfth cranial nerves producing paralysis of the vagal, glossal, and other nerves and the tongue on the same side. Usually a result of injury. Report this disorder with ICD-9-CM code 352.6. *Synonym(s): Collet-Sicard syndrome, vagohypoglossal syndrome.*

vagotomy Division of the vagus nerves, interrupting impulses resulting in lower gastric acid production and hastening gastric emptying. Used in the treatment of chronic gastric, pyloric, and duodenal ulcers that can cause severe pain and difficulties in eating and sleeping.

vagus nerve stimulation Treatment of partial-onset seizures in which spinal electrodes are implanted around the left vagus nerve and connected to an infraclavicular generator pack. The vagus nerve is stimulated at regular time intervals or upon demand. *Synonym(s): VNS.*

VAIN Vaginal intraepithelial neoplasia. Dysplasia in the epithelial cells of the vagina. VAIN has three stages: VAIN I is low-grade, affecting the outer third of the surface layer of the vagina; VAIN II, high-grade, affecting the outer two thirds of the surface; and VAIN III, high-grade, affecting full thickness. VAIN III is also known as carcinoma in situ of the vagina. All three grades are considered precancerous. VAIN I and VAIN II are reported with ICD-9-CM code 623.0 and VAIN III is reported with 233.31. If complicating pregnancy, labor, or delivery, report with a code from ICD-9-CM subcategory 654.7.

VALE Visual acuity, left eye.

Valentine's test Three glass test using three vials of the same stream of urine to determine contents of the anterior urethra, bladder, ureters, and seminal vesicles.

value code Two-digit code with an associated numerical amount used to report information necessary to process a claim. Value codes represent payments received, lab readings, newborn weights, and various other types of data.

value-added network Vendor of electronic data interchange data communications and translation services. *Synonym(s): VAN.*

valve Fold or membrane within a body canal or passageway that prevents backflow of fluids running through it.

V-Z

valve prolapse syndrome "Mid-late" systolic click due to massive protrusion of mitral valvular leaflet in left atrial cavity. Report this disorder with ICD-9-CM code 424.0. *Synonym(s): Barlow's syndrome.*

valvectomy Excision of a valve.

valvotomy Cutting through stenosed cardiac valve leaflets or cusp to relieve or repair the obstruction caused by scar tissue and inflammation. Report according to the specified valve. *Synonym(s): valvulotomy.*

valvuloplasty Surgical repair of a valve.

VAN Value-added network.

van Buchem's syndrome Multiple fractures and bowing of all extremities, thickening of skull bones, and osteoporosis. Report this disorder with ICD-9-CM code 733.3.

Van Den Bergh test Test comparing serum or plasma to bilirubin.

van der Hoeve's syndrome Blue sclera, little growth, brittle bones, and deafness. Report this disorder with ICD-9-CM code 756.51.

van der Hoeve-Halbertsma-Waardenburg syndrome Eyebrow or upper or lower eyelid sags. Report this disorder with ICD-9-CM code 270.2. *Synonym(s): Mendes syndrome, ptosis-epicanthus syndrome, van der Hoeve-Waardenburg-Gualdi syndrome, Waardenburg-Kleinvan syndrome.*

van Neck-Odelberg syndrome Disease of growth centers, especially at the top of the femur, in which the epiphyses is replaced by new calcification. Report this disorder with ICD-9-CM code 732.1.

Van Slyke method Test checks for amino-acid nitrogen.

vanillylmandelic acid Organic findings indicative of pheochromocytoma or neuroblastoma. A urine test for vanillylmandelic acid measures catecholamines or catecholamine metabolites (degradation products). Used to diagnose and monitor treatment of pheochromocytomas and neuroblastomas, the lab test for vanillylmandelic acid is reported with CPT code 84585. *Synonym(s): VMA 3-Methoxy-4-Hydroxymandelic Acid 24-hour urine.*

vanishing twin syndrome Diagnosed twin pregnancy in which one fetus disappears, resulting in only one fetus being delivered. The mother's body may reabsorb the vanished twin or it may be reincorporated in the placenta. This condition is reported with a code from ICD-9-CM subcategory 651.3, and is believed to be caused by an insufficient amount of human chorionic gonadotropin, or hCG, the hormone that supports pregnancy.

VAP Ventilator-associated pneumonia.

VaporTrode Brand name electrode delivering high-density electrical current for removal of prostate tissue in transurethral resection, reported with CPT code 52601.

Vaqta Brand name hepatitis A vaccine provided in a single-dose vial or syringe. Supply of Vaqta is reported with CPT codes 90632 and 90633; administration is reported separately. Need for vaccination is reported with ICD-9-CM code V05.3.

VAR Various routes of administration.

VARE Visual acuity, right eye.

variant Creutzfeldt-Jakob disease Fatal brain disease believed to be caused by the same prion agent responsible for bovine spongiform encephalopathy (mad cow disease) in cattle. Characterized by unusually long incubation periods that may last years, classic signs and symptoms include psychiatric and behavioral disturbances, impaired sensation, and delayed neurological signs. Report this disorder with ICD-9-CM code 046.11.

varicella-zoster Contagious viral infection causing rash with pustules and fever. This condition is reported with ICD-9-CM codes 052.0-052.9. *Synonym(s): chickenpox.*

varices Enlarged, dilated, or twisted turning veins. *NCD Reference: 100.10.*

Varicocele

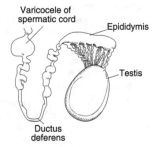

varicocele Abnormal dilation of the veins of the spermatic cord in the scrotum, reported with ICD-9-CM code 456.4. *Synonym(s): scrotal varices.*

varicose vein Abnormal, permanently distended or stretched vein.

Varigrip Brand name spinal instrumentation system that attaches to the lamina without requiring pedicle screws. It provides multidirectional support, and allows for extension attachments to the thoracic spine.

Varivax Brand name varicella virus vaccine provided in a single-dose vial. Supply of Varivax is reported with CPT code 90716; administration is reported separately. The need for vaccination is reported with ICD-9-CM code V05.4.

V-Z

vas deferens Duct that arises in the tail of the epididymis that stores and carries sperm from the epididymis toward the urethra.

vascular Pertaining to blood vessels.

vascular insufficiency Inadequate blood flow and oxygenation.

vascular insufficiency syndrome Complete or partial block of the superior mesenteric artery with symptoms of vomiting, pain, blood in the stool, and distended abdomen. Results in bowel infarction. Report this disorder with ICD-9-CM code 557.1. *Synonym(s): Wilkie's syndrome.*

vascular splanchnic syndrome Visceral circulation syndrome. Report this disorder with ICD-9-CM code 557.0.

vascular tree Contiguous or branching vessels that arise from a major first order vessel of origin.

vascularization Surgically induced development or growth of vessels in a tissue; the process of blood vessel generation.

vasectomy Surgical procedure involving the removal of all or part of the vas deferens, usually performed for sterilization or in conjunction with a prostatectomy. When performed separately, report CPT code 55250. *NCD Reference: 230.3.*

vaso- Relating to blood vessels.

vasoconstrictor Substance that causes blood vessels to narrow and lessens the chance of hemorrhage.

vasodilator Substance that causes blood vessels to dilate or open wider and increase blood flow.

vasomotor Relationship of the nerves and muscles that cause blood vessels to constrict or dilate.

vasomotor acroparesthesia syndrome Paresthesia of the tips of the extremities or attacks of tingling resulting from nerve compression at several levels, and cyanosis. May result in gangrene of the affected areas. Report this disorder with ICD-9-CM code 443.89. *Synonym(s): Nothnagel's syndrome.*

vasomotor syndrome Symptoms in a moving limb including pain tension, and weakness but absent at rest. Caused by occlusive arterial diseases of the limbs. Report this disorder with ICD-9-CM code 443.9. *Synonym(s): Charcot's syndrome.*

vasospasm Contractions or hypertonic irritability of blood vessels resulting in periodic narrowing of the vessel lumen.

vasovagal syndrome Fall in blood pressure, slow pulse, and convulsions. Believed to be sudden stimulation of the vagal nerve by receptors in the heart, carotid sinus, or aortic arch. Report this disorder with ICD-9-CM code 780.2. *Synonym(s): Gower's syndrome.*

VASS Vacuum assisted sock system. Vacuum pump system used with an artificial limb to reduce fluid fluctuation in the residual limb thereby improving the gait of the patient. It is considered by many payers to be investigational. VASS is reported with HCPCS Level II code L5781 or L5782.

VAT Vestibular autorotation test. Computerized test to measure nystagmus using active head movements. There is no specific nystagmus code for VAT. VAT is considered investigational.

VATER Vertebral, anal, tracheal, esophageal, and renal anomalies.

Vater-Pacini bodies Connective tissue containing lamellae and sensory tissue at nerve endings.

VATS Video-assisted thoracic surgery. Less invasive technique than open thoracic surgery for various procedures on the heart and lungs. The surgeon typically gains access to the chest cavity using trocars (slender tube-like instruments), through which an endoscope and the surgical instruments are passed. The patient's internal organs can then be viewed intraoperatively on a monitor.

VAX-D Vertebral axial decompression. Treatment modality utilizing pelvic or cervical traction and a specialized table that permits application of the traction for symptomatic pain relief associated with lumbar disc problems. VAX-D is considered investigational and is not covered by Medicare; individual commercial insurance policies may vary. *NCD Reference: 160.16.*

VBAC Vaginal birth after cesarean section. Because of the uterine incision made for cesarean section, the mother has a higher risk for complications when delivering a subsequent infant vaginally. Delivery codes for those expecting to deliver vaginally after a previous C-section are in CPT code range 59610-59622. A patient who has had a previous C-section is assigned a code from ICD-9-CM category 654.2 in addition to a code from category 660.2 when that previous cesarean delivery resulted in a uterine scar causing obstructed labor.

V-Z

VBG

VBG is the acronym for
vertical band gastroplasty

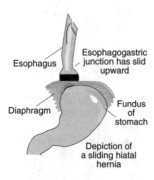

Esophagus
Esophagogastric
junction has slid
upward

Diaphragm
Fundus
of
stomach

Depiction of
a sliding hiatal
hernia

A band is placed to reduce
the perceived volume of the
stomach to suppress eating
in obese patients

VCU

VCU is the acronym for
voiding cystourethrogram

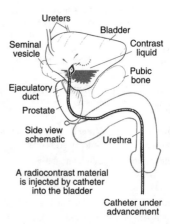

Ureters
Bladder
Seminal
vesicle
Contrast
liquid
Pubic
bone
Ejaculatory
duct
Prostate
Side view
schematic
Urethra

A radiocontrast material
is injected by catheter
into the bladder
Catheter under
advancement

VBG Vertical banding gastroplasty. Treatment for obesity in which an adjustable band is placed to restrict filling of the stomach. Open VBG is reported with CPT code 43842 and ICD-9-CM procedure code 44.69. Laparoscopic VBG is reported with CPT code 43775 and ICD-9-CM procedure code 44.68. Report the appropriate obesity and BMI codes to support medical necessity of VBG. *NCD Reference: 100.1.*

VC Vena cava.

VCF Vertebral compression fracture, reported with ICD-9-CM code 733.13.

VCG Vectorcardiogram.

vCJD Variant Creutzfeldt-Jakob disease, reported with ICD-9-CM code 046.11.

VCU Voiding cystourethrogram. X-ray image of the bladder and urethra during urination, reported with CPT code 51600 for the injection procedure and 74455 for the imaging and radiological supervision and interpretation. *Synonym(s): voiding urethrocystography.*

VCUG Voiding cystourethrogram. X-ray examination of the bladder and urethra to evaluate voiding function. Liquid contrast material is instilled into the bladder via a catheter while x-rays are made before, during, and after this process and again as the patient voids. This procedure is useful in detecting reflux, rupture of the bladder, or obstructions or strictures of the urethra. VCUG is reported with ICD-9-CM procedure code 87.76 and CPT codes 51600 or 51605 and 74455. *Synonym(s): delayed cystogram.*

VD Venereal disease.

VDH Valvular disease of the heart.

VDO Varus derotational osteotomy.

VDRL Venereal disease report.

VDRR Vitamin D resistant rickets.

VE Voluntary effort.

vector Carrier of illness from one host to another, such as biting flies and ticks. Generally, the carrier is not ill or symptomatic.

VEF Ventricular ejection fraction. Heart function test.

vegetative endocarditis Endocardial inflammation associated with the presence of fibrinous clots (vegetations) forming on the ulcerated surfaces of the valves. Report this condition with ICD-9-CM code 421.0.

V-Z

VEGF Vascular endothelial growth factor. Naturally occurring substance in the body responsible for the growth of new blood vessels (neovascularization). VEGF helps the body to heal; however, VEGF may stimulate growth of abnormally fragile vessels in the retina that are prone to leakage. This leakage causes scarring in the macula and eventually leads to loss of central vision. VEGF is also used as a treatment for coronary artery disease. VEGF is injected directly into the heart. This therapy is still in clinical trials. *Synonym(s): therapeutic angiogenesis.*

vein Vessel through which oxygen-depleted blood passes back to the heart.

Velban See vinblastine.

Velbe See vinblastine.

VELCADE Brand name injectable chemotherapeutic drug used as a third-line treatment for multiple myeloma and in treatment of non-small cell lung cancer. Supply of VELCADE is reported with HCPCS Level II code J9041 and its administration is reported with CPT code 96409 or ICD-9-CM procedure code 99.25. Note that the volume of medication covered in the supply code is 0.1 mg. For a typical 3.5 mg single-dose vile of VELCADE, the total number of billing units would be 35. *Synonym(s): bortezomib.*

velopharyngeal Soft palate and the pharynx.

velopharyngeal insufficiency Congenital or acquired condition in which closure between the mouth and nose is not possible due to a weakened or improperly formed soft palate (velum). Report ICD-9-CM code 750.29 if the condition is congenital and 528.9 if it is acquired.

Velsar See vinblastine.

vena cava Main venous trunk that empties into the right atrium from both the lower and upper regions, beginning at the junction of the common iliac veins inferiorly and the two brachiocephalic veins superiorly.

vena cava interruption Procedure that places a filter device, called an umbrella or sieve, within the large vein returning deoxygenated blood to the heart to prevent pulmonary embolism caused by clots. Report vena cava interruption with ICD-9-CM procedure code 38.7 and CPT code 37620.

vena cava syndrome Obstruction of the vena cava. Report this disorder with ICD-9-CM code 459.2.

Vena Tech filter Brand name, permanent, umbrella-shaped filter implanted in the vena cava and designed to trap small clots of blood or plaque before they reach the lungs and cause pulmonary embolism. The filter is inserted intraluminally, usually through the femoral or jugular veins. Placement of a Vena Tech filter is reported with CPT code 37620. Radiological supervision and interpretation of filter placement is reported with CPT code 75940.

veneer In dentistry, restoration that is cemented to the front (facial) surface of a tooth. Also refers to a layer of tooth-colored material made of composite, porcelain, ceramic, or acrylic resin, used to construct crowns or pontics and attached by direct fusion, cementation, or mechanical retention.

venipuncture Piercing a vein through the skin by a needle and syringe or sharp-ended cannula or catheter to draw blood, start an intravenous infusion, instill medication, or inject another substance such as radiopaque dye.

venography Radiographic study of the veins.

venotomy Incision or puncture of a vein.

venous Relating to the veins.

Ventak Prizm Brand name implantable cardioverter defibrillator system.

ventilating tube Tiny, delicate tube placed in the ear through an incision in the eardrum that provides a drainage route to help reduce middle ear infections.

ventilator-associated pneumonia Subtype of hospital-acquired pneumonia in patients who have been on mechanical ventilation by endotracheal or tracheostomy tube for 48 hours or more. Diagnosis is most accurately achieved by quantitative culture and microscopic examination of secretions from the lower respiratory tract. Since these patients are already critically ill, mortality rate is high. Report ventilator-associated pneumonia with ICD-9-CM diagnosis code 997.31, with an additional code to identify the organism, if specified.

ventricular assist device Temporary measure used to support the heart by substituting for left and/or right heart function. The device replaces the work of the left and/or right ventricle when a patient has a damaged or weakened heart. A left ventricular assist device (VAD) helps the heart pump blood through the rest of the body. A right VAD helps the heart pump blood to the lungs to become oxygenated again. Catheters are inserted to circulate the blood through external tubing to a pump machine located outside of the body and back to the correct artery. Report VAD with CPT codes 33975-33980 and 0048T. *Synonym(s): VAD. NCD Reference: 20.9.*

ventricular septal defect Congenital cardiac anomaly resulting in a continual opening in the septum between the ventricles that, in severe cases, causes oxygenated blood to flow back into the lungs, resulting in pulmonary hypertension. *Synonym(s): VSD.*

ventricular tachycardia Excessively rapid ventricular rhythm of the heart, usually more than 150 beats per minute, with an origin beat generated in the ventricle, commonly from atrioventricular dissociation. Ventricular tachycardia is reported with ICD-9-CM code 427.1. *Synonym(s): V tach, VT.*

V-Z

ventriculocisternostomy Surgically created communication established between a lateral ventricle and the cisterna magna for drainage of cerebrospinal fluid in hydrocephalus. *Synonym(s): Stookey-Scarff procedure, Torkildsen's operation, ventriculocisternal shunt.*

ventriculogram Interventional procedure that demonstrates the contractility of the cardiac ventricles by serial recording of the distribution of intravenously injected radionuclide or that of radiographic contrast medium injected through an intracardiac catheter.

ventriculomyotomy Incision into the ventricular musculature of the heart.

ventriculoperitoneal shunt Most common surgery for relief of hydrocephalus, in which a channel is created using plastic tubing to drain excess fluid off the brain from the cerebral ventricle into the peritoneum.

Ventritex Brand name automatic implantable cardioverter-defibrillator (AICD) with a transvenous lead.

ventro- *1)* Relating to the abdomen. *2)* Anterior surface of the body.

VEP Visual evoked potentials. Stimulation of the retina and optic nerve to evaluate the visual nervous system pathways, performed to confirm a diagnosis of multiple sclerosis, detect subclinical optic neuritis, or to evaluate optic disease including pseudotumor cerebri, amblyopia, or injury. It can also be performed during optic nerve surgery. VEP is reported with CPT code 95930. *Synonym(s): VER, visual evoked response.*

VEPTR Brand name vertical expandable prosthetic titanium rib. An expandable rib implanted in pediatric patients to treat thoracic insufficiency syndrome (TIS). VEPTR helps straighten the spine and separate ribs so that the lungs can grow and expand with enough air to breathe properly. The length of the device can be adjusted through an incision in the patient's back as the patient grows.

Verbiest's syndrome Symptoms in a moving limb including pain, tension, and weakness but absent at rest. Caused by occlusive arterial diseases of the limbs. Report this disorder with ICD-9-CM code 435.1. *Synonym(s): Charcot's syndrome.*

verbigeration See cataphasia.

verification of eligibility Process by which the payer or provider determines that the beneficiary is currently enrolled in a plan and that the requested services are covered by the plan.

Verisyse Brand name intraocular lens that can correct vision in patients who are not candidates for LASIK or other corneal corrective surgeries. With Verisyse, a corrective lens is placed in the patient's eye between the cornea and the iris. Verisyse is usually not covered by medical insurance, since it is considered a cosmetic vision-correction surgery.

Vermilion Border

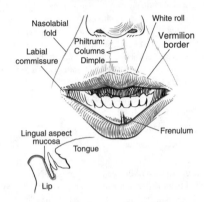

vermilion border Red margin of the upper and lower lip that commences at the exterior edge of the intraoral labial mucosa, and extends outward, terminating at the extraoral labial cutaneous junction.

Vernet's syndrome Unilateral lesions of the ninth, tenth, eleventh, and twelfth cranial nerves producing paralysis of the vagal, glossal, and other nerves and the tongue on the same side. Most usually result of injury. Report this disorder with ICD-9-CM code 352.6. *Synonym(s): Collet-Sicard syndrome.*

verruca Benign, viral, warty skin lesion with a rough, nipple-like surface. Report this condition with a code from ICD-9-CM subcategory 078.1. *Synonym(s): wart.*

vertebra Any one of the 33 bones composing the spinal column, generally having a disc-shaped body, two transverse processes, and a spinal process centered posteriorly. Vertebrae are connected by the laminae between them and are attached to the body by pedicles, forming an enclosed, protective ring around the vertebral foramen through which the spinal cord runs.

vertebral axial decompression Treatment modality utilizing pelvic or cervical traction and a specialized table that permits application of the traction for symptomatic pain relief associated with lumbar disc problems. VAX-D is considered investigational and is not covered by Medicare; individual commercial insurance policies may vary. *Synonym(s): VAX-D.*

V-Z

Vertebral Body

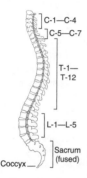

vertebral body Disc-shaped portion of a vertebra that is anteriorly located and bears weight.

Vertebral Column

vertebral column Thirty-three bones that house the spinal cord, consisting of seven cervical vertebrae, 12 thoracic vertebrae, five lumbar vertebrae, five fused vertebrae in the sacrum, and four fused vertebrae in the coccyx.

vertebral corpectomy Removal of the body of a vertebra, most often performed for decompression of the spinal cord in cervical myelopathy and spinal stenosis. Once the vertebral body and discs have been removed, a bone graft is performed to preserve the structural integrity of the spine.

vertebral foramen Space between the vertebral body and vertebra arch that contains the spinal cord.

vertebral interspace Non-bony space between two adjacent vertebral bodies that contains the cushioning intervertebral disk.

vertebroplasty Minimally invasive procedure for treatment of vertebral compression fractures in which orthopedic cement is injected percutaneously into the fractured vertebrae. Report vertebroplasty with ICD-9-CM procedure code 81.65 or a code from CPT range 22520-22522. *Synonym(s): percutaneous vertebroplasty, PV.*

verteporfin Intravenous drug that is light activated and approved for treatment of age-related macular degeneration. Supply is reported with HCPCS Level II code J3396. *NCD Reference: 80.3.*

vertigo Sensation of movement, either of one's own body or the environment rotating or spinning, due to a disturbance of the inner ear, vestibular centers, or pathways in the central nervous system. This condition often causes nausea and vomiting. Vertigo as a symptom is reported with ICD-9-CM code 780.4; however, ICD-9-CM does provide several cause-specific vertigo codes.

vesical fistula Abnormal communication between the bladder and another stricture.

vesicant Intravenous chemotherapy or other agents that have the potential to cause significant tissue damage and necrosis if they leak (extravasate) outside the vein and infiltrate into the tissue around the IV site. Report this occurrence with ICD-9-CM code 999.81 for chemotherapy and 999.82 for other vesicant agent.

vesico- Relating to the bladder.

vesicoureteral reflux Urine passage from the bladder back up into the ureter and kidneys that can lead to bacterial infection and an increase in hydrostatic pressure, causing kidney damage. Vesicoureteric reflux is reported with a code from ICD-9-CM subcategory 593.7. *Synonym(s): VUR.*

vesicourethral obstruction Blockage of the bladder neck or outlet preventing proper outflow of urine. It may be caused by contracture or stenosis due to radiation, injury, catheterization, infection, cancer, impaction, or a disease compressing the bladder neck in either sex. Males are more often affected due to benign prostatic hypertrophy or prostate cancer. Vesicourethral obstruction is reported with ICD-9-CM code 596.0.

vesicovaginal fistula Abnormal communication between the bladder and the vagina that is the most common genital fistula, often with urinary leakage causing skin irritation of the vulva and thighs, or total incontinence.

vesiculectomy Removal of one or both of the seminal vesicles through an incision in the lower abdomen or the perineum, reported with CPT code 55650.

vesiculotomy Incision of one or both of the seminal vesicles, the paired glands that lie behind the urinary bladder and produce fluid that is mixed with the semen. If the procedure does not require extensive dissection, report with CPT code 55600; if extensive, report 55605.

vestibule of the ear Oval-shaped cavity in the middle of the inner ear canals (bony labyrinth) that connects with the cochlea and semicircular canals.

V–Z

vestibule of the mouth Mucosal and submucosal tissue of the lips and cheeks within the oral cavity, not including the dentoalveolar structures.

vestibuloplasty Surgical procedure in which the vestibule of the mouth is deepened for the purpose of increasing the height of the alveolar ridge. Depending on the location and complexity of the surgery, vestibuloplasty is reported with CPT code 40840 or with a code from range 40842-40845.

vestigal Remains or remnant of a structure occurring in the fetal stage of growth.

VF *1)* Ventricular fibrillation. *2)* Visual field.

VFL Vinflunine.

VFR Voiding flow rate.

VGH Very good health.

VGM Vein graft myringoplasty.

VH-IVUS Virtual histology intravascular ultrasound, reported with an ICD-9-CM procedure code from category 00.2.

VI Cranial nerve that exits on the surface of the brainstem and enervates the lateral rectus muscle, which abducts the eye.

viability Ability to live, develop, grow, or survive after birth.

Viarox Brand name compression stockings. Supply of Viarox stockings by the pair is reported with HCPCS Level II code A6534 or A6535.

vibrio cholerae Acute infection of the entire bowel due to vibrio cholerae. Genus of gram negative, anaerobic, rod-shaped, mobile bacteria divided into six serogroups. It presents with profuse diarrhea, cramps, and vomiting. The rice water diarrhea produced by the cholera enterotoxin results in severe dehydration, electrolyte imbalance, and death. It is spread through ingestion of food or water contaminated with feces of infected persons and is still prevalent in countries with poor socioeconomic conditions. Cholera is the acute infectious enteritis caused by this class of bacteria, reported with ICD-9-CM codes 001.0-001.9; suspected carrier, V02.0; exposure to or contact with, V01.0; and prophylactic vaccination against, V03.0. Until recently cholera has only been diagnosed with bacterial stool culture or other advanced scientific method, rarely available in the prevalent area of disease. Recently a dipstick method (CPT code 87450) has become available for early detection. *Synonym(s): chelora.*

vibrio parahaemolytics Species of Vibrio bacteria most often responsible for food poisoning with gastroenteritis secondary to eating raw or improperly cooked seafood, occurring frequently in Japan. Reported with ICD-9-CM code 005.4.

vibrio vulnificus Species of Vibrio bacteria that ferment lactose and cause food poisoning with septicemia and cellulitis due to eating raw or improperly cooked seafood that can be fatal to those with pre-existing liver disease. Reported with ICD-9-CM code 005.81.

ViCPs Vi capsular polysaccharide, a type of typhoid vaccine. Report the appropriate CPT intramuscular injection code as the primary procedure and supply of ViCPs secondarily, with CPT code 90691. The need for immunization is reported with ICD-9-CM code V03.1.

Vicq D'Azyr operation Temporary tracheostomy, reported with CPT codes 31600-31605 or ICD-9-CM facility code 31.1.

video display tube syndrome Chronic neck and back pain developing from sitting at a computer. Report this disorder with ICD-9-CM code 723.8. *Synonym(s): VDT.*

Villaret's syndrome Unilateral lesions of the ninth, tenth, eleventh, and twelfth cranial nerves producing paralysis of the vagal, glossal, and other nerves and the tongue on the same side. Most usually result of injury. Report this disorder with ICD-9-CM code 352.6. *Synonym(s): Collet-Sicard syndrome.*

villonodular synovitis Inflammation of the synovial membrane due to excessive synovial tissue formation, especially in the knee.

Vimpat Brand name injectable antiepileptic drug indicated for the treatment of partial-onset seizures. Approved for use as an add-on therapy in patients 17 years of age or older, Vimpat may also be sold under the generic name of lacosamide and is reported with HCPCS Level II code C9254.

VIN Vulvar intraepithelial neoplasia. Dysplasia in the epithelial cells of the vulva. VIN has three stages: VIN I is low-grade, affecting the outer third of the surface layer of the vulva; VIN II, high-grade, affecting the outer two thirds of the surface; and VIN III, high-grade, affecting full thickness. VIN III is also known as carcinoma in situ of the vulva. All three grades are considered precancerous. VIN I and VIN II are reported with ICD-9-CM code 624.8 and VIN III is reported with 233.32. If complicating pregnancy, labor, or delivery, report with a code from ICD-9-CM subcategory 654.8.

vinblastine Injectable chemotherapeutic agent used in the treatment of a number of malignancies, including that of the breast, bladder, and testicles. It is also used to treat Hodgkin's and non-Hodgkin's lymphoma and melanoma. Supply is reported with HCPCS Level II code J9360.

vinblastine sulfate See vinblastine.

vincaleukoblastine See vinblastine.

vinorelbine tartrate Injectable chemotherapeutic agent used to treat specific types of malignancies, including

V-Z

breast and non-small cell lung cancer. Supply is reported with HCPCS Level II code J9390.

Vinson-Plummer syndrome Condition in middle-aged women with hypochromic anemia, marked by cracks or fissures at the corners of the mouth, painful tongue, and dysphagia due to esophageal stenosis or webs. Report this disorder with ICD-9-CM code 280.8. *Synonym(s): Kelly syndrome, Paterson-Brown-Vinson syndrome, Plummer-Vinson syndrome.*

violation Disregard or abuse of the laws, rules, or guidelines, knowingly or unknowingly resulting in receipt of inappropriate reimbursement.

VIP Vasoactive intestinal peptide, reported with CPT code 84586.

virgule In typography, a forward slash. For example, the slash between and/or. The Institute for Safe Medication Practices discourages the use of virgules in documentation or prescriptions.

virilism syndrome Mature masculine somatic characteristics by a prepubescent male, girl, or woman. This syndrome may show at birth or develop later as result of adrenocortical dysfunction. Report this disorder with ICD-9-CM code 255.2. *Synonym(s): virilizing adrenocortical hyperplasia syndrome.*

virtual colonoscopy Computed tomographic colonography. For screening, report CPT code 74263. For diagnostic CT colonoscopy, report 74261 or 74262. *Synonym(s): CT colonoscopy.*

virtual private network Technical strategy for creating secure connections, or tunnels, over the Internet. *Synonym(s): VPN.*

Virtuoso ICD Brand name implantable cardioverter defibrillator.

viscera Large interior organs enclosed within a cavity, generally referring to the abdominal organs.

visceral larval migrans syndrome Prolonged migration of nematode larvae in the viscera, which can cause hypereosinophilia, hepatomegaly, and pneumonitis. Report this disorder with ICD-9-CM code 128.0.

viscero- Relating to the abdominal organs.

visceromegaly Enlargement of the internal organs in the abdomen, such as the liver, spleen, stomach, kidneys, or pancreas.

Visian Brand name Collamer lens implanted to correct nearsightedness. The lens is a phakic IOL, classified as such because the eye retains its natural lens when the Visian lens is implanted. This procedure would be considered cosmetic in nature.

Visilex Brand name polypropylene mesh specifically designed for laparoscopic hernia repair.

VISION Vital information system to improve outcomes in nephrology.

vision Ability of the eye to receive, resolve, and transmit light images to the occipital lobe in the brain where the light sensation is interpreted.

VISTAKON Brand name extended-wear, soft contact lens for treatment of near- and far-sightedness, astigmatism, or presbyopia. Supply is reported with HCPCS Level II codes V2520-V2523.

visual disorientation syndrome Cortical paralysis of visual fixation, optic ataxia, and disturbance of visual attention. Eye movements are normal. Report this disorder with ICD-9-CM code 368.16. *Synonym(s): Balint's syndrome, Holmes' syndrome, Riddoch's syndrome.*

visual function screening Determination of visual acuity, ocular alignment, field of vision, and color vision. Report this screening with CPT code 99172.

Visudyne See verteporfin.

vit Vitamin (followed by specific letter).

vital signs Pulse, respiration, and temperature.

Vitality Brand name implantable cardioverter defibrillator system.

vitamin B6 deficiency syndrome Deficiency-caused syndrome exhibiting gastrointestinal disturbance, erythema, nervous disorders, and mental disturbances. Report this disorder with ICD-9-CM code 266.1. *Synonym(s): Pellagra syndrome.*

vitelliform dystrophy Rare autosomal dominant form of macular degeneration, with symptoms occurring in early childhood, anywhere from ages 3 to 15 years. A mass of fatty material appears as a striking yellowish, orange yolk-like (vitelline) lesion under the retinal pigment epithelium in the macula, which then progresses through different stages over years. The break-up of this mass, which often ruptures, is referred to as the scrambled-egg stage and causes vision loss. Fluid and yellow deposits from the ruptured cyst spread throughout the macula. The macula and the underlying retinal pigment epithelium begin to atrophy, with possible development of a choroidal neovascular membrane, causing vision loss as central vision deteriorates to about 20/100 late in life. This disease does not always affect both eyes equally. Report this disease with ICD-9-CM code 362.76. *Synonym(s): Best's disease, vitelliform macular degeneration.*

vitelliform macular degeneration Rare autosomal dominant form of macular degeneration, with symptoms occurring in early childhood, anywhere from ages 3 to 15. A mass of fatty material appears as a striking yellowish, orange yolk-like (vitelline) lesion under the retinal pigment epithelium in the macula, which then progresses through different stages over years. The break-up of this mass, which often ruptures, is referred to as the scrambled-egg stage and causes vision loss.

V-Z

Fluid and yellow deposits from the ruptured cyst spread throughout the macula. The macula and the underlying retinal pigment epithelium begin to atrophy, with possible development of a choroidal neovascular membrane, causing vision loss as central vision deteriorates to about 20/100 late in life. This disease does not always affect both eyes equally. Report this disease with ICD-9-CM code 362.76. **Synonym(s):** *Best's disease, vitelliform dystrophy.*

vitiligo   Chronic, progressive, pigmentary anomaly of the skin, usually manifested by white patches devoid of pigment surrounded by a hyperpigmented border.

vitreal lamina   Transparent inner layer of the choroid that comes in contact with the pigmented layer of the retina. **Synonym(s):** *basal lamina, Bruch's membrane, complexus basalis choroideae, lamina basalis choroideae.*

vitreous   Clear gel filling the posterior segment of the eye and functioning as a refractive component in vision and as a method of maintaining pressure in the posterior segment.

vitreous humor   Clear gel filling the posterior segment of the eye that functions as a refractive component in vision and as to maintain pressure in the posterior segment.

vitreous opacities   Particles of cellular debris within vitreous gel material of the eye. They appear as streaks, strings, dots, spider webs, and bugs that seem to be in front of the eye, but are actually casting a shadow on the retina from within the vitreous. Report vitreous opacities with ICD-9-CM code 379.24. **Synonym(s):** *vitreous floaters.*

vitreous prolapse   Slipping of vitreous out of its normal position within the space between the retina and the lens. Report this condition with ICD-9-CM code 379.26.

Vivotif   Brand name oral typhoid vaccine provided in a four-capsule package. Report the appropriate CPT administration code as the primary procedure and supply of Vivotif secondarily, with CPT code 90690. The need for immunization is reported with ICD-9-CM code V03.1.

VLAT   Visual laser ablation of trigone. Treatment for bladder inflammation.

VLB   Vincaleukoblastine. See vinblastine.

VLBW   Very low birth weight. Prematurity generally referring to a newborn weighing 1,000 to 2,499 grams. These infants are generally born after 32 weeks' gestation, spend time in the newborn intensive care unit, and are at higher risks for long-term effects of prematurity. This condition is reported with a code from ICD-9-CM subcategory 765.1 and a second code from subcategory 765.2 to report the completed weeks of gestation.

VLCD   Very low calorie diet.

VLDL   Very low density lipoprotein.

VM-26   Teniposide. Chemotherapy drug.

VMA   Vanillylmandelic acid. Organic findings indicative of pheochromocytoma or neuroblastoma. A urine test for vanillylmandelic acid measures catecholamines or catecholamine metabolites (degradation products). Used to diagnose and monitor treatment of pheochromocytomas and neuroblastomas, the lab test for vanillylmandelic acid is reported with CPT code 84585. **Synonym(s):** *vanillylmandelic acid 3-Methoxy-4-Hydroxymandelic Acid 24-hour urine.*

VMD   Vitelliform macular dystrophy. Genetic dominant disorder that presents in childhood with a lesion on the macula and progresses to affect the retina and vision. VMD is reported with ICD-9-CM code 362.76. **Synonym(s):** *Best's disease.*

VML   Very malignant leanings.

VMPAC   Verbal Motor Production Assessment for Children. Speech evaluation for patients ages 3 to 12.

VMST   Visual motor sequencing test.

VNS   Vagus nerve stimulator. Implanted neurostimulator treating seizures and chronic or recurrent major depression. Hospitals report the supply of the generator with HCPCS Level II code C1767; supply of the lead is reported with C1778. **NCD Reference:** *160.18.*

VO   Verbal order.

VO2   Maximum oxygen consumption.

vocational rehabilitation   Services or training provided to people with physical or mental impairments in order to prepare them to enter or re-enter the workforce. Report encounters for vocational rehabilitation with ICD-9-CM code V57.22.

Vodder method   Rhythmic strokes applied lightly to the skin to reduce lymphedema by improving the lymphatic circulatory system. Lymphedema is reported with ICD-9-CM code 457.1 when an acquired chronic condition; postmastectomy lymphedema is reported with 457.0; and hereditary edema of the legs is reported with 757.0. **Synonym(s):** *manual lymph drainage, MLD.*

Vogt's syndrome   Spastic diplegia with athetosis and pseudobulbar paralysis found with a lesion of the caudate nucleus and putamen. Report this disorder with ICD-9-CM code 333.71.

Vogt-Koyanagi (-Harada) syndrome   Uveomeningitis marked by patchy depigmentation of hair, eyebrows, and lashes. Retinal detachment, deafness and tinnitus may also result. Report this disorder with ICD-9-CM code 364.24.

Vogt-Spielmeyer disease   Juvenile type of neuronal ceroid lipofuscinosis or amaurotic familial idiocy. This disease is an inherited disorder in which the body stores excessive amounts of lipofuscin, the pigment that remains after damaged cells are broken down and digested, resulting in progressive nervous tissue damage, vision loss, and fatality. Vogt-Spielmeyer disease manifests between ages 5 and 10 with excessive neural tissue lipofuscin storage causing massive loss of brain tissue with accompanying cerebral and retinal decay. Death usually occurs within another 10 or 15 years. Report this disease with ICD-9-CM code 330.1.

voiding EMG Voiding electromyography. Procedure performed on patients with voiding dysfunctions in which the physician places a pad or needle in the anal or urethral sphincter and measures the electrical activity of the sphincter muscles with the bladder filled and during emptying. This procedure is reported with CPT codes 51784 and 51785.

voiding pressure study Voiding pressure produced by the bladder and the resultant flow of urine is determined.

volar Palm of the hand (palmar) or sole of the foot (plantar).

Volkmann's contracture Shortening of the muscles in the fingers or wrist due to injury near the elbow or vascular damage.

volume *1)* Number of services performed. *2)* Number of patients. *3)* Number of patients in a DRG during a specific time.

volume depletion Depletion of total body water.

Volvulus

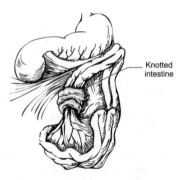

Knotted intestine

volvulus Twisting, knotting, or entanglement of the bowel on itself that may quickly compromise oxygen supply to the intestinal tissues. A volvulus usually occurs at the sigmoid and ileocecal areas of the intestines. Volvulus is reported with ICD-9-CM code 560.2.

vomer Flat bone that forms the lower, posterior portion of the nasal septum.

von Bechterew-Strümpell syndrome Rheumatoid inflammation of vertebrae. Report this disorder with ICD-9-CM code 720.0.

von Graefe's syndrome Progressive external ophthalmoplegia, a slowly progressive bilateral myopathy only affecting the muscles around the eye, including lids. Paralysis of the muscles around the eye results. Report this disorder with ICD-9-CM code 378.72.

von Hippel-Lindau syndrome Formation of multiple angiomas on the retina. Report this disorder with ICD-9-CM code 759.6.

von Recklinghausen's disease Autosomal dominant inherited condition with developmental changes in the nervous system, muscles, bones, and skin, producing coffee colored spots of pigmented skin (cafe au lait spots), and multiple soft tumor neurofibromas distributed over the entire body. *Synonym(s): neurofibromatosis.*

von Schroetter's syndrome Stress thrombosis of the subclavian or axillary vein. Report this disorder with ICD-9-CM code 453.89.

von WIllebrand's disease Congenital disease marked by abnormal blood coagulation caused by deficient blood factor VII. Symptoms include excess or prolonged bleeding. Report this disorder with ICD-9-CM code 286.4.

VOR Vestibulo-ocular response. Reflexive eye movements assessed following the placement of cold water in one ear.

Vorbeireden Symptom of providing the approximate answer or talking past the point, or at cross purposes as seen in the Ganser syndrome. A form of factitious illness that is also associated with malingering or brain injuries.

VOSS Visual observation shivering score.

VOYAGER OTW or RX Brand name coronary dilatation catheter used in percutaneous intraluminal balloon angioplasty as a treatment approach for blocked coronary arteries. The procedure is reported with CPT code 92982 for one vessel and 92984 for each additional vessel. If performed with atherectomy, 92995 would be reported, with 92996 for each additional vessel. Inpatient procedures would be reported with ICD-9-CM procedural codes 00.40-00.43 and 00.66.

voyeurism Repetitively seeking out situations in which the individual looks at unsuspecting people who are either naked, in the act of disrobing, or engaging in sexual activity that may stimulate sexual excitement of the observer, frequently with orgasm.

VP *1)* Voiding pressure study. Voiding pressure produced by the bladder and the resultant flow of urine is determined. A transducer is placed in the bladder to measure urine flow rate and pressure during emptying of the bladder, reported with CPT code 51728 or 51729. Intra-abdominal voiding pressure studies test the amount of straining necessary to void and reported with code 51797. *2)* HCPCS Level II modifier for use with CPT codes, identifying an aphakic patient. Aphakia is the

V-Z

absence of a lens in the eye. This modifier has no effect on Medicare reimbursement. **3)** Variegate porphyria. Genetic hepatic porphyria most often seen in white South Africans. A deficiency in protoporphyrinogen oxidase causes acute attacks similar to those found in AIP, as well as skin photosensitivity. VP is reported with ICD-9-CM code 277.1.

VP-16   Etoposide. Chemotherapy drug.

VPB   Ventricular premature beat.

VPC   Ventricular premature contraction.

VPL   Ventro-posterolateral.

VPN   Virtual private network.

VPRC   Volume of packed red cells.

VPT   Vibration perception threshold. Ability to distinguish vibrations, as measured as a noninvasive evaluation of peripheral sensory neuropathy, usually in diabetic patients. Nerve damage from vibration also can occur in patients with prolonged exposure to vibration in the workplace. Testing with a VPT meter can be reported with CPT new technology code 0107T. As a new technology, reimbursement for this service may vary from payer to payer.

VRA   Visual reinforcement audiometry. A test in which a child older than six months is observed for responses to sound because the child is too young to cooperate in a more standard hearing exam. The test is reported with CPT code 92579.

VS   *1)* Vesicular sound. *2)* Vital signs.

VSA   Vital signs absent.

VSD   Ventricular septal defect.

VSW   Ventricular stroke work.

VT   Ventricular tachycardia. Excessively rapid ventricular rhythm of the heart, usually more than 150 beats per minute, with an origin beat generated in the ventricle, commonly from atrioventricular dissociation. VT is reported with ICD-9-CM code 427.1. **Synonym(s):** *V tach.*

VTG   Volume thoracic gas.

vulva   Area on the female external genitalia that includes the labia majora and minora, mons pubis, clitoris, bulb of the vestibule, vaginal vestibule and orifice, and the greater and lesser vestibular glands.

vulvectomy   Surgical removal of all or part of the vulva, often performed to treat malignant or premalignant lesions. Lymph nodes may be removed at the same time. Vulvectomy is reported with CPT codes 56620-56640. **Synonym(s):** *Bassett's operation.*

vv   Veins

VW   Vessel wall.

V-Y operation   Plastic surgery technique that is used to cover defects or wounds on surface areas of the body and also to lengthen some anatomic structures. An incision is made in a V pattern and the flap is then approximated to cover the defect area as a Y shape. V-Y operation is used in many types of repairs and reconstructions, such as skin defects, nasal deformities, perianal or perineal areas after tumor resection or necrotizing fasciitis, fingertip amputations, and penile elongation in cases of hidden penis.

VZIG   Varicella-zoster immune globulin. VZIG is administered to people who have been exposed to varicella zoster (chicken pox) but have not developed symptoms of the disease. Because of its limited supply, its administration has been limited to immunocompromised patients. Supply of VZIG is reported with CPT code 90396 and administration is reported with the appropriate injection code. The need for VZIG is reported with ICD-9-CM code V01.71.

VZV   Varicella zoster virus. Virus causing chickenpox. Codes for chickenpox and its complications are found under ICD-9-CM category 052.

w   With.

w/   With.

W/C   Wheelchair.

w/HSBH   Warmed heelstick blood gas.

w/o   Without.

Waardenburg-Klein syndrome   Eyebrow or upper or lower eyelid sags. Report this disorder with ICD-9-CM code 270.2. **Synonym(s):** *Mendes syndrome, van der Hoeve-Halbertsma-Waardenburg syndrome.*

Wagner (-Unverricht) syndrome   Polymyositis occurring with characteristic skin changes that include a rash on the upper eyelids with edema, a rash on the forehead, neck, shoulders, trunk, and arms, and papules on the knuckles. Report this disorder with ICD-9-CM code 710.3. **Synonym(s):** *Petges-Clegat syndrome, Unverricht-Wagner syndrome.*

WAGR syndrome   Wilms' tumor, aniridia, gonadoblastoma, mental retardation syndrome. Rare genetic predisposition to eye abnormalities, mental retardation, and cancer of the kidney and testes or ovaries. There is no diagnosis code specific to the syndrome. Report Wilms' tumor with ICD-9-CM code 189.0 and the other manifestations as appropriate.

waiver of liability   Provision established by Medicare to protect beneficiaries and physicians from liability when services are denied as inappropriate or medically unnecessary. Under the provision, if the Medicare beneficiary knew or should have known that the services billed for were not covered, the beneficiary is liable for paying for the services. If neither the beneficiary nor the hospital knew or reasonably could have been expected to know that the services were not covered, Medicare is liable for paying the claim. If the provider should have

V-Z

known and the beneficiary is protected from liability, then liability falls with the provider, and the hospital cannot bill the beneficiary for services other than deductibles and coinsurance amounts, even though no Medicare payment has been made. Beneficiaries who do not know that services were noncovered are protected from liability when the services are not reasonable and/or necessary (including adverse level of care determinations) and when custodial care is involved.

WAK Wearable artificial kidney.

Waldenström's syndrome Increase in macroglobulins in the blood. Has symptoms of hyperviscosity such as weakness, fatigue, bleeding disorders, and visual disturbances. Report this disorder with ICD-9-CM code 273.3.

Waldenström-Kjellberg syndrome Condition in middle-aged women with hypochronic anemia, marked by cracks or fissures at the corners of the mouth, painful tongue, and dysphagia due to esophageal stenosis or webs. Report this disorder with ICD-9-CM code 280.8.

Walker-Warburg syndrome Genetically linked sideroblastic anemia present from birth, reported with ICD-9-CM code 285.0. **Synonym(s):** Pagon syndrome.

wall motion study Evaluation for cardiac wall motion abnormalities using echocardiography, MRI, CT, and/or radionuclide imaging techniques, either at rest or during exercise or pharmacologic-induced stress. Deficient inward movement of the left ventricular wall during systole may occur with conditions such as dilated cardiomyopathy, ischemic heart disease, and end-stage valvular disease. Types of insufficient movement include no systolic inward motion (akinesis), outward systolic bulging (dyskinesis), and diminished inward motion (hypokinesis).

Walsh modified radical prostatectomy Radical prostatectomy resects the rectum and surrounding tissue.

Washington Publishing Company Company that publishes the X12N HIPAA implementation guides and the X12N HIPAA data dictionary that also developed the X12 Data Dictionary, and that hosts the EHNAC STFCS testing program. **Synonym(s):** WPC.

Wasserman test Test for syphilis.

waste Spend or use federal funds carelessly.

water load test Test to diagnose inappropriate levels of antidiuretic hormone (ADH). ADH promotes reabsorption of water from the kidneys back into the circulation, hence the decreased formation of urine. Patients with an increased amount of ADH will not respond with increased urine output when increasing their fluid intake. For the water load test, the patient is given a set amount of water for each kilogram of body weight and then output is measured over the next few hours to see if values increase normally.

water retention syndrome Fluid overload caused by electrolyte and acid-base imbalance. Report this disorder with ICD-9-CM code 276.69.

Water's view Posterolateral (PA) radiographic view of the face with cephalad angulation, useful for evaluation of sinus disease and facial trauma. **Synonym(s):** occipitomental view.

Waterhouse (-Friderichsen) syndrome Acute fulminating meningococcal septicemia occurring in children below 10 years of age. Symptoms include vomiting, cyanosis, diarrhea, purpura, convulsions, and circulatory collapse. The patient will often display meningitis and hemorrhaging into the adrenal glands. Report this disorder with ICD-9-CM code 036.3.

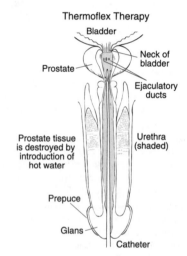

Thermoflex Therapy

Bladder

Neck of bladder

Prostate

Ejaculatory ducts

Prostate tissue is destroyed by introduction of hot water

Urethra (shaded)

Prepuce

Glans

Catheter

water-induced thermotherapy Therapeutic elevation of body temperature between 107.6 and 113.0 degrees Fahrenheit.

watermelon stomach Dilated veins in the stomach that may resemble the markings on a watermelon. If bleeding is not present, report watermelon stomach with ICD-9-CM code 537.82. If bleeding is present, report 537.83. **Synonym(s):** gastric antral vascular ectasia, GAVE.

Waterston procedure Type of aortopulmonary shunting done to increase pulmonary blood flow. The ascending aorta is anastomosed to the right pulmonary artery. Report Waterston procedure with ICD-9-CM procedure code 39.0 and CPT code 33755.

WB Whole blood.

WBC White blood count.

WBRT Whole brain radiation therapy.

wc Wheelchair.

WC Wheelchair.

WCC Well child care.

WD Well-developed.

W-D Wet to dry (dressings).

weakness syndrome Hypersomatic disorder with no indefinable pathology. Report this disorder with ICD-9-CM code 300.5.

web syndrome Dysplasia of the fingernails and toenails, hypoplasia of the patella, iliac horns, thickening of the glomerular lamina densa, and a flask-shaped femur. Report this disorder with ICD-9-CM code 756.89.

Weber's syndrome Paraplegia and anesthesia over half or part of the body. Caused by lesions in the brain or spinal cord. Report this disorder with ICD-9-CM code 344.89. *Synonym(s): Avellis syndrome, Babinski-Nageotte syndrome, Benedikt's syndrome, Brown-Sequard syndrome, Cestan-Chenais syndrome, Cestan's syndrome, Foville's syndrome, Gubler-Millard syndrome, Jackson's syndrome, Weber-Leyden syndrome.*

Weber's test Evaluation of hearing loss by holding a vibrating tuning fork against the forehead. This test is usually part of the physical exam portion of evaluation and management services and is not reported separately on the claim.

Weber-Christian syndrome Relapsing febrile nodular nonsuppurative panniculitis with development of nodules that spread centrifugally with erythematous borders and clearing centrally to form pigmented plaques. Report this disorder with ICD-9-CM code 729.30.

Weber-Cockayne syndrome Dwarfism with a precociously senile appearance, pigmentary degeneration of the retina, optic atrophy, deafness, sensitivity to sunlight, and mental retardation. Report this disorder with ICD-9-CM code 757.39.

Weber-Dimitri syndrome Formation of multiple angiomas in the skin of the head and scalp. Report this disorder with ICD-9-CM code 759.6. *Synonym(s): Kalischer's syndrome.*

Weber-Gubler syndrome Paraplegia over half or part of the body. Caused by lesions in the brain or spinal cord. Report this disorder with ICD-9-CM code 344.89. *Synonym(s): Avellis syndrome, Babinski-Nageotte syndrome, Benedikt's syndrome, Brown-Sequard syndrome, Cestan-Chenais syndrome, Cestan's syndrome, Foville's syndrome, Gubler-Millard syndrome, Jackson's syndrome, Weber-Leyden syndrome.*

Weber-Osler (-Rendu) syndrome Small telangiectasias and dilated venules that develop slowly on the skin and mucus membranes of the lips, tongue, nasopharynx, tongue, and the face. Report this disorder with ICD-9-CM code 448.0.

wedge Standard type of block or absorber used in radiation therapy, used to manipulate the radiation dose given to the patient.

wedge excision Surgical removal of a section of tissue that is thick at one edge and tapers to a thin edge. CPT code(s) used will be based on the anatomical site listed in documentation.

WEDI Work group on electronic data interchange.

Wedl cells Balloon cells on the posterior lens surface causing posterior subcapsular cataract. Report this condition with ICD-9-CM code 366.02.

weekly treatment management services Radiation therapy treatment visits are paid based on weekly time periods. Five radiation therapy sessions (fractions) make up a weekly service. A patient may have more than one radiation therapy visit in one day (e.g., two visits equal two fractions). However, treatment for multiple sites during a single visit is classified as one fraction.

Wegener's granulomatosis Uncommon, chronic necrotizing granulomatous inflammation of the respiratory tract manifested by sinus pain and purulent nasal discharge.

Wegener's syndrome Necrotizing granulomatous vasculitis involving the upper and lower respiratory tracts, which is thought to be a hypersensitivity to unknown antigens. Report this disorder with ICD-9-CM code 446.4.

weighting Assigning more worth to a fee based on the number of times it is charged, weighting the resource-based relative value fees for an area.

Weill-Marchesani syndrome Abnormally round and small lens, short stature, and brachydactyly. Report this disorder with ICD-9-CM code 759.89.

Weingarten's syndrome Transient infiltrations of lungs by eosinophilia, resulting in night coughing, fever, and dyspnea. Report this disorder with ICD-9-CM code 518.3.

Weiss-Baker syndrome Stimulation of an overactive carotid sinus, causing a marked drop in blood pressure, which, in turn, may stop or block the heart. Report this disorder with ICD-9-CM code 337.01. *Synonym(s): Carotid sinus syndrome, Charcot-Weiss-Baker syndrome.*

Weissenbach-Thibierge syndrome Systemic disorder of the connective tissue marked by induration and thickening of the skin, with circulatory and organ changes. May reside in the face and hands for some time. Also includes Raynaud's phenomenon and, in some cases, esophageal problems. Report this disorder with ICD-9-CM code 710.1.

well-baby care Medical services, immunizations, and regular provider visits considered routine for an infant.

Wenckebach phenomenon Second degree atrioventricular block in which progressive lengthening

V-Z

of the atrioventricular conduction time, or a series of steadily increasing P-R intervals, precedes periodic dropping of one or more beats. This phenomenon is reported with ICD-9-CM code 426.13. **Synonym(s):** *Mobitz type I.*

Werlhof-Wichmann syndrome Small number of platelets in circulating blood, causing bruising. Report this disorder with ICD-9-CM code 287.39.

Wermer's syndrome Tumors in more than one endocrine gland, including the pancreatic islets and parathyroid glands. This syndrome is inherited. Report this disorder with ICD-9-CM code 258.01.

Werner's syndrome Accelerated aging in adults from an autosomal recessive trait, marked by sclerodermal skin changes with muscular atrophy, aged appearance including baldness, and a predisposition for diabetes mellitus. This syndrome is reported with ICD-9-CM code 259.8.

Wernicke's syndrome Thiamine deficiency, disturbances in ocular motility, pupillary alterations, nystagmus, and ataxia with tremors. Organic toxic psychosis often coexists. Most often due to alcoholism. Report this disorder with ICD-9-CM code 265.1. **Synonym(s):** *Gayet-Wernicke syndrome.*

Wertheim hysterectomy Radical operation for uterine carcinoma includes excising a portion of the vagina and lymph nodes.

Wertheim's operation Abdominal hysterectomy in which lymphatics, the cervix, and part of the vagina is removed. It is typically performed to treat cervical cancer. Wertheim's operation is reported with CPT code 58210 or ICD-9-CM facility code 68.6.

West Nile virus Virus spread to humans through the bite of an infected mosquito, first noted in the United States in 1999 and a focus of concern for the Centers for Disease Control. West Nile infections usually create mild symptoms, but in 1 percent of the population, central nervous system involvement increases morbidity. Mosquitoes are carriers that become infected when they feed on infected birds. Report this virus with a code from ICD-9-CM subcategory 066.4. **Synonym(s):** *WNV.*

Westergren test Test determines the sedimentation rate of red blood cells in fluid blood by mixing venous blood with an aqueous solution of sodium citrate and allowing it to stand for measured periods of time.

Westphal-Strüempell disease Rare, progressive, chronic disease caused by an inherited copper metabolism defect that results in the poisonous accumulation of copper in certain organs and tissues, such as the brain, kidneys, cornea, and liver. The disease causes cirrhosis, brain degeneration with progressive neurological dysfunction, and pigmented Kayser-Fleischer corneal ring. Report this condition with

ICD-9-CM code 275.1. **Synonym(s):** *familial hepatitis, hepatolenticular degeneration, Kinnier Wilson's disease, pseudosclerosis of Westphal, Westphal-Strümpell syndrome, Wilson's syndrome, Wilson's disease.*

wet brain syndrome Chronic alcohol dependence that is both a psychological and physical state, resulting from excessive alcohol consumption. Characterized by behavioral and other responses that always include a compulsion to ingest alcohol on a continuous or periodic basis in order to experience its psychological effect, and sometimes to avoid the discomfort of its absence. Report this disorder with a code from ICD-9-CM range 303.90-303.93. **Synonym(s):** *alcohol dependence syndrome.*

wet feet syndrome Blotchy cyanosis, increased sweating, paresthesia, and edema. Caused by hypothermia. Report this disorder with ICD-9-CM code 991.4. **Synonym(s):** *immersion foot, trench foot.*

wet macular degeneration New vessel formation in the oxygen-deprived tissues feeding the retina. This neovascularization results in tiny, delicate vessels that break easily, causing leakage, hemorrhaging, swelling, and damage to surrounding tissue, and accounts for 10 percent of all cases of macular degeneration in the United States. Report this condition with ICD-9-CM code 362.52. **Synonym(s):** *disciform senile macular degeneration, exudative senile macular degeneration, neovascular macular degeneration.*

WG Work group.

Wharton's ducts Salivary ducts below the mandible.

wheezing Whistling sound upon respiration.

WHFO Wrist-hand-finger orthotic.

whiplash syndrome Acute cervical sprain caused by hyperextension of the neck (C4-C5) during an accident, usually in an automobile. Report this disorder with ICD-9-CM code 847.0.

V-Z

Whipple Procedure

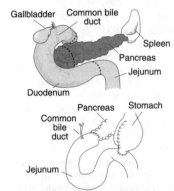

A portion of the pancreas closest to the duodenum is resected along with the entire length of the duodenum. The distal portion of the stomach is resected (usually along with the duodenum) and the gallbladder is removed. A length of jejunum is pulled up and the pancreas remnant is anastomosed to it or, it is sutured closed without pancreatojejunostomy. The distal stomach is sewn end-to-side to the jejunum and the common bile duct is attached as well

Whipple procedure   Pancreaticoduodenectomy (removal of gallbladder, part of the duodenum, and the head of the pancreas) performed to treat pancreatic cancer or chronic pancreatitis. Whipple procedure is reported with CPT code 48150 or 48152 or inpatient ICD-9-CM procedure code 52.7.

Whipple's syndrome   Radical removal of the head of the pancreas, duodenum, and distal third of the stomach. Report this disorder with ICD-9-CM code 040.2.

whistle tip catheter   Catheter design with a lateral and terminal opening.

whistleblower   Individual who discloses misconduct by a provider and may be eligible for monetary returns if the misconduct involves financial misconduct as determined on a case-by-case basis.

whistling face syndrome   Deviation of hands and face, with protrusion of lips as in whistling, sunken eyes, and small nose. Report this disorder with ICD-9-CM code 759.89. *Synonym(s): Freeman-Sheldon syndrome.*

whitehead hemorrhoidectomy   Two circular incisions above and below hemorrhoidal veins pull down normal mucosa for suturing to anal skin.

Whitman astragalectomy   Removal of cartilage of the talus.

WHO   World Health Organization. International agency comprising UN members to promote the physical, mental, and emotional health of the people of the world and to track morbidity and mortality statistics worldwide. WHO maintains the International Classification of Diseases (ICD) medical code set.

whooping cough   Acute, highly contagious respiratory tract infection caused by *Bordetella pertussis* and *B. bronchiseptica*. Characteristic paroxysmal cough.

WHZ   Wheeze.

wick catheter   Device used to monitor interstitial fluid pressure, and sometimes used intraoperatively during fasciotomy procedures to evaluate the effectiveness of the decompression.

Widal (-Abrami) syndrome   One of anemic syndromes caused by exposures to trauma, poisons, and other causes that decreases the number of red blood cells. Report this disorder with ICD-9-CM code 283.9. *Synonym(s): Dyke-Young syndrome, Hayem-Widal syndrome.*

WIFC   Widely invasive follicular carcinoma.

WIHS   Women's Interagency HIV Study. Consortium producing data on the effect of HIV on women's health across the nation. WIHS is funded by several government agencies, including the National Cancer Institute and the National Center for Research Studies.

Wilkie's syndrome   Complete or partial block of the superior mesenteric artery with symptoms of vomiting, pain, blood in the stool, and distended abdomen. Results in bowel infarction. Report this disorder with ICD-9-CM code 557.1.

Wilkinson-Sneddon syndrome   Non-inflammatory intimal hyperplasia of medium sized vessels. Report this disorder with ICD-9-CM code 694.1.

Willan-Plumbe syndrome   Eruption of circumscribed, discrete, reddish, silvery-scaled maculopapules on the knees, elbows, scalp, and trunk. Report this disorder with ICD-9-CM code 696.1.

willingly   Performing actions deliberately or intentionally.

Willi-Prader syndrome   Rounded face, almond-shaped eyes, strabismus, low forehead, hypogonadism, hypotomia, mental retardation and an insatiable appetite. Report this disorder with ICD-9-CM code 759.81.

Wilms' tumor   Malignant tumor of the kidney that develops rapidly from embryonic elements and occurs unilaterally or bilaterally in children before age 5 and rarely in older years. Wilms' tumor is reported with ICD-9-CM code 189.0.

Wilson's disease   Rare, progressive, chronic disease caused by an inherited copper metabolism defect that results in the poisonous accumulation of copper in certain organs and tissues, such as the brain, kidneys, cornea, and liver. The disease causes cirrhosis, brain degeneration with progressive neurological dysfunction, and pigmented Kayser-Fleischer corneal ring. Report this condition with ICD-9-CM code 275.1. **Synonym(s):** *familial hepatitis, hepatolenticular degeneration, Kinnier Wilson's disease, pseudosclerosis of Westphal, Westphal-Struempell disease, Wilson's syndrome.*

Wilson's syndrome Rare, progressive, chronic disease caused by an inherited copper metabolism defect that results in the poisonous accumulation of copper in certain organs and tissues, such as the brain, kidneys, cornea, and liver. The disease causes cirrhosis, brain degeneration with progressive neurological dysfunction, and pigmented Kayser-Fleischer corneal ring. Report this condition with ICD-9-CM code 275.1. **Synonym(s):** *Westphal-Strümpell syndrome.*

Wilson-Mikity syndrome Pulmonary insufficiency in newborn babies, especially those with low birth weight with hypercapnia and cyanosis of rapid onset during the first month of life and resulting frequently in death. Report this disorder with ICD-9-CM code 770.7.

winged catheter Indwelling urethral catheter with wing-like projections on the end for retention within the bladder.

winking syndrome Tic motor disorder not otherwise specified. Report this disorder with ICD-9-CM code 307.20.

Winograd Specific type of wedge resection utilizing a "D" shaped excision of the nail root usually performed on the toenails. Report this procedure with CPT code 11765.

WISC Wechsler Intelligence Scale for Children.

Wiskott-Aldrich syndrome Immunodeficiency shown by eczema, thrombocytopenia, and recurrent pyogenic infection. Patients suffer an increased susceptibility to infection with encapsulated bacteria. Report this disorder with ICD-9-CM code 279.12.

WIT

WIT is the acronym for water induced thermotherapy

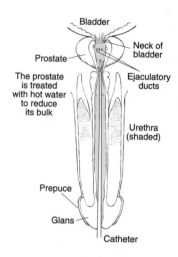

The prostate is treated with hot water to reduce its bulk

Prostate tissue is destroyed by introduction of hot water

WIT Water-induced thermotherapy. Minimally invasive treatment of benign prostatic hyperplasia (BPH) by introducing heated (60ºC) water into the prostatic urethra by means of a special heat-transmitting balloon catheter. The precisely controlled heated water destroys a predictable amount of tissue, which is reabsorbed into the body, and the obstructed urethra is reopened. WIT is an outpatient procedure requiring only topical anesthesia. WIT is reported with CPT code 55899.

withdrawal reaction of childhood or adolescence Emotional disturbance in children chiefly manifested by a lack of interest in social relationships and indifference to social praise or criticism.

withhold Percentage of payment to providers held by an HMO until the cost of referral or services has been determined. If the provider goes over the amount determined appropriate, the HMO keeps that amount.

WJG Widers-Jongsma-van Ginneken (pacemaker model).

Wk Week.

WKD Wilson-Kimmelstiel disease.

WKI Wakefield Inventory.

WKS Wernicke-Korsakoff syndrome.

WLQ Work limitation questionnaire.

WLS Wet lung syndrome.

WM Waldenström's macroglobulinemia.

V-Z

WMFT Wolf Motor Function Test.

WMP Warm moist packs.

WMT Word Memory Test.

WMX Whirlpool, massage, and exercise.

WN Well-nourished.

WNE West Nile encephalitis.

WNL Within normal limits.

Woake's syndrome Polyp-like growths that hamper sinus function. Report this disorder with ICD-9-CM code 471.1. *Synonym(s): polypoid sinus degeneration.*

Wolff-Parkinson-White syndrome Pre-excitation associated with paroxysmal tachycardia or atrial fibrillation with a short P-R interval on EKG and an early delta wave. The normal conduction pathway is bypassed. This syndrome is reported with ICD-9-CM code 426.7. *Synonym(s): anomalous atrioventricular excitation, pre-excitation syndrome, WPW syndrome.*

wolhynia fever Moderately severe disease borne by body lice and relatively common among the homeless. The onset of symptoms is sudden, with high fever, severe headache, back and leg pain, and a fleeting rash. Recovery takes a month or more. Relapses are common. Report this condition with ICD-9-CM code 083.1. *Synonym(s): shin bone fever, trench fever.*

WOP Without pain.

word deafness Developmental delay in the comprehension of speech sounds.

work conditioning Work-related, intensive, goal-oriented treatment program specifically designed to restore an individual's systemic, neuromusculoskeletal (strength, endurance, movement, flexibility, and motor control), and cardiopulmonary functions to restore the client's physical capacity and function so the client can return to work.

work hardening Highly structured, goal-oriented, individualized treatment program designed to return the person to work by using real or simulated work activities to restore physical, behavioral, and vocational functions.

workers' compensation State-governed system designated to administer and regulate the provision and cost of medical treatment and wage losses arising from a worker's job-related injury or disease, regardless of who is at fault. In exchange, the employer is protected from being sued.

workforce Under HIPAA, employees, volunteers, trainees, and other persons under the direct control of a covered entity, whether or not they are paid by the covered entity.

Workgroup for Electronic Data Interchange Health care industry group that lobbied for HIPAA A/S, and that has a formal consultative role under the HIPAA legislation. WEDI also sponsors the strategic national implementation process (SNIP). *Synonym(s): WEDI.*

working aged Patient or spouse, older than age 65, eligible for group health insurance through employment or the employment of his or her spouse. Under these circumstances, Medicare would be the secondary payer.

World Health Organization International agency comprising UN members to promote the physical, mental, and emotional health of the people of the world and to track morbidity and mortality statistics worldwide. WHO maintains the International Classification of Diseases (ICD) medical code set. *Synonym(s): WHO.*

wound Injury to living tissue often involving a cut or break in the skin.

wound repair Surgical closure of a wound is divided into three categories: simple, intermediate, and complex. *simple repair:* Surgical closure of a superficial wound, requiring single layer suturing of the skin epidermis, dermis, or subcutaneous tissue. *intermediate repair:* Surgical closure of a wound requiring closure of one or more of the deeper subcutaneous tissue and non-muscle fascia layers in addition to suturing the skin; contaminated wounds with single layer closure that need extensive cleaning or foreign body removal. *complex repair:* Repair of wounds requiring more than layered closure (debridement, scar revision, stents, retention sutures).

WPC Washington Publishing Company.

WPFM Wright peak flow meter.

WPPSI Wechsler Preschool and Primary Scale of Intelligence.

WPW Wolff-Parkinson-White syndrome.

WR *1)* Wasserman reaction. *2)* Wrist.

wraparound plan Insurance or health plan coverage for copays and deductibles not covered under a member's base plan.

WRAT Wide Range Achievement Test.

wrist drop Inability to extend the hand, which droops permanently at the wrist, due to extensor muscle paralysis. Report this condition with ICD-9-CM code 736.05. *Synonym(s): carpoptosis, hand drop.*

WRUED Work-related upper extremity disorder.

WSEP Williams syndrome in early puberty.

Wt Weight.

WT1 Wilm's tumor 1 protein.

WT2 Wilm's tumor 2 protein.

WTHD Wish to hasten death.

X Cranial nerve, also known as the vagus nerve, affecting the pharynx, larynx, and trachea, it also extends to the esophagus, lungs, heart, and colon.

X12 ANSI-accredited group that defines EDI standards for health care. Most of the electronic transactions standards mandated or proposed under HIPAA are X12 standards.

X12 148 "First Report of Injury." This standard could eventually be included in the HIPAA mandate.

X12 270 "Health Care Eligibility and Benefit Inquiry" transaction. Version 4010 of this transaction has been included in the HIPAA mandates.

X12 271 "Health Care Eligibility and Benefit Response" transaction. Version 4010 of this transaction has been included in the HIPAA mandates.

X12 274 "Provider Information" transaction.

X12 275 "Patient Information" transaction. This transaction is expected to be part of the HIPAA claim attachments standard.

X12 276 X12 "Health Care Claims Status Inquiry" transaction. Version 4010 of this transaction has been included in the HIPAA mandates.

X12 277 X12 "Health Care Claim Status Response" transaction. Version 4010 of this transaction has been included in the HIPAA mandates. This transaction is also expected to be part of the HIPAA claim attachments standard.

X12 278 X12 "Referral Certification and Authorization" transaction. Version 4010 of this transaction has been included in the HIPAA mandates.

X12 811 X12 "Consolidated Service Invoice & Statement" transaction.

X12 820 X12 "Payment Order & Remittance Advice" transaction. Version 4010 of this transaction has been included in the HIPAA mandates.

X12 831 X12 "Application Control Totals" transaction.

X12 834 X12 "Benefit Enrollment & Maintenance" transaction. Version 4010 of this transaction has been included in the HIPAA mandates.

X12 835 X12 "Health Care Claim Payment & Remittance Advice" transaction. Version 4010 of this transaction has been included in the HIPAA mandates.

X12 837 X12 "Health Care Claim or Encounter" transaction. This transaction can be used for institutional, professional, dental, or drug claims. Version 4010 of this transaction has been included in the HIPAA mandates.

X12 997 X12 "Functional Acknowledgment" transaction.

X12 IHCEBI & IHCEBR X12 "Interactive Healthcare Eligibility & Benefits Inquiry (IHCEBI)" and "Response (IHCEBR)" transactions. These are being combined and converted to UN/EDIFACT Version 5 syntax.

X12 IHCLME X12 "Interactive Healthcare Claim" transaction.

X12 Standard X12 standard that has been approved since the most recent release of X12 American National Standards. Since a full set of X12 American National Standards is released only about once every five years, it is the X12 standards that are most likely to be in active use. These standards were previously called "draft standards for trial use."

X12/PRB X12 Procedures Review Board.

X12F Subcommittee of X12 that defines EDI standards for the financial industry. This group maintains the X12 811 [generic] "Invoice" and the X12 820 [generic] "Payment & Remittance Advice" transactions, although X12N maintains the associated HIPAA implementation guides.

X12J Subcommittee of X12 that reviews X12 work products for compliance with the X12 design rules.

X12N Subcommittee of X12 that defines EDI standards for the insurance industry, including health care insurance.

X12N/SPTG4 HIPAA Liaison Special Task Group of the Insurance Subcommittee (N) of X12. This group's responsibilities have been assumed by X12N/TG3/WG3.

X12N/TG1 Property & Casualty Task Group (TG1) of the Insurance Subcommittee (N) of X12.

X12N/TG2 Health Care Task Group (TG2) of the Insurance Subcommittee (N) of X12.

X12N/TG2/WG1 Health Care Eligibility Work Group (WG1) of the Health Care Task Group (TG2) of the Insurance Subcommittee (N) of X12. This group maintains the X12 270 "Health Care Eligibility & Benefit Inquiry" and the X12 271 "Health Care Eligibility & Benefit Response" transactions, and is also responsible for maintaining the IHCEBI and IHCEBR transactions.

X12N/TG2/WG10 Health Care Services Review Work Group (WG10) of the Health Care Task Group (TG2) of the Insurance Subcommittee (N) of X12. This group maintains the X12 278 "Referral Certification and Authorization" transaction.

X12N/TG2/WG12 Interactive Health Care Claims Work Group (WG12) of the Health Care Task Group (TG2) of the Insurance Subcommittee (N) of X12. This group maintains the IHCLME "Interactive Claims" transaction.

X12N/TG2/WG15 Health Care Provider Information Work Group (WG15) of the Health Care Task Group (TG2) of the Insurance Subcommittee (N) of X12. This group maintains the X12 274 "Provider Information" transaction.

X12N/TG2/WG19 Health Care Implementation Coordination Work Group (WG19) of the Health Care Task Group (TG2) of the Insurance Subcommittee (N) of X12. This is now X12N/TG3/WG3.

Z-V

X12N/TG2/WG2 Health Care Claims Work Group (WG2) of the Health Care Task Group (TG2) of the Insurance Subcommittee (N) of X12. This group maintains the X12 837 "Health Care Claim or Encounter" transaction.

X12N/TG2/WG3 Health Care Claim Payments Work Group (WG3) of the Health Care Task Group (TG2) of the Insurance Subcommittee (N) of X12. This group maintains the X12 835 "Health Care Claim Payment & Remittance Advice" transaction.

X12N/TG2/WG4 Health Care Enrollments Work Group (WG4) of the Health Care Task Group (TG2) of the Insurance Subcommittee (N) of X12. This group maintains the X12 834 "Benefit Enrollment & Maintenance" transaction.

X12N/TG2/WG5 Health Care Claims Status Work Group (WG5) of the Health Care Task Group (TG2) of the Insurance Subcommittee (N) of X12. This group maintains the X12 276 "Health Care Claims Status Inquiry" and the X12 277 "Health Care Claim Status Response" transactions.

X12N/TG2/WG9 Health Care Patient Information Work Group (WG9) of the Health Care Task Group (TG2) of the Insurance Subcommittee (N) of X12. This group maintains the X12 275 "Patient Information" transaction.

X12N/TG3 Business Transaction Coordination and Modeling Task Group (TG3) of the Insurance Subcommittee (N) of X12. TG3 maintains the X12N business and data models and the HIPAA Data Dictionary. This was formerly X12N/TG2/WG11.

X12N/TG3/WG1 Property & Casualty Work Group (WG1) of the Business Transaction Coordination and Modeling Task Group (TG3) of the Insurance Subcommittee (N) of X12.

X12N/TG3/WG2 Healthcare Business and Information Modeling Work Group (WG2) of the Business Transaction Coordination and Modeling Task Group (TG3) of the Insurance Subcommittee (N) of X12.

X12N/TG3/WG3 HIPAA Implementation Coordination Work Group (WG3) of the Business Transaction Coordination and Modeling Task Group (TG3) of the Insurance Subcommittee (N) of X12. This was formerly X12N/TG2/WG19 and X12N/SPTG4.

X12N/TG3/WG4 Object-Oriented Modeling and XML Liaison Work Group (WG4) of the Business Transaction Coordination and Modeling Task Group (TG3) of the Insurance Subcommittee (N) of X12.

X12N/TG4 Implementation Guide Task Group (TG4) of the Insurance Subcommittee (N) of X12. This group supports the development and maintenance of X12 implementation guides, including the HIPAA X12 IGs.

X12N/TG8 Architecture Task Group (TG8) of the Insurance Subcommittee (N) of X12.

Xact Brand name carotid stent system.

xanthelasma Small, yellow tumors of the eyelid, usually appearing near the nose. Seen in patients with high blood-fat levels and in the elderly.

xanthochromia Yellowish discoloration, usually referring to cerebrospinal fluid or skin. In cerebrospinal fluid, xanthochromia is seen following a subarachnoid hemorrhage. The fluid takes on a yellow cast, the result of lysis of blood. As a finding, xanthochromia in spinal fluid would be reported with ICD-9-CM code 792.0. In the skin, xanthochromia may be an indication of jaundice.

XC In surgical documentation, a cross clamp.

Xe Xenon (isotope mass of xenon 133).

Xeloda Brand name pharmaceutical for treatment of colorectal or metastatic breast cancer. Xeloda is an oral medication. Supply is reported with HCPCS Level II codes J8520 and J8521. *Synonym(s): capecitabine.*

xeno- Relating to a foreign substance.

xenograft Tissue that is harvested from one species and grafted to another. Pigskin is the most common xenograft for human skin and is applied to a wound as a temporary closure until a permanent option is performed. Report xenografting of skin with CPT codes 15400-15421.

xenon arc photocoagulator Device that produces a multiwavelength light that is optically focused to heat eye tissue, causing it to seal.

xenotransplantation Use of live, nonhuman animal cells, tissues, and organs grafted into humans, such as porcine skin grafts derived from pigs (CPT codes 15400 and 15401).

xero- Indicates a dry condition.

xerostomia Dry mouth due to lack of saliva, reported with ICD-9-CM code 527.7.

XFS Exfoliation syndrome. Ocular disorder characterized by the production and accumulation of a flakey, fibrillar extracellular material in the eye that can lead to glaucoma. Most cases of unilateral glaucoma are associated with XFS, reported with ICD-9-CM code 366.11, and any resultant glaucoma, with 365.52. *Synonym(s): exfoliative syndrome, pseudoexfoliation syndrome.*

XI Cranial nerve on the surface of the medulla that conveys motor control signals to the sternomastoid and trapezius muscles.

Xigris See drotrecogin alfa (activated).

XII Cranial nerve emerging from the medulla and responsible for motor commands of the tongue muscles.

xiphopagus Monozygotic (identical) twins who are joined at the abdomen. Report this abnormality with ICD-9-CM code 759.4. *Synonym(s): omphalopagus.*

XLS Excimer laser system.

XM Cross match.

XML Extensible Markup Language.

XO syndrome Short stature, webbed neck, congenital heart disease, mental retardation, and other symptoms. Report this disorder with ICD-9-CM code 758.6. *Synonym(s): Turner's syndrome.*

XR Extremely rare.

x-ray Images of the bones and internal organs obtained by sending small amounts of radiation through the body, leaving a shadow-like image of internal structures.

XRBT External beam radiotherapy.

XRT External radiotherapy.

XSTOP Brand name titanium implant intended to lift the spinous processes of the lumbar spine and reduce symptoms of neurogenic intermittent claudication secondary to stenosis. XSTOP consists of a spacer assembly and a wing assembly. XSTOP application would be reported with CPT unlisted code 22899 in addition to appropriate osteotomy, corpectomy, or diskectomy codes.

XYNTHA Brand name injectable recombinant antihemophilic factor indicated for surgical prophylaxis and control and prevention of bleeding episodes in patients with hemophilia A. Report supply with HCPCS Level II code J7185.

YDV Yeast-derived hepatitis B vaccine.

Yellofins Brand name stirrups used during laparoscopic surgery.

yellow vernix syndrome Syndrome marked by placental dysfunction, infarction, and insufficiency. Report this disorder with a code from ICD-9-CM subcategory 656.7. *Synonym(s): placental dysfunction.*

yersinia enterocolitica Species of gram-negative, facultative anaerobes responsible for yersiniosis, a form of acute gastroenteritis that can lead to mesenteric lymphadenitis in children with subsequent arthritis, and septicemia in adults. Yersinia enterocolitica is reported with ICD-9-CM code 008.44.

YF-Vax Brand name yellow fever vaccine provided in a single-dose or five-dose vial. Report the appropriate CPT subcutaneous injection code as the primary procedure and supply of YF-Vax secondarily, with CPT code 90717. The need for immunization is reported with ICD-9-CM code V04.4.

y-o Year-old.

YOB Year of birth.

YOD Year of death.

YPLL Years of potential life lost before age 65.

YTD Year to date.

Zahorsky's syndrome Vesicular pharyngitis caused by Coxsackie virus. Report this disorder with ICD-9-CM code 074.0.

ZEEP Zero end-expiratory pressure.

Zeis gland Sebaceous gland attached directly to an eyelash follicle. Hordeolum, also known as a stye, is an infection of a Zeis gland. If external, a hordeolum is reported with ICD-9-CM code 373.11; internal is reported with 373.12. Digital expression of the infected Zeis gland is reported with the appropriate level E/M code.

Zeitgeber In sleep disorder medicine, a cue that identifies time and influences biological rhythm (e.g., light, noise, or physical activity).

Zellweger syndrome Rare autosomal recessive disorder presenting with enlarged liver, high levels of copper and iron in the blood, polycystic kidneys, jaundice, lack of muscle tone, and abnormal craniofacial characteristics. Zellweger syndrome results in death in early infancy. Report this syndrome with ICD-9-CM code 277.86. *Synonym(s): cerebrohepatorenal syndrome.*

Zenith AAA graft Brand name endovascular graft for abdominal aortic aneurysm (AAA) repair made of polyester and steel.

Zephir system Brand name for temporary anterior cervical stabilization system including bone plates and screws.

ZHC Zajdela hepatoma cell.

zidovudine Oral or intravenous antiviral for the treatment of human immunodeficiency virus (HIV) that causes AIDS. Zidovudine is used with other antiretrovirals to prevent HIV transmission by pregnant women to the baby, for health care workers with needle stick exposure, and in some rape cases. Its supply is reported with HCPCS Level II code J3485 or S0104. *Synonym(s): azidothymine.*

Ziere's syndrome Acute hepatitis or cirrhosis of the liver associated with alcoholism. Report this disorder with ICD-9-CM code 571.1.

ZIFT Zygote intrafallopian transfer.

Zilver stent Brand name, self-expanding iliac artery stent currently approved by the FDA for investigational use.

Zinacef See cefuroxime sodium.

Zollinger-Ellison syndrome Peptic ulceration with gastric hypersecretion, tumor of the pancreatic islets, and hypoglycemia. Report this disorder with ICD-9-CM code 251.5. *Synonym(s): Ellison-Zollinger syndrome.*

zonules Fibers that connect the ocular lens to the ciliary body and hold it in position, relaxing and contracting to

V-Z

allow the lens to increase or decrease its curvature to alter its refraction.

Zoophilia Sexual or anal intercourse with animals.

Zostavax Brand name live vaccine to reduce the risk of shingles and postherpetic neuralgia caused by the latent varicella zoster virus. Supply of the vaccine is reported with CPT code 90736, and its administration is reported with 90471. **Synonym(s):** *varicella zoster vaccine.*

ZPIC Zone Program Integrity Contractor. CMS newly created entity currently being transitioned to replace the existing Program Safeguard Contractors (PSC). These contractors will be responsible for ensuring the integrity of all Medicare-related claims under Parts A and B (hospital, skilled nursing, home health, provider, and durable medical equipment claims), Part C (Medicare Advantage health plans), Part D (prescription drug plans), and coordination of Medicare-Medicaid data matches (Medi-Medi).

Zygoma

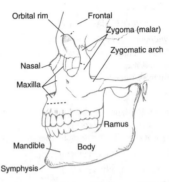

zygoma Zygomatic process of the temporal bone that creates the cheekbone.

zygomatic arch Part of the temporal bone of the skull that forms the prominence of the cheek.

zygote Fertilized ovum or the cell created after the union of a male and female gamete.

Z-plasty

Any of a wide variety of scar revision techniques may be employed. A Z-plasty may be used to lengthen or break up the scar line. Revision also serves to neutralize contractures that occur along the scar line

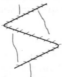

Example of a common Z-plasty where flaps are rotated to break scar line

z-plasty Plastic surgery technique used primarily to release tension or elongate contractured scar tissue in which a Z-shaped incision is made with the middle line of the Z crossing the area of greatest tension. The triangular flaps are then rotated so that they cross the incision line in the opposite direction, creating a reversed Z.

ZSRDS Zung Self-Rating Depression Scale.

Zuelzer-Ogden syndrome Folate-deficiency anemia caused by a drug, congenital, dietary, or other reason. Report this disorder with ICD-9-CM code 281.2.

Metric Conversion Tables

An Illustration of Weight

The following weights are used for fifth digits in ICD-9-CM categories 764 Slow fetal growth and fetal malnutrition and 765 Disorder relating to short gestation and unspecified low birthweight.

0	unspecified (weight)		
1	less than 500 grams	17.87 oz.	Less than 1.1 pounds
2	500 – 749 grams	17.86 – 26.75 oz.	1.11 – 1.67 pounds
3	750 – 999 grams	26.78 – 35.6 oz.	1.68 – 2.23 pounds
4	1,000 – 1,249 grams	35.71 – 44.6 oz.	2.24 – 2.78 pounds
5	1,250 – 1,499 grams	44.64 – 53.5 oz.	2.79 – 3.34 pounds
6	1,500 – 1,749 grams	53.6 – 62.4 oz.	3.35 – 3.9 pounds
7	1,750 – 1,999 grams	62.5 – 71.4 oz.	3.91 – 4.5 pounds
8	2,000 – 2,499 grams	71.43 – 89.25 oz.	4.51 – 5.58 pounds
9	2,500 grams and over	89.28 oz.	Greater than 5.6 pounds

An Illustration of Lesion Size

The following graph illustrates the size of lesions and incisions outlined in CPT.

= 2 centimeters

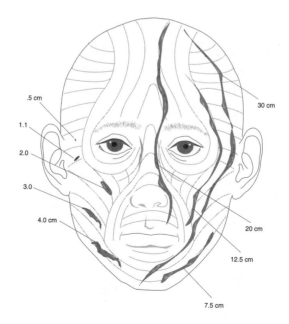

Not to scale

Measures of Length

Micrometers	Millimeters	Centimeters	Meters	Feet	Inches
1	0.001	10^{-4}			0.000039
10^3	1	10^{-1}		0.00328	.03937
10^4	10	1	0.01	0.03281	0.3937
254,000	25.4	2.54	0.0254	0.0833	1
	304.8	30.48	0.3048	1	12
10^6	10^3	10^2	1	3.2808	39.37
914,400	914.40	91.44	0.9144	3	36
10^9	10^6	10^5	10^3	3280.8	
			1609.0	5280.0	

Measures of Weight

Grains	Drams	Ounces	Pounds	Milligrams	Grams	Kilograms
1	0.0366	0.0023	0.00014	64.8	0.0648	0.000065
27.34	1	0.0625	0.0039		1.772	0.001772
437.5	16	1	0.0625		28.350	0.028350
7,000	256	16	1		453.5924	0.453592
0.0154				1	0.001	
15.4324	0.05648	0.0353	0.002205	1000	1	0.001
15,432.358	564.32	35.27	2.2046		1000	1

Conversions to Celsius

Fahrenheit	Celsius	Fahrenheit	Celsius
50	10.0	103	39.4
55	12.7	104	40.0
60	15.5	105	40.5
65	18.3	106	51.1
70	21.1	107	41.6
75	23.8	108	42.2
80	26.6	109	42.7
85	29.4	110	43.3
90	32.2	111	43.8
91	32.7	112	44.4
92	33.3	113	45.0
93	33.8	114	45.5
94	34.4	115	46.1
95	35.0	116	46.6
96	35.5	117	47.2
97	36.1	118	47.7
98.6	37.0	119	48.3
99	37.2	120	48.8
100	37.7	212	100
101	38.3		
102	38.8		